Thomson Delmar Learning's

CLINICAL MEDICAL ASSISTING

3rd Edition

Thomson Delmar Learning's

CLINICAL MEDICAL ASSISTING

3rd Edition

Wilburta Q. Lindh, MA
Marilyn S. Pooler, RN, MA, MEd
Carol D. Tamparo, CMA, PhD
Barbara M. Dahl, CMA, CPC

THOMSON
DELMAR LEARNING

Australia Canada Mexico Singapore Spain United Kingdom United States

THOMSON

DELMAR LEARNING

Thomson Delmar Learning's Clinical Medical Assisting, Third Edition
by Wilburta Q. Lindh, Marilyn S. Pooler, Carol D. Tamparo, and Barbara M. Dahl

Vice President, Health Care Business Unit:
William Brottmiller

Editorial Director:
Matthew Kane

Acquisitions Editor:
Rhonda Dearborn

Developmental Editor:
Sarah Duncan

Editorial Assistant:
Debra Gorgos

Marketing Director:
Jennifer McAvey

Marketing Coordinator:
Kimberly Duffy

Technology Director:
Laurie K. Davis

Technology Project Manager:
Mary Colleen Liburdi

Technology Project Coordinator:
Carolyn Fox

Production Director:
Carolyn Miller

Production Manager:
Barbara A. Bullock

Production Editor:
Jack Pendleton

Project Editor:
Natalie Pashoukos

Printed in Canada
2 3 4 5 6 7 8 XXX 09 08 07 06

For more information, contact
Thomson Delmar Learning,
5 Maxwell Drive,
Clifton Park, NY 12065

Or find us on the World Wide Web at
http://www.delmarlearning.com

Library of Congress Cataloging-in-Publication Data
ISBN 1-4018-8132-7

Notice to the Reader

CONTENTS

ABOUT THE AUTHORS

Wilburta (Billie) **Q. Lindh,** MA, holds professor emerita status at Highline Community College, Des Moines, Washington. She is the former program director and consultant to the Medical Assistant Program at Highline Community College and the 2000 Outstanding Faculty Member of the year. Lindh is a member of the SeaTac Chapter of the American Association of Medical Assistants (AAMA) and has lectured at AAMA seminars on the importance of communication. She is coauthor of *Therapeutic Communications for Allied Health Professions* published by Thomson Delmar Learning. She also coauthored *The Radiology Word Book* and *The Ophthalmology Word Book*, texts frequently used by transcriptionists, and is the medical assistant chapter author for *Guide to Careers in the Health Professions*.

Marilyn S. Pooler, RN, MA, MEd, is a professor in medical assisting. She taught for more than 25 years at Springfield Technical Community College in Springfield, Massachusetts, and served as Department Chairperson for several years. She has served on the Certifying Board of the AAMA Task Force for test construction and was a site surveyor for the AAMA for many years. Pooler has been a speaker at numerous local and state medical assisting meetings and seminars, emphasizing the importance of education, certification, and recertification of medical assistants. For a number of years, Pooler was a member of the executive board of the Northeast Association of Allied Health Educators. Pooler presently works in Health Services at Baypath College, Longmeadow, Massachusetts, at Baystate Medical Associates in Springfield, Massachusetts, in the gastroenterology clinic and for the Center for Business and Technology at Springfield Technical Community College, where she teaches refresher courses to medical assistants, licensed practical nurses, and registered nurses.

Carol D. Tamparo, CMA, PhD, served as a medical assistant instructor for 24 years and as program director for medical assisting for 15 years at Highline Community College in Des Moines, Washington. She was the Dean of Business and Allied Health programs at Lake Washington Technical College in Kirkland, Washington, for 4 years and currently is president of the Lake Washington College Foundation. She is the coauthor of *Therapeutic Communications for Health Professionals; Medical Law, Ethics, & Bioethics for Ambulatory Care*; and *Diseases of the Human Body*. She is a member of the SeaTac Chapter of AAMA and volunteers as a CASA advocate (*guardian ad litum*) in the King County Court System. She resides in Des Moines, Washington, with her husband, Tom.

Barbara M. Dahl, CMA, CPC, has dedicated her professional life to the recognition and advancement of medical assisting through quality education, increased public awareness, legislative compliance, and positive professional enhancement. She is a tenured faculty member at Whatcom Community College in Bellingham, Washington, and has been the Medical Assisting Program Coordinator and Department Chair since 1991. She is an active member of the Whatcom County Chapter of Medical Assistants, Washington State Society of Medical Assistants, AAMA, and the Washington State Medical Assisting Educators. She is a former chapter and state president and has served on and chaired many committees on the chapter, state, and national levels. She was instrumental in designing the AAMA Excel award-winning WSSMA Web site and continues to serve as the state Web master. Through the years she has acquired a wealth of knowledge and understanding about the professional and legal aspects of medical assisting, particularly in relation to the Washington State HCA law. She is also a member of the American Association of Professional Coders and is a founding member of the Whatcom Professional Coders, for which she has served as president. She proctors both the AAMA and the AAPC examinations. She has been an educational presenter/speaker at both Washington and Oregon state conferences and at Oregon State's Leadership Retreat.

ACKNOWLEDGMENTS

The authors personally acknowledge the following people:

To my husband, who continually supports and assists in so many ways, thank you. To my family for support and encouragement, and to Laura Lindh, who provided expertise for some chapters, thank you. To the students, graduates, and fellow colleagues who challenge me to stay current with skills and up-to-date with technology, thank you.

Billie Q. Lindh, MA

Thanks to my friends who were very supportive of my efforts, and a special thanks to my husband, Jud, for his patience and understanding during this endeavor.

Marilyn S. Pooler, RN, MA, MEd

Many thanks to those who believed that this edition was necessary and who recognized the abilities of each of its authors. Thanks to my husband, Tom, who was very patient during this undertaking and helped in numerous ways. To Billie, Marilyn, and Barbara, thanks for being such supportive and top-notch authors. Thanks to Barbara Murray for input and suggestions. Thanks to all the Delmar staff who make this text what it is.

Carol D. Tamparo, CMA, PhD

This writing experience has been exciting and humbling at the same time. I most definitely have received more than I have given. Mostly I have learned about myself. Having spent so many years educating and training medical assisting students, I am so astounded that I have helped produce a product that will serve as a learning tool for medical assisting students everywhere. I thank my students for all their patience and assistance; they are an absolute wealth of ideas! Much thanks to my college administrators for their endorsements. I thank my family for all their support, especially my husband, Ed, for his faith in my abilities and for fixing me breakfast, lunch, and dinner on those many Saturdays while I was glued to the computer; my son, Nik, for his amazing work on the workbook competencies; my former student, Sheila Atwater, and colleague, Sheri Greimes, for their generosity in sharing their laboratory expertise; my good friend and colleague, Lisa Carter, for her emotional support, excellent medical business acumen, and friendship. I thank the other authors, Billie, Carol, and Marilyn, for listening to my ideas and mentoring me through my first real writing experience. I also thank Sarah Duncan, my developmental editor, for her wise and calming nature that kept me reasonable and grounded during this writing experience. Most of all, though, I thank God that this project is finished! (And for blessing me with this unique and never-to-be-forgotten opportunity.)

Barbara M. Dahl, CMA, CPC

A sincere thank you to Joanne Cerrato, former coauthor, for her many invaluable contributions to the formation of the first edition of this text.

A sincere thank you to the medical assisting students at Whatcom Community College and at the following facilities for their assistance with the art program in this book: Madrona Medical Group and Bellingham Walk-in Clinic.

REVIEWERS

Julie L. Akason, RN, BSN
Department Head of Medical Assisting
Argosy University/Twin Cities
Eagan, MN

Diana E. Alagna, RN
Certified Phlebotomy Instructor
Medical Assisting Program Director
Branford Hall Career Institute
Southington, CT

Carole Berube, MA, MSN, BSN, RN
Professor Emerita in Nursing
Medical Assisting Program Faculty
Bristol Community College
Fall River, MA

Norma Bird, MEd, CMA
Medical Assisting Program Director/Instructor
Idaho State University College of Technology
Pocatella, ID

Michelle Blesi, CMA
Medical Assisting Program Director/Instructor
Century College
White Bear Lake, MN

Cheryl H. Bordwine, BS, HCA NCICS
Medical and Business Instructor
Texas School of Business
Friendswood, TX

David Bruce Drumm, PCMA, ASB, AE
Medical Department Coordinator
Computer Learning Network
Mechanicsburg, PA

George Fakhoury, MD, DORCP, CMA
Academic Program Manager, Healthcare
Heald College
San Francisco, CA

Deborah Fox, CAHI/CMA
Medical Assisting Program Supervisor
Porter and Chester Institute
Wethersfield, CT

Jeanette Goodwin, BSN CMA
Medical Assisting Program Chair
Southeast Community College
Lincoln, NE

Michaelea Holten, CRTT, NCMA
Medical Assisting Program Director
Pioneer Pacific College
Portland, OR

Diane M. Klieger, RN, MBA, CMA
Medical Assisting Program Director
Pinellas Technical Education Centers-SP
St. Petersburg, FL

Gerry Landes, CMA
Medical Assisting Department Chair
Bryman College
Everett, WA

Renee Levert, MA
Allied Health Manager
Kaplan Higher Education
Roswell, GA

Claire E. Maday-Travis, MA, MBA, CPHQ
Allied Health Program Director
The Salter School
Wooster, MA

Joseph E. McCann, BA, LVN (Ret)
Instructor
San Antonio College
San Antonio, TX

Tanya Mercer, BS, RN, RMA
Allied Health Curriculum Developer
KAPLAN Higher Education
Roswell, GA

Brigitte Niedzwiecki, RN, MSN
Medical Assistant Program Director
Chippewa Valley Technical College
Eau Claire, WI

Margaret O. Noirjean, RN, BSN
Instructor
Dakota County Technical College
Rosemount, MN

Deborah Odegaard, BS, CMA
Instructor, Medical Assistant Program
Des Moines Area Community College
Ankeny, IA

D. J. Overbey, RN, CCRC
Medical Assisting Program Director
Virginia College at Austin
Austin, TX

Nanciann Rosier, MEd, BSEd
Medical Assisting Technology Instructor
Ohio University Lancaster Campus
Lancaster, OH

Trevor Smith, DC, DAHom, FASA
Instructor
National College of Business & Technology
Nashville, TN

Stephanie J. Suddendorf, CMA, AAS
Medical Assistant Program Director
Minnesota School of Business/Globe College
Minneapolis, MN

Lori Warren, MA, RN, CPC, CCP, CLNC
Medical Department Co-Director
Spencerian College
Louisville, KY

Prior Edition Reviewers

Kaye Acton
Director of Medical Assisting Program
Alamance Community College
Graham, NC

Magdalena Andrasevits, NRCMA
Medical Assistant Program Director
Sanford-Brown College
North Kansas City, MO

Joseph DeSapio, RMA
Director of Facility and Library Resources
Medical Assisting Instructor
Ultrasound Diagnostic School
New York, NY

Eleanor K. Flores, RN, BSN, MEd
Briarwood College
Southington, CT

Tova Green
IVTC Fort Wayne
Fort Wayne, IN

Karen Jackson, NR-CMA
Medical Program Chair
Education America, Dallas Campus
Garland, TX

Barbara G. Kalfin, BS, AAS, CMA-C
Medical Assisting Extern Coordinator
Instructor, Medical Assisting Program
City College
Ft. Lauderdale, FL

Theresa Offenberger, PhD
Professor of Medical Assisting
Cuyahoga Community College
Cleveland, OH

Agnes Pucillo, LPN
Medical Assisting Program Director
Ultrasound Diagnostic School
Iselin, NJ

Patricia Schrull, RN, MBA, MEd, CMA
Program Director, Medical Assisting Program
Lorain County Community College
Elyria, OH

Janet Sesser, BS Ed. Admin., RMA, CMA
Corporate Director of Education, Allied Health
High-Tech Institute, Inc.
Phoenix, AZ

Kimberly A. Shinall, RN
President and CEO
KAS Enterprises
Virginia Beach, VA

Lois M. Smith, RN, CMA
Arapahoe Community College
Golden, CO

Susan Sniffin
Suffolk Community College
Great Neck, NY

Alisa M. Tetlow, RMA
Medical Assistant Program Director
Ultrasound Diagnostic School
Philadelphia, PA

Nina Thierer
Tidewater Technical Institute
Virginia Beach, VA

Fred Valdes, MD
Medical Department Chairman
City College
Ft. Lauderdale, FL

Sujana Wardell, RMA, RPT (AMT), AS
Program Director for Clinical and Administrative Medical Assisting
San Joaquin Valley College, Visalia Campus
Visalia, CA

Sally Wooten
Whitman Education Group
Miami, FL

Terri Wyman, CMA
Director of Health Information Specialties
Ultrasound Diagnostic School
Springfield, MA

LIST OF PROCEDURES

PREFACE

The world of health care has changed rapidly over the past few years, and as medical assistants, you will be called on to do more and respond to an increasing number of clinical responsibilities. Now is the time to equip yourself with the skills you will need to excel in the field. Now is the time to maximize your potential, expand your base of knowledge, and dedicate yourself to becoming the best multifaceted, multiskilled medical assistant that you can be.

The new edition of *Thomson Delmar Learning's Clinical Medical Assisting* will guide you on this journey. This text is part of a dynamic learning system that also includes a student software CD, workbook, and online materials. Together, this learning package includes coverage of the entry-level competencies identified by the Accrediting Bureau of Health Education Schools (ABHES) and the Commission on Accreditation of Allied Health Education Programs (CAAHEP), and maps to the standards defined by American Association of Medical Assistants' (AAMA's) Role Delineation Study and American Medical Technologists' (AMT's) Registered Medical Assistant Competency Inventory.

You will find that this edition provides you with more opportunities to use your critical thinking skills, through case studies, question boxes, scenarios, and features that tie directly to *Thomson Delmar Learning's Skills and Procedures and Critical Thinking for Medical Assistants DVD Series*. You will also see that the text responds to the growing need to learn about softer skills such as professionalism, as well as practical skills, including how to comply with Health Insurance Portability and Accountability Act (HIPAA) regulations and deal with privacy issues on the job.

How the Text Is Organized

Thomson Delmar Learning's Clinical Medical Assisting, 3rd edition, presents a logical, in-depth review of all clinical competencies required of today's multiskilled medical assistants—*in full color!*

- **Section I, General Procedures (Chapters 1 through 9),** provides the groundwork for understanding the role and responsibilities of the medical assistant. Topics include the medical assisting profession, the health care team, history of medicine, therapeutic communications, coping skills for the medical assistant, legal and ethical issues, and emergency procedures and first aid. New in Section I: Additional information about AMT, RMA,

CMAS, and ABHES; Introduction of Integrative Medicine and Alternative Therapies; Mechanisms for making ethical decisions; Provider level CPR; New procedure: Identifying Community Resources.

- **Section II, Clinical Procedures (Chapters 10 through 32),** gives you a thorough understanding of all clinical, diagnostic, and laboratory procedures important to today's ambulatory care settings. Topics include medical asepsis, medical history, vital signs and measurements, physical examination, obstetrics and gynecology, pediatrics, male reproductive system, gerontology, body systems, assisting with minor surgery, diagnostic imaging, rehabilitation medicine, nutrition, pharmacology, medication calculations, ECG, safety guidelines, venipuncture, hematology, urinalysis, microbiology, and specialty tests. New in Section II: Safety needles and lancets; Principles of IV Therapy; Order of Draw; Syringe Technique; Removal of non–CLIA-waived procedures; New procedures, including: wet prep and KOH prep, pulse oximetry, multiple channel ECG, and obtaining a capillary specimen for transport using a Microtainer.
- **Section III, Professional Procedures (Chapters 33 through 36),** examines the role of the medical assistant as office and human resources manager and provides tools and techniques to use when preparing for externship, medical assisting credentials, and employment. New in Section III: Management styles; Risk Management; CMA and RMA certification process; E-résumés.
- **Glossary** includes definitions of all key terms, with related chapter numbers indicated.
- **Student Software CD** includes StudyWARE with quizzes and activities, as well as the Critical Thinking Challenge, which presents real-life scenarios in which you must use your critical thinking skills to choose the most correct action in response to the situation.

How Each Chapter Is Organized

All chapters include similar features and presentation and function as building blocks to a comprehensive medical assisting education. However, each chapter is also a self-contained module and can be studied in any order or independently of other chapters in the text.

Features include:

- **Key terms, chapter outline,** and **objectives** to help identify important concepts and provide direction for the chapter
- **Featured Competencies,** which map the chapter material to ABHES and CAAHEP competencies
- An **introduction** with a real-life **scenario**
- **Spotlight on Certification** for CMA, RMA, and CMAS examinations
- **Graphic icons, photographs,** and **figures** in full-color to illustrate the text discussion
- **Procedures** with step-by-step instructions, rationales, and **charting examples**
- **Patient Education, HIPAA,** and **Critical Thinking** boxes
- **Case Studies** with critical thinking questions
- **Study for Success** checklist to provide a track for learning and reviewing the material
- **Summary** to assess and reinforce concepts learned in the chapter
- **Review Questions,** in multiple choice and critical thinking short answer formats
- **Web Activities** for exploration and research using the Internet
- **The DVD Hook-Up,** tying the chapter material to *Thomson Delmar Learning's Critical Thinking and Skills and Procedures DVD Series*
- **References/Bibliography** for further study

EXTENSIVE TEACHING/ LEARNING PACKAGE

The complete supplements package helps instructors efficiently manage time and resources and helps students to develop the necessary skills and competencies required by the demanding profession of medical assisting.

Student Workbook

The workbook helps you learn and reinforce the essential competencies needed to become a successful, multiskilled medical assistant. Each chapter includes:

- Pre-test and post-test
- Vocabulary builder exercises and word games
- Learning review in true/false, matching, and fill-in-the-blank style questions
- Certification review
- Case studies
- Competency Assessment checklists

  Student Workbook, ISBN 1-4018-8133-5

Instructor's Resource Manual

The Instructor's Resource Manual is a dynamic teaching tool to help you plan the course and implement activities by chapter. It contains the following features:

- Instructor Tips and Strategies for teaching, lesson planning, and evaluation
- How to incorporate the book in your classroom
- Chapter Overviews, Lesson Plans, Activities
- Printed Test Bank and Answers
- Answers to Review Questions and Case Studies
- Answers to Workbook Questions
- Grids mapping the text content to ABHES and CAAHEP competencies and certification exams

Instructor's Resource Manual, ISBN 1-4018-8134-3

WebTutor Advantage

Designed to complement the book, WebTutor is an online classroom management tool that takes your course beyond the classroom wall. WebTutor is a content-rich, Web-based teaching and learning aid that reinforces and helps clarify complex concepts; it is available on WebCT and Blackboard platforms. WebTutor provides rich communication and course management tools, including a Course Calendar, Chat, E-Mail, Threaded Discussions, Web Links, and a White Board. It also includes additional content, including:

- Learning Links explore health care topics through research on the Internet
- Critical Thinking Questions and Case Studies with DVD clips
- Discussion Questions and Quizzes for each chapter
- Unit Tests, Section Tests, and a comprehensive Final Exam
- PowerPoint presentation with DVD clips

WebTutor Advantage on WebCT, ISBN 1-4018-8129-7

WebTutor Advantage on Blackboard,
ISBN 1-4018-8130-0

WebTutor Toolbox

With WebTutor Toolbox, you get the same rich communication tools and funcionality of this Web-based teaching and learning aid. Chapter components include objectives, advance preparation, and FAQs.

WebTutor Toolbox on WebCT, ISBN 1-4180-3104-6

WebTutor Toolbox on Blackboard, ISBN 1-4180-3103-8

HOW TO USE THIS BOOK

Thomson Delmar Learning's ***Clinical Medical Assisting, 3rd edition,*** contains many features that make it an easy-to-use learning system. They include:

Chapter Outline

At the beginning of each chapter, you will find an outline of all major headings. Review these headings of topic areas before you study the chapter. They are a road map to your understanding.

Key Terms

All key terms are listed at the beginning of each chapter. Within the text, the term is always boldfaced at its first occurrence for easy identification. Turn to the glossary for definitions of all key terms.

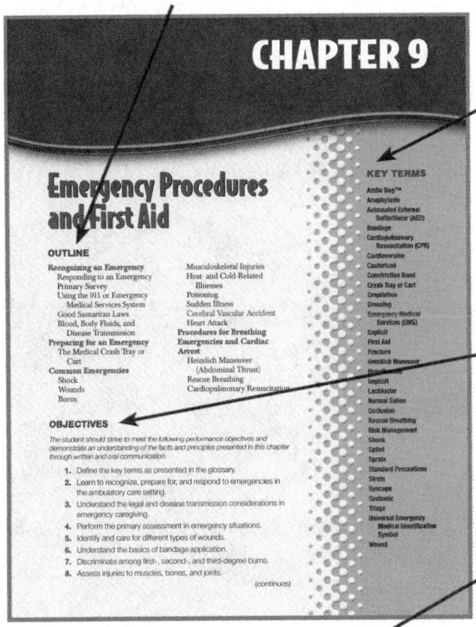
CHAPTER 9

Emergency Procedures and First Aid

OUTLINE

Recognizing an Emergency
Responding to an Emergency
Primary Survey
Using the 911 or Emergency Medical Services System
Good Samaritan Laws
Blood, Body Fluids, and Disease Transmission
Preparing for an Emergency
The Medical Crash Tray or Cart
Common Emergencies
Shock
Wounds
Burns
Musculoskeletal Injuries
Heat- and Cold-Related Illnesses
Poisoning
Sudden Illness
Cerebral Vascular Accident
Heart Attack
Procedures for Breathing Emergencies and Cardiac Arrest
Heimlich Maneuver (Abdominal Thrust)
Rescue Breathing
Cardiopulmonary Resuscitation

OBJECTIVES

The student should strive to meet the following performance objectives and demonstrate an understanding of the facts and principles presented in this chapter through written and oral communication.

1. Define the key terms as presented in the glossary.
2. Learn to recognize, prepare for, and respond to emergencies in the ambulatory care setting.
3. Understand the legal and disease transmission considerations in emergency caregiving.
4. Perform the primary assessment in emergency situations.
5. Identify and care for different types of wounds.
6. Understand the basics of bandage application.
7. Discriminate among first-, second-, and third-degree burns.
8. Assess injuries to muscles, bones, and joints.

(continues)

KEY TERMS

Ambu Bag™
Anaphylaxis
Automated External Defibrillator (AED)
Bandage
Cardiopulmonary Resuscitation (CPR)
Cardioversion
Cauterized
Constriction Band
Crash Tray or Cart
Crepitation
Dressing
Emergency Medical Services (EMS)
Explicit
First Aid
Fracture
Heimlich Maneuver
Implicit
Lackluster
Normal Saline
Occlusion
Rescue Breathing
Risk Management
Shock
Splint
Sprain
Standard Precautions
Strain
Syncope
Systemic
Triage
Universal Emergency Medical Identification Symbol
Wound

Objectives

Performance objectives test your knowledge of the key facts presented in the chapter. Use these objectives, together with review questions, to test your understanding of the chapter's content.

Spotlight on Certification

This feature maps the chapter material to the content outlines of the RMA, CMA, and CMAS certifying examinations to help you prepare to obtain medical assistant credentials.

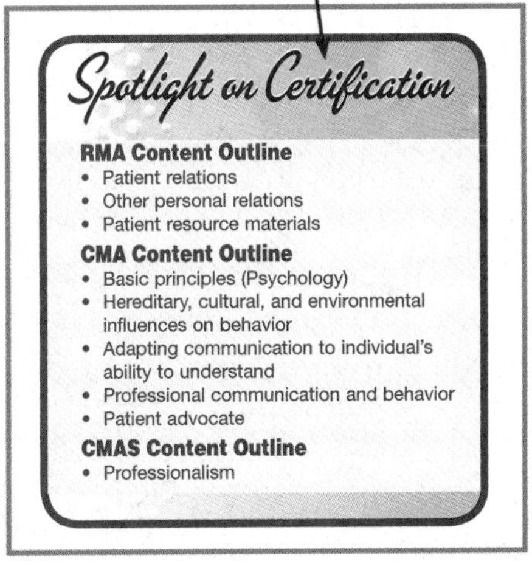
Spotlight on Certification

RMA Content Outline
- Patient relations
- Other personal relations
- Patient resource materials

CMA Content Outline
- Basic principles (Psychology)
- Hereditary, cultural, and environmental influences on behavior
- Adapting communication to individual's ability to understand
- Professional communication and behavior
- Patient advocate

CMAS Content Outline
- Professionalism

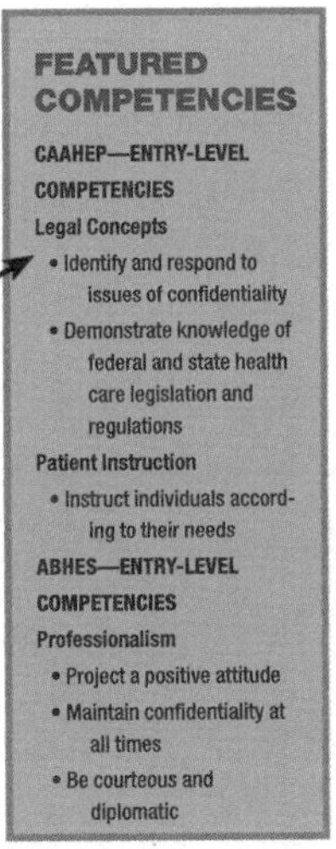
FEATURED COMPETENCIES

CAAHEP—ENTRY-LEVEL COMPETENCIES

Legal Concepts
- Identify and respond to issues of confidentiality
- Demonstrate knowledge of federal and state health care legislation and regulations

Patient Instruction
- Instruct individuals according to their needs

ABHES—ENTRY-LEVEL COMPETENCIES

Professionalism
- Project a positive attitude
- Maintain confidentiality at all times
- Be courteous and diplomatic

Featured Competencies

Entry-Level Competencies defined by ABHES and CAAHEP are listed at the beginning of each chapter to focus on the skills and functions that medical assistants will need to perform on the job.

Patient Education

This feature helps all current and future medical assistants anticipate patient concerns and provides sound suggestions for effective patient communication.

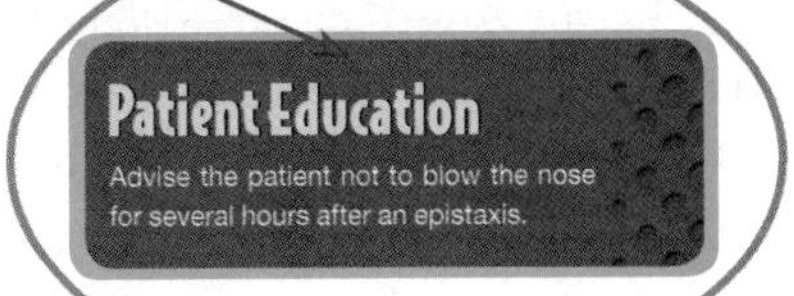
Patient Education

Advise the patient not to blow the nose for several hours after an epistaxis.

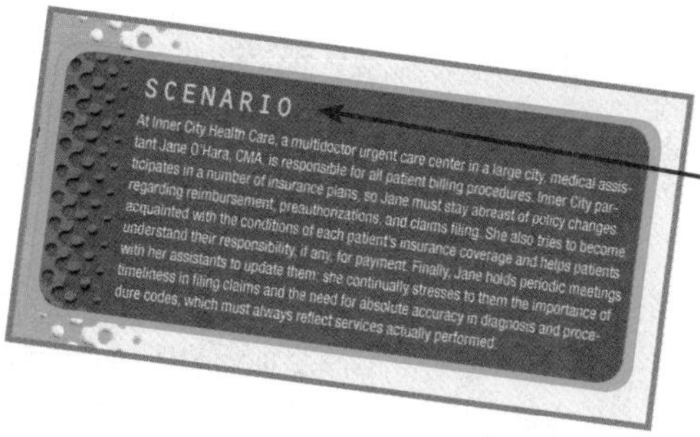
SCENARIO

At Inner City Health Care, a multidoctor urgent care center in a large city, medical assistant Jane O'Hara, CMA, is responsible for all patient billing procedures. Inner City participates in a number of insurance plans, so Jane must stay abreast of policy changes regarding reimbursement, preauthorizations, and claims filing. She also tries to become acquainted with the conditions of each patient's insurance coverage and helps patients understand their responsibility, if any, for payment. Finally, Jane holds periodic meetings with her assistants to update them; she continually stresses to them the importance of timeliness in filing claims and the need for absolute accuracy in diagnosis and procedure codes, which must always reflect services actually performed.

Real-Life Scenarios

The introduction in each chapter includes an overview of the material *and* a real-life scenario. Through these scenarios you will come to understand some of the stimulating challenges faced by medical assistants and gain insight into how these challenges are overcome.

Procedures

Step-by-step procedures are conveniently grouped together at the end of each chapter. They give step-by-step instruction on all important administrative, clinical, and general competencies as defined by AAMA and AMT.

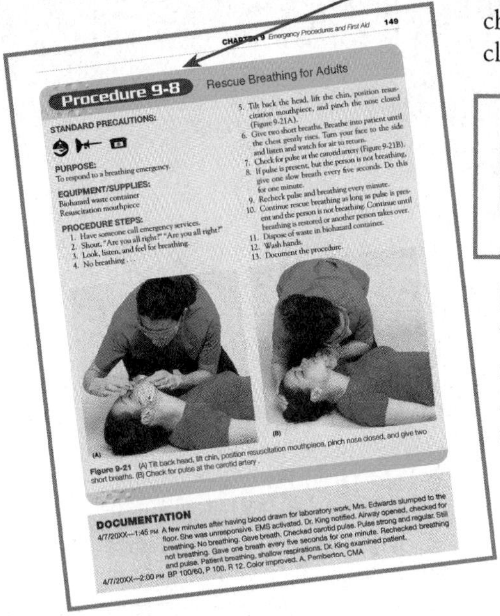

Critical Thinking

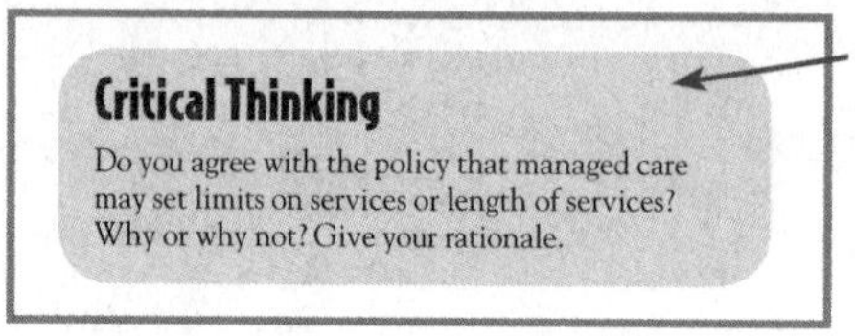

Topical questions sprinkled throughout the chapter are designed to stimulate critical thinking for discussion and emphasize skills necessary for medical assissting.

HIPAA

These boxes highlight important information relating to the Health Insurance Portability and Accounting Act of 1996 to help you comply with regulations and deal with privacy issues on the job.

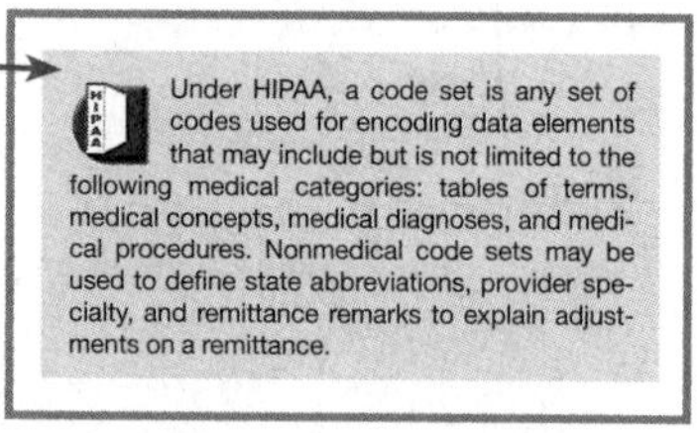

Under HIPAA, a code set is any set of codes used for encoding data elements that may include but is not limited to the following medical categories: tables of terms, medical concepts, medical diagnoses, and medical procedures. Nonmedical code sets may be used to define state abbreviations, provider specialty, and remittance remarks to explain adjustments on a remittance.

Case Studies

The case studies with accompanying review questions encourage a problem/solution approach. Use the case studies to put your knowledge into practice and arrive at a deeper understanding of the profession.

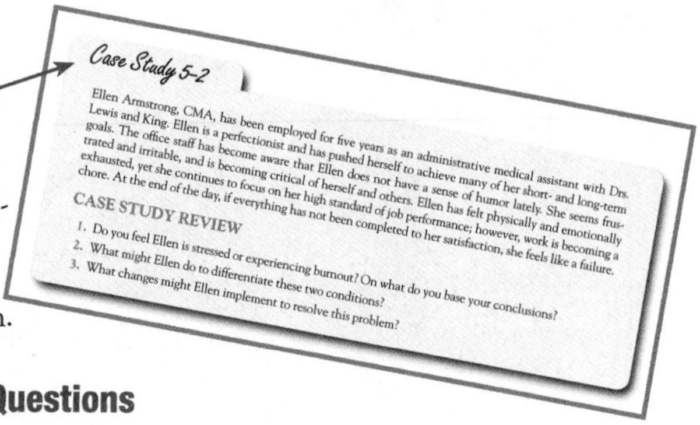

Study for Success

Before the activities at the end of each chapter, use this feature as a checklist to help focus and track your study of the material.

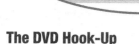

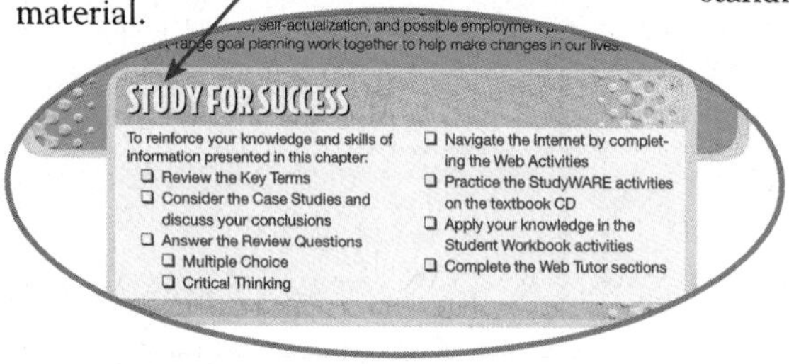

Review Questions

Test your comprehension of the chapter with structured multiple choice questions and open-ended critical thinking questions that require you to combine an understanding of chapter material with your personal insight and judgment.

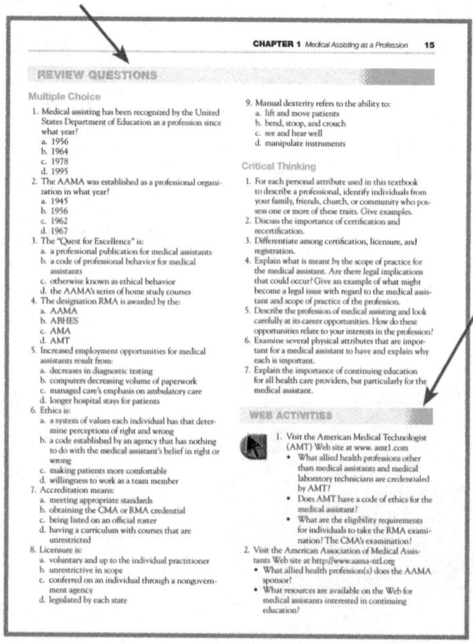

Web Activities

This feature at the end of each chapter gives you practice navigating the Internet and using it as a research tool by suggesting online activities.

The DVD Hook-Up

This tool provides synopses and scene references for *Thomson Delmar Learning's Critical Thinking and Skills and Procedures for Medical Assisting DVD Series* to show real-world application of the chapter material. Critical thinking questions can facilitate thought-provoking discussion and the DVD journal summary encourages you to share your ideas and grasp important issues that come up in the medical office.

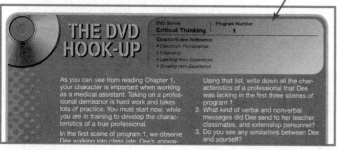

HOW TO USE THE STUDENT SOFTWARE CD

The Critical Thinking Challenge

You are on a three-month externship in a medical office. You will be confronted with a series of situations in which you must use your critical thinking skills to choose the most appropriate action in response to the situation.

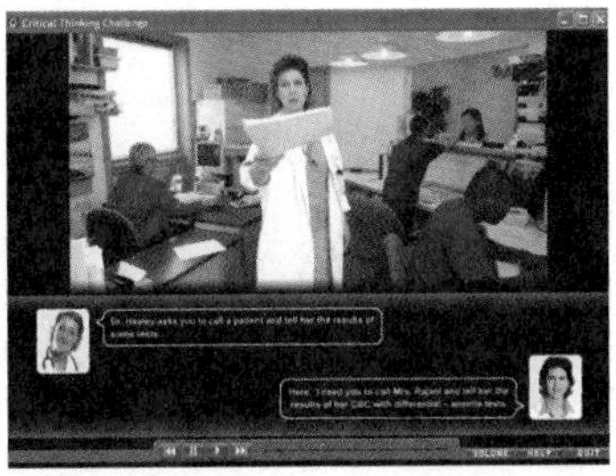

You may consult with members of the office staff and document resources to help you choose the best action, but not all of these resources will be available at all times or always offer helpful advice.

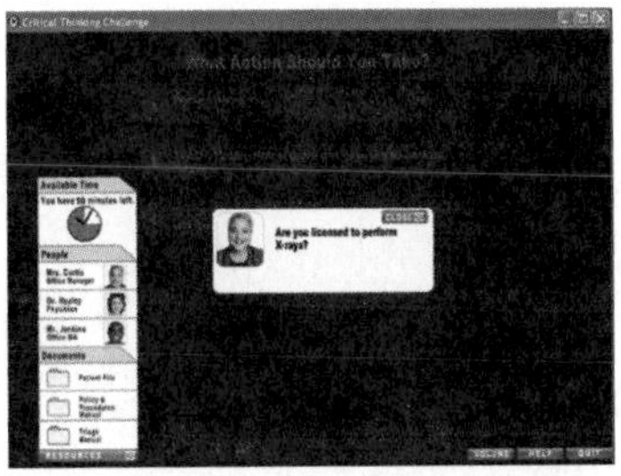

Your decisions will be evaluated in three categories: how your decisions affect the practice, the patient, and your career.

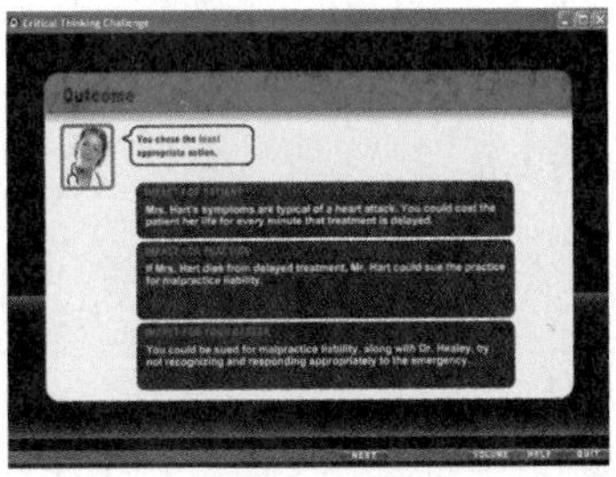

Your goal is to be hired by Dr. Healey's office as a full-time medical assistant. However, if you show a lack of critical thinking skills that threatens the well-being of the practice and the patients, Dr. Healey will terminate your externship and you will have to start over.

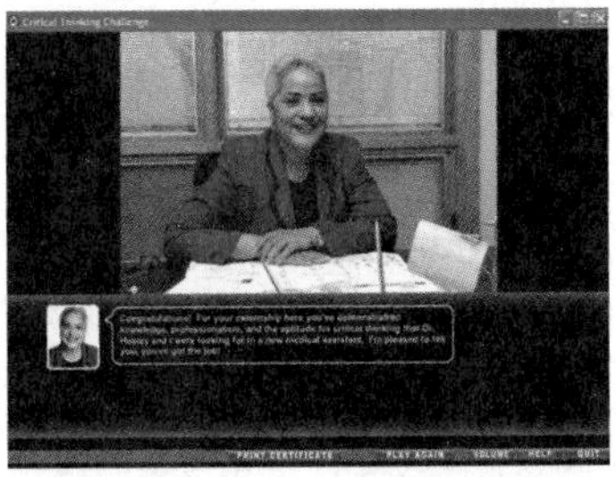

StudyWARE™

StudyWARE™ is interactive software with learning activities and quizzes to help you study key concepts and test your comprehension. The activity and quiz content corresponds with each unit in the book.

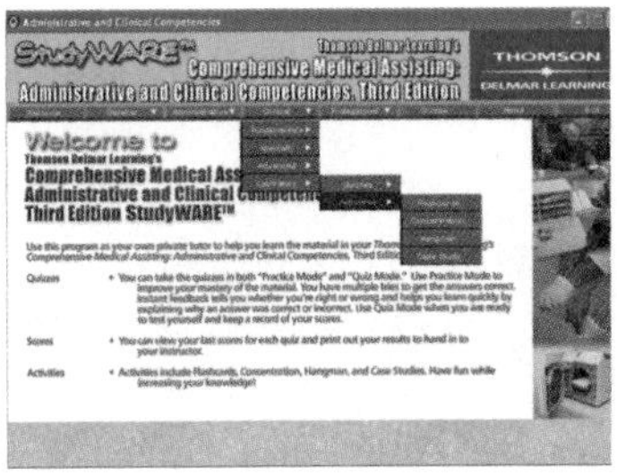

Each unit contains Multiple Choice, True/False, and Fill-in-the-Blank quizzes that can be taken in practice mode, which gives immediate feedback after each question, or in quiz mode, which allows your score for each quiz to be stored or printed.

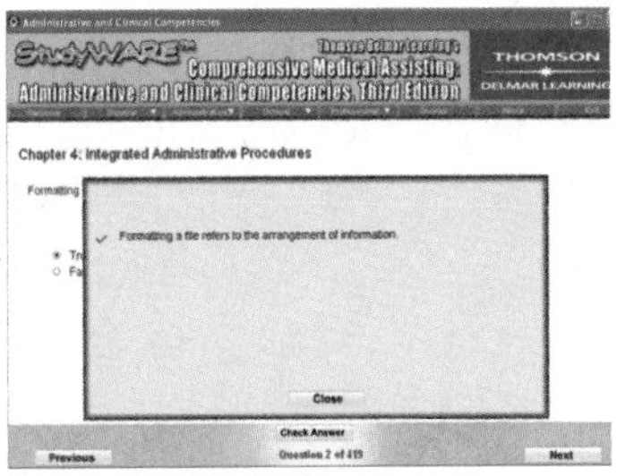

The activities within each unit include Flash Cards, Concentration, Hangman, Case Studies, and Championship Games.

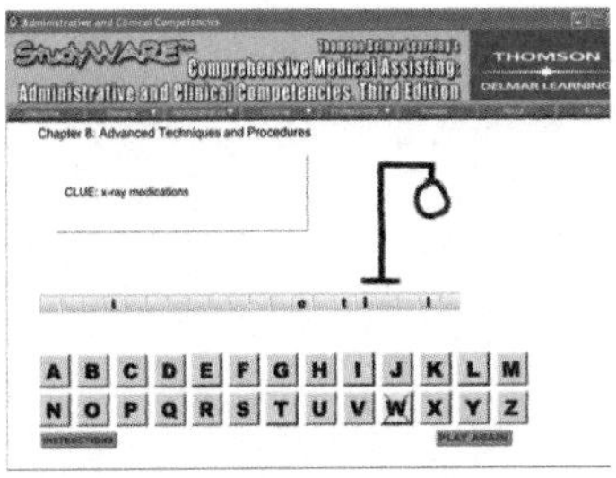

Medical Terminology Audio Library

Practice your pronunciation and recognition of medical terms using the Audio Library. You may search for terms by word or body system. Once you've selected a word, it is pronounced correctly and defined on the screen.

UNIT 1
Introduction to Medical Assisting and Health Professions

CHAPTER 1

Medical Assisting as a Profession

OUTLINE

Personal Attributes of the Professional
- Empathy
- Attitude
- Dependability
- Initiative
- Flexibility
- Desire to Learn
- Physical Attributes
- Ability to Communicate
- Ethical Behavior

Historical Perspective of Medical Assisting

American Association of Medical Assistants
- Accreditation
- Certification
- Continuing Education

American Medical Technologist
- Certification

Education of the Professional Medical Assistant
- Preparation for Externship
- Educational Institutions

Career Opportunities

Regulation of Health Care Providers
- Scope of Practice

OBJECTIVES

The student should strive to meet the following performance objectives and demonstrate an understanding of the facts and principles presented in this chapter through written and oral communication.

1. Define the key terms as presented in the glossary.
2. Identify and discuss nine personal attributes that are important for a professional medical assistant to possess.
3. Discuss the history of medical assisting.
4. Describe the American Association of Medical Assistants and list its three major functions.
5. Discuss the role of the American Medical Technologists Association in credentialing of Medical Assistants.

(continues)

KEY TERMS

Accreditation
Ambulatory Care Setting
Attribute
Bachelor's Degree
Certification
Certified Medical Assistant (CMA)
Competency
Compliance
Credentialed
Cultivate
Dexterity
Diploma
Disposition
Empathy
Externship
Facilitate
Improvise
Integrate
Internship
License
Licensure
Litigious
Practicum
Professionalism
Proprietary
Registered Medical Assistant (RMA)
Scope of Practice

FEATURED COMPETENCIES

CAAHEP—ENTRY-LEVEL COMPETENCIES

Professionalism

- Project a professional manner and image
- Demonstrate initiative and responsibility
- Work as a member of a health care team
- Prioritize and perform multiple tasks
- Adapt to change
- Promote the CMA credential
- Enhance skills through continuing education

Legal Concepts

- Perform within legal and ethical boundaries
- Recognize professional credentialing criteria

ABHES—ENTRY-LEVEL COMPETENCIES

Professionalism

- Project a positive attitude
- Maintain confidentiality at all times
- Be a "team player"
- Be cognizant of ethical boundaries
- Exhibit initiative
- Adapt to change
- Evidence a responsible attitude
- Conduct work within scope of education, training and ability

Communication

- Be attentive, listen and learn
- Professional components
- Allied health professions and credentialing

OBJECTIVES (continued)

6. Explain accreditation, certification, and continuing education as they pertain to the professional medical assistant.
7. Identify the importance of the accreditation process to an educational institution.
8. Recall two methods to obtain recertification.
9. List five means of obtaining continuing education units.
10. Describe the certifying agency that certifies medical assistants as registered medical assistants.
11. Describe the externship experience.
12. Recall two criteria for the selection of externship sites.
13. List three benefits of externship to student and site.
14. Describe the profession of medical assisting and analyze its career opportunities in relationship to your interests.
15. Differentiate among certification, licensure, and registration.
16. State the importance of understanding the scope of practice for the medical assistant.

SCENARIO

A group of high school freshmen have come to tour the medical assisting class and laboratory areas. The Program Director of Medical Assisting is showing the students around the department. The Program Director then takes them into the medical assisting laboratory where the senior medical assistant students are there practicing their clinical skills. Each senior student pairs up with a high school freshman, and each pair talks about medical assisting, with the medical assistant students answering questions the others may have. The medical assistant students are in uniform as part of their preparation to go into various health care agencies to do their externship or practicum. The medical assistant students look professional, clean, fresh, and motivated. They tell the high school students about medical assisting and describe the personal and physical attributes desirable for those who want to become medical assistants. They explain the importance of these attributes, as well as what duties a professional medical assistant performs and what education is needed to pursue a career in medical assisting.

Throughout the question and answer discussions, the senior medical assistant students and the program director stress the importance of ethics, empathy, attitude, dependability, and teamwork as favorable attributes. Individuals seeking a career in medical assisting should develop and maintain these attributes.

INTRODUCTION

Historically, medical science has been fascinating to most people. Perhaps you have been drawn to medical assisting because you too are intrigued by medicine and want to learn about advances in health care and become involved in providing care to patients. More than likely you have a desire to help others.

Medical assistants have always played an integral role in physicians' offices and ***ambulatory care settings*** *such as clinics and urgent care facilities, where health care services are offered on an outpatient basis. And now more than ever, because of the explosion of knowledge and high technology in medicine, medical assistants are involved in an ever-widening scope of clinical and administrative duties. With the medical assistant's expanded role has come the responsibility to become a well-educated and highly competent professional dedicated to providing the highest quality of health care.*

Consumers of health care have become increasingly aware, primarily through the media, of the availability of the latest advances, techniques, and discoveries in medicine. They realize that they have a right to have health care provided to them by educated, skilled, and competent professionals.

As you study to become a medical assistant, it is important for you to understand what a professional is. According to Merriam-Webster's Collegiate Dictionary, *10th edition, it is "one who has acquired a specialized body of knowledge, skills, and attitudes." You will practice* ***professionalism*** *as you learn the technical and ethical standards of this profession.*

You will learn to ***integrate,*** *or unify, your desire and need to help others with the knowledge, skills, and attitudes you acquire through your studies. By blending all of these, you will be able to provide patients with the best health care possible and will learn what it means to be a professional medical assistant.*

PERSONAL ATTRIBUTES OF THE PROFESSIONAL

There are certain characteristics or personal qualities that medical assistants should strive to cultivate. These are the **attributes** that identify a true professional; when caring for patients, these qualities should come from the heart. They will enable the patient to trust you, the caregiver.

Empathy

To have **empathy** means to consider the patient's welfare and to be kind. It means stepping into the patient's place, discovering what the patient is experiencing, and then recognizing and identifying with those feelings.

Medical assistants should treat patients as they themselves would want to be treated. A visit to the doctor's office is often a time of fear and anxiety. Apprehension can be allayed tremendously when patients realize that their caregiver understands their feelings and desires to make their lives more pleasant and comfortable. See Figure 1-1.

It is important to realize that patients' health problems can have a profound effect on you, the medical assistant. By maintaining a balanced outlook, medical assistants can safeguard themselves from becoming too emotionally involved with patients' problems. Empathy is extremely important in the health care profession; however, emotionalism can cloud one's judgment.

Attitude

A friendly, warm **disposition** and a sense of humor will help patients feel more at ease. A sincere affection for people can be conveyed by actions that **facilitate** open and honest communication. Your attitude should radiate genuine interest.

On occasion, difficult patients can test the tolerance level of the most experienced medical assistant because they seldom seem to be content with the care or services received. But no matter what the circumstances, patients should never be treated with disinterest or in an unfriendly manner. The medical assistant should always be pleasant and courteous.

When giving care to patients, do so unrestricted by your concerns about their attitudes, disease, race, religion, economic status, or sexual orientation.

As a member of the health care delivery team, the medical assistant needs to be cooperative and supportive

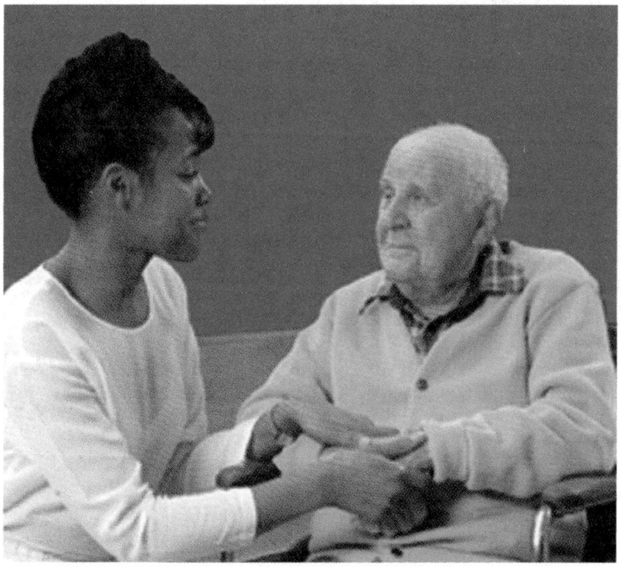

Figure 1-1 The medical assistant should have a friendly disposition and communicate empathy for the patient.

of all other members, working with the team in an honest, open manner while keeping in mind the patient's right to privacy and confidentiality.

Dependability

When providing for a patient's well-being, it is important to focus attention on activities in the office or clinic environment that will demonstrate that you are well-organized, accurate, and responsive to patients' needs.

Being dependable means that employer and coworkers rely on the medical assistant to be respectful of them, of patients, and of equipment and materials. Other members of the health care team will expect you to be accountable for the duties and responsibilities you undertake. A dependable person interacts with coworkers in a supportive manner, is punctual, and limits absences from work.

Initiative

The willingness and ability to work independently shows initiative. A person with initiative is observant, notices work that needs to be done, and then takes action to complete those tasks without being told to do them. Employer and coworkers must be able to count on one another to anticipate patients' needs and be attentive to work that needs to be accomplished. The successful medical assistant will be ready to pitch in and recognize when others need assistance.

By asking appropriate questions and seeking information that will improve performance, medical assistants will demonstrate that they have the foresight and the "get up and go" needed to complete the numerous and varied tasks of the ambulatory care environment.

Flexibility

The ability to be adaptable is a trait that serves all professionals well. When caring for ill people, unexpected situations arise daily, and medical assistants must be able to respond to a variety of situations (many of them emergencies and unanticipated) without losing a sense of equilibrium. Finding solutions to problems and developing alternative action plans demonstrates flexibility. To **improvise,** or solve problems that arise either routinely or spontaneously, is a characteristic worth nurturing.

Desire to Learn

A willingness to continually learn and grow is the mark of a true professional. With the growing technology in medicine, there is an ongoing necessity for constant learning. Medical assistants must be dedicated to high standards of performance, which can be accomplished by showing a desire to acquire information and by constantly updating their knowledge and skills. Keeping abreast of the latest diseases, treatments, procedures, and techniques can be achieved in a variety of ways, such as college courses, seminars, workshops, reading, and simply by being observant. The sharper the power of observation, the more the medical assistant will learn from physician, employer, and coworkers.

Physical Attributes

Appearance is important in patients' perceptions of the delivery of their care. Imparting the look of a professional requires an appearance that is clean and fresh and wholesome; in general, an appearance that reflects good health habits (Figure 1-2). Good personal hygiene practices (daily shower, deodorant), weight control, and healthy-looking skin, hair, teeth, and nails all contribute to a professional appearance. Rest, good nutrition, regular exercise, and recreation all promote good health.

Female medical assistants should wear only appropriate light daytime makeup. For the safety of both the professional and the patient, no necklaces or dangling earrings should be worn. The only jewelry worn should be single earposts or wedding rings. Hair should be neat and off the collar. Fingernails should be short and manicured. Male medical assistants should be clean-shaven and have short hair. The only jewelry worn should be a wedding ring. Colognes, perfumes, and aftershave should

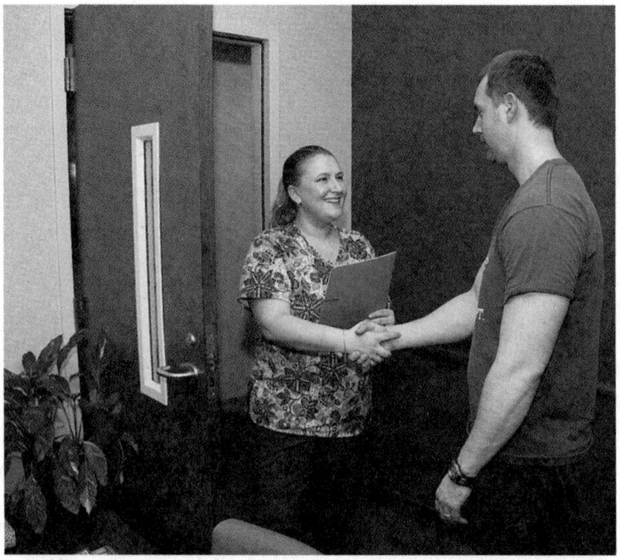

Figure 1-2 A professional, neat appearance makes patients feel at ease with their health care provider.

not be worn at work. Body piercings and tattoos should not be visible.

Patient care can place physical demands on medical assistants. Lifting and moving patients is often required, and the use of correct body mechanics will help minimize injuries to the back. Although every reasonable accommodation is made for physically challenged medical assistants, to be mobile without assistance is important because medical assistants move about throughout the day while performing tasks and procedures. It is frequently necessary to bend, stoop, kneel, and crouch, especially when filing and retrieving patients' records, and for other tasks as well. Most procedures require that medical assistants have the ability to hear and see well for the accurate completion of tasks (Figure 1-3). Listening to blood pressures, taking a medical history, observing patients, performing phlebotomy, and identifying microorganisms under a microscope are some of the routine tasks and procedures performed daily in a medical facility.

Manual **dexterity** is also needed for manipulating certain instruments and for entering data using a computer.

Ability to Communicate

It is important that medical assistants learn to develop the ability to communicate well verbally and nonverbally with patients, staff, and other professionals.

Compliance with the physician's treatment plan is important for a positive outcome of patients' illnesses (Figure 1-4). Also, patients will feel more comfortable and less threatened in a medical office or ambulatory center that encourages staff to keep them informed.

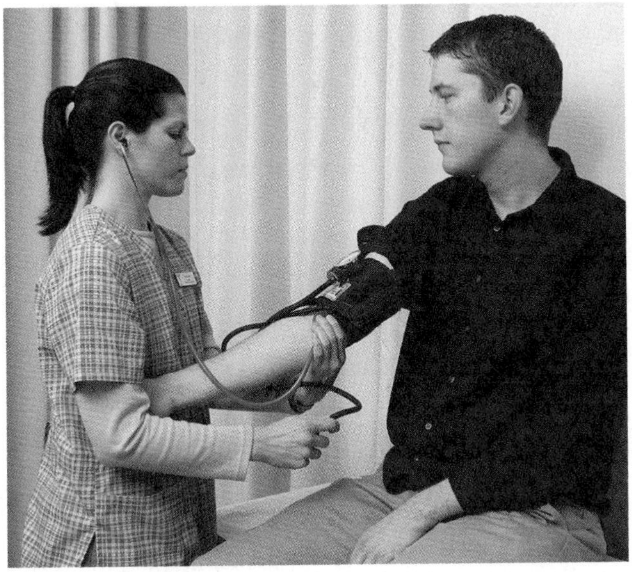

Figure 1-3 Measuring blood pressure is a task that requires the medical assistant to see and hear well.

Critical Thinking

Of all the personal attributes that your text describes, which do you think is your most developed attribute? Give an example of that attribute that comes from your daily life.

Ethical Behavior

No discussion about personal attributes is complete without the mention of ethics. Ethics is a system of values each individual has that determines perceptions of right and wrong. Our life experiences mold this set of values, which is considered a personal code of ethics.

Medical ethics govern medical conduct or that behavior practiced as health care providers. These ethics involve relationships with patients, their families, fellow professionals, and society in general. Good ethical behavior will have a positive impact on the profession of medical assisting and on the medical community as well. By adhering to the medical assistants' Code of Ethics, we endeavor to elevate the profession to a position of dignity and respect. (A more in-depth discussion of this Code of Ethics can be found in Chapter 8.)

The personal qualities of empathy, healthy attitude, dependability, initiative, flexibility, the desire to learn, a wholesome physical presence, the ability to communicate well, and ethical behavior are some of the characteristics that most professionals have and that medical assistants

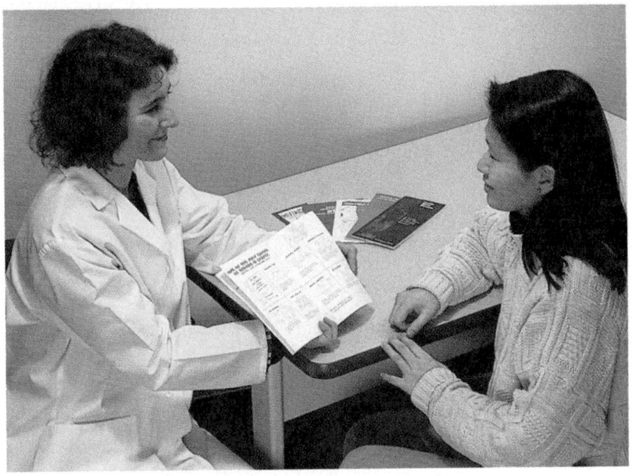

Figure 1-4 Patient education requires skill in communicating instructions to patients in language appropriate to their needs.

should strive to develop. When entering into the profession of medical assisting, it is important to learn more about these and other qualities and to begin to **cultivate** and refine them.

HISTORICAL PERSPECTIVE OF MEDICAL ASSISTING

Historically, when physicians began their practices, it was common for them to hire individuals and train them on the job. Physicians originally hired nurses, but eventually they came to realize that nurses alone could not perform the variety of duties that are required in medical offices and ambulatory care centers. The nurse's role was limited to assisting the physician with clinical procedures, whereas the medical assistant's role was and is much broader and includes a large number of activities, procedures, and responsibilities, both administrative and clinical.

Today, with a much more informed patient comes the need for educated and credentialed medical assistants. In addition, in today's **litigious** atmosphere, which makes health care providers vulnerable to malpractice suits, most employers recognize the importance of employing medical assistants who are professionally prepared through formal education. Physicians want knowledgeable and dependable medical assistants so they can focus their time and attention on the medical decisions, treatments, and techniques for which they have been educated and licensed. This leaves the medical assistant to assist the physician in the operation and management of the practice.

It was in 1978 that the profession of medical assisting was formally recognized by the United States Department of Education. Twenty-four years before this official recognition of the profession, a group of medical assistants gathered to establish a professional organization. With support, encouragement, and guidance from the American Medical Association (AMA), the American Association of Medical Assistants (AAMA) was founded in 1956 (Figure 1-5). The first president of the organization was Maxine Williams.

AFFILIATE OF THE
AMERICAN ASSOCIATION
OF MEDICAL ASSISTANTS

CERTIFIED MEDICAL ASSISTANTS:
HEALTHCARE'S MOST VERSATILE PROFESSIONALS

Figure 1-5 Logo of the American Association of Medical Assistants, a professional organization founded in 1956. (Courtesy of the American Association of Medical Assistants.)

In 1991, the AAMA's board of trustees approved the current definition of medical assisting:

> Medical Assisting is an allied health profession whose practitioners function as members of the health care delivery team and perform administrative and clinical procedures.

AMERICAN ASSOCIATION OF MEDICAL ASSISTANTS

The AAMA has three major purposes:

1. Accreditation
2. Certification
3. Continuing education

Accreditation and certification standards were developed by the AMA and the AAMA through the Commission on Accreditation of Allied Health Education Programs (CAAHEP) for schools wishing assurance that their medical assistant programs are of the highest quality and satisfy CAAHEP criteria.

Accreditation

The AAMA works jointly with the AMA to define the essential components and appropriate standards of quality that educational institutions offer in their medical assistant curriculum. The United States Department of Education has approved the AAMA/AMA as an **accreditation,** or approving, body for educational programs for medical assistants. A medical assisting program that is accredited meets the standards as outlined in the *Standards and Guidelines for an Accredited Education Program for the Medical Assistant*. *Standards* are the minimum standards of quality used in accrediting programs that prepare individuals to enter the medical assisting profession. On-site review teams evaluate the program's **compliance** with, or adherence to, the standards. All aspects of programs seeking accreditation status undergo scrutiny to ascertain the program's quality and to ensure continued compliance with the standards.

Certification

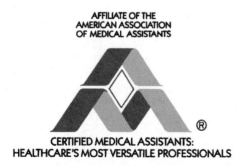

As the profession grew and developed, some states came to require special licensure or certification to perform certain tasks; in other states, health professionals were challenged by the skill and broad spectrum of the medical assistant's ability. To defend medical assistants whose right to practice clinical procedures was being challenged, the AAMA responded at their 1995 convention with the following policy, which became effective February 1, 1998:

> that any candidate for the AAMA Certification Examination be a graduate of a CAAHEP-accredited medical assisting program. This requirement would become effective February 1, 1998. Anticipated benefits of the recommendation are to: (1) safeguard the quality of care to the consumer; (2) ensure the CMA's role in the rapidly evolving health care delivery system; and (3) continue to promote the identity and stature of the profession.

Certification is voluntary, not mandatory, for medical assistants to practice, although the AAMA strongly urges those who are eligible to take the national certification examination. The examination measures professional **competency** at job entry level. Successful completion of the examination earns the individual the status of being certified and of being known as a **certified medical assistant (CMA).** The initials follow the individual's name. Conferring of the CMA status is referred to as being **credentialed** (Figure 1-6). It signifies recognition of competency by having attained a certain level of knowledge and skill.

The examination is offered twice yearly simultaneously at more than 200 test sites across the United States. In October 2004, a third examination was added on a trial basis. If, as anticipated, there is a demonstrated need for the third examination, the AAMA will consider making it permanent.

Recertification of the credential must be undertaken within five years from the date of certification to maintain current status as a CMA. Two routes are available to recertify. One is by accumulating approved continuing education units, and the other is by taking the certification examination again.

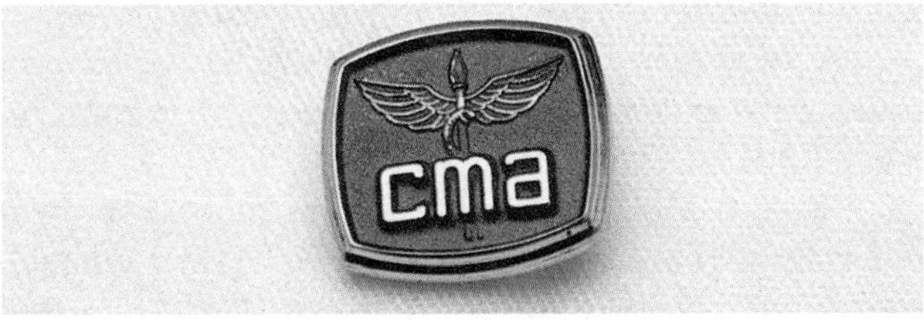

Figure 1-6 Certified medical assistant (CMA) pin awarded by the American Association of Medical Assistants on successful completion of the national certification examination.

The status of a medical assistant's credentials (whether current or not current) is a public record available at the AAMA executive office, 20 N. Wacker Dr., Suite 1575, Chicago, IL 60606-2963; 1-800-228-2262, www.AAMA-WTL.org. The AAMA Board of Trustees approved a policy change at the association's 1999 annual convention in Nashville. Effective January 1, 2003, all certified medical assistants who are employed or seeking employment *must* have current status as a CMA to use the credential. The mandatory current status for use of the CMA designation protects patients, employers, and the medical assistant's right to practice. Certification and recertification attest to the medical assistant's desire for professional development.

At one time, the credentials CMA-A (Certified Medical Assistant, Administrative), CMA-C (Certified Medical Assistant, Clinical), CMA-AC (Certified Medical Assistant, Administrative and Clinical), and CMA-Ped (Certified Medical Assistant, Pediatrics) were awarded to candidates who successfully passed specialty examinations in addition to the basic CMA examination.

Although these specialty examinations have been phased out for newly graduated medical assistants, current medical assistants who have already earned these specialty credentials can maintain them and continue to be recertified through the Continuing Education Hours method. Currently, there are approximately 95,000 CMAs in the United States.

Continuing Education

The AAMA vigorously encourages continuing education for all medical assistants. This can be accomplished through various means such as educational meetings, seminars, workshops, conventions, and the "Quest for Excellence," AAMA's series of home study courses for continuing education credit.

Membership in the AAMA is tri-level: local, state, and national. Educational meetings are held regularly at local and state meetings and conventions. The annual AAMA national convention provides an excellent forum for attaining knowledge through its educational offerings and for networking with other medical assistants.

Continuing an education is a lifelong process and serves as testimony to a commitment to professionalism.

AMERICAN MEDICAL TECHNOLOGIST

Founded in 1939, the American Medical Technologist (AMT) is a national certification and professional membership association that represents 27,000 allied health care individuals. Its purpose is to certify and credential medical assistants, clinical laboratory personnel, allied health instructors, dental assistants, medical administrative specialists, and others. In 1972, the AMT established the certification examination for medical assistants. The designation of **registered medical assistant (RMA)** is conferred on those individuals who successfully pass the examination (Figures 1-7A and B).

The Accrediting Bureau of Health Education Schools (ABHES) accredits private postsecondary institutions and programs that prepare individuals for entry into the profession of medical assisting. In 1991, ABHES spun off from the AMT and became a separate entity.

Certification

The AMT has its own committees, conventions, bylaws, state chapters, officers, registrations, and certification examinations.

RMA is a voluntary credential for the profession of medical assisting. RMA credentials are national, and examinations are given throughout the United States in both computerized and paper and pencil format. The exam consists of 200–210 multiple choice questions, covering general, administrative, and clinical areas. Voluntary means that neither the federal government nor most states require a medical assistant to be either certified or registered to practice the profession. Most employers, however, prefer to employ credentialed medical assistants. Most physicians desire hiring employees with the credentials because they recognize that doing so safeguards the quality of patient care and reduces the risk for liability issues for themselves.

RMAs have been active in legislation to protect medical assistants, assuring improvement in medical assistant education and providing for continuing education opportunities.

(A)

(B)

Figure 1-7 (A) Logo of the American Medical Technologists. (B) Logo of Registered Medical Assistant. (Courtesy of American Medical Technologists.)

Another profession that the AMT certifies is the Medical Administrative Specialist (MAS). Individuals who successfully pass the AMT certification examination are conferred with the credential of Certified Medical Administrative Specialist (CMAS). The CMAS exam is given in both computerized and paper and pencil format. The exam consists of 200–210 multiple choice questions.

An MAS serves an important role in the hospital, clinic, or medical office. The MAS is competent in a multitude of skills such as medical records management, coding and billing for insurance, practice finance management, information processing, and fundamental management practices. The MAS also is familiar with the clinical and administrative concepts that are required to coordinate office functions in the health care setting.

Graduating from a program accredited by either CAAHEP or ABHES has significant benefits, such as proof that the student has completed a program that meets national standards, recognition of their education by their professional peers, and eligibility for AMT credentialing exams.

Some medical assistants may choose to attain both RMA and CMAS credentials.

It is important to remember that credentialing, whether through the AAMA (CMA) or AMT (RMA), is evidence to employers and patients alike that you want the profession of medical assisting to be recognized and promoted. Also, credentials safeguard patients, because you will deliver health care at the highest quality with the most current techniques and procedures. Credentials help secure the medical assistant's role in the health care field.

For more information, call 1-800-275-1268 or write to AMT, 710 Higgins Rd., Park Ridge, IL 60068, or access their Web site, at: www.amt1.com.

EDUCATION OF THE PROFESSIONAL MEDICAL ASSISTANT

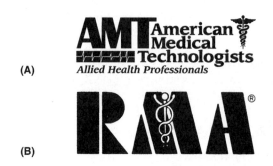

Formal education of medical assistants takes place in community and junior colleges, as well as in **proprietary** schools. The AAMA has established educational requirements for program directors to follow for their programs to be considered accredited. These requirements were previously known as the Developing A CUrriculuM (DACUM) Analysis. In 1997, in coordination with the National Board of Medical Examiners, educators, and practicing CMAs, the AAMA developed the Medical Assistant Role Delineation Chart, which is the occupational analysis of the medical assisting profession, (see Appendix B to review this chart). In addition, the entry-level competencies that must be mastered by students in academic programs and the *Standards* (formerly "Essentials") *and Guidelines for an Accredited Education Program for the Medical Assistant* are revised to reflect the findings of the Role Delineation Study. On graduation, the student will receive a **diploma** or certificate of completion.

Educational institutions seeking accreditation for a medical assisting program must develop the curricula to these *Standards and Guidelines* to ensure the highest quality medical assistant education and employment preparedness.

Although not a complete list, some of the administrative, general (transdisciplinary), and clinical courses include those shown in Table 1-1.

Another aspect of an educational medical assisting program is the **externship,** a period when students participate in a **practicum.** This provides an excellent opportunity to apply theory to practice.

TABLE 1-1 TYPICAL ADMINISTRATIVE, GENERAL, AND CLINICAL COURSES IN AN ACCREDITED MEDICAL ASSISTING PROGRAM

Administrative Courses
Computer Applications
Manual Recording of Patients' Data
Scheduling Appointments
Maintaining Medical Records
Word Processing/Keyboarding
Billing/Collections/Managing Patients' Accounts
Coding/Insurance Claims
Telephone Triage
Personnel Management
General Courses
Anatomy and Physiology
Medical Terminology
Human Diseases
Patient Education
Medical Law and Ethics
Clinical Courses
Infection Control
Pharmacology/Administration of Medications
Assisting Techniques/Physical Examination
Assisting with Minor Surgery
Basic Laboratory Procedures/Routine Blood and Urine Testing
Cardiopulmonary Resuscitation and First Aid

Preparation for Externship

Externship, practicum, and **internship** are all terms used to define the transition period between the classroom and actual employment. An externship is planned and supervised by a coordinator from the medical assisting program and the health care facility that agrees to become a partner in the education and employability of the student.

Externship Sites. Sites for externship are chosen carefully to ensure that a variety of experiences is available for the student. The sites should provide the student with adequate administrative, clinical, and general experiences. The staff at the various sites must be willing to make a commitment to the medical assistant's education by spending appropriate time observing and instructing the student.

Benefits of Externship. The externship experience is mutually beneficial to the student and staff at the health care facility that is providing the educational experiences.

Some of the benefits to the student are the opportunity to:

- Apply classroom knowledge and skill in a real-world medical setting
- Recognize improvement in performance and knowledge
- Understand that there may be more than one acceptable method of performance
- Begin to establish a network of support through colleagues

Some of the benefits to the externship site are:

- Greater alertness of staff because of their educational responsibilities to the student
- Opportunity for staff to observe students who will soon be seeking employment
- Possibility that staff will learn more about the profession of medical assisting

Critical Thinking

Patients and physicians desire professional medical assistants who have had the benefit of a formal education to work for them. Discuss the impact of this education on patients and employers. Why is it important to both groups?

Educational Institutions

Educational institutions that confer associate or bachelor degrees require general education courses for graduation in addition to the administration and clinical courses.

There are four-year institutions of higher learning that offer a **bachelor's degree** to medical assistants who have graduated with an associate's degree from a community or junior college. The graduate is accepted as a third-year student and can obtain a bachelor's degree in such areas as health care management or health care facility administrator.

Because there is a demand for medical assistant educators, some experienced medical assistants take education courses to become allied health educators.

CAREER OPPORTUNITIES

Medical assistants have been described as health care's most versatile, multifaceted professionals. That medical assistants possess a broad scope of knowledge and skills makes them ideal professionals for any ambulatory care setting. Indeed, because of such versatility, medical assistants find employment in a variety of settings: offices, clinics, hospitals, medical laboratories, insurance companies, government agencies, pharmaceutical companies, and educational institutions. Although the range of employment opportunities continues to grow, in the past decade, about four of five medical assistants were employed in physicians' offices and clinics. About one in five worked in offices of other health care practitioners, such as chiropractors, optometrists, and podiatrists. There are other career opportunities available to the medical assistant. Some medical assistants work as phlebotomists, coding specialists, medical laboratory assistants, and CMASs. The outlook for employment for medical assistants is promising. According to the AAMA, there are currently 1.3 million medical assistants in the work force. The United States Department of Labor Bureau of Statistics listed medical assisting as one of the fastest growing allied health professions for the years 1998–2012.

Increased employment opportunities for medical assistants result from the increased medical needs of an aging population, growth in the number of health care practitioners and their desire to hire the most qualified person for the task, increased diagnostic testing, greater volume and complexity of paperwork and computer information, managed care's emphasis on ambulatory care, and the insurance-mandated shorter stay of patients in hospitals.

REGULATION OF HEALTH CARE PROVIDERS

One way health care providers can be regulated is through the process of credentialing. Credentialing recognizes health care providers who are professionally and technically competent. Recognition comes from professional associations, certifying agencies, and the state or federal government. Regulation ensures:

- Competence of health care providers
- A minimum standard of knowledge, training, and skill
- The limiting of the performance of certain procedures to a specific occupation

Licensure, certification, and registration are three kinds of regulations/credentialing. See Table 1-2.

Scope of Practice

Medical assisting is not licensed as a profession; however, some states require that medical assistants be graduates of an accredited medical assisting program to work as medical assistants.

Two examples of licensed professions are medicine and nursing. A **license** regulates the activities of these

TABLE 1-2 COMPARISON OF REQUIREMENTS FOR CERTIFICATION, LICENSURE, AND REGISTRATION

	Certification	Licensure	Registration
Practice Requirement	Voluntary	Mandatory	Voluntary
Conferred by	Nongovernmental agency or professional association	Legislated by each state	Professional association
	If qualified and meets requirements	If qualified and meets requirements	Listed on an official roster
	Must pass national examination	Must pass state examination	Passing examination not always required
How restrictive	Used by most professional associations	Most restrictive	Least restrictive

professions by enacting laws that specify educational requirements and by defining the **scope of practice.** A license is conferred on an individual who successfully completes specialized educational requirements and successfully passes an examination administered by the state in which the individual resides. The state grants a license to that individual to practice medicine or nursing. Licensure forbids anyone who is not licensed from performing activities that are designated by that particular license. For example, the law states that the physician's license allows diagnosing and prescribing treatment. If someone were to diagnose or prescribe without a license, that individual would be committing an illegal act and would be practicing medicine without a license, which is considered a felony.

There are state laws that govern the practice of medicine and nursing (medical practice acts, nursing practice acts), and many states have acts that give physicians the right to delegate certain clinical procedures to qualified allied health professionals. Because medical assistants are not required to be licensed, they are allowed to perform clinical procedures only under the supervision of the physician or other licensed health care professional who is granted the right and who delegates the specific clinical procedures to them.

In some states, including California, Washington, and others, unlicensed health care providers are required to have authorization from the state to perform allergy testing and venipuncture and to give injections. A registration fee and mandatory training are required. In such circumstances, medical assistants or other health care providers would be breaking the law if they performed these procedures without registration and training.

In some states, authorization is required for unlicensed health care providers to expose patients to X-rays.

Medical assistants do not perform procedures for which they have not been educated and trained. The AAMA's Role Delineation Chart (see Appendix B) is an excellent reference source that identifies which clinical, administrative, and general (transdisciplinary) procedures medical assistants are educated to perform. However, because of the variability of state statutes, the medical assistant would be wise to check with the AAMA or AMT if in doubt about the legality of certain clinical procedures.

Critical Thinking

A medical assistant relates to a patient on the telephone that her symptoms are "probably the flu" and to "take over-the-counter cough syrup" for her cough. Is this an appropriate or inappropriate action for the medical assistant to take? Discuss your answer and explain why you came to your decision.

SUMMARY

Progress has been made in the advancement of the profession of medical assisting since the first group of medical assistants gathered to become organized and formed the AAMA. For example, the number of certified medical assistants has exceeded 95,000 and continues to grow since certification began in 1963. The total number of medical assistants in the work force is approximately 1.3 million, and employment opportunities continue to grow. Educational requirements have become increasingly important. The AAMA and the AMT continue to promote standards of excellence for its members, encouraging continuing education and awarding continuing education credits to members of AAMA and AMT via various means.

All of these factors are evidence of a strong professional perspective and should offer encouragement and support to any student or graduate of medical assisting.

Becoming a professional is a gradual process and cannot be learned in its entirety from a textbook. The challenge of becoming a professional medical assistant will require open-mindedness and a desire for continued learning and education, certification and recertification of the CMA or RMA credential, and professional involvement through organizational participation.

As the scope of work done by medical assistants broadens and medical assistants seek and require formal education, the professional medical assistant will gain additional respect and be in even greater demand. Medical assistants must continuously pursue excellence, which is the hallmark of all professional behavior.

STUDY FOR SUCCESS

To reinforce your knowledge and skills of information presented in this chapter:

- ❑ Review the Key Terms
- ❑ Answer the Review Questions
  - ❑ Multiple Choice
  - ❑ Critical Thinking
- ❑ Navigate the Internet and complete the Web Activities
- ❑ Practice the StudyWARE activities on the textbook CD
- ❑ Apply your knowledge in the Student Workbook activities
- ❑ Complete the Web Tutor sections
- ❑ View and discuss the DVD situations

REVIEW QUESTIONS

Multiple Choice

1. Medical assisting has been recognized by the United States Department of Education as a profession since what year?
   a. 1956
   b. 1964
   c. 1978
   d. 1995
2. The AAMA was established as a professional organization in what year?
   a. 1945
   b. 1956
   c. 1962
   d. 1967
3. The "Quest for Excellence" is:
   a. a professional publication for medical assistants
   b. a code of professional behavior for medical assistants
   c. otherwise known as ethical behavior
   d. the AAMA's series of home study courses
4. The designation RMA is awarded by the:
   a. AAMA
   b. ABHES
   c. AMA
   d. AMT
5. Increased employment opportunities for medical assistants result from:
   a. decreases in diagnostic testing
   b. computers decreasing volume of paperwork
   c. managed care's emphasis on ambulatory care
   d. longer hospital stays for patients
6. Ethics is:
   a. a system of values each individual has that determine perceptions of right and wrong
   b. a code established by an agency that has nothing to do with the medical assistant's belief in right or wrong
   c. making patients more comfortable
   d. willingness to work as a team member
7. Accreditation means:
   a. meeting appropriate standards
   b. obtaining the CMA or RMA credential
   c. being listed on an official roster
   d. having a curriculum with courses that are unrestricted
8. Licensure is:
   a. voluntary and up to the individual practitioner
   b. unrestrictive in scope
   c. conferred on an individual through a nongovernment agency
   d. legislated by each state
9. Manual dexterity refers to the ability to:
   a. lift and move patients
   b. bend, stoop, and crouch
   c. see and hear well
   d. manipulate instruments

Critical Thinking

1. For each personal attribute used in this textbook to describe a professional, identify individuals from your family, friends, church, or community who possess one or more of these traits. Give examples.
2. Discuss the importance of certification and recertification.
3. Differentiate among certification, licensure, and registration.
4. Explain what is meant by the scope of practice for the medical assistant. Are there legal implications that could occur? Give an example of what might become a legal issue with regard to the medical assistant and scope of practice of the profession.
5. Describe the profession of medical assisting and look carefully at its career opportunities. How do these opportunities relate to your interests in the profession?
6. Examine several physical attributes that are important for a medical assistant to have and explain why each is important.
7. Explain the importance of continuing education for all health care providers, but particularly for the medical assistant.

WEB ACTIVITIES

1. Visit the American Medical Technologist (AMT) Web site at www. amt1.com
   - What allied health professions other than medical assistants and medical laboratory technicians are credentialed by AMT?
   - Does AMT have a code of ethics for the medical assistant?
   - What are the eligibility requirements for individuals to take the RMA examination? The CMA's examination?
2. Visit the American Association of Medical Assistants Web site at http://www.aama-ntl.org
   - What allied health profession(s) does the AAMA sponsor?
   - What resources are available on the Web for medical assistants interested in continuing education?

THE DVD HOOK-UP

DVD Series	Program Number
Critical Thinking	**1**

Chapter/Scene Reference
- *Classroom Performance*
- *Externship*
- *Learning from Supervisors*
- *Growing from Experience*

As you can see from reading Chapter 1, your character is important when working as a medical assistant. Taking on a professional demeanor is hard work and takes lots of practice. You must start now, while you are in training to develop the characteristics of a true professional.

In the first scene of program 1, we observe Dee walking into class late. Dee's appearance is in total disarray and her attitude is poor. Even though Dee promised her teacher that she would work on her professional characteristics, Dee enters her externship with the same attitude that she possessed in school. After Dee speaks with her externship supervisor, she starts to realize that her teacher is right, and that she does need to develop her professional skills if she is going to succeed as a medical assistant.

1. This chapter lists characteristics that are important to possess as a professional. Using that list, write down all the characteristics of a professional that Dee was lacking in the first three scenes of program 1.
2. What kind of verbal and nonverbal messages did Dee send to her teacher, classmates, and externship personnel?
3. Do you see any similarities between Dee and yourself?

DVD Journal Summary

After watching the designated scenes from program 1, write a paragraph in your journal that summarizes what you learned from watching these scenes. What kind of verbal and nonverbal messages do you typically send to your classmates? What will you do to improve other people's impressions of your professional characteristics?

REFERENCES/BIBLIOGRAPHY

American Association of Medical Assistants, Executive Office, 20 N. Wacker Dr., Chicago, IL 60606.

American Medical Technologists, Allied Health Professions, 710 Higgins Rd., Park Ridge, IL 60068.

Balasa, D. (2000). Securing the future for medical assistants to practice. *Professional medical assistant*, January/February 2000, 6–7.

Merriam-Webster (2002). *Merriam-Webster's collegiate dictionary* (11th ed.). Springfield, MA: Author.

CHAPTER 2

Health Care Settings and the Health Care Team

OUTLINE

OBJECTIVES

The student should strive to meet the following performance objectives and demonstrate an understanding of the facts and principles presented in this chapter through written and oral communication.

1. Define the key terms as presented in the glossary.
2. Analyze the benefits and limitations of working in the different health care settings.
3. Assess the role and impact of managed care in the health care environment.
4. Identify and describe the three primary medical management models.
5. Describe the function of the health care team.

(continues)

KEY TERMS

Acupuncture
Ambulatory Care Setting
Fringe Benefits
Health Maintenance Organization (HMO)
Homeopathy
Independent Physician Association (IPA)
Integrative Medicine
Managed Care Operation
Preferred Provider Organization (PPO)
Triage

FEATURED COMPETENCIES

CAAHEP—ENTRY-LEVEL COMPETENCIES

Legal Concepts

- Perform within legal and ethical boundaries
- Demonstrate knowledge of federal and state health care legislation and regulations

ABHES—ENTRY-LEVEL COMPETENCIES

- Be a "team player"
- Be impartial and show empathy when dealing with patients
- Serve as liaison between physician and others
- Allied health professions and credentialing

OBJECTIVES (continued)

6. Discuss the role of the medical assistant in the health care team.
7. List and describe a minimum of 12 physician specialists.
8. List and describe a minimum of three alternative health care specialists.
9. List and describe a minimum of 12 allied health professionals.
10. Compare and contrast the types of nurses.
11. Critique alternative therapies and discuss their role in today's health care setting.

SCENARIO

You always had thought you wanted to be a medical assistant and work in a clinic where you would see a variety of patients. But after discussing this chapter in class, you are really intrigued with becoming an emegency medical technician. What kind of research can you do to make certain you have chosen the right path? Consider working hours, rate of pay, patient contact, required schooling, and job availability.

INTRODUCTION

There are few professions in our society as rich and complex as the health care profession. Particularly in recent years, the health care environment has been very much in flux as the profession seeks ways to provide quality care while containing costs. This effort to curtail costs has resulted in the rise of managed care, which, in turn, has spawned a number of medical models such as health maintenance organizations (HMOs) and preferred provider organizations (PPOs), two well-known managed care entities.

Many other types of physician networks and alliances are also being established as providers merge to give patients the best of care whereas controlling their costs. Ambulatory care settings, where services are provided on an outpatient basis, have become increasingly pivotal to consumer health care as insurers direct dollars away from hospitals and toward outpatient care.

Just as the medical setting continues to evolve to meet new societal needs, health care technology is ever-changing. Health care is a dynamic, stimulating industry that requires the medical assistant and other professionals to constantly develop new skills if they are to contribute to the team effort. The range of skills within the health care team is astonishing, and includes physicians, or medical doctors, in more than 25 specialties, an increasing number of nontraditional alternative practitioners licensed to practice, and more than 20 kinds of allied health professionals.

AMBULATORY HEALTH CARE SETTINGS

Although medical assistants may work in a number of different environments, including laboratories or hospitals, most are employed in an **ambulatory care setting** such as a medical office (either a solo-physician or group practice), an urgent or primary care center, or a managed care organization such as an HMO.

Often, the medical assistant will choose to work in one setting rather than another based on interests, personality, and work preferences. For instance, the individual practice may provide medical assistants with the opportunity to use their full array of skills, whereas in urgent care centers, the work of the medical assistant may be more specialized in nature.

FORMS OF MEDICAL PRACTICE MANAGEMENT

Medical assistants employed in ambulatory care settings or medical offices and clinics are likely to see three major forms of medical practice management: sole proprietorships, partnerships, and corporations.

Whatever form of management is chosen by physicians, they are responsible for the employees that serve with them. (Refer to the discussion of *respondeat superior* in Chapter 7.) Physician–employers and their medical assistants must have the kind of healthy working relationship where mutual trust and respect are apparent. The physician must understand the skill level of the medical assistant, and the medical assistant must feel secure enough to ask any necessary questions or admit any errors. Critical errors are often made when this trust does not exist between employer and employee. This causes a breakdown in the delivery of the best health care for patients.

Sole Proprietorships

In the past, many physicians preferred a solo practice. A solo practice entitles the physician or sole proprietor to hold exclusive right to all aspects of the medical practice or sole proprietorship, including profits and debts. If the business fails, the sole proprietor's personal property may also be attached.

A sole proprietorship may employ other physicians to participate in the practice. The employed physician(s) would be entitled to any employee **fringe benefits** such as health insurance and paid vacation, but the solo practitioner is not so entitled.

Partnerships

When two or more physicians join together under a legal agreement to share in the total business operations of the practice, a partnership is formed. Several physicians who share a facility and practice medicine are often referred to as a group. Partners share income, expenses, debt, equipment, records, and personnel according to a predetermined agreement. Partners are liable for only their own actions, but may be liable for the whole amount of the partnership debts.

Corporations

Physicians may form a corporation, usually referred to as a professional service corporation. The physician shareholders are considered employees of the corporation. A corporation allows income and tax advantages to all employees. A variety of fringe benefits can be offered to the employees, which may include pension, profit-sharing plans, medical expense reimbursement, and life, health, and disability insurance. These benefits are separate from salary. Another advantage is that professional employees of a corporation are liable only for their own acts, and personal property cannot be attached in litigation. A sole proprietor may incorporate if the practice is large enough.

The health maintenance organization (HMO) is one type of corporation in which physicians often practice. Basically, physicians are employees of the HMO and are paid by various methods; physicians in the HMO usually serve as the primary care physician (PCP). In this situation, a referral from the PCP may be necessary before a patient can see a specialist or allied health professional.

Figure 2-1 Different forms of medical practice management.

Medical assistants should also recognize the three major forms of medical practice management and how they affect salary, benefits, and liability issues (Figure 2-1).

Individual and Group Medical Practices

For years, the most common form of medical office was the individual physician or group practice. This model competes with a variety of other models such as urgent care centers and HMOs, but many medical assistants still find the individual or group practice a challenging place of employment.

Individual Practices. In the individual practice, also called the solo practice, one primary physician sees and treats all patients. Although this type of arrangement is limited in the number of people it can serve, many patients feel secure in this kind of health care setting because they come to know and trust their doctor. Because they always see the same doctor, they feel their health care is being managed in a personal way. The solo-physician practice, however, can be an expensive arrangement, because one doctor must undertake the costs of office space, equipment, and personnel.

Group Practices. Group practices are attractive arrangements where two or more physicians can share the costs of space, equipment, and personnel. The advantages of a group practice are not solely economic, however; physicians learn from and consult one another, and patients receive the benefit of this exchange of information and knowledge. Often, a group practice may have more than one office and some employees may be asked to travel between sites to cut overhead. Group practices may also be formed to offer specialized care, such as oncology or women's health care.

In most group practices, patients may request that they see the same physician for all appointments, although sometimes patients are assigned to the next available doctor. For emergencies, group practices have the staff and flexibility to ensure that there is always a doctor on call.

Most medical practices are still groups of three or four doctors, but in the most recent past a trend shows a return to one- and two-doctor practices. Merritt, Hawkins, and Associates, a staffing and recruiting firm in Texas, reports that physicians in two-person partnerships increased from 9% in 1998 to 22% in 2002. In the same period, physicians placed in group settings decreased from 53% to 41%. A consulting firm in California, Professional Management and Marketing, reports that solo start-ups have increased fivefold in the last three years.

This trend seems to be led by some primary care physicians who learned firsthand that a bigger practice may not always be better. Many physicians in small groups allowed large practice management firms to acquire their assets and manage the business side of their practice. In some cases, these practice management firms were sold to even larger practice management companies that eventually went bankrupt, forcing them to shed all their practices. This dilemma left physicians with no recourse except to start over. Therefore, a number of physicians are returning to the **preferred provider organization (PPO),** where physicians network to offer discounts to employers and other purchasers of health insurance and agree to discounted fees for services.

Urgent Care Centers

Urgent care centers are usually private, for-profit centers that provide services for primary care, routine injuries and illnesses, and minor surgery. Sometimes laboratory services and a radiology department are located on the premises. Physicians and other health care professionals in the center are often salaried employees, not owners who share in the profits, and often are associated with other medical facilities.

The pace in most urgent care centers is brisk, and typically a number of doctors are working at one time. Patients are usually requested to make appointments, but drop-ins are accepted in some centers, especially for emergencies.

Because these centers often see a higher volume of patients, usually for a lower cost than the traditional solo-physician or small group practice, some experts predict that urgent care centers will continue to grow in popularity.

Managed Care Operations

Health maintenance organizations, or **HMOs,** are probably the most familiar **managed care operation.** Originally, HMOs were designed to provide a full range of health care services under one roof. More recently, the HMO without walls has become established, which is typically a network of participating physicians within a defined geographic area.

Originally, the HMO with walls was conceived to provide patients with comprehensive health care services at one facility. Today, as managed care and managed competition sweep the health care industry, other arrangements include the preferred provider organization (PPO), where physicians network to offer discounts to employers and other purchasers of health insurance, and the **Independent Physician Association (IPA),** of which the members agree to treat patients for an agreed-upon fee.

The Impact of Managed Care in the Health Care Setting

The emergence of managed care in today's society provides new administrative and clinical challenges to members of the health care team as they struggle to provide the best health care while working within limitations often imposed by insurance carriers. Virtually all health care settings, whether they are individual practices or urgent care centers, are experiencing the impact of managed care, where physicians network and compete to serve patients better and more cost-efficiently.

Under managed care, critics charge, health care dollars have grown scarce, physicians must strive to provide the same quality for reduced reimbursement, preapprovals must be obtained for many services, and some services may be denied because they are not considered cost-effective.

Critical Thinking

Do you agree with the policy that managed care may set limits on services or length of services? Why or why not? Give your rationale.

Clinically, managed care may set limits on services or length of services. Second opinions are encouraged and sometimes required. In some systems, the patient selects a primary care physician, who is considered the gatekeeper and who must provide a referral for specialist care. Critics of managed care point out that restricting or denying services may lead to an increase in professional liability.

Administratively, paperwork and documentation have become increasingly important to ensure proper reimbursement. Although it is the patient's responsibility to understand the conditions of the insurance policy, these are often difficult to understand or interpret. The medical staff must be fully aware of when a preapproval or treatment plan is required, when a second opinion is necessary for reimbursement, and of other clauses and restrictions that affect care and reimbursement for care.

At the same time, although managed care is challenging even the most resilient of providers, the very real need to keep costs down has also generated considerable creativity and energy among the health care profession as physicians seek to use technology more efficiently; as they collaborate on new, cost-effective delivery methods; and as everyone involved in health care—insurers, providers, and patients—works together to contain costs by emphasizing prevention and lifestyle changes.

THE HEALTH CARE TEAM

In every kind of health care setting, the team concept is critical to the quality of patient care. A primary care physician is most likely the main source of health care for patients. From time to time, however, a specialist will be sought or recommended. A number of different allied health professionals, including the medical assistant, will supply additional health care as ordered by the physician. Increasingly, patients are looking outside traditional medicine for portions of their health care. A study published by the *New England Journal of Medicine* in 1993 indicated that more than one third of the adult population chose alternative over conventional forms of medical treatment. In 2001, the World Health Organization (WHO) estimated that between 65% and 80% of the world's population relied on alternative medicine as their primary health care source. One third of all medical schools in the United States now have courses in alternative medicine, and many people in the United States seem to desire a more "natural" approach to health care whenever possible. Although alternative care may not be covered by medical insurance, traditional and nontraditional health care practices are nonetheless blending in many areas.

In whatever manner health care is sought, all members of the health care team must communicate, sometimes in person and sometimes just through the medical history and record, with one another to ensure quality patient care. Note Patient Education box for another major member of the health care team.

The Role of the Medical Assistant

In the ambulatory care setting, a critical allied health professional is the medical assistant. The medical assistant, performing both administrative and clinical tasks under the direction of the physician, is an important link between patient and physician. The medical assistant serves in many capacities—receptionist, secretary, office manager, bookkeeper, insurance coder and biller, sometimes transcriptionist, patient educator, and clinical assistant. The latter requires the medical assistant to be able to administer injections and perform venipuncture, prepare patients for examinations, assist the physician with examinations and special procedures, and perform electrocardiography and various laboratory tests. Medical assistants **triage** and assess patient needs when scheduling appointments and tests. However, although medical assistants have a broad range of responsibilities, it is critical that they perform only within the scope of their training and personal capabilities and always function within ethical and legal boundaries and state statutes.

Because medical assistants are often the patient's first contact with the facility and its physicians, a positive attitude is important. They must be excellent communicators, both verbally and nonverbally, and project a professional image of themselves and their physician-employer. Medical assistants who believe in their work, who are proud of their career, and who convey compassion and caring provide a positive experience for patients who may be ill or in a great deal of discomfort.

The Title "Doctor"

The public is often confused by the title *doctor*. The term implies an earned academic degree of the highest level in a particular area of study. Physicians have earned the MD, or Doctor of Medicine, degree. In the medical field, the abbreviation *Dr.* is used and the title *doctor* is addressed to the person qualified by education, training, and licensure to practice medicine.

Other medical degrees include the Doctor of Osteopathy (DO), Doctor of Dentistry (DDS), Doctor of Optometry (OD), Doctor of Podiatric Medicine (DPM),

Patient Education

Continually remind your patients of the important role they carry in their own health care. *Only your patients* know exactly what happens to their bodies and minds in any particular illness. *Only your patients* know if their pain is too much to bear. *Only your patients* know whether they will remain on any treatment regimen established. *Only your patients* know if they are already embracing some alternative form of treatment. *Only your patients* know how much financial burden they can handle for health care. In initial interviews and pre-physician preparations, ask your patients questions that encourage them to tell you what is happening, whether they are coping, and how their particular problem affects their daily lives. Listen to them carefully. Do not rush or second-guess their responses. Be mindful of the special needs of elderly patients and individuals for whom English is their second language. They are likely unfamiliar with taking a major role in their own health care. Always remember to be therapeutic and observe nonverbal cues. Empower your patients to be a member of their own health care team.

CRITICAL THINKING: Discuss with a peer what action might be taken when patients refuse all opportunities to be a member of their own health care team. How might you encourage patients to take even a small part in their own health care? How would major decisions be made?

Doctor of Chiropracty (DC), and Doctor of Naturopathy (ND).

In nonmedical disciplines, the persons who have achieved a doctorate conferred by a college or university include the Doctor of Education (EdD) and the Doctor of Philosophy (PhD). Both the EdD and PhD have several areas of specialty.

Health Care Professionals and Their Roles

Medical Doctors. A doctorate degree in medicine and a license to practice allows a person to diagnose and treat medical conditions. The doctor of medicine candidate will attend four years of medical school after receiving a bachelor's degree. Newly graduated MDs enter into a residency program that is three to seven years of additional training and education depending on the specialty chosen. This residency comes under the direct supervision of senior physician educators. Family practice, internal medicine, and pediatrics require a three-year residency; general surgery requires a five-year residency. Some refer to the first year of residency as an internship; the American Medical Association (AMA) no longer uses this term, however. At this point, many physicians choose to be board certified, which is optional and voluntary. Certification assures the public that the doctor's knowledge, experience, and skills in a particular specialty have been tested and deemed qualified to provide care in that specialty. Doctors can be certified through 24 specialty medical boards and in 88 subspecialty fields. See Table 2-1 for a partial listing of these fields.

Physicians must still obtain a license to practice medicine from a state or jurisdiction of the United States in which they are planning to practice. They apply for the permanent license after completing a series of examinations and completing a minimum number of years of graduate medical education. Doctors must continue to receive a certain number of continuing medical education (CME) requirements per year to ensure that the doctor's knowledge and skills are current. CME requirements vary by state, professional organizations, and hospital staff organizations.

Osteopathy. Osteopaths are generally recognized as equal to medical doctors in all respects. The Doctor of Osteopathy, or DO, is a fully qualified physician licensed to perform surgery and prescribe medication. The training and education is quite similar to that of the MD. Osteopathic medicine was established in 1874 by Dr. Andrew Taylor Still, who was one of the first physicians to study the attributes of good health to better understand the process of disease. He identified the musculoskeletal system as a key element of health, and encouraged preventive medicine, eating properly, and keeping fit. The education of an osteopath includes a four-year undergraduate degree plus four years of medical school. After graduation from

TABLE 2-1 SELECTED MEDICAL AND SURGICAL SPECIALTIES

Specialties	Title of Doctor	Description
Allergy and Immunology	Allergist and Immunologist	Evaluates diseases/disorders of the immune system and problems related to asthma and allergy
Dermatology	Dermatologist	Evaluates disorders/diseases of skin, hair, nails, and related tissues
Family Practice	Family Practitioner	Treats the whole family from infancy to death
Internal Medicine	Internist	Provides comprehensive care, practices preventive care, treats long-term and chronic conditions
Obstetrics and Gynecology	Obstetrician and Gynecologist	Provides care to pregnant women, delivers babies, treats disorders/diseases of reproductive system
Ophthalmology	Ophthalmologist	Provides comprehensive care of the eye and its structures and offers vision services
Otolaryngology	Otolaryngologist	Treats diseases/disorders of the ears, nose, and throat
Pediatrics	Pediatrician	Treats diseases/disorders of children and adolescents; monitors growth and development of children
Psychiatry and Neurology	Psychiatrist and Neurologist	Diagnoses and treats patients with mental, emotional, or behavioral disorders
General Surgery	Surgeon	Operates to repair or remove diseased or injured parts of the body
Colon and Rectal	Colorectal Surgeon	Operates to remove or repair diseased colon and rectal areas of the body
Neurological	Neurosurgeon	Treats conditions of the nervous systems, often through surgery
Plastic	Plastic Surgeon	Repairs and reconstructs physical defects; provides cosmetic enhancements
Thoracic	Thoracic Surgeon	Performs surgery on the respiratory system, chest, heart, and cardiovascular system
Urology	Urologist	Treats diseases/disorders of the urinary tract

medical school, a DO can choose to practice in any of the 18 American Osteopathic Association specialty areas, requiring from two to six years of additional training. Approximately 65% of all osteopathic physicians practice in primary care areas such as family practice, pediatrics, obstetrics/gynecology, and internal medicine. DOs must pass a state licensure examination and maintain currency in their education. Most patients will find little difference between an MD and a DO. However, doctors of osteopathy also will be able to incorporate osteopathic manipulative treatment (OMT) in their treatment of patients as deemed helpful.

Integrative Medicine and Alternative Health Care Practitioners

Many **integrative medicine** and alternative health care practitioners also carry the title *doctor*, but they have a different training regimen than required for the MD or DO. The training is highly specialized and specific; and when licensed, these professionals are allowed to diagnose and treat medical conditions.

As mentioned earlier, alternative therapies are increasingly being perceived as complements to traditional health care in a form of integrative medicine. In this text, three broad disciplines are identified: chiropractic, naturopathy, and Oriental medicine/acupuncture.

Chiropractic. Chiropractic is a branch of the healing arts that gives special attention to the physiological and biochemical aspects of the body's structure and includes procedures for the adjustment and manipulation of the articulations and adjacent tissues of the human body, particularly of the spinal column. Chiropractic is a drug-free, nonsurgical science that does not include pharmaceuticals or surgery.

The roots of chiropractic care may be traced back to the beginning of recorded time. Writings from China and Greece written in 2700 B.C. and 1500 B.C. mention spinal manipulation and maneuvering of the lower extremities to ease lower back pain. Daniel David Palmer founded the chiropractic profession in the United States in 1895. Throughout the twentieth century, doctors of chiropractic gained legal recognition and licensure in all 50 states.

Doctors of chiropractic (DC) complete four to five years of study at an accredited chiropractic college. The curriculum includes a minimum of 4,200 hours of classroom, laboratory, and clinical experience. About 555 hours are devoted to adjustive techniques and spinal analysis. This specialized education must be preceded by a minimum of 90 hours of undergraduate courses focusing on science. On successful completion of their education and training, doctors of chiropractic must also pass the national board examination and all examinations or licensure requirements identified by the particular state in which the individual wishes to practice.

Doctors of chiropractic frequently treat patients with neuromusculoskeletal conditions, such as headaches, joint pain, neck pain, lower back pain, and sciatica. Chiropractors also treat patients with osteoarthritis, spinal disk conditions, carpal tunnel syndrome, tendonitis, sprains, and strains. Chiropractors also may be found treating a variety of other conditions such as allergies, asthma, and digestive disorders. There are obstacles to chiropractors in some areas, however, because states vary in what they authorize chiropractors to practice and may limit their ability to practice **homeopathy** or **acupuncture** or to dispense or sell dietary supplements.

Naturopathy. Naturopathy, often referred to as "natural medicine," is based on the belief that the cause of disease is violation of nature's laws. The goal of the naturopath is to remove the underlying causes of disease and to stimulate the body's natural healing processes. Naturopathic treatments may include fasting, adhering to natural food diets, taking vitamins and herbs, tissue minerals, counseling, homeopathic remedies, manipulation of the spine and extremities, massage, exercise, naturopathic hygienic remedies, acupuncture, and applications of water, heat, cold, air, sunlight, and electricity. Most of these treatment methods are used to detoxify the body and strengthen the immune system.

In the United States, a Doctor of Naturopathy (ND) or Doctor of Naturopathic Medicine (NMD) will receive education, training, and credentials from a full-time naturopathy college. The full-time education includes two years of science courses and two years of clinical work. Naturopaths are currently licensed to practice in 11 states, and other states are considering licensure. In many states, naturopaths practice independently and unlicensed, or they practice under the direction of a physician.

Oriental Medicine and Acupuncture. Oriental medicine is a comprehensive system of health care with a history of more than 3,000 years. Oriental medicine includes acupuncture, Chinese herbology and bodywork, dietary therapy, and exercise based on traditional Oriental medicine principles. This form of health care is used extensively in Asia and is rapidly growing in popularity in the West.

Oriental medicine is based on an energetic model rather than the biochemical model of Western medicine. The ancient Chinese recognized a vital energy behind all life-forms and processes called *qi* (pronounced "chee"). Oriental healing practitioners believe that energy flows along specific pathways called meridians. Each pathway is associated with a particular physiological system and internal organ. Disease is the result of deficiency or imbalance of energy in the meridians and their associated physiological systems. Acupuncture points are specific sites along the meridians. Each point has a predictable effect on the vital energy passing through it. Modern science has measured the electrical charge at these points, corroborating the locations of the meridians. Traditional Oriental medicine uses an intricate system of pulse and tongue diagnosis, palpation of points and meridians, medical history, and other signs and symptoms to create a composite diagnosis. A treatment plan then is formulated to induce the body to a balanced state of health.

The World Health Organization (WHO) recognizes acupuncture and traditional Oriental medicine's ability to treat many common disorders, including the following disorders:

- *Gastrointestinal disorders:* food allergies, peptic ulcer, chronic diarrhea, constipation, indigestion, anorexia, gastritis
- *Urogenital disorders:* stress incontinence, urinary tract infections, and sexual dysfunction
- *Gynecological disorders:* irregular, heavy, or painful menstruation; premenstrual syndrome (PMS); and infertility
- *Respiratory disorders:* emphysema, sinusitis, asthma, allergies, and bronchitis
- *Neuromusculoskeletal disorders:* arthritis; migraine headaches; neuralgia; insomnia; dizziness; and low back, neck, and shoulder pain
- *Circulatory disorders:* hypertension, angina pectoris, arteriosclerosis, and anemia
- *Eye, ear, nose, and throat disorders:* otitis media, sinusitis, and sore throats
- *Emotional and psychological disorders:* depression; anxiety; and addictions to alcohol, nicotine, and drugs
- *Pain:* elimination or control of pain for chronic and painful debilitating disorders

In the hands of a comprehensively trained acupuncturist, patients will not find acupuncture painful. Sterile, very fine, flexible needles about the diameter of a human hair are used in treatment. Practitioners may also recommend herbs, dietary changes, and exercise together with lifestyle changes.

Training for acupuncture and Oriental medicine may be obtained in schools and colleges accredited by the Accreditation Commission for Acupuncture and Oriental Medicine. There is a minimum of two years of undergraduate study required, and some colleges prefer applicants to have a bachelor's degree. Most of these specialized programs are three years and on completion graduates are conferred with a Masters in Acupuncture and Oriental Medicine (MAOM) or a Masters in Acupuncture (MA) degree. Nearly all states regulate the practice of acupuncture and Oriental medicine, either through licensure or a ruling by the Board of Medical Examiners. It is likely that passing a national certification examination or other testing procedure is required before licensure. Many doctors (MDs, DOs, DCs, and NDs) have become qualified to perform acupuncture and to use Oriental medicine in their practices through additional education and training.

Future of Integrative Medicine

There was a time when chiropractors were not accepted by the medical establishment and had difficulty with licensure. Naturopaths, acupuncturists, and Oriental medicine practitioners face similar challenges, and states vary greatly in their regulations of any form of alternative medicine.

The road may be bumpy for alternative practitioners, but their numbers are increasing rapidly. By 2010, the number of chiropractors is projected to double, and the number of naturopaths is expected to triple. Oriental medicine practitioners, including acupuncturists already licensed in 42 states and in the District of Columbia, are likely to grow even more. This latter fact is partially attributed to the Asian American population that is expected to increase by as much as 95% by 2010. Managed care health plans are offering increased access to alternative medicine clinicians, mostly because of the ability to expand patient choices at a lower cost. It is expected that states will broaden their licensure to increased numbers of well-educated and trained alternative practitioners.

Neither the growth in the number of alternative medicine practitioners nor the laws and insurance practices that facilitate their access by patients likely would have occurred without broad public acceptance of alternative and complementary medicine. Americans seem quite willing to pay out-of-pocket expenses for alternative forms of treatment such as massage therapy, aromatherapy, biofeedback, guided imagery, hydrotherapy, hypnotherapy, and homeopathy. Furthermore, there are many patients seeking a more integrated form of medicine that occurs when primary care physicians are willing to refer to an alternative practitioner and vice versa. See Table 2-2 for a brief description of a few alternative modalities that fairly easily integrate with traditional medical practices.

ALLIED HEALTH PROFESSIONALS AND THEIR ROLES

In the health care team, allied health professionals bring specific educational backgrounds and a broad array of skills to the medical environment. Medical assistants are considered allied health professionals. Table 2-3 lists some of the allied health professionals recognized by the Commission on Accreditation of Allied Health Education Programs (CAAHEP) and the Accrediting Bureau of Health Education Schools (ABHES).

As a medical assistant, you may not work directly with all the identified allied health care professionals, but you are likely to have contact with many of them by telephone and written or electronic communication. Knowledge of the roles these health professionals play enables you to interact more intelligently with all members of the health care team.

In addition to the professionals listed in Table 2-3, you may encounter some or all of the following health care professionals in daily patient care.

TABLE 2-2 SELECTED ALTERNATIVE MEDICINE MODALITIES

Acupressure: A massage technique that applies pressure to specific acupuncture-like points on the body; pressure encourages the flow of vital energy *(qi)* along the meridian pathways. It is used to control chronic pain, migraine headaches, and backaches.
Aromatherapy: The inhalation and bodily application of essential oils from aromatic plants to relax, balance, rejuvenate, restore, or enhance the body's mind and spirit. It strengthens the self-healing process by indirect stimulation of the immune system.
Biofeedback: Biofeedback machines gauge internal bodily functions and help patients tune in to these functions and identify the triggers that evoke symptoms. Relaxation can be taught to relieve the symptoms.
Guided Imagery: Uses images or symbols to train the mind to create a definitive physiological or psychological effect; relieves stress and anxiety and reduces pain.
Homeopathy: Healing that claims highly diluted doses of certain substances can leave an energy imprint in the body and bring about a cure. Homeopathic remedies are made from naturally occurring plant, animal, or mineral substances and are manufactured by pharmaceutical companies under strict guidelines.
Hydrotherapy: Hydrotherapy uses the buoyancy, warmth, and effects of water and its turbulence to speed recovery after surgery and to reduce pain and stress, spasm and discomfort. It is especially beneficial for work- or sports-related injuries and arthritis.
Hypnotherapy: Hypnotherapy facilitates communication between the right and left sides of the brain with the patient in a state of focused relaxation when the subconscious mind is open to suggestions. It is currently used to help people lose weight, stop smoking, reduce stress, and relieve pain, anxiety, and phobias.
Massage: Massage reduces stress, manages chronic pain, promotes relaxation, and increases circulation of the blood and lymph. Hand stroking on the body helps patients become more familiar with their pain.

TABLE 2-3 SELECTED ALLIED HEALTH PROFESSIONS

Occupation	Abbreviations	Job Description
Anesthesiologist Assistant	AA	Performs preoperative tasks, performs airway management and drug administration for induction and maintenance of anesthesia during surgery under direction of a licensed and qualified anesthesiologist
Athletic Trainer	AT	Provides a variety of services including injury prevention, recognition, immediate care, treatment, and rehabilitation after athletic trauma
Clinical Laboratory Technician *Associate Degree*	CLT	Performs all routine tests in a medical laboratory and is able to discriminate and recognize factors that directly affect procedures and results. Works under direction of pathologist, physician, medical technologist, or scientist
Diagnostic Medical Sonographer	DMS	Provides patient services using medical ultrasound under the supervision of a physician
Electroneurodiagnostic Technologist	EEG-T	Possesses the knowledge, attributes, and skills to obtain interpretable recordings of a patient's nervous system functions
Emergency Medical Technician—Paramedic	EMT-P	Recognizes, assesses, and manages medical emergencies of acutely ill or injured patients in prehospital care settings, working under the direction of a physician (often through radio communication)
Health Information Administrator	RRA	Manages health information systems consistent with the medical, administrative, ethical, and legal requirements of the health care delivery system
Health Information Technician	ART	Possesses the technical knowledge and skills necessary to process, maintain, compile, and report patient data
Medical Assistant	MA	Functions under the supervision of licensed medical professionals and is competent in both administrative/office and clinical/laboratory procedures
Medical Illustrator	MI	Creates visual material designed to facilitate the recording and dissemination of medical, biological, and related knowledge through communication media
Occupational Therapist	OT	Educates and trains individuals in the application of purposeful, goal-oriented activity in the evaluation, diagnosis, and treatment of loss of ability to cope with the tasks of daily living and impairment caused by physical injury, illness, or emotional disorder, congenital or developmental disability; or the aging process
Ophthalmic Medical Technician or Technologist	OMT	Assists ophthalmologists to perform diagnostic and therapeutic procedures
Personal Trainer	PT	Develops activity plans for each individual that integrates a complete approach to fitness and wellness through exercise, strength training, and proper diet
Physician Assistant (includes Surgeon's Assistant)	PA	Practices medicine under the direction and responsible supervision of a Doctor of Medicine or Osteopathy; performs diagnostic, therapeutic, preventive, and health maintenance services in any setting in which the physician renders care
Radiographer	RT(R)	Provides patient services using imaging modalities, as directed by physicians qualified to order and perform radiologic procedures
Respiratory Therapist	RRT	Applies scientific knowledge and theory to practical clinical problems of respiratory care
Surgical Technologist	ST	Works as an integral member of the surgical team, which includes surgeons, anesthesiologists, registered nurses, and other surgical personnel delivering patient care and assuming appropriate responsibilities before, during, and after surgery

Health Unit Coordinator

Health unit coordinators (HUCs) perform nonclinical patient care tasks for the nursing unit of a hospital. This profession requires a self-motivated, mature individual who can handle the stress and hectic pace of coordinating personnel and their duties at the nurses' station. Also called unit secretary, administrative specialist, ward clerk, or ward secretary, a health unit coordinator receives on-the-job training with an emphasis on administrative office skills.

Medical Laboratory Technologist

Medical laboratory technologists (MLTs) physically and chemically analyze, as well as culture, urine, blood, and other body fluids and tissues. They work closely with physician specialists such as oncologists, pathologists, and hematologists. Knowledge of specimen collection, anatomy and physiology, biochemistry, laboratory equipment, asepsis, and quality control is essential. The American Society of Clinical Pathology (ASCP) is a professional organization that oversees credentialing

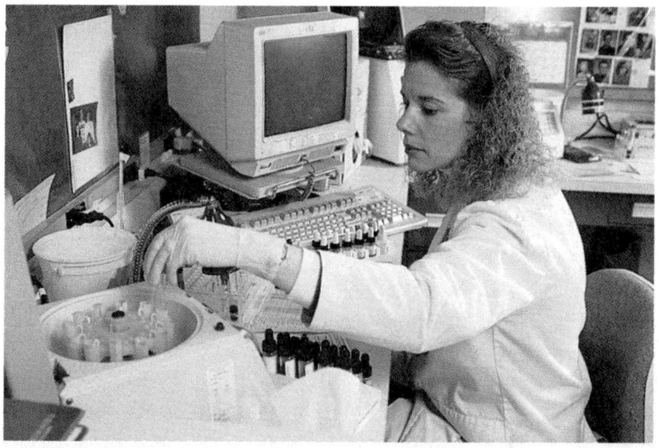

Figure 2-2 Medical laboratory personnel performing blood analysis. (Courtesy of Foote Health Systems.)

and education in the medical laboratory professions. See Figure 2-2.

Nurses

Neither ABHES nor CAAHEP is responsible for nurse education or accreditation, but they are listed here as a major participant in health care. Nurses are licensed by the state in which they practice. Although nurses' education and training are oriented to bedside care, some are employed in medical offices as clinical assistants, especially in offices where surgery is performed. Nurses play a number of roles on the health care team.

Registered Nurse. In the United States, registered nurses (RNs) are professionals who have completed at a minimum, a two-year course of study at a state-approved school of nursing and passed the National Council Licensure Examination (NCLEX-RN). Employment settings most often include hospitals, convalescent homes, clinics, and home health care.

Licensed Practical Nurse. A licensed practical nurse (LPN) is a professional trained in basic nursing techniques and direct patient care. LPNs practice under the direct supervision of an RN or physician and are employed in similar settings to RNs. Training includes completion of a state-approved program in practical nursing and successful completion of a national licensure examination.

Nurse Practitioner. Sometimes referred to as an Advanced Registered Nurse Practitioner (ARNP), a nurse practitioner (NP) is an RN who, by advanced education (usually a master's degree) and clinical experience in a branch of nursing, has acquired expert knowledge in a specific medical specialty. Nurse practitioners are employed by physicians in private practice or in clinics, and sometimes practice independently, especially in rural areas. ARNPs may or may not be licensed to prescribe medications.

Registered Dietitian

Registered dietitians (RDs) have specialized training in the nutritional care of groups and individuals and have successfully completed an examination of the Commission on Dietetic Registration. Dietitians assist patients in regulating their diets. Although they are typically employed in hospitals and clinics, they can also be found working with the public in personal nutritional counseling. Education includes a bachlor's degree with a major in dietetics, food and nutrition, or food service systems management in addition to completion of an approved internship.

Pharmacist

Pharmacists (RPh) are licensed by each state to prepare and dispense all types of medications, as well as medical supplies related to medication administration. They may practice in hospitals, medical centers, and pharmacies. The minimum training for a pharmacist is a five-year bachelor's degree; some pharmacists pursue a Doctor of Pharmacy degree (PharmD), which is offered by major universities in the United States.

Pharmacy Technician

Pharmacy technicians assist the pharmacist with preparation and administration of medications, as well as perform receptionist and billing duties. In hospitals, nursing homes, and assisted living facilities, their responsibilities may include reading patient charts and preparing and delivering medications to patients. Pharmacists must check all orders before delivery. The technician can copy the information about the prescribed medication onto the patient's profile. Professional certification of pharmacy technicians varies from state to state and is administered by state pharmacy associations. See Figure 2-3.

Phlebotomist

Phlebotomists (LPTs) are trained in the art of drawing blood for diagnostic laboratory testing. Phlebotomists are also referred to as laboratory liaison technicians. Phlebotomists may be nationally certified and are employed in medical clinics, hospitals, and laboratories. Training consists of one to two semesters in a community college program or on-the-job training.

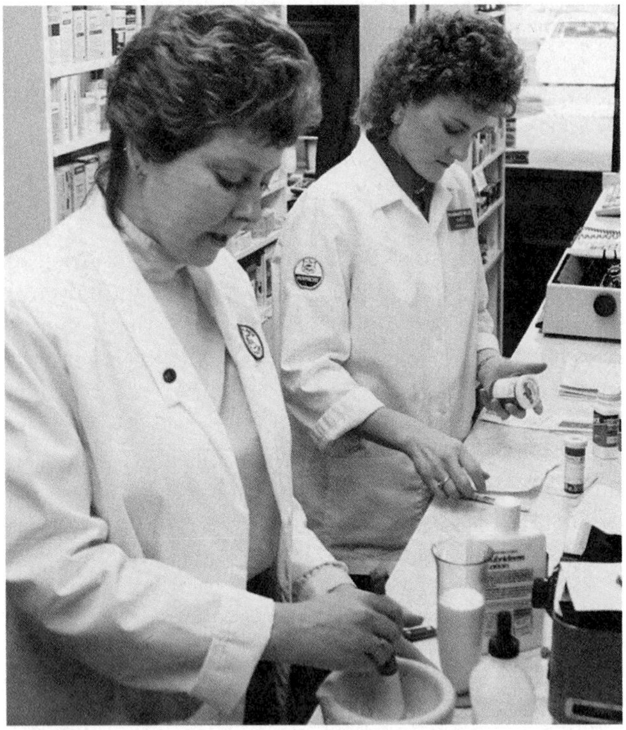

Figure 2-3 Pharmacy technician working with pharmacist in preparing medications. (Courtesy of the Michigan Pharmacists Association and the Michigan Society of Pharmacy Technicians.)

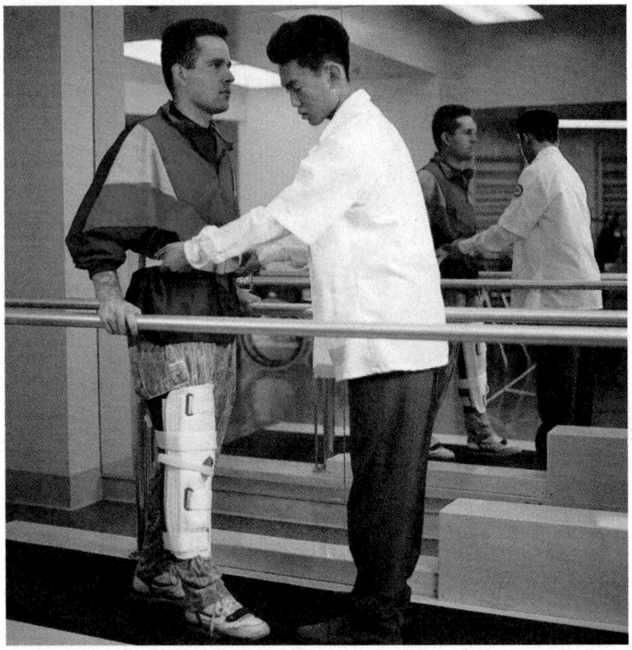

Figure 2-4 Physical therapist working with a patient requiring physical rehabilitation.

Physical Therapist

Physical therapists (PTs) are licensed professionals who assist in the examination, testing, and treatment of physically disabled or challenged people. They also assist in physical rehabilitation of patients after an accident, injury, or serious illness using special exercises, application of heat or cold, *ultrasound* therapy, and other techniques. Educational requirements for a PT are a minimum of a four-year bachelor's degree (Bachelor of Science) or a special certificate course after obtaining the Bachelor of Science in a related field. PTs must also successfully complete a state licensure examination. See Figure 2-4.

Physical Therapy Assistant

Physical therapy assistants (PTAs) are trained to use and apply physical therapy procedures, such as exercise, and physical agents under the supervision of a physical therapist. The PTA has earned an Associate of Science degree from an accredited program and must pass a licensure or registry examination in selected states.

THE VALUE OF THE MEDICAL ASSISTANT TO THE HEALTH CARE TEAM

With their broad range of competencies in both administrative and clinical areas, medical assistants are increasingly valued as health care team members. Medical assistants are the great communicators, serving as liaison between physician and hospital staff and between physician and any number of allied and other health professionals. Because they are the first providers to see or speak with patients, they undertake responsibility for directing, informing, and guiding patient care while establishing a professional and caring tone for the entire health care team. The value of a competent, professional, compassionate medical assistant is immeasurable in today's fast-paced and challenging health care environment.

Case Study 2-1

The number of sole proprietors and small partnerships may be increasing.

CASE STUDY REVIEW

1. What role has managed care had in this event?
2. Describe the impact, if any, this fact has on quality health care.

Case Study 2-2

You are the medical assistant for a family practice physician, Bill Claredon, who is close to retirement. He is much adored by all his patients, but he thinks alternative medicine is outright quackery. Marjorie Johns, a patient with debilitating back pain, tells you she is seeing an acupuncturist and is taking less and less of her prescribed medications. You quietly mention that to Dr. Claredon before he enters the examination room to see Marjorie. He glares at you with disgust at the information and is quite agitated when he enters the examination room. Describe the discussion that you think will occur between Dr. Claredon and Marjorie. If Marjorie is unhappy when she is ready to leave the facility, is there anything you can do or say to help her? Can you do anything to help Dr. Claredon?

SUMMARY

The health care environment is a dynamic service that changes rapidly in response to new technology and societal needs. In an effort to reduce the cost of health care, managed care will continue to have a profound impact on all health care settings. A strong health care team is critical in the health care setting, as primary care physicians, specialists of all disciplines, alternative care practitioners, and allied and other health professionals collaborate on the best way to provide integrative medicine and quality patient care. In almost any health care environment, but especially the ambulatory care setting, the medical assistant is a vital link in the team and is responsible for a range of responsibilities, both clinical and administrative.

STUDY FOR SUCCESS

To reinforce your knowledge and skills of information presented in this chapter:

- ❑ Review the Key Terms
- ❑ Consider the Case Studies and discuss your conclusions
- ❑ Answer the Review Questions
  - ❑ Multiple Choice
  - ❑ Critical Thinking
- ❑ Navigate the Internet and complete the Web Activities
- ❑ Practice the StudyWARE activities on the textbook CD
- ❑ Apply your knowledge in the Student Workbook activities
- ❑ Complete the Web Tutor sections
- ❑ View and discuss the DVD situations

REVIEW QUESTIONS

Multiple Choice

1. Medical assistants are mostly employed in:
   a. hospitals
   b. nursing facilities
   c. ambulatory care settings
   d. insurance companies
2. A health maintenance organization is one kind of:
   a. managed care operation
   b. individual practice
   c. sole proprietorship
   d. hospital
3. With its emphasis on controlling costs, managed care is likely to affect:
   a. only hospitals
   b. all health care settings
   c. only physicians in private practice
   d. only patients
4. The health care team:
   a. should exclude the patient as part of the team
   b. is only important in the hospital setting
   c. is made up of physicians and nurses
   d. includes physicians, nurses, allied health care professionals, patients, and integrative medicine practitioners
5. Integrative health care approaches:
   a. are increasingly accepted as complementary to traditional health care
   b. are always covered by insurance
   c. are seldom approved for licensure
   d. are not important to understand
6. A medical assistant permitted by law to draw blood for diagnostic laboratory testing performs a procedure similar to those performed by a:
   a. health unit coordinator
   b. health information technician
   c. phlebotomist
   d. respiratory therapist
7. The distinct difference between the PA and the MA is that the PA:
   a. draws blood and gives injections
   b. practices medicine
   c. performs diagnostic services
   d. both b and c
8. Physicians just establishing their practice often seek to work with another physician in the same field. When expenses and profits are shared, this form of management is called a/an:
   a. HMO
   b. corporation
   c. sole proprietor
   d. group or partnership
9. Managed care may be identified as care that:
   a. offers unlimited services
   b. forbids second opinions
   c. establishes a primary care physician as gatekeeper
   d. offers protection to physicians against liability
10. An alternative approach to medicine that treats patients using thin, flexible needles is called:
    a. acupuncture
    b. naturopathy
    c. chiropractic
    d. homeopathy

Critical Thinking

1. Evaluate the different health care settings and discuss the pros and cons of working in each setting.
2. From a patient's point of view, which health care setting do you think offers the most benefits? Why?
3. Review the three forms of medical management models. Which is probably the most advantageous from the physician's point of view? From the medical assistant's point of view? Justify your responses.
4. Recall a few types of allied health professionals and, working in small groups, create scenarios in which the medical assistant needs to coordinate patient care with two or three allied professionals.
5. Identify as many reasons as you can for why patients might be seeking alternative approaches to traditional medicine. Explain your choices.
6. Compare Doctors of Osteopathy and Chiropractic. When and why might one be selected over the other?
7. Discuss the validity of licensure or national certification for health care practitioners.

WEB ACTIVITIES

1. American Board of Medical Specialties (http://www.abms.org): Use this site to review details of the specialties. What does board certified mean? Identify those for whom you would most enjoy working and give your reasons.
2. Natural Healers (http://www.naturalhealers.com): Scan this Web site for a listing of most alternative therapy modalities. Select one modality and identify the schools/colleges where education is available and what kind of credentialing is necessary to practice the modality.

3. http://www.integrativemedicine.org identifies a Web site that may prove helpful for health care professionals. It is a membership site, but access is available for introduction and explanation of services. Identify two or three reasons that make this site beneficial to anyone embracing integrative medicine.
4. American Osteopathic Association (http://www.osteopathic.org): After you visit this Web site, discuss the role of the osteopath as a primary care physician in today's health care structure.
5. American Medical News (http://www.amednews.com): This is a newspaper for American's physicians. Find and identify as many articles as you can that discuss how physicians and alternative therapy practitioners identify their roles, where they merge, and where they conflict.
6. American Chiropractic Association (http://www.amerchiro.org): Locate two colleges that educate and train chiropractors. Determine the tuition and cost of each.
7. If you have doubts about alternative medicine, you might want to view the following Web site: http://www.quackwatch.org. It is helpful to research as many thoughts on a subject as possible. Examine the validity of the Web site and whether any biases are evident.

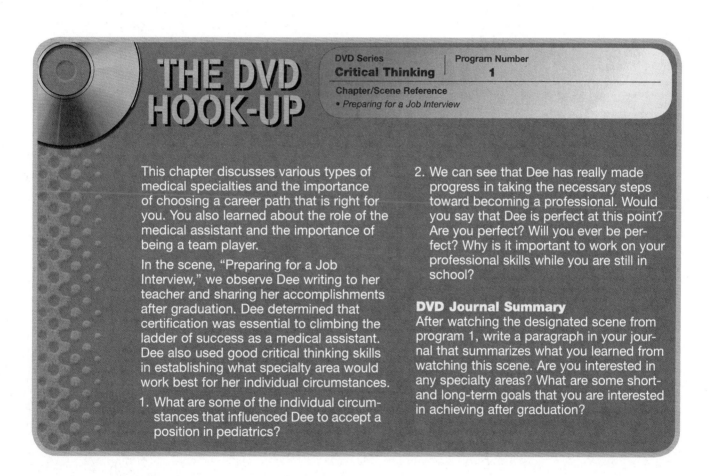

THE DVD HOOK-UP

DVD Series: **Critical Thinking** | Program Number: **1**

Chapter/Scene Reference
- *Preparing for a Job Interview*

This chapter discusses various types of medical specialties and the importance of choosing a career path that is right for you. You also learned about the role of the medical assistant and the importance of being a team player.

In the scene, "Preparing for a Job Interview," we observe Dee writing to her teacher and sharing her accomplishments after graduation. Dee determined that certification was essential to climbing the ladder of success as a medical assistant. Dee also used good critical thinking skills in establishing what specialty area would work best for her individual circumstances.

1. What are some of the individual circumstances that influenced Dee to accept a position in pediatrics?
2. We can see that Dee has really made progress in taking the necessary steps toward becoming a professional. Would you say that Dee is perfect at this point? Are you perfect? Will you ever be perfect? Why is it important to work on your professional skills while you are still in school?

DVD Journal Summary

After watching the designated scene from program 1, write a paragraph in your journal that summarizes what you learned from watching this scene. Are you interested in any specialty areas? What are some short- and long-term goals that you are interested in achieving after graduation?

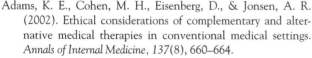

REFERENCES/BIBLIOGRAPHY

Adams, K. E., Cohen, M. H., Eisenberg, D., & Jonsen, A. R. (2002). Ethical considerations of complementary and alternative medical therapies in conventional medical settings. *Annals of Internal Medicine, 137*(8), 660–664.

American Board of Medical Specialties. (2000). *Approved ABMS specialty boards & certificate categories*. Evanston, IL: Author.

Eisenberg, D. M., Cohen, M. H., Hrbek, A., Grayzel, J., Van Rompay, M. I., & Cooper, R. A. (2002). Credentialing complementary and alternative medical providers. *Annals of Internal Medicine, 137*(12), 965–973.

Frenkel, M. A., & Borkan, J. M. (2003). An approach for integrating complementary-alternative medicine into primary care. *Family Practice, 20*(3), 324–332.

Health professions career & education directory (2004–2005). (2004). Chicago, IL: American Medical Association.

Tamparo, C. D., & Lewis, M.A. (2005). *Diseases of the human body* (4th ed.). Philadelphia: F.A. Davis Publishers.

Triveri, Jr., L., & Anderson, J. W. (2002). *Alternative medicine. The definitive guide* (2nd ed.). Berkeley, CA: Celestial Arts.

CHAPTER 3

History of Medicine

OUTLINE

Cultural Heritage in Medicine
Medical Specialists in History
History of Medical Education
History of Attitudes toward Illness
Historical Medical Treatments
Significant Contributions to Medicine
Frontiers in Medicine

OBJECTIVES

The student should strive to meet the following performance objectives and demonstrate an understanding of the facts and principles presented in this chapter through written and oral communication.

1. Define the key terms as presented in the glossary.
2. Discuss the effects of culture on medicine.
3. Identify the role of religion, magic, and science in medicine's history.
4. Describe how attitudes toward illness are manifested today.
5. Identify a minimum of three previously used common medical treatments.
6. Recall a minimum of three theories/practices of ancient medicine that are still prevalent today.
7. Name and describe the historical roles of medical specialists.
8. Discuss the role of women in medicine.
9. Trace the progression of medical education.
10. Name at least five significant contributions to medicine.
11. Identify a minimum of three recent developments in medicine.

KEY TERMS

Allopathic
Asepsis
Bubonic Plague
Malaria
Moxibustion
Pharmacopoeia
Pluralistic (Pluralism)
Septicemia
Typhus (Typhoid)
Yellow Fever

SCENARIO

You may recall your mom putting a mentholated salve on your chest when you had a cold. Your cousins had to take a spoonful of cod-liver oil each night before they went to bed. Grandma made chicken soup with homemade noodles when you had the flu. An apple a day, mustard plaster for the chest, hot or cold steam in a room, and many more are medical practices of years gone by. Many still stand, however, and from them others have developed. Interestingly, medicine has a rich history, and every culture exhibits that history differently. The more you know and understand of that history and its various cultural influences, the more effective and therapeutic will be your communication with patients.

INTRODUCTION

A historical overview of medicine must do more than identify a series of contributions by physicians. It must remind us that more than one discipline and more than one philosophy have contributed to medicine. This is perhaps more true now than ever as our world becomes smaller and our society becomes increasingly ***pluralistic,*** *ethnically, culturally, and religiously.*

CULTURAL HERITAGE IN MEDICINE

Today's health professional will give care to individuals of varied cultures who hold differing philosophical beliefs toward medicine. The informed and caring health professional will recognize that a person's culture and ethnic heritage play an enormous role in any kind of health care. For example, if the patient's cultural experience leans toward a more natural, nonmedical form of health care, treating the patient with prescription drugs will necessitate an explanation and rationale for the use of medications. Otherwise, the patient may refuse to take all or part of the medications, thus hindering recovery. It would be better to seek a treatment for the patient that embraces both the health care professional's desire to heal and the individual's wish to respect cultural tradition.

In every society, medicine has been an important element for its people. From the earliest time, culture was an important influence on medicine, and modern day medicine is in many ways a reflection of this diverse and rich heritage.

It is certain that religion, magic, and science all played a vital part in the history of medicine. Religion was important because it was perceived that certain gods were to be called on for a cure through ceremonies, prayers, and sacrifices. Magic was practiced because it was such an important part of many societies and was seen as an essential ingredient to chase away evil spirits. The importance of science was demonstrated in the use of plants and minerals for medicinal purposes. The use of plants and minerals is found throughout medicine's history. Unearthed clay tablets reveal hundreds of plants, minerals, and animal substances used for medicinal purposes in ancient Mesopotamia and Babylon. The Chinese **pharmacopoeia** was rich in the use of herbs.

Skeletal remains of prehistoric cultures show advanced stages of arthritis, a nearly toothless jaw, and only a 20- to 40-year life span for humans. Skull bones reveal round holes referred to as trephination, believed necessary to release the evil spirits thought to be causing a person's illness. Mesopotamian cultures believed that illness was a punishment by the gods for violation of a moral code. Ancient Egyptians believed the body was a system of channels for air, tears, blood, urine, sperm, and feces. All the channels were thought to come together in the rectum, and were believed to become easily clogged. Thus, emetics, enemas, and purges of the anus were common treatments. In ancient India, plastic surgery was practiced. Punishment for adultery was cutting off the nose, therefore allowing physicians many opportunities to practice and refine the art of nose reconstruction.

The ancient Chinese cultures examined and carefully monitored the pulse in each wrist. It was believed that the pulse had hundreds of characteristics important in medical treatment. There were five methods of treatment to bring a person back to the right track. They were:

1. Cure the spirit.
2. Nourish the body.

Critical Thinking

Are there any indications today that moral behavior, or lack of it, may be the cause of disease and illness? Give examples.

3. Give medications.
4. Treat the whole body.
5. Use acupuncture and moxibustion.

Acupuncture is the piercing of the skin by very thin, flexible needles into any of 365 points along 12 meridians that transverse the body and transmit the active life force called "qi" (pronounced "chee") (Figure 3-1). Each of these spots is related to a particular organ. **Moxibustion** requires the use of a powdered plant substance that is made into a small mound on the person's skin and then burned, usually raising a blister.

Even today's **allopathic,** or traditional, physicians would agree that the first four methods of treatment from Chinese culture are excellent guidelines for health care.

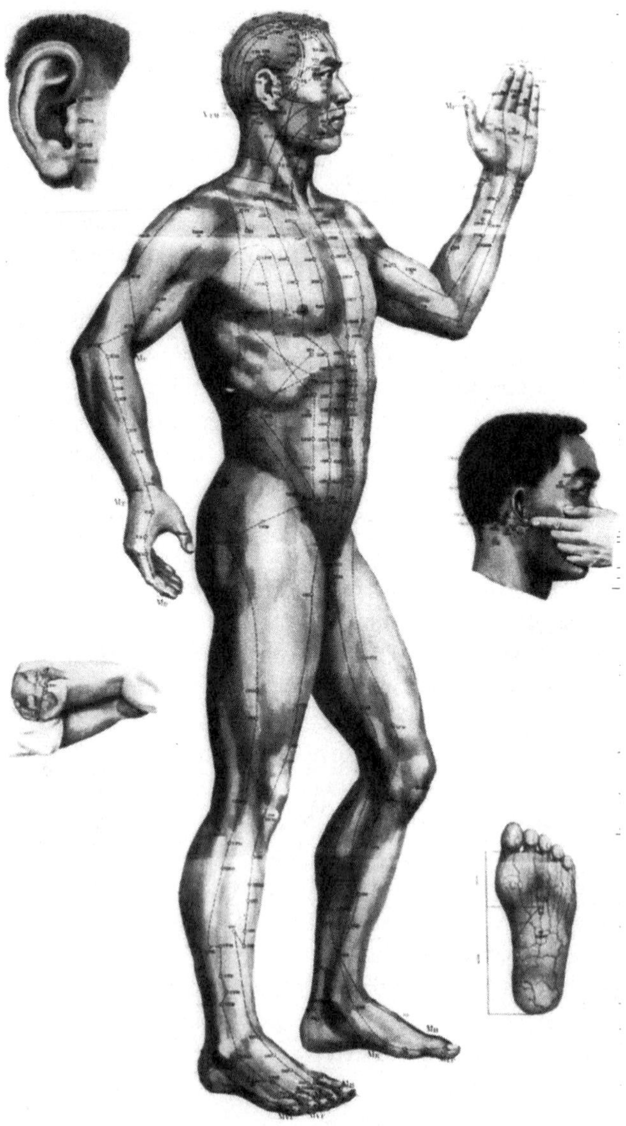

Figure 3-1 Chinese acupuncture points and meridians. (Courtesy of the World Health Organization.)

There also is an increasing awareness that acupuncture has a valid place in allopathic medicine, especially for the control of some types of pain.

MEDICAL SPECIALISTS IN HISTORY

Medicine's history gives early evidence of many "specialists" in the healing arts. They were known by various names—witch doctors, medicine men and women, shamans or healing priests, and physicians. These healers were more than ancestors of the modern physician, however, for they performed many functions that involved the welfare of the entire community or village. By today's standards, they were considered to be equivalent to spiritual advisers, social workers, counselors, and teachers.

Whereas women were accepted as healers in primitive societies, later cultures reduced their status to that of being allowed to care only for women and to assist in childbirth. In any culture that granted women only secondary status, women were also considered unqualified to become physicians. In Chinese culture, the first reference to a female physician mentioned by name is in documents from the Han dynasty (206 B.C.–A.D. 220). In Muslim society, the reluctance of Arabic physicians to violate social taboo and touch the genitals of female strangers further encouraged relegating the practice of obstetrics and gynecology to midwives.

Women were not accepted as medical doctors in Western culture until the nineteenth and twentieth centuries. Italy granted women the status earlier than other cultures. In the United States, the first female physician was Elizabeth Blackwell, who was awarded her degree in 1849. Although she was snubbed by the public, she soon earned the respect of her colleagues. When she refused to be absent from class when the male reproductive system was discussed, her fellow male students supported her actions.

From the earliest times, it appears that some payment was expected for medical services rendered. In many instances, the payment was dependent on the status of the physician, as well as the patient. At the same time, some cultures punished a physician who was not successful in treatment by forcing that physician to treat only those too poor to pay.

HISTORY OF MEDICAL EDUCATION

During the rise of Christianity, emphasis was placed on the soul rather than the body; therefore, early Christian monks held great control over medicine. This is evidenced by St. Benedict of Nursia (480–554), who forbade the study of medicine. The care of the sick was encouraged, but only through prayer and divine intervention. Thus, Christ's healing mission was institutionalized in a fashion that was to control medical care almost completely for the next 500 years, until the seventh century.

At that time, however, the religion of Islam moved to preserve the classical learning that had been achieved in medicine, and practitioners were not only able to return to the same methods as those practiced by earlier Greek and Roman cultures, but medical study was now encouraged.

Medical education in established universities began in the ninth century. These universities included Salerno in southern Italy, the University of Montpelier in southern France, and the University of Paris. By the time the Renaissance was at its height in the midfifteenth century, the physician had become licensed, was receiving great status, and was attending the ill in a velvet bonnet and fur-trimmed cloak.

Art and science were more closely related during the Renaissance than at any other period. Michelangelo (1475–1564) spent years on careful human dissection, and this anatomical detail is evident in his paintings in the Sistine Chapel in the Vatican in Rome. Leonardo da Vinci (1452–1519) made anatomical preparations from which he produced drawings representing the skeletal, muscular, nervous, and vascular systems. His accurate sketch of the spinal vertebrae went undiscovered for more than 100 years.

HISTORY OF ATTITUDES TOWARD ILLNESS

Various attitudes prevailed toward the ill person. A sick person might be excused from daily activity, but was likely to be shunned if the disease was believed to be a punishment by the gods for mortal sin. This forced isolation may well have been beneficial to the community. In contrast, touching by Jesus was an important component of healing, as was the faith of the individual involved. The New Testament parable of the Good Samaritan helped establish a nexus between the early church and a concern for the sick. It was believed that though the body might be wasted and foul with disease, the purity of the soul guaranteed life everlasting. This was unlike the pagan religions that tended to abandon individuals thought to be ill because they were in disfavor with the gods.

Native Americans had various feelings about illness. The ill were treated with kindness among the Navaho and Cherokee, and some who recovered from serious illness were considered to have extraordinary powers. However, if a tribe was faced with famine, suicide by the aged and infirm was considered the highest form of bravery. The Eskimos put their older adults unprotected onto ice floes. Neither the Romans nor the Greeks treated the hopelessly ill or deformed, and unwanted infants were disposed of quickly or left to die.

Some of these attitudes are seen even today. The Western medical community and the consumers it serves are heatedly debating the right to choose life or death and the ethics and legality of physician-assisted suicide, which is acceptable in many other cultures. Even with our vast knowledge of medicine and the disease process, many individuals are still fearful of any illness they do not understand or that they perceive as threatening their health—AIDS is a good example. This fear is often accompanied by public ill treatment of the individuals suffering from certain diseases. For example, Cuba quarantines everyone who tests positive for human immunodeficiency virus (HIV) infection, even if they show no signs of illness.

HISTORICAL MEDICAL TREATMENTS

The writings of ancient Egypt reveal that when a woman suspected she was pregnant, she urinated over a mixture of wheat and barley seeds combined with dates and sand. If any of the grains sprouted, she was surely pregnant. If the wheat grew, she would have a boy. If the barley grew, it would be a girl. Urine is still used in modern tests to determine pregnancy.

During the Ming dynasty (1368–1644), Chinese medicine seemed to reach its peak. This is the time that Li Shih-chen wrote his Pen ts'ao kang mu, "The Great Herbal." This pharmacopoeia summarizes what was known of herbal medicine up to the late sixteenth century, describing in detail more than 1,800 plants, animal substances, minerals, and metals, together with their medicinal properties and applications.

Early medical treatments were often crude. For a sore throat, a physician might mix barley water, vinegar, and mulberry syrup for a gargle. Someone suffering with rheumatism might be given a prescription of chopped mice, lynx claws, and elk hooves. Rhubarb, senna, bitter apple, turpentine, camphor, and mercury were among the physicians' staples. Some physicians washed the instruments used in treating the ill; others scoffed at such a practice. **Malaria,** diphtheria, tuberculosis, **typhoid,** and dysentery were commonplace. Leprosy was prevalent; and venereal diseases were rife. Smallpox was frequent in villages; sometimes the sufferer would be placed in a meat pickling vat and fumigated. The death toll from such diseases was particularly high among children. Finally, in the eighteenth century, Edward Jenner made a great contribution to the prevention of disease by discovering a method of vaccination against smallpox.

Critical Thinking

What steps are taken today in hospitals and in ambulatory care settings to prevent the spread of harmful bacteria and viruses? What steps do you personally take?

Medicine progressed rapidly during the nineteenth century. Two important discoveries occurred: anesthesia to alleviate pain during surgery, and the realization that some bacteria cause disease. Once it had been proved that certain bacteria were causes of diseases and were transmissible agents responsible for contagion, greater care was taken to prevent that transmission. **Asepsis** became important to reduce the risk for infection. The Hungarian physician and obstetrician Ignaz Philipp Semmelweis (1818–1865) was able to prove that physicians who came from an autopsy directly to the care of postpartum women, without scrubbing their hands and washing instruments, carried infection with them that often caused puerperal fever (**septicemia** after childbirth) and death to the new mothers.

The names of Louis Pasteur (1822–1895), Joseph Lister (1827–1912), and Robert Koch (1843–1910) are familiar to all bacteriologists. Louis Pasteur has sometimes been referred to as the father of preventive medicine as the result of his work in recognizing the relationship between bacteria and infectious disease (Figure 3-2). Joseph Lister revolutionized surgery because of his belief in Pasteur's theory of using carbolic acid as an antiseptic spray. He insisted that all instruments and physicians' hands be washed with the solution. Robert Koch used the culture-plate method for isolating bacteria and demonstrated how cholera was transmitted by food and water. His discovery changed the way health departments cared for persons with infectious disease.

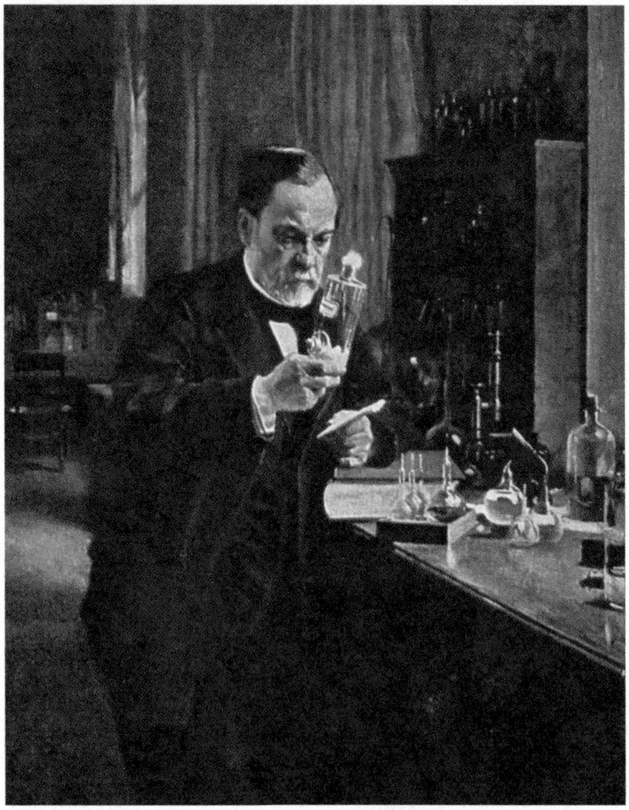

Figure 3-2 Louis Pasteur, the father of preventive medicine.

Fortunately, early in the twentieth century, society was finally liberated from many of the infectious and epidemic diseases that had scourged the human race for millennia. Smallpox vaccinations became common, and causes of **yellow fever, typhus,** and **bubonic plague** were determined. Life expectancy increased. Tuberculosis became less frequent. In 1922, Frederick G. Banting and a medical student, Charles Best, were able to isolate and inject insulin into a 14-year-old boy who was dying of diabetes. Two weeks later, the boy was alive and alert. By 1923, insulin was available for general sale in pharmacies throughout the world. Antibiotics were discovered and the Salk and Sabin vaccines were found for poliomyelitis.

The first electrocardiogram machine was invented in 1903. George Papanicolaou discovered cancer cells in 1928, the same year penicillin was discovered by Alexander Fleming. Penicillin, however, required further development, which was accomplished by Howard Florey and Ernst Chain, and was finally brought into production in 1945. C. Walton Lillehei performed the first successful open-heart surgery in 1952. Dr. Christian Barnard performed the first human heart transplant in 1967. Advancing technology enabled medicine to march steadily forward.

Yet, as we enter the twenty-first century, we are quite aware of the limitations of modern medicine. AIDS is a reminder that plagues are still possible. In developing countries torn with war and strife, cholera causes the deaths of thousands simply because there is no proper sanitation. In the microbial world, there are new, drug-resistant strains of malaria, tuberculosis, and other diseases that are not responding to known treatments. The challenge of medicine is as strong today as it was 100 years ago.

Critical Thinking

Do you agree with the statement: "The challenge of medicine is as strong today as it was 100 years ago"? Identify your reasoning and give examples.

SIGNIFICANT CONTRIBUTIONS TO MEDICINE

Hippocrates (c. 460–c. 377 B.C.) is the physician most frequently recalled from the Greek culture. It is not known why his name surfaces above all other Greek physicians, for some were surely just as prominent. His writings, however, have contributed much to today's medical culture. Hippocrates is remembered by many for his well-known Hippocratic Oath, which established guidelines for a physician's practice of medicine. Although few physicians swear to this oath today when they embark on their medical career, it is still recognized for its validity and wisdom. There are various translations of the Hippocratic Oath, but all communicate the same fundamental message.

It would be impossible to identify all the other individuals who made significant contributions to medicine in this text. However, Table 3-1 lists several notable individuals in the history of medicine.

FRONTIERS IN MEDICINE

There has been phenomenal growth in medicine in the past two decades. Only a few advances are mentioned here. Much better imaging leading to much better diagnosis is now available. Where exploratory surgery might have been

TABLE 3-1 IMPORTANT PERSONS AND EVENTS IN THE HISTORY OF MEDICINE

Moses (1205 B.C.)	Advocate of health rules in Hebrew religion
1000 B.C.	Beginnings of Ancient Chinese medicine
Hippocrates (460–377 B.C.)	Greek physician; "father of medicine"
Chang Chung-ching (168–196)	Chinese physician; called the Hippocrates of China
1368–1644	Chinese medicine reaches its peak
Andreas Vesalius (1514–1564)	Brussels physician; wrote first anatomical studies
Anton van Leeuwenhoek (1632–1723)	Dutch lens grinder; discovered lens magnification
John Hunter (1728–1793)	Founder of scientific surgery
Edward Jenner (1749–1823)	Developed smallpox vaccine
Rene Laennec (1781–1826)	Invented the stethoscope
Samuel Hahnemann (1755–1843)	German physician; established homeopathy
Ignaz Semmelweis (1818–1865)	Introduced hand washing to prevent childbed fever
W. T. G. Morton (1819–1868)	U.S. physician; introduced ether as anesthetic
Louis Pasteur (1822–1895)	"Father of bacteriology"
Florence Nightingale (1820–1910)	Founder of modern nursing
Elizabeth Blackwell (1821–1910)	First female physician in the United States
Clara Barton (1821–1912)	Started the American Red Cross in 1881
Joseph Lister (1827–1912)	Laid the groundwork on asepsis
Andrew Taylor (1828–1917)	Established the first school of osteopathy in 1892
Daniel David Palmer (1845–1913)	Founded chiropractic profession in Iowa in 1895
Elizabeth G. Anderson (1836–1917)	First female physician in Great Britain
Frederick G. Banting (1891–1941)	Isolated and injected insulin for diabetes treatment in 1922
1903	First electrocardiogram machine invented
Robert Koch (1843–1910)	Bacteriologist; developed culture-plate method
Wilhelm Roentgen (1845–1923)	Discovered X-rays (roentgenograms)
George Papanicolaou (1883–1962)	Discovered cancer cells in 1928
Sir Alexander Fleming (1881–1955)	Discovered penicillin in 1928
Albert Schatz (1920–2005)	Discovered streptomycin in 1943; cure for tuberculosis
1945	Penicillin brought into production
Paul Zoll (1911–1999)	Created the first heart pacemaker in 1952
C. Walton Lillehei (1918–1999)	Performed first successful open-heart surgery in 1952
John Gibbon (1903–1973)	First heart–lung machine used for surgery (1953)
Joseph Murray (1919–)	First person-to-person kidney transplant in 1954
Christian Barnard (1922–2001)	First human heart transplant performed in 1967
Ian Wilmut (1944–)	Cloned a Finn Dorset sheep called Dolly in 1996
1990–2000	Human genome map created by team of scientists
2000–present	Adult stem cells used in treatment of disease

THE OATH OF HIPPOCRATES

I swear by Apollo Physician and Aesculapius and Hygeia and Panacea and all the gods and goddesses, making them my witnesses, that I will fulfill according to my ability and judgment this oath and this covenant:

To hold him who has taught me this art as equal to my parents and to live my life in partnership with him, and if he is in need of money to give him a share of mine, and to regard his offspring as equal to my brothers in male lineage and to teach them this art—if they desire to learn it—without fee and covenant; to give a share of precepts and oral instruction and all the other learning to my sons and to the sons of him who has instructed me and to pupils who have signed the covenant and have taken an oath according to the medical law, but to no one else.

I will apply dietetic measures for the benefit of the sick according to my ability and judgment; I will keep them from harm and injustice.

I will neither give a deadly drug to anybody if asked for it nor will I make a suggestion to this effect. Similarly, I will not give to a woman an abortive remedy. In purity and holiness I will guard my life and my art.

I will not use the knife, not even on sufferers from stone, but will withdraw in favor of such men as are engaged in this work.

Whatever houses I may visit, I will come for the benefit of the sick, remaining free of all intentional injustice, of all mischief, and in particular of sexual relations with both female and male persons, be they free or slaves.

performed in the past to determine a diagnosis, noninvasive ultrasound, CT scans, and MRIs assist in diagnosis now. People who have worn glasses or contact lenses for many years are turning to laser eye surgery and implantable lenses.

Recently, surgeons performed the first successful human larynx transplant. Consider the implications of the AIDS saliva test that creates a needle-free way to test for HIV. Needleless injections are now possible. There is a flu prevention inhaler and an osteoporosis pill.

Since 2000 there has been successful use of adult stem cells in the treatment of some diseases. Adult bone marrow stem cells are able to produce multiple tissues, and adult stem cells from various organs of the body have shown amazing abilities to develop into healthy tissue. Adult stem cells can be stimulated to form insulin-secreting pancreatic cells, to repair eye retina damage, and to stimulate growth in children with bone disease. There is the possibility that the adult stem cells will also be able to treat Parkinson's disease and other degenerating neural disorders. In the meantime, the political debate continues over the use of human embryonic stem cells.

Experimentation with aromatherapy indicates that some aromas actually improve brain function. Research has shown that individuals suffering from dementia often respond favorably to the odor of freshly roasted coffee and bread baking. Inhaling the scents of green apple, banana, and peppermint stimulates positive feelings. It is thought that with aromatherapy we will soon accelerate learning and speed up rehabilitation for people who have had a stroke.

Who can possibly predict what the future will bring in medicine?

Case Study 3-1

You are a male physician on call in your hospital's emergency department when a woman, five months pregnant, is brought in. She is hemorrhaging. Her husband shuns you and demands a female physician. You quickly realize this couple is Muslim. Role-play this scenario with a classmate. How can you solve the dilemma? Consider the possibility that your only female physician is out of the country on vacation.

Case Study 3-2

Your physician–employer, Dr. Anne Shea, an internist in Southern California, is considering renting office space to an acupuncturist and a naturopath, because many of her patients often seek treatment from both. Dr. Shea believes her practice can be integrated, therefore allowing patients one-stop treatment for their illnesses. As the medical assistant and office manager, you are asked to participate in a meeting of all three practitioners to discuss guidelines for the clinic. What questions will you ask the group?

SUMMARY

Medicine's history leaves us with a rich heritage and a sound basis for the future of health care. Medical history continues to be in the making today. For example, research in gene manipulation has the potential benefit of being able to reverse the progression of many debilitating diseases. One day we will look on medical discoveries of this decade and be impressed by how much further medicine has advanced.

STUDY FOR SUCCESS

To reinforce your knowledge and skills of information presented in this chapter:

- ❑ Review the Key Terms
- ❑ Consider the Case Studies and discuss your conclusions
- ❑ Answer the Review Questions
  - ❑ Multiple Choice
  - ❑ Critical Thinking
- ❑ Navigate the Internet and complete the Web Activities
- ❑ Practice the StudyWARE activities on the textbook CD
- ❑ Apply your knowledge in the Student Workbook activities
- ❑ Complete the Web Tutor sections
- ❑ View and discuss the DVD situations

REVIEW QUESTIONS

Multiple Choice

1. A pharmacopoeia is:
   a. a book describing drugs and their preparation
   b. an ancient religious rite used in medicine
   c. a source of magic
   d. used only by twentieth-century physicians
2. At one time, women were typically allowed to use their health care skills to:
   a. cure everyone in society
   b. care only for women and to assist in childbirth
   c. become physicians
   d. care only for older adults
3. An accurate sketch of the spinal vertebrae was created during the Renaissance by:
   a. Leonardo da Vinci
   b. Michelangelo
   c. early Christian monks
   d. Louis Pasteur
4. Hippocrates is a Greek physician often called:
   a. the founder of scientific surgery
   b. the inventor of the smallpox vaccine
   c. the father of medicine
   d. the father of preventive medicine

5. The first woman physician in the United States was:
   a. Florence Nightingale
   b. Clara Barton
   c. Elizabeth Anderson
   d. Elizabeth Blackwell
6. The physician who introduced hand washing to prevent childbed fever was:
   a. Joseph Lister
   b. John Hunter
   c. Ignaz Semmelweis
   d. Edward Jenner
7. Medicine was greatly influenced by:
   a. Greek and Chinese physicians
   b. Culture and science
   c. Religion and magic
   d. b and c

Critical Thinking

1. With a group of peers, identify the effects of culture on today's medicine.
2. How does the role of a medical specialist today compare to the role of a medical specialist in the past? Consider both similarities and dissimilarities.
3. You are the medical assistant. Your physician–employer has just prescribed opiates for a young Asian woman suffering from migraine headaches. You overhear the young woman arguing with her mother who thinks that she should take nonaddictive Chinese herbs. What, if anything, would you do?
4. Discuss with a peer the role of women in medicine today. What difficulties, if any, might a female physician face today? Compare today's difficulties with those of female health care practitioners 100 years ago.
5. Using the example of aromatherapy use in Frontiers in Medicine, identify any new frontiers using integrative medicine that you know about or have seen used in patient treatment.
6. Breakthroughs in medicine often have been realized through accident or a number of trial and error experiments. Human experimentation is also often necessary. Discuss the need for continued research, funding for research and experimentation, and how patients might often be involved.
7. From your personal experience and observations, identify ways in which physicians (both nontraditional and traditional) have been paid for their services. What major changes in the payment process have been evidenced in the last decade?

WEB ACTIVITIES

The World Wide Web is an ideal place to seek evidence of new and emerging technologies in medicine. One such avenue is "Medical Breakthroughs" reported by Ivanhoe Broadcast News, Inc. Identify at least two or three recent discoveries you find particularly interesting from your research on the Web.

1. Do an Internet search using the keywords "penicillin discovered" to find some interesting sites. Determine the reasons it took so long to put penicillin into production. What kind of hurdles do new medications face today before they are available on the market to consumers and patients?
2. Two physicians reviewed many medical discoveries to determine the 10 greatest discoveries in the history of Western medicine. Using the keywords "medicine's ten greatest discoveries," identify the names of the two physicians. How many discoveries were researched? What do these physicians name as the "greatest medical achievement of all time"? Are all 10 of the discoveries listed in this text? The two physicians are betting on cures for two ailments in the future. Name them. Have the cures been found?
3. Access the Internet to compare/contrast medical schools and universities in the United States with medical universities in China. What major differences do you note? Are there any similarities?

REFERENCES/BIBLIOGRAPHY

Fenster, J. M. (2003). *Mavericks, miracles, and medicine*. New York: Carroll & Graf Publishers.

Lewis, M. A., & Tamparo, C. D. (2002). *Medical law, ethics, and bioethics for ambulatory care* (5th ed.). Philadelphia: F.A. Davis.

Lyons, A. S., & Petrucelli II, J. R. (1978). *Medicine: An illustrated history*. New York: Harry N. Abrams, Inc.

Warden, C. D. (1986). *Health care in the 1980s from a consumer's perspective*. Unpublished doctoral dissertation, Union Graduate School, Seattle, WA.

UNIT 2
The Therapeutic Approach

CHAPTER 4

Therapeutic Communication Skills

OUTLINE

Importance of Communication
Biases and Prejudices
The Communication Cycle
- The Sender
- The Message
- The Receiver
- Feedback

Listening Skills
Types of Communication
Verbal Communication
- The Five Cs of Communication

Nonverbal Communication
- Facial Expression
- Territoriality
- Posture
- Position
- Gestures and Mannerisms
- Touch

Congruency in Communication
Cultural Influence on Therapeutic Communication
- Establishing Cross-Cultural Communication
- Cultural Brokering
- Maslow's Hierarchy of Needs

Community Resources
Technology and Communication
Roadblocks to Therapeutic Communication
Defense Mechanisms
Therapeutic Communication in Action
- Interview Techniques
- Telephone Techniques

OBJECTIVES

The student should strive to meet the following performance objectives and demonstrate an understanding of the facts and principles presented in this chapter through written and oral communication.

1. Define the key terms as presented in the glossary.
2. Identify the importance of communication.
3. List and define the four basic elements of the communication cycle.
4. Identify the four modes or channels of communication most pertinent in our everyday exchange.
5. Discuss the importance of active listening in therapeutic communication.

(continues)

KEY TERMS

Active Listening
Bias
Body Language
Buffer Words
Closed Questions
Clustering
Compensation
Congruency
Cultural Brokering
Decode
Defense Mechanism
Denial
Displacement
Encoding
Hierarchy of Needs
Indirect Statements
Interview Techniques
Kinesics
Masking
Open-Ended Questions
Perception
Prejudice
Projection
Rationalization
Regression
Repression
Roadblocks
Sublimation
Therapeutic Communication
Undoing

FEATURED COMPETENCIES

CAAHEP—ENTRY-LEVEL COMPETENCIES

Patient Care

- Perform telephone and in-person screening

Professional Communications

- Recognize and respond to verbal communications
- Recognize and respond to nonverbal communications
- Demonstrate telephone techniques

Patient Instruction

- Instruct individuals according to their needs
- Identify community resources

ABHES—ENTRY-LEVEL COMPETENCIES

Communication

- Be attentive, listen, and learn
- Be impartial and show empathy when dealing with patients
- Adapt what is said to the recipient's level of comprehension
- Serve as liaison between physician and others
- Use proper telephone techniques
- Interview effectively
- Use appropriate medical terminology
- Recognize and respond to verbal and non-verbal communication
- Principles of verbal and nonverbal communication
- Adaptation for individualized needs

Administrative Duties

- Locate resources and information for patients and employers

OBJECTIVES (continued)

6. Differentiate between the terms *verbal* and *nonverbal communication.*
7. Analyze the five Cs of communication, and describe their effectiveness in the communication cycle.
8. Demonstrate the following body language or nonverbal communication behaviors: facial expressions, territoriality, position, posture, gestures/mannerisms, and touch.
9. Identify and explain congruency in communication.
10. Discuss the use of Maslow's hierarchy of needs in therapeutic communication.
11. Recall at least four influences on therapeutic communication related to culture, and describe four common biases/prejudices in today's society.
12. Recall at least three steps to building trust with culturally diverse patients.
13. Discuss cultural brokering and its use in medical facilities.
14. Discuss communication modification for electronically transmitted messages.
15. Recall eight significant roadblocks to therapeutic communication.
16. List and describe seven common defense mechanisms.
17. Compare/contrast closed questions, open-ended questions, and indirect statements.
18. List four tools or considerations when communicating on the telephone.
19. Demonstrate the correct way to speak into the mouthpiece of a telephone by answering an incoming call and closing a telephone conversation.

SCENARIO

In the two-doctor office of Drs. Lewis and King, four medical assistants constantly interact with patients, allaying their concerns, scheduling their appointments, instructing them on medications, and helping them understand their insurance coverage. On any given day, office manager Marilyn Johnson, CMA, is greeting patients warmly as they arrive for their appointments. Some patients, such as Anna and Joseph Ortiz, are new to the practice. Marilyn's warm manner puts them at ease. Other patients, such as Martin Gordon, who has prostate cancer, may be depressed and anxious. Marilyn tries to create an environment where they feel free to share their concerns and anxieties.

While Marilyn is busy with patients, administrative medical assistant Ellen Armstrong, CMA, is on the telephone, scheduling appointments, answering patient questions, and making decisions about what calls need priority attention. Ellen projects a warm, courteous presence over the telephone; she maintains her composure, even when faced with difficult calls, and tries always to ask the right questions of callers in a nonthreatening manner.

INTRODUCTION

Of all the tasks and skills required of the medical assistant in the ambulatory care setting, none is quite so important as communication. Communication is the foundation for every action taken by health care professionals in the care of their patients. Because medical assistants are often the liaison between patient and physician, it is critical to be aware of all the complexities of the communication process.

Everyday, Marilyn, Ellen, and the two clinical medical assistants at the offices of Drs. Lewis and King face many communication challenges. This chapter describes effective communication principles, applies those principles to face-to-face communication, as well as telephone communication, and describes the basic roadblocks to communication. The key word to all communication in the medical setting is therapeutic. *In all conversations with patients, the more therapeutic the conversation, the more satisfied the patient will be with the care provided.*

IMPORTANCE OF COMMUNICATION

Therapeutic communication differs from normal communication in that it introduces an element of empathy into what can be a traumatic experience for the patient. It imparts a feeling of comfort in the face of even the most horrific news about the patient's prognosis. The patient is made to feel validated and respected. Therapeutic communication uses specific and well-defined professional skills.

Communication in the health care setting is the foundation of all patient care and is of the utmost importance. Communication must be in nontechnical language the patient can understand, delivered with feeling for the patient's emotional situation and state of mind, yet it still must be technically accurate. The medical staff must be alert to the patient's state of stress and whether defense mechanisms have taken over to the extent that the patient has "tuned out" and is no longer communicating with the staff.

Patients seeking an ambulatory care service look for medical professionals with technical skills and a clinical staff capable of communicating with them. Questions frequently asked by individuals seeking a new physician and clinic include: "Will the doctor talk with me so that I understand?" "Will the doctor listen to what I have to say?" and "Can I talk to the doctor honestly and openly?" The answer to all of these questions needs to be "yes." This chapter discusses these issues and presents some specific techniques for therapeutic communication.

Spotlight on Certification

RMA Content Outline

- Patient relations
- Other interpersonal relations

CMA Content Outline

- Basic principles (Psychology)
- Defense mechanisms
- Recognizing and responding to verbal and nonverbal communication
- Professional communication and behavior
- Evaluating and understanding communication
- Services available

CMAS Content Outline

- Professionalism
- Communication

BIASES AND PREJUDICES

Personal preferences, biases, and prejudices will enter into many physician–patient relationships. Such biases affect the types of communication possible. When individuals are not aware of their biases or prejudices, hostile attitudes may prevail.

For therapeutic communication to take place, biases must be examined, a person's comfort level with each bias determined, and measures taken to ensure that a hostile attitude is not present. **Bias** is defined as a slant toward a particular belief. **Prejudice** is defined as an opinion or judgment that is formed before all the facts are known; prejudice is a preconceived and unfavorable concept. Common biases and prejudices in today's society include:

1. A preference for Western style medicine
2. Choosing physicians according to gender
3. Prejudice related to a person's sexual preference
4. Discrimination based on race or religion
5. Hostile attitudes toward people with different value systems than one's own

Critical Thinking

Define in your own words the terms *bias* and *prejudice*. Now identify one bias and one prejudice that you have. How will these impact your ability to respond therapeutically in the medical setting? What steps can you take to become more accepting of the uniqueness of others, thereby improving therapeutic communication?

6. A belief that people who cannot afford health care should receive less care than someone who can pay for full services

Medical assistants must recognize such biases and prejudices so that their own culture with its biases does not prevent them from responding therapeutically in communications with patients. Such recognition requires being aware of the differences among human beings and willingly accepting the uniqueness of each person.

THE COMMUNICATION CYCLE

All communication, whether social or therapeutic, involves two or more individuals participating in an exchange of information. The communication cycle involves sending and receiving messages even when unconsciously aware of them.

Four basic elements are included in the communication cycle. They are: (1) the sender, (2) the message and a channel or mode of communication, (3) the receiver, and (4) feedback (Figure 4-1).

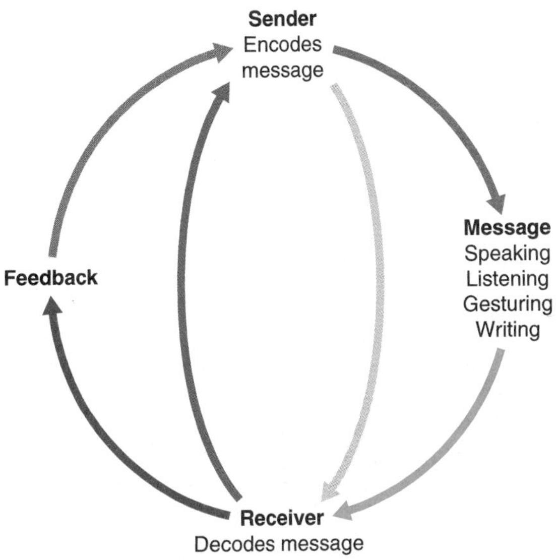

Figure 4-1 The communication cycle and channels of communication.

The Sender

The sender begins the communication cycle by **encoding** or creating the message to be sent. This is an important step, and much care should be taken in formulating the message. Before creating the message, the sender must observe the receiver to determine the complexity of the words to be used within the message, the receiver's ability to interpret the message, and the best channel by which to send the message.

The Message

The message is the content being communicated. The message must be understood clearly by the receiver. Various levels of complexity in communication are used depending on the ability of the receiver to recognize and understand the words contained within the message. Children do not have the vocabulary base or the cognitive skills to communicate and understand at the same level as adults. The health of the receiver also must be considered. A patient who is experiencing stress or in pain may find it difficult to concentrate on the message. If the patient is of a different nationality or culture from the sender, verbal communication may require special skill. When visual or hearing acuity is impaired, another challenge must be surmounted.

The four modes of communication, also called channels of communication, most pertinent in our everyday exchange include: (1) speaking, (2) listening, (3) gestures or body language, and (4) writing. These modes or channels are affected by our physical and mental development, our culture, our education and life experiences, our impressions from models and mentors, and in general by how we feel and accept ourselves as individuals. Each mode or channel of communication has its appropriateness and must be considered when formulating the message.

The Receiver

The receiver is the recipient of the sender's message. The receiver must **decode,** or interpret, the meaning of the message. The primary sensory skill used in verbal communication is listening. It is hard work to concentrate and listen. When decoding the message, the receiver must be aware that not only the spoken words, but the tone and pitch of the voice and the speed at which the words are spoken carry meaning and must be evaluated.

> The idea of minimum necessary access to protected health information (PHI) is important to job performance. HIPAA requires that a reasonable effort be made to limit access to PHI to only what is necessary to accomplish the intended purposes of the use, disclosure, or request. The information accessed must fit the needs of the job description and nothing more. Employees must be careful to not discuss PHI with those outside the scope of their work. For example, a Certified Medical Administrative Specialist scheduling appointments does not need to know the diagnosis after the patient has been seen by the physician.

Feedback

Feedback takes place after the receiver has decoded the message sent by the sender. Feedback is the receiver's way of ensuring that the message that is understood is the same as the message that was sent. Feedback also provides an opportunity for the receiver to clarify any misunderstanding regarding the original message and to ask for additional information.

LISTENING SKILLS

A vital part of feedback in the communication cycle is listening. A good listener is alert to all aspects of the communication cycle—the verbal and nonverbal message, as well as verification of the message through appropriate feedback.

Active listening is one method used in therapeutic communication. In this technique, the received message is sent back to the sender, worded a little differently, for verification from the sender.

> Sender: "How can I possibly pay this fee when I have no insurance?"
>
> Receiver: "You're worried about paying your bill?"

The preceding example illustrates how the receiver is able to validate the sender's concerns at the same time the message is checked for accuracy. The door is then left open for a therapeutic response, such as:

> Sender: "Our bookkeeper will be glad to work out a payment plan with you that will fit your resources."

Active listening involves listening with a "third ear," that is, being aware of what the patient is *not* saying or picking up on hints to the real message by observing body language. The health care professional should have three listening goals:

- To improve listening skills sufficiently so that patients are heard accurately
- To listen either for what is *not* being said or for information transmitted only by hints
- To determine how accurately the message has been received

So many health professionals try to "fix" everything with a recommendation, a prescription, even advice. Sometimes, none of those things is necessary. The patient simply needs someone to listen, to acknowledge the difficulty, and to remember that the patient is not helpless in finding a solution to the problem.

Skill in communication takes years of practice and frequent review. It will never become perfect; we can only hope that we will become better at it with each passing day. Communication is and always will be the basis for any therapeutic relationship (Tamparo & Lindh, 2000).

TYPES OF COMMUNICATION

We communicate by what we say, and also by our tone of voice, body movements, and facial expressions. The following paragraphs present the aspects of verbal and nonverbal communication. The importance of maintaining consistency between verbal and nonverbal messages also is stressed.

VERBAL COMMUNICATION

Verbal communication takes place when the message is spoken. However, one must keep in mind that unless the words have meaning, and unless the sender and the receiver apply the same meaning to the spoken words, verbal communication may be misunderstood. If, for example, you overhear a conversation in a language foreign to you, you are indeed a witness to verbal communication, but you may not understand the message. To have any meaning, the spoken word must be understood by all parties of the communication (Tamparo & Lindh, 2000).

The Five Cs of Communication

In the book *Professional Development*, Mary Wilkes and C. Bruce Crosswait (1995) identify the five Cs of Communication in business. They are: (1) complete, (2) clear, (3) concise, (4) courteous, and (5) cohesive. These five Cs apply equally well in health care professions.

Complete. The message must be complete, with all the necessary information given. The medical assistant cannot expect the patient to be compliant if all the instructions are not given and understood.

Clear. The information given in the message must also be clear. The use of eye contact enhances clarity. Health care professionals must be able to articulate by using good diction and by enunciating each word distinctly. The patient must be allowed time to process the message and verify its meaning. The message must also be heard to promote understanding.

Concise. A concise message is one that does not include any unnecessary information. It should be brief and to the point (Figure 4-2). Patients must not be overloaded with technical terms that may not be understood or that tend to distract them by diverting their attention away from the balance of the message.

Courteous. Courtesy is important in all aspects of communication. It only takes a moment to acknowledge a patient with a smile or by name. Knocking on the examination room door before entering validates the patient's right to privacy and builds self-esteem.

When a patient must be placed on hold on the telephone, thank the patient for waiting. Try not to keep the patient waiting too long if you must find information.

Remember to be courteous to colleagues in the office. Good working relationships and professionalism are always enhanced by simple courtesy.

Cohesive. A cohesive message is organized and logical in its progression. The cohesive message does not ramble and does not jump from one subject to another. The patient should be able to follow the message easily. The medical assistant should always allow time to summarize detailed messages and use responding skills to verify that the patient fully understands the message.

Patient Education

Sensitive medical assistants will encourage patients to verbalize their concerns. The ability to ask questions in a nonprobing way and to elicit patient response is an important function in any ambulatory care setting, because it is critical to know a patient's history, current medications, and other relevant data.

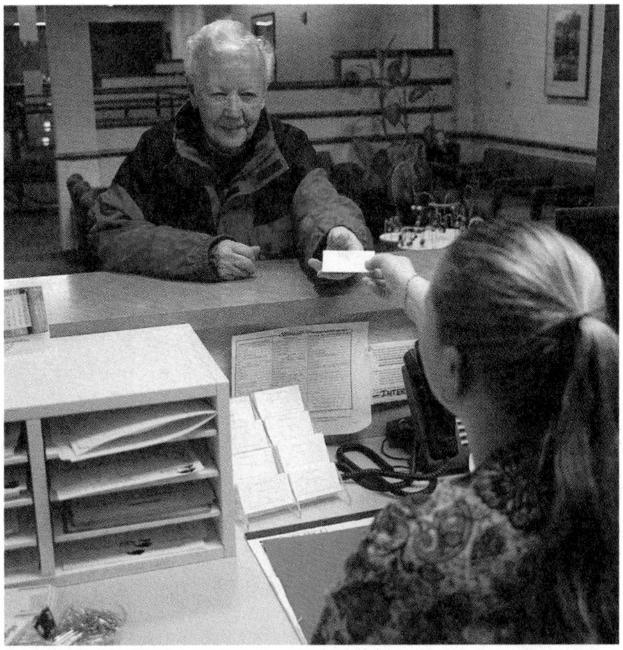

Figure 4-2 To say to the patient after greeting her by name, "I've completed an appointment card to remind you of your next appointment, Tuesday at 2:00 PM," is an example of a concise message that is brief and to the point.

When communicating within the health professions, keep in mind the following:

1. Good communication skills are necessary in establishing rapport with patients.
2. Patients feel respected and validated when called by their full name, such as Mary O'Keefe or Mrs. O'Keefe.
3. Patients should be encouraged to verbalize their feelings.
4. Patients should be given technical information in a manner that they can understand.
5. Patients should be allowed to make practical application to their personal health needs.

NONVERBAL COMMUNICATION

Verbal communication alone is not always adequate in conveying the message being sent. In most instances, more than one mode or channel of communication is used. Nonverbal communication, often referred to as **body language,** includes the unconscious body movements, gestures, and facial expressions that accompany speech. The study of body language is known as **kinesics** (Figure 4-3).

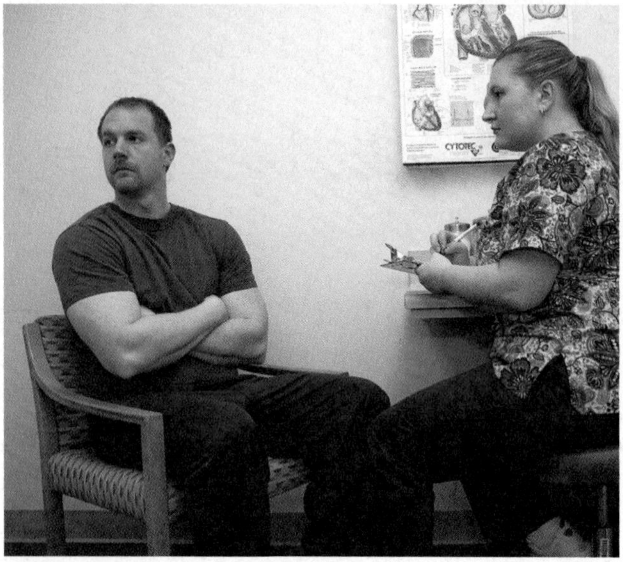

Figure 4-3 Body language can communicate more than spoken words.

Nonverbal communication is the language we learn first. It is learned seemingly automatically when infants learn to return a smile or respond to touches on the cheek. Much of our body language is a learned behavior and is greatly influenced by the primary caregivers and the culture in which we are raised.

Feelings and emotions are communicated most often through nonverbal means. The body expresses its true repressed feelings using body language. Most of the negative messages we communicate are also expressed nonverbally and usually are unintentional. Experts tell us that 70% of communication is nonverbal. The tone of voice communicates 23% of the message—only 7% of the message is actually communicated by the spoken word (Wilkes & Crosswait, 1995).

Facial Expression

Facial expression is considered one of the most important and observed nonverbal communicators. Each facet or aspect of the anatomy of the face sends a nonverbal message.

Often expressions of joy and happiness or sorrow and grief are reflected through the eyes. The anatomy of the eyes does not change, but the movements of the structures surrounding the eyes enhance or magnify the message being communicated.

Children are told it is not polite to stare at people. It is acceptable to stare at animals in the zoo or art objects in the museum, but not at humans. Staring is dehumanizing and is often interpreted as an invasion of privacy.

The medical assistant must learn not to stare when patients present with ailments that make them "look" different. Patients such as these are individuals who have needs, who perhaps feel pain and discomfort, and who have decreased self-esteem and value. These feelings will only be amplified if the medical assistant and other health professionals are unable to "see" them as humans. A lack of eye contact may also be viewed as avoidance or disinterest in being involved.

The movements of the eyebrow indicate many nonverbal cues as well. Surprise, puzzlement, worry, amusement, and questioning are often nonverbal messages reflected by the position of the eyebrow. Wrinkling of the forehead sends similar messages.

Cultural influences affect customs and different forms of facial expressions. It is important to remember that there are many cross-cultural similarities in body language, but there are also many differences. Various cultures denote different meanings to various gestures. If your patient is from another culture, never assume that gestures used hold the same meaning for the patient as they do for you. For example, some cultures believe that prolonged eye contact is rude and an invasion of privacy, whereas others consider it a sign of intimacy. Some people stare at the floor when concentrating or thinking through a process. Other cultures avoid eye contact to display modesty, whereas others feel eye contact expresses hostility or aggression. It is important to understand the cultures of the patients treated in the facility in which you are employed.

Territoriality

Territoriality is the distance at which we feel comfortable with others while communicating. In the classroom, for example, students claim their territory the first day of class. The area is well defined by using books and papers, or by placing the arm, hand, or chair on boundary lines. When another invades the territory, a shift in body position or the use of eye contact sends the message, "This is my area." Individuals may feel threatened when others invade their personal space without permission. Some examples of comfortable personal space for U.S. culture are as follows:

- Intimate: touching to 6 inches
- Personal: 1½ to 4 feet
- Social: 4 to 12 feet
- Public: 12 to 15 feet

As with facial expressions, territoriality or personal space will be handled differently by various cultures. For example, there is no word for privacy in the Japanese language. Population numbers require crowding together publicly, as well as privately. Public crowding is often viewed as a sign of warmth and pleasant intimacy in Japan. In the private home, several generations may live together; however, each considers this space to be his own and resents intrusion into it.

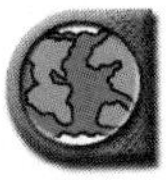

Arabs like to touch their companions, to feel and to smell them. To deny a friend your breath is to be ashamed. When two Arabs talk to each other, they look each other in the eyes with great intensity. U.S. businessmen often end a business arrangement with a handshake; however, American Indians may view a handshake as an act of aggression or an offensive behavior. Each culture has its own distinct nonverbal communication cues.

The medical assistant may perform many invasive tasks during the course of an office visit. Examples include taking vital signs or giving injections, both of which require touching the patient. It is beneficial to explain procedures that invade another's space before beginning the procedure so that it will not be perceived as threatening. This helps to empower the patient by involving the patient in the decision-making process and builds a sense of trust in the medical assistant.

Posture

Like territoriality, posture is important to allied health care professionals. Posture relates to the position of the body or parts of the body. It is the manner in which we carry ourselves, or pose in situations. We tend to tighten up in threatening or unknown situations and to relax in nonthreatening environments. Those who study kinesics believe that a posture involves at least half the body, and that the position can last for nearly five minutes.

When the patient is seated with the arms and legs crossed, the message of closure or being opinionated may be relayed. In contrast, sitting in a chair relaxed with the hands clasped behind the head indicates an attitude of being open to suggestions. Slumped shoulders may signal depression, discouragement, or, in some cases, even pain.

Position

Position, the physical stance of two individuals while communicating, is a key factor to consider while communicating with the patient. Most physician–patient relationships use the face-to-face communication arrangement. When speaking with a patient, the physician or medical assistant will want to maintain a close but comfortable position, enabling observation of all cues being sent, both verbal and nonverbal (Figure 4-4).

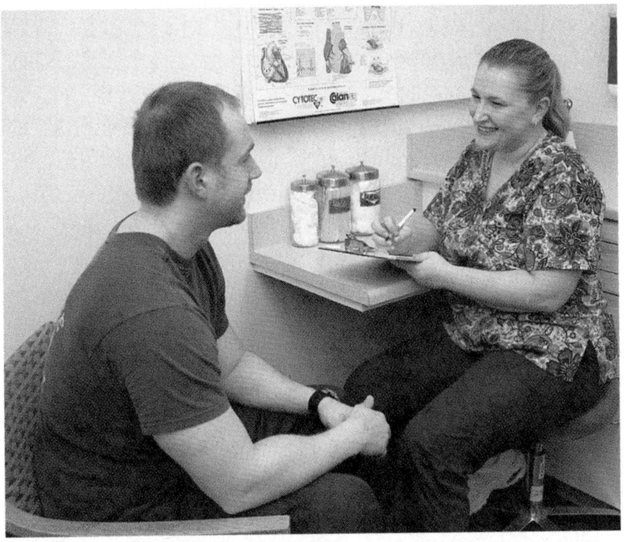

Figure 4-4 Positive posture and position encourage therapeutic communication.

Standing over a patient can convey a message of superiority, and too much distance between the two parties may be interpreted as avoidance or exclusivity. Generally, leaning toward the patient expresses warmth, caring, interest, acceptance, and trust. Moving away from the patient may be interpreted as dislike, disinterest, boredom, indifference, suspicion, or impatience.

Whenever possible, it is best to have a chair in the examination room and to have the patient seated comfortably in the chair to begin the communication cycle. The medical assistant or physician can sit on a stool that can be moved easily toward the patient. This arrangement aids the patient in feeling valued, listened to, and cared for as a fellow human being.

Gestures and Mannerisms

Most of us use gestures and mannerisms when we "talk" with our hands. This form of body language may be useful in enhancing the spoken word by emphasizing ideas, thus creating and holding the attention of others.

Touch

Touch is a powerful tool that communicates what cannot be expressed in words. Its appropriateness in the patient/health professional relationship has well-defined boundaries and requires the use of good judgment on the part of the professional. Infants who are not touched, cuddled, and loved do not grow and develop as those who receive these reassuring gestures. Children of Vietnamese, Cambodian, Hmong, or Thai families traditionally consider the head to be the site of the soul. During conversation and patient assessment, avoid touching the patient's head unless it is necessary for the examination. Southeast Asian clients may fear bodily intrusion; therefore, physical examination and treatment procedures should be explained carefully and completely before they are performed. The touch that communicates caring, sincerity, understanding, and reassurance is usually welcomed and considered to be a therapeutic response. Most patients will understand and accept the touching behavior as it relates to the medical setting; however, we must remember that not all patients are comfortable with touch. Whenever the patient is not comfortable with touch, ask permission and create as safe and reassuring an environment as possible.

CONGRUENCY IN COMMUNICATION

Using some keys to successful communication promotes effective communication. There must be **congruency** between the verbal and nonverbal communication. Shaking your head NO while saying YES verbally sends a mixed message. In most cases, the nonverbal messages will be accepted as the intended message.

It is also important to remember that most nonverbal messages are sent in groups of various forms of body language. The grouping of nonverbal messages into statements or conclusions is known as **clustering. Masking** involves an attempt to conceal or repress the true feeling or message. The perceptive professional will be aware of all these messages.

Perception as it relates to communication is the conscious awareness of one's own feelings and the feelings of others. To be most useful and therapeutic as health professionals, we must first explore our own feelings and appreciate and accept ourselves.

Learning to use perception involves the ability to sense another's attitudes, moods, and feelings. It takes practice and experience to develop and use this skill effectively. Being attentive to other professionals and observing their use of perception will yield insight into its usefulness and provide an example to emulate. A word of caution—the use of perception may easily be misinterpreted, especially when going with your feeling or assessment of what is happening regarding the patient. Always follow perceived assessments with verbal validation before assuming your perception of the circumstance is correct.

Nonverbal communication is easily misinterpreted. Careful observation for congruency between verbal and nonverbal communication, and clustering nonverbal cues being sent into nonverbal statements will strengthen our ability to interpret the message accurately.

CULTURAL INFLUENCE ON THERAPEUTIC COMMUNICATION

For true therapeutic communication to take place, the influence of culture must be considered. Cultural influences include one's ethnic heritage, geographic location and background, genetics, age, sex, economics, educational experiences, life experiences, and value systems.

Any or all of these influences may exhibit themselves when health care is sought by patients. A patient's ethnic heritage may indicate a slant toward the Eastern influence in medicine as opposed to the traditional Western style more commonly taught in the United States today. Geographic location and background may indicate that a person is more comfortable with a family physician in a small clinic than one in a large metropolitan multispecialty practice.

Age and sex are factors with a strong influence on communication. How and when do you communicate with a young child? What do you communicate to that child? How do you impress upon an older gentleman who has taken little medications throughout his lifetime that he now must take his pill everyday? In a culture where the husband is the authority, how does the doctor discuss with the female patient the inadvisability of another pregnancy at this time?

The influence of economics may reveal a discomfort if the office staff and patients have a different perception about how billing is managed and when and how payment is expected. A discussion of billing and payment procedures at the first office visit or before a major procedure will be beneficial to all concerned parties.

Educational and life experiences will, in part, determine how patients react to their care. Patients with family members being treated for a chronic illness will have more knowledge and understanding of that illness in their own lives. Individuals who have already suffered a great deal of loss and grief in their lives may handle the information of a life-threatening illness more calmly than someone who has experienced little grief.

Establishing Cross-Cultural Communication

Before cross-cultural communication or any therapeutic communication can begin, the patient must first be willing to discuss his or her health care issues, listen to the professional's questions, and give honest answers to those questions. The patient must trust the professional. Several steps to building trust include:

- Risk/Trust: The need for the helping professional to build an atmosphere of trust, making it easier for the patient to risk expressing feelings and attitudes about the problem, is essential. Trust has to be earned. Remember to promise no more than you can deliver, be honest, and carefully and thoroughly explain procedures and policies. Answer all questions truthfully and honestly.

- Empathy: Empathy is the ability to accept another's private world as if it were your own. Empathy communicates identification with and understanding of another's situation. It states, "I'm available to walk this road with you."
- Respect: Respect values another person and considers him or her as a special individual. It is important to respect the patient's personal space, to provide privacy, and to use his or her full name and title when appropriate.
- Genuineness: This means being real and honest with others. The health care professional must be able to communicate honestly with others, while being careful not to blame or condemn.
- Active listening: Active listening involves verbal and nonverbal clues that send the message you are completely involved in the communication. Sit facing the patient with no barriers, such as a desk, between you. Lean toward the patient slightly to convey genuine concern and interest. Establish and maintain appropriate eye contact to elicit interest and concern. Maintain an open, relaxed posture to establish a nonthreatening environment for the patient. Listen carefully to the words the patient uses to describe problems, and use those terms rather than medical terminology when discussing symptoms.

Cultural Brokering

Cultural brokering is "the act of bridging, linking, or mediating between groups or persons through the process of reducing conflict or producing change" (National Center for Cultural Competence, Georgetown University Center for Child and Human Development, Georgetown University Medical Center, 2004). A cultural broker serves as a go-between, or one who advocates on behalf of another individual or group within the health care community. The 2000 Census indicates the projected demographic trends in the United States are more complex than ever measured previously. The belief systems related to health, healing, and wellness are diverse, with many cultural variations in the perception of illness and disease and their causes. Cultural brokers respect the values of diverse cultures and health care systems and are knowledgeable of both. They are able to overcome any existing language barriers, so that everyone understands each other clearly. The goal of the Cultural Broker Project is to increase the capacity of health care and mental health programs to design, implement, and evaluate culturally and linguistically competent service delivery systems. Cultural and linguistic competence have been determined to be fundamental in the goal of eliminating racial and ethnic disparities in health care. The project also defines the values, characteristics, areas of awareness, knowledge, and skills required of a cultural broker. The Cultural Broker Project is tailored to the needs and preferences of health care settings of the communities served by the program.

Cultural brokers may assume the role of medical interpreter. An interpreter is one who takes the spoken message in one language and converts it to another language. Interpreters do not provide word-to-word equivalence, but rather focus on the accurate expression of equivalent meaning. They serve as communicators and liaisons between the patient and the provider in health care facilities. If an interpreter is necessary, it is important to remember to speak directly to the patient, not the interpreter. If English is the second language or a heavy accent is involved, speaking clearly and slowly can greatly enhance communication.

In some cases, a family member may serve as the interpreter. This may not be the best solution, because the family member may not understand the medical terminology. It would also be difficult for a family member to be the one to share a life-threatening diagnosis or a poor prognosis.

Patient Education

Do not assume that a patient who does not speak English, or does not speak it fluently, is stupid, does not understand, and cannot pay.

Maslow's Hierarchy of Needs

Abraham Maslow is considered the founder of humanistic psychology and is most well known for his **hierarchy of needs** (Figure 4-5). *Webster's Dictionary* defines hierarchy as "a group of persons or things arranged in order of rank, grade, class etc." According to Maslow's theory, human needs could be grouped into five levels. He also theorized that each level of need must be satisfied before one could move on to the next level.

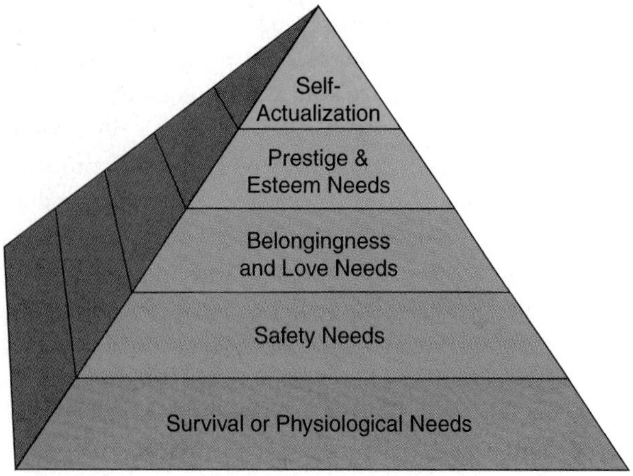

Figure 4-5 Maslow's hierarchy of needs.

The needs in the first level include physiologic or survival needs. These needs include food, water, and air to breathe—homeostasis for the body. The second level includes needs of safety and security; that is, the need for security, stability, and protection. Everyone has the desire to be free from fear and anxiety. Safety needs also include the need for structure, law and order, and limits.

The third level involves belonging and love needs. This level of need involves both giving and receiving affection. Additional words that express our connectedness are roots, origins, peers, friends, family, neighborhood, territory, clan, class, and gang. We have a basic animal tendency to herd, flock, join, and belong.

The fourth level, prestige and esteem needs, come from a basic need for a stable, healthy self-respect for ourselves and others. There is the desire for achievement, strength, and confidence. Also, there is the need for recognition, prestige, reputation, status, and even fame. Satisfaction of these needs leads to feelings of self-confidence and worth. The final level is self-actualization. In this stage, we are at our peak, doing what truly fits us. It is an achievement of potential.

Individuals may move back and forth from one need to another depending on circumstances.

Critical Thinking

An established patient arrives 20 minutes early for his appointment. He is in obvious pain and discomfort and tells the receptionist, "I can't sleep, I can't eat, and I can't go to work today." Which of Maslow's stages most accurately describes this patient? What actions should the medical assistant take to assist this patient?

Understanding this hierarchy helps to assess a patient's needs. If the most basic of needs are not met, it is highly unlikely that a patient can be successful with any treatment protocol. Keeping this hierarchy in mind will help to facilitate therapeutic communication.

COMMUNITY RESOURCES

There may be circumstances in which a patient will need a referral to a community resource. These resources range from the more simple acts of arranging with Meals on Wheels to deliver a hot meal daily to making complex arrangements for skilled nursing facilities or hospice care. The medical assistant will need to know the patient's name, address, and telephone number, as well as the particular resource needed, the diagnosis, and the reason for the service.

It is helpful to have a list of community resources readily available. The list may be computerized, or hard-copy information may be filed in a notebook. The information should be put into categories for ease in locating it quickly. See Procedure 4-1 for steps in developing a Community Resource Reference.

TECHNOLOGY AND COMMUNICATION

Face-to-face communication is the mode of choice in most physician offices today. However, technological devices are becoming more and more accepted as a means of communication. Technology-mediated communication and a greater reliance on cyberspace technology will greatly affect communication in the twenty-first century. Examples of new technologies in medical offices include interactive videoconferencing, clinical e-mail, automated routing units, instant messaging, paging systems, and physician digital assistants (PDAs).

Do these new communication methods change the communication cycle? There is still a message, a sender, a receiver, and feedback. What changes is the way in which the message is encoded and decoded. The content of the message will be examined for credibility rather than one's dress, eye contact, facial expression, vocal inflection, and posture. Technology does not convey emotions nearly as well as face-to-face or even telephone conversations. Another factor to consider is that your composed message may not look like what your reader sees. The software and hardware that you use for composing, sending, sorting, downloading, and reading may be completely different from what your recipient uses. Modifications to the format may change the intended emphasis or meaning of the message.

There are several advantages for the use of e-mail rather than postal mail (commonly referred to as "snail mail"). E-mail is less expensive and faster than mailing a letter. Because the turnaround time can be so fast, e-mail is more conversational than traditional paper-based media. An e-mail transmission is less intrusive than a telephone call and less bother than a fax. When one uses e-mail transmissions, differences in location and time zone are less of a problem.

ROADBLOCKS TO THERAPEUTIC COMMUNICATION

Being sensitive to patients' unique personalities and needs will enable the health care professional to avoid **roadblocks** to communication (Table 4-1).

It must be the concern of each health care professional to facilitate communication by encouraging and enabling patients to express themselves honestly without fear. Roadblocks close communication and prevent quality care of the total person.

DEFENSE MECHANISMS

When patients are frightened, ashamed, guilty, or threatened, they often will resort to defense mechanisms as a means of avoiding injury to their ego. We all use them to some limited extent, but they become harmful when they result in a breakdown in therapeutic communication. Failure by the patient to face problems often results in inability to provide satisfactory treatment on the part of the medical practitioner. Recognizing common defense mechanisms enables the medical staff to minimize the triggering event and to communicate more effectively.

Defense mechanisms are defined as behavior that is used to protect the ego from guilt, anxiety, or loss of esteem. Employment of defense mechanisms is most often unconscious to the person using them. It is the body's way of seeking relief from uncomfortable or painful reality. A mentally healthy person uses defense mechanisms to put a problem on hold until sufficient time has passed to permit him or her to address it without unacceptable emotional pain. Excessive use of defense mechanisms or failure to address a problem even after sufficient time has elapsed is a sign of a mental health issue.

Defense mechanisms are usually readily apparent to the disaffected observer; however, they are difficult to analyze without knowledge of the motive behind the behavior. The following paragraphs describe some commonly observed defense mechanisms.

Regression is an attempt to withdraw from an unpleasant circumstance by retreating to an earlier, more secure stage of life. It is usually used when the person feels powerless to affect the events causing the pain; it can be thought of as a desperation move. A toddler's regression to bed-wetting or soiling himself or herself shortly after a new baby arrives in the family is an example of this defense mechanism. Use of a security blanket by an adult or child when faced with something that disrupts his or her life is another example.

Denial is refusal to accept painful information that is readily apparent to others. This defense mechanism commonly is encountered in the case of a person being diagnosed with a disease such as cancer or experiencing the death of a close family member or associate. Denial has a devastating effect on communication. The person will not hear what you say, but will quite frequently acknowledge what you are saying. Careful attention to what the person is saying will reveal that he or she does not accept his or her situation and is not mentally conscious that it is happening. Denial is often the first stage of an emotional response after a traumatic event. The next stage is anger toward the event, the medical staff,

TABLE 4-1 ROADBLOCKS TO COMMUNICATION

Roadblock	Example
Reassuring clichés	"Don't worry, Mr. McKay, about not having a job; you'll find another one really soon."
Moralizing/lecturing	"If you were smart, Mrs. Johnson, you'd lose fifty pounds and you wouldn't have such a problem with your diabetes and hypertension."
Requiring explanations	"Why would you not want to have chemotherapy, Mr. Gordon? Seeing your wife die of cancer should surely make you want to seek treatment."
Ridiculing/shaming	"Ha, ha, Mr. Gordon! It's not *prostrate*—it's prostate cancer."
Defending/contradicting	"Mr. Marshal, I assure you the physician is *very busy*. He will not see you until he has finished with his other patients."
Shifting subjects	"Yes, Mrs. Jover, your work is very interesting, but I must ask you to sign this permission form to test for HIV."
Criticizing	"Mrs. O'Keefe, why in the world would you stay with an abusive husband?"
Threatening	"There is no way you will get rid of this cough if you do not stop smoking, Mr. Fowler."

God, or others. The stage after anger is frequently depression. A mentally healthy person eventually reaches the final stage of acceptance.

Repression is similar to denial, but it is a totally unconscious reaction. In the case of repression, the person seems to experience temporary amnesia. It is the mind's way of defending itself from mental trauma by forgetting or wiping things out of the conscious memory. A child unconsciously forgetting to tell parents that he or she got into trouble at school is an example. The fear associated with the event becomes overwhelming, causing the mind to forget. Repression should not be confused with outright lying. In severe cases, repression can be related to mental illness.

Projection is attributing unacceptable desires, impulses, and thoughts falsely to others to avoid acknowledging they are actually the person's own experiences. It is a means of defending against feelings or urges the person does not want to admit they are experiencing. A mother who abuses her child might accuse the medical assistant of being rough with the child while performing patient assessment to conceal her feelings of wanting to throttle the child. Projection is an indication of mental illness.

Sublimation is the channeling of a socially unacceptable behavior into a socially acceptable behavior. An overly aggressive person directed to play football to relieve their aggression is an example. Constructive behavior is substituted for destructive behavior.

Displacement is the unconscious transfer of unacceptable emotions, thoughts, or feelings from one's self to a more acceptable external substitute. A patient who is angry with the doctor for some reason slams the door as he or she leaves the clinic.

Compensation is a conscious or unconscious overemphasizing of a characteristic to offset a real or imagined deficiency. This defense mechanism involves substituting strength for a weakness and may be viewed as healthy. An example is the young boy whose physical stature keeps him from being a football star, so he compensates by achieving an academic award.

Rationalization is the mind's way of making unacceptable behavior or events acceptable by devising a rational reason. The purpose of rationalization is to avoid embarrassment or guilt, or to avoid obeying a directive. The rational reason is usually a stretch of the truth and can be quite apparent to disinterested individuals. An example is the patient who tells the doctor that he or she did not take his or her blood pressure medication because he or she did not have enough time before leaving for work. The medication easily could have been taken at home or at work. Most people rationalize things to some extent, but excessive rationalization may be construed as unhealthy.

Undoing is actions designed to make amends or to cancel out inappropriate behavior. Showering the abused person with gifts to compensate for unacceptable actions that took place in the past is an example.

THERAPEUTIC COMMUNICATION IN ACTION

The following sections identify the proper communication techniques that the medical assistant should use as part of the two most important communication functions they perform: patient interview techniques and telephone techniques.

Interview Techniques

All health professionals must be adept at **interview techniques**—knowing how to encourage the best communication between themselves and the patient. It is important to remember that an unequal relationship exists between the health professional and the patient. The health professional, whether it be the physician or the medical assistant, is in the power position and has a great deal of control over the patient. Therefore, it is important to equalize the relationship as much as possible. That is the reason why some professionals use the term *client* rather than *patient*.

Early in the interview, the patient must feel comfortable enough to risk being honest with the health professional. The health professional must build an atmosphere of trust by showing concern for the patient. A gentle touch and a warm, caring facial expression may be all that is necessary. Always be honest and genuine in your responses to patients. Be sympathetic and empathic and create an environment that is free of hypocrisy.

When the medical assistant is interviewing the patient for the chief complaint, it is important to listen with a "third" ear. Listen to what the patient is not saying but is apt to exhibit through nonverbal communication.

You might choose to share your observation of the nonverbal message with the patient, thus encouraging the patient to verbalize more freely. When feelings are shared, validate and acknowledge those feelings through such statements as "I understand your distress." You can verify the communication by reflecting or paraphrasing what the patient has said.

You will be asking **closed questions** during the interview. Closed questions can be answered with a simple yes or no.

"Are you still taking your medication?"
"Are you in pain now?"

You will also use **open-ended questions** with the patient. These questions encourage therapeutic communication because the patient is required to verbalize more information.

> "What kind of help will you have at home during your recovery?"
> "How are you coming along on this diet?"

Indirect statements will also prove helpful in facilitating therapeutic communication. An indirect statement will elicit a response from a patient without the patient feeling questioned.

> "Tell me what you've been doing since you retired."
> "I'd like to know more about your exercise program."

Refer to Chapter 11 for additional information related to patient interviewing.

Telephone Techniques

It often has been said that the telephone is the lifeline of the physician's office. Communication over the telephone requires understanding on the part of each communicator (Figure 4-6).

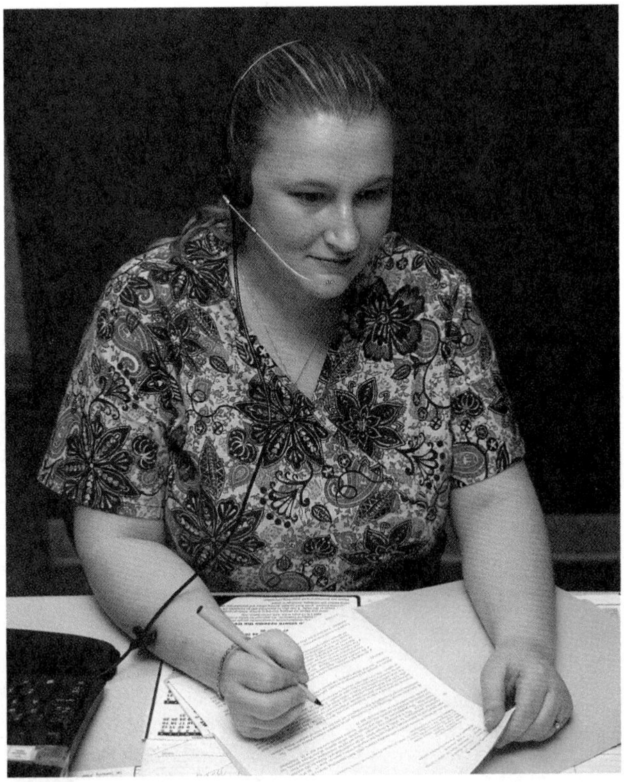

Figure 4-6 When communicating over the telephone, listen with full attention to make certain the message sent and received is correct.

Each medium uses the proper tools to get the job done. Speaking on the telephone is much like a conversation between two blindfolded individuals. The facial expressions cannot be seen, there is no eye contact, and there is no visual feedback. The listener will interpret mood by the tone, the pacing of voice, and the words spoken. When speaking on the telephone, quick conclusions are drawn. Often, we jump to conclusions, and the communication is misinterpreted.

The old, cold, aloof, formal business greeting comes across like frostbite in the medical office setting. It sounds curt, bored, and uncaring. Think of welcoming a new acquaintance into your home, then practice the same characteristics when speaking on the telephone. Speak clearly, use words that will be easily understood, and ask questions to verify that the patient has understood the message being conveyed.

Concentrate on enunciating and being understood. If you hear, "What? I didn't understand you. I can't hear you," slow down and speak a little louder with distinct enunciation directly into the mouthpiece. The mouthpiece should be held one to two inches away from the mouth. Project your voice at the mouthpiece, and then project another foot further. Your voice is the delivery system for your words and thoughts. Speak with confidence and conviction.

Have you ever called an office and had the firm name clipped off? The name of the office is important. To avoid clipping off the office name, practice using buffer words. **Buffer words** are expendable; if you clip them off, at least the office name remains intact. Use buffer words before the office name and before you identify yourself. "Good morning, this is Inner City Health Care. This is Walter, how may I help you?" *Good morning* and *this is* are buffer words.

All the techniques for effective face-to-face communication must be more intentionally observed when the communication is over the telephone because you cannot see the person with whom you are speaking. You must listen with full attention to make certain that the message sent and received is correct.

To close a telephone conversation to schedule an appointment, for example, consider the following:

1. Use the patient's name if it can be done without announcing the name to persons in the reception area.
2. Confirm the date and time of the appointment.
3. Identify the physician if there is more than one physician in the office.
4. Give any specific instructions that may be necessary.
5. Say good-bye.

The following Health Insurance Portability and Accountability Act (HIPAA) guidelines should be followed when communicating information to patients by telephone:

- Determine whether the patient has requested confidential communications. The office policy and procedure manual should provide guidelines for making this determination.
- If the patient has not requested protected health information (PHI), the patient should simply be called at the normal phone number contained in their records. If the patient has requested PHI and has provided an alternate telephone number, care must be taken to ensure that only the alternate number is called.
- The caller should identify himself or herself by name, identify the medical practice where he or she is employed, and ask to speak with the intended person.
- If the patient is not available, it is acceptable to leave a live or recorded message asking the patient to return the call. It is important, however, that the message does not contain any medical information and does not mention the purpose of the call. If the name of the practice indicates the nature of the call, do not disclose the name.
- When the patient is contacted, it is acceptable to discuss their medical information over the phone. Test results and other PHI must not be given to anyone other than the patient or a person designated as the patient's representative.

Procedure 4-1 Identifying Community Resources

PURPOSE:

To have a list of community resources readily available for referral to patients.

EQUIPMENT/SUPPLIES:

Computer and printer

Following is a list of information sources to consider when beginning to put together a Community Resource Reference:

- Local Public Health Department
- Internet
- Community service numbers in the local telephone directory
- State/federal agencies
- Visiting nurses
- Counselor/social workers at local hospitals
- Nursing home associations
- Local charities

PROCEDURE STEPS:

1. Determine the type of information to be in your database. RATIONALE: Only resources useful to your specific office should be maintained to save time and space.
2. Contact the sources listed previously and request any listings they may have. RATIONALE: This will save time.
3. Search the Internet using your favorite search engine. Enter under the city, state, and community resources. You may have to modify the subject of your search to obtain the desired resources. RATIONALE: This is an effective way to access information quickly.
4. Develop a database on your computer so you can search easily for the resource when needed by a patient and simply print it out. You may wish to have a notebook with the information printed and indexed, so other office staff can simply copy a page for a patient. Your data should include as many resources for assistance as you can find for each type of resource. RATIONALE: To have a listing of community resources readily available for office use.

Case Study 4-1

It is a typically active day at the offices of Drs. Lewis and King. Despite the three emergencies in the early afternoon and the full schedule of patients, everything is running smoothly with Dr. Lewis, and the entire staff is responding quickly but thoroughly to patient concerns.

At 4:00 PM, another emergency patient arrives; at the same time, Jim Marshal, an architect in a downtown firm, comes in early for a routine appointment and demands to be seen immediately. Jim, a regular patient, has a history of being difficult and impatient; being a bit arrogant, he tends to put his needs first. However, Dr. Lewis is occupied with another patient. It is critical to treat the patient with the emergency as soon as possible, and Jim is half an hour early.

Joe Guerrero, CMA, the office's administrative and clinical medical assistant, calmly asks Mr. Marshal to please wait until his scheduled appointment time. When he threatens to leave, Joe explains to Mr. Marshal that there are two patients ahead of him, but that the doctor will see him at his scheduled appointment time.

CASE STUDY REVIEW

1. What communication roadblocks did medical assistant Joe Guerrero avoid in reacting to Jim Marshal's demands to see the doctor?
2. With another student, role-play the scenario, with one student taking the role of patient and one student the role of the medical assistant. Identify roadblocks to communication imposed by the patient. How is the medical assistant using the five Cs of communication to deal with the situation?
3. Do you think the medical assistant reacted appropriately? What else could he have done? What should he *not* do in this situation?

Case Study 4-2

You have learned in this chapter that communication has not been successful until the cycle is complete. Consider the following scenario:

An 82-year-old woman with moderate dementia and a hearing impairment is brought to the surgeon's office for a follow-up appointment after hip replacement surgery. The woman's daughter accompanies her. The goal of the appointment is to make certain the hip is healing nicely and to discuss precautions before the patient returns to her assisted-living apartment. Almost immediately, the conversation is directed toward the daughter because it is so much easier to explain to her what should be done.

CASE STUDY REVIEW

1. What might the staff do to help the patient understand the following?
   - Use the walker consistently.
   - Shoes must be leather tennis shoe type or uniform style; consider Velcro closure as opposed to laces that have to be tied.
   - Do not wear pantyhose.
   - You will not be able to walk your dog on a leash.
2. Should the patient be left out of the conversation? Should the daughter be included?
3. In cases such as these, is something other than verbal communication indicated?

SUMMARY

Throughout this text you are reminded of the importance of effective communication techniques. Good communication takes practice. Use the techniques identified in this chapter with your family and with your peers. Watch for roadblocks, be aware of defense mechanisms, and remember the five Cs of communication.

STUDY FOR SUCCESS

To reinforce your knowledge and skills of information presented in this chapter:

- ❑ Review the Key Terms
- ❑ Practice the Procedure
- ❑ Consider the Case Studies and discuss your conclusions
- ❑ Answer the Review Questions
  - ❑ Multiple Choice
  - ❑ Critical Thinking
- ❑ Navigate the Internet by completing the Web Activities
- ❑ Practice the StudyWARE activities on the textbook CD
- ❑ Apply your knowledge in the Student Workbook activities
- ❑ Complete the Web Tutor sections
- ❑ View and discuss the DVD situations

REVIEW QUESTIONS

Multiple Choice

1. Culture influences which of the following?
   a. biases and prejudices
   b. ethnic heritage, age, and sex
   c. educational and life experiences and value systems
   d. b and c only
2. In the cycle of communication, encoding means:
   a. deciphering a message
   b. creating the message to be sent
   c. sending the message
   d. receiving the message
3. Body language:
   a. is used to express feelings and emotions
   b. is not as important as verbal communication
   c. only makes up 7% of the message
   d. is only used in Eastern cultures
4. A comfortable social space is defined as:
   a. touching to 6 inches
   b. 1½ feet to 4 feet
   c. 12 to 15 feet
   d. 4 to 12 feet
5. A reassuring cliché is:
   a. a way of calming down a patient
   b. a means of rationalizing a decision
   c. a roadblock to communication
   d. always useful in daily communications
6. Redirecting a socially unacceptable impulse into one that is socially acceptable is an example of which of these defense mechanisms?
   a. sublimation
   b. rationalization
   c. projection
   d. displacement
7. When using an open-ended question with a patient, we expect:
   a. a yes or no answer
   b. him or her to tell us the truth
   c. a response that permits the patient to elaborate
   d. only the right answers
8. Buffer words:
   a. help us get through the day
   b. are meant to soothe a patient's feelings
   c. are expendable words used in answering a telephone call
   d. are important in face-to-face communication

Critical Thinking

1. A 15-year-old girl awaiting a sports physical examination says that she is overweight and has pimples. How will you respond therapeutically?
2. Bill, who is 28 years old, comes for his annual checkup. When reviewing his social data sheet, you discover he is now living in an apartment and has a

new phone number. He mumbles to you that his wife left him and won't let him see the kids. How will you respond therapeutically?

3. You try to be gentle and gracious with Edith. She is fragile and difficult to please. While positioning her for a radiograph, she sneers and says, "You are about the roughest person who ever cared for me." How will you respond therapeutically, and how will you control your body language?
4. When you report to Herb that his cholesterol is quite high and that the doctor wants to discuss medication and diet, he responds, "That is impossible; you must have made some mistake." Which defense mechanism is Herb using? How will you respond therapeutically?
5. How might the unequal relationship between physician and client/patient impact therapeutic communication?

WEB ACTIVITIES

Select three cultures of particular interest to you personally and search the World Wide Web for information regarding these cultures and communication traditions. How might this new information be applied to the physician whose clientele is primarily made up of these cultures? How might this new knowledge benefit a medical assistant employed in this type of setting?

THE DVD HOOK-UP

DVD Series	Program Number
Critical Thinking	**2**

Chapter/Scene Reference

- *Introduction*
- *Forms of Communication*
- *Professional Communication*

(Skip: Communicating with Patients and Communication on the Telephone)

- *Communicating with Special Populations*

In this chapter, you learned the importance of positive communication and what distractions can impede the communication process. You also learned the importance of nonverbal communication and how it is not necessarily what you say, but rather how you say it, that leaves the strongest impression on others.

Program 2 of Critical Thinking deals with many of the same issues that are listed in this chapter. We observed the effects of body language in the communication process. Communicating with special populations also was addressed. We learned the office's responsibility in providing an interpreter for our deaf patients and how we can better serve our blind patients. We also learned about managing the angry patient.

1. What are some benefits to being bilingual?
2. What is one mistake that many people make when working with blind patients?
3. What is the best approach to take when dealing with an angry patient?

DVD Journal Summary

Write a paragraph that summarizes what you learned from watching the designated scenes from today's DVD program. How do you feel about working with patients from different cultures? Are you the type of person who gets angry when conversing with other people who are angry? What steps will you take to deal with an angry patient or coworker?

REFERENCES/BIBLIOGRAPHY

Blair, G. M. (January 23, 2000). *Conversation as communication*. Retrieved from http://www.ee.ed.ac.uk/~gerard/Management/art7.html

Luckmann, J. (2000). *Transcultural communication in health care*. Clifton Park, NY: Thomson Delmar Learning.

National Center for Cultural Competence, Georgetown University Center for Child and Human Development, Georgetown University Medical Center. (Spring/Summer 2004). Bridging the cultural divide in health care settings: The essential role of cultural broker programs. Washington, DC: Author.

Taber's cyclopedic medical dictionary. (19th ed.). (2004). Philadelphia: F. A. Davis.

Tamparo, C. D., & Lindh, W. Q. (2000). *Therapeutic communications for health professions*. Albany, NY: Delmar.

Webster's new twentieth century dictionary. (2nd ed.). (1983). New York: New World Dictionaries/Simon and Schuster.

Wilkes, M., & Crosswait, C. B. (1995). *Professional development: The dynamics of success*. San Diego: Harcourt Brace Jovanovich.

CHAPTER 5

Coping Skills for the Medical Assistant

OUTLINE

OBJECTIVES

The student should strive to meet the following performance objectives and demonstrate an understanding of the facts and principles presented in this chapter through written and oral communication.

1. Define the key terms as presented in the glossary.
2. Differentiate between stress and stressors.
3. Describe Hans Selye's General Adaptation Syndrome theory.
4. Identify several approaches to managing stress in the ambulatory care setting.
5. Identify three characteristics associated with burnout in the workplace.
6. Describe the four stages of burnout.
7. List a minimum of five ways to reduce the risk for burnout.
8. Differentiate between long-range and short-range goals.

KEY TERMS

Burnout
Goal
Inner-Directed People
Long-Range Goals
Outer-Directed People
Parasympathetic Nervous System
Self-Actualization
Short-Range Goals
Stress
Stressors
Sympathetic Nervous System

FEATURED COMPETENCIES

ABHES—ENTRY-LEVEL COMPETENCIES

Professionalism

- Be a "team player"
- Adapt to change
- Conduct work within scope of education, training, and ability

SCENARIO

At the office of Drs. Lewis and King, there are four full-time medical assistants who collaborate to make the office run smoothly, both administratively and clinically. One day a month, though, office manager Marilyn Johnson, CMA, is out of town, leaving Ellen Armstrong, CMA, the administrative medical assistant, in charge of a busy reception area and an ever-ringing telephone.

On these days, Ellen is particularly careful to organize her work so that things run as they should. She organizes some work the night before, she sets priorities so that she is confident that the critical work will get done, and she tries to maintain her calm by taking a short break every couple of hours to review new needs that have come up during the day. Although Ellen cannot anticipate every emergency, she does try to influence the situation rather than let events control her.

INTRODUCTION

Even in the most well-managed ambulatory care setting, medical assistants and other health providers are likely to feel the effects of stress from time to time. They may be overworked on certain days, they may face difficult patient situations, and they may find that the administrative and paperwork load is getting ahead of them.

This chapter helps today's busy, multifaceted medical assistant pinpoint the symptoms of stress and provides ideas for coping with stress as it occurs. The better equipped the medical assistant is to confront and solve the sources of stress, the less likely stressors will become so overwhelming as to lead to burnout on the job. Goal setting, recognizing one's limitations and potentials, setting priorities, and keeping a balanced perspective can work together to reduce stress and enable the medical assistant to take pleasure in working with patients and colleagues.

WHAT IS STRESS?

The body's response to mental and physical change is termed **stress.** Adaptive behavior patterns we assume in response to real physical threats or emotional effects result in either eustress, positive feelings; or distress, negative feelings. Moving to a new city or receiving a promotion usually are perceived as positive events, whereas going through a divorce or losing a job are conversely negative events; however, each of these events can result in inducing stress in the body. These events are called **stressors.**

According to Hans Selye, who first conceived the theory of nonspecific reaction as stress, the body does not differentiate positively and negatively induced stress. It is only the level of the stress and its duration that affect the body. Some stress is beneficial and adds anticipation and a feeling of "being alive," for example, when we experience a roller coaster ride or bungee jump off a cliff. The short-lived adrenaline rush brings the world into sharper focus and enhances our lives. Short-duration stress is beneficial and helps us focus on details, achieve difficult goals, and perform at our best. When we have a last-minute rush in the office or are hurrying to get an assignment finished for school, we are experiencing short-duration stress. Short-duration stress is experienced when the telephone rings, the examination rooms are full, and the physician is called to the hospital on an emergency. Immediately, the body's stress mode is activated and adrenaline is produced, enabling you to make quick judgements and decisions, to be organized and efficient, and to accomplish tasks within minimal time limits.

Longer duration stress, normally associated with negative events, can be harmful to the body, resulting in illness such as headaches, insomnia, allergies, cancer, acute indigestion, stomach ulcers, hypertension, blood clots, stroke, and immune system disorders. Psychologically, the body also is influenced by long-term stress. Onsets of depression and anxiety, as well as eating problems resulting in weight loss or gain, are associated with the body's psychological response to stress. Anorexia and bulimia are common eating disorders attributed to long-term stressful events. Long-duration stress can also affect our ability to think clearly, and objectivity may be impaired. Physical symptoms of these emotional effects may include cigarette smoking, obesity, lack of interest, and excessive sexual activity.

Adaptation to Stress

The body's response to stress goes back to early human development. That response was designed to help humans survive whatever they were experiencing that caused a fearful response. The **sympathetic nervous system** prepared the body for "fight or flight" to allow humans the best chance of survival. The brain inhibits short-term memory, promotes long-term memory, and releases hormones such as adrenaline into the bloodstream. The respiration rate becomes more rapid, blood flow increases, red and white blood cells are released by the spleen, the immune system is altered to allow immune-boosting bodies to be sent to the body. Blood vessels in the skin are contracted to minimize blood loss from wounds, blood vessels in the muscles dilate to increase circulation, and fluids are diverted from nonessential locations; the metabolism rate is diminished to permit all available energy to be focused on the event that triggered the fight-or-flight response.

All of these caveman responses to stress are with us today, even though they may no longer be needed in the twenty-first century. The symptoms of headache, stomach ache, diarrhea, cold clammy hands, heart palpitations, indigestion, and short-term memory loss that we experience are the result of our body's reaction to stressors that has been developed over millennia. Short term, these responses are not harmful, and the body's **parasympathetic nervous system** returns to normal after the stressor has been removed. Long term, these responses are harmful to the body. See Figure 5-1 for an illustration of the adaptive stages related to stress.

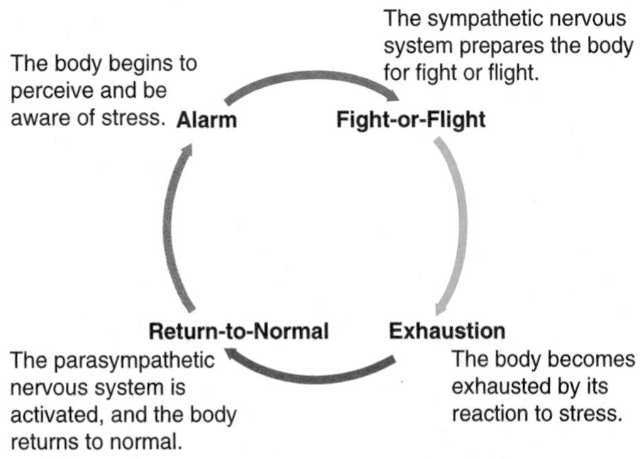

Figure 5-1 Hans Selye's General Adaptation Syndrome (GAS) theory proposes that four stages are involved in adapting to stress.

MANAGEMENT OF STRESS

Stress cannot be prevented; in fact, life would be dull without short-term stress. Anticipating the birth of a child, planning an upcoming wedding, or graduating from school are all stressful changes, albeit pleasant ones, that make life interesting. Long-term stressful situations are not desirable, but the situations leading to them can be managed if we understand the causes. Some causes of long-term stress are:

- *Powerlessness:* inability to control expectations, workload, and duties; feelings of frustration and panic because of schedules
- *Round peg in square hole:* not suited for the position you hold
- *Traumatic events on the job:* not emotionally prepared for trauma involved in the job
- *Environmental:* physical conditions such as noise, lighting, or temperature influence work
- *Management style:* your manager's style causes uproar or instability in work demands
- *Failure to satisfy needs:* job conditions do not permit achievement of Maslow's needs (see Chapter 4 for information related to Maslow's hierarchy of needs)

Requesting that you have a written job description can control powerlessness. You will then know the duties and responsibilities, and you will not experience sudden change when you least expect it. A job description will also help to avoid some of the instability resulting from a manager who is too sanguine or manages from one crisis to another. If you know what your job entails, you can anticipate the events and take action to prevent a crisis.

Planning and prioritization can help to avoid panic and reduce stress when faced with the inevitable situation of too much work and too little time. A job that looks

Critical Thinking—Practice in Time Management Analysis

List all of the tasks you do in a typical day. Beside each task write down how many minutes/hours you spend on each task. At the conclusion of the exercise, draw a histogram showing the percentage of each day spent on each task. This will quickly show where you spend most of your time. How could you save time? Develop a plan to reduce time spent in nonproductive, unessential activities.

impossible can be broken down into elements that are manageable. Prioritization of the smaller elements and proceeding without wasting time procrastinating usually results in getting the job finished in the allotted time or at least with a minimum amount of stress.

Managing your lifestyle also becomes part of stress management. Finding time to relax and divert your mind from the worries of the job is an effective tool in managing stress. Instead of working during lunch to solve a problem, taking a break away from the problem will reduce the stress to the point that you will actually increase your productivity. This is probably a good time to discuss worry. Worry is defined as undue concern for problems over which you have no control. Worry causes stress, yet it does nothing to resolve the problem causing your worry. Therefore, just remembering this definition and thinking about it every time you are inclined to worry will help you to stop worrying and actually will help you become more focused and better able to resolve the stressful event.

Mental attitude plays a role in tolerance to stress. Individuals who can focus on the positive can offset the depression often associated with stress. Identifying what is being accomplished versus focusing on what is not being accomplished or what does not meet your expectations is what is meant by focusing on the positive. Maintaining an active social network that allows you to discuss your problems is also quite helpful. The network should not include persons of negative personality who have common problems. This situation is likely to have as its outcome a "complain session."

Physical condition affects your body's tolerance to stress. Maintaining a regular sleep cycle, eating a proper diet, and getting regular exercise contribute to improving your body's tolerance to stressors (Figure 5-2). Stress can affect sleep and appetite, but intentionally not getting enough sleep or not eating a balanced diet makes you more susceptible to stress in the first place. Anything that "bugs" you contributes to stress. Some people believe that soft background music will reduce stress, but for a job requiring intense concentration, any distraction contributes to stress. Clothes or shoes that are uncomfortable can "bug" you and contribute to stress. The color of the walls in your office can contribute to stress. If the color "bugs" you, it will contribute to stress. Telephone interruptions can result in a stressful situation. All of these "minor" things that contribute to stress are manageable and should be considered as part of a plan to manage stress. See Table 5-1 for suggested techniques for reducing stress at work.

Maintaining a good interpersonal relationship with fellow employees or fellow students and faculty is important to achieving a satisfying work or school experience. Before a strong interpersonal relationship is established with others, a positive self-attitude is needed. The choices we make effect our positive attitude. Making positive decisions will affect our school and work environment, and hence the level and duration of stress experienced. Following are choices we all make in our lives:

- To be respectful of others
- To be a diligent worker

Critical Thinking—Checking Your Success-Oriented Attitude

Select three attitude attributes for which you are quite negative and develop a plan of action to make them more positive. Implement your plan; after two weeks, review whether your actions have impacted the stress level associated with that activity.

Negative Attributes	20%	40%	60%	80%	100%	Positive Attributes
Bored						Enthusiastic
Unhappy						Joyful
Never						Can do
Lethargic						Energetic
Cut corners						Honest
Out of control						Under control
Lack of confidence						Confident
Selfish						Selfless
Unyielding						Flexible
Loner						Part of a group
Know it all						Open to suggestion

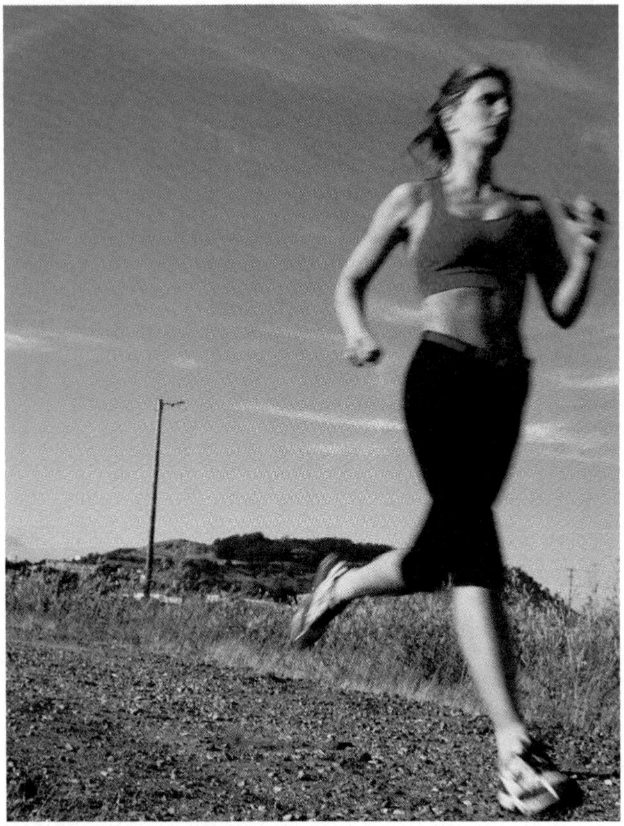

Figure 5-2 Regular exercise in some form improves the body's tolerance to stress.

- To be willing to learn
- To be honest
- To be willing to assume responsibility for actions
- To express appropriate humor
- To have an attitude of humility

TABLE 5-1 TECHNIQUES FOR REDUCING STRESS AT WORK
• Stretch or change positions. • Slowly roll your head from side to side and forward and back. • Slowly rotate your shoulders forward and backward several times. • Turn away from the computer, or close your eyes for several seconds. • Walk around and deliver charts or laboratory specimens, and so on. • Stand or sit tall and take a few deep breaths. • Meditate for 30 seconds. • Know your limits and be aware of your body's needs.

- To be goal directed
- To understand Maslow's needs

By anticipating how an organization can cause stress, we can be prepared and minimize its effects. Following are common causes of stress in an organization:

- *Low salary:* Salary plays an important role in our needs. It leads to frustration if we believe it is too low, and this contributes to a negative attitude. Positive job conditions can overshadow low salary; however, if combined with other negative feelings, it is an overpowering cause of stress.
- *Little opportunity for career growth:* This reason results in frustration and leads to stress and burnout.
- *Overspecialization:* This problem results in the employee never seeing the overall picture and receiving little or no satisfaction from his or her work.
- *Workload:* Continual work level beyond your capability to complete it results in frustration, and ultimately burnout.
- *Job complexity versus skill level:* Expectation to perform beyond your skill level leads to long-term stress.
- *Responsibility delineation:* Lack of delineation of responsibility leads to continual questioning of whom is responsible for what job, and ultimately to frustration.

Critical Thinking—Self-Evaluation

- List several situations in your life that are stressful. Select the *one* that is most stressful.
- List as many things as possible about the situation that make it stressful to you.
- How would you change each of the things you have listed to make them less stressful?
- List the things you "could do" to effect the changes you listed.
- Rank the items in your "could do" list in terms of achievability.
- Select one or two of the items that are achievable and discuss them with a classmate. Now attempt to put them into practice for a week. Report back to your classmate on how effective these items were in reducing stress in your life.

- *Organization size:* Some individuals can get lost in a large organization.
- *Discrimination:* This illegal activity leads to bad feelings and frustration.
- *Poor time management skills:* The inability to prioritize and manage time effectively can lead to work overload.
- *Technological changes:* Change, even good changes, can cause stress.
- *Not being in control of your situation:* Lacking control leads to frustration.

WHAT IS BURNOUT?

Burnout is the result of stress and frustration, principally brought about by unrealistic expectations. Fatigue and exhaustion resulting from trying to meet unrealistic expectations compound it. Because burnout is so damaging, it needs to be discussed as a unique topic.

Stages of Burnout

Burnout has four stages:

- *Honeymoon:* love your job and have unrealistic expectation placed on you either by your manager or by yourself if you are a perfectionist; take work home and look for all the work you can get, cannot say "no" to accepting additional work
- *Reality:* begin to have doubts you can meet expectations; feel frustrated with your progress, work harder to meet expectations; begin to feel pulled in many directions; may not have a role model to follow, and established guidelines may not be defined
- *Dissatisfaction:* loss of enthusiasm; try to escape frustrations by binges of one sort or another, drinking, partying, shopping, or excessive eating or sex; fatigue and exhaustion develop.
- *Sad state:* depression, work seems pointless, lethargic with little energy, consider quitting, and look on yourself as a failure; represents full-blown burnout.

All of these stages are part of the process leading to burnout. The honeymoon stage might seem desirable, and it is pleasant, however, the seeds of the illness are present in the unrealistic expectations and the workaholic attitude of the employee. Unless these causes are eliminated, the progression to full burnout is assured.

Burnout in the Workplace

Burnout happens to people who previously were enthusiastic and bursting with energy and new ideas when first hired on the job or beginning a new experience. When individuals with a high need to achieve do not reach their goals, they are apt to feel angry and frustrated. Failing to recognize these signs as symptoms of burnout, they may throw themselves even more fully into work-related goals. Unless there is some type of revitalization outside of the workplace, burnout occurs.

Three characteristics associated with burnout in the workplace include:

- *Role Conflict:* When employees have conflicting responsibilities, they feel pulled in many directions. The perfectionist tries to do everything equally well without setting priorities. Fatigue and exhaustion associated with burnout begin to set in after time.
- *Role Ambiguity:* The employee does not know what is expected and how to accomplish it because there may not be a role model to follow or ask, or established guidelines to follow.
- *Role Overload:* If the employee cannot say no and continues to accept more responsibility than they can handle, burnout is sure to set in.

What to Do If You Are Burned Out

When you recognize the signs and symptoms of burnout, it is time to do some self-analysis by asking yourself some hard questions. Recall and analyze when you began feeling so tired and unable to relax and enjoy your work. Have you always been a perfectionist? Have you always had a higher need than most of your peers to do a job well? Are you irritable toward coworkers or patients? At what point did you lose your sense of humor? Do you always see work as a chore? Are you so intensely striving to achieve your goals that if you do not succeed you consider yourself a failure? Are you physically and emotionally exhausted?

The next step is to make some changes.

- Make a list of negative words or phrases that you most often use. Now replace the negatives with more neutral words or phrases.
- Create some job diversity for yourself. Drive to work via a different route; enter the building through a different door; change your work routine slightly; change your start time.
- Become creative. Redecorate your area.

Critical Thinking

Negative attitudes combined with low pay are a formula for burnout. Why?

- Establish some long- and short-term realistic goals and write them down.
- Take care of yourself; change your eating habits; exercise more; get more sleep.
- Renew friendships; go to lunch with coworkers; laugh with them.
- Implement time management techniques.
- Delegate responsibility to others who are capable.

Prevention and Recovery from Burnout

All of the techniques used for stress management are applicable for prevention and recovery from burnout. Following are the basic steps that need to be taken by a person who experiences burnout:

- Get some rest and relaxation away from the job for as long as is practical.
- Develop outside interests and an active social life.
- Set realistic goals for your life and your job.
- Negotiate a job description with your manager that has achievable expectations.
- Do not take work home.
- Develop time management techniques.
- Take steps to achieve regular sleep habits, nutritious diet, and physical exercise.
- Concentrate on thinking positively regarding job success.

GOAL SETTING AS A STRESS RELIEVER

Do you direct your life, or do you allow others to influence and make decisions for you? **Outer-directed people** let events, other people, or environmental factors dictate their behavior. By contrast, **inner-directed people** decide for themselves what they want to do with their lives. Laurence Peter, author of *The Peter Principle*, states, "If you don't know where you are going, you will end up somewhere else" (Wilkes & Crosswait, 1995).

Discoveries prove that goal-oriented employees are more effective and assertive than colleagues with no goals or future objectives. Recognizing the value of goal planning, many employers arrange planning sessions or seminars to encourage goal setting as a practical application for coping with stress and burnout and to develop career objectives. If your employer does not offer these outlets, seek your own seminars for goal setting. Such an activity not only "centers" you in your current employment, but helps you clearly picture your future plans and hopes.

What is a **goal?** According to *Merriam-Webster's Collegiate Dictionary*, a goal is "the result or achievement toward which effort is directed." To reach a desired goal, a person must implement planning together with a sincere desire to work hard. Skill in goal setting allows the medical assistant to clarify what must be accomplished and to develop a strategic plan to successfully achieve the goal.

A goal must be specific, challenging, realistic, attainable, and measurable. Specific goals are focused and have precise boundaries. A goal that is challenging creates enthusiasm and interest in achievement. Realistic goals are practical or beneficial for the present and for future **self-actualization.** An attainable goal refers to the fact that the goal is possible to fulfill. Measurable goals achieve some form of progress or success. By reflecting on the process, one is encouraged to establish additional goals.

Long-range goals are achievements that may take three to five years to accomplish. Long-range goals give direction and definition to our lives and serve to keep us "on track" so to speak. Much discipline, perseverance, determination, and hard work will be expended in accomplishing long-range goals. Some adjustment and readjustment to your goals may be necessary, however. The rewards of goal achievement include satisfaction, pride, a sense of accomplishment, and a job well done.

Short-range goals take apart long-range goals and reassemble the required activities into smaller, more manageable time segments. The time segments may be daily, weekly, monthly, quarterly, or yearly periods.

As a graduate and new employee, one of your long-range goals might be to become the office manager in the ambulatory care setting in which you are currently employed. You may wish to attain this goal within the next three to five years; by breaking it into three longer range goals and a series of short-range goals, you will be able to measure progress and feel a sense of accomplishment. Examples of long- and short-range goals might include:

Long-range goal 1:

To become proficient in all back-office clinical skills during the first year of employment.

Short-range goals necessary to achieve this:

- Practice accuracy and proficiency when performing tasks and skills.
- Practice efficiency by planning ahead for the equipment and supplies needed for each task performed.
- Evaluate your progress on a regular basis, and identify areas that need improvement.

Long-range goal 2:

To add front-office administrative tasks and skills to your routine during the second year of employment.

Short-range goals necessary to achieve this:

- Practice accuracy and proficiency when performing all front-office tasks and skills.
- Practice efficiency by planning ahead for the equipment and supplies needed for each task performed.
- Evaluate your progress on a regular basis, and identify areas that need improvement.

Long-range goal 3:

To begin to focus on office management during the third year of employment.

Short-range goals necessary to achieve this:

- Develop a procedure manual for all back- and front-office tasks and skills.
- Enroll in office management classes.
- Focus on team-building skills.

By the fourth year, you will be ready to move into the office manager position.

Long- and short-range goals work together to help make changes in our lives. Goals keep life interesting and give us something for which to strive. We can all reach goals successfully with some planning, hard work, discipline, and dedication.

Case Study 5-1

Ellen Armstrong, CMA, is an administrative medical assistant with Drs. Lewis and King. This is her first job. She is just two years out of school, and she is trying to learn everything she can to achieve her long-range goal of becoming office manager at this or some other ambulatory care setting.

Ellen has a great deal in her favor, for she is good with patients, both face-to-face and over the telephone. She is not daunted by the complexity of administrative work her job requires. Ellen knows she has a great deal yet to learn and, although she is a bit intimidated by her, Ellen looks to Marilyn Johnson, CMA, the office manager, for guidance and advice.

CASE STUDY REVIEW

1. How would you advise Ellen to go about achieving her long-term goal of office manager?
2. What are some of the short-term goals Ellen should set? Why are short-term goals important to her success?
3. Besides learning on the job, what else can Ellen do to achieve her goal?

Case Study 5-2

Ellen Armstrong, CMA, has been employed for five years as an administrative medical assistant with Drs. Lewis and King. Ellen is a perfectionist and has pushed herself to achieve many of her short- and long-term goals. The office staff has become aware that Ellen does not have a sense of humor lately. She seems frustrated and irritable, and is becoming critical of herself and others. Ellen has felt physically and emotionally exhausted, yet she continues to focus on her high standard of job performance; however, work is becoming a chore. At the end of the day, if everything has not been completed to her satisfaction, she feels like a failure.

CASE STUDY REVIEW

1. Do you feel Ellen is stressed or experiencing burnout? On what do you base your conclusions?
2. What might Ellen do to differentiate these two conditions?
3. What changes might Ellen implement to resolve this problem?

SUMMARY

Stress is very much a part of the medical profession. Each individual working in a medical career experiences consecutive days of demanding, emotionally and physically draining interactions with patients and staff members. This highly technical and ever-changing career requires its professionals to maintain a high level of skill and training and to be familiar with the newest technology.

Goal setting is one approach to reducing stress and burnout and promoting a sense of pride in the workplace, self-actualization, and possible employment promotion. Both long-range and short-range goal planning work together to help make changes in our lives.

STUDY FOR SUCCESS

To reinforce your knowledge and skills of information presented in this chapter:

- ❑ Review the Key Terms
- ❑ Consider the Case Studies and discuss your conclusions
- ❑ Answer the Review Questions
  - ❑ Multiple Choice
  - ❑ Critical Thinking
- ❑ Navigate the Internet by completing the Web Activities
- ❑ Practice the StudyWARE activities on the textbook CD
- ❑ Apply your knowledge in the Student Workbook activities
- ❑ Complete the Web Tutor sections

REVIEW QUESTIONS

Multiple Choice

1. Which answer is *not* true about stress?
   a. It does not occur suddenly.
   b. It has physical and emotional effects on the body.
   c. It may be positive or negative on its effects on the body.
   d. It is the body's response to change.
2. Hans Selye's General Adaptation Syndrome theory proposes that adaptation to stress occurs in how many stages?
   a. 2 stages
   b. 3 stages
   c. 4 stages
   d. 5 stages
3. Which is *not* a stage in the General Adaptation Syndrome?
   a. fight-or-flight
   b. exhaustion
   c. burnout
   d. alarm
4. Signs and symptoms of burnout include all of the following *except:*
   a. emotional and physical exhaustion
   b. hair-trigger display of emotion
   c. feelings of accomplishment and pride in work
   d. irritability and impatience
5. Long-range goals are easy to achieve if:
   a. they are not too challenging
   b. they are divided into a series of short-range goals
   c. they don't involve too much hard work
   d. you never change or adjust them

Critical Thinking

1. You have just graduated from a two-year medical assisting program and have been hired by a pediatric practice as a receptionist. The practice is busy with many telephone calls daily and many new patients who need charts created and information entered into the database. While in school you learned that you enjoyed the laboratory and clinical work much more than the front-office procedures. How do you think this position will impact your short- and long-term stress?
2. Identify two long-range goals you personally would like to attain within the next five years. How will you achieve these goals?
3. After you have been on the job for five years, you begin to recognize signs of burnout. How will you manage these symptoms?

WEB ACTIVITIES

Search the World Wide Web for additional information on burnout in the workplace. Compile your information into a report for your instructor. Be sure to include a bibliography identifying your Web sources.

REFERENCES/BIBLIOGRAPHY

Keir, L., Wise, B. A., & Krebs, C. (2003). *Medical assisting: Administrative and clinical competencies* (5th ed.). Clifton Park, NY: Thomson Delmar Learning.

Merriam-Webster's collegiate dictionary (10th ed.). (1994). Springfield, MA: Merriam-Webster.

Stress. (September 2001). Retrieved from http://www.reutershealth.com/wellconnected/doc31.html. Accessed April 5, 2005.

Stress management. (2000). Retrieved from http://www.ivf.com/stress.html. Accessed April 5, 2005.

Tamparo, C. D., & Lindh, W. Q. (2000). *Therapeutic communications for allied health professions*. Albany, NY: Delmar.

What you need to know about stress management. (2004). Retrieved from http://stress.about.com/cs/workplacestress/a/?once=true&. Accessed May 16, 2005.

Wilkes, M., & Crosswait, C. B. (1995). *Professional development: The dynamics of success*. San Diego: Harcourt Brace Jovanovich.

CHAPTER 6

The Therapeutic Approach to the Patient with a Life-Threatening Illness

KEY TERMS

Durable Power of Attorney for Health Care
Living Will
Physician's Directive
Psychomotor Retardation

OUTLINE

Life-Threatening Illness
Cultural Perspective on Life-Threatening Illness
Choices in Life-Threatening Illness
The Range of Psychological Suffering
The Therapeutic Response to the Patient with HIV/AIDS
The Therapeutic Response to the Patient with Cancer
The Therapeutic Response to the Patient with End-Stage Renal Disease
The Stages of Grief
The Challenge for the Medical Assistant

OBJECTIVES

The student should strive to meet the following performance objectives and demonstrate an understanding of the facts and principles presented in this chapter through written and oral communication.

1. Define the key terms as presented in the glossary.
2. Describe possible patient perspectives when facing a life-threatening illness.
3. Define "life-threatening" illness.
4. Discuss cultural manifestations of life-threatening illness.
5. Identify the strongest cultural influence in the life of a patient.
6. List at least four choices to be made when facing a life-threatening illness.
7. Briefly describe the use of living wills and physician directives.

(continues)

FEATURED COMPETENCIES

CAAHEP-ENTRY-LEVEL COMPETENCIES

Professional Communications

- Recognize and respond to verbal communications
- Recognize and respond to nonverbal communications

Patient Instructions

- Identify community resources

ABHES—ENTRY-LEVEL COMPETENCIES

Professionalism

- Exhibit initiative
- Adapt to change
- Be courteous and diplomatic

Communication

- Be attentive, listen and learn
- Be impartial and show empathy when dealing with patients
- Adapt what is said to the recipient's level of comprehension
- Serve as a liaison among physician and others
- Recognize and respond to verbal and nonverbal communication

Legal Concepts

- Use appropriate guidelines when releasing records or information

Competency Components

- Seek patient's written authorization for release of any medical information

Psychology

- Recognize cultural influences on behavior
- Help patients adjust to illness

Instruction

- Instruct patients with special needs

OBJECTIVES (continued)

8. Discuss the range of psychological suffering that accompanies life-threatening illnesses.
9. Discuss additional concerns/fears when the life-threatening illness is AIDS, cancer, or end-stage renal disease.
10. Recall a number of challenges faced by the medical assistant when caring for people with life-threatening illnesses.

SCENARIO

You have seen the medical reports and agonize with your physician who must tell Suzanne Markis, a long-time patient, when she comes in today that she has inoperable pancreatic cancer. When she arrives, you treat her as you normally would, making certain she suspects nothing from you. When she emerges from the physician's room, you make certain to meet her, take her arm, and ask if you can call someone for her. You do not present her with a bill or make another appointment at this time. You recognize that anything you say probably will not be remembered, so you focus entirely on this patient and her immediate needs. In a day or two, as instructed by your physician–employer, you will make a phone call to set up an appointment for Suzanne and anyone she might want present at her visit with the physician so any questions can be answered.

You remind yourself to have Suzanne sign the necessary paperwork defining any designees she might identify to receive her medical information.

INTRODUCTION

Everything you learned in Chapter 4 regarding therapeutic communications is heightened and considered more difficult when the patient has a life-threatening illness. If you were told today that your life would probably be shortened because of a serious illness, your perspective would likely change. What was important yesterday may mean little or nothing now. Something that meant nothing to you yesterday suddenly takes on great importance to you now. It is essential for the medical assistant to remember this difference in perspective and what is likely to be important to patients with a life-threatening illness.

It also must be remembered that no two individuals respond to a life-threatening illness in the same way. Some respond with denial and act as if the information had never been shared with them. Others alter their lives radically and drastically change their priorities. Still others quietly continue their lives changing little outwardly but recognize that their choices may now be limited (Figure 6-1).

LIFE-THREATENING ILLNESS

A life-threatening illness is not easily defined. Some will use the word *terminal;* others refuse to use that word because they believe it removes any hope from the situation. Also, what is life-threatening for one individual may not be for another. For our purposes, life-threatening is used to imply a life that in all probability will be shortened because of a serious or debilitating illness or disease. It may be defined as death that is imminent; it may be defined in terms of a serious illness that one will battle for many years but will ultimately shorten his or her life.

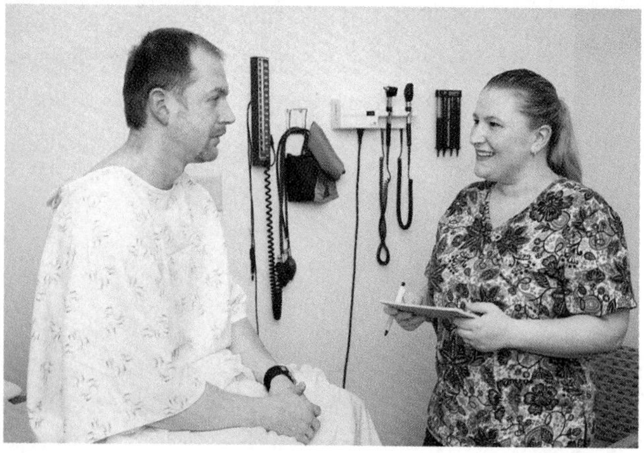

Figure 6-1 Establishing a caring and trusting relationship can help the patient come to terms with a life-threatening illness.

Cultural Perspective on Life-Threatening Illness

Strong cultural manifestations will be seen in the treatment of a life-threatening illness and for anyone facing death. Culture is defined as how we live our lives, how we think, how we speak, and how we behave. Cultures can be accepting, denying, or even defying of death. Death can be considered either as the end of existence or as a transition to another state of being or consciousness. Death can be considered as profane or sacred. In some cultures, a life-threatening illness may be viewed or referred to as a "slow-motion" death because of degenerative diseases that often exhaust the resources and emotions of patients and their families.

Some cultures prefer that the life-threatening illness not be shared with the patient in the beginning, but with the family who helps to prepare the patient for the inevitable. A few cultures generally do not seek care for an illness until it is quite advanced; this practice can make pain management and treatment more difficult or impossible in some cases. Some cultures surround the person who is ill with great attention, never leaving the person alone. Other cultures view the illness as something that must be removed from the body, perhaps even believing

Spotlight on Certification

RMA Content Outline

- Patient relations
- Other personal relations
- Patient resource materials

CMA Content Outline

- Basic principles (Psychology)
- Hereditary, cultural, and environmental influences on behavior
- Adapting communication to individual's ability to understand
- Professional communication and behavior
- Patient advocate

CMAS Content Outline

- Professionalism

that the individual has been given this illness because of some past sin or transgression.

Pain is viewed in the same manner. Some cultures believe it is to be endured quietly without complaint; others believe there is to be no pain, and family members will go to great lengths to have health care providers relieve the pain. When questioning a patient about the pain level, it must be within a cultural perspective. For example, cultures with an Asian influence are more likely to describe pain in general terms related to the imbalance of the body than in terms of "piercing, intermittent, or throbbing" or on a scale of 1 to 10.

It must also be remembered that the strongest influence in managing any life-threatening illness in the life of the patient is *not* the health care team; it is the family and those closest to the patient. Therefore, great care must be taken to determine and understand the patient's cultural perspective as much as possible, and the patient must be given great respect. Often, the cultural influence may contradict the standard of care preferred by the health care provider. It is better to understand the culture and work within it than to deny it and continually work against the patient's belief system and influence of family.

CHOICES IN LIFE-THREATENING ILLNESS

Many choices are available to a patient with a life-threatening illness, but many decisions are to be made, also. The urgency of the decisions will depend, in part, on possible life expectancy. Sometimes these decisions may seem contrary to recommended medical intervention.

Patients have the right to choose or to refuse treatment in most cases. Some rush into a treatment protocol only to discover later that their choices have brought them pain, disability, and expense far beyond what originally was assumed. Although it is the health care professional's goal to heal, if healing is not likely or possible, patients ought not to be "urged" into treatment protocols that are likely to be contrary to their personal wishes for the sake of treatment only.

Although health care professionals seem less comfortable with death than they are with saving life, there are some issues appropriate to discuss with patients especially when facing life-threatening illness. Those issues include the following:

1. Alternative methods of treatment should be discussed, as well as the outcome if no treatment is sought. At some point, many patients will want to know *all* the treatment protocols that are feasible. This is a logical time to discuss any alternative therapies or integrative medicine that have shown success. Explanations should be made in language that the patient can understand. Illustrations and diagrams can be beneficial. Referrals might be made to integrative medicine practitioners, and patients are to be encouraged to discuss any chosen alternative therapies with their primary care physician. Patients may also ask what happens if no treatment is chosen. This question can be difficult for health care providers who are anxious to provide some form of treatment for patients, but patients may have a number of reasons not to seek treatment. Sometimes treatment alternatives the patient may consider are not within the realm of recognized medical acceptability, but it is better to have that discussion than to ignore the possibility. Remember the earlier statement indicating that family members and friends bring more influence to bear than does the health care professional.
2. Discussion of pain management and treatment is essential. The major fears patients have in facing life-threatening illness are pain and loss of independence. A frank discussion of pain control and how that can be accomplished can alleviate a fair amount of concern. Physicians should be ready to discuss loss of independence related to any life-threatening illness, or make a referral to someone who can be helpful. Patients have concerns such as wanting to know how long before the disease takes its toll, how long can they drive, what kind of care or assistance will be necessary, can they remain in their own home, and how long before they must have someone make decisions for them.
3. A **durable power of attorney for health care** allows an individual to make decisions related to health care when the patient is no longer able to do so. In the best of circumstances, this document will carry out the decisions the patient has already made in a **living will** or **physician's directive** regarding terminal conditions and whether to prolong life. Advances in medicine allow patient's lives to be sustained even when they are unlikely to recover from a persistent and vegetative state. The living will and the durable power of attorney for health care allow patients to make decisions before becoming incapacitated or whether life-prolonging medical or surgical procedures are to be continued, withheld, or withdrawn, as well as if or when artificial feeding and fluids are to be used or withheld. The living will and the durable power of attorney for health care documents are legal in all 50 states. Although states may vary somewhat

in the wording of these documents, they provide the same overall benefit to patients. (See Chapter 7 for more information.) The federal government passed the Patient Self-Determination Act in 1990 giving all patients receiving care in institutions receiving payments from Medicare and Medicaid written information about their right to accept or refuse medical or surgical treatment. The act also requires that patients be given information about their options to create living wills and to appoint someone to act on their behalf in making health care decisions (durable power of attorney for health care). Any documents of this nature that the patient has should be copied in the medical chart that goes with the patient when admitted to the hospital. At any time the patient makes a change in such a document, the old document is to be replaced with the new one.

4. Finances are to be considered. What will insurance cover (if there is insurance)? Who makes the decisions in a managed care environment? What family resources can or will be used? Finances are no one's favorite subject, especially physicians. However, such a discussion is important. Often, patients fear not being able to meet their financial obligations and leaving large debts to surviving family members almost as much as the life-threatening illness itself. As a medical assistant, you can help patients understand the parameters of their health insurance and any restrictions there might be on particular illnesses or treatments. Can medical insurance be canceled if employment pays a portion of the health insurance and the patient is no longer able to work? If there is a life insurance policy, help patients determine if any portion of the policy can be used for end-of-life expenses. Any services you can provide to the patient or family members in relieving the financial stress can bring great relief to everyone involved.
5. Emotional needs of the patient and family members are important. Emotional support is vital when dealing with a life-threatening illness. Health care professionals will want to determine where that support comes from for the patient. Should a support group be suggested for the patient and family members? For some patients and families, an individual giving spiritual guidance is seen as a member of the family and a member of the health care team. For others, no spiritual influence is recognized or sought.

It is not the responsibility of the health care professionals treating the individual with life-threatening illness to provide all these services, but a health care professional who raises these issues for patients and families to deal with is more closely in tune with a patient's power in the illness.

THE RANGE OF PSYCHOLOGICAL SUFFERING

The range of suffering associated with a life-threatening illness is extensive. Patients feel extreme distress. Anxiety and depression are common. At the time of diagnosis, patients' responses may include denial, numbness, and inability to face the facts. Sadness, hopelessness, helplessness, and withdrawal often are exhibited.

The range of psychological suffering leads to physical symptoms, such as tension, tachycardia, agitation, insomnia, anorexia, and panic attacks. The physician may be so intent on treating the physical ramifications of the illness that the psychological suffering is mostly ignored.

Relationships of individuals with a life-threatening illness often change. Close friends may feel uncomfortable with someone who is dying. Some fear touching or caressing the dying and become aloof and distant. However, new friendships can often be made as well, if patients meet others with the same or similar life-threatening issues and help maintain each other's self-esteem. Relationships are important because they provide support and encouragement beyond any other source. Patients experience a loss of self-esteem when they are ill, are in pain, and have a body that is failing them. When self-image is lost, patients feel useless, see themselves as burdens, and have difficulty accepting help from anyone. The psychological effect of this "loss of self" can even hasten death.

It is often helpful to encourage patients to set goals for themselves. These can be small goals such as walking around the block, eating all their dinner, and connecting with a friend. The goals may also be much larger, such as staying alive until a son graduates from college, or putting all financial matters in order for surviving family members. Personal goals give the patient something other than their illness to plan for and work toward.

Careful listening to patients and seeking clues for what *may not* be said is essential for the medical assistant and support staff caring for patients. Putting yourself in their shoes and asking what would be helpful is often beneficial. Be ready with a list of community resources that may benefit patients at this time.

It is not the intention of this chapter to specifically identify the many life-threatening illnesses and their particular needs. However, three threatening illnesses are identified in the following sections with some specific information.

THE THERAPEUTIC RESPONSE TO THE PATIENT WITH HIV/AIDS

Patients testing positive for human immunodeficiency virus (HIV) and those with acquired immune deficiency syndrome (AIDS) feel great stress from the infection, the disease, and the fear of other life-threatening illnesses. Persons with HIV infection may have only a short time before the onset of AIDS; others may have a much longer period. AIDS is a disease that can have many periods of fairly good health and many periods of serious near-death illnesses. Recent developments in the treatment of HIV infection and AIDS help patients to live longer, but their lives are greatly compromised because of their suppressed immune system.

In some cases, guilt develops about past behavior and lifestyles, or the possibility of having transmitted the disease to others. Members of the gay community or individuals addicted to intravenous drugs who are at high risk for the disease may also be estranged from their family's support system. Individuals with HIV infection may feel added strain if this is the first knowledge their families have of any high-risk behaviors they have that are associated with the transmission of the disease. When the disease is contracted by individuals who feel they are protected or safe from the disease, anger is paramount. HIV has affected mostly individuals who are relatively young. Thus, they are not as likely to have substantial financial resources or permanent housing. Treating HIV is expensive, and many patients have little or no insurance coverage.

Patients with HIV may experience central nervous system involvement. Forgetfulness and poor concentration may be followed by **psychomotor retardation,** or the slowing of physical and mental responses, decreased alertness, apathy, withdrawal, and diminished interest in work. Some patients later experience confusion and progressive impairment of intellectual function or dementia. When HIV-infected patients contract other opportunistic diseases, those symptoms are experienced as well.

A complex criteria determines when a patient's illness is identified as AIDS rather than HIV infection. Some physicians prefer not to use the term *AIDS;* rather, they discuss the illness as early or later stage HIV infection. Many physicians in the United States and around the world use the term *AIDS* when patients' CD4 counts (healthy T4 lymphocytes) decline to less than 200. (The average healthy individual will have CD4 lymphocyte counts of 800–1,500.) Many developing countries in the world, however, are unable to measure the CD4 counts. AIDS is then diagnosed by the symptoms and any immunodeficient illnesses the patients have. Using only a CD4 count for diagnosis can be quite discouraging for patients who monitor those counts quite closely. Also, a patient's CD4 count can decrease dramatically into the "AIDS zone" one time, and then increase in sufficient numbers to move the patient back into HIV infection another time. Allied health professionals will need to take the lead from their physician–employers.

Critical Thinking

What can be done to help individuals with HIV to cope with their emotional roller coaster?

THE THERAPEUTIC RESPONSE TO THE PATIENT WITH CANCER

The first reaction patients with cancer usually have is the fear of loss of life. Patients think, "Cancer equals death. Am I going to die?" After that, issues begin to differ for each person. Some may choose no treatment and allow life to take its course. Most, however, will wonder about what treatment to choose, how to make that choice, and how effective will it be. Many patients are empowered by taking a major role in the decision making related to their cancer. Research can be helpful in studying the many options that may be available in treatment. The fact is that many patients diagnosed with cancer will die, whereas others diagnosed will live many years after diagnosis and treatment.

The three most likely treatments for cancer are surgery, radiation, and chemotherapy. Often, treatment is a combination of the three. Patients can experience serious side effects from both radiation and chemotherapy. Alternative practitioners have shown that meditation or acupuncture can help relieve the side effects for some patients. Loss of hair, nausea, vomiting, and pain are quite disconcerting to patients trying to cope. The American

Critical Thinking

Many individuals in the end stages of both AIDS and cancer have lost their image of themselves. Their bodies have been diminished; they may have lost a great deal of weight from the disease or gained much weight from medications taken. They may have no hair. They may have lost their ability to speak or to control bodily functions. What can you do or say to help them feel like a human being?

Cancer Society (http://www.cancer.org) has a number of resources for patients.

The most common signs and symptoms of advanced cancer are weakness, loss of appetite and weight, pain, nausea, constipation, sleepiness or confusion, and shortness of breath. Make certain your patients understand your physician's willingness to relieve and treat these symptoms. Even when there is "nothing more to do" related to the cancer, there is still "much to do" to maintain comfort and to give patients the chance to do the things that are meaningful to them and their families.

THE THERAPEUTIC RESPONSE TO THE PATIENT WITH END-STAGE RENAL DISEASE

Loss of kidney (renal) function leads to serious illness known as end-stage renal disease (ESRD). When the kidneys fail completely, patients cannot live for long unless they receive dialysis or a kidney transplant. A successful kidney transplant relieves the person of kidney failure. However, there are not enough transplants for every person who needs one, and not all transplants are appropriate or successful. Dialysis is the name of the process of artificially replacing the main functions of the kidneys—filtering blood to remove wastes. Choosing dialysis as a treatment plan can sustain life for years and is covered by Medicare, but it does have complications that burden patients and their caregivers.

Depending on age, a patient's general health, and other circumstances, some patients will opt not to have dialysis and to let death come from kidney failure. The by-products of the body's chemistry accumulate in renal failure and cause an array of symptoms. Mild confusion and disorientation are common. Upsetting hallucinations or agitation can occur. Certain minerals concentrated in the blood can cause muscle twitching, tremors, and shakes. Some patients experience mild or severe itching. Appetite decreases early, and there can be rapid, shallow breathing. Many patients with kidney failure pass little or no urine. Fluid overload results in edema, or swelling of the body, particularly of the legs and abdomen. Patients with some urine output may live for months even after stopping dialysis. People with no urine output are likely to die within a week or two. Patients will lose energy and become sleepy and lethargic. Typically, patients slip into a deeper sleep and gradually lose consciousness. Kidney failure has a reputation for being a gentle death.

Life-threatening illnesses are family illnesses. There are primary (the person suffering from the illness) and secondary (family and friends) patients. Stress on a spouse or partner is enormous as they think about taking over the other person's role and as they try to deal with their own feelings. Patients and their families and friends cannot avoid feeling angry. The situation is tragic and, in some instances, might have been avoided (for example, a long-time smoker dying of lung cancer). There needs to be time to grieve. Depression is common among patients with life-threatening illness and warning signs should be reported to the physician. Remember that how patients live their last days is just as important as the numbers on the laboratory reports.

The Stages of Grief

There are a number of different philosophies on grief and the stages patients are apt to experience when they know their lives are about to end, but none is so widely known as that of Dr. Elisabeth Kubler-Ross, who was one of the first to conduct research and determine possible stages of grief. Those stages are:

Denial—"This *cannot* be happening to me."

Anger—"Why is this happening to me?"

Bargaining—"Okay, but only if I can just watch my last child graduate from college."

Depression—"I feel sad, blue, and prefer not to be around anyone."

Acceptance—"If this must be, then I am ready."

Dr. Kubler-Ross reminds health care professionals that not all patients go through all five stages; some patients go through all five stages many, many times, and still others get stuck in one stage, usually the denial stage. Grief and dying is personal. No two patients will follow the same pattern. The stages are identified so that you can be more aware of what is happening in the process to both the patients and their loved ones. Clashes are likely among family members and patients when they are in different stages.

THE CHALLENGE FOR THE MEDICAL ASSISTANT

As a medical assistant, you face the challenge of caring for people with a life-threatening illness; you must comfort those who face great suffering and death. You will become a source of information for patients and their support members. You must be particularly sensitive

Critical Thinking

What steps would you personally take to make certain you do not burnout from caring for patients with a life-threatening illness?

and respectful toward individuals who may be viewed as social pariahs. You will have to examine your own beliefs, lifestyle, and biases. You must be comfortable treating all patients, no matter what the illness is or how it was contracted.

As well as assisting your physician–employer in providing the best possible medical care, many nonmedical forms of assistance may be required by patients suffering from a life-threatening illness. You may need to make referrals to community-based agencies or service groups. Health departments, social workers, trained hospice volunteers, and AIDS volunteers may also be helpful to you, your patients, and their families.

The best therapeutic response to the patient with a life-threatening illness will build on the person's own culture and coping abilities, capitalize on strengths, maintain hope, and show continued human care and concern. Patients may want up-to-date information on their disease, its causes, modes of transmission, treatments available, and sources of care and social support. Be prepared to recommend support groups where patients can discuss their feelings and express their concerns. Treat patients with concern and compassion and assure them everything will be done to provide continuity of care and relief from distress. Patients may be encouraged to call on clergy for spiritual support.

Case Study 6-1

The extended family of Wong Lee is concerned about his illness and his care. Chronic obstructive pulmonary disease (COPD) has ravaged his body. He is on oxygen all the time now. He wants to remain at home to die; his family wants that, too. The family has been with him and has been involved in his care plan all along. Yet you are still uncertain of how much information to give to members of his expanded family when they call.

CASE STUDY REVIEW

1. Are the questions the extended family members raise intended to harm or help Mr. Lee?
2. Is there a durable power of attorney for health care in place?
3. Which, if any, of the family's desires are related to the culture?
4. What can you and your physician–employer suggest to be of help to everyone involved?

Case Study 6-2

Inner City Health Care, a multidoctor urgent care center in a large city, has a large roster of patients, some of whom have AIDS. Although clinical medical assistant Bruce Goldman tries not to be, sometimes he is nervous about assisting with patients who are gay. When Bill Swartz is seen by the physician for a change in a mole on his calf, Bruce does his best to interact in a professional manner even though Bill is gay. After this patient exchange, Bruce Goldman decides it is time to deal with his prejudices against gay and lesbians, as well as his fear of AIDS and all patients with AIDS.

CASE STUDY REVIEW

1. Although Bruce Goldman may not admit it, he is fearful of AIDS. What should he know about HIV transmission that may reduce his fears?
2. In the future, Bruce would like to be more open and supportive when he is dealing with an HIV-infected patient. What are some of the things he can do to help patients?
3. What are some things Bruce can do to reduce wariness regarding patients who are gay?

SUMMARY

Medical assistants must be aware that when caring for patients with a life-threatening illness, having even the slightest fear of death can undermine the ability to respond professionally, with empathy and support. If you feel yourself losing the ability to be helpful, it is time to briefly step aside. This does not mean withdrawal from your position or refusal to care for your patients. It means that you do whatever is necessary so that your perspective is not lost. It may mean taking a day off from work to "fill up your psyche" and to give yourself a rest. If the ambulatory care setting has an abundance of patients with life-threatening illnesses, it may require that you spend some time in a support group of your own so that you are better able to cope. Never be afraid to feel sad or weep with your patients. It is better to sense their pain and, at times, feel the pain with them, than it is to be so clinically objective you miss their true needs.

STUDY FOR SUCCESS

To reinforce your knowledge and skills of information in this chapter:

- ❑ Review the Key Terms
- ❑ Consider the Case Studies and discuss your conclusions
- ❑ Answer the Review Questions
  - ❑ Multiple Choice
  - ❑ Critical Thinking
- ❑ Navigate the Internet and complete the Web Activities
- ❑ Practice the StudyWARE activities on the textbook CD
- ❑ Apply your knowledge in the Student Workbook activities
- ❑ Complete the Web Tutor sections
- ❑ View and discuss the DVD situations

REVIEW QUESTIONS

Multiple Choice

1. When a practice treats patients with HIV/AIDS, cancer, or ESRD, it is important for medical assistants to:
   a. warn other patients about the dangers of transmission
   b. segregate these patient reception areas from other patient areas
   c. be supportive and free of prejudice
   d. deny any information to patients regarding the seriousness of the illness
2. The Patient Self-Determination Act:
   a. allows a patient to have a choice of physicians
   b. ensures a patient's right to accept or refuse treatment
   c. gives patients the right to formulate advance directives
   d. all of the above
   e. only b and c
3. The strongest influence on a patient with a life-threatening illness is:
   a. the physician
   b. the hospital
   c. the family
   d. the patient
4. Life-threatening illness may be defined as:
   a. a life shortened because of serious illness or disease
   b. death that is imminent
   c. serious illness to battle for many years but may shorten life
   d. all of the above
5. Culture may be defined in part as:
   a. how we choose a friend
   b. how we think and live our lives
   c. how we select a medication
   d. all of the above

6. Therapeutic communication with a patient with a life-threatening illness:
   a. is no different than communicating with any patient
   b. is heightened and considered more difficult
   c. is left to nonmedical support staff
   d. comes naturally and requires no special skill
7. Cultural influence may in part determine:
   a. when/how to involve family members
   b. whether spiritual support is sought
   c. how the illness and its pain is managed
   d. all of the above
8. Durable power of attorney for health care:
   a. enables someone other than the patient to make only health care decisions
   b. enables someone other than the patient to make any decisions for the patient
   c. makes certain that patients' financial responsibilities are met
   d. makes certain an attorney's wishes are followed
9. The confusion, disorientation, and mental deficiency seen in some patients with life-threatening illness:
   a. may make communication difficult or impossible
   b. is a good reason for a durable power of attorney for health care
   c. is made easier if patients expressed earlier their desires in a physician's directive
   d. all of the above
10. Effective pain management may depend on:
    a. patient's medical insurance
    b. family wishes and patient's needs
    c. professional nursing criteria
    d. all of the above

Critical Thinking

1. Research other sections in this text that discuss end-of-life legal documents. Describe additional information you find.
2. Discuss with a friend what cultural influences might affect each of you if you were facing a life-threatening illness. What choices would each of you make?
3. List common psychological reactions people might have from learning they have a life-threatening illness.
4. List the advantages/disadvantages of the physician directives available.
5. Discuss with a nurse or a nursing student in your school how nurses deal with the psychological suffering in patients with a life-threatening illness.
6. Discuss with a classmate your concerns in dealing with patients with a life-threatening illness. Would you choose to work where you seldom lost a patient to a life-threatening illness? If so, what are your reasons?
7. Research the agencies available in your community that can provide support for people and family members facing life-threatening illness.
8. At Inner City Health Care, Dr. Ray Reynolds is known for his compassion and great warmth toward people. On difficult days at the center, this attitude holds him in good stead. Sometimes, he tends to take on the more challenging cases: patients with life-threatening diseases, often young people with AIDS who should be in the prime of their lives. Clinical medical assistant Wanda Slawson always tries to learn from Dr. Reynolds' example. Although she is quieter and not as outgoing as Dr. Reynolds, Wanda hopes to be both courteous and comforting to patients, especially those who are anxious. She makes it a point to help patients discover a new way to cope with debilitating diseases. What resources might she use?
9. Teri Montague, RMA, is the office manager for a pediatric oncologist. In the past several months there seem to have been more patient deaths than usual. She notices that the entire staff seems "low and a little depressed." She discusses this concern with her physician–employer, Dr. Anita Glenn. The decision is made to close the office for a 2-hour lunch on Wednesday. The lunch will be catered, and a very good friend of Dr. Glenn will be invited to join everyone. Dr. Penny Hein has a PhD in psychosocial nursing and years of experience in grief counseling. Teri and Dr. Glenn believe she can give everyone some helpful information. Is this a good plan? Why or why not?

THE DVD HOOK-UP

DVD Series
Critical Thinking

Program Number
2

Chapter/Scene Reference
- *Communicating with Patients*

This chapter introduces you to the concept of using a therapeutic approach when working with patients.

In the designated DVD clip, we observed Mrs. Smith become quite anxious about her abnormal mammogram results. We also observed how Gwen, the medical assistant, addressed Mrs. Smith's concerns.

1. Do you feel that Gwen demonstrated a therapeutic approach toward Mrs. Smith's concern over her abnormal mammogram results?
2. List some gestures that Gwen used that illustrated her concern and compassion toward the patient.
3. Did Gwen overstep her boundaries as a medical assistant when she discussed the mammogram results with Mrs. Smith, or do you think that Gwen was trying to help the patient understand what the physician had already explained?

DVD Journal Summary

Write a paragraph that summarizes what you learned from watching the designated scene from today's DVD program. Did you empathize with Mrs. Smith regarding her anxiety over her abnormal mammogram? What will you do when you are faced with similar challenges in the industry? Do you think that you could ever work in an oncology practice? Why or why not?

WEB ACTIVITIES

1. Using your favorite search engine, key in American Cancer Society and look for statistics for the current year. Pay particular attention to the area reporting how long patients survive after diagnosis. What are the major changes in the last two years?
2. Many sites will come on your screen when you search for end-stage renal disease (ESRD). Seek out the site that identifies the six warning signs of kidney and urinary tract diseases. Identify the functions of the kidneys and what happens in ESRD. How many people in the U.S. population have ESRD?
3. Using search words "HIV Today" will take you to an AEGIS site that includes the latest press releases and statistics on AIDS. Browse around a bit. In what countries of the world is AIDS the greatest threat? Did you find a fact sheet providing a list of opportunistic infections related to AIDS? Print copies of a resource or two that might help patients.
4. Using the World Wide Web can be challenging, especially if you find more that 270,000 sites to browse. That is what you will find if you key in "Helping the Dying." Choose a couple of the topics that are especially helpful to you or might help other students studying this chapter. Write a brief paragraph on each.

REFERENCES/BIBLIOGRAPHY

Lewis, M., & Tamparo, C. (2002). *Medical law, ethics, and bioethics for ambulatory care*. Philadelphia: F. A. Davis Company.

Purnell, L., & Paulanka, B. (1998). *Transcultural health care: A culturally competent approach*. Philadelphia: F. A. Davis Company.

Tamparo, C., & Lindh, W. (2000). *Therapeutic communications for health professionals*. Clifton Park, NY: Thomson Delmar Learning.

UNIT 3
Responsible Medical Practice

CHAPTER 7

Legal Considerations

OUTLINE

Sources of Law
- Statutory Law
- Common Law
- Criminal Law
- Civil Law

Administrative Law
- Title VII of the Civil Rights Act
- Federal Age Discrimination Act
- Uniform Anatomical Gift Act
- Regulation Z of the Consumer Protection Act
- Occupational Safety and Health Act
- Controlled Substances Act
- Americans with Disabilities Act
- Family and Medical Leave Act
- Health Insurance Portability and Accountability Act

Contract Law
- Termination of Contracts

Tort Law
- Medical Practice Acts
- Standard of Care
- Risk Management

Informed Consent
- Implied Consent
- Consent and Legal Incompetence

Civil Litigation Process
- Subpoenas
- Discovery
- Pretrial Conference
- Trial
- Statute of Limitations

Public Duties
- Reportable Diseases/Injuries
- Abuse
- Good Samaritan Laws

Physician's Directives
- Living Wills
- Durable Power of Attorney for Health Care

OBJECTIVES

The student should strive to meet the following performance objectives and demonstrate an understanding of the facts and principles presented in this chapter through written and oral communication.

1. Define the key terms as presented in the glossary.
2. List and briefly describe the five sources of law.
3. Compare/contrast civil and criminal law.
4. Identify the three major areas of civil law that directly affect the medical profession.

(continues)

KEY TERMS

Administer
Administrative Law
Agent
Alternative Dispute Resolution (ADR)
Arbitration
Civil Law
Common Law
Constitutional Law
Contract Law
Criminal Law
Defendant
Deposition
Discovery
Dispense
Doctrine
Durable Power of Attorney for Health Care
Emancipated Minor
Expert Witness
Expressed Contract
Felony
Implied Consent
Implied Contract
Incompetence
Informed Consent
Interrogatory
Libel
Litigation
Malfeasance
Malpractice
Mature Minor
Mediation
Medically Indigent
Minor
Misdemeanor
Misfeasance
Negligence
Noncompliant
Nonfeasance

(continues)

KEY TERMS (continued)

Patient Self-Determination Act (PSDA)
Plaintiff
Precedents
Prescribe
Risk Management
Slander
Statutory Law
Subpoena
Tort
Tort Law

FEATURED COMPETENCIES

CAAHEP—ENTRY-LEVEL COMPETENCIES

Patient Care

- Maintain medication and immunization records

Legal Concepts

- Identify and respond to issues of confidentiality
- Perform within legal and ethical boundaries
- Demonstrate knowledge of federal and state health care legislation and regulations

ABHES—ENTRY-LEVEL COMPETENCIES

Professionalism

- Maintain confidentiality at all times
- Be cognizant of ethical boundaries
- Conduct work within scope of education, training, and ability

Legal Concepts

- Use appropriate guidelines when releasing information
- Follow established policy in initiating or terminating medical treatment

(continues)

OBJECTIVES (continued)

5. Recall at least seven of the nine administrative law acts important to the medical profession.
6. Compare/contrast administering, prescribing, and dispensing of controlled substances.
7. Describe the measures to take for disposal of controlled substances.
8. Recall the three main goals of HIPAA.
9. Explain the differences between expressed and implied contracts.
10. Identify the three main reasons for the physician/patient contract to be terminated.
11. Define and give examples of torts.
12. List and describe the 4Ds of negligence.
13. Discuss what constitutes battery in the ambulatory care setting.
14. Describe the two forms of defamation of character and how it might occur.
15. Recall how medical assistants can help to maintain a patient's privacy.
16. Identify at least 10 practices to help in risk management.
17. Discuss informed consent and its importance.
18. Compare/contrast the types of minors.
19. Outline the necessary steps in civil litigation and how a medical assistant might be involved.
20. Discuss how and when subpoenas are used.
21. Recall the special considerations for patients related to issues of confidentiality, the statute of limitations, public duties, and AIDS.
22. Describe procedures to follow in reporting abuse.
23. Discuss Good Samaritan laws.
24. Identify various forms of physician's directives.
25. Recall maintenance of advanced directives in the ambulatory care setting.
26. Discuss HIPAA regulations for confidentiality in physician's directives.

SCENARIO

Gwen, the office manager in Dr. Gold's office, is reviewing legal concerns in a staff meeting. Even though each employee is well aware of privacy, confidentiality, and the many ways their actions are legally binding, Gwen has noticed occasional carelessness creeping into their busy activities. Employees are reminded of how far their voices may carry in a phone conversation with a patient, they review placement of patients' medical charts for Dr. Gold, and they discuss how to protect confidentiality in filing insurance claims.

FEATURED COMPETENCIES (continued)

- Dispose of controlled substances in compliance with government regulations
- Maintain licenses and accreditation
- Monitor legislation related to current healthcare issues and practices
- Perform risk management procedures

Spotlight on Certification

RMA Content Outline
- Licensure, certification, registration
- Principles of medical ethics
- Ethical conduct
- Legal responsibilities

CMA Content Outline
- Displaying professional attitude
- Performing within ethical boundaries
- Maintaining confidentiality
- Licenses and accreditation
- Legislative
- Physician–patient relationship
- Patient advocate

CMAS Content Outline
- Legal and Ethical Considerations
- Professionalism
- Confidentiality
- Risk Management and Quality Assurance

INTRODUCTION

The law as it relates to health care has grown increasingly complex in the last decade. The agendas of federal and state governments include an investigation of quality health care, a desire to control health care costs (whereas hoping to ensure equitable access to health care), and an interest in protecting the patient. A full discussion of health law requires several volumes; therefore, the aim of this chapter is awareness of the law and its implications and establishment of sound practices and procedures to both safeguard patient rights and protect the health care professional.

SOURCES OF LAW

Law is a binding custom or ruling for conduct that is enforceable by an agency assigned that authority. The highest authority in the United States is the U.S. Constitution. Adopted in 1787, this document provides the framework for the U.S. government. The Constitution includes 27 amendments, 10 of which are known as the Bill of Rights. This authority is sometimes referred to as **constitutional law.** The U.S. Constitution calls for three branches of the federal government:

- Executive branch: the President, Vice President (elected by U.S. citizens), Cabinet officers, and various other departments of the federal government
- Legislative branch: members of the U.S. Senate, the House of Representatives (elected by U.S. citizens), and the staffs of individual legislators and legislative committees.
- Judicial branch: the courts, including the U.S. Supreme Court, Courts of Appeals for the nine judicial regions, and District Courts

Laws enacted at the federal level are called acts or laws. An example is Title XIX of Public Law established in 1967 to provide health care for the **medically indigent.** This program is known as Medicaid.

Statutory Law

Constitutions in the 50 states identify the rights and responsibilities of their citizens and identify how their state is organized. States have a governor as the head and state legislatures (both elected by the state's citizens), as well as their own court systems with a number of levels. The body of laws made by states is known as **statutory law.** All powers that are not conferred specifically on the federal government are retained by the state, yet states vary widely in their interpretation of that power. State law cannot override the power of any laws defined in the U.S. Constitution or its amendments.

Common Law

Common law is not so easily defined, but is essential to understanding law in the United States. Common law was developed by judges in England and France over many centuries and was brought to the United States with the early settlers. Common law is often called judge-made law. The law consists of rulings made by judges who base their decisions on a combination of a number of factors: (1) individual decisions of a court, (2) interpretation of the U.S. Constitution or a particular state constitution, and (3) statutory law. These decisions become known as **precedents** and often lay down the foundation for subsequent legal rulings.

Criminal Law

Criminal law addresses wrongs committed against the welfare and safety of society as a whole. Criminal law affects relationships between individuals and between individuals and the government. Another term that might be used to describe a criminal act is **malfeasance.** Malfeasance is conduct that is illegal or contrary to an official's obligation. Criminal offenses generally are classified into the basic categories of a **felony** or a **misdemeanor** that are specifically defined in statutes.

Felonies are more serious crimes and include murder, larceny or thefts of large amounts of money, assault, and rape. Punishment for a felony is more serious than for a misdemeanor. A convicted felon cannot vote, hold public office, or own any weapons. Felonies often are divided into groups such as first degree (most serious), second degree, and third degree. Sentences are generally for longer than one year and are served in a penitentiary. Misdemeanors are considered lesser offenses and vary from state to state. Punishment may include probation or a time of service to the community, a fine, or a jail sentence in a city or county facility. Misdemeanors also can be divided into groups or classifications, such as A, B, or C class misdemeanors, denoting the seriousness of the crime (Class A is the most serious).

For a person to be found guilty of a crime, a judge or jury must prove the evidence against the individual "beyond a reasonable doubt." In a criminal case, charges are brought against an individual by the state with the intent of preventing any further harm to society. For example, a physician practicing medicine without a proper license may be subject to criminal action by the courts for endangering a patient's life.

Civil Law

Civil law affects relationships between individuals, corporations, government bodies, and other organizations. Terms that may be used in civil law are **misfeasance,** referring to a lawful act that is improperly or unlawfully executed, and **nonfeasance,** referring to the failure to perform an act, official duty, or legal requirement. The punishment for a civil wrong is usually monetary in nature. When a charge is brought against a **defendant** in a civil case, the goal is to reimburse the **plaintiff** or the person bringing charges with a monetary amount for suffering, pain, and any loss of wages. Another goal might be to make certain the defendant is prevented from engaging in similar behavior again. In civil law, cases need to show that a "preponderance of the evidence" is more than likely true against the defendant. The most common forms of civil law that directly affect the medical profession are **administrative law, contract law,** and **tort law.**

ADMINISTRATIVE LAW

Administrative law establishes agencies that are given power to specialize and enact regulations that have the force of law. The Internal Revenue Service is an example of an administrative agency that enacts tax laws and regulations. Health care professionals are bound by federal administrative law through the Medicare and Medicaid program rules administered by the Social Security Administration.

There are a number of other regulations in administrative law governing physicians and their employees. It is important that medical assistants be informed of legislation and any federal or state regulations that are critical to patients and the medical profession. Membership and attendance at meetings of professional organizations supporting the medical professions is a good way to remain current in health care issues. Identified here with a brief description are additional administrative acts, some of which also are referred to in other chapters in this textbook.

Title VII of the Civil Rights Act

Title VII of the Civil Rights Act of 1964 protects employees from sexual harassment. The office of Equal Employment Opportunities Commission (EEOC) guidelines make the employer strictly liable for the acts of supervisory employees, as well as for some acts of harassment by coworkers and clients. A written policy on sexual harassment detailing inappropriate behavior and stating specific steps to be taken to correct an inappropriate situation should be established. The policy should include: (1) a statement that harassment is not tolerated, (2) a statement that an employee who feels harassed needs to bring the matter to the immediate attention of a person designated in the policy, (3) a statement about the confidentiality of any incidents and specific disciplinary action against the harasser, and (4) the procedure to follow when harassment occurs.

Federal Age Discrimination Act

The Federal Age Discrimination Act of 1967 states that an employer with 15 or more employees must not discriminate in matters of employment related to age, sex, race, creed, marital status, national origin, color, or disabilities. Some states are more restrictive in their law and identify employers with eight or more employees. Valid reasons to decline applicants include: (1) health issues that may interfere with the safe and efficient performance of the job, (2) unavailability for the work schedule of the particular job, (3) insufficient training or experience to perform the duties of the particular job, and (4) someone else is better qualified.

Uniform Anatomical Gift Act

The Uniform Anatomical Gift Act of 1968 allows persons 18 years or older and of sound mind to make a gift of all or any part of their body (1) to any hospital, surgeon, or physician; (2) to any accredited medical or dental school, college, or university; (3) to any organ bank or storage facility; and (4) to any specified individual for education, research, advancement of medical/dental science, therapy, or transplantation. The gift may be noted in a will or by signing, in the presence of two witnesses, a donor's card. Some states allow these statements on the driver's license.

Regulation Z of the Consumer Protection Act

Regulation Z of the Consumer Protection Act of 1967, referred to as the Truth in Lending Act, requires that an agreement by physicians and their clients for payment of medical bills in more than four installments must be in writing and must provide information on any finance charge. This act is enforced by the Federal Trade Commission. These guidelines are often seen in prearrangements for surgery or prenatal care and delivery in fee-for-service plans, because patients may not be able to pay the entire fee in one payment.

Occupational Safety and Health Act

The Occupational Safety and Health Act (OSHA) of 1967 is a division of the U.S. Department of Labor. Its mission is to ensure that a workplace is safe and has a healthy environment. Penalties can be quite high for repeated and willful violations assessed by OSHA. These guidelines make certain that all employees know what chemicals they are handling, know how to reduce any health risks from hazardous chemicals that are labeled 1 to 4 for severity, and have Material Safety Data Sheets (MSDSs) listing every ingredient in the product. Other sections of this law protecting medical assistants and patients are detailed in additional chapters. They include Clinical Lab Improvement Amendments of 1988 (CLIA) (see Chapter 26), Blood-borne Pathogens Standard of July 1992 (see Chapter 10), and the Needle Stick Prevention Amendment of 2001 (see Chapter 10).

Controlled Substances Act

The Controlled Substances Act of 1970 became effective in 1971. The act is administered by the Drug Enforcement Administration (DEA) under the auspices of the U.S. Department of Justice. The Controlled Substances Act lists controlled drugs in five schedules (I, II, III, IV, and V) according to their potential for abuse and dependence, with Schedule I having the greatest abuse potential and no accepted medical use in the United States. This act and the U.S. Code of Federal Regulations regulate individuals who administer, prescribe, or dispense any drug listed in the five schedules. Every physician who **administers, prescribes,** or **dispenses** any controlled substance must be registered with the DEA. The DEA supplies a form for registration and mandates that renewal occurs every three years.

A physician who only prescribes Schedule II, III, IV, and V controlled substances in the lawful course of professional practice is not required to keep separate records of those transactions. Physicians who regularly administer controlled substances in Schedules II, III, IV, and V or who dispense controlled substances are required to keep records of each transaction.

An inventory must be taken every two years of all stocks of the substances on hand. The inventory must include: (1) a list of the name, address, and DEA registration number of the physician; (2) the date and time of the inventory; and (3) the signatures of the individuals taking the inventory. This inventory must be kept at the location identified on the registration certificate for at least two years. All Schedule II drug records must be maintained separate from all other controlled substance records. These records must be made available for inspection and copying by duly authorized officials of the DEA. Some states are even more restrictive than the federal requirements.

Any necessary disposal of controlled substances, usually occurring when they become outdated or when a physician's practice is closed, requires specific action. The physician's DEA number and registration certificate should be returned to the DEA. Specific guidelines for destruction of the controlled substances will need to be

> **Critical Thinking**
>
> Identify the type of doctors or medical specialties most likely to prescribe and dispense controlled substances.

obtained from the nearest divisional office for the DEA. Using the Internet, search using the words "Controlled Substances Act of 1970" for a listing of sites providing more information. You will find a listing of drugs in each of the five schedules that change from time to time as new drugs come on the market and are classified.

Americans with Disabilities Act

The Americans with Disabilities Act (ADA) of 1990 prohibits discrimination of individuals who have physical or mental disabilities from accessing public services and accommodations, employment, and telecommunications. A disability implies that a physical or mental impairment substantially limits one or more of an individual's major life activities. ADA is identified in five titles. Title I, enforced by the EEOC, prohibits discrimination in employment (see Chapter 34 for further details). Essentially, Title I requires a potential employer to identify and prove that certain disabilities cannot be accommodated in performing the job requirements. Individuals who formerly abused drugs and alcohol and those who are undergoing rehabilitation also are covered by the ADA and cannot be denied employment because of their history of substance abuse.

Titles II, III, and IV mandate disabled individuals access to public services, public accommodations, and telecommunications. ADA protects persons with HIV infection or AIDS, making certain they cannot be refused treatment by health care professionals because of their health status. Generally speaking, health care professionals with HIV infection or AIDS cannot be kept from providing treatment either, unless that treatment could be found to be a significant risk to others. Title V covers a number of miscellaneous issues such as exclusions from the definition of "disability," retaliation, insurance, and other issues. The ADA law applies to businesses with at least 15 employees, but some states have more stringent laws.

Family and Medical Leave Act

The Family and Medical Leave Act (FLMA) of 1993 is important for large ambulatory care centers and hospitals. FLMA requires all public employers and any private employer of 50 or more employees to provide up to 12 weeks of job-protected, unpaid leave each year for the following reasons: (1) birth and care of the employee's child, or placement for adoption or foster care of a child; (2) care of an immediate family member who has a serious health condition; and (3) care of the employee's own serious health issue. Employees must have been employed for at least 12 months and have worked at least 1,250 hours in the 12 months preceding the beginning of the FMLA leave.

Health Insurance Portability and Accountability Act

The Health Insurance Portability and Accountability Act (HIPAA) of 1996 requires the Department of Health and Human Services to adopt national standards for electronic health care transactions. The law also requires the adoption of privacy and security standards to protect an individual's identifiable health information. The goal of HIPAA is also to assist in making health insurance more affordable and accessible to individuals by protecting health insurance coverage for workers and their families when they change or lose their jobs.

HIPAA law is identified in seven titles. They are summarized briefly as follows:

I. Health Insurance Access, Portability, and Renewal: Increases the portability of health insurance, allows continuance and transfer of insurance even with preexisting conditions, and prohibits discrimination based on health status.
II. Preventing Health Care Fraud and Abuse: Establishes a fraud and abuse system and spells out penalty if either event is documented; improves the Medicare program through establishing standards; establishes standards for electronic transmission of health information.
III. Tax-Related Provisions: Promotes the use of medical savings accounts (MSAs) used for medical expenses only. Deposits are tax-deductible for self-employed individuals who are able to draw on the accounts for medical expenses.
IV. Group Health Plan Requirements: Identifies how group health care plans must plan for portability, access, and transferability of health insurance for its members.
V. Revenue Offsets: Details how HIPAA changed the Internal Revenue Code to generate more revenue for HIPAA expenses.
VI. General Provisions: Explains how coordination with Medicare-type plans must be carried out to prevent duplication of coverage.
VII. Assuring Portability: Ensures employee coverage from one plan to another; written specifically for health insurance plans to ensure portability of coverage.

As of April 14, 2004, all covered health care entities were to have been in compliance of HIPAA's regulations. Each time a newly formed agency with regulations to practice appears, there is concern about how to comply and what costs will be involved. However, once the electronic codes and transactions for electronic filing of health insurance claims have been identified and put in place, the required security and privacy of all patient information is not as complex. If medical facilities and physician practices have been consistently diligent about protecting patient confidentiality, complying with HIPAA is not difficult. Many helpful Web sites are available simply by keying in HIPAA and having your favorite search engine identify sites. Look for a site that explains or summarizes this public law. You will see mention of HIPAA throughout this text as identified by the HIPAA icon as shown on the left.

CONTRACT LAW

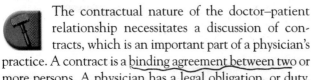

The contractual nature of the doctor–patient relationship necessitates a discussion of contracts, which is an important part of a physician's practice. A contract is a binding agreement between two or more persons. A physician has a legal obligation, or duty, to care for a patient under the principles of contract law. The agreement must be between competent persons to do or not to do something lawful in exchange for a payment.

A contract exists when the patient arrives for treatment and the physician accepts the patient by providing treatment. An example of a valid contract occurs when a patient calls the office or clinic to make an appointment for an annual physical examination. Assuming both physician and patient are competent, and that the physician performs the lawful act of the physical examination and the patient pays a fee, all aspects of the contract exist.

There are two types of contracts: expressed and implied. An **expressed contract** can be written or verbal and will specifically describe what each party in the contract will do. A written contract requires that all necessary aspects of the agreement be in writing. An **implied contract** is indicated by actions rather than by words. The majority of physician–patient contracts are implied contracts. It is not required that the contract be written to be enforceable as long as all points of the contract exist. An implied contract can exist either by the circumstances of the situation or by the law. When a patient reports a sore throat and the physician does a throat culture to diagnose and treat the ailment, an implied contract exists by the circumstances. An implied contract by law exists when a patient goes into anaphylactic shock and the physician administers epinephrine to counteract shock symptoms. The law says that the physician did what the patient would have requested had there been an expressed contract.

For a contract to be valid and binding, the parties who enter into it must be competent; therefore, the mentally incompetent, the legally insane, individuals under heavy drug or alcohol influences, infants, and some minors cannot enter into a binding contract.

Medical assistants are considered **agents** of the physicians they serve, and as such must be cautious that their actions and words may become binding for their physicians. For example, to say that the doctor can cure the patient may cause serious legal problems when, in fact, a cure may not be possible.

Termination of Contracts

A broken contract or breach of contract occurs when one of the parties does not meet contractual obligations. A physician is legally bound to treat a patient until:

- The patient discharges the physician
- The physician formally withdraws from patient care
- The patient no longer needs treatment and is formally discharged by the physician

Patient Discharges Physician. When the patient discharges the physician, the physician should send a letter to the patient to confirm and document the termination of the contract. The notice should be sent by certified mail with return receipt requested. Keep a copy of the letter in the patient's record (Figure 7-1).

LEWIS & KING, MD
2501 CENTER STREET
NORTHBOROUGH, OH 12345

January 6, 20XX

CERTIFIED MAIL

Jim Marshal
76 Georgia Avenue
Millerton, TX 43912

Dear Mr. Marshal:

This will confirm our telephone conversation today in which you discharged me as your attending physician in your present illness. In my opinion your condition requires continued medical supervision by a physician. If you have not already done so, I suggest that you employ another physician without delay.

You may be assured that after receiving a written request from you, I will furnish the physician of your choice with information regarding the diagnosis and treatment which you have received from me.

Very truly yours,

Winston Lewis

Winston Lewis, MD
WL:ea

Figure 7-1 Letter confirms physician's discharge by the patient.

Inner City Health Care
222 S. First Avenue
Carlton, MI 11666

May 9, 20XX

CERTIFIED MAIL

Lenny Taylor
260 Second Street
Carlton, MI 11666

Dear Mr. Taylor:

You will recall that we discussed our physician-patient relationship in my office on May 6, 20XX.

Your son, George Taylor, and Bruce Goldman, my medical assistant were also present. As you know, the primary difficulty has been your failure to cooperate with the medical plan for your care.

While it is unfortunate that our relationship has reached this stage, I will no longer be able to serve as your physician. I will be available to you on an emergency basis only until June 10, 20XX. Meanwhile, you should immediately call or write the Medical Society, 123 Omega Drive, Carlton, MI 11666, Tel. 123-456-7899 and obtain a list of gerontologists. Any delay could jeopardize your health, so please act quickly.

Your physical (and/or mental) problems include: hypertensive heart disease, decreased kidney function, and arteriosclerosis. You could have additional medical problems that may also require professional care. Once you have found a new physician have him or her call my office. I will be happy to discuss your case with the physician assuming your care, and will transfer a written summary of your case to them upon the receipt of a written request from you to do so.

Thank you for your anticipated cooperation and courtesy.

Very truly yours,

James Whitney

James Whitney, MD
JW:kr

Figure 7-2 Letter reiterates "for the record" the physician's decision to withdraw from the case discussed during a previous meeting with patient.

Physician Formally Withdraws from the Case. To avoid any charges of abandonment, the physician should formally withdraw from the case when, for example, the patient becomes **noncompliant** or the physician feels the patient can no longer be served. Again, notice should be sent to the patient by certified mail with return receipt requested and a copy of the notice should be filed in the patient's record (Figures 7-2 and 7-3).

Inner City Health Care
222 S. First Avenue
Carlton, MI 11666

December 5, 20XX

CERTIFIED MAIL

Rhoda Au
41 Academy Road
Carlton, MI 11666

Dear Ms. Au:

I find it necessary to inform you that I am withdrawing further professional medical service to you because of your persistent refusal to follow my medical advice and treatment.

Since your condition requires medical attention, I suggest that you place yourself under the care of another physician without delay. If you so desire, I shall be available to attend you for a reasonable time after you have received this letter, but in no event later than January 7, 20XX. This should give you sufficient time to select a physician from the many competent practitioners in this area.

You may be assured that, upon receiving your written request, I will make available to the physician of your choice your case history and information regarding the diagnosis and treatment which you have received from me.

Very truly yours,

Mark Woo

Mark Woo, MD
MW:kr

Figure 7-3 Letter notifies patient of physician's withdrawal as attending physician.

The Patient No Longer Needs Treatment. Unless a formal discharge or withdrawal has occurred, a physician is obligated to care for a patient until the patient's condition no longer requires treatment.

TORT LAW

A **tort** is a wrongful act, other than a breach of contract, resulting in injury to one person by another.

Medical Practice Acts

Each state has medical practice acts that regulate the practice of medicine with the intent of protecting its citizens from harm. These statutes govern licensure, standards of care, professional liability and negligence, confidentiality, and torts. Medical assistants sometimes are asked to maintain their employer's records of continuing education for license renewal and to process the renewal at the proper time. In some states, the renewal may be done on-line if the license is active and in good standing.

States also may regulate personnel who are employed in the ambulatory care setting. Generally, medical assistants perform their duties and responsibilities under the direct supervision of the physician or doctor, and therefore are governed by Medical Practice Acts or the Board of Medical Examiners. Medical assistants employed and supervised by independent nurse practitioners are governed by the Nurse Practice Act and the Board of Nursing. Also, some states require that medical assistants be licensed or certified to perform any invasive procedures. Other states require additional training in radiology for the medical assistant to be able to take radiographs. Furthermore, some states are so strict in their regulations that medical assistants mostly perform clerical functions and noninvasive clinical duties.

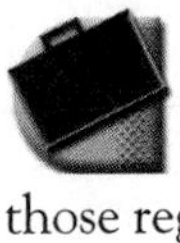

Certainly, medical assistants desiring to use their skills must be aware of state regulations and always perform only within the scope of those regulations. Medical assistants should be as diligent about maintaining their certification, registration, and licensure as physicians and doctors and should monitor any legislation that pertains to licensure or certification.

Standard of Care

To better understand torts, we must consider the standard of care and the four Ds of negligence. Physicians, medical assistants, and all health care providers have the responsibility and duty to perform within their scope of training and to always do what any reasonable and prudent health care professional in the same specialty or general field of practice would do. That is what is expected of every physician when a contact is made by a patient. Failure to do what any reasonable and prudent health care professional would do in the same set of circumstances can be seen as a breach of the standard of care.

Negligence is defined as the failure to exercise the standard of care that a reasonable person would exercise in similar circumstances. Negligence occurs when someone experiences injury because of another's failure to live up to a required duty of care. This is a primary cause of malpractice suits. **Malpractice** is professional negligence.

Four Ds of Negligence. The four elements of negligence, sometimes called the 4 Ds, are:

1. Duty: duty of care
2. Derelict: breach of the duty of care
3. Direct cause: a legally recognizable injury occurs as a result of the breach of duty of care
4. Damage: wrongful activity must have caused the injury or harm that occurred

If an individual has knowledge, skill, or intelligence superior to that of a layperson, that individual's conduct must be consistent with that status. Medical assistants are held to a high standard of care by virtue of their skills, knowledge, and intelligence. As professionals, medical assistants are required to have a standard minimum level of special knowledge and ability. This is what is known as duty of care.

The Medical Assistant's Role in Negligence. Medical assistants may commit a tort that may result in **litigation.** If it can be proven that the injury resulted from the medical assistant (or other health care professional) not meeting the standard of care governing their respective professions, then litigation is a possibility. If, however, the medical assistant (or other health care professional) commits a wrongful act but the patient experiences no injury or harm, then no tort exists. If, for example, the medical assistant changes a wound dressing, breaks sterile technique, and the patient suffers a severely infected wound, the medical assistant has committed a tort and can be held liable, and legal action can be taken. In contrast, if the medical assistant changes a wound dressing, breaks sterile technique, and the patient's wound does not become infected, no harm has occurred, and a tort does not exist. If a medical assistant fails to report to the physician an abnormal result on a blood test that causes the physician to fail to make an early diagnosis of a disease, the assistant's omission of an act has caused a breach in the standard of care.

There are two major classifications of torts: intentional and negligent. Intentional torts are deliberate acts of violation of another's rights. Negligent torts are not deliberate and are the result of omission and commission of an act. Malpractice is the unintentional tort of professional negligence; that is, a professional either failed to act in a reasonable and prudent manner and caused harm to the patient or did what a reasonable and prudent person would not have done and caused harm to a patient.

There are two Latin terms that can be used to describe aspects of negligence. These are known as **doctrines.** *Res ipsa loquitur*, or "the thing speaks for itself," is the term used in cases that involve situations such as a nick made in the bladder when the surgeon is performing a hysterectomy. The negligence is obvious. The other doctrine, *respondeat superior*, "let the master answer," expresses that physicians are responsible for their employees' actions. If a medical assistant violates the standard of care, therein lies the basis for a suit of medical malpractice. For example, the medical assistant used the incorrect solution to clean the patient's wound and the patient sustained injuries to the wound. The physician–employer can be sued under the doctrine of *respondeat superior* because the physician–employer is responsible for the acts of employees committed in the scope of their employment. The medical assistant also can be sued because individuals are responsible for their own actions.

Risk Management

Some common areas of negligence may result in torts when adherence to the standard of care has not been carried out; practicing good **risk management** makes the medical assistant and the physician–employer less vulnerable to litigation.

Following are some ways to avoid incidents that may lead to litigation:

- Perform only within the scope of your training and education.
- Comply with all state and federal regulations and statutes.
- Keep the office or clinic safe and equipment in readiness.
- Never leave a patient unattended; if you must leave, pass the responsibility for the patient's care on to another individual.
- Keep all patient information confidential.
- Follow all policies and procedures established for the office or clinic.
- Document fully only facts; formally document withdrawing from a case and discharging clients.
- Log telephone calls and return calls to clients within a reasonable time frame.
- Follow up on missed or canceled appointments.
- Never guarantee a cure or diagnosis, and never advise treatment without a physician's order.
- Secure informed consent as necessary.
- Do not criticize other practitioners.
- Explain any appointment delays.
- Be particularly watchful with patients who have special needs, such as the elderly, pediatric patients, and those with physical and emotional disabilities.
- Report any error that may have occurred to your physician–employer.

Critical Thinking

Identify the suggestions in the previous column that are most likely not performed if the staff in the ambulatory care setting find themselves overworked, overwhelmed, and behind. What might be done to prevent carelessness brought on by such circumstances?

Some specific examples of common torts that can occur in the office or clinic are battery, defamation of character, and invasion of privacy.

Battery. The basis of the tort of battery is unprivileged touching of one person by another. A patient must consent to being touched. When a procedure is to be performed on a patient, the patient must give consent in full knowledge of all the facts. It does not matter whether the procedure that constitutes the battery improves the patient's health. Patients have the right to withdraw consent at any time.

One example of battery is when a medical assistant insists on giving the patient an injection the physician ordered for the patient even though the patient refuses the injection. Another example can be seen when a physician performs additional surgery beyond the original procedure (the surgeon performed a hysterectomy, for which consent was given, but is liable for battery for removing an abdominal nevus from the patient's abdomen without consent). It does not matter that the physician does not charge for the additional procedure. It also does not matter if the patient would have given consent if asked in advance.

Defamation of Character. The tort of defamation of character consists of injury to another person's reputation, name, or character through spoken or written words for which damages can be recovered. Two kinds of defamation are **libel** and **slander.** Libel is false and malicious writing about another, such as in published materials, pictures, and media. An example can be seen when the medical assistant writes in the patient's record, "Mr. O'Keefe's wife and her negative attitude appear to be the cause of his ulcer." A copy of Mr. O'Keefe's records were later sent to a new physician who reviewed the record and reads the remarks quoted by the medical assistant.

Slander is false and malicious spoken words. Slander can be seen in the following comment directed by a patient toward the physician, "Dr. Woo is incompetent. He should have his license revoked." The statement is overheard by the office receptionist and other patients waiting in the reception area.

For a tort of defamation of character (either libel or slander) to exist, a third party must see or hear the words and understand their meaning.

Invasion of Privacy. Invasion of privacy is another kind of tort. It includes unauthorized publicity of patient information, medical records being released without the patient's knowledge and permission, and patients receiving unwanted publicity and exposure to public view. For example, if a minor unmarried girl has been examined for possible pregnancy, and the medical assistant telephones the girl's home and inadvertently gives the laboratory results to someone other than the patient, her privacy has been invaded. A second situation exists when persons other than those providing care and performing examinations and procedures (essential or nonessential personnel) are allowed to be present without the patient's consent. Yet another example of the patient's right to privacy being violated is when the patient is asked to walk from the examination room across the hall to a treatment room while wearing only a patient gown in full view of other patients and personnel.

Medical assistants and other health care professionals should:

- Close a door, pull a curtain, or provide a screen when looking at, handling, or examining the patient
- Expose only body parts necessary for treatment (drape the patient, exposing only the part that is being treated)
- Discuss patients with no one except those individuals involved in the patient's care, and then discuss only those aspects of care that relate to the needs of the patient

It is not an invasion of privacy to disclose information required by a court order **(subpoena)** or by statute to protect the public health and welfare, as in the reporting of violent crime.

INFORMED CONSENT

Documentation of **informed consent** becomes an important part of the patient care process. Every patient has a right to know and understand any procedure to be performed. The patient is to be told in language easily understood:

1. The nature of any procedure and how it is to be performed
2. Any possible risks involved, as well as expected outcomes of the procedure
3. Any other methods of treatment and those risks
4. Risks if no treatment is given

It is the responsibility of the health care provider to make certain the patient understands. If an interpreter is necessary, the physician must procure one.

Often, consent forms will be signed if there is to be a surgical or invasive procedure performed (Figure 7-4). The medical assistant may be asked to witness the patient's signature and may be expected to follow through on any of the physician's instructions or explanations, but is not expected to explain the procedure to the patient. The signed consent form is kept in the medical chart, and a copy also is given to the patient.

Implied Consent

Two circumstances related to consent are worth mentioning at this point. **Implied consent** occurs when there is a life-threatening emergency, or the patient is unconscious or unable to respond. The physician, by law, is allowed to give treatment without a signed consent. Implied consent also occurs in more subtle ways. The patient who rolls up a shirtsleeve for the medical assistant to take a blood pressure reading is implying consent to the procedure by the action taken.

Consent and Legal Incompetence

Consent for treatment is not valid if the patient is legally incompetent to give consent. Legal **incompetence** means that a patient is found by a court to be insane, inadequate, or to not be an adult. In such instances, consent must be obtained from a parent, a legal guardian, or the court on behalf of the patient. Consent for treatment may be given only by the natural parent or legal guardian as determined by the court for a **minor** child. A minor is a person who has not reached the age of majority (18–21 years old), depending on the laws of each state. Generally, a minor is considered unable to give effective consent for medical treatment; therefore, without proper consent from parents or guardians, medical professionals can be held liable for battery if medical treatment is given. Exceptions to this rule are in cases of emergency and for mature and **emancipated minors.** Emancipated minors are younger than 18 years who are free of parental care and are financially responsible, married, become parents, or join the Armed Forces. **Mature minors** are persons, usually younger than 18 years, who are able to understand and appreciate the nature and consequences of treatment despite their young age. Nearly every state allows minors to give consent for treatment for pregnancy, drug or alcohol addiction, and sexually transmitted disease. Some states have passed legislation that name minors as statutory adults at 14 years old for the purpose of receiving medical care. In these states, minors may consent and

CONSENT TO
OPERATION, ADMINISTRATION OF ANESTHETICS AND
RENDERING OF OTHER MEDICAL SERVICES

1. I hereby authorize and direct Dr. ______________________________, my physician, and whomever he/she designates as his/her assistants (associates and/or resident physicians), to perform upon (state name of patient or myself)______________________________
The following procedures: ______________________________
____
____

If any unforeseen condition arises in the course of this operation for the physician's judgment to perform procedures in addition to or different from those now contemplated, I further request and authorize him/her to do whatever he/she deems advisable and necessary in these circumstances. Such additional services may include, but are not limited to, the administration and maintenance of anesthesia and the performance of services involving pathology and radiology.

2. The following information has been explained to me to the degree that I wish to have it discussed:
   - The nature and character of the proposed treatment or procedure;
   - The anticipated results;
   - Possible recognized alternative methods of treatment, including non-treatment;
   - Recognized serious possible risks, complications, and anticipated benefits involved in proposed and alternative treatments, including non-treatment.

   My questions have been answered to my satisfaction. I acknowledge that no guarantee, warrantee, or assurance has been made as to the results or cure that may be obtained.

3. Federal Regulations (21 CFR Part 821) require manufacturers to track certain medical devices, and assist the U.S. Food and Drug Administration (FDA) with notification to individuals in the event that a certain medical device presents serious health risks. I authorize and agree to the release of my contact information to the manufacturer: ______________________________ for this tracking purpose only. I understand that the manufacturer may notify me, if necessary, of important safety information about my medical device, and may release my information to the FDA if ordered to do so. I understand that this consent is valid for the life of the medical device.

Any sections below that do not apply to the proposed treatment may be crossed out. The patient must initial any section crossed out.

4. I consent to the administration of blood and blood products if deemed medically necessary. I understand that all blood and blood products involve the risk of allergic reaction, fever, hives, and in rare circumstances infectious diseases such as hepatitis and HIV/AIDS. I understand that precautions are taken by the blood bank in screening donors and in matching blood for transfusion to minimize those risks.

5. I hereby consent to the disposal or use for research purposes any tissues, parts, or products of conception, which may be removed.

6. I authorize and agree to the presence of observers during my surgical procedure. These observers may include persons other than the medical staff that are considered appropriate by my health care provider during my care and treatment. The purpose of these individuals observing would be for instruction and medical study.

I certify that I have read this form and understand its contents.

____
PATIENT NAME & ID #

____
Signature of Patient or Legally Responsible Party

____
Relationship to patient, if not signed by patient

____
Signature of Witness

____
Printed Name of Witness

Date______________ Time______________ a.m. / p.m.

MRD: HOSP1
DISTRIBUTION: 1-**WHITE** – CHART 2-**CANARY** – PATIENT COPY

Figure 7-4 Model formal consent for treatment form.

Critical Thinking

Identify problems that may occur in the ambulatory care setting when a minor seeks treatment for drug or alcohol addiction or a sexually transmitted disease, or is determined to be pregnant. What is the role of the medical assistant?

be protected by confidentiality and privacy even though their parents or legal guardians may still be financially responsible for their medical bills.

Questions of ability to give consent related to minors and emancipated minors often must be determined on a case-by-case basis because state statutes vary. Placing a telephone call to the state attorney general's office can help clarify issues, questions, and concerns that involve consent and treatment of minors.

CIVIL LITIGATION PROCESS

Despite all the best efforts of health care professionals and their employees, litigation can occur. Litigation is the process of taking a lawsuit or a criminal case through the courts. It is helpful to understand the steps taken for civil litigation to occur. The greatest amount of any litigation seen in the ambulatory care setting occurs when relationships between individuals break down for one reason or another. When this happens, the party, or plaintiff, bringing the action, usually a patient, seeks an attorney who agrees to bring the complaint to the courts. The physician, or defendant, is summoned to court. This summons or subpoena notifies the physician of the plaintiff's suit and allows the defendant to file an answer with the court.

Subpoenas

A portion of a medical record or the entire medical record may be subpoenaed or the physician and health care provider (*subpoena duces tecum*) may be subpoenaed to testify in court, or both may be subpoenaed. The subpoena is an order from the court naming the specific date, time, and reason to appear. The staff in the ambulatory care setting usually will have ample time to make certain the record is current and complete before its inclusion in court. Out of courtesy, the physician will notify patients whose records have been subpoenaed. If, for any reason, the patient does not want the record released, the physician must call for legal advice on how to respond to the subpoena.

Certain records, because of their sensitive nature, may require more than a subpoena to be released. These include records related to sexually transmitted diseases, including AIDS and HIV testing; mental health records; substance abuse records; and sexual assault records. For the courts to have access to these records, a court order is required in some states.

HIPAA law requires clinics to identify in written policies and procedures what information they will release regarding patients. Before patient information is released, the following must be identified: (1) the purpose or need for the information, (2) the nature or extent of the information to be released, (3) the date of the authorization, and (4) the signature(s) of the person(s) authorized to give consent. Release only what the subpoena or court order specifically requests rather than releasing the entire medical record. Many practitioners keep a patient's consent information in a specific section of the medical record for quick referral and to demonstrate HIPAA compliance.

The care taken with subpoenas and court orders for certain information is to assure patients of confidentiality. The information in the medical record, including the information a patient shared with the physician and medical assistant, is private.

No patient information can be given to another (another physician, patient's attorney, insurance company, federal or state agency) without the expressed written consent of the patient. Care must be exercised at all times to ensure that the patient's right to confidentiality is not breached. For example, information given to unauthorized personnel associated with the physician's or clinic's practice in regard to the patient's condition or financial status regarding payment of bills violates the patient's right to confidentiality. Likewise, when discussing issues over the telephone that can be overheard, such as the patient's account being turned over to a collection agency, the patient's right to confidentiality has been violated.

There are certain disclosures of information about a patient's conditions and suspected illnesses that are required by law. Legally required disclosures are necessary when the public needs to know certain information for its safety and welfare. The disclosures supersede the patient's right to privacy and confidentiality. See "Public Duties" in this chapter.

Discovery

A time of **discovery** follows the subpoenas. This is the time in which both parties are allowed access to all the information and evidence related to the case. Rules of discovery vary from state to state, but may include the following:

1. An **interrogatory** is a written set of questions that can come from either the plaintiff or the defendant

that must be answered, under oath, and within a specific time period.

2. A **deposition** is oral testimony taken with a court reporter present in a location agreed on by both parties. Both attorneys are usually present when depositions are taken.

Medical assistants may be asked to respond to an interrogatory or may be deposed by the plaintiff's attorney. The defendant's attorney will provide specific instructions in both situations. Because both are done under oath, honesty is an absolute. The medical assistant may be asked to refer to certain documents, recall specific information, or identify documentation in a medical record.

Expert Witnesses. Physicians and members of their staff may be called to testify in court to the standard of care. In such a case, they are usually considered **expert witnesses.** An expert witness is one who has enough knowledge and experience in a field to be able to testify to what is the reasonable and expected standard of care. Expert witnesses are expected to tell what they know to be fact and are best counseled to use lay terms rather than complicated medical language. The goal is for jurors and judges to understand the nature of any medical information shared. Visual aids, charts, and computer simulations often are used to illustrate or clarify testimony given by expert witnesses.

Pretrial Conference

A pretrial conference is generally held close to the trial date to decide if there is just cause for the suit, to make certain that both parties are ready, and to determine if there might be an out-of-court settlement. If a trial seems imminent, **alternative dispute resolution (ADR)** may be suggested. **Mediation** allows a neutral facilitator to help the two parties settle their differences and come to an acceptable solution. If no settlement is reached, the case can still look to the court for satisfaction. **Arbitration** allows the neutral party to settle the dispute. This arbitration can be binding or nonbinding. In binding arbitration, both parties agree at the outset to accept the neutral party's decision as final. In nonbinding arbitration, the case can look to the court for settlement. ADR saves money, time, and adverse publicity that can come from a trial.

Trial

A trial can be held before a judge or a judge and a jury. When the trial begins, opening statements outlining the details of the case are made by both sides. The plaintiff's attorney calls witnesses to produce evidence first. This is known as direct examination. In cross examination, the defendant's attorney questions the witness. When the plaintiff's case is finished, the defendant presents the case in the same manner. When all the information has been presented, the case is turned over for judgment.

If the plaintiff's case is successful, the judge or jury may award a specific amount of money or damages. The judge will instruct a jury regarding the kinds of damages that can be considered in that state. A number of states have placed limits on monetary awards in malpractice cases. If the defendant's case is successful, the case is dismissed. After a court decision, the party that has lost the case can begin an appeal process. The appeal requests an opinion from higher courts that reviews cases usually on the basis of a faulty legal process or action.

Figure 7-5 outlines the civil case process.

Statute of Limitations

No discussion of negligence, malpractice, or medical records is complete without a brief statement regarding the statute of limitations that will, in part, determine how long medical records are kept. Generally, all records should be retained until after the statute has run, usually three to six years. Statutes of limitations most commonly begin at the time a negligent act was committed, when the act was discovered, or when the care of the patient and the patient–physician relationship ended. It is easy to understand why many physicians choose to keep their records indefinitely.

State and federal statutes set maximum time periods during which certain actions can be brought or rights enforced; there is a time limit for individuals to initiate legal action. The statute of limitations varies from one jurisdiction to another and a lawsuit may not be brought after the statute of limitations has run. For example, in the Commonwealth of Massachusetts, the statute of limitations for an act of medical malpractice committed on an adult is three years. If harm to a patient resulted from a medical assistant administering the wrong dose of medication to a patient in Massachusetts, a lawsuit must be brought within three years from the time the medication error was made, with the three years commencing at the time the negligent act was committed.

PUBLIC DUTIES

Reportable Diseases/Injuries

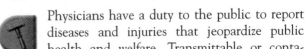

Physicians have a duty to the public to report diseases and injuries that jeopardize public health and welfare. Transmittable or contagious diseases and injuries resulting from knife or gunshot are examples; these must be reported to the appropriate authorities. This is done without the patient's consent

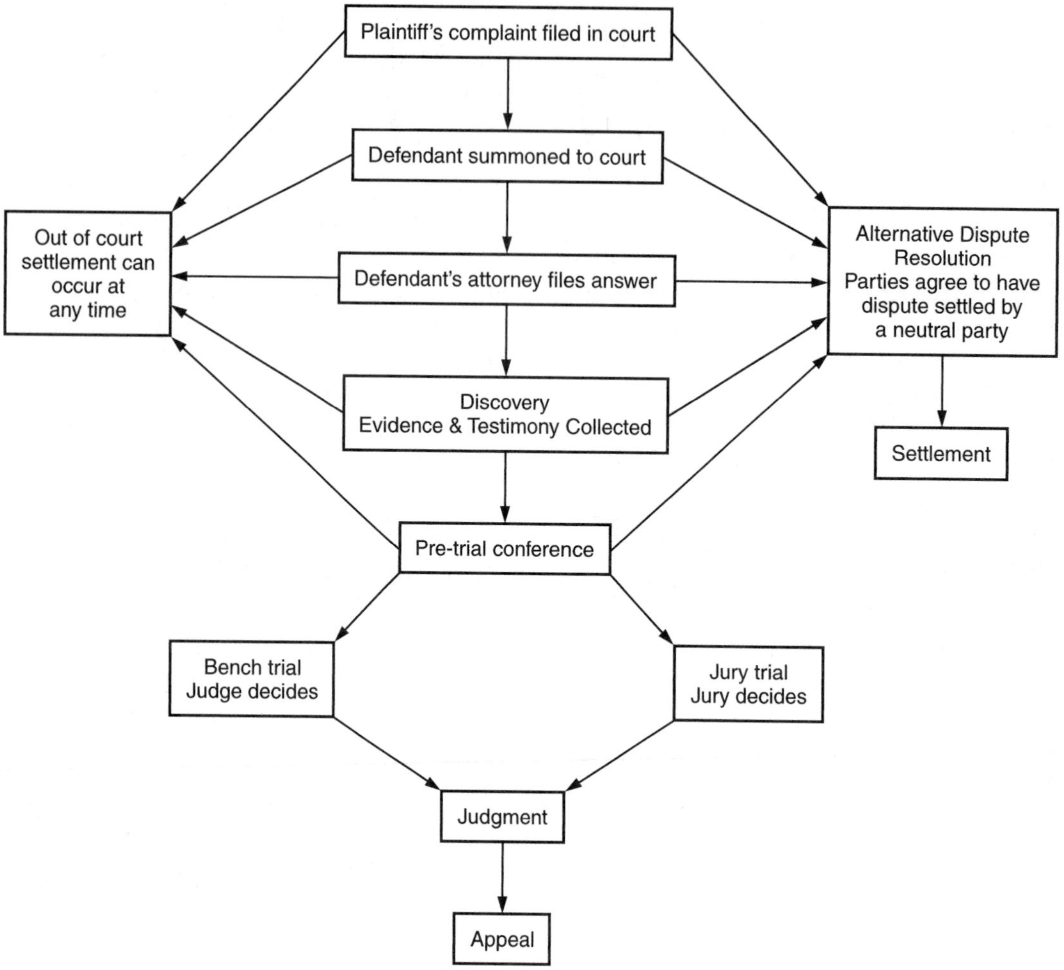

Figure 7-5 Civil litigation process.

because it is required by law. When reporting, it is important to do so properly and according to the laws of the state in which one is employed. Knowledge of which illnesses, injuries, and conditions to report, to whom to report, and the appropriate forms to submit is essential. Copies of all information must be kept for the office or clinic.

Medline Plus, a Web site sponsored by the U.S. National Library of Medicine and the National Institutes of Health, has an excellent site connected to the Medline Encyclopedia identifying guidelines for reportable diseases. Local, state, and national agencies such as the Centers for Disease Control and Prevention require such diseases to be reported when diagnosed by doctors or laboratories. States may vary in the diseases that require reporting, but their lists are likely to include the basic list provided on-line at http://www.nlm.nih.gov. Some diseases require written reports. Others require reporting by telephone; they include rubeola (measles) and pertussis (whooping cough). Still others ask only for the number of cases to be reported. Such reporting is beneficial to society and all health care managers in tracking and preventing illness. The list changes from time to time as new diseases occur and are diagnosed.

Other generally required facts to report include births, deaths, childhood immunizations, rape, and abuse toward a child, elder, or domestic partner.

Some states have laws specific to the release of information relative to mental or psychological treatment, human immunodeficiency virus testing, acquired immune deficiency syndrome diagnosis and treatment, sexually transmitted diseases, and chemical substance abuse.

Local or state health departments can provide lists of diseases and injuries to report and will also provide the appropriate forms.

Abuse

Child abuse, domestic violence, and elder abuse are becoming more common in our society. As a result, patients experiencing such abuse may be seen in the ambulatory care setting. In all cases of abuse, medical records hold valuable information if a court procedure ensues. Careful documentation is critical. State laws are fairly specific in mandates to report child abuse, but laws related to elder abuse and domestic violence are not as detailed. In any case, the rights of victims must be protected.

Child Abuse. The law mandates, or requires, that physicians and health care professionals, teachers, social workers, and certain others who suspect child abuse report the incident to the proper authorities. Confidentiality in the physician–patient relationship does not exist when children are abused. If a person has a reason to suspect abuse and reports the abuse to the police, and in the case of child abuse to the child protective agency, this individual is protected against liability as a result of making the report. Failure to report could result in criminal or civil penalties. Usually, the Child Protective Unit of the State Department of Social Services is called to investigate suspected cases of child abuse. Some injuries that are commonly seen in child abuse are bruises, welts, burns, fractures, and head injuries. Evidence of neglect or intimidation also may be seen.

If a suspicion of abuse exists, the physician and health care professional should:

- Treat the child's injuries
- Send the child to the hospital for further treatment when necessary
- Inform parents of the diagnosis and that it will be reported to the police and social services agency
- Notify the child protective agency (keep phone number posted)
- Document all information
- Provide court testimony if requested

Elder Abuse. Elder abuse may consist of neglect, physical abuse, punishment, physical restraint, or abandonment. Examples are seen when elders are overmedicated or undermedicated, physically restrained, intimidated by shouting or profanity, sexually abused, neglected or abandoned, or in any other way have their rights and dignity violated. The person reporting the abuse is generally a health care professional, and the reporting agency is most likely one of a social service or welfare nature.

Domestic Violence. Incidents of spousal abuse have escalated since the 1970s. The battered women's syndrome is a significant problem. The violence of it is a criminal act, and failure to report it may be considered a misdemeanor in some states. Victims of domestic violence should be treated as soon as possible after the assault so as to preserve evidence for legal purposes. In the United States, domestic violence is a crime. Domestic violence, however, is considered acceptable behavior in many cultures, even in the United States. Some cultures believe the woman is chattel, or property, of her spouse, that she has no rights or authority, and that she must submit to her husband's, brother's, or father's demands. A woman who manages to come to the ambulatory care setting with signs of domestic violence is courageous. She probably is extremely frightened also, because she knows that reporting the violence puts her at increased risk for continued violence, and even death in some instances. Make certain there are community resources readily available for these women, even if they choose to stay in the abusive situation. In many cases, the abused patient's options are so few that leaving is more frightening than staying in the abusive relationship. Do not pass judgment on these women; they desperately need your understanding and your compassion. Your understanding and compassion is perhaps the only door through which they might feel comfortable enough to enter to leave the abusive relationship.

Good Samaritan Laws

Most states have laws regarding the rendering of first aid by health care professionals at the scene of an accident or sudden injury. Good Samaritan laws, although not always clearly written, encourage physicians and health care professionals to provide medical care within the scope of their training without fear of being sued for negligence. In an emergency situation, medical assistants cannot be held liable should an injury result from some form of first aid rendered or from first aid they omitted to render as long as they acted in a reasonable way within the scope of their knowledge. Medical assistants and other health care professionals with skills in cardiopulmonary resuscitation (CPR) who are present when CPR is needed must perform the procedure on the victim or otherwise could be declared negligent. Emergencies that arise in the ambulatory care setting generally are not covered by Good Samaritan laws.

PHYSICIAN'S DIRECTIVES

Medical assistants in the ambulatory care setting will be asked to attach physician's directives or living wills to patients' charts (Figure 7-6). These directives are legal documents in which patients indicate their wishes in the case of a life-threatening

Washington
Health Care Directive

Directive made this____________day of ________________________, ______________.
(date) *(month)* *(year)*

I, ____,
(name)

having the capacity to make health care decisions, willfully and voluntarily make known my desire that my dying shall not be artificially prolonged under the circumstances set forth below, and do hereby declare that:

(a) If at any time I should be diagnosed in writing to be in a terminal condition by the attending physician, or in a permanent unconscious condition by two physicians, and where the application of life-sustaining treatment would serve only to artificially prolong the process of my d… I direct that such treatment be withheld or withdrawn, and that I be
permitted to die naturally. I understand by usi … ble and irreversible
condition caused by injury, disease, or illness … death within a
reasonable period in accordance with accept … -sustaining treatment
would serve only to prolong the process of dy … anent unconscious
condition means an incurable and irreversible … asonable medical
judgment as having no reasonable probabilit … vegetative state.

(b) In the absence of my ability to give … atment, it is my
intention that this directive shall be honored … f my legal right to
refuse medical or surgical treatment and I ac … son is appointed to
make these decisions for me, whether throu … that the person be
guided by this directive and any other clear e …

(c) If I am diagnosed to be in a termin … check one):

- ❑ I DO want to have artificially provid …
- ❑ I DO NOT want to have artificially …

(d) If I have been diagnosed as pregn … irective shall have no
force or effect during the course of my pregr …

(e) I understand the full import of this … make the health care
decisions contained in this directive.

(f) I understand that before I sign this … ge the wording of this
directive and that I may add to or delete fro … be consistent with
Washington State law or federal constitutional law to be legally valid.

(g) It is my wish that every part of this directive be fully implemented. If for any reason any part is held invalid, it is my wish that the remainder of my directive be implemented.

(h) I make the folllowing additional instructions regarding my care:

Signed:____

City, County, and State of Residence:____________________________

____

The declarer has been personally known to me and I believe him or her to be capable of making health care decisions.

Witness:____

Witness:____

Figure 7-6 Health Care Directive (Washington State sample). Compassion & Choices Federation makes legally recognized documents available for interested persons. (Reprinted by permission of Compassion & Choices Federation, 6312 SW Capitol Hwy., #415, Portland, OR 97239.)

illness or serious injury. Such documents should always accompany the patients to the hospital for any treatment or care. They may be updated from time to time, and the patient can ask to rescind such a document at any time. Medical assistants must remember that these documents reflect the choices of their patients and are to be respected as such.

Living Wills

Living wills are necessary because advances in medicine allow medical professionals to sustain life even if the individual will not recover from a persistent vegetative state. Persons who prefer not to remain in that state can use the living will to make decisions about life support and direct others to implement their wishes in that regard. The living will allows individuals to indicate to family and health care professionals whether life-prolonging medical or surgical procedures are to be continued, withheld, or withdrawn, and if artificial feeding and fluids are to be used or withheld. The living will allows individuals to make this decision before incapacitation.

To be valid, the proper and particular form, different in each state, must be used, and it must be lawfully executed. States vary in the number of witnesses required and whether a Notary Public is required for those signatures. The form goes into effect when provided to a patient's health care provider *and* when the patient is no longer capable of making health care decisions. Examples of incapacity may include permanent unconsciousness, life-threatening illness in the latter stages, or inability to communicate. The U.S. Legal Forms Web site (http://USlegalforms.com) has samples of living wills for all 50 states and the District of Columbia under the heading "Living Will Forms."

Durable Power of Attorney for Health Care

Another document seen in the ambulatory care setting is the **durable power of attorney for health care** or Designation of Health Care Surrogate (Figure 7-7). This document allows a patient to name another person as the official spokesperson for the patient should the patient be unable to make health care decisions. The documents may allow another person to manage finances and personal matters (durable power of attorney) or just to make medical decisions.

Every state has different versions of the physician's directive. The American Bar Association has a section on their Web site (www.abanet.org) on "Law for Older Americans" and "Health Care Advance Directives" that is useful in answering many questions. Also, the Web site for the Compassion in Dying Federation (http://www.compassionindying.org; located in Portland, OR) is quite helpful. Individuals wishing to have their choices known should they suffer from severe dementia may execute a document similar to the sample in Figure 7-8. The "Alzheimer's Provision" may be included in the Living Will document as well.

In 1991, the federal government passed the **Patient Self-Determination Act (PSDA),** which applies to all health care institutions receiving payments from Medicare and Medicaid. PSDA requires that all adults receiving health care from these institutions be given the opportunity to provide information about their wishes in an advanced directive.

Copies of advance directives are to be provided to patients' physicians so they can be transferred to a hospital or nursing facility as necessary. Any named agent should have a copy, and family members also may have a copy.

Patient Education

Because of increased awareness of confidentiality as a result of HIPAA, medical assistants can be helpful by suggesting that any family member(s) who might be involved and need to know about the patient's care be indicated in the patient's chart with a signed release from the patient. There have been examples recently of adult children of elder adults who were either not informed when their ailing parent was taken to emergency services in another state, or were unable to get any information about their parent from a hospital or physician even though a durable power of attorney for health care was in place. If that directive does not go with the patient, no information can be given. For that reason, it is suggested that patients may want to keep a wallet card containing a notice of the advance directive, any appointed agent named, and any family member(s) who is allowed information.

Washington Durable Power of Attorney for Health Care

I understand that my wishes as expressed in my living will may not cover all possible aspects of my care if I become incapacitated. Consequently, there may be a need for someone to accept or refuse medical intervention on my behalf, in consultation with my physician. Therefore,

I, ____,
as principal, designate and appoint the person(s) listed below as my attorney-in-fact for health care decisions.

First Choice: Name: ______________________________

Address: ______________________________

City/State/Zip Code: ______________________________

____

Telephone Number: ______________________________

If the above person is unable, unavailable, or unwilling to serve, I designate:

Second Choice: Name: ______________________________

Address: ______________________________

City/State/Zip Code: ______________________________

____

Telephone Number: ______________________________

1. This Power of Attorney shall take effect upon my incapacity to make my own health care decisions, as determined by my treating physician and one other physician, and shall continue as long as the incapacity lasts or until I revoke it, whichever happens first.

2. The powers of my attorney-in-fact under this Power of Attorney are limited to making decisions about my health care on my behalf. These powers shall include the power to order the withholding or withdrawal of life-sustaining treatment if my attorney-in-fact believes, in his or her own judgment, that is what I would want if I could make the decision myself. The existence of this Durable Power of Attorney for Health Care shall have no effect upon the validity of any other Power of Attorney for other purposes that I have executed or may execute in the future.

3. In the event that a proceeding is initiated to appoint a guardian of my person under RCW 11.88, I nominate the person designated as my first choice (on page 1) to serve as my guardian. My second choice (on page 1) will serve as my guardian if the first person is unable or unwilling.

4. I make the following additional instructions regarding my care:

By signing this document, I indicate that I understand the purpose and effect of this Durable Power of Attorney for Health Care.

Dated this ______________ day of ______________________, 20________.
(date) *(month)* *(year)*

Signed: ______________________________

The person named as principal in this document is personally known to me. I believe that he/she is of sound mind, and that he/she signed this document freely and voluntarily.

Witness: ______________________________

Witness: ______________________________

Figure 7-7 Durable Power of Attorney for Health Care (Washington State sample). (Reprinted by permission of Compassion & Choices Federation, 6312 SW Capitol Hwy., #415, Portland, OR 97239.)

The "Alzheimer's Provision"

Most advance directives become operative only when a person is unable to make health care decisions and is either "permanently unconscious" or "terminally ill." There is usually no provision that applies to the situation in which a person suffers from severe dementia but is neither unconscious nor dying.

The following language can be added to any Living Will. There it will serve to advise physicians and family of the wishes of a patient with Alzheimer's disease or other forms of dementia.

> **If I am unconscious and it is very unlikely that I will ever become conscious again, I would like my wishes regarding specific life-sustaining treatments, as indicated on the attached document entitled "My Particular Wishes," to be followed.**
>
> **If I remain conscious but have a progressive illness that will be fatal and the illness is in an advanced stage, and I am consistently and permanently unable to communicate, swallow food and water safely, care for myself and recognize my family and other people, and it is very unlikely that my condition will substantially improve, I would like my wishes regarding specific life-sustaining treatments, as indicated on the attached document entitled "My Particular Wishes," to be followed.**
>
> **If I am unable to feed myself while in this condition, I do/do not (circle one) want to be fed.**

I hereby incorporate this provision into my durable power of attorney for health care, living will, and any other previously executed advance directive for health care decisions.

____________________________________ ____________

Signature Date

Figure 7-8 Compassion & Choices "Alzheimer's Provision" applies to the situation when a person has severe dementia but is neither unconscious nor dying. (Reprinted by permission of Compassion & Choices Federation, 6312 SW Capitol Hwy., #415, Portland, OR 97239.)

Case Study 7-1

Three weeks ago, Dr. King treated a new patient, Boris Bolski, for lower back pain, which the patient believed was the result of consistent heavy lifting at his job. Medical assistant Joe Guerrero assisted Dr. King during the examination and, today, both Joe and Dr. King were served with subpoenas by Mr. Bolski's attorney. Mr. Bolski is alleging that unsafe conditions at his workplace caused severe strain on his back, and he is suing his employer for damages. Dr. King and Joe Guerrero were called as expert witnesses to a civil hearing; Joe, especially, is a bit nervous about this, because he has never been on the witness stand in court and is not sure what is expected of him.

CASE STUDY REVIEW

1. How will Mr. Bolski's medical record help Joe answer questions at the hearing?
2. What information should Joe gather to be prepared to testify?
3. As an expert witness, what is Joe expected to communicate to the judge in this case?

Case Study 7-2

Wanda Hanson is working on a part-time basis in Hudson, Florida as an administrative medical assistant on the phone desk in the Emergency Department at Hudson Community Hospital when a frantic long-distance call is received. The caller is Larry Nelson from Cheyenne, Wyoming. He received a call from the nursing home where his 95-year-old mother was living informing him that she was taken by ambulance to your hospital. Larry wants to know if Muriel Nelson has arrived and what her condition is. You are aware of a patient's right to privacy, confidentiality, and the new HIPAA regulations. You observed Mrs. Nelson arrive at the emergency department quite incoherent and confused.

CASE STUDY REVIEW

1. What can Wanda tell Mr. Nelson, especially after noting that no records were with the elderly Mrs. Nelson when she arrived at the hospital?
2. What information would Wanda need from Mr. Nelson before complying to his request?
3. How can Wanda put Mr. Nelson at ease? What can Wanda do to help?

SUMMARY

Changing societal values have contributed to an increase of lawsuits in medical practice. Patients are more aware than ever of their rights, especially those of confidentiality and the right to privacy, consent, and records ownership. They are likely to seek redress when they perceive their rights have been violated.

A healthy relationship between physicians and patients and between medical assistants and patients, as well as respect for the patient's rights, reduces the likelihood of a lawsuit.

Additional knowledge of the laws that regulate medical and business practices in your state is necessary to be in compliance. Sources of information regarding state and federal laws can be obtained from the state medical society, the physician's liability insurance company, the state medical assistant society, the state attorney general's office, the Internet, or the public library.

STUDY FOR SUCCESS

To reinforce your knowledge and skills of information presented in this chapter:

- ❑ Review the Key Terms
- ❑ Consider the Case Studies and discuss your conclusions
- ❑ Answer the Review Questions
  - ❑ Multiple Choice
  - ❑ Critical Thinking
- ❑ Navigate the Internet and complete the Web Activities
- ❑ Practice the StudyWARE activities on the textbook CD
- ❑ Apply your knowledge in the Student Workbook activities
- ❑ Complete the Web Tutor sections
- ❑ View and discuss the DVD situations

REVIEW QUESTIONS

Multiple Choice

1. The type of contract that most often exists between physician and patient is:
   a. expressed
   b. implied
   c. privileged
   d. civil
2. The administrative law act that prohibits discrimination, has five sections, and is enforced by the EEOC is called the:
   a. Controlled Substances Act
   b. Federal Age Discrimination Act
   c. Americans with Disabilities Act
   d. Health Insurance Portability and Accountability Act
3. Slander is defamation through:
   a. spoken statements that damage an individual's reputation
   b. written statements that damage a person's reputation
   c. written falsehoods about an individual
   d. a, b, and c
4. Occasionally, a physician will be sued for the negligence of an employee, even though the physician is not guilty of any negligent act. This is done on the basis of the doctrine of:
   a. *res ipsa loquitur*
   b. *respondeat superior*
   c. proximate cause
   d. contract law
5. The standard of care expected of a physician is held by the courts to mean:
   a. on a par with all other physicians engaged in the same medical specialty anywhere
   b. reasonable, attentive, diligent care comparable with other physicians of the same specialty in the same or similar community
   c. the best possible under the circumstances
   d. the same as the national norm
6. Physician's directives:
   a. allow patients to direct how their billing is to be handled
   b. are designed to encourage physicians to render first aid in an emergency
   c. direct physicians based on a patient's wishes in life-threatening circumstances
   d. are not considered legal documents
7. A subpoena:
   a. is a court order requesting data, an appearance in court, or both
   b. is sufficient to enforce a release of any type medical record or information
   c. may be ignored without consequences
   d. allows the person being served to select a specific date or time to appear
8. The 4 Ds of negligence are:
   a. duty, danger, damage, and disaster
   b. derelict, direct cause, damage, and danger
   c. danger, direct cause, damage, disaster
   d. duty, derelict, direct cause, damage
9. Emancipated minors:
   a. are considered adults and can consent to treatment
   b. live on their own and are self-supporting
   c. may be married or serve in the military
   d. all of the above
   e. only b and c
10. Torts:
    a. include battery, defamation of character, invasion of privacy
    b. are always intentional in nature
    c. do not require that harm has occurred
    d. do not include malpractice

Critical Thinking

1. Chris is a 6-year-old girl who Dr. King treated for a broken leg. Chris' parents fail to follow Dr. King's treatment plan for Chris. What, if any, action can Dr. King take? What is the legal term for this situation?
2. Marijuana is presently listed as a Schedule I controlled substance and is identified by the DEA as having "no accepted medical use in the United States." As of May, 2005, eleven states have passed legislation allowing patients to use marijuana to alleviate pain, nausea, and other symptoms without fear of prosecution. Discuss the issue of the state's power overriding the federal administrative law. Can you recall what other legal battle recently occurred between the federal and state jurisdictions that involved the U.S. Attorney General in physician-assisted suicide? How was that issue resolved?
3. Jaime arrived in the clinic having sustained a serious laceration at his construction site. Dr. Woo ordered Demerol R 100 mg. 1.m - stat, which Wanda, the medical assistant, administers. Dr. Woo determines surgery is required. Should a consent form be prepared? If so, by whom, and what should be included?
4. Do you have a living will or a physician's directive? Why or why not? Identify to a family member or a loved one what your wishes might be if you were seriously injured in an accident and were still in what appears to be an irreversible coma after 10 months.
5. Discuss the medical assistant's obligations in regard to public duties.
6. What is the Good Samaritan law? What must a medical assistant and any other health care

professional remember when giving first aid at the scene of an accident?

7. Describe three types of abuse. Tell what your role as a medical assistant is when Juanita brings her 3-year-old son Henry to the clinic. Henry has bruises on his face and chest and appears quite frightened when you approach him. While you prepare Henry for the pediatrician's examination, Juanita's answers to your questions seem evasive.

WEB ACTIVITIES

1. Research the American Bar Association Web site (http://www.abanet.org). How often should an advance directive be renewed or reviewed, or is such renewal necessary? Is an advance directive valid when you cross state lines?
2. Using the Internet, determine if or when a medical clinic might be required to follow the federal guidelines of the Family and Medical Leave Act (FMLA). Identify reasons to follow the FMLA guidelines.
3. Using your favorite search engine, key in the words "Medical Malpractice Awards." A number of sites will appear. Has a national limit been set on malpractice awards? What makes this topic a political one? Identify those who favor malpractice award limits and also those who oppose these limits.
4. Research the World Wide Web for the statute of limitations related to claims injuries. What is the time span in your state?

THE DVD HOOK-UP

DVD Series: **Critical Thinking** | Program Number: **3**

Chapter/Scene Reference
- *Licensing and Scope of Practice*
- *Regulating Agencies OSHA, DEA, and CMS*

This chapter deals with legal considerations that must be adhered to when working in the medical industry. One of the most important legal responsibilities that you have as a medical assistant is to stay within the boundaries of your scope and training as a medical assistant.

In one of the scenes listed above, Barb, the office manager, reprimands Eileen for administering a Demerol injection. Eileen states that the doctor ordered her to give the injection, which is why she gave it. The office manager tells Eileen that medical assistants are not allowed to give controlled substances in that particular state. Eileen replies that she didn't know she could not give controlled substances, and that she gave controlled substances in the last office that she worked. Barb reminds Eileen that the information was posted in the office's procedures manual that she was suppose to have read at the time of orientation. Barb told Eileen that she had no other choice but to document this error in her personal record.

1. Why did Barb take such a hard approach with Eileen? What steps does Barb need to take in the future? What responsibility does the doctor have?
2. How could Eileen have avoided this awkward situation?
3. What will you do if a physician orders you to perform a procedure that medical assistants are not allowed to perform?

DVD Journal Summary

Write a paragraph that summarizes what you learned from watching the designated scenes from today's DVD program. What steps will you take to make certain that you know what medical assistants can and cannot do in the state in which you practice?

REFERENCES/BIBLIOGRAPHY

American Bar Association. Health Care Advance Directives. Retrieved from http://www.abanet.org. (Public Documents). Accessed April 4, 2005.

American Bar Association. Law for older Americans. Retrieved from http://www.abanet.org. Accessed April 4, 2005.

Balasa, D. A. (May/June 2004). Legal environment differs under independent nurse practitioners. *CMA TODAY,* Vol. 37, Issue 3, 24–25.

Compassion & Choices. The Alzheimer's Provision. Retrieved from http://compassionindying.org. Accessed May 23, 2005.

Compassion & Choices. Washington Durable Power of Attorney for Health Care. Retrieved from http://compassionindying.org. Accessed May 23, 2005.

Flight, M. (2004). *Law, liability and ethics for medical office professionals* (4th ed.). Clifton Park, NY: Thomson Delmar Learning.

Krager, D., & Krager, C. (2005). *HIPAA for medical office personnel.* Clifton Park, NY: Thomson Delmar Learning.

Lewis, M. A., & Tamparo, C. D. (2002). *Medical law, ethics, and bioethics for ambulatory care* (5th ed.). Philadelphia: F. A. Davis.

CHAPTER 8

Ethical Considerations

OUTLINE

Ethics
- Principle-Centered Leadership
- Five Ps of Ethical Power
- Ethics Check Questions

Bioethics

Keys to the AAMA Code of Ethics

Ethical Guidelines for Doctors
- Advertising
- Confidentiality
- Medical Records
- Professional Fees and Charges
- Professional Rights and Responsibilities
- Abuse

Bioethical Dilemmas
- Allocation of Scarce Medical Resources
- Abortion and Fetal Tissue Research
- Genetic Engineering/ Manipulation
- Artificial Insemination/ Surrogacy
- Dying and Death
- HIV and AIDS

OBJECTIVES

The student should strive to meet the following performance objectives and demonstrate an understanding of the facts and principles presented in this chapter through written and oral communication.

1. Define the key terms as presented in the glossary.
2. Identify two reasons for Codes of Ethics.
3. Discuss the eight characteristics of principle-centered leadership.
4. Describe the five Ps of ethical power.
5. Recall the ethics check questions.
6. Relate the five principles of the AAMA code to patient care in the ambulatory care setting.
7. Discuss the ethical guidelines for doctors, giving at least four examples.
8. Restate the dilemmas encountered by the following bioethical issues: (a) allocation of scarce medical resources; (b) abortion and fetal tissue research; (c) genetic engineering/manipulation; (d) artificial insemination/surrogacy; (e) dying and death; (f) HIV and AIDS.

KEY TERMS

Bioethics
Cryopreservation
Ethics
Genetic Engineering
Macroallocation
Microallocation
Surrogate

FEATURED COMPETENCIES

CAAHEP—ENTRY-LEVEL COMPETENCIES

Communications

- Recognize and respond to verbal communications
- Recognize and respond to nonverbal communications

Legal Concepts

- Identify and respond to issues of confidentiality
- Perform within legal and ethical boundaries
- Document appropriately
- Demonstrate knowledge of federal and state health care legislation and regulations

ABHES—ENTRY-LEVEL COMPETENCIES

Professionalism

- Project a positive attitude
- Maintain confidentiality at all times
- Be a "team player"
- Be cognizant of ethical boundaries
- Evidence a responsible attitude
- Be courteous and diplomatic
- Conduct work within scope of education, training, and ability

Communication

- Be impartial and show empathy when dealing with patients
- Serve as liaison between physician and others
- Recognize and respond to verbal and nonverbal communication

(continues)

SCENARIO

On occasion, ethical dilemmas occur because patients are unsure of the role of the medical assistant. For example, the medical assistants of Inner City Health Care are truly multidisciplinary and have a range of administrative and clinical skills. However, patients sometimes think of them as nurses who have an entirely different set of skills. Although most of the medical assistants gently correct patients and make it a point to practice only within their area of expertise, occasionally newer members of the medical assistant staff may feel more "important" when patients regard them as nurses or physicians' assistants.

A few weeks ago, medical assistant Liz Corbin, who is in her early 20s, was taken aback when Walter Seals, the office manager, spoke up about Liz's tendency to let patients assume she was a nurse. Although Liz never deliberately intended to mislead patients, she never corrected them about their misconceptions. Walter pointed out that to present a good example of the medical assisting profession, Liz should gently but firmly help patients understand that she was a medical assistant with a specific range of skills that complemented, but did not substitute for, nursing skills.

FEATURED COMPETENCIES (continued)

- Professional components
- Allied health professions and credentialing

Administrative Duties

- Schedule and monitor appointments
- Use physician fee schedule

Legal Concepts

- Determine needs for documentation and reporting
- Use appropriate guidelines when releasing records or information
- Maintain licenses and accreditation
- Monitor legislation related to current healthcare issues and practices

INTRODUCTION

It is impossible in today's world to function as a medical assistant without an awareness of the impact of ethics and bioethics on health care. Just as an understanding of the law and working within the law is vital information for the medical assistant, it is equally important to understand ethics and bioethics.

From Chapter 7, you have come to realize that there are many circumstances and situations that occur in health care that are guided and directed by state and federal laws. You, personally, are expected to be above reproach in all your actions in this regard. You must also work with your employer and other members of the health care team to assure that each member of the staff functions within the law—protecting both patients and providers.

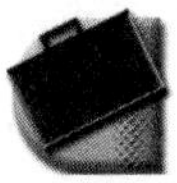

Ethics plays a huge role in such an endeavor. To function ethically demands that you never function outside the law. Ethics, however, demands something more—ethics calls for honesty, trustworthiness, integrity, confidentiality, and fairness. To function ethically, you must know yourself well and understand weaknesses and any vulnerabilities that might prevent you from acting ethically.

The scenario described earlier is just one situation in which medical assistants may need to reflect on their actions and be sure that they are acting ethically and within the range of their skills. Medical assistants also need to recognize the warning signs that they, or some other staff member, may be about to breach a code of ethics. Often, this kind of breach occurs when one has, or seeks to have, too much power; when one attempts to take on too much authority; and when one has too little knowledge and experience. When a breach seems about to occur, the individuals involved should be encouraged to step back and review their actions and the likely consequences of those actions.

ETHICS

Traditionally, **ethics** is defined in terms of what is considered right or wrong. Sometimes ethics is referred to as "morals." Professional organizations often identify their ethics in "codes," or a set of principles and guidelines. Physicians, through the American Medical Association (AMA), have established such a code of ethics called the Principles of Medical Ethics. This code can be reviewed by accessing the AMA Web site (http://www.ama-assn.org/ama/pub/category/2512.html). The Code of Medical Ethics Current Opinions with Annotations is published every two years; this document provides up-to-date information on a number of ethical dilemmas. Medical assistants have a code of ethics and a creed. The AAMA Mission Statement, AAMA Medical Assistant Code of Ethics, and AAMA Medical Assistant Creed appear on the AAMA Web site (http://www.aama-ntl.org). Clicking on the Mission Statement, Code, and Creed will identify these statements for you in an interesting fashion.

There are more than 50 differing codes of ethics for professional organizations, and most are related to medicine. There are seven ethical codes that relate to the entire world. These include such famous codes as the Declaration of Geneva, Declaration of Helsinki, and the International Code of Medical Ethics. A listing of these codes is found by searching the Internet for "world medical ethics codes." Another fascinating Web site identifies the characteristics of Traditional Chinese Medical Ethics when you use the Internet to search for "Chinese Medical Ethics." Chinese medical ethics emphasizes self-cultivation and personal ethics of practitioners rather than a strict organizational code of ethics.

Codes of ethics bring standards of moral and ethical behavior together in one place. They assist organizations and individuals in putting words to their expected behaviors and actions. There is a benefit to such codes when they become reminders to everyone regarding their conduct. Codes also can have a limiting affect, however. For instance, if an organization does not have a code of ethics, is that organization viewed as unethical? When one answers that question, there also comes the understanding that having a code of ethics does not necessarily create an ethical organization.

Medical assistants and medical professionals are asked to balance personal and professional areas of their lives in the middle of constant pressure and crises. At the same time, the quality of one's personal life is going to be shown in the quality of their service to others in their professional life. To be effective in the medical profession, there needs to be maturity in both the personal and the professional selves that creates the utmost of ethical conduct and professionalism.

Principle-Centered Leadership

Stephen R. Covey, author of *The 7 Habits of Highly Effective People* and *Principle-Centered Leadership*, has identified eight characteristics of principle-centered leaders. Leaders who know themselves and understand their principles more easily abide by a code of ethics. Consider the following questions as guides to how you might perform ethically in a medical setting.

Are you continually learning? Are you seeking training, taking classes, listening to others, learning from your peers? Are you curious? Do you realize that developing new knowledge and skills is a lifelong endeavor?

Are you service-oriented? Do you see your life as a mission rather than a career? Are you generally a nurturing individual who seeks service in the medical field? Can you see yourself working alongside a coworker and pulling together with that person toward a goal? Can you put yourself in the place of others?

Do you radiate positive energy? Are you cheerful, pleasant, optimistic, and positive? Is your spirit hopeful? If it is, you carry a positive energy field that allows you to neutralize or sidestep a negative energy source. Are you aware of your energy field and its impact on those around you? Do you see yourself as a peacemaker or one that can create harmony to undo negative energy?

Do you believe in other people? Can you keep from labeling, stereotyping, or prejudging other people? Can you believe in the unseen potential of others? Can you keep from overreacting to negative behaviors and criticism? Can you put aside any grudges?

The final three characteristics of principle-centered leaders identified in Covey's *7 Habits of Highly Effective People* are more personal but can help you maintain an understanding of yourself and how you might make ethical decisions in the medical field, and appear below.

Do you lead a balanced life? Do you keep up with current affairs and events? Do you know what is happening in the medical field and how that affects you? Do you have at least one confidant with whom you can be transparent? Are you physically active within your limits of age and health? Do you enjoy yourself? Do you have a good sense of humor? Are you open to communication?

Do you see life as an adventure? Are you able to rediscover persons each time you meet them? Are you interested in others? Do you listen well? Are you flexible and unflappable? Does your security come from within rather than from without?

Are you synergistic? Synergy is what happens when the whole of something is greater than the sum of its parts. Do you know your weaknesses? Can you complement your weaknesses with the strength of others on the team? Can you work hard to improve most situations? Are you trusting? Can you separate the person from the problem?

Do you exercise for self-renewal? In this element, Mr. Covey identifies four dimensions of the human personality that need exercise: physical, mental, emotional, and spiritual dimensions. How do you keep your body in shape? How do you keep your mind alert? Do patience, unconditional love, and accepting responsibility for your own actions keep you emotionally healthy? Do you have a way to meditate, pray, or "draw away" for a period to "fill up your spirit"?

These questions and your response to them can give you insight into your ability to function ethically and to be successful in the world of medicine.

Five Ps of Ethical Power

Kenneth Blanchard and Norman Vincent Peale, wrote a simple, but powerful little book called *The Power of Ethical Management*. In it they discuss the "Five Ps of Ethical Power." The five Ps are as follows:

Purpose: Understand your objective or your purpose. Your purpose may change from time to time, but it is something that requires you to behave in a way that makes you feel good about yourself.

Pride: Have pride in what you do. Feel good about yourself and your accomplishments. Nurture your self-esteem while remaining humble. Be proud to be a medical assistant.

Patience: It takes time to create an atmosphere where your objective can be obtained. Strive to believe that no matter what happens, everything is going to work out. Expect results from yourself and your work, but refrain from demanding it "now."

Persistence: To act in an ethical manner means to strive to act in that manner all the time, not just when you want to or it seems easy to do. Winston Churchill said, "Never! Never! Never! Never! Give Up!" That is what persistence is. If you make a mistake,

Critical Thinking

With a peer, identify one or more examples in your life when you truly did not give up on attaining your goals. Describe what you learned from that experience. How might "never giving up" help in your pursuit of a career?

admit it, correct it, learn from the mistake, and move on, but never give up.

Perspective: Keep your life and your purpose in perspective. Find time each day to maintain balance in your life (perhaps looking again at the eight characteristics of principle-centered individuals). Plan some quiet time, some fun time, but certainly some reflective time. The constant pressure and the crises will become overwhelming without keeping perspective.

Ethics Check Questions

Finally, those striving to act in an ethical manner can perform a little test each time they have a question about ethics. This, too, comes from Blanchard and Peale. The questions to ask are: (1) Is it legal? Is it against the law or any company policy? (2) Is it balanced? Is this the best possible approach for all concerned? Does it promote a win–win situation? (3) How will it make me feel about myself? Will I feel good if my decision is published in a newspaper? Will my family and coworkers be proud of my decision?

Ethics are not easy. Performing ethically is hard work. Being ethical means determining who you are and how you will act. Laws are more clearly defined than ethics, but acting in an unethical manner can cause as much pain and difficulty as can acting illegally. The ideas of Covey, Blanchard, and Peale give guidance, thoughts to ponder, and perhaps goals to reach. Keep them in mind as you review the next section.

Spotlight on Certification

RMA Content Outline

- Principles of medical ethics
- Ethical conduct

CMA Content Outline

- Displaying professional attitude
- Performing within ethical boundaries
- Maintaining confidentiality
- Legislation
- Physician–patient relationship

CMAS Content Outline

- Legal and Ethical Considerations
- Professionalism
- Confidentiality

BIOETHICS

Bioethics brings the entire focus of ethics into the field of health care and into those ethical issues dealing with life. Never before in the history of medical care has bioethics been such a topic of concern. In the past, most bioethical decisions were made by physicians and esteemed members of the medical or legal profession. However, advancing technology giving patients and consumers numerous choices regarding their health care causes each one of us to take an active role in bioethics.

Medical assistants will encounter ethical and bioethical issues across the lifespan. In Figure 8-1, a few issues are identified for contemplation and discussion. Issues of bioethics common to every medical clinic are the allocation of scarce medical resources, abortion and fetal tissue research, genetic engineering or manipulation, and the many choices surrounding life, dying, and death.

For medical assistants to fully comprehend a discussion of ethics and bioethics, review of the Code of Ethics of AAMA (Figure 8-2) is beneficial.

KEYS TO THE AAMA CODE OF ETHICS

Medical assistants should consider the more salient points in the AAMA Code of Ethics and ask themselves the following questions:

A. *Render service with full respect for the dignity of humanity.*
   - Will I respect every patient even if I do not approve of his or her morals or choices in health care?
   - Will I honor each patient's request for information and explain unfamiliar procedures?
   - Will I give my full attention to acknowledging the needs of every patient?
   - Will I be able to accept the indigent, the physically and mentally challenged, the infirm, the physically disfigured, and the persons I simply

A FEW ISSUES FOR CONTEMPLATION AND DISCUSSION

Infants

- In premature, deformed, or severely disabled infants, ethical issues include the decision to provide or withhold treatment. Health care professionals and parents are not always in agreement. Central to this issue, also, is the expense involved in certain treatments and deciding who pays the cost of treatment, because insurance usually does not.
- Vulnerability of infants can lead to issues of negligence, abuse, or rejection. Parents also are vulnerable because they may be unable to cope with the needs of the entire family.

Children

- Children who are ill-fed, housed, educated, and clothed exhibit great needs for preventive, curative, and rehabilitative health care. Obesity in children is becoming a serious issue.
- Minors with sexually transmitted diseases can seek treatment without the parents' knowledge. Treatment also must be offered without parental consent to pregnant, infected, or addicted minors.
- Child abuse presents an ethical dilemma, especially when a child confides physical, sexual, or emotional abuse to a health care worker but does not want the information divulged. Health care professionals, as mandated reporters, must report suspected child abuse. Will the child/patient view this as a violation of confidence or suffer dire consequences as a result of the reported abuse?

Adolescents

- Adolescents as young as 14 to 18 years of age may seek abortion without parental knowledge or consent. Is this a violation of parents' right to medical information regarding their children? Or should the adolescent, fearful of parental reaction, have the right to decide?
- The adolescent's growing autonomy, need for independence, changing values, and desire for peer acceptance lead to a number of ethical issues that may involve the health care environment. These include the adolescent's decision to be sexually active, to use birth control, to protect against sexually transmitted diseases, and to use drugs and alcohol.

Adults

- Many low-income women do not have sufficient access to prenatal care, which has proven to be a cost-saving medical measure that is critical to the health of both mother and infant.

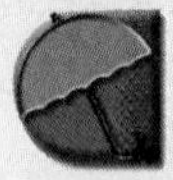

- As employers seek to reduce the cost of health insurance benefit programs, many individuals and families are finding themselves shifted from one insurance program to another, leaving them with little or no continuity of care. Also, in some managed care programs, adults may receive medical services from a number of health care professionals with whom they have no opportunity to establish an ongoing physician-patient relationship.
- Even with a physician's directive or a living will, a dying patient's wishes may not be followed. Technological advances in medicine have created a situation where patients may not be able to exercise a choice in the death issue.

Senior Adults

- Dementia is a common problem that is physically and financially exhausting for the caregiver, who is usually a spouse or adult child. How do caregivers cope with their own needs and the needs of dependent adults? Often, the elderly may reject nursing home placement, and there may be limited funds for such long-term and specialized care.
- Elderly patients have the right to maintain dignity and privacy, but their dependency on others may deprive them of these basic rights.
- Physician-assisted suicide for terminally ill patients is a prominent issue in our society, especially when elderly patients sense a total loss of dignity.
- Oregon, the only state with voter-approved assisted dying legislation was threatened when the Attorney General John Ashcroft ruled physicians who used controlled substances to assist patients in dying would face federal prosecution. May 26, 2004 the Ninth Circuit Court of Appeals confirmed a lower court ruling that Oregon's law was valid and beyond the scope of Ashcroft's Department of Justice. Some believe the ruling is destined for the U.S. Supreme Court.

Figure 8-1 Ethical issues across the life span. (Compiled by Carol D. Tamparo, CMA, PhD, and Marilyn Pooler, RN, MEd.)

AAMA CODE OF ETHICS

The Code of Ethics of AAMA shall set forth principles of ethical and moral conduct as they relate to the medical profession and the particular practice of medical assisting.

Members of AAMA dedicated to the conscientious pursuit of their profession, and thus desiring to merit the high regard of the entire medical profession and the respect of the general public which they serve, do pledge themselves to strive always to:

A. render service with full respect for the dignity of humanity;
B. respect confidential information obtained through employment unless legally authorized or required by responsible performance of duty to divulge such information;
C. uphold the honor and high principles of the profession and accept its disciplines;
D. seek to continually improve the knowledge and skills of medical assistants for the benefit of patients and professional colleagues;
E. participate in additional service activities aimed toward improving the health and well-being of the community.

(A)

CREED

I believe in the principles and purposes of the Profession of Medical Assisting.
I endeavor to be more effective.
I aspire to render greater service.
I protect the confidence entrusted to me.
I am dedicated to the care and well-being of all people.
I am loyal to my employer.
I am true to the ethics of my profession.
I am strengthened by compassion, courage, and faith.

(B)

Figure 8-2 (A) American Association of Medical Assistants (AAMA) Code of Ethics. (B) AAMA Creed. (Copyright by the American Association of Medical Assistants, Inc. Revised October, 1996.)

do not like as equal and valid human beings with an equal right to service?

B. *Respect confidential information obtained through employment unless legally authorized or required by responsible performance of duty to divulge such information.*
   - Will I refrain from needless comments to a colleague regarding a patient's problem?
   - Will I refrain from discussing my day's encounters with patients with my family and friends?
   - Will I always protect a patient's chart and everything in it from unnecessary observation?
   - Will I keep patients' names and the circumstances that bring them to my place of employment confidential?

C. *Uphold the honor and high principles of the profession and accept its disciplines.*
   - Am I proud of serving as a medical assistant?
   - Will I always perform within the scope of my profession, never exceeding the responsibility entrusted to me?
   - Will I encourage others to enter the profession and always speak honorably of medical assistants?

D. *Seek to continually improve the knowledge and skills of medical assistants for the benefit of patients and professional colleagues.*
   - Will I always be willing to learn new skills, to update my skills, and seek improved methods for assisting the physician in the care of patients?
   - Will I keep my credentials current and valid?
   - Can I always remember that I am a member of a group of broad-based health care professionals, and that my goal is to complement rather than to compete with that team?

E. *Participate in additional service activities aimed toward improving the health and well-being of the community.*
   - Will I be able to serve in the community where I reside and work to further quality health care?
   - Will I promote preventive medicine?
   - Will I practice good health care management for myself, being a model for others to follow?

ETHICAL GUIDELINES FOR DOCTORS

It is fairly common for each professional group of medical practitioners to have their own code of ethics. The AMA's Code of Medical Ethics and the "Current Opinions with Annotations of the Council on Ethical and Judicial Affairs" was mentioned earlier. The American Chiropractic Association has a Code of Ethics identified in six sections. Other practitioners may consider their mission and policies to be their code of ethics. Some have no specific written code of ethics, but rather call on their practitioners to refer to their culture as one based on ethics, mutual respect, and moral evaluation when ethical decisions are made. There are many similarities in these statements on ethics that are important for patients and medical employees.

Advertising

Physicians and professional people traditionally have not advertised; however, it is not illegal or unethical to do so if claims made are truthful and not misleading. Advertisements may include credentials of physicians and a description of the practice, kinds of services rendered, and how fees are determined. Managed care agencies may advertise their services and the names of participating physicians.

Confidentiality

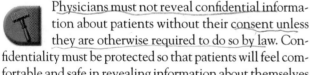

Physicians must not reveal confidential information about patients without their consent unless they are otherwise required to do so by law. Confidentiality must be protected so that patients will feel comfortable and safe in revealing information about themselves that may be important to their health care. The following list contains examples of the kinds of reports that allow or require health professionals to report a confidence.

- A patient threatens another person and there is reason to believe that the threat may be carried out.
- Certain injuries and illnesses *must* be reported. These include injuries such as knife and gunshot wounds, wounds that may be from suspected child abuse, communicable diseases, and sexually transmitted diseases.
- Information that may have been subpoenaed for testimony in a court of law.

When in doubt, it is always recommended that a physician have the patient's permission to reveal any confidential information.

Extra caution must be taken to protect the confidentiality of any patient's data that are kept on a computer database. As few people as possible should have access to the computer data, and only authorized individuals should be permitted to add or alter data. Adequate security precautions must be used to protect information stored on a computer.

Medical Records

The medical chart and the information in it are the property of the physician and the patient. No information should be revealed without the patient's consent unless required by law. The record is confidential. Physicians should not refuse to provide a copy of the record to another physician treating the patient so long as proper authorization has been received from the patient. Also, physicians should provide a copy of the record or summary of its contents if a patient requests it. A record cannot be withheld because of an unpaid bill.

On a physician's retirement or death, or when a practice is sold, patients should be notified and given ample time to have their records transferred to another physician of their choice.

Professional Fees and Charges

Illegal or excessive fees should not be charged. Fees should be based on those customary to the locale and should reflect the difficulty of services and the quality of performance rendered. Fee splitting (a physician splits the fee with another physician for services rendered with or without the patient's knowledge) in any form is unethical. Physicians may charge for missed appointments (if patients have first been notified of the practice) and may charge for multiple or complex insurance forms. Physicians and their employees must be diligent to assure that only the services actually rendered are charged or indicated on the insurance claim. Only what is documented in the patient's chart is to be billed.

Increasingly, there are a number of physicians who now refuse any insurance payments and operate strictly on a cash only basis. Some others charge a yearly fee to care for a family, providing all services necessary at that flat fee. Physicians, upset by the rules and regulations of insurance, find this method of payment creates a simpler form of medical practice. Physicians and patients alike will be discussing the ethics of such a move for some time. Although physicians may choose whom they wish to serve, the cash only basis makes it difficult for low-income families and the poor.

Professional Rights and Responsibilities

As stated earlier, physicians may choose whom to serve, but may not refuse a patient on the basis of race, color, religion, national origin, or any other illegal discrimination. It is unethical for physicians to deny treatment to HIV-infected individuals on that basis alone if they are qualified to treat the patient's condition. Once a physician takes a case, the patient cannot be neglected or refused treatment unless official notice is given from the physician to withdraw from the case.

Patients have the right to know their diagnoses, the nature and purpose of their treatment, and to have enough information to be able to make an informed choice about their treatment protocol. Physicians should inform families of a patient's death and not delegate that responsibility to others.

Physicians should expose incompetent, corrupt, dishonest, and unethical conduct by other physicians to the disciplinary board. It is unethical for any physician to treat patients while under the influence of alcohol, controlled substances, or any other chemical that impairs the physician's ability.

Physicians who know they are HIV positive should refrain from any activity that would risk the transmission of the virus to others.

Any activity that might be regarded as a "conflict of interest" (for example, a physician holding stock in a pharmaceutical company and prescribing medications only from that company) should be avoided. Financial interests are not to influence physicians in prescribing medications, devices, or appliances.

Abuse

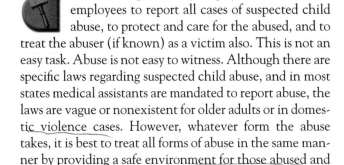

It is the responsibility of physicians and their employees to report all cases of suspected child abuse, to protect and care for the abused, and to treat the abuser (if known) as a victim also. This is not an easy task. Abuse is not easy to witness. Although there are specific laws regarding suspected child abuse, and in most states medical assistants are mandated to report abuse, the laws are vague or nonexistent for older adults or in domestic violence cases. However, whatever form the abuse takes, it is best to treat all forms of abuse in the same manner by providing a safe environment for those abused and seeking treatment for the abused and the abuser.

BIOETHICAL DILEMMAS

Guidelines for bioethical issues are even harder to define than are guidelines for ethics, because each of the bioethical issues calls on us to make decisions that directly affect a person's life. In some instances, the bioethical issue requires a choice about who lives and requires a definition of the quality of life. Such dilemmas are difficult, if not impossible, to approach from a neutral point of view even though medical assistants should strive not to impose their own moral values on patients or coworkers.

Allocation of Scarce Medical Resources

The issue faced daily by health care workers is the allocation of scarce medical resources. Even with the government's attempts at health care reform, medical resources still are not available to everyone. When the receptionist determines who receives the only available appointment in a day, when patients are turned away because they have no insurance or financial resources to pay for services, when Medicare/Medicaid patients are denied services because of low return from state and federal insurance programs, scarce medical resources are being denied.

Weightier decisions might include who gets the surgery, a kidney transplant, or the experimental bone marrow transplant. These allocations are being made and will continue to require decisions on the part of the health care team. As recent as the 2004 national meeting of the AMA, a proposal was made suggesting that physicians refuse treatment to lawyers and their family members or any patients who "threaten" a lawsuit if treatment is unsuccessful. The proposal did not pass, but it came from frustrated physicians trying to spotlight the access problems caused by professional liability cases. Rationing of health care may become more widespread as managed care operations try to achieve a balance between providing access to care while still curtailing costs.

Decisions made by Congress, health systems agencies, and insurance companies are termed **macroallocation** of scarce medical resources. Decisions made individually by physicians and members of the health care team at the local level are termed **microallocation** of scarce resources. No matter what the level, physicians and medical assistants will be involved.

Abortion and Fetal Tissue Research

It appears these issues associated with abortion and fetal tissue research will be with us for quite some time. Although the law is specific on abortion guidelines as set forth in *Roe v. Wade*, there is a continual challenge in the courts of its validity. Some states are more restrictive in how and if abortions might be performed in the second and third trimesters of pregnancy. However, the law stipulates that a woman has a right to an abortion in the first trimester without interference from regulations in any state.

A physician must decide whether to perform abortions within the legal parameters and under what circumstances. A physician cannot be forced to perform abortions, nor can any employee be forced to participate or assist the physician to perform an abortion. Employees not wishing to participate in abortions are advised to seek employment where they are not performed.

There are many unanswered ethical questions related to abortion that make it difficult for health care professionals. Should abortion be considered a form of birth control? If not, should birth control be readily available to all who seek it regardless of age? Should insurance pay for birth control? Is it ethical to deny a woman on welfare an abortion whereas providing one to a woman who either has money for the procedure or whose insurance pays for it? And, of course, the major unanswered question that must be determined by every physician is: When does life begin?

The abortion issue raises another bioethical issue—fetal tissue research and transplantation. Fetal tissue research, as early as the 1950s, led to the development of polio and rubella vaccines. Today, fetal cells hold promise for medical research into a variety of diseases and medical conditions, including Alzheimer's disease, Huntington's disease, spinal cord injury, diabetes, and multiple sclerosis. There is some research to indicate that fetal retinal transplants may be a successful treatment for macular degeneration, which is the leading cause of old-age blindness in the United States. This issue is also political, as well as bioethical, and it changes with each major political shift in our government. Fetal tissue research gets caught up in the pro-life forces, also. About half of the states have laws regulating fetal research. Some ban the research using aborted fetuses. Federal law prohibits the sale of fetal tissue and requires all federally funded fetal tissue research projects to comply with state and local laws. Fetal tissue research is not to be used to encourage women to have abortions; rather, the tissue would be available only after a decision had already been made regarding abortion.

Genetic Engineering/Manipulation

So much is possible today in the area of **genetic engineering** and new discoveries increasingly are being seen. This biotechnology can be used in the diagnosis of disease, production of medicines, forensic documentation (DNA used in solving crimes), and for research. Some reasons to continue study in this area include to determine if anything can be done to prevent or cure some 4,000 recognized genetic disorders and major diseases that have large genetic components. Who among us would not want to be free of certain illnesses? But at what cost? How far do we go in genetic engineering? Would we prefer a society where everyone is healthy and beautiful? If it is determined that a fetus suffers from a serious defect, should abortion be encouraged? If we manipulate the genes before implantation, are we playing God? If fertilization takes place *in vitro,* is discarding defective embryos a reasonable and presumed choice?

Artificial Insemination/Surrogacy

For many individuals, artificial insemination is the only means by which they can conceive a child. Physicians are called on to perform artificial insemination for couples, single women, or lesbians who want a child. If artificial insemination is performed, it is recommended that the signed consent of each party involved be obtained. It is also recommended that physicians practicing AID (artificial insemination by donor), use many donors for semen, and that meticulous screening be performed before the insemination.

Surrogacy is another bioethical issue. Men have been used as **surrogates,** or substitutes, for decades with the practice of artificial insemination, but society seems to have a more difficult time accepting surrogate mothers who are artificially inseminated by a donor and carry the fetus to term for another parent. Gay men seek surrogates who are able to provide them a child who represents half their genetic makeup. How should the rights of each individual in the exchange be protected? For many of these issues, there is little protection or guidance under the law; therefore, physicians and their employees must make decisions on the basis of their own belief systems.

Artificial insemination and surrogacy were viewed as experimental and quite controversial just 20 years ago. Today, however, the procedures are widely practiced and available. Both artificial insemination and surrogacy are costly and can become legal tangles for all involved if careful steps are not taken.

Critical Thinking

When fertilization occurs outside the womb, additional embryos are stored and saved for future use. How long should they be stored? To whom do they belong? What happens if no one wants those embryos later? Should they be destroyed, given to some other hopeful parent, or used for research?

Dying and Death

Patients are making more choices regarding their own death. We all have the right to direct health care professionals regarding our death in the case of a life-threatening illness. Through a living will or a physician's directive, we can mandate that life support systems be removed. Review Chapter 7. Sometimes, patients make these decisions before physicians are ready to remove the life support. Other times, physicians can determine when a case is hopeless far quicker than the patient or the patient's family. What should be done then? When a physician is committed to sustaining life, it is difficult to make decisions to terminate life. Oregon, the only state to pass a physician-assisted suicide law has had great difficulties maintaining and putting the law into practice, partly because of a challenge by the United States Attorney General. Oregon voters have held firm, however, and so far the Attorney General has been unsuccessful in overturning the voters' wishes.

Choices available to patients who are dying always cause us to ask ourselves what is "quality of life"? Although the answer to that question is different for everyone, it is a question often in conflict with today's medical technology that can, in many instances, keep a patient alive much longer than the patient might prefer. The benefits of advanced technology will continue to be weighed against what many consider the right to die with dignity and a minimum of medical intervention.

HIV and AIDS

The general public's fear of AIDS has caused some serious bioethical issues. Patients who may suspect they have HIV or AIDS should be tested for the virus. Their confidentiality must be protected as much as possible because individuals with AIDS often face loss of employment, medical insurance, and even loss of family and friends. It is unethical to deny treatment to individuals because they test positive for HIV.

Although individuals with HIV/AIDS must be protected, so must the public. Therefore, if physicians suspect that an HIV-seropositive patient is infecting an unsuspecting individual, every attempt should be made to protect the individual at risk. Health professionals must first encourage the infected person to cease endangering any person. Second, if the patient refuses to notify the person at risk or wishes the physician to notify the person, the physician can contact authorities. Many states and cities have Partner Notification Programs that will anonymously notify the patient at risk, keeping the source confidential. The program informs them that it has been brought to their attention that they are a "person at risk" and provides them with free testing. Third, the physician can notify the person at risk.

Case Study 8-1

Harley Navarro is a new medical assistant in a busy internist's clinic. Harley is nervous and fairly intimidated by the other medical assistants who are female and have many years of experience. He is especially hesitant to ask for assistance or admit that he is having a problem. Twice today he was unable to get a good blood pressure reading on patients. One patient was very obese, and the other kept trying to carry on a conversation with him.

CASE STUDY REVIEW

1. If Harley's behavior does no harm to the patient, has he acted unethically? Illegally?
2. What might the office manager do if she senses Harley's lack of certainty?
3. Discuss the role of female and male medical assistants working together and how they might complement each other.

Case Study 8-2

Liz Corbin is a medical assistant in the fertility clinic of a large metropolitan medical clinic and hospital. Liz really likes her job and is delighted when parenthood is made possible for many of those seeking the clinic's advanced technology. The clinic also stores and maintains the unused frozen embryos that result from artificial insemination. She is a little alarmed when her physician–employer informs her that four of the embryos are to be destroyed. The physician has been unable to contact the owners (now parents of more than one child from artificial insemination) for directions, and space for storage is limited. The physician instructs Liz to destroy the embryos.

CASE STUDY REVIEW

1. Liz is rather hesitant to comply with her physician's orders, so she does a little research. She discovers that most fertility clinics ask couples using **cryopreservation** to decide early in the process how to handle their excess embryos. The choices are: (1) discard the embryos, (2) donate anonymously to other infertile couples, and (3) donate to scientific research. What might Liz do to influence the clinic's policy?
2. Can anything be done to ensure that couples do not abandon their embryos?
3. If embryos are given to other infertile couples, how is a decision made on who should have them?

SUMMARY

As medical technology continues to advance, a greater need for ethical guidelines will be necessary. Physicians and health care professionals at all levels must stay abreast of the issues and carefully consider all aspects before making any decision.

Medical assistants must, however, keep the following legal and ethical guidelines in mind: (1) always practice within the law; (2) preserve the patient's confidentiality; (3) maintain meticulous records; (4) obtain informed, written consent; (5) do not judge patients whose belief system differs from yours.

STUDY FOR SUCCESS

To reinforce your knowledge and skills of information in this chapter:

- ❑ Review the Key Terms
- ❑ Consider the Case Studies and discuss your conclusions
- ❑ Answer the Review Questions
  - ❑ Multiple Choice
  - ❑ Critical Thinking
- ❑ Navigate the Internet and complete the Web Activities
- ❑ Practice the StudyWARE activities on the textbook CD
- ❑ Apply your knowledge in the Student Workbook activities
- ❑ Complete the Web Tutor sections
- ❑ View and discuss the DVD situations

REVIEW QUESTIONS

Multiple Choice

1. Typically, ethics has been defined in terms of:
   a. what is right and wrong
   b. whether an action is legal
   c. the expedient thing to do
   d. professionalism in the workplace
2. Bioethics has to do with:
   a. biological reproduction
   b. the act of artificial insemination
   c. genetic engineering
   d. ethical issues that deal with life and health care
3. The AAMA Code of Ethics:
   a. is concerned with principles of ethical and moral conduct
   b. defines the duties the medical assistant can perform
   c. is intended for physicians only
   d. applies only to patient rights
4. When a physician or medical assistant suspects child abuse, they should:
   a. give the parent a warning
   b. report it to the proper authorities
   c. not impose their values on the parents
   d. give the child some hints on how to protect against abuse
5. When a patient has HIV:
   a. it is ethical for the physician not to provide treatment
   b. it is unethical for the physician not to provide treatment
   c. other patients should be warned of the possibility of infection
   d. all friends and family members of the patient should be notified
6. A copy of a medical record may be granted to:
   a. a physician the patient is being referred to
   b. a physician's attorney when subpoenaed or released by patient
   c. the patient
   d. all of the above
   e. only a and b
7. The eight characteristics of principle-centered leaders originates from the following author:
   a. James R. Jones
   b. Steven R. Covey
   c. Francis H. Ambrose
   d. Jason N. Diamond
8. The five Ps of ethical power are:
   a. Personality, performance, purpose, pride, patience
   b. Purpose, patience, perfection, personality, procrastination
   c. Patience, purpose, pride, persistence, perspective
   d. Purpose, pride, patience, perfection, perspective
9. Which of the following is true?
   a. A physician can choose whom to serve.
   b. A physician may charge for completing multiple and complex insurance claims.
   c. Physicians and their employees cannot be forced to perform abortions.
   d. All of the above
   e. None of the above
10. You are most likely to make ethical decisions correctly when:
   a. you have a clear picture of the situation
   b. you leave emotion out of the decision as much as possible
   c. you understand your weaknesses and vulnerabilities
   d. honesty and integrity are hallmarks of your entire life
   e. all of the above

Critical Thinking

1. In your own words, define ethics and bioethics.
2. A physician observes another physician put a patient at risk while under the influence of alcohol and does nothing about it. What would constitute ethical behavior?
3. A physician refuses to accept any more Medicaid patients for medical care. Is this the physician's right? Is it ethical? Why or why not?
4. A medical assistant whispers to the receptionist, "There goes the guy with AIDS." How should the receptionist view this behavior?
5. The services reported on the insurance claim are more complex than those actually rendered. Is this ethical or unethical? State your reasons.
6. The physician refuses to perform a legal abortion. Do you consider this an ethical issue? Why?
7. A physician performs artificial insemination for a lesbian couple; however, the medical assistant refuses to participate or assist the physician. What are the ramifications of the medical assistant's behavior? Do you believe the medical assistant has a right to refuse?
8. Referring to Figure 8-1, select an ethical issue with which you may have had some personal experience. Now, form a small group, with each student leading a discussion on a different issue.

WEB ACTIVITIES

1. Using the World Wide Web, print out the latest issue of the AMA Principles of Medical Ethics. Compare that with the AAMA Code of Ethics. Do you find this comparison helpful in more clearly understanding ethics, responsibility, and professionalism? Give your reasons.
2. Using the Web site given at the beginning of this chapter, select one additional code of ethics to compare with the AMA Principles and the AAMA Code. What are the similarities?
3. Using your favorite Internet search engine, key in two or three of the bioethical issues and do a small-scale review of items listed. From your research, identify at least three ethical/bioethical questions for your class to discuss.

THE DVD HOOK-UP

DVD Series: **Critical Thinking** | Program Number: **3**

Chapter/Scene Reference
- *Ethical Practice*

In this chapter, you learned about the importance of ethical behavior when working in the medical field. Ethics are not laws, but rather a set of morals or principles to which we adhere.

In the designated DVD clip, we observed Jen talking to Sarah about a patient that has diabetes. Jen feels that the patient has complications with her diabetes because she makes poor choices in her eating habits. Barb, the supervisor, overhears the conversation and talks to Jen and Sarah about the importance of being compassionate as health care providers. Even though this clip does not deal with some of the more noted ethical issues such as fetal tissue research or genetic engineering, judging the patient is a violation of ethical behavior and probably one of the more typical ethical issues that you will struggle with as a medical assistant.

1. As a medical assistant, you will make observations about your patients that can be helpful to the physician. What was inappropriate in the way Jen handled her observations?
2. Diseases such as emphysema, obesity, and diabetes can all be the result of unhealthy life styles. How will you as a medical assistant keep from judging a patient's actions or lifestyle that have resulted in illness?

DVD Journal Summary

Write a paragraph that summarizes what you learned from watching the designated scenes from today's DVD program. Ethical dilemmas may involve anyone in the medical office. For example, what would you do if you smelled alcohol on a coworker? What if you suspect the coworker is abusing alcohol? Are you obligated to say something? To whom? Why or why not?

REFERENCES/BIBLIOGRAPHY

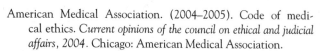

American Medical Association. (2004–2005). Code of medical ethics. *Current opinions of the council on ethical and judicial affairs, 2004*. Chicago: American Medical Association.

Blanchard, K., & Peale, N. V. (1988). *The power of ethical management*. New York: William Morrow and Company, Inc.

Covey, S. R. (1991). *Principle-centered leadership*. New York: Simon & Schuster.

Flight, M. (2004). *Law, liability, and ethics for medical office personnel* (4th ed.). Clifton Park, NY: Thomson Delmar Learning.

Lewis, M. A., & Tamparo, C. D., (2002). *Medical law, ethics, and bioethics for ambulatory care* (5th ed.). Philadelphia: F. A. Davis.

CHAPTER 9

Emergency Procedures and First Aid

OUTLINE

Recognizing an Emergency
- Responding to an Emergency
- Primary Survey
- Using the 911 or Emergency Medical Services System
- Good Samaritan Laws
- Blood, Body Fluids, and Disease Transmission

Preparing for an Emergency
- The Medical Crash Tray or Cart

Common Emergencies
- Shock
- Wounds
- Burns
- Musculoskeletal Injuries
- Heat- and Cold-Related Illnesses
- Poisoning
- Sudden Illness
- Cerebral Vascular Accident
- Heart Attack

Procedures for Breathing Emergencies and Cardiac Arrest
- Heimlich Maneuver (Abdominal Thrust)
- Rescue Breathing
- Cardiopulmonary Resuscitation

OBJECTIVES

The student should strive to meet the following performance objectives and demonstrate an understanding of the facts and principles presented in this chapter through written and oral communication.

1. Define the key terms as presented in the glossary.
2. Learn to recognize, prepare for, and respond to emergencies in the ambulatory care setting.
3. Understand the legal and disease transmission considerations in emergency caregiving.
4. Perform the primary assessment in emergency situations.
5. Identify and care for different types of wounds.
6. Understand the basics of bandage application.
7. Discriminate among first-, second-, and third-degree burns.
8. Assess injuries to muscles, bones, and joints.

(continues)

KEY TERMS

Ambu Bag™
Anaphylaxis
Automated External Defibrillator (AED)
Bandage
Cardiopulmonary Resuscitation (CPR)
Cardioversion
Cauterized
Constriction Band
Crash Tray or Cart
Crepitation
Dressing
Emergency Medical Services (EMS)
Explicit
First Aid
Fracture
Heimlich Maneuver
Hypothermia
Implicit
Lackluster
Normal Saline
Occlusion
Rescue Breathing
Risk Management
Shock
Splint
Sprain
Standard Precautions
Strain
Syncope
Systemic
Triage
Universal Emergency Medical Identification Symbol
Wound

FEATURED COMPETENCIES

CAHEEP—ENTRY-LEVEL COMPETENCIES

Patient Care

- Recognize and respond to emergencies
- Coordinate patient care information with other health care providers

Professionalism

- Demonstrate initiative and responsibility
- Work as a member of the health care team
- Prioritize and perform multiple tasks
- Treat all patients with compassion and empathy

Legal Concepts

- Comply with established risk management and safety procedures

ABHES—ENTRY-LEVEL COMPETENCIES

Professionalism

- Exhibit initiative
- Conduct work within scope of education, training and ability

Clinical Duties

- Recognize emergencies
- Perform first aid and CPR
- Prepare and administer medications as directed by physician

Legal Concepts

- Perform risk management procedures

OBJECTIVES (continued)

9. Describe heat- and cold-related illnesses.
10. Describe how poisons may enter the body.
11. Recall the eight types of shock.
12. Define a cerebral vascular accident.
13. Describe the signs and symptoms of a heart attack.
14. Demonstrate proficiency in Heimlich maneuver, rescue breathing, and cardiopulmonary resuscitation (CPR).

SCENARIO

Inner City Health Care, which is located in Carlton, Michigan, has its share of cold, snowy winters, and when the temperature drops near freezing, that snow sometimes turns to ice. Last night, as Clinical Medical Assistant Wanda Slawson, CMA, was leaving for the evening, she noticed a woman from an adjacent office slip and fall in the parking lot. Wanda immediately went over to the woman to lend assistance and saw that, in falling, the woman had cut the palm of her hand. Apparently, she had tried to break her fall with her hand only to sustain a wound that was now bleeding moderately. Fortunately, Wanda knew that one of the physicians was still in the office and she led the woman back to the building, reassuring her along the way. Once in the office, Wanda assisted Susan Rice, the physician, to examine the wound. After determining that sutures were not needed, Dr. Rice and Wanda cleansed the wound, applied a dry, sterile dressing, and covered it with an elastic bandage. The patient was instructed to call her physician first thing in the morning.

INTRODUCTION

Although the ambulatory care setting is primarily designed to see patients under nonemergency conditions, occasionally the physician will need to administer emergency care, and the medical assistant will be called on to assist the physician in this care. For the medical assistant who may need to triage or assess the patient's condition, the first and most critical step in responding to an emergency is developing the skill to recognize when emergency measures should be taken.

Whereas some emergencies can be treated in the office, others cannot, and the medical assistant must know when to call for outside help. If the emergency occurs in the ambulatory care setting, the physician usually provides immediate care. It is possible, however, that the medical assistant may be the first emergency caregiver should the physician be out of the office. The medical assistant also may be called on to provide care in an emergency outside of the office environment.

This chapter acquaints the medical assistant with types of emergency situations that may occur either inside or outside of the office. However, this chapter is merely an introduction to emergency topics and does not substitute for first aid and cardiopulmonary resuscitation (CPR) instruction taught either through the college curriculum or through the American Red Cross, the American Heart Association, the American Safety and Health Institute, or the National Safety Council. These hands-on classes are vital teaching tools, and all medical assistants should take them on a regular basis to continually update their skills.

RECOGNIZING AN EMERGENCY

An emergency is considered any instance in which an individual becomes suddenly ill and requires immediate attention. Most emergencies develop quickly and usually without warning. They can occur unexpectedly at any time to anyone. Some may be gradual, as seen with dehydration or slow blood loss, and become an emergency over time. Some common signs that an individual has an emergency include unusual noises, such as yelling, moaning, or crying. A person may appear to be behaving strangely when choking or if having difficulty breathing. To recognize when an emergency exists, it is important to have sharp senses of hearing, sight, and smell and be acutely sensitive to any unusual behaviors.

In the ambulatory care setting, medical assistants may encounter a range of emergency situations requiring first-aid techniques. **First aid** is designed to render immediate and temporary emergency care to persons injured or otherwise disabled before the arrival of a physician or transport to a hospital or other health care agency.

Spotlight on Certification

RMA Content Outline

- Body systems
- Disorders of the body
- First aid procedures

CMA Content Outline

- Performing telephone and in-person screening
- Preplanned action (Emergencies)
- Assessment and triage
- Establishing and maintaining an airway
- Identifying and responding (First Aid)
- Signs and symptoms
- Management (First Aid)

CMAS Content Outline

- Medical Office Emergencies

Emergency situations can be minor or severe and can include:

- Stroke
- Wounds
- Bleeding
- Burns
- Shock
- Fractures
- Poisoning
- Sudden illnesses such as fainting/falling
- Illnesses related to heat and cold
- Heart attack
- Choking and breathing crises

Some of these situations will be life-threatening; all will require immediate care. In either case, it is critical to remain calm, to follow the emergency policies and procedures established by the ambulatory care setting, and to be well-versed in first-aid and CPR techniques. The patient should not be further endangered.

HIPAA

Patient confidentiality must be maintained during an emergency situation, as it must at all times. Sometimes, when a situation is urgent and the patient is having trouble breathing, bleeding heavily, having a severe allergic reaction, or any other kind of emergency, in your eagerness to assist the patient, your voice when talking to other health care providers may be overheard by other patients. Be certain other patients cannot hear any conversations. Privacy must be maintained when faxing information to the emergency department. Also be cautious when speaking on the telephone. Do not give out information to a patient's family or to other practitioners without the patient's consent. Be cautious to keep the patient's anonymity protected.

Responding to an Emergency

Once it has been determined that an emergency exists, it is essential to act quickly. Before making any decisions about how to proceed, it is necessary to assess the nature of the situation. Does it include respiratory or circulatory failure, severe bleeding, burns, poisoning, or severe allergic reaction?

Sometimes, it is possible that more than one type of care must be administered. In this case, it is necessary to **triage** the situation, which is a method of prioritizing treatment. When an individual experiences more than one illness or injury, care must be given according to the severity of the situation. When two or more patients present with emergencies simultaneously, triage also determines which patient is treated first. The main principle of triage states that absence of heartbeat and breath and severe bleeding are immediate life threats. See Table 9-1 for the common ordering of triage situations.

To identify the nature of the emergency and respond effectively, it is critical that the patient be assessed. If the patient is conscious, ask for personal identification and identification of next of kin. Try to obtain information about symptoms being experienced to identify the problem. Always check for a **universal emergency medical identification symbol** (Figure 9-1) and accompanying identification card, which will describe any serious or life-threatening health problems that the patient has. Quickly observe the patient's general appearance, including skin color and size and dilation of pupils. Check pulse and blood pressure.

Primary Survey

If the patient is unresponsive, it is critical to assess the ABCs, which include:

- Airway
- Breathing
- Circulation

To assess whether the unresponsive patient is breathing and to determine if there is an open airway, place your face close to the patient's face and look, listen, and feel. Look at the patient's chest and notice whether the chest rises and falls with breathing. Listen for air entering and leaving the nose and mouth and feel for moving air.

If the individual is not breathing, first open the airway by either tilting the head and lifting the chin (Figure 9-2A); or by the jaw-thrust maneuver, which involves

TABLE 9-1 EXAMPLES OF TRIAGE SITUATIONS

First Priority	Next Priority	Least Priority
Airway and breathing problems	Second-degree burns not on the neck and face	Fractures (simple)
Cardiac arrest	Major or multiple fractures	Minor injuries
Severe bleeding that is uncontrolled	Back injuries	Sprains, strains
Head injuries	Severe eye injuries	
Poisoning		
Open chest or abdominal wounds		
Shock		
Second- and third-degree burns		

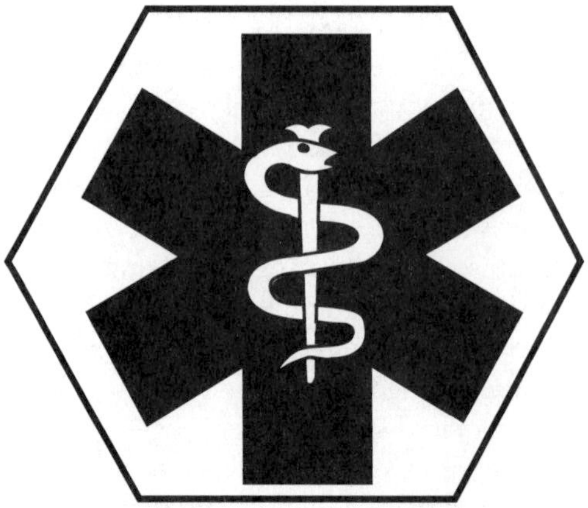

Figure 9-1 The universal emergency medical identification symbol.

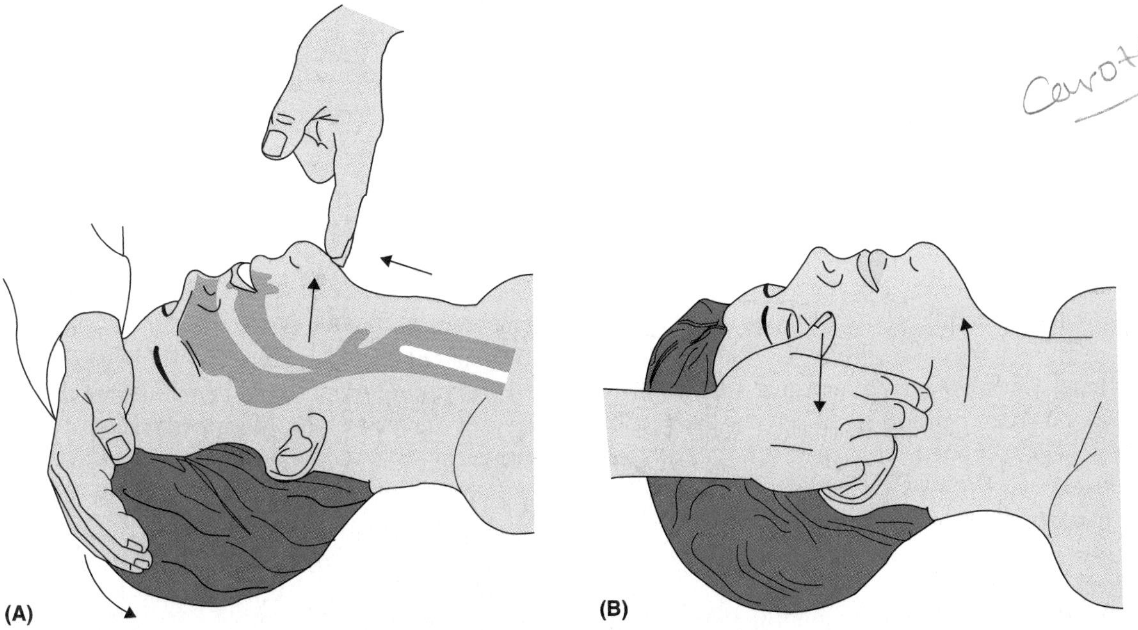

(A) (B)

Figure 9-2 If the individual is not breathing, first open the airway (A) by tilting the head and lifting the chin, or (B) by the jaw-thrust maneuver, which involves placing both thumbs on the patient's cheekbones and placing the index and middle fingers on both sides of the lower jaw.

placing both thumbs on the patient's cheekbones and placing the index and middle fingers on both sides of the lower jaw (see Figure 9-2B). **CAUTION:** Do not attempt to tilt the head and lift the chin when the patient has a head, neck, or spinal cord injury.

If the patient still does not breathe after the airway has been opened, rescue breathing must be performed (discussed later in this chapter).

To assess circulation, check for the presence of a pulse at the carotid artery on the side of the neck below the ear. If no pulse is present, the patient may be in cardiac arrest and must be given CPR. Use of an **automated external defibrillator (AED)** may be necessary (see Chapter 25). CPR techniques are discussed in detail later in this chapter.

Patient Education

Alert patients to the importance of carrying the universal emergency medical identification symbol and its accompanying identification card if the patient suffers from severe heart disease, diabetes, or has other life-threatening illnesses or allergies.

Using the 911 or Emergency Medical Services System

The **Emergency Medical Services (EMS)** system is a local network of police, fire, and medical personnel who are trained to respond to emergency situations. Other community experts and volunteers also act as resources in an EMS system. In many communities, the network is activated by calling 911. Even when preliminary emergency care is provided by the ambulatory care physician, the patient may still need to be transported to a hospital for follow-up care. It is also possible that the physician may not be equipped to deliver the type of emergency care required, in which case, one person should call for EMS help while another stays with the patient until help arrives. Never leave a seriously ill or unconscious patient unattended.

While waiting for EMS to arrive, continuously check the patient for the following signs: (1) degree of responsiveness, (2) airway/breathing ability, (3) heartbeat (rate and rhythm), (4) bleeding, and (5) signs of shock. Monitor vital signs. Keep patient warm and lying down. If there are no head injuries, the legs can be elevated on pillows.

Good Samaritan Laws

When delivering or assisting in delivering emergency care, the medical assistant may be concerned about professional liability. Most states have enacted Good Samaritan laws, which provide some degree of protection to the health care professional who offers first aid.

Most Good Samaritan laws provide some legal protection to those who provide emergency care to ill or injured persons. However, when medical assistants or any other individuals give care during an emergency, they must act as reasonable and prudent individuals and provide care only within the scope of their abilities. Remember that a primary principle of first aid is to prevent further injury.

Although Good Samaritan laws give some measure of protection against being sued for giving emergency aid, they generally protect *off-duty* health care professionals. Also, conditions of the law vary from state to state. As part of establishing emergency care guidelines, every ambulatory care setting should understand the **explicit** and **implicit** intent of the Good Samaritan law in its state. See Chapter 7 for more information on legal guidelines.

Blood, Body Fluids, and Disease Transmission

When providing emergency care, medical assistants should always protect themselves and the patient from infectious disease transmission. Serious infectious diseases, such as hepatitis B (HBV), hepatitis C (HCV), and HIV can be transmitted through blood and body fluids (see Chapter 10 for more detailed information).

By establishing and following strict guidelines, the risk for contracting or transmitting an infectious disease while providing emergency care is greatly reduced.

- Always wash hands thoroughly before (if possible) and after every procedure.
- Use protective clothing and other protective equipment (gloves, gown, mask, goggles) during the procedure.
- Avoid contact with blood and body fluids, if possible.
- Do not touch nose, mouth, or eyes with gloved hands.
- Carefully handle and safely dispose of soiled gloves and other objects.

Refer to Chapter 10 for more information on standard precautions. **Standard precautions** were issued by the Centers for Disease Control and Prevention (CDC) in 1996 and combine many of the basic principles of universal precautions with techniques known as body substance isolation. These augmented 1996 guidelines represent the standard in infection control and are intended to protect both patients and health care professionals.

PREPARING FOR AN EMERGENCY

Emergencies are unexpected but can and should be anticipated and prepared for in the ambulatory care setting. Being properly prepared assures that the office has the materials and resources needed to respond to emergencies.

An in-office handbook of policies and procedures should be developed and should be familiar to all staff members. Telephone numbers for the local emergency medical services (often this is 911) and the poison control center should be posted and kept in an established place so that there is no delay in calling for outside assistance. Materials and supplies should be maintained in proper inventory. All personnel should be trained in the basics of first aid and CPR, so that every staff member can respond to or assist the physician in providing care. Proper documentation should be completed after any emergency situation. The office environment itself should be a safe one and as accident-proof as possible. Wipe up spills to avoid falls on a slippery floor, keep corridors free of clutter, and keep medications out of sight. These basic **risk management** techniques will help medical personnel focus on giving emergency care and also will protect the facility from possible litigation.

The Medical Crash Tray or Cart

Every health care facility should have a **crash tray or cart,** with a carefully controlled inventory of supplies and equipment (Figure 9-3). These first-aid supplies should be kept in an accessible place, and the inventory should be routinely monitored to assure that all supplies are replaced and that all medications are up to date and have not reached their expiration dates.

A smaller practice may require only a portable tray for emergency and first-aid supplies; larger urgent care centers may respond more frequently to emergencies, and thus may need a cart that can hold a larger inventory and variety of supplies. Whether a tray or cart is used, supplies should be customized to the facility and the type of emergencies frequently encountered. Remember that only physicians can order medications or treatment.

Following is a brief list of some common supplies found on most trays and carts. Also see Chapter 23 "Basic

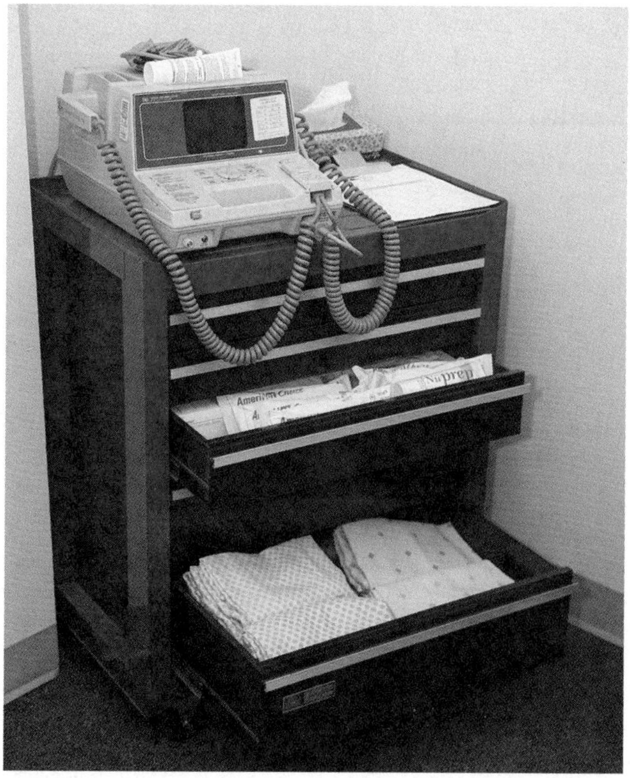

Figure 9-3 Medical crash cart with defibrillator.

Pharmacology" for more information on supplies and medications.

General supplies:

- Adhesive and hypoallergenic tape
- Alcohol wipes
- Bandage scissors
- Bandage material
- Blood pressure cuff (standard, pediatric, large)
- **Constriction band**
- Defibrillator
- Dressing material
- Gloves
- Hot/cold packs
- Intravenous (IV) tubing
- Needles and syringes for injection
- Orange juice for diabetics (refrigerated)
- Penlight (with extra batteries)
- Personal protective equipment
- Stethoscope

Emergency medications	**Uses**
Activated charcoal	Poisonings
Aspirin	Fever, heart attack
Atropine	Slow heartbeat
Dextrose	Insulin reaction
Diazepam*	Antianxiety
Diphenhydramine	Antihistamine
Dopamine	Increases blood pressure
Epinephrine	Constricts blood vessels, increases blood pressure
Glucagon	Insulin reaction
Insulin	Hyperglycemia
Lidocaine	Local anesthetic, IV for cardiac arrhythmia
Nitroglycerin tablets, patches	Chest pain from angina pectoris
Phenobarbital*	Sedative
Verapamil	Hypertension, angina pectoris, irregular heartbeat, tachycardia
Xylocaine, Marcaine	Local anesthetics

*Controlled substance—must be kept in locked cabinet.

Respiratory supplies:

- Airways of all sizes for nasal and oral use
- **Ambu bag™**
- Bulb syringe for suction
- Oxygen mask
- Oxygen tank

This list represents just some of the supplies to be found on a well-stocked crash cart or tray. The type and list of supplies should always be overseen by facility physicians and tailored to the emergency demands of the practice. The medical assistant should be familiar with the equipment and medication on the crash cart or tray. Practice "drills" simulating various emergency situations are helpful for preparing staff members for actual emergencies.

COMMON EMERGENCIES

Included in this discussion of common emergencies are shock, wounds, burns, musculoskeletal injuries, heat- and cold-related illnesses, poisoning, sudden illness, cerebral vascular accident, and heart attack.

Shock

When a severe injury or illness occurs, shock is likely to develop. **Shock** is basically a condition in which the circulatory system is not providing enough blood to all parts of the body, causing the body's organs to fail to function properly.

Shock is always life threatening, and EMS should be activated. The body's attempt to compensate for a massive injury or illness, especially those involving the heart and lungs and severe bleeding, often lead to other problems. During shock, several things occur.

- The heart becomes unable to pump blood properly.
- Consequently, the body's cells, tissues, and organs do not get enough oxygen, which is carried by the blood.
- The body tries to compensate by sending blood to critical organs and reducing the flow of blood to arms, legs, and skin.

Signs and Symptoms of Shock. Learn to recognize the signs and symptoms of shock.

- Patient may be restless or feel irritable.
- Weakness, dizziness, thirst, or nausea may occur.
- Breathing may be shallow and rapid.
- Skin is cool, clammy, and pale.
- Pulse is weak and rapid.
- Blood pressure is low.
- Area around the lips, eyes, and fingernails may turn cyanotic (blue) from lack of oxygen.
- The patient may be confused or become suddenly unconscious, or both.
- Dilated pupils and **lackluster** eyes are obvious.

Types of Shock. There are eight major types of shock, including respiratory, neurogenic, cardiogenic, hemorrhagic, anaphylactic, metabolic, psychogenic, and septic. See Table 9-2 for a description of each.

Treatment for Shock. A person suffering from shock needs immediate medical attention. Call for outside emergency help first, then care for the patient until help arrives. **CAUTION:** Shock requires immediate medical help. Shock is progressive, and if not treated immediately, most types can be life threatening. Once shock reaches a certain point, it is irreversible.

To care for a patient in shock, follow these procedures:

- Lie the patient down. This minimizes pain and decreases stress on the body.
- Loosen clothing.
- Check for an open airway.

TABLE 9-2 EIGHT TYPES OF SHOCK WITH DESCRIPTIONS

Type of Shock	Description
Respiratory	Trauma to the respiratory tract (trachea, lungs) that causes a reduction of oxygen and carbon dioxide exchange. Body cells cannot receive enough oxygen.
Neurogenic	Injury or trauma to the nervous system (spinal cord, brain). Nerve impulse to blood vessels impaired. Blood vessels remain dilated and blood pressure decreases.
Cardiogenic	Myocardial infarction with damage to heart muscle; heart unable to pump effectively. Inadequate cardiac output. Body cells not receiving enough oxygen.
Hemorrhagic	Severe bleeding or loss of body fluid from trauma, burns, surgery, or dehydration from severe nausea and vomiting. Blood pressure decreases, thus blood flow is reduced to cells, tissues, and organs.
Anaphylactic	Results from reaction to substance to which patient is hypersensitive or allergic (allergen extracts, bee sting, medication, food). Outpouring of histamine results in dilation of blood vessels throughout the body, blood pressure decreases and blood flow is reduced to cells, tissue, and organs.
Metabolic	Body's homeostasis impaired; acid–base balance disturbed (diabetic coma or insulin shock); body fluids unbalanced.
Psychogenic	Shock caused by overwhelming emotional factors; i.e., fear, anger, grief. Sudden dilation of blood vessels results in fainting because of lack of blood supply to the brain. In most cases, not life-threatening unless it leads to physical trauma as a result of a fall.
Septic	An acute infection, usually **systemic,** that overwhelms the body (for example, toxic shock syndrome). Poisonous substances accumulate in bloodstream and blood pressure decreases, impairing blood flow to cells, tissues, and organs.

- Check breathing.
- Control any external bleeding.
- Help the patient maintain normal body temperature. A blanket over and under the patient can help avoid chilling. Do not overheat.
- Reassure the patient.
- Elevate the legs about 12 inches, unless you suspect head injury, spinal injuries, or broken bones involving the hips or legs.
- Do not give the patient anything to eat or drink.
- Ascertain that outside help has been called and stay with the patient until help arrives.
- Monitor vital signs.

Wounds

Typically, **wounds** are classified as open wounds or closed wounds. In the closed wound, there is no break in the skin; a bruise, contusion, and hematoma are common closed wounds. An open wound represents a break in the skin and can be classified as an abrasion, avulsion, incision, laceration, or puncture wound.

Closed Wounds. Most closed wounds do not present an emergency situation. If there is pain and swelling, the application of a cold compress can be effective. Protect the patient's skin by placing a cloth beneath the source of cold; apply the compress for 20 minutes, then remove for 20 minutes; continue for 24 hours. Then apply heat 20 minutes on and 20 minutes off for the next 24 hours. A common procedure for treating closed wounds is to RICE or MICE it.

RICE
- *Rest*
- *Ice*
- Compression
- *Elevation*

MICE
- Motion or Movement
- *Ice*
- Compression
- *Elevation*

Recently, some physicians, especially those who treat sport injuries, advocate motion or movement as a means of treating a closed wound injury. They also advise ice, compression (elastic bandage), and elevation (MICE). Check with the physician.

Some closed wounds, such as hematomas, can be dangerous and may cause internal bleeding. If the patient is in severe pain and was subject to an injury caused by high impact, call for help and keep the patient comfortable until the help arrives. Watch for symptoms of shock and monitor vital signs.

Open Wounds. Open wounds can be minor tears in the skin or more serious skin breaks, but all open wounds represent an opportunity for microorganisms to gain entry and cause an infection. Some major open wounds may involve heavy bleeding, which will need to be controlled, probably by suturing. A tetanus injection is indicated for an open wound if the patient has not had a booster in the last 7 to 10 years. See Chapter 10 for immunization information.

There are five common types of open wounds:

1. *Abrasions* are a superficial scraping of the epidermis. Because nerve endings are involved, they can be painful. However, they are not usually serious, unless they cover a large area of the body. Administer first aid by cleaning the area carefully with soap and water, apply an antiseptic ointment if prescribed by a physician, and cover with a dressing.
2. In an *avulsion*, the skin is torn off and bleeding is profuse. Avulsion wounds often occur at exposed parts: fingers, toes, ear. First, control bleeding (see Procedure 9-1) if necessary. Then clean the wound. If there is a skin flap, reposition it. Apply a dressing, then bandage as necessary. Note that pieces of the body may be torn away. If possible, save the body part, keep moist, and transport with the patient.
3. *Incisions* are wounds that result from a sharp object, such as a knife or piece of glass. Incisions may need sutures. The wound must be cleaned with soap and water and a dressing applied.
4. *Lacerations* tear the body tissue and can be difficult to clean; therefore, care must be taken to avoid infection. If there is not severe bleeding, which in itself is a cleansing mechanism, these wounds may need to be soaked in antiseptic soap and water to remove debris. If there is severe bleeding, it must be controlled immediately (see Procedure 9-1). Lacerations with severe bleeding usually need suturing.
5. *Punctures* pierce and penetrate the skin and may be deep wounds while appearing insignificant. Usually, external bleeding is minimal, but the patient should be assessed for internal bleeding. Because a puncture wound is deep, the risk for infection is great and the patient should be advised to watch for signals of infection, such as pain, swelling, redness, throbbing, and warmth.

Use of Tourniquets in Emergency Care. In the past, tourniquets were regularly used in the field to control hemorrhaging from an extremity when all other attempts to control bleeding were unsuccessful. However, because tourniquet application was meant to completely stop blood flow, many times this complete lack of blood flow resulted in the death of the arm or leg. Often, the affected extremity needed to be amputated.

To remedy this situation, a "constriction band" was substituted for the tourniquet and is now widely used. The constriction band is made of a material similar to that used in the tourniquet. When the band is applied to an extremity to control bleeding, it is applied tightly enough to stem the rapid loss of blood but loosely enough to allow a small amount of blood to continue to flow. A pulse should be felt distally to the constriction band. The use of the constriction band applied in this manner allows a blood supply to the remainder of the extremity unlike the tourniquet, which cuts off all blood flow. See Chapter 19 for information on wounds and minor surgery.

Dressings and Bandages. When a patient presents with an open wound, after the physician has treated the wound, it is critical to dress and bandage it properly to curtail infection. Covering of the wound is accomplished by a series of **dressings** and **bandages.**

Typically, dressings are sterile gauze pads placed directly on the wound; they often have nonstick, sterile surfaces, but they are absorbent and will soak up blood and protect the wound from microorganisms. They are often made of a gauze-type material.

Bandages, which are nonsterile, are placed over the dressing. They hold the dressing in place and are made to conform to the area to be covered. Sometimes, as in a Band-Aid®, the dressing and bandage are combined. Roller bandages, such as those made of elastic, can be placed over a dressing and used to help control bleeding or swelling.

Kling gauze, a type of gauze that stretches and clings as it is applied, and roller bandages, long strips of soft material wound on itself, are other types of bandage materials.

Bandages and their applications can take many shapes and forms, depending on the type of injury and the injury site. In all cases, a bandage must be secure, but not constricting. Avoid too tight or too loose a wrap.

- Spiral bandages are useful for injuries to the arms or legs (Figure 9-4).
- A figure-eight bandage will hold the dressing in place on a wound on the hand or wrist, knee, or ankle (Figure 9-5).
- Fingers, toes, arms, and legs can also be bandaged using a tubular gauze bandage (Figures 9-6, 9-7, and 9-8). Using a cylindrical applicator, a quantity of gauze is stretched over the wound site.
- Commercial arm slings are used to support injured or fractured arms (Figure 9-9). To apply, support the injured arm above and below the injury site while applying the sling.

Burns

Most burns are commonly caused by heat, chemicals, explosions, and electricity. Critical burns can be life threatening and require immediate medical care. Accord-

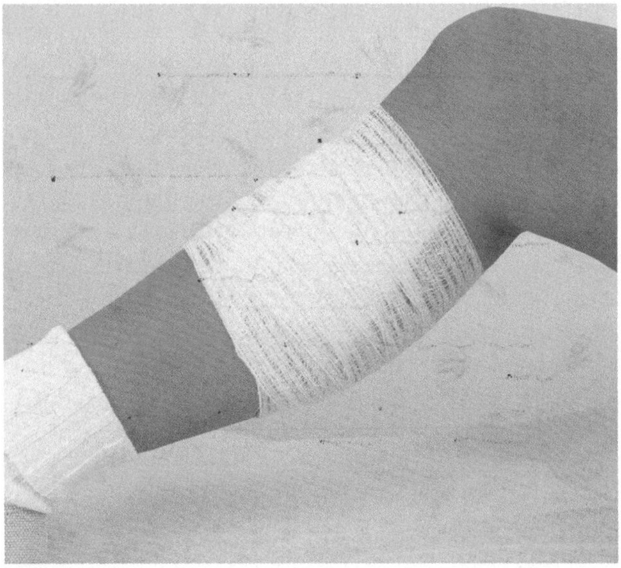

Figure 9-4 The spiral bandage is an option for arm and leg injuries.

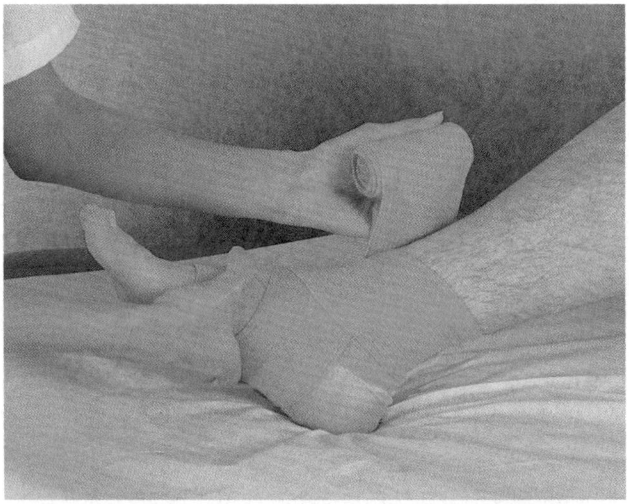

Figure 9-5 An elastic figure-eight bandage holds dressings in place or can be used for immobilization as with an ankle sprain.

ing to the American Red Cross, critical burns have the following characteristics:

- Involve breathing difficulty
- Cover more than one body part
- Involve the head, neck, hands, feet, or genitals
- Involve any burns to a child or older adult (other than minor burns)

To distinguish critical from minor burns, it is important to understand the degrees of burns and what they mean.

First-, Second-, and Third-Degree Burns. First-degree burns are superficial burns that involve only the top layer of skin. The skin appears red, feels dry, is warm to the touch, and is painful. First-degree burns usually heal in a week or so with no permanent scarring.

In a second-degree burn, the skin is red and blisters are present. The healing process is slower, usually a month, and some scarring may occur. Second-degree burns affect the top layers of the skin, are very painful, and may take three to four weeks to heal. Some scarring may occur.

Third-degree burns are the most serious, affecting or destroying all layers of skin. It is not unusual for fat, muscles, bones, and nerves to be involved. These burns look charred or brown. There may be great pain or, if nerve endings are destroyed, the burn may be painless. Victims of third-degree burns must receive immediate medical attention both for the burn and for shock. Of serious con-

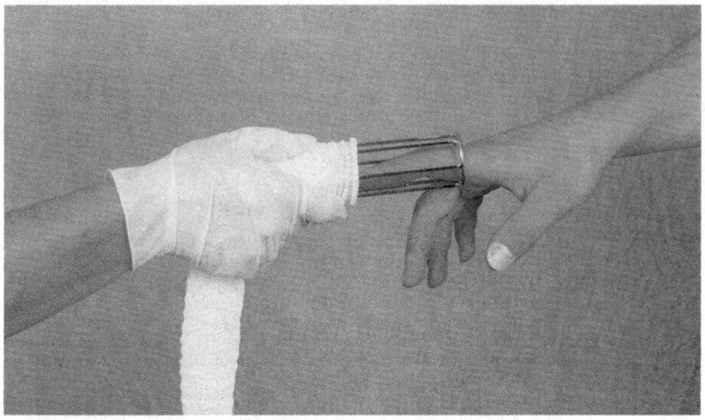

Figure 9-6 There are several types and sizes of tubular gauze applicators, including plastic, solid metal, and metal cage applicators; the metal cage is shown here. All applicators use a seamless elastic gauze bandage (also available in various sizes) that slides over the applicator. The applicator with the gauze then fits over the appendage to be wrapped.

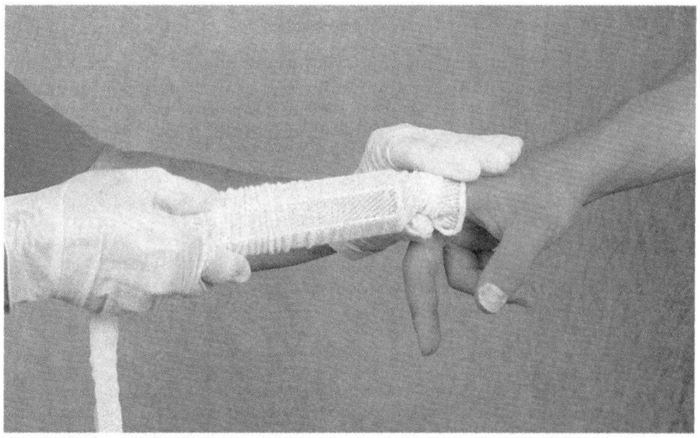

Figure 9-7 The gauze bandage is stretched over the appendage by pulling the applicator away from the base of the appendage. At the same time, the bandage should be held in place at the appendage base with the other hand.

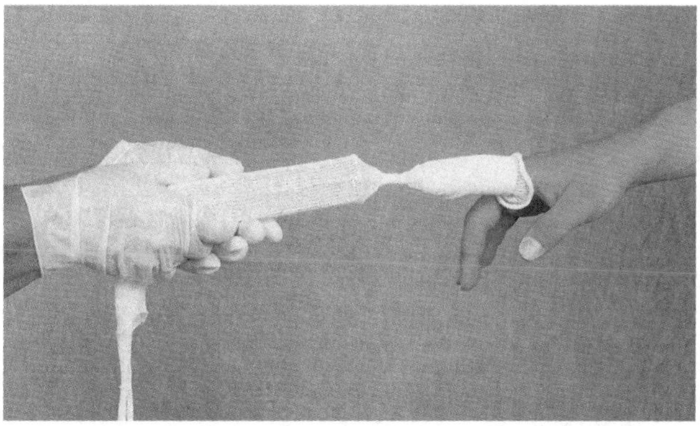

Figure 9-8 Once the applicator has been pulled off the finger, a layer of the bandage will remain on the appendage. To apply another layer, the applicator is again fitted over the finger and a new layer is applied in the same manner as before.

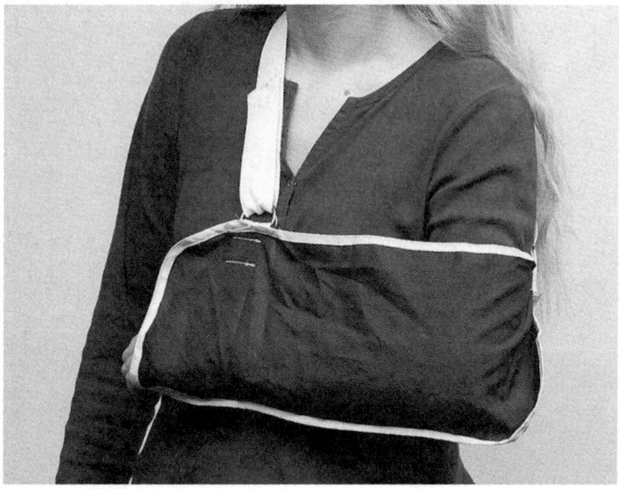

Figure 9-9 A commercial sling is used to support injured or fractured arms.

cern with a third-degree burn is the likelihood of infection and the amount of fluid loss. Scarring can result in loss of body function. Skin grafts may be necessary.

Figure 9-10 shows the relative penetration level of each degree of burn into the skin and underlying structures.

General Guidelines for Caring for Burns. Treatment for burns depends on the type of agent causing the burn. General treatment strategies for any degree of burn include the following:

- Cool the burn with large amounts of cool normal saline, or water if saline is unavailable.
- Cover the burn with a sterile dressing if one is available and burn is minor. Otherwise, cover the burn with a sheet or other smooth textured cloth for a burn over a large area of the body.
- Be sure the patient is protected from being either chilled or overheated.

However, it is important to follow these guidelines:

- Do not apply ice or ice water to a burn.
- Do not touch a burn, except with a sterile dressing.
- Do not clean a severe burn, break blisters, or use any kind of ointment.
- Do not remove pieces of clothing that may be sticking to the burn.

First Aid for Burns. First aid for burns is outlined in Table 9-3.

Types of Burns. Most burns are caused by heat; however, burns can also be caused by chemicals, electricity, and solar radiation.

Chemical Burns. Chemical burns can occur in the workplace or even in the home with "ordinary" household chemicals. To stop the burning process, you must remove the chemical from the skin. Have someone call an ambu-

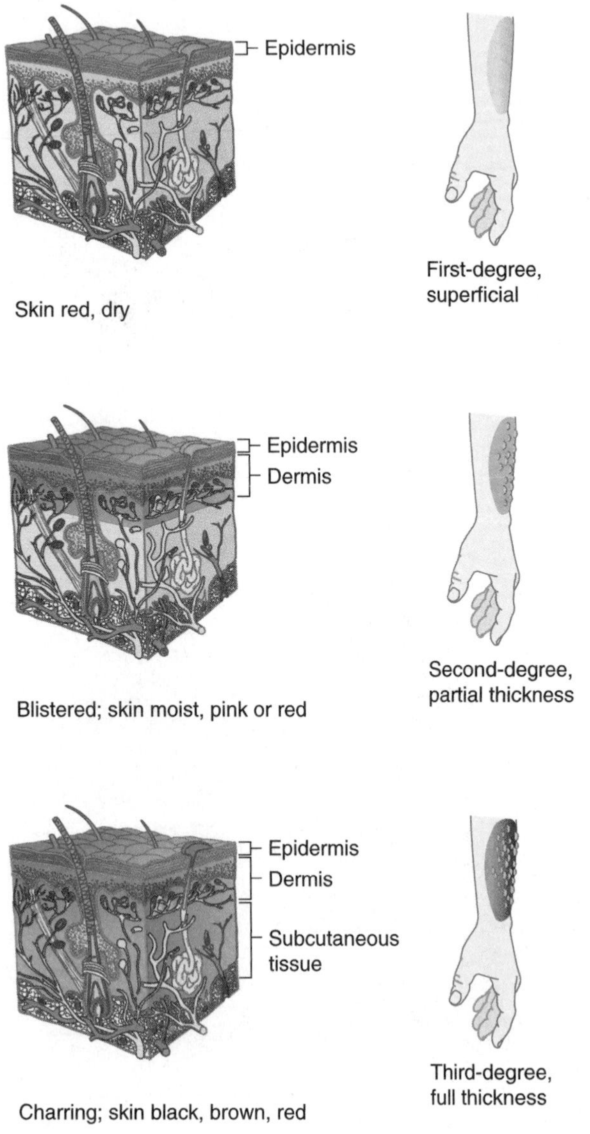

Figure 9-10 Classification of burn injuries.

Patient Education

Some burns can be prevented. Advise patients who insist on sunbathing to protect themselves against harmful rays by using a sunscreen and avoiding the sun between 10 AM and 2 PM.

Patient Education

Advise patients not to run should their clothing catch on fire. They should fall to the ground or wrap themselves in a blanket or rug and roll on the ground to extinguish the flames.

lance while you flush the skin or eyes with cool water. Remove any clothing contaminated by the chemicals unless they adhere to the skin. If clothing clings to the skin, it can be cut with scissors. Do not attempt to pull clothing away from a burned area.

Electrical Burns. Electrical burns can be caused by power lines, lightning, or faulty electrical equipment in the home or workplace. *It is important to remember never to go near a patient injured by electricity until you are sure the power has been shut off, because you*

TABLE 9-3 FIRST AID FOR BURNS

First-Degree Burn Response Guide

Questions	Responses	Action to Take	Rationale
Is skin reddened without blisters?	YES ⇨	Submerge in cool **normal saline** or water 2–5 minutes. ⇨	Stops burning process.
NO ⇩			
Does area involve: • hands? • feet? • genitals? • face?	YES ⇨	Have patient come to office. ⇨	These are potential danger areas and require evaluation by the physician.
NO ⇩			
Is patient: • elderly? • very young?	YES ⇨	Have patient come to office. ⇨	These groups are susceptible to burn complications.
NO ⇩			
Consult physician.			Physician has final decision whether patient is seen.

Second-Degree Burn Response Guide

Questions	Responses	Action to Take	Rationale
Is skin reddened with blisters or splitting of the skin?	YES ⇨	Submerge in cool normal saline or water 10–15 minutes if skin is intact. Use compresses if skin is broken. Do not break blisters. Do not use anesthetic creams or sprays. ⇨	Stops burning process. If blisters are broken, can allow infection in burn. Creams or spray may slow healing process and increase severity of a burn.
NO ⇩			
Does area involve: • hands? • feet? • genitals? • face?	YES ⇨	Have patient come to office or go to the emergency department. ⇨	These are potentially dangerous areas and require medical attention.
NO ⇩			
Is the area involved larger than a child's hand?	YES ⇨	Have patient come to office or go to the emergency department. ⇨	Burns of this size are susceptible to complications.
NO ⇩			
Is patient experiencing trouble breathing?	YES ⇨	Patient should go to emergency department. ⇨	There may be swelling of the airways because of heat and noxious fumes.
NO ⇩			
Consult physician.			Physician has final decision whether patient is seen.

(continues)

TABLE 9-3 FIRST AID FOR BURNS (continued)

Third-Degree Burn Response Guide

Questions	Responses	Action to Take	Rationale
Is skin gray, black, or charred appearing? Can muscle, fat, or bone be seen in wound?	YES ⇨	Call EMS immediately. Do not apply cold; do not remove burnt clothing from burn area. ⇨	Life-threatening emergency that requires prompt attention.
NO ⇩			
Is patient experiencing: • pallor • loss of consciousness? • shivering?	YES ⇨	Patient in shock: • call EMS. • maintain airway. • maintain body temp. • elevate feet if appropriate. • monitor breathing. • may need oxygen and intravenous fluids while waiting for EMS to arrive. ⇨	Need to control shock caused by fluid loss.
NO ⇩			
Consult physician.			Physician has final decision whether patient is seen.

could be injured. If there is a downed line, call the power company and EMS.

A victim of an electricity burn may be suffering from two burns: one where the power entered the body, and one where it exited. Often, the burns themselves may be minor. Of more serious consequence are the possibilities of shock, breathing difficulties, and other injuries. CPR often is needed in this situation.

Solar Radiation. Most "sunburns," although not advisable or good for the skin, represent minor burns. If the patient has a severe burn, however, he or she should see a physician who will cover the burn area to reduce infection and protect the patient against chill.

Musculoskeletal Injuries

Most injuries to muscles, bones, and joints are not life threatening, but they are painful and, if not properly treated, can be disabling. Some injuries, such as those to the spinal cord, can be quite serious and can result in paralysis. These injuries are not typically seen in the ambulatory care setting.

Types of Injuries. A **sprain** is an injury to a joint, often an ankle, knee, or wrist, that involves a tearing of the ligaments. Some sprains are minor and heal quickly; others are more severe, include swelling, and may not heal properly if the patient continues to put stress on the sprained joint. Signs of a sprain are rapid swelling, discoloration at the site, and limited function. Many times it is difficult to determine whether the patient has sustained a sprain or a fracture because the degree of pain may not be a true indicator of the patient's injury. As with most closed wounds, treating the injury with the RICE or MICE method is beneficial, and determined by the physician's choice.

A **strain** results from the overuse or stretching of a muscle or group of muscles, as with improper lifting or moving heavy objects. Applications of ice and heat (as described for treatment of sprains), as well as rest, are indicated for treatment of strains.

Dislocations are painful and involve the separation of a bone from its normal position. These usually occur from the kind of wrenching motion that might result from a fall, automobile accident, or sports injury.

Fractures involve a break in a bone and can be caused by a fall, by a blow, from bone disease, or from sports injuries. There are several types of fractures, but all are classified as either open or closed fractures. An open fracture involves an open wound and is characterized by a protruding bone. In a closed fracture, the skin is not broken. Signs and symptoms that occur with a fracture may include swelling, discoloration, pain, deformity, and immobility of the body part. It is not unusual for patients to tell you that they heard the bone break or that they sensed a grating feeling. **Crepitation** is the term that describes the grating sensation experienced or heard when bone fragments rub together. Fractures are further defined as follows:

- Incomplete or greenstick: fracture in which the bone has cracked, but the break is not all the way through; frequently seen in children

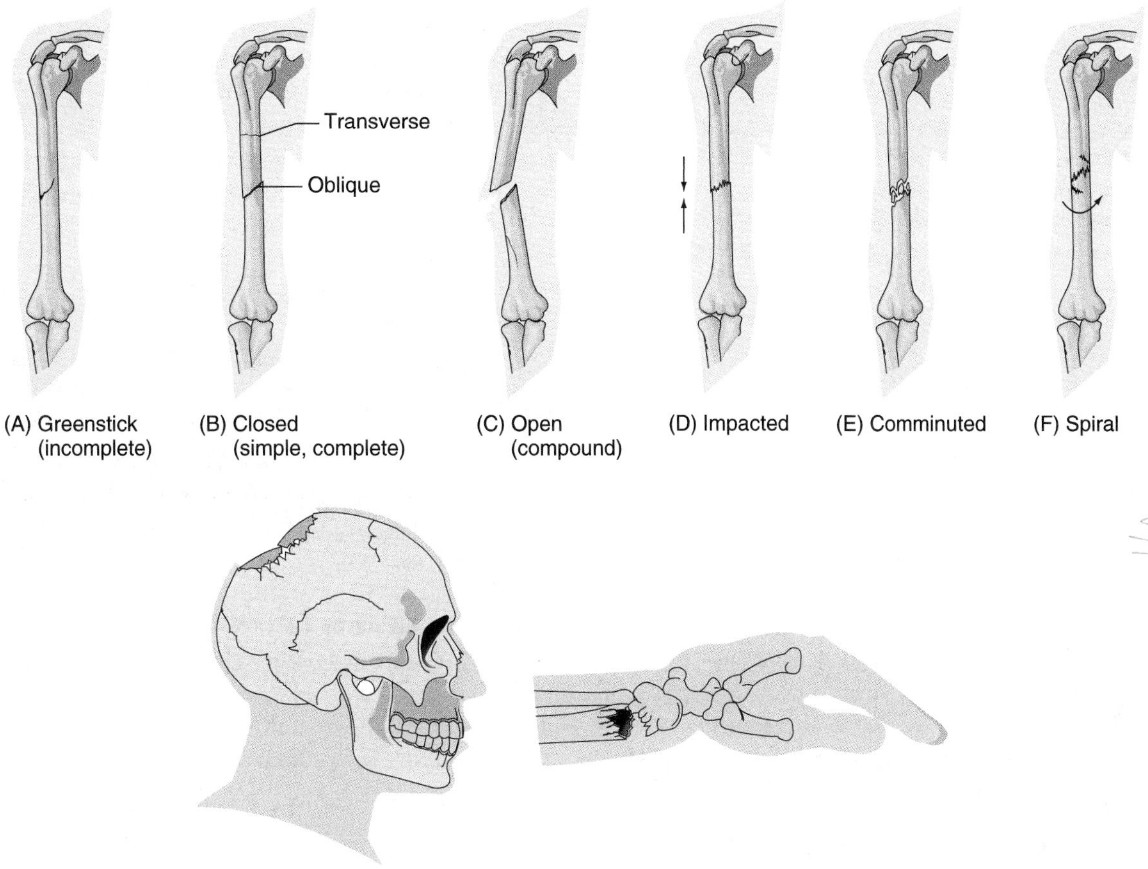

Figure 9-11 Types of fractures.

- Simple: complete bone break in which there is no involvement with the skin surface
- Compound: fracture in which the bone protrudes though the skin surface, creating the possibility of infection
- Impacted: fracture in which the broken ends are jammed into each other
- Comminuted: more than one fracture line and several bone fragments are present
- Spiral: fracture that occurs with a severe twisting action, causing the break to wind around the bone
- Depressed: fracture that occurs with severe head injuries in which a broken piece of skull is driven inward
- Colles: fracture often caused by falling on an outstretched hand; involves the distal end of the radius and results in displacement, causing a bulge at the wrist

See Figure 9-11 for examples of these fractures.

Assessing Injuries to Muscles, Bones, and Joints. Sometimes it is difficult to determine the extent of an injury, especially in closed fractures. There are some assessment techniques to call on, however, to gauge the seriousness of an injury.

- Note the extent of bruising and swelling.
- Pain is a signal of injury.
- There may be noticeable deformity to the bone or joint.
- Use of the injured area is limited.
- Talk to the patient: What was the cause of the injury? What was the sound or sensation at the time of injury?

Caring for Muscle, Bone, and Joint Injuries. Most injuries to muscles, bones, and joints are treated in a similar way; some require rest, some motion, elevation of the injured part, immobilization, and the application of ice to the injury.

After calling for outside care (always check for life-threatening symptoms, such as breathing difficulties, bleeding, or head, neck, or back injuries), it is important to immobilize the injured area if the patient must be moved. EMS personnel use a variety of **splints** to immobilize bones and joints. See Procedure 9-2 for splinting an arm in the ambulatory care setting.

Heat- and Cold-Related Illnesses

The condition of patients who have been subject to extreme heat and cold can deteriorate rapidly, and either a heat- or cold-related illness can result in death. Individuals especially vulnerable to extreme exposures include the very young and very old, individuals who must work out of doors, and people who suffer from poor circulation.

Heat-Related Illnesses. Illnesses related to heat, in increasing degree of severity, include heat cramps, heat exhaustion, and heat stroke. Heat cramps, the least serious, involve cramping in the legs and abdomen caused by excessive body exposure or exercise in hot weather. Heat cramps should be considered a signal to stop, slow down, rest in a cool place, and drink plenty of water. Salt tablets should not be taken. The individual should lightly stretch the muscles. Heat cramps can progress to heat exhaustion or heat stroke, both of which are more serious conditions.

Heat exhaustion, often experienced by people who work or exercise in extreme heat, is a more serious reaction and is signaled by exhaustion, cold and clammy skin, profuse sweating, headache, and general weakness. The individual should come out of the heat immediately, apply cool, wet towels, and slowly drink cool water. The physician will advise the patient not to resume activity in the heat.

Heat stroke is the least common but the most dangerous of heat-related illnesses and requires immediate medical attention. Heat stroke is characterized by red, dry, hot skin; an abnormal, weak pulse; and breathing that is shallow and fast. In heat stroke, the body systems are extremely taxed. EMS should be alerted; until they arrive, stay with the patient, watch for breathing problems, and attempt to reduce body temperature by applying cool, wet towels or sheets.

Cold-Related Illnesses. Exposure to extreme cold for prolonged periods can lead to frostbite or hypothermia.

Frostbite, which typically affects the extremities such as fingers, toes, ears, and nose, involves the freezing of exposed body parts. Symptoms include skin that becomes off-color, is cold, or takes on a waxy appearance. Severity can range from the superficial (frostnip) to more penetrating stages, which may require amputation.

Individuals with frostbite need immediate medical attention. To care for frostbitten extremities, warm the area of injury by wrapping clothing or blankets around the affected body part. Be careful in handling the frozen part. It is best to have the patient transported as soon as possible to emergency care. This type of facility is better able to properly rewarm the frozen part, preventing further tissue damage.

Hypothermia is a serious illness in which the body temperature decreases to a perilously low level. It can result in death if the individual does not receive care and if the progression of hypothermia is not reversed. Hypothermia occurs when a person falls through the ice or is exposed to cold temperatures, for example, after getting lost in the woods while hiking. Symptoms include shivering, cold skin, and confusion.

After checking for breathing problems and alerting EMS, care for the patient. Make the individual comfortable, provide a source of warmth, such as a blanket, and *gradually* warm the body. If clothing is wet or cold, remove and put on dry clothing. In extreme cases, it may be necessary to provide rescue breathing (discussed later in this chapter).

Poisoning

Poisons can enter the body in four ways:

- *Ingestion*. Ingested poisons enter the body by swallowing. Swallowed poisons may include medications, plant material, household chemicals, contaminated foods, and drugs.
- *Inhalation*. Poisons are inhaled into the body in poorly ventilated areas where cleaning fluids, paints and chemical cleaners, or carbon monoxide may be present.
- *Absorption*. Poisons absorbed through the skin include plant materials such as poison oak or ivy, lawn care products such as chemical pesticides, and other chemical powders or liquids.
- *Injection*. Drug abuse is the most common cause of injected poisons. The stingers of insects inject poisons into the body and can be extremely dangerous and can lead to anaphylactic shock in allergic individuals.

Whenever a patient calls regarding poisoning or there is a suspicion of poisoning, call the local poison control center or the local emergency number and ask for advice. Telephone numbers of the poison control center should be posted in a familiar and accessible place.

Patient Education

Remind patients who are parents of young children to remove any potential sources of poisoning from their homes or to keep them in locked cabinets. Also advise them to include the nearby poison control center in their list of emergency phone numbers. They should also keep activated charcoal on hand.

The treatment for poisoning will vary according to the source of the poisoning and must be tailored to the specific incident. The physician will have advised staff regarding specific poisoning antidotes. Generally, do not give the patient anything to eat or drink; try to determine what poison the patient was exposed to and, if ingested, how much was taken; if the patient vomits, save some of the vomitus for analysis.

If prescribed by a physician or recommended by the poison control center, medication used to treat poisoning is activated charcoal, which is used to absorb certain swallowed poisons.

Insect Stings. The medical assistant in the ambulatory care setting is likely to receive a number of calls every summer from patients who have been stung by insects, typically yellow jackets, hornets, honeybees, or wasps. In the nonallergic patient, the sting is likely to result in localized swelling and tenderness and slight redness. The physician will recommend that these localized symptoms be managed with a topical cream and oral antihistamines. Swelling can be significant and cause for serious concern if the sting occurred in a vulnerable area of the body such as the mouth or tongue. Swelling in these locations can be frightening and dangerous because it can impair breathing. An antihistamine, administered as soon as possible after the sting, may help to curtail symptoms somewhat. Treatment for insect stings in nonallergic individuals consists of removing the stinger by scraping it off with the edge of something rigid such as a credit card or your fingernail. Tweezers can cause more venom to be dispersed into the patient's body tissues, so this method should not be used. Wash the area with soap and water, apply a cold pack to the site, and watch for a possible severe reaction.

The individual who experiences an allergic reaction or hypersensitivity to a sting needs to be seen immediately, because in severe cases a sting may induce an anaphylactic reaction that can lead to death. If allergic, individuals who have been stung are likely to experience symptoms within a half hour of the incident. Symptoms are generalized throughout the body and may include hives, itching, and lightheadedness, and may progress to difficulty breathing, faintness, and eventual loss of consciousness.

Patient Education

Advise all patients with known allergic reactions to be particularly careful when working or playing outdoors. Insects are not usually aggressive until their nests are approached; however, often these nests are not easy to detect, and an individual may approach one without being aware of its presence. Patients with allergies to insects should always wear shoes when outside, wear light-colored clothing, preferably with long sleeves and pant legs, look before taking a sip from a beverage when outdoors, and inspect lawn areas, shrubbery, and building walls periodically for evidence of stinging insect nests.

For individuals with known allergic reactions, the physician will prescribe epinephrine, which patients should carry with them and self-inject should they not be able to get immediate emergency care. EPIPEN is a brand of epinephrine to self-inject. The patient should then seek immediate emergency treatment. For individuals who present at the ambulatory care setting with an apparent allergic reaction to a sting, the physician will prescribe epinephrine, an antihistamine, and corticosteroids if necessary. Attempt to allay patient apprehension and monitor vital signs while waiting for EMS personnel to arrive.

Sudden Illness

Sudden illness is, by definition, an unexpected occurrence. Although the cause of the illness may be inexplicable, it is important to respond sensibly and responsibly within the parameters of knowledge and resources.

Sudden illnesses include, but are not limited to, fainting, seizures, diabetic reaction, and hemorrhage.

Fainting. Also known as **syncope,** fainting involves a loss of consciousness, caused by an insufficient supply of blood to the brain. Loss of consciousness may simply be the result of a fainting episode, or it may indicate a more serious medical problem such as diabetic coma or shock. A fall during a fainting incident may result in bodily harm.

If a patient in the office or clinic "feels faint," indicated by lightheadedness, weakness, nausea, or unsteadiness, have the individual lie down or sit down with head level with the knees. This may prevent a fainting episode.

If a patient faints, gradually lower the patient to a flat surface, loosen any tight clothing, check breathing and for any life-threatening emergencies, and apply cool compresses to forehead. Elevate the legs if there is no back or head injury. If vomiting occurs, place the patient on his or her side. Although fainting is typically not serious in itself, 911 or EMS may need to be called because the problem may be indicative of a more complex medical condition.

Seizures. Seizures or convulsions occur when normal brain functioning is disrupted, which can occur for a variety of reasons including fever, disease such as diabetes, infection, or injury to the brain. Epilepsy is a common cause of convulsions. Involuntary spasms or contractions of muscles characterize seizures.

To the onlooker, seizures look frightening and painful, which may lead inexperienced individuals to try to stop the seizure when they see it occurring in another individual. A patient experiencing a seizure should never be restrained; simply care for the victim of a seizure with compassion and medical understanding. The goal is to protect the patient from self-injury during the episode. Also, do not force anything between the patient's clenched teeth—individuals experiencing seizures cannot "swallow" their tongues.

Most patients will recover from a seizure in a few minutes. During the seizure, protect the patient from injury, cushion the patient's head, and roll the patient to the side if any fluid is in the mouth. After the seizure subsides, calm and comfort the patient.

If a patient is known to regularly have seizures, and the patient's seizure subsides in a matter of minutes, EMS personnel usually do not need to be summoned. Repeated seizures during the same time frame, however, dictate a call to emergency services, as does any seizure if the patient is diabetic, pregnant, injured, or does not regain consciousness after the incident.

Diabetes. Diabetes is defined by the American Diabetes Society as the "inability of the body to properly convert sugar from food into energy."

Under normal functioning, the body produces a hormone called insulin, which transports sugars into body cells. In some cases, the body does not produce insulin at all or does not produce enough; this results in diabetes.

Diabetes occurs in two major types:

- Type I, or insulin-dependent diabetes
- Type II, or noninsulin-dependent diabetes, which usually occurs in adults; in type II, the body produces insulin in insufficient quantities

Complications from diabetes, which you may encounter in a medical office or clinic setting, include diabetic coma (acidosis) and insulin shock or reaction. The physician will prescribe either insulin or glucose before the patient is transported to the hospital. Both are serious emergencies that require immediate EMS assistance. See Table 9-4 for common causes and symptoms of diabetic coma or insulin shock.

Hemorrhage. The different sources of bleeding determine the seriousness of hemorrhage, or bleeding.

External Bleeding. External bleeding includes capillary, venous, and arterial bleeding. Capillary bleeding, often from cuts and scratches, usually clots without first-aid measures. Bleeding from a vein, which is characterized by dark red blood that flows steadily, needs to be controlled quickly (see Procedure 9-1) to avoid excessive blood loss. Bleeding from an artery produces bright red bleeding that spurts from the wound; this is the most serious type of bleeding and occurs when an artery is punctured or severed. Like venous bleeding, arterial bleeding requires immediate emergency care, because serious loss of blood and profound irreversible shock can quickly ensue.

Epistaxis, or nosebleed, may be the result of breathing dry air for a long period; result from injury or blowing the nose too hard; caused by high altitudes; caused by hypertension (high blood pressure); or result from overuse of medications such as aspirin and anticoagulants.

To control nosebleeds, seat the patient, elevate the patient's head, and pinch the nostrils for at least 10 min-

Patient Education

Advise the patient not to blow the nose for several hours after an epistaxis.

TABLE 9-4 CAUSES AND SYMPTOMS OF DIABETIC COMA AND INSULIN SHOCK

Diabetic Coma or Acidosis		Insulin Shock or Reaction	
Causes	Too little insulin, too much to eat, infections, fever, emotional stress	Causes	Too much insulin or oral hypoglycemic drug, too little to eat, an unusual amount of exercise
Symptoms	Skin: Dry and flushed	Symptoms	Skin: Moist and pale
	Behavior: Drowsy		Behavior: Often excited
	Mouth: Dry		Mouth: Drooling
	Thirst: Intense		Thirst: Absent
	Hunger: Absent		Hunger: Present
	Vomiting: Common		Vomiting: Usually absent
	Respiration: Exaggerated, air hungry		Respiration: Normal or shallow
	Breath: Fruity odor of acetone		Breath: Usually normal
	Pulse: Weak and rapid		Pulse: Full and pounding (gives patient feeling of heart pounding)
	Vision: Dim		Vision: Diplopia (double)
	Blood glucose greater than 200 mg/100 ml		Low blood glucose level (40–70 mg/100 ml or less)
First aid	Keep patient warm	First aid	If conscious, give patient sugar or any food containing sugar (fruit juice, candy, crackers)
	Obtain medical help immediately		Obtain medical help immediately

utes. Assist the patient to sit with head tilted forward so blood running down the back of the throat will not be swallowed. If bleeding cannot be controlled, the physician may request that you activate EMS. The patient's nostril may need to be **cauterized** or a gauze packing inserted.

Internal Bleeding. Internal bleeding may be minor or serious depending on the cause of the injury. A contusion, or bruise, will result in minor internal bleeding. A sharp blow may induce severe internal bleeding.

Because there is no visible blood flow, it is important to recognize other symptoms of internal bleeding. Symptoms are similar to those of shock and include a rapid and weak pulse, low blood pressure, shallow breathing, cold and clammy skin, dilated pupils, dizziness, faintness, thirst, restlessness, and a feeling of anxiety. There may be pain, tenderness, or swelling at the injury site. The abdomen may be boardlike.

If internal bleeding is suspected, ask another staff member to call EMS; until they arrive, stay with the patient and take measures to prevent shock. Monitor vital signs.

Cerebral Vascular Accident

The common term for a cerebral vascular accident (CVA) is stroke. A stroke is the result of a ruptured blood vessel in the brain; it can also be caused by the **occlusion** of a blood vessel or by a clot. Both these situations can result in blood spilling over brain cells and depriving them of oxygen, causing them to die. Symptoms of a stroke include numbness in face, arm, and leg on one side of the body; loss of vision; severe headache, mental confusion; slurred speech; nausea; vomiting; and difficulty in breathing and swallowing. Paralysis may be present. If a patient is suspected of having a stroke, call EMS, loosen tight clothing, lie the patient down, and keep him or her comfortable. Position the patient's head to facilitate the flow of secretion from the mouth to avoid choking and maintain an open airway. Do not give anything by mouth and monitor vital signs. Immediate emergency care is critical for all individuals experiencing strokes. If the stroke is caused by a clot that blocks blood flow, drugs may be able to protect the individual from permanent injury. Rapid transport to the hospital is important for treatment to be instituted as soon as possible. Treatment with the clot-dissolving drug must be given within a certain time frame after onset of symptoms for it to be effective.

Heart Attack

Heart attack, also known as myocardial infarction, is usually caused by blockage of one or more of the coronary arteries. Symptoms include tightness of the chest, pain radiating down one or both arms, or pain radiating into the left shoulder and jaw. Other signs include rapid and weak pulse, excessive perspiration, agitation, nausea, and cold and clammy skin. Heart attack symptoms in a woman may or may not be similar to those experienced by a man. Women may have symptoms such as abdominal discomfort, burning sensation in the chest, discomfort or pain in the lower chest or back, unexplained sudden fatigue, sweating, and breathlessness.

If you suspect the patient is experiencing a heart attack, contact EMS immediately, loosen tight clothing, and keep the patient comfortable. Prepare to give oxygen and other medications such as aspirin, as directed by the physician. Monitor vital signs. If the patient experiences an episode of cardiac fibrillation, **cardioversion** or defibrillation may be necessary with an automatic external defibrillator. See Chapter 25. Prepare to begin CPR if necessary.

PROCEDURES FOR BREATHING EMERGENCIES AND CARDIAC ARREST

Breathing or respiratory emergencies occur for a variety of reasons, including choking, shock, allergies, and other illnesses or injuries such as drowning and electrical shock. When an individual stops breathing, artificial or rescue breathing must be given quickly, for without a constant supply of oxygen, brain damage or death will occur.

When the breathing problem is accompanied by cardiac arrest, the rescue breathing must be accompanied by chest compressions. This is known as **cardiopulmonary resuscitation (CPR).** Cardiac emergencies may occur in the medical office because of the large number of patients who have heart disease.

The procedures that follow will help you respond to breathing emergencies in your clinic or office until EMS arrives. The techniques vary for conscious and unconscious individuals, and for adults, children, and infants. These procedures are for review purposes only; it is essential that every medical assistant attain provider-level CPR certification and take first-aid training courses as stated in the curriculum content of CAAHEP Standards and Guidelines. Frequent refresher courses and recertification in CPR are necessary.

> **Patient Education**
>
> Teach patients to perform the abdominal thrust when they are alone and choking. To perform the Heimlich maneuver when alone, use the fist or thrust against a chair back or any other hard object of adequate height that reaches just below the navel. See Figure 9-14.

Heimlich Maneuver (Abdominal Thrust)

A common cause of breathing difficulty results from choking. If an individual signals distress from choking, assist the patient in coughing up the object (Figures 9-12 and 9-13). If the patient cannot cough up the object, and the breathing airway is becoming completely blocked, act immediately. It is apparent that the airway is becoming blocked when the patient cannot cough or speak and the patient uses the universal sign for choking.

Have someone call an ambulance while you perform abdominal thrusts, known as the **Heimlich maneuver.** Patients can be taught to give themselves abdominal thrusts if they are alone and choking (Figure 9-14).

Procedures 9-3, 9-4, 9-5, 9-6, and 9-7 describe how to perform the Heimlich maneuver for adults, children,

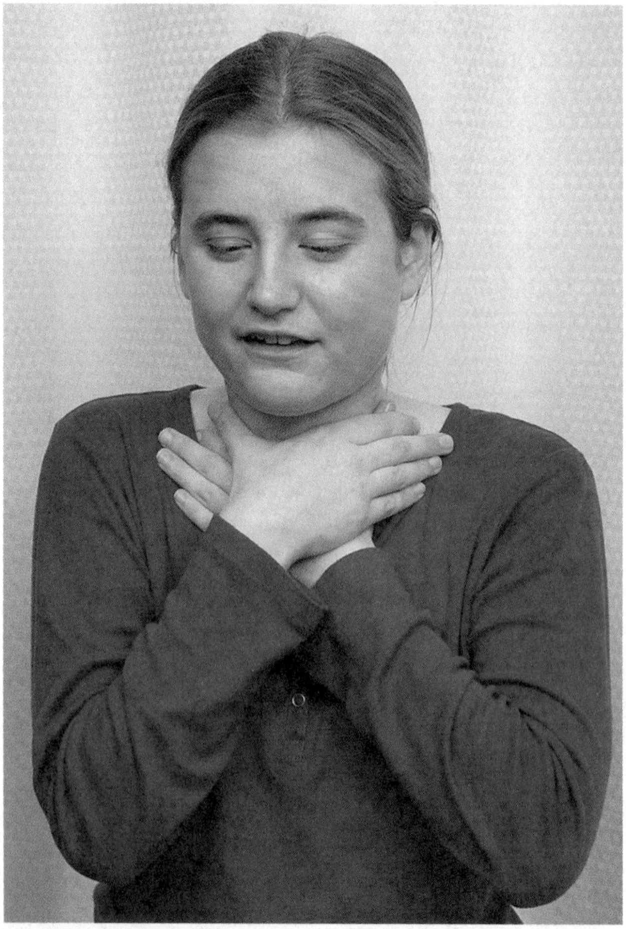

Figure 9-12 Universal sign for choking.

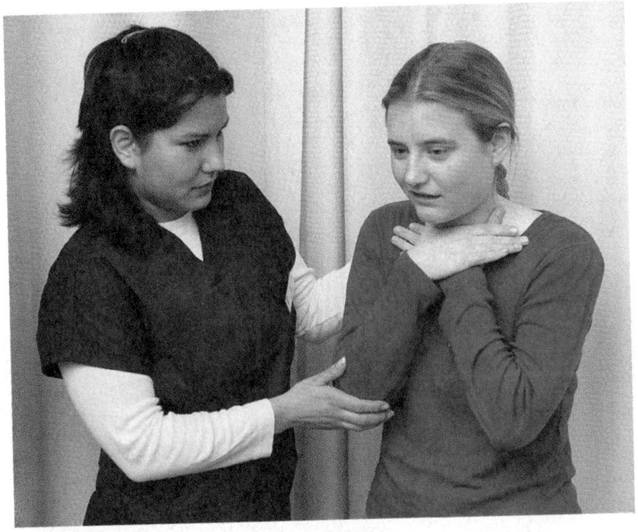

Figure 9-13 Assist the patient in coughing up an object by encouraging continuous coughing.

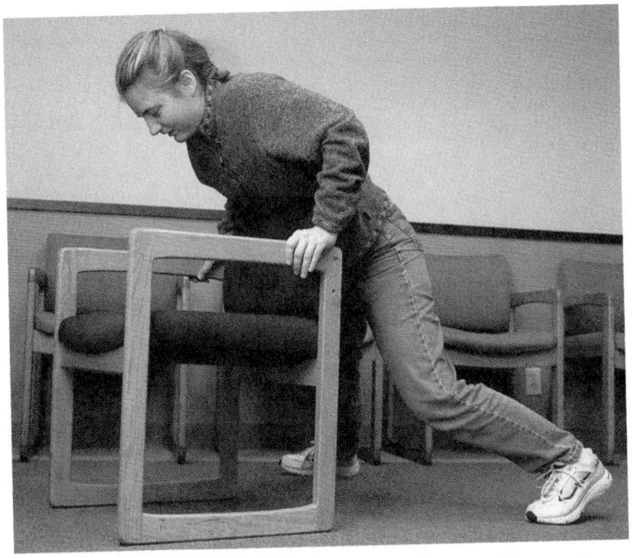

Figure 9-14 If alone, individuals can self-administer the Heimlich maneuver by using the back of a chair or similar hard object.

and infants. These reflect the American Red Cross latest updates, effective July 2000.

Rescue Breathing

Individuals in respiratory arrest require immediate emergency care. **Rescue breathing,** previously called mouth-to-mouth resuscitation, provides oxygen to the patient until emergency personnel arrive.

When performing rescue breathing procedures in the ambulatory care setting, it is recommended that resuscitation mouthpieces be used and that direct mouth-to-mouth (i.e., with no personal protective equipment) resuscitation never be used.

Procedures for rescue breathing differ for adults, children, and infants. See Procedures 9-8, 9-9, and 9-10.

Cardiopulmonary Resuscitation

The combination of rescue breathing and chest compressions is known as CPR. Alone, CPR cannot save an individual from cardiac arrest—it represents preliminary care until advanced medical help is available to the heart attack victim. See Procedures 9-11, 9-12, and 9-13.

When performing CPR, the rule is that you do not stop until

- another trained person can take over,
- EMS arrives and takes over care of the patient,
- you are physically exhausted and not able to continue, or
- the environment becomes unsafe for any reason.

Procedure 9-1 Control of Bleeding

STANDARD PRECAUTIONS:

PURPOSE:
To control bleeding from an open wound.

EQUIPMENT/SUPPLIES:
Sterile dressings
Sterile gloves
Mask and eye protection
Gown
Biohazard waste container

PROCEDURE STEPS:
1. Wash hands.
2. Assemble equipment and supplies.
3. Apply eye and mask protection and gown if splashing is likely to occur.
4. Put on gloves.
5. Apply dressing and press firmly (Figure 9-15A).
6. If bleeding continues, elevate arm above heart level (Figure 9-15B).
7. If bleeding still continues, press adjacent artery against bone (Figure 9-15C). Notify the physician if bleeding cannot be controlled.

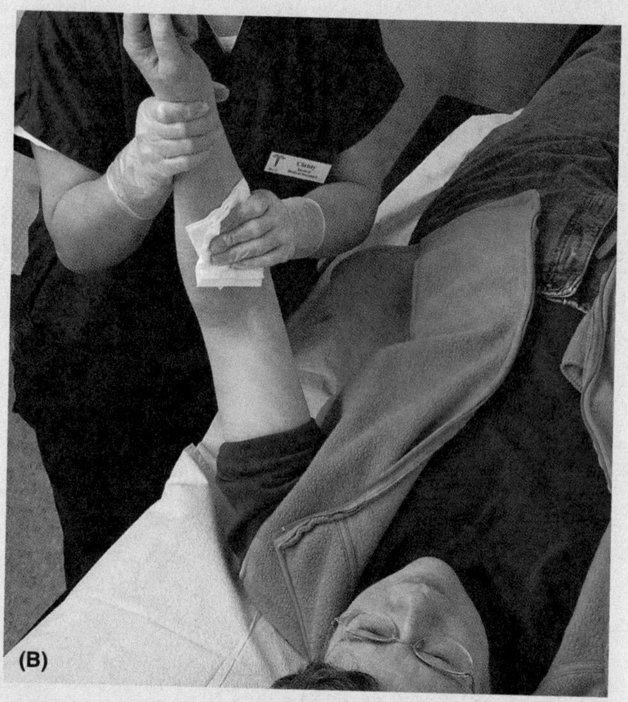
(B)

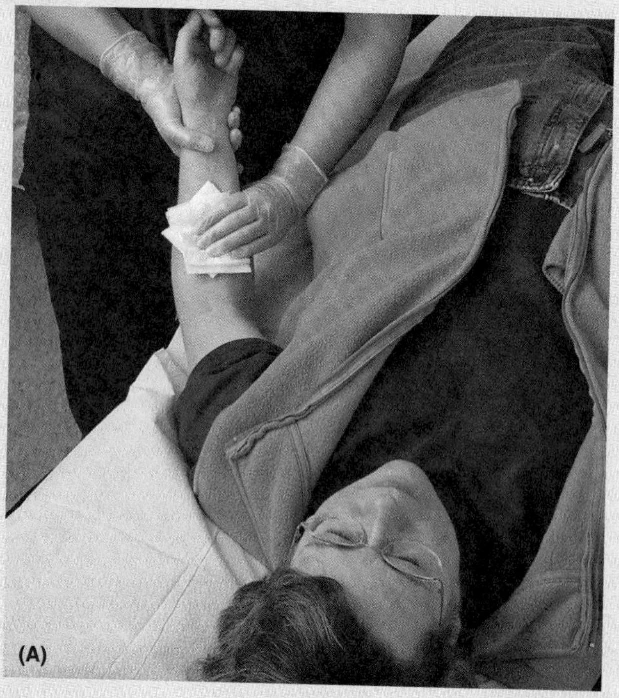
(A)

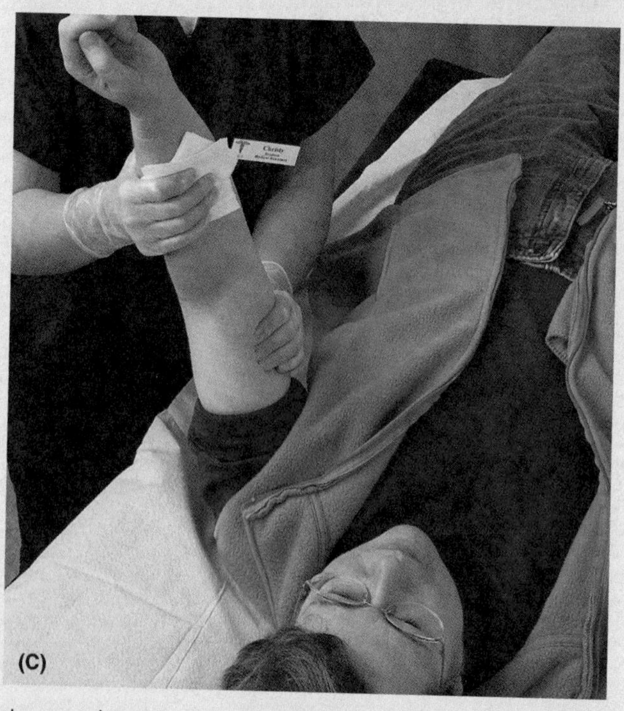
(C)

Figure 9-15 (A) Apply dressing and press firmly. (B) Elevate arm above heart level. (C) Press artery against bone.

(continues)

Procedure 9-1 (continued)

8. Apply pressure bandage over the dressing.
9. Dispose of waste in biohazard container.
10. Remove gloves, dispose of in biohazard container.
11. Wash hands.
12. Document procedure.

CAUTION: If wound is large and bleeding is not controlled, the patient may go into hemorrhagic shock. Be prepared to call EMS immediately.

DOCUMENTATION

4/4/20XX—10:00 AM Patient sustained small (1 cm) laceration on inside left forearm. Bleeding moderately. Pressure dressing applied to wound, left arm elevated above heart level. Bleeding continued. Pressure applied to brachial artery. Pressure bandage applied over dry sterile dressing. Bleeding seems to have subsided. BP 118/74, P 92. Dr. King notified. W. Slawson, CMA

Procedure 9-2 Applying an Arm Splint

STANDARD PRECAUTIONS:

PURPOSE:
To immobilize the area above and below the injured part of the arm to reduce pain and prevent further injury.

EQUIPMENT/SUPPLIES:
Thin piece of rigid board; cardboard can be used if necessary
Gauze roller bandage

PROCEDURE STEPS:

1. Place the padded splint under the injured area.
2. Hold the splint in place with gauze roller bandage. Pad gaps between arm and board (wrist) with gauze pads or other soft material.
3. After splinting, check circulation (note color and temperature of skin, color of nails, check pulse) to ascertain that the splint is not too tightly applied.
4. A sling can be applied to keep the arm elevated, which increases comfort and reduces swelling.
5. Wash hands.
6. Document the procedure.

DOCUMENTATION

4/4/20XX—2:00 PM Splint applied to right arm above and below injured area. Sling applied for comfort. Nail beds pink, hand warm, radial pulse easily palpated. Seen by Dr. Woo. J. Guerro, CMA

Procedure 9-3 Abdominal Thrusts for a Conscious Adult

STANDARD PRECAUTIONS:

PURPOSE:
To open up a blocked airway.

EQUIPMENT/SUPPLIES:
None needed

PROCEDURE STEPS:

1. Victim cannot cough, speak, or breathe.
2. Call 911.
3. Place the thumb side of your fist against the middle of the abdomen, just above the umbilicus and below the xiphoid process.
4. Grasp your fist with your other hand and give quick upward thrusts (Figure 9-16).
5. Repeat the procedure until the patient coughs up the object. If the person becomes unconscious, perform abdominal thrusts for an unconscious individual (see Procedure 9-4).
6. Wash hands.
7. Document the procedure.

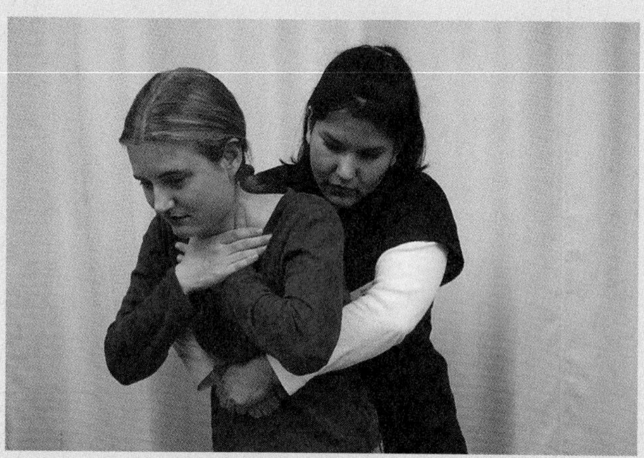

Figure 9-16 Grasp your fist with your other hand and give quick thrusts.

DOCUMENTATION

4/4/20XX—4:00 PM Patient was choking and coughing. Made the universal sign for choking with hands. Became unable to cough, speak, or breathe. Abdominal thrusts given several times. Patient coughed up a large piece of chicken. Breathing easily, color of skin good. BP 130/90, P 100. States she was very frightened but feels much better now. K. Hanson, CMA

Procedure 9-4 Abdominal Thrusts for an Unconscious Adult or Child

STANDARD PRECAUTIONS:

PURPOSE:
To open up a blocked airway in an unconscious victim.

EQUIPMENT/SUPPLIES:
Gloves
Resuscitation mouthpiece
Biohazard waste container

PROCEDURE STEPS:
1. Have someone call emergency services.
2. Put on gloves if available.
3. Lie person on back. Open victim's mouth and look for foreign object. Position resuscitation mouthpiece. Tilt back person's head (Figure 9-17A).
4. Give two breaths (Figure 9-17B).
5. If air will not go in, retilt head to try to give two breaths again. If air will not go in, give 15 abdominal thrusts.
6. Find hand position on breastbone 2 inches above xiphoid and compress 2 inches deep. (For child, give five abdominal thrusts, 1½ inches deep.)
7. Lift the jaw, look for object, and sweep it out of the mouth with finger, if seen (Figure 9-17C).
8. Tilt back the head, lift the chin, and give breaths again slowly. Continue giving breaths and thrusts, looking for object and sweeping it out if seen. Continue breathing until breaths go in. If the airway is cleared and victim does not begin to breathe on his or her own, prepare to perform CPR (see Procedure 9-11).
9. Check carotid pulse.
10. Dispose of waste in biohazard container.

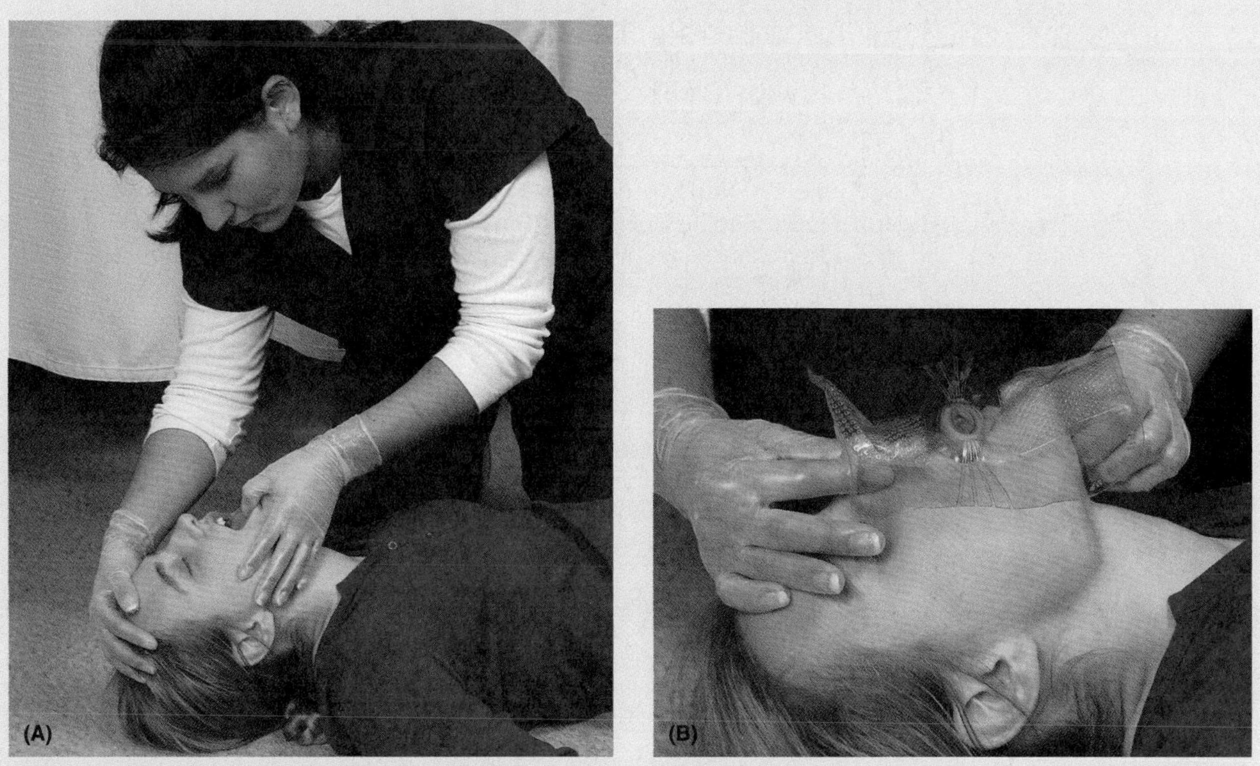

Figure 9-17 (A) Tilt back head. (B) Give breaths.

(continues)

Procedure 9-4 (continued)

11. Remove gloves, dispose of in biohazard container, and wash hands.
12. Monitor vital signs.
13. Document the procedure.

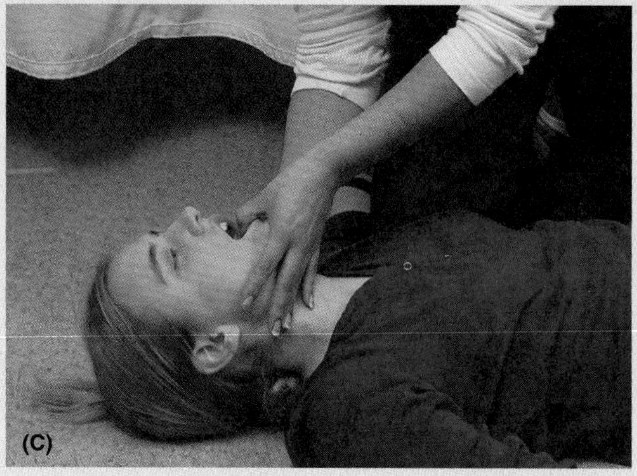

Figure 9-17 (C) Lift jaw and sweep out mouth.

DOCUMENTATION

4/5/20XX—9:00 AM While doing abdominal thrusts to a choking patient, the victim suddenly collapsed to the floor and lost consciousness. EMS notified by W. Slawson, CMA. No foreign object seen in mouth. Head tilted, breaths given, no air went into victim's body. Retilted head, gave two more breaths, and still no air could get through. Apparent foreign object in throat. Abdominal thrusts given, mouth swept, and large piece of apple found and removed. Breaths entered nose and throat easily, and patient regained consciousness and was breathing easily on own. BP 154/88, P 120, R 24. Color good. Advised to see her physician.

4/5/20XX—9:30 AM Blood Pressure recheck 144/82, P 102, R 20. K. Hanson, CMA

Procedure 9-5 Abdominal Thrusts for a Conscious Child

STANDARD PRECAUTIONS:

PURPOSE:
To open up a blocked airway.

EQUIPMENT/SUPPLIES:
None needed

PROCEDURE STEPS:
1. Place the thumb side of your fist against the middle of the child's abdomen, just above the umbilicus and below the xiphoid process (Figure 9-18A).
2. Grasp your fist with your other hand. Give quick upward thrusts (Figure 9-18B). Repeat the procedure until the object is expelled or until the patient loses consciousness (see Heimlich maneuver for unconscious child, Procedure 9-4).
3. Wash hands.
4. Document the procedure.

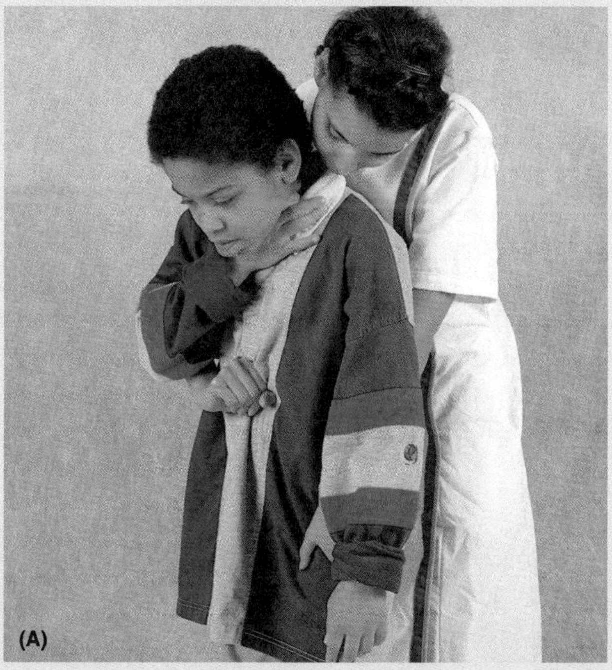
(A)

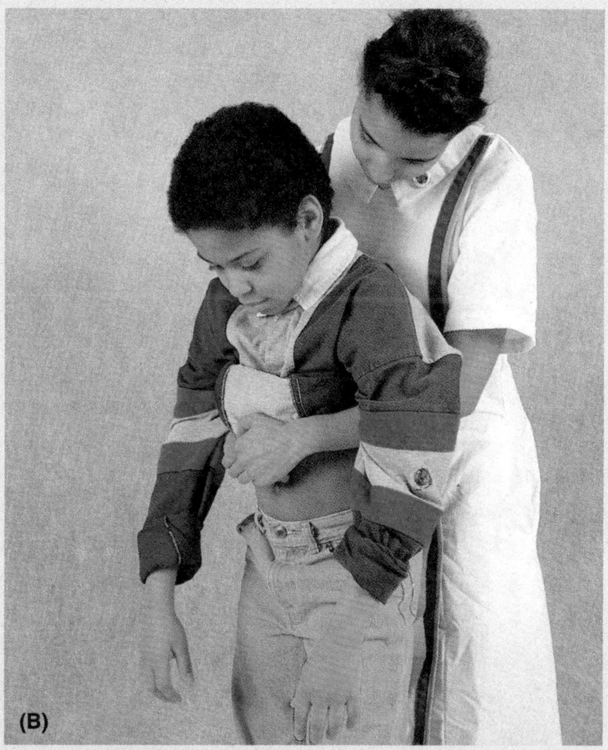
(B)

Figure 9-18 (A) Place the thumb side of your fist against the middle of the abdomen, just above the umbilicus and below the xiphoid process. (B) Grasp your fist with your other hand and give quick upward thrusts.

DOCUMENTATION

4/5/20XX—11:30 AM Child began choking while running with a hard candy in his mouth. Abdominal thrusts performed five to six times, and the candy was expelled onto the floor. Breathing easily. Color good. Dr. King notified. K. Hanson, CMA

Procedure 9-6 Back Blows and Chest Thrusts for a Conscious Infant Who Is Choking

STANDARD PRECAUTIONS:

PURPOSE:
To open up a blocked airway and assist a conscious infant who is choking, and cannot cough, cry, or breathe.

EQUIPMENT/SUPPLIES:
None needed

PROCEDURE STEPS:

1. Call 911.
2. With the infant face down on your forearm, give five back blows between the infant's shoulder blades with the heel of your hand (Figure 9-19A).
3. Position the infant face up on your forearm.
4. Give five chest thrusts ½ to 1 inch deep, on about the center of the breastbone (Figure 9-19B).
5. Look in the infant's mouth for the object. Repeat the back blows and chest thrusts and look for object until the infant begins to breathe on own. If the infant becomes unconscious, use back blow and chest thrust techniques for unconscious infants (see Procedure 9-7).
6. Activate EMS if unconscious.
7. Wash hands.
8. Document the procedure.

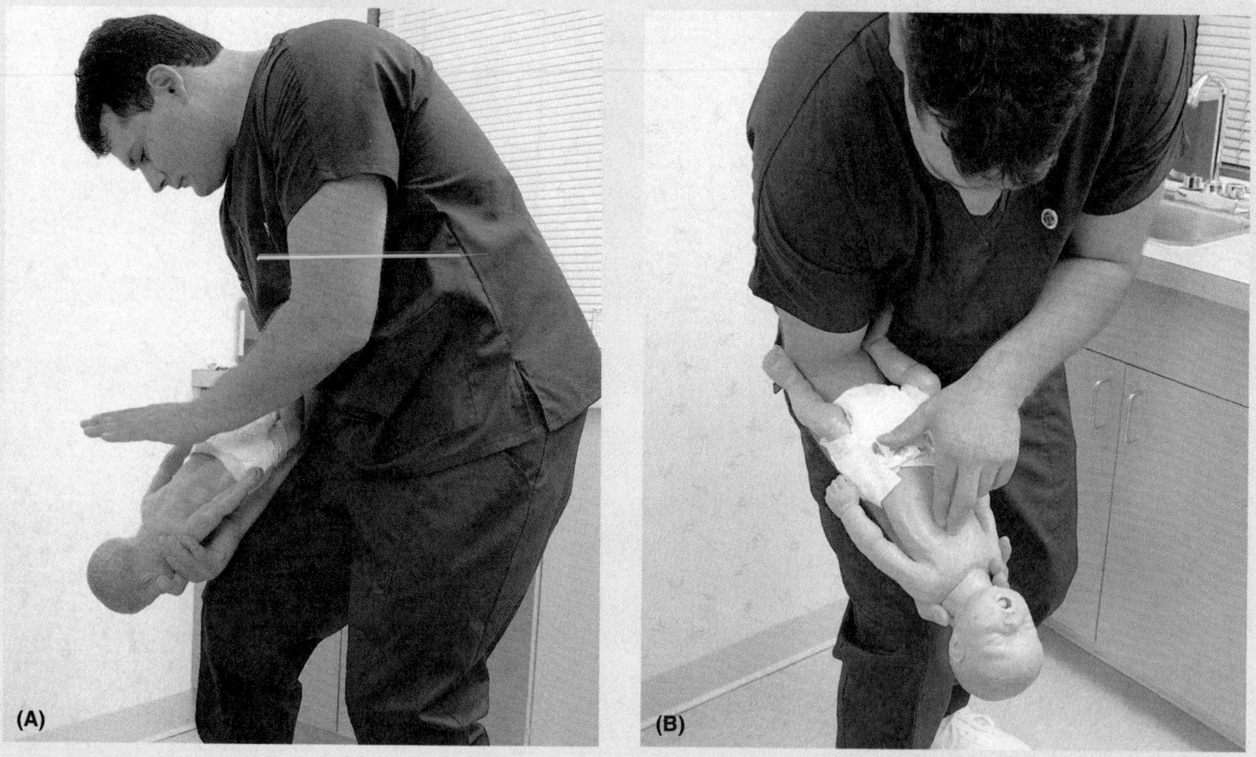

Figure 9-19 (A) With the infant face down on your forearm, give five back blows. (B) With the infant face up on your forearm, give five chest thrusts.

DOCUMENTATION

4/6/20XX—1:30 PM Baby appears to be choking. Back blows and chest thrusts given. Baby began to cry and forced object out of her mouth. Cried forcefully and color returned to pink. Checked by Dr. King. C. McInnis, CMA

Procedure 9-7 Back Blows and Chest Thrusts for an Unconscious Infant

STANDARD PRECAUTIONS:

PURPOSE:

To open up a blocked airway.

EQUIPMENT/SUPPLIES:

Gloves
Resuscitation mouthpiece

PROCEDURE STEPS:

1. Have someone call emergency services.
2. Don gloves. Tap the infant gently to check for consciousness.
3. Gently tilt back the infant's head. Do not hyperextend (Figure 9-20A).
4. Listen and watch for breathing.
5. Apply resuscitation mouthpiece. Give two breaths, covering infant's nose and mouth with your mouth (Figure 9-20B).
6. If air will not go in, retilt head, attempt to give breaths again.
7. If breaths still will not go in, give five chest compressions ½ to 1 inch deep.
8. Lift jaw and tongue and check for object. If you see the object, sweep it out (Figure 9-20C).
9. Tilt back head and give one breath again.

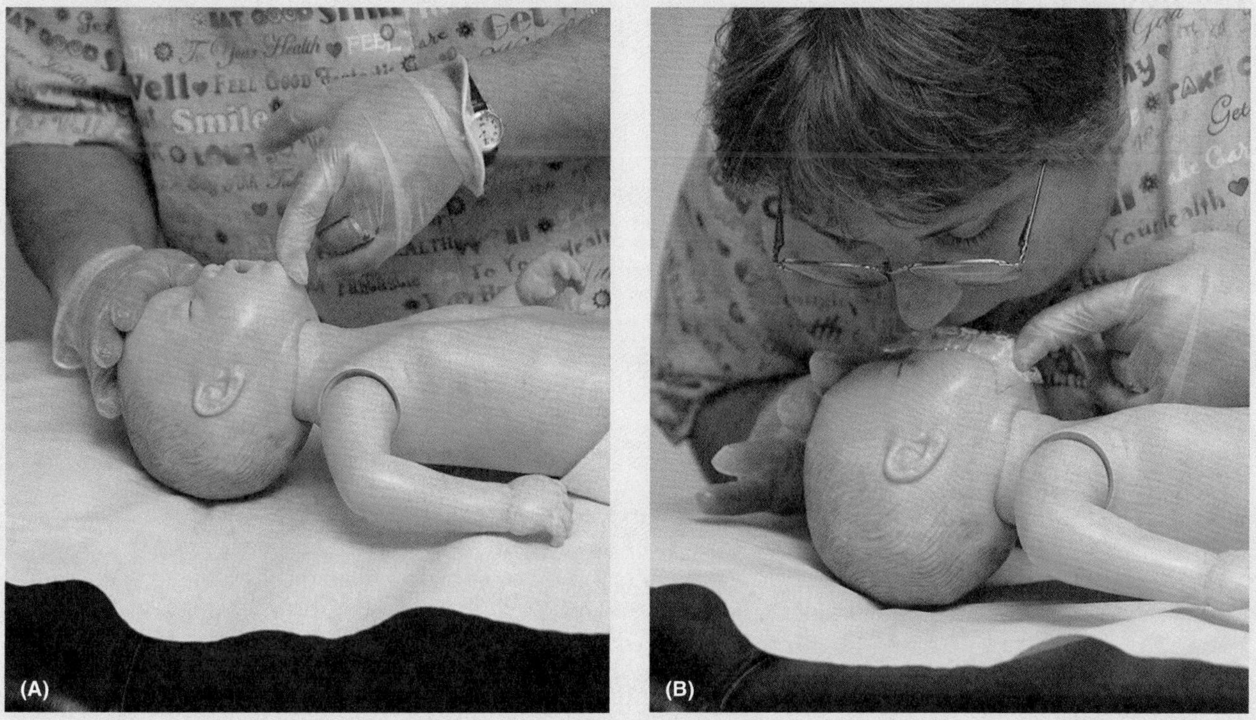

Figure 9-20 (A) Gently tilt back head. (B) Give two breaths, covering the infant's nose and mouth.

(continues)

Procedure 9-7 (continued)

10. Repeat breaths and five chest compressions, and check for object until breaths go in. If the infant does not begin to breathe on his or her own, prepare to perform CPR.
11. Remove gloves. Wash hands.
12. Document the procedure.

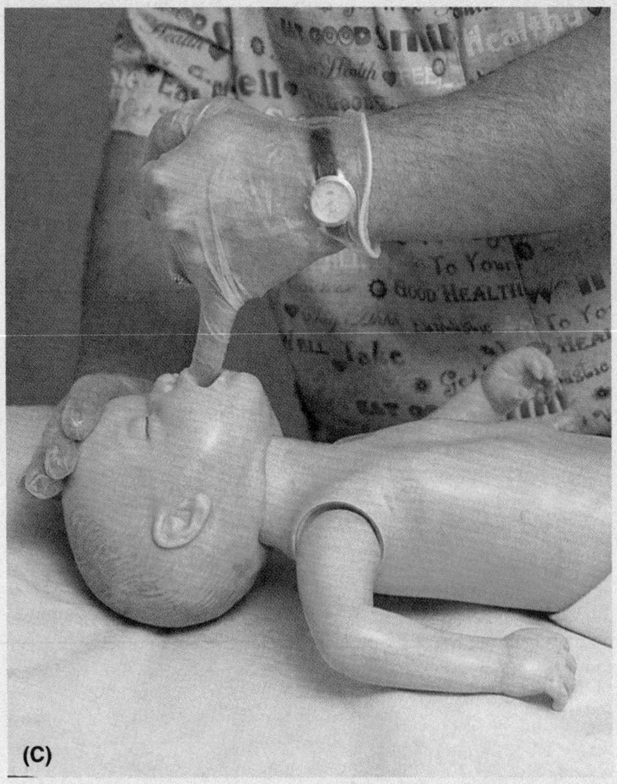

Figure 9-20 (C) Lift jaw and tongue. Check for object and, if seen, sweep out.

DOCUMENTATION

4/6/20XX—3:00 PM Mother stated that while her 1½-year-old was playing with a toy on the reception room floor, she noticed that the baby fell over, looked blue, wasn't breathing, and was limp. EMS activated. Dr. King notified. Baby unresponsive. Looked into baby's mouth, no object seen. Breaths given. Would not go in. Retilted head and two more breaths given. Still unable to get air into baby. Chest compressions given (½–1 inches deep). Breaths and compressions continued for about two minutes. Baby suddenly coughed up a small object. Crying and breathing on her own. Color pink, does not seem in distress. Seen and examined by Dr. King. W. Slawson, CMA

Procedure 9-8 Rescue Breathing for Adults

STANDARD PRECAUTIONS:

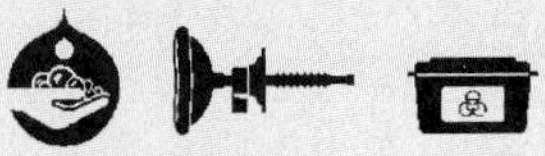

PURPOSE:

To respond to a breathing emergency.

EQUIPMENT/SUPPLIES:

Biohazard waste container
Resuscitation mouthpiece

PROCEDURE STEPS:

1. Have someone call emergency services.
2. Shout, "Are you all right?" "Are you all right?"
3. Look, listen, and feel for breathing.
4. No breathing . . .
5. Tilt back the head, lift the chin, position resuscitation mouthpiece, and pinch the nose closed (Figure 9-21A).
6. Give two short breaths. Breathe into patient until the chest gently rises. Turn your face to the side and listen and watch for air to return.
7. Check for pulse at the carotid artery (Figure 9-21B).
8. If pulse is present, but the person is not breathing, give one slow breath every five seconds. Do this for one minute.
9. Recheck pulse and breathing every minute.
10. Continue rescue breathing as long as pulse is present and the person is not breathing. Continue until breathing is restored or another person takes over.
11. Dispose of waste in biohazard container.
12. Wash hands.
13. Document the procedure.

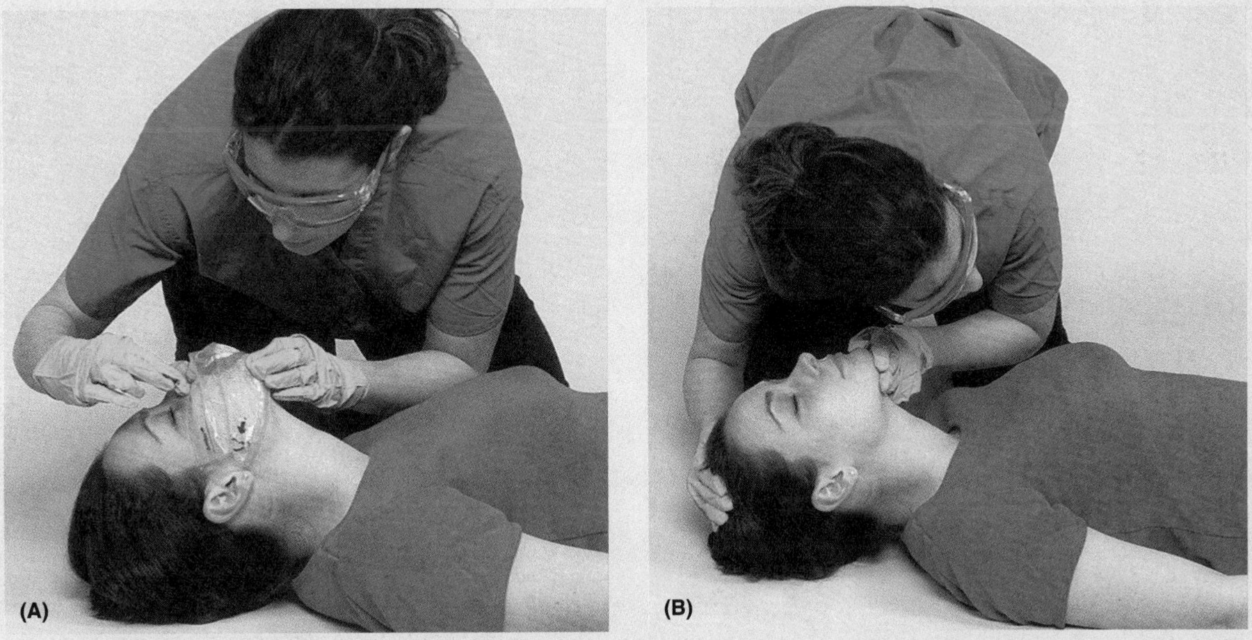

Figure 9-21 (A) Tilt back head, lift chin, position resuscitation mouthpiece, pinch nose closed, and give two short breaths. (B) Check for pulse at the carotid artery .

DOCUMENTATION

4/7/20XX—1:45 PM A few minutes after having blood drawn for laboratory work, Mrs. Edwards slumped to the floor. She was unresponsive. EMS activated. Dr. King notified. Airway opened, checked for breathing. No breathing. Gave breath. Checked carotid pulse. Pulse strong and regular. Still not breathing. Gave one breath every five seconds for one minute. Rechecked breathing and pulse. Patient breathing, shallow respirations. Dr. King examined patient.

4/7/20XX—2:00 PM BP 100/60, P 100, R 12. Color improved. A. Pemberton, CMA

Procedure 9-9 Rescue Breathing for Children

STANDARD PRECAUTIONS:

PURPOSE:
To respond to a breathing emergency.

EQUIPMENT/SUPPLIES:
Gloves
Resuscitation mouthpiece

PROCEDURE STEPS:

1. Have someone call emergency services.
2. Don gloves.
3. Tilt back the head, lift the chin, position the resuscitation mouthpiece, pinch the nose closed, and give two short breaths (Figure 9-22A). If air does not go in, retilt head and breathe again.
4. Check for a pulse at the carotid artery (Figure 9-22B).
5. If pulse is present, but the child is not breathing, give one slow breath every three seconds. Do this for one minute.
6. Recheck pulse and breathing every minute.
7. Continue rescue breathing as long as pulse is present but the child is not breathing.
8. Remove gloves. Wash hands.
9. Document the procedure.

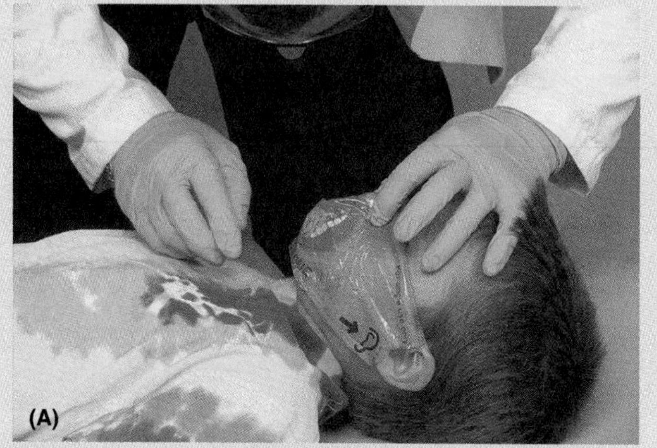
(A)

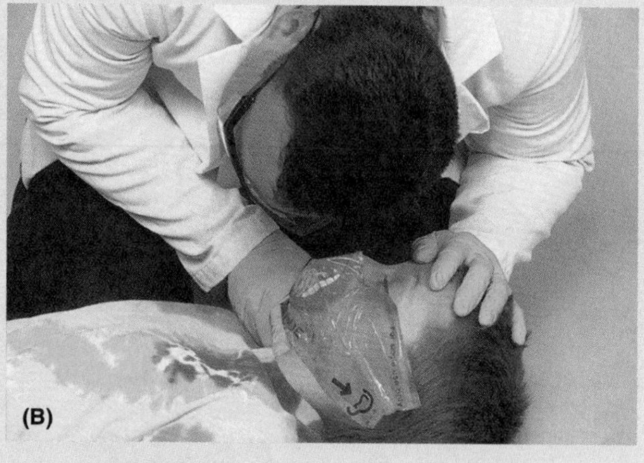
(B)

Figure 9-22 (A) Tilt back head, lift chin, position resuscitation mouthpiece, pinch nose closed, and give two short breaths. (B) Check for pulse at the carotid artery.

DOCUMENTATION

4/9/20XX—4:30 PM Seven-year-old JR was in the clinic today for his scheduled allergy desensitization injection. About 5–10 minutes after the injection, JR became weak, pale, and sweaty. He fell to the floor and was unresponsive. Rescue breathing began after activating EMS. Dr. Woo notified. After opening the airway, two slow breaths were given and after finding a carotid pulse, one breath was given every three seconds. JR began to breathe shallow breaths. Examined by Dr. Woo. EMS arrived, stabilized JR, and took him to the emergency department. C. McInnis, CMA

Procedure 9-10 Rescue Breathing for Infants

STANDARD PRECAUTIONS:

PURPOSE:

To respond to a breathing emergency.

EQUIPMENT/SUPPLIES:

Gloves
Resuscitation mouthpiece

PROCEDURE STEPS:

1. Have someone call emergency services.
2. Don gloves.
3. Tilt back the head (Figure 9-23A).
4. Position resuscitation mouthpiece. Seal your lips tightly around the infant's nose and mouth (Figure 9-23B).
5. Give two slow breaths. Breathe into the infant until the chest rises.
6. Check for a pulse at the brachial artery (Figure 9-23C).
7. If pulse is present, but infant is not breathing, give one slow breath every three seconds. Do this for one minute.
8. Recheck pulse and breathing every minute (Figure 9-23D).
9. Continue rescue breathing as long as pulse is present but the infant is not breathing.
10. Remove gloves. Wash hands.
11. Document the procedure.

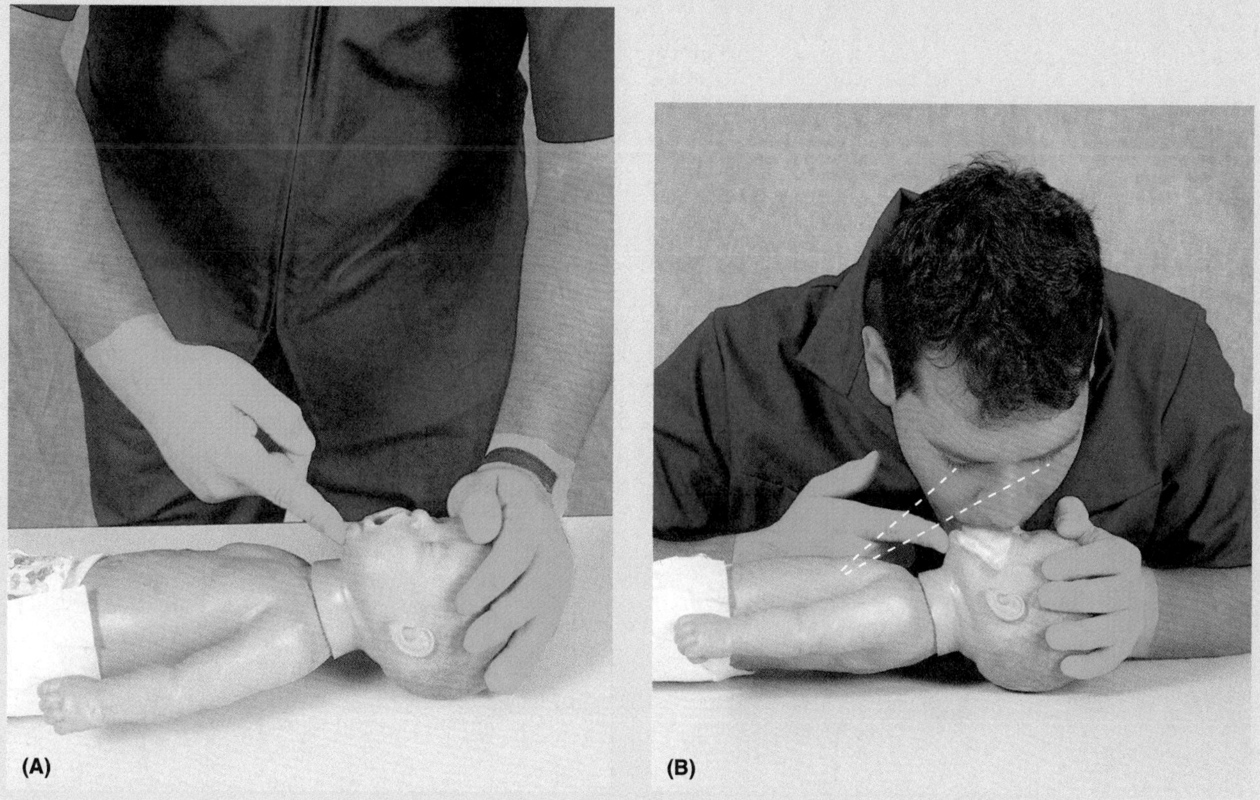

Figure 9-23 (A) Tilt back head. (B) Position resuscitation mouthpiece. Seal lips around nose and mouth and give two slow breaths.

(continues)

Procedure 9-10 (continued)

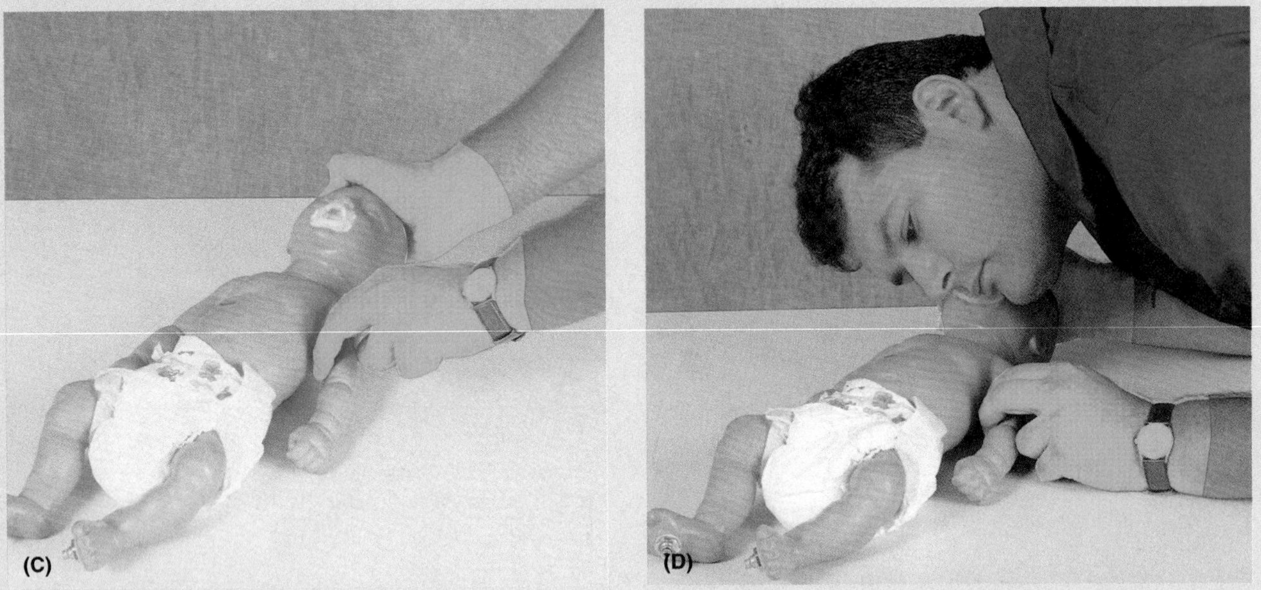

Figure 9-23 (C) Check for pulse at the brachial artery. (D) Recheck pulse and breathing every minute.

DOCUMENTATION

4/7/20XX—2:45 PM Six-month-old Samantha is seen by Dr. Woo in the pediatric clinic because she has “croup.” T 102°F, P 124, R 32. While being examined by Dr. Woo, Samantha suddenly stops breathing. EMS activated. Rescue breathing begun. Two slow breaths given, pulse checked, and found pulse to be present. Breaths given every three seconds. Samantha began breathing after about three minutes of rescue breathing. Dr. Woo wants baby admitted to the hospital. Arrangements made with Gulf Shore Hospital. W. Slawson, CMA

Procedure 9-11 CPR for Adults

STANDARD PRECAUTIONS:

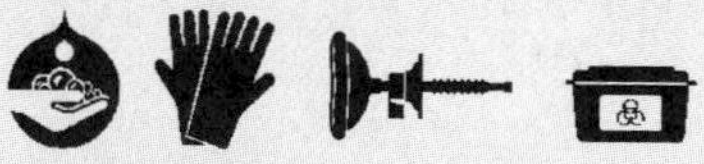

PURPOSE:

To respond to a breathing and cardiac arrest emergency.

EQUIPMENT/SUPPLIES:

Biohazard waste container
Resuscitation mouthpiece
Gloves

PROCEDURE STEPS:

Ask, "Are you OK?" If no response:

1. Have someone call emergency services.
2. Put on gloves if available.
3. Tilt back head and lift chin.
4. Look, listen, and feel for breathing for 10–15 seconds. If the patient is not breathing, keep the airway open, pinch the nose, position the mouthpiece, seal your mouth over the device, and give two breaths through the mouthpiece into the patient's lungs.
5. Check the pulse at the carotid artery for 10 seconds. If the patient has a pulse, continue rescue breathing. If the patient does not have a pulse, start chest compressions.
6. After locating the area on the abdomen two inches above the xiphoid (Figure 9-24A), position your shoulders over your hands and compress the chest about 2 inches 15 times (Figure 9-24B).
7. Give two slow breaths, holding the nose (Figure 9-24C).
8. Do 3 more sets of 15 compressions and two breaths.
9. Check the pulse and breathing for about 10 seconds.

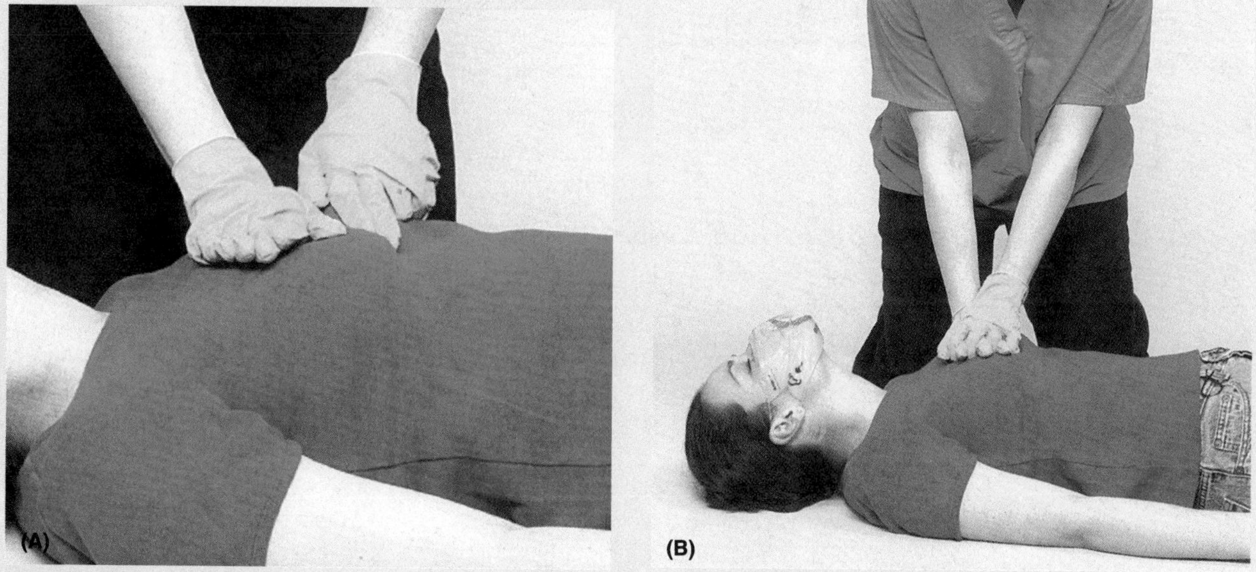

Figure 9-24 (A) Tilt back head and lift chin. Locate hand on the breastbone two inches above xiphoid process. (B) Position your shoulders over your hands and compress the chest 15 times.

(continues)

Procedure 9-11 (continued)

10. If there is no pulse or breathing, continue sets of 15 compressions and 2 breaths.
11. Use AED (Figure 9-25).
12. Dispose of waste in biohazard container.
13. Remove gloves, dispose of in biohazard container, and wash hands.
14. Document the procedure.

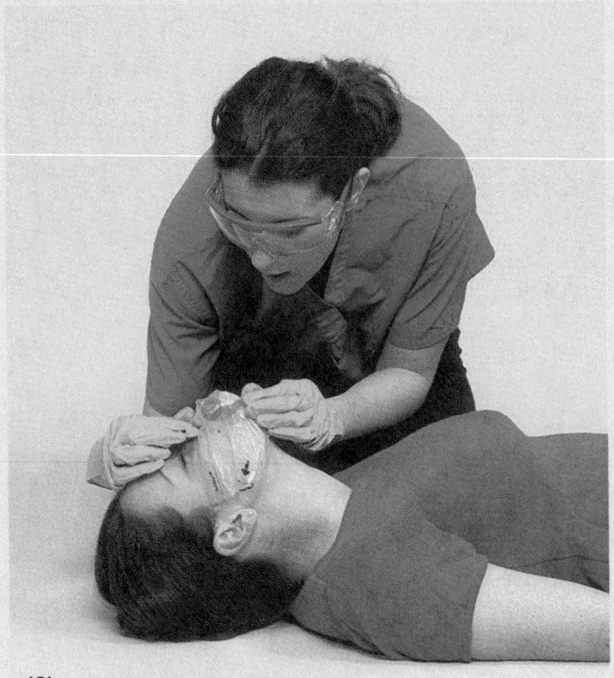

(C)

Figure 9-24 (C) Give two slow breaths, holding nose.

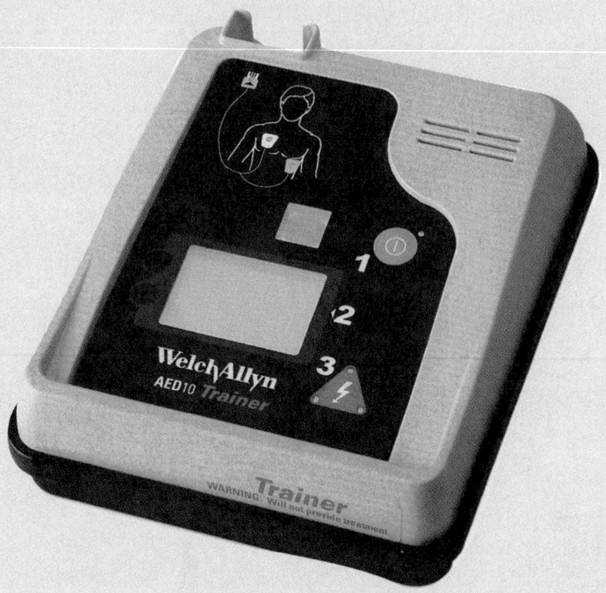

Figure 9-25 Automatic external defibrillator (AED). (Courtesy of Welch-Allyn.)

DOCUMENTATION

4/8/20XX—11:20 AM Fifty-four-year-old patient complaining of severe chest pain radiating down left arm and up into jaw. Nitroglycerin given sublingually. BP 100/70, P 116, R 28. Electrocardiography performed. Examined by Dr. Long. Suddenly patient stopped breathing. EMS activated. Two breaths given. Carotid pulse palpated and not present. CPR started. Fifteen chest compressions and two breaths given for four rounds. Pulse and breathing rechecked. Neither pulse nor breathing present. CPR continued. Oxygen given, automated electronic defibrillator (AED) used on patient. Patient's pulse returned. BP 90/60, P 100 (weak), R 8. Adrenalin given subcutaneously by Dr. Long. EMS arrived and stabilized patient for transport to emergency department. G. Burns, CMA

Procedure 9-12 CPR for Children

STANDARD PRECAUTIONS:

PURPOSE:

To respond to a cardiac arrest emergency in a child.

EQUIPMENT/SUPPLIES:

Gloves
Resuscitation mouthpiece

PROCEDURE STEPS:

1. Put on gloves.
2. Tap child to check consciousness level. Activate EMS.
3. Tilt head; look, listen, and feel for breathing. If there is no breathing, give two slow breaths. Check carotid artery for pulse.
4. Locate one hand on the breastbone and one hand on the forehead to maintain an open airway. Use heel of hand only above notch of xiphoid. Position your shoulders over the child's chest and compress the chest 1½ inches for five times (Figure 9-26A).
5. Position resuscitation mouthpiece. Give one slow breath, while pinching the nose (Figure 9-26B).
6. Repeat cycles of five compressions and one breath for about one minute.
7. Check the pulse and breathing for about 5 seconds (Figure 9-26C).

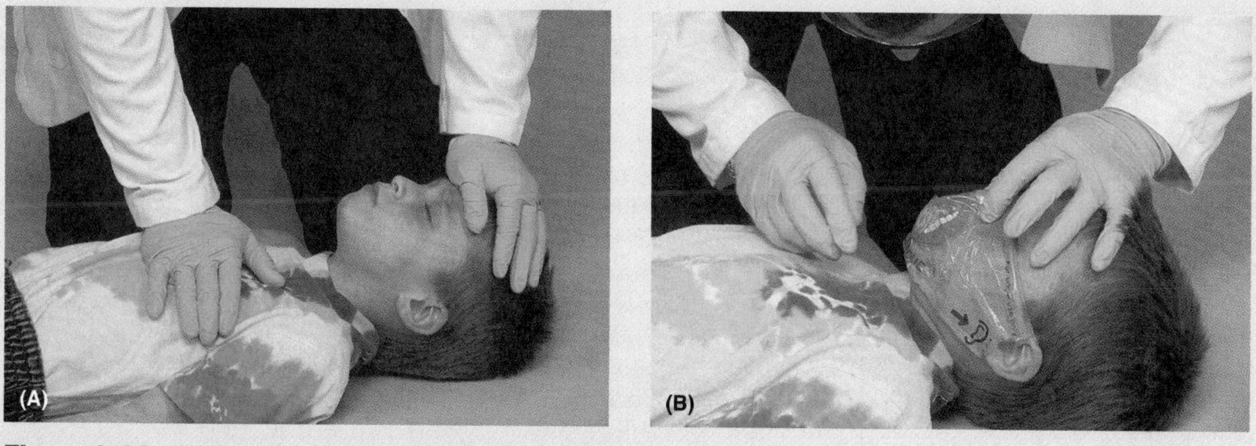

Figure 9-26 (A) Position your shoulders over the child's chest and compress the chest five times. (B) Give one slow breath, holding the nose.

(continues)

Procedure 9-12 (continued)

8. If there is no pulse, continue sets of five compressions and one breath.
9. Recheck the pulse and breathing every few minutes.
10. If child is 8 years or older and is 55 pounds, use AED.
11. Remove gloves. Wash hands.
12. Document the procedure.

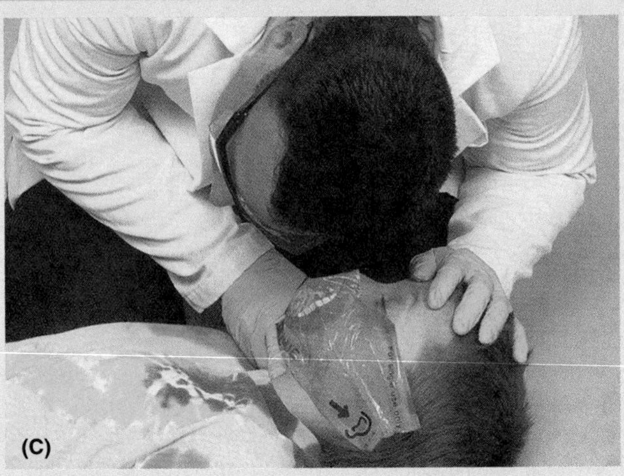

Figure 9-26 (C) Check pulse and breathing for 5 seconds.

DOCUMENTATION

4/8/20XX—3:20 PM Eight-year-old Sam was given allergy desensitization injection. Within four to five minutes, he collapsed. Checked for breathing, and it was absent. Two breaths given, carotid checked. Both absent. Dr. King notified and examined patient. EMS activated and CPR begun. Sets of one breath to five chest compressions continued for approximately three to four minutes. Patient began to move slightly. Shallow breathing and weak carotid pulse felt. BP 70/40, P 116 (weak), R 12 (shallow). Adrenaline, Benadryl, and oxygen given by Dr. Woo. Patient transported to emergency department after stabilization. C. McInnis, CMA

Procedure 9-13 CPR for Infants

STANDARD PRECAUTIONS:

PURPOSE:
To respond to a cardiac arrest emergency in an infant.

EQUIPMENT/SUPPLIES:
Gloves
Resuscitation mouthpiece

PROCEDURE STEPS:

1. Don gloves.
2. Gently tap the infant to determine consciousness level. Have someone activate EMS.
3. Tilt head. Look, listen, and feel for breathing. If there is no breathing, position resuscitation mouthpiece and give two slow breaths, covering mouth and nose. Check brachial artery for pulse for 5–10 seconds.
4. Find your finger position on the center of the sternum between the nipples.
5. Compress the infant's chest five times about ½–¾ inch.
6. Give one slow breath (Figure 9-27A).
7. Repeat cycles of five compressions and one breath for one minute.
8. Recheck brachial pulse and breathing for about 5–10 seconds (Figure 9-27B).
9. If there is no pulse, continue cycles of five compressions and one breath.
10. Recheck the pulse and breathing every few minutes.
11. Remove gloves. Wash hands.
12. Document the procedure.

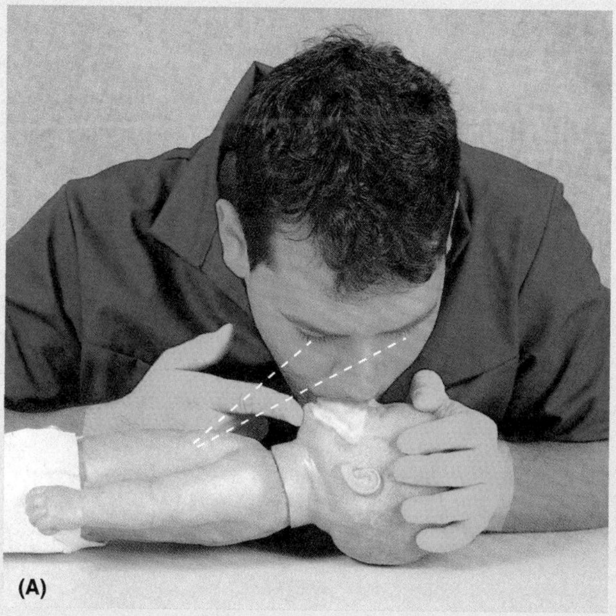

(A)

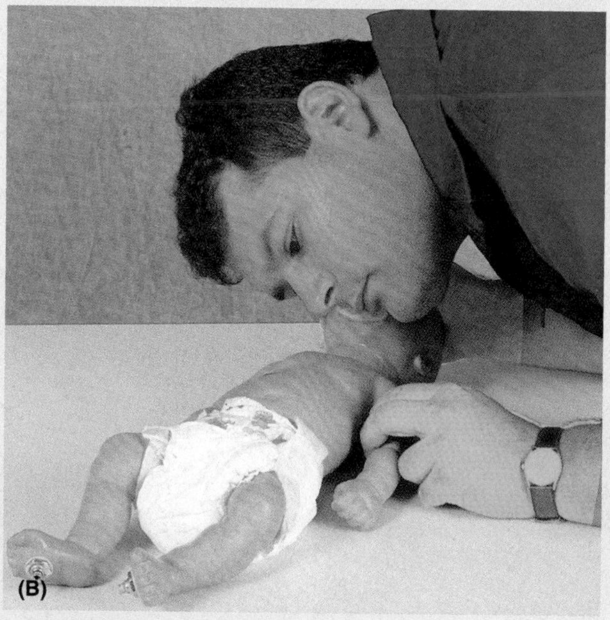

(B)

Figure 9-27 (A) Give one slow breath. (B) Recheck brachial pulse and breathing for 5–10 seconds.

DOCUMENTATION

4/8/20XX—4:30 PM Infant unresponsive. Mother states, "I think she was bitten by a spider." No breathing, no pulse. CPR began after activating EMS. Dr. Woo examined infant and directed CPR be resumed. One breath and five chest compressions given for about one minute. Rechecked patient in one minute. Still no pulse, no respirations. No blood pressure. Oxygen, adrenaline, and Benadryl administered by Dr. Woo. CPR continued. EMS arrived and stabilized infant with IVs and oxygen and transported infant and mother to emergency department. E. Nagle, CMA

Case Study 9-1

Annette Samuels, a regular patient at Inner City Health Care, is walking her dog one morning, stops to rest on a grassy knoll, and notices a wasp on her arm. She brushes it away, unthinkingly, and then realizes it has stung her. She receives two more stings and suddenly notices she is at a nest site. Annette is now a half-hour walk from home but is not really concerned because she has never had an allergic reaction to a wasp sting. However, a few minutes into her walk, her palms become itchy, her ears start to burn, and she feels light-headed. She is not having difficulty breathing. She is determined to get home and she does, at which point she notices she is covered with hives. She calls Inner City Health Care to ask: Should she come in?

CASE STUDY REVIEW

1. Wanda Slawson, CMA, is triaging calls the morning Annette is stung. What questions should she ask Annette?
2. Because Annette obviously is having a hypersensitive or an allergic reaction, she is advised to seek emergency care immediately. What first-aid measures might be taken?
3. What advice about precautions against getting stung again should Wanda give Annette?

Case Study 9-2

Abigail Johnson has arrived at Inner City Health Care for her scheduled appointment. As she checks in with Bruce Goldman, the medical assistant, she reports feeling nauseated, having some pressure in her chest, and being short of breath.

CASE STUDY REVIEW

1. What immediate actions should Bruce take to respond to Mrs. Johnson's complaints?
2. What equipment/supplies/medications should be ready and available for Dr. Lewis?
3. Because of the possibility of myocardial infarction, what action would Dr. Lewis direct Bruce to take after Mrs. Johnson has been stabilized?
4. What patient education can Bruce use in this situation?

SUMMARY

Although many of the emergencies covered in this chapter may never be seen by the medical assistant in the ambulatory care setting, it is nonetheless important to develop a broad base of information about the various types of potential emergency situations. This knowledge gives the medical assistant the confidence and the preparation to manage the emergencies that do occur with speed, accuracy, and understanding until outside emergency help arrives. Staff will need to assess their response to emergencies on a continual basis. Was protocol followed? Were there difficulties in the delivery of care? Were staff and equipment prepared and ready to deal with these potentially life-threatening situations? Staff meetings should be held to discuss these and other questions that may have arisen and to allow staff the opportunity to talk about any fears or concerns they might have. It must be stressed that this chapter is at best an introduction to the topic of emergency procedures and first aid; it is essential medical assistants in all ambulatory care settings, whether large or small, enroll in a Red Cross, American Heart Association, American Safety and Health Institute, or National Heart Association first-aid and CPR program, attain provider level CPR, and take refresher courses to update skills.

STUDY FOR SUCCESS

To reinforce your knowledge and skills of information presented in this chapter:

- ❑ Review the Key Terms
- ❑ Practice any Procedures
- ❑ Consider the Case Studies and discuss your conclusions
- ❑ Answer the Review Questions
  - ❑ Multiple Choice
  - ❑ Critical Thinking
- ❑ Navigate the Internet and complete the Web Activities
- ❑ Practice the StudyWARE activities on the textbook CD
- ❑ Apply your knowledge in the Student Workbook activities
- ❑ Complete the Web Tutor sections
- ❑ View and discuss the DVD situations

REVIEW QUESTIONS

Multiple Choice

1. Good Samaritan laws:
   a. are designed to protect the public
   b. protect non–health care professionals
   c. require that all individuals providing assistance act within the scope of their knowledge and training
   d. protect health care professionals on the job
2. First-degree burns:
   a. are the most serious and penetrate all layers of skin
   b. affect only the top layer of skin
   c. often leave scar tissue
   d. usually take more than a month to heal
3. A fracture in which the bone protrudes through the skin is called:
   a. greenstick fracture
   b. compound fracture
   c. depressed fracture
   d. comminuted fracture
4. To control a nosebleed, it is important to:
   a. have the patient lie down
   b. tilt the patient's head back
   c. tilt the patient's head forward
   d. call 911 immediately
5. Another name for a heart attack is:
   a. cerebral vascular accident
   b. cardiac arrest
   c. angina pectoris
   d. myocardial infarction

Critical Thinking

1. Sixteen-year-old Cindy Roland, a patient newly diagnosed with seizures caused by epilepsy, came into the office for a follow-up appointment today. She approached the reception desk and said she can see flashing bright lights in both eyes and that she feels "weird." The receptionist alerted the

medical assistant, who immediately responded to the patient.
   a. What actions should the medical assistant take?
   b. Is there a significance to the flashing bright lights? Explain.
   c. Address strategies the medical assistant can use to educate Cindy about her disease. Discuss at least five topics to include when teaching patients and others about epilepsy.
2. Mrs. Williams, a 75-year-old patient, came to the office today for a routine follow-up appointment for her diabetes. She suddenly collapsed onto the floor of the reception area.
   a. What immediate steps did the medical assistant take to provide care for this patient in distress?
3. Define the purpose of a crash cart or tray and compile a list of the major supplies and medications it should contain.
4. Describe shock and tell how and why it is important to prevent a patient from going into shock.
5. Recall three types of bandages and give examples of their use.
6. Describe the difference between first-, second-, and third-degree burns.
7. Recall and describe the four ways that poisons may enter the body.
8. What is a hemorrhage? What kinds of bleeding may the medical assistant encounter? What are the symptoms of each?
9. Explain when and why Heimlich maneuver, rescue breathing, and CPR techniques are performed.
10. Explain steps to take if a patient has a laceration on the hand with moderate to heavy bleeding.

WEB ACTIVITIES

1. Search the Internet for sites and resources on the Emergency Medical Services (EMS) System. Are there any cities or towns within 100 miles of your place of residence that do not use the EMS System?
2. What sites can you recommend to patients and their families who are looking for first-aid information about diabetes and heart attack?
3. What organizations could you use to search for information that deals with first aid for convulsions?
4. Search the Internet for information regarding first aid for insect stings.
5. What sites are available for information about poisonings?

REFERENCES/BIBLIOGRAPHY

The American National Red Cross. (2001). *Staywell*. St. Louis, MO: Mosby-Year Book, Inc.

Taber's cyclopedic medical dictionary (21st ed.). (2003). Philadelphia: F. A. Davis.

THE DVD HOOK-UP

DVD Series: **Skills Based Series** | Program Number: **8**

Chapter/Scene Reference
- *Triaging Phone Emergencies*

In this chapter, you learned about proper techniques to follow during emergency situations. In the designated DVD clip, we observed the medical assistant (MA) screening a call from a mother whose child was experiencing an asthma attack. The MA used a triage manual to assist her in screening the call accurately. With the aid of the triage manual, the MA instructs the mother to call the EMS. The mother refuses to call the EMS and decides to bring the child into the office. The mother hangs up the phone before the doctor gets a chance to speak with her. The next scene shows the mother bringing the child into the office in respiratory distress. The MA and physician work together as a team to get the patient's breathing stabilized.

1. Do you think that it was wise of the MA to take the extra time to ask screening questions once the mother stated that the child was having an asthma attack? Why or why not?
2. Why is it necessary for you to follow an approved triage manual if you are put into the role of screening patient calls?
3. Why was it important to get the patient's phone number at the beginning of the call?

DVD Journal Summary

Write a paragraph that summarizes what you learned from watching the designated scene from today's DVD program. What are some things you can do to help you know how to respond to emergencies before they happen?

UNIT 4
Integrated Clinical Procedures

CHAPTER 10

Infection Control, Medical Asepsis, and Sterilization

OUTLINE

KEY TERMS

Acquired Immunodeficiency Syndrome (AIDS)
Acyclovir
Airborne Transmission
Amniocentesis
Amoebic Dysentery
Anorexia
Antibodies
Antigen
Asepsis
Aspirate
Barrier
Biohazard
Bloodborne
Bloodborne Pathogen
Carrier
Caustic
Cell-Mediated Immunity
Cirrhosis
Communicable
Contact Transmission
Contaminate
Contracting
Coryza
Debris
Declination Form
Disinfection
Documentation
Droplet Transmission
Endemic
Endoscopy
Engineering Controls
Epidemic
Epidemiology
Epistaxis
Excoriated
Excretion
Expectorate
Exudate
Fomite
Gross Contamination
Human Immunodeficiency Virus (HIV)

(continues)

KEY TERMS (continued)

Humoral Immunity
Immune System
Immunity
Immunoglobulins
Immunosuppressed
Incinerate
Infection Control
Infectious Agent
Infectious Waste
Inflammatory Response
Invasive Procedures
Isolation
Isolation Categories
Jaundice
Jet Injection
Lesion
Leukorrhea
Lochia
Lumbar Puncture
Lymphadenopathy
Macular
Malaise
Malaria
Manifest
Medical Asepsis
Menses
Microorganism
Morbidity
Morphology
Mortality
Normal Flora
Opportunistic Infections
Palliative
Pandemic
Papular
Paracentesis
Parenteral
Pathogen
Phlebotomy
Preexisting
Purulent
Regulated Waste
Resistance
Sanitization
Scabies
Scoop Technique
Secretion
Severe Acute Respiratory Syndrome (SARS)
Sharps
Sodium Hypochlorite
Solvent
Spill Kit
Sputum
Standard

(continues)

OBJECTIVES

The student should strive to meet the following performance objectives and demonstrate an understanding of the facts and principles presented in this chapter through written and oral communication.

1. Define the key terms as presented in the glossary.
2. Define and state the critical importance of infection control in the ambulatory care setting.
3. Outline the six links in the chain of infection.
4. Define the five classifications of infectious microorganisms.
5. Recall and elaborate on the four phases the immune system uses to defend against infectious disease.
6. State the four stages of infectious diseases.
7. Recall at least five infectious diseases, their agents of transmission, and their symptoms.
8. Compare the routes of transmission of AIDS and hepatitis B and C and discuss the risk for infection from needlestick.
9. Describe the purpose of Standard Precautions and give six examples of ways health care providers should practice Standard Precautions.
10. Differentiate among the three types of Transmission-Based Precautions, defining what they are and how they are applied.
11. List eight types of body fluids and give an example of each.
12. Describe personal protective equipment.
13. Recognize five situations in which exposure to a patient's blood can occur, and discuss why Standard Precautions are important.
14. Describe proper disposal of infectious waste.
15. List human fluids that may contain HIV, HBV, and HCV.
16. Define medical asepsis.
17. Define surgical asepsis.
18. Compare and contrast medical asepsis and surgical asepsis.
19. State four methods of sterilization.
20. List supplies and equipment necessary to achieve surgical asepsis when using an autoclave.
21. Explain competent wrapping and operation of the autoclave.
22. State storage measures and expiration periods for autoclaved materials.

KEY TERMS (continued)

Standard Precautions
Surgical Asepsis
Thermolabile
Thoracentesis
Transmission
Transmission-Based Precautions
Trichomoniasis
Ultrasonic Cleaner
Undifferentiated
Universal Precautions
Vaccine
Vector
Vesicular
Virulence
Work Practice Controls

FEATURED COMPETENCIES

CAAHEP—ENTRY-LEVEL COMPETENCIES

Fundamental Procedures

- Perform hand washing
- Wrap items for autoclaving
- Perform sterilization techniques
- Dispose of biohazardous materials
- Practice Standard Precautions

Patient Care

- Maintain medication and immunization records

ABHES—ENTRY-LEVEL COMPETENCIES

Clinical Duties

- Apply principles of aseptic techniques and infection control
- Wrap items for autoclaving
- Perform sterilization techniques
- Dispose of biohazardous materials
- Practice Standard Precautions

SCENARIO

At Inner City Health Care, a multiphysician urgent care center, medical assistant Bruce Goldman, CMA, assumes responsibility for all infection control measures taken in the ambulatory care setting. In addition to his daily responsibilities related to medical and surgical asepsis, Bruce also makes it a point to stay current with infection control principles. Recently, Bruce attended a workshop about infection control. The Centers for Disease Control and Prevention (CDC) discussed Standard Precautions and Transmission-Based Precautions. When Bruce receives information on any form of infection control, he makes it a point to become thoroughly familiar with the guidelines and to share his knowledge with other urgent care staff.

INTRODUCTION

Infectious diseases have plagued humans since the beginning of time. Recent scientific advances have changed our thoughts and behaviors regarding infectious disease. Advances such as antibiotic therapy and vaccination have significantly reduced risks for mortality from some previously fatal or debilitating infectious diseases. Infectious diseases that once were highly feared because of their likelihood of causing premature death are now preventable or treatable, causing us to forget the ***virulence*** *and destructive potential of epidemics of infectious disease. The presence of acquired immunodeficiency syndrome (AIDS) as an incurable and fatal infectious disease (although people are living with HIV for many years), as well as* ***severe acute respiratory syndrome (SARS),*** *Mad Cow, and bird flu, have caused the world to realize the enduring impact of pathogens on the human race.*

Although these medical advances have reduced the incidence of ***mortality*** *and* ***morbidity*** *from infectious diseases, humans must never underestimate the potential of resurgent infectious diseases. Tuberculosis has been the single leading cause of death in the history of humankind, yet was drastically reduced with the discovery of antituberculosis drugs. Today, however, the tuberculosis organism may be found that has adapted to the drugs, thereby becoming resistant to our only line of defense. Medical assistants must pay close attention to the prevention of infectious diseases.*

This chapter addresses the principles of the process of infection and control measures for use in ambulatory care settings. Because medical assistants deal directly with patients and other health care professionals, stringent adherence to the principles can greatly reduce ***transmission,*** *or spread, of infectious disease. Continuous reliance on infection control measures ensures a clinical environment that is as safe as possible for employees, patients, and families. When infection control principles are not followed, infectious diseases may be transmitted to self, coworkers, or patients. The goals of infection control are to limit the presence of* ***infectious agents,*** *to create barriers against transmission, and to decrease the risk to others for contracting infectious diseases. These goals can be achieved through medical asepsis and sterilization, by observation of all Standard Precautions and Transmission-Based Precautions set forth by the CDC, and the Occupational Safety and Health Administration (OSHA) guidelines.*

Spotlight on Certification

RMA Content Outline

- Asepsis
- Sterilization

CMA Content Outline

- Legislation
- Principles of infection control
- Equipment preparation and operation
- Principles of operation
- Safety precautions

CMAS Content Outline

- Asepsis in the Medical Office

IMPACT OF INFECTIOUS DISEASES

Since the discovery of the germ theory by Louis Pasteur and Robert Koch in the nineteenth century, we have seen dramatic changes in global mortality and morbidity statistics from infectious diseases. Many scientists devoted their professional lives to the quest for the prevention and cure of infectious diseases, which were the main cause of death in earlier centuries. In developed countries, deaths from such diseases as tuberculosis, pneumonia, and smallpox have been significantly reduced because of pharmacologic agents such as antibiotics and **vaccines.** Antibiotic agents were widely introduced during World War II, reducing deaths from traumatic wound infections. Edward Jenner is credited with the discovery of the first vaccine to protect against smallpox. Because of the vaccine, smallpox is considered to have been eradicated worldwide.

Epidemiology is the science that studies the history, cause, and patterns of infectious diseases. This field of medicine is credited to a Japanese bacteriologist in the late nineteenth century who correlated incidences of bubonic plague with rat infestation. Recent epidemiological studies have traced infectious diseases such as AIDS from the inception of the epidemic. The future of studies in infectious diseases will focus on increasing the pharmacologic war against infectious diseases.

Reliance only on treatment of infectious disease does not address the crucial step in the spread of infectious diseases; that is, of prevention, or **infection control.** Emerging issues related to infectious diseases involve microorganisms that are resistant to present technology, **bloodborne pathogen** transmission, increased **immunosuppressed** populations, and global access to infection control and treatment. Developed countries become accustomed to antiinfectious medications, clean water, and laws that protect the public from infectious agents found in food and other consumables. These safety measures may not be present in other locations where political or economic factors limit access to infection control measures.

In the future, drug-resistant infectious diseases will place greater emphasis on prevention because there may never be a safe and universally effective drug for all infectious diseases.

Study of the history of infectious diseases allows us to realize the impact these diseases have on the lifestyles of people in various cultures. Infectious diseases such as AIDS and other sexually transmitted diseases have differing levels of social or cultural impact. Medical assistants should be aware of facts regarding the infectious process of specific diseases to reduce cultural isolation for the patient and to dispel myths regarding infectious diseases. See Chapter 6.

THE PROCESS OF INFECTION

Infectious diseases are caused by pathogenic microorganisms that are capable of causing disease. **Microorganisms** are microscopic living creatures capable of reproduction and transmission in specific circumstances. **Pathogens** are microorganisms that can cause infectious disease. Although all pathogens are capable of causing disease, not all microorganisms cause disease. Many microorganisms are necessary for human, animal, and plant life survival. In the absence of microorganisms, life would not be possible. The term **normal flora** is used to recognize the beneficial role of microorganisms in certain parts of the body, in which microorganisms normally occupy space and use nutrients, thus retarding the potential of pathogenic growth in that specific body area. A fundamental concept in the study of infectious disease is that similar steps or phases occur in all infectious diseases; however, each specific microorganism causes unique characteristics and alterations in the process of infection. Medical assistants must apply the theoretical process of infectious disease growth and transmission to relate to specific pathogens. The goal is to reduce transmission and incidence of infectious diseases in patients, employees, and families.

Growth Requirements for Microorganisms

For microorganisms to survive and thrive, a suitable environment must be available to them. Following is a list of growth requirements for microorganisms:

- Oxygen: an aerobic microorganism needs oxygen to live; most pathogenic microorganisms need oxygen to survive
- Lack of or no oxygen: an anaerobic microorganism needs little or no oxygen to live; two examples are tetanus and gas gangrene
- Moisture: microorganisms grow well in a moist environment; the body provides moisture
- Nutrition: the body supplies plenty of nutrients
- Temperature: the body's temperature of approximately 98.6°F is an optimum temperature for growth of microorganisms
- Darkness: the body's cavities and organs provide darkness
- Neutral or slightly alkaline pH: the body's fluids are neutral when in a healthy state

Through the understanding of the optimum growth requirements for microorganisms to proliferate, elimination of any or all of the factors helps keep microorganisms from causing infection.

CHAIN OF INFECTION

For infectious diseases to spread, several necessary steps must occur. These steps, or links, are known as the "chain of infection." Each link or step in the infectious process must occur for the spread of infection to take place. Infection control is based on the fact that the transmission of infectious diseases will be prevented when any of the levels in the chain are broken or interrupted (Figure 10-1). The steps are:

1. Infectious agent
2. Reservoir
3. Portal of exit
4. Means of transmission
5. Portal of entry
6. Susceptible host

Infectious Agents

Infectious agents are microorganisms that can be grouped into five classifications: viruses, bacteria, fungi, parasites, and rickettsia. For an infection to occur, an infectious agent must be present. When infectious diseases are identified according to the specific disease-causing microorganism, the disease may be prevented with the use of antiinfective drugs or infection control practices. Each of the five classifications of infectious microorganisms will be explored.

Virus. Viruses are pathogens that require a living cell for reproduction and activity. These microorganisms are

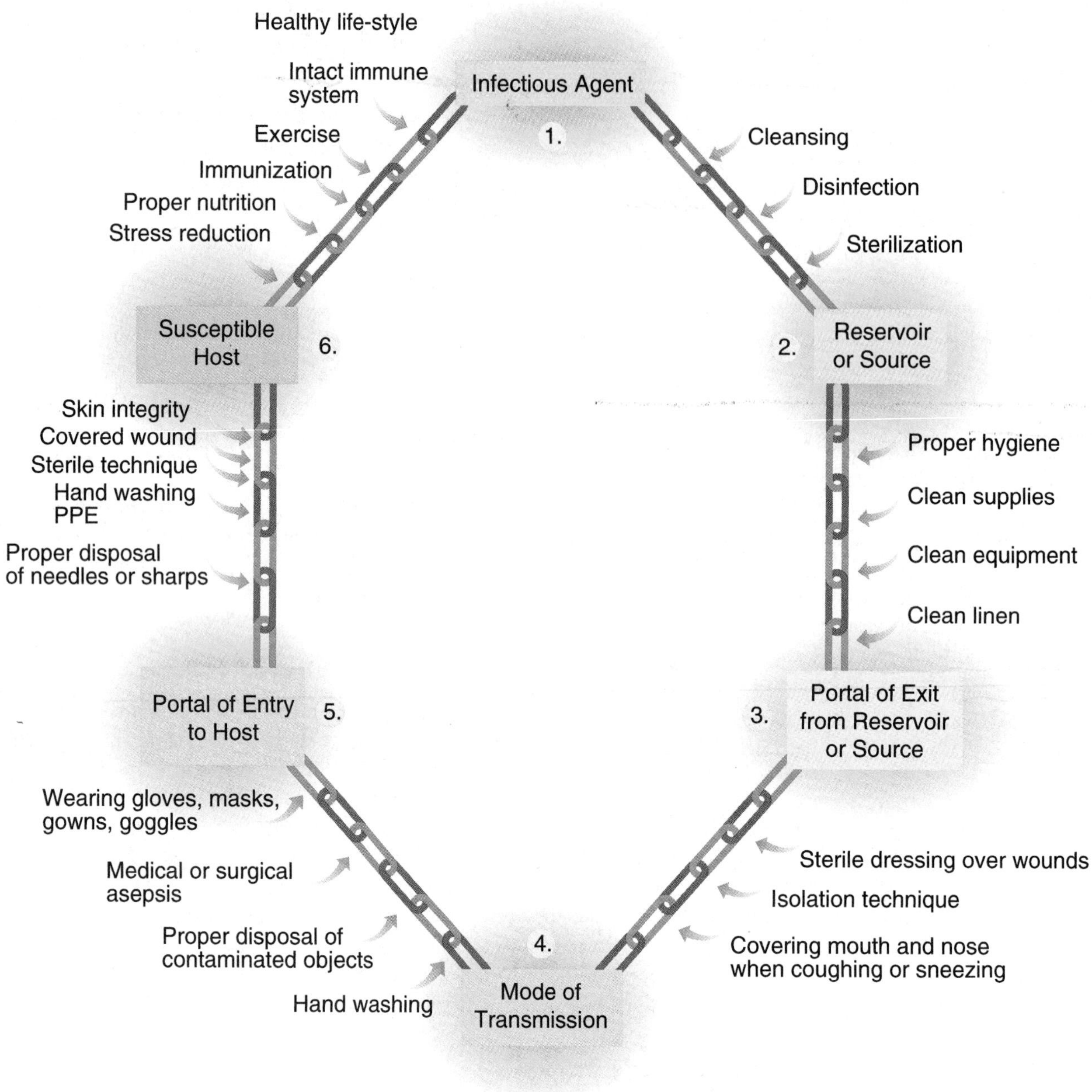

Figure 10-1 Health care worker's interventions used to break the chain of infection transmission.

considered intracellular parasites, because they must live inside cells to multiply. They do so by altering particles of genetic material, such as DNA (deoxyribonucleic acid) or RNA (ribonucleic acid). Because viruses live inside cells, they are protected against agents such as chemical disinfectants. To survive, viruses have a notable characteristic of being able to change specific characteristics over time. For instance, viruses can adapt to their environment so they remain resistant to efforts to limit their growth. Viral infections have only a few pharmacologic treatment agents, and usually these agents are **palliative** because they only relieve symptoms of the disease instead of curing the infection. Some viral infections can be prevented by vaccination.

Bacteria. Bacteria are single-celled microorganisms that live in tissues rather than in body cells and are identified by characteristic shapes, or **morphology.** Bacteria may also be grouped according to ability to accept laboratory staining agents. Gram-negative bacteria stain visibly red

TABLE 10-1 EXAMPLES OF SOME INFECTIOUS BACTERIAL DISEASES

Disease	Infectious Agent	Mode of Transmission
Anthrax	Bacillus anthracis	Inhalation
Botulism (food poisoning)	Clostridium botulinum	Ingestion
Chlamydia (sexually transmitted disease)	Chlamydia trachomatis	Sexual contact
Clostridial myonecrosis (Gas gangrene)	Species of gram-positive clostridia	Wound entry
Escherichia coli	Gram-negative bacilli	Ingestion, wound entry
Gonorrhea (sexually transmitted disease)	Neisseria gonorrhoeae	Sexual contact
Legionnaires disease (pneumonia)	Legionella pneumophila	Inhalation
Meningococcal meningitis	Neisseria meningitidis, Streptococcus pneumoniae, or Haemophilus influenzae	Direct contact, inhalation
Nosocomial (hospital-acquired) infection	Gram-negative bacteria	Normal flora transmitted during illness/ procedures; opportunistic pathogens transmit during debilitated condition
Pneumococci	Streptococcus pneumoniae	Respiratory (inhalation)
Pulmonary tuberculosis	Mycobacterium tuberculosis	Inhalation
Samonellosis (food poisoning)	Salmonella	Ingestion
Shigellosis (bacillary dysentery, diarrhea)	Shigellae	Fecal-oral
Staphylococcal infection (abscesses, food poisoning, urinary tract infections)	Staphylococci	Direct contact, ingestion, inhalation, bloodborne, vectors (animals)
Streptococcal infection (strep throat, otitis media, pneumonia)	Hemolytic streptococci (usually beta-hemolytic group A)	Inhalation
Syphilis (sexually transmitted disease)	Treponema pallidum	Sexual contact
Tetanus (lockjaw)	Clostridium tetani	Wound entry
Tuberculosis	Mycobacterium tuberculosis	Inhalation
Typhoid fever (enteric fever)	Salmonella typhi	Fecal-oral

under the microscope, whereas gram-positive bacteria stain purple. The bacteria that do not accept stain are considered spores, which are bacteria with a covering that protects them from many chemical disinfectants and higher levels of heat. The three classifications of bacteria are cocci (sphere or dot shaped); bacilli (rod shaped); and spirilla (spiral shaped). Bacteria are either pathogenic or nonpathogenic. Nonpathogenic bacteria normally reside on the skin of humans and in mucous membrane areas of the body. These are known as *normal flora*. Nonpathogenic bacteria use nutrients and occupy space, competing with the pathogenic bacteria. When nonpathogenic bacteria are reduced, the opportunity exists for pathogenic organisms to take over and cause infectious disease. A common cause of the reduction of nonpathogenic microorganisms is the use of antiinfectious drugs. Examples of some bacterial pathogens are listed in Table 10-1.

Fungi. Fungi are microorganisms that may be unicellular (single-cell) or multicellular (many cells). Mushrooms and molds are examples of fungi that are nonpathogenic. Pathogenic fungi cause athlete's foot, ringworm, and candida infections. Other pathogenic fungi include histoplasmosis and toxoplasmosis, which are fungal infections spread through the air from infected fowl and bird waste.

Parasites. Organisms that live in or on another organism are classified as parasites. They may be single-celled or multicelled. Examples include protozoa (single-cell microscopic organisms that cause **malaria, amoebic dysentery,** and **trichomoniasis**); metazoa (multicellular organisms that cause pinworms, hookworms, and tapeworms); and ectoparasites (multicellular organisms that live superficially on another host, such as lice and **scabies**).

Rickettsiae. Rickettsiae are intracellular parasites, similar to the virus. However, they are larger than viruses and can be seen under conventional microscopes after staining procedures. These microorganisms are susceptible to antibiotic therapy. Examples of rickettsiae infections include typhus (transmitted by the body louse); Lyme disease (transmitted by ticks); and Rocky Mountain Spotted Fever (transmitted by ticks). Characteristic of rickettsia infections is a skin rash caused by the rickettsia invading the small blood vessels. This appears on the skin as a small hemorrhagic rash.

Reservoir

The second link in the chain of infection is the reservoir or location of the infectious agent. Reservoirs are people, equipment, supplies, water, food, and animals or insects (known as vectors). Methods of infection control in the reservoir link include hand washing, environmental hygiene, disinfection, sterilization, and maintenance of employee health standards, such as annual tuberculosis skin testing.

Portal of Exit

Although the infectious agent is housed or living in the reservoir, it must leave the reservoir to infect another person. The portal of exit is the method by which an infectious agent leaves the reservoir. Microorganisms may leave the human body with normally occurring body fluids, such as **excretions, secretions,** skin cells, respiratory droplets, blood, or any body fluid. The portal of exit may be continuous, such as with respiratory droplets, or dependent on the body fluid exiting the body under unusual circumstances, such as when blood leaves the body during a surgical procedure or phlebotomy.

Standard Precautions and **Transmission-Based Precautions** are infection control methods based on the knowledge that exiting infectious diseases can be spread to others. These precautions attempt to control the spread of infectious diseases as infectious agents exit the reservoir.

Means of Transmission

The means of transmission are specific ways in which microorganisms travel from one place (reservoir) to another (susceptible host). Transmission depends on the characteristics of the microorganisms. Types of routes of transmission include:

- Direct contact (touching the **exudate** from a person with an infected wound)
- Airborne transmission (inhaling the microorganism into the susceptible host's respiratory system)
- Bloodborne transmission (infected blood enters susceptible host)
- Ingestion (eating or drinking contaminated items)
- Indirect contact (microorganism on a **fomite,** a nonliving object such as a table or piece of equipment that can absorb and transmit infection)
- **Vector** (a carrier of disease, usually an insect)

Infection control measures in the ambulatory care area specifically address the transmission stage of the process of infection.

Methods that reduce the transmission of pathogens include adherence to Standard and Transmission-Based Precautions, hand washing, sanitization, disinfection, and sterilization. Methods of infection control are used in food handling, water and sewage processing, and child care.

Portal of Entry

After transmission, the infectious agent must enter another person, or a susceptible host. The portal of entry allows the agent access to the next person. Common entrance sites to the human body include broken skin, mucous membranes, and systems of the body exposed to the external environment, such as the respiratory, gastrointestinal, and reproductive systems. Breathing in airborne microorganisms allows infectious diseases to be spread to the lungs. Eating or drinking contaminated water is a cause of gastrointestinal infectious diseases. Sexually transmitted diseases spread through vaginal, oral, and anal intercourse. Care of patients with infectious diseases includes careful consideration of infection control to limit further spread of the microorganism. Methods such as sterile wound care, transmission-based precautions, and **aseptic** technique limit the transmission of infectious microorganisms. The portals of exit and entry need not be the same for infection to be transmitted.

Susceptible Host

Finally, infectious microorganisms must enter another person who is susceptible. This means that the person is able to contract the pathogenic organism. The susceptible host is therefore not resistant or immune to the organism. Causes of susceptibility include the presence of other diseases, immunosuppression (weakened immune system), surgical procedures, trauma, or the absence of immunity to the specific microorganism. Susceptibility of a person depends on several factors, including:

1. Number and specific type of pathogen
2. Duration of exposure to the pathogen
3. General physical condition
4. Psychological health status
5. Occupation or lifestyle environment
6. Presence of underlying diseases or conditions
7. Youth or advanced age (young and old at greater risk)

The goal of infection control at this link in the chain of infection is to identify patients at risk for suscep-

Critical Thinking

Identify and describe the steps in the chain of infection.

tibility, treat their underlying conditions if possible, and isolate them from those reservoirs that could be hazardous to the susceptible person.

THE BODY'S DEFENSE MECHANISMS FOR FIGHTING INFECTION AND DISEASE

The Body's Natural Barriers

The body has many natural barriers and defenses in place to help us avoid exposure to pathogens and infection.

These barriers can be categorized under physical/mechanical, chemical, and cellular factors. Physical/mechanical factors include eyelashes and eyebrows, cilia (tiny hairs in the respiratory tract), and barriers such as eyelids, and skin/mucous membranes. Chemical barriers include tears, sweat, mucus, saliva, gastrointestinal secretions, and vaginal secretions. Cellular barriers are also called body defenses and consist of our white blood cells, which defend us from infection in many ways in our tissues, bloodstream, and lymphatic system. The cellular defenses are explained in more detail in the following two sections.

Inflammatory Response

Inflammation is the body's natural way of responding when invaded by a pathogen or trauma. Inflammation is a nonspecific response, meaning that it can occur with any threat to the body, not just in reaction to a particular pathogen. Inflammation can occur even without a pathogen regardless of whether the agent is pathogenic, trauma, a foreign body, or extremes in temperature. If a pathogen is present, the body goes through a distinct process in an attempt to destroy and eliminate the pathogenic microorganisms and their by-products and, if that is not possible, to restrict the amount of damage done.

The cardinal signs of inflammation are redness, heat, swelling, and pain. These symptoms may be slight, almost unnoticed, or quite evident. Remember, inflammation is a natural response and does not indicate infection. The two should not be confused. Inflammation can occur without infection, but infection does not occur without inflammation.

The steps in the inflammatory process are:

- Local dilation of blood vessels increases blood flow to injured (infected) area causing redness or heat.
- Plasma moves into the tissue causing swelling and pain due to pressure on nerve endings.
- White blood cells move into injured tissue to fight infection and phagocytes destroy invading pathogens.

After destruction of the pathogen, tissue repair can begin. If the **inflammatory response** is not effective, the specific immune response is necessary.

Indications that an inflammatory process is inadequate are: (1) the accumulation of **purulent** matter in the area (due to destroyed pathogens, white blood cells, and body cells); (2) lymph node enlargement (swollen glands); and (3) septicemia may result because pathogens have spread to the bloodstream.

Immediate antibiotic therapy is indicated in these circumstances because of the inadequacy of the inflammatory response.

The Immune System and Immunity

To fight infectious diseases, our bodies are equipped with several effective physical and chemical **barriers** such as the skin, mucous membranes, body excretions and secretions, and a complex, highly specific **immune system.** The immune system's purpose is to protect against pathogens and abnormal cell growth. The system is composed of various cells that collectively recognize, subdue, attack, and eliminate pathogens. The two types of immune responses include cell-mediated immunity and humoral immunity. **Cell-mediated immunity** is usually involved in attacks against viruses, fungi, organ transplants, or cancer cells. This type of immunity does not produce antibodies. **Humoral immunity** produces antibodies that are capable of killing microorganisms and of recognizing the pathogen in the future. Generally, both types of immune responses occur in four phases:

1. *Recognition of the invader*. The immune system is equipped with cells that identify agents, pathogens, and abnormal cell growth as foreign substances. Macrophages and helper T cells recognize foreign invaders, whether they are pathogens, cancer cells, or transplanted tissues.
2. *Growth of defenses, which allows for multiplication of helper T cells and B cells*. After foreign substance recognition, the immune system alerts T and B cells

to multiply and move to the site of the foreign substance. In cell-mediated immunity, activation of helper T cells means that the T cells are specifically oriented to a unique **antigen,** a substance such as bacteria the body recognizes as foreign. Activated T cells divide, forming memory T cells and killer T cells. In humoral immunity, activated B cells are antigen specific and divide into memory B cells and plasma cells.

3. *Attack against the infection*. Cell-mediated immunity uses killer T cells and macrophages to phagocytize, or engulf and destroy the pathogens. Humoral plasma cells have the ability to produce specific **antibodies** that lock on to specific antigens, which prevents the disease-producing characteristics of the pathogen from forming. These antibodies are called **immunoglobulins** and they render the pathogen unable to reproduce or continue growth.
4. *Slowdown of the immune response after death of the infectious agent*. After the death of the foreign substance, the immune response is halted. T and B cells return to normal levels, and in the case of humoral immunity, the presence of antibody production causes the immune system to resist the specific infectious pathogen in future contacts with the pathogen.

Susceptibility to some infectious diseases is closely linked to the person's unique resistance, or immunity. **Immunity** means the ability of the body to resist specific pathogens and their toxins. **Resistance** occurs after an exposure to a pathogen, which is the antigen–antibody reaction. This natural body defense to fight infectious disease occurs gradually and over time as pathogens and other foreign substances such as antigens enter the human body. When the antigen enters the body, the immune system recognizes the antigen as foreign and attempts to contain and subdue the foreign invader. Specific chemical antibodies to the antigen are produced by B cells, which attempt to prevent the antigen from further growth. After the completion of the stages of that infectious disease, the body retains the ability to produce antibodies in response to that specific microorganism or antigen. Therefore, immunity can last for some length of time, possibly to provide lifetime protection against specific infectious microorganisms. Several forms of immunity can occur in response to specific antigens:

- Naturally acquired active immunity results from contracting an infectious agent and experiencing either an acute or subclinical infectious disease. This immunity is permanent.
- Artificially acquired active immunity is achieved after administration of vaccines. This immunity is semi-permanent to permanent.
- Naturally, congenitally acquired passive immunity occurs when antibodies pass to a fetus from the mother providing short-term immunity for the newborn. This immunity is temporary.
- Artificially acquired passive immunity may be achieved through administration of ready-made antibodies, such as gamma globulin, used to treat or prevent infectious diseases. This immunity is temporary.

Our defenses against diseases can be categorized as specific and nonspecific. Specific defenses include those things that protect us against a specific pathogen, whereas nonspecific defenses are not so particular. Some examples of specific defenses are:

- *Vaccines/Immunizations:* designed for specific pathogen
- *Antibodies:* created against a specific pathogen
- *Tetanus shot:* protects individuals from tetanus
- *Active immunities:* created against a specific pathogen
- *Globulin:* antibodies for exposure to a specific pathogen

Some examples of nonspecific defenses are:

- *Tears:* contain chemical harmful to a variety of pathogens
- *Skin:* creates a barrier against many different pathogens
- *Saliva:* contains chemicals harmful to a variety of pathogens
- *Species resistance:* being human protects us from many diseases to which other animals are susceptible

Immunization. Immunizing individuals against specific infectious diseases provides immunity with active or passive vaccines (see Tables 10-2 and 10-3). Most of the severe childhood communicable diseases can be prevented. The U.S. Department of Health and Human Services has estimated that about 80% of U.S. preschoolers younger than 2 years are fully vaccinated according to recommended schedules. Several factors influence vaccination rates, such as access to health care, cost of vaccinations, and irregularity or confusion in maintaining young children on the recommended schedule. There are pockets within large cities of significant numbers of under-immunized children. A substantial number of these children are minority children. An outbreak could cause an **epidemic** of diseases that are preventable with vaccines (see Chapter 15).

There is a movement by parents and caregivers that is resisting the mandated childhood immunizations even though all states have immunization requirements for school admission. These groups want state laws changed and feel that they, as parents and caregivers, should be allowed to decide if they want their children immunized.

Exemptions from mandated immunizations are allowed in all states if there are medical reasons. Some states will exempt children for religious reasons, and some on philosophical grounds.

In general, children would more likely suffer greater complications associated with childhood diseases than from the immunizations given to prevent them. Because most of the vaccinations are administered in ambulatory health care settings, medical assistants may have the responsibility to administer, document, and monitor immunizations (Chapter 15).

There are various classifications of vaccines, depending on the method of immune stimulation:

1. *Live attenuated (changed) pathogens*. These pathogens stimulate the body's own antibody production. However, the patient does not contract the infectious disease (or only a mild or subclinical case) because the pathogen has been altered in some mechanical or chemical means by the manufacturer. Examples of live attenuated pathogens include measles and varicella.
2. *Pathogenic toxins*. Some pathogens produce toxins (poisonous substances) that can stimulate antibody production. Examples of toxin vaccines include tetanus and diphtheria.
3. *Killed pathogens*. Inactivated pathogens stimulate antibody production; however, several vaccines may be required to provide sustained protection. Examples include pertussis, rabies, and poliomyelitis.

STAGES OF INFECTIOUS DISEASES

Depending on the specific pathogen causing an infectious disease, several stages occur from the time of exposure until full recovery and the absence of infection. These stages are often predictable and offer guidelines for patient education and treatment opportunities.

Incubation Stage

The incubation stage is the interval of time between exposure to a pathogenic microorganism and the first appearance of signs and symptoms of the disease. Some infectious diseases have short incubation stages, whereas other infections have lengthy stages, lasting for years. If an exposure to an infectious agent occurs, the patient will **manifest** the disease if the patient's immune system cannot contain the agent. If therapeutic medications are available, it can help to prevent disease progression. Not all infectious agents are treatable or preventable.

Prodromal Stage

The prodromal stage is the initial stage of the disease. It is characterized by common, general complaints of illness, such as **malaise** and fever. It is the interval between the earliest symptoms and the appearance of fever or rash that suggest an impending disease process is occurring.

Acute Stage

Disease processes reach their peak during the acute stage. Symptoms are fully developed and can often be differentiated from other specific symptoms. Treatment modalities are useful to reduce patient discomfort, to reduce possibilities of debilitation and adverse effects, and to promote healing and recovery.

The inflammatory process is the body's natural defensive reaction to the invasion by a foreign substance such as a pathogen, and it is in this acute state that the response is evident.

Declining Stage

Patient symptoms begin to subside or wane during the declining stage. The infectious disease remains, however, though the patient will demonstrate improving levels of health. It is often during the declining phase of an illness when patients begin to feel better that they prematurely discontinue taking the antibiotic that may have been prescribed. This premature discontinuance can result in microorganisms becoming resistant to antibiotics. It is important to educate our patients in the proper use of antibiotics.

Convalescent Stage

Recovery and recuperation from the effects of a specific infectious disease are called the convalescent stage. The patient regains strength and stamina. The overall goal

TABLE 10-2 RECOMMENDED ADULT IMMUNIZATION SCHEDULE BY VACCINE AND AGE GROUP
UNITED STATES • 2003–2004

Legend: For all persons in this group · Catch-up on childhood vaccinations · For persons with medical/exposure indications

VACCINE / AGE	19-49 YEARS	50-64 YEARS	65 YEARS & OLDER
Tetanus, Diphtheria (Td)*	1 dose booster every 10 years		
Influenza	1 dose annually	1 dose annually	
Pneumococcal (polysaccharide)	1 dose		1 dose
Hepatitis B*	3 doses *(0, 1–2, 4–6 months)*		
Hepatitis A	2 doses *(0, 6–12 months)*		
Measles, Mumps, Rubella (MMR)*	1 dose if measles, mumps or rubella vaccination history is unreliable; 2 doses for persons with occupational or other indications		
Varicella*	2 doses *(0, 4–8 weeks)* for persons who are susceptible		
Meningococcal (polysaccharide)	1 dose		

* Covered by the Vaccine Injury Compensation Program. For information on how to file a claim, call **1-800-338-2382**. Please also visit **www.hrsa.osp.gov/vicp**. To file a claim for vaccine injury, write: U.S. Court of Federal Claims, 717 Madison Place, NW, Washington, DC 20005. Telephone 202-219-9657.

This schedule indicates the recommended age groups for routine administration of currently licensed vaccines for persons 19 years of age and older. Licensed combination vaccines may be used whenever any components of the combination are indicated and the vaccine's other components are not contraindicated. Providers should consult the manufacturers' package inserts for detailed recommendations.

Report all clinically significant post-vaccination reactions to the Vaccine Adverse Event Reporting System (VAERS). Reporting forms and instructions on filing a VAERS report are available by calling **1-800-822-7967** or from the VAERS website at **www.vaers.org**.

For additional information about the vaccines listed above and contraindications for immunization, please visit the National Immunization Program Website at **www.cdc.gov/nip** or call the National Immunization Hotline, **1-800-232-2522** (English) or **1-800-232-0233** (Spanish).

APPROVED BY THE ADVISORY COMMITTEE ON IMMUNIZATION PRACTICES (ACIP) AND
ACCEPTED BY THE AMERICAN COLLEGE OF OBSTETRICIANS AND GYNECOLOGISTS (ACOG)
AND THE AMERICAN ACADEMY OF FAMILY PHYSICIANS (AAFP)

CDC National Immunization Hotline:
800-232-2522 ENGLISH • **800-232-0233** ESPAÑOL

DEPARTMENT OF HEALTH & HUMAN SERVICES • USA

CDC SAFER • HEALTHIER • PEOPLE™

Department of Health and Human Services
Centers for Disease Control and Prevention

TABLE 10-3 RECOMMENDED ADULT IMMUNIZATION SCHEDULE BY VACCINE AND MEDICAL AND OTHER INDICATIONS UNITED STATES • 2003–2004

UNITED STATES • 2003-2004

Legend: For all persons in this group · Catch-up on childhood vaccinations · For persons with medical/exposure indications · Contraindicated

Medical Conditions ▼ / Vaccine ►	Tetanus-Diphtheria (Td)*	Influenza	Pneumococcal (polysaccharide)	Hepatitis B*	Hepatitis A	Measles, Mumps, Rubella (MMR)*	Varicella*
Pregnancy		A					
Diabetes, Heart Disease, Chronic Pulmonary Disease, Chronic Liver Disease, including Chronic Alcoholism		B	C		D		
Congenital Immunodeficiency, Leukemia, Lymphoma, Generalized Malignancy, Therapy with Alkylating Agents, Antimetabolites, Radiation or Large Amounts of Corticosteroids			E				F
Renal Failure/End Stage Renal Disease, Recipients of Hemodialysis or Clotting Factor Concentrates			E	G			
Asplenia, including Elective Splenectomy and Terminal Complement Component Deficiencies		H	E, I, J				
HIV Infection			E, K			L	

A. For women without chronic diseases/conditions, vaccinate if pregnancy will be at 2nd or 3rd trimester during influenza season. For women with chronic diseases/conditions, vaccinate at any time during the pregnancy.

B. Although chronic liver disease and alcoholism are not indicator conditions for influenza vaccination, give 1 dose annually if the patient is age 50 years or older, has other indications for influenza vaccine, or if the patient requests vaccination.

C. Asthma is an indicator condition for influenza but not for pneumococcal vaccination.

D. For all persons with chronic liver disease.

E. For persons < 65 years, revaccinate once after 5 years or more have elapsed since initial vaccination.

F. Persons with impaired humoral immunity but with intact cellular immunity may be vaccinated. *MMWR* 1999; 48 (RR-06):1-5.

G. Hemodialysis patients: Use special formulation of vaccine (40 ug/mL) or two 1.0 mL 20 ug doses given at one site. Vaccinate early in the course of renal disease. Assess antibody titers to hep B surface antigen (anti-HBs) levels annually. Administer additional doses if anti-HBs levels decline to <10 milliinternational units (mIU)/ mL.

H. There are no data specifically on risk of severe or complicated influenza infections among persons with asplenia. However, influenza is a risk factor for secondary bacterial infections that may cause severe disease in asplenics.

I. Administer meningococcal vaccine and consider Hib vaccine.

J. Elective splenectomy: vaccinate at least 2 weeks before surgery.

K. Vaccinate as close to diagnosis as possible when CD4 cell counts are highest.

L. Withhold MMR or other measles containing vaccines from HIV-infected persons with evidence of severe immunosuppression. *MMWR* 1998; 47 (RR-8):21-22; *MMWR* 2002; 51 (RR-02):22-24.

of this stage is that the patient is returned to the original state of health.

DISEASE TRANSMISSION

When providing patients with health care, medical assistants run the risk for **contracting,** or acquiring, an infection from pathogens that are causing patients' illnesses. Such pathogens are viruses, bacteria, fungi, and others that can be found in patients' blood and body fluids. In medical offices, ambulatory care centers, and hospitals, many ill patients are seen everyday. Pathogens can be easily transmitted to another person if care is not taken to prevent such an occurrence.

Consistent use and adherence to infection control measures significantly reduce the risk for disease transmission. The CDC recommends that health care providers consider each patient to be potentially infectious for AIDS, hepatitis B and C, and other bloodborne pathogens and to routinely and conscientiously apply the techniques of Standard Precautions as a means of infection control.

Infectious diseases are caused by unique infectious agents, are characterized by various symptoms, are transmitted by differing means, and have unique treatments and prognoses. Medical assistants must recognize the unique characteristics of specific infectious diseases to prevent their transmission and help patients suffering from these infections. Table 10-4 classifies several common infectious diseases by critical components. When patients have contracted an infectious disease or are exposed to the risk for transmission, patient education plays an important role in infection control. Although a family member may have an infectious disease, proper training and education may protect other family members and close contacts.

Medical assistants are in a unique position to educate patients and the public about disease control. These measures become even more important with the increase in drug-resistant pathogens. All health care professionals must consistently and diligently use every infection control measure available, as well as teach our patients to do the same.

HUMAN IMMUNODEFICIENCY VIRUS AND HEPATITIS B AND C

A great deal of attention has been focused on the **human immunodeficiency virus (HIV)** that causes AIDS, and yet there remains no cure for the disease, although great advances have been made. With the focus on AIDS, other potentially life-threatening and fatal illnesses seem less dangerous. In reality, hepatitis B and C are examples of other diseases that place health care providers at great risk for serious illness or death. Acute viral hepatitis deserves close attention.

HIV/AIDS

AIDS is caused by a bloodborne virus, HIV. The viral infection directly affects the immune response. The HIV is responsible for T cell destruction; T cells are the white blood cells that provide immunity.

HIV is carried in semen, blood, and other body fluids, and the virus can penetrate mucous membranes. Once inside the body, the reduced number of helper T cells leaves the patient vulnerable to a wide range of infections and malignancies. The infections that the patient contracts can be devastating. Many people are living for many years with HIV. When people are positive for HIV infection, their T-cell counts must be regularly and closely monitored, and they must live their lives with careful consideration toward preventing opportunistic infections. If their T-cell count decreases to less than 200, they are considered to have AIDS. There is no curative treatment for HIV infections, but there are antiviral drugs such as lamivudine, azidothymidine, zidovudine, stavudine, and others that are used to slow cell processes and weaken cell protein, which is important in the virus's reproduction.

Acute Viral Hepatitis Diseases

In any of the acute viral hepatitis diseases, the liver becomes inflamed, and hepatic cells can be destroyed. Healthy persons can regenerate cells, but older adult patients usually cannot. There are several types of viral hepatitis, hepatitis A (HAV), hepatitis B (HBV), hepatitis C (HCV), hepatitis D (HDV), and hepatitis E (HEV). HAV, HBV, and HCV are the more common viruses; HDV and HEV are less common.

Symptoms of HCV. Infection with HCV is a progressive disease that can become chronic. Individuals can carry the virus in their blood for the rest of their lives. Many individuals do not realize that they are infected; therefore, they can transmit the virus to others. HCV is usually a chronic disease that damages the liver and causes **cirrhosis** and liver failure.

According to former Surgeon General Koop, there are 5 million people in the United States infected with HCV, yet it is a disease relatively unknown to the general public. Koop claims that "hepatitis C may surpass the death rate of AIDS if it is not contained."

Individuals at risk for HCV include those who had a blood transfusion before July 1992. Improved blood tests for HCV became available at that time.

TABLE 10-4 EXAMPLES OF SOME COMMON INFECTIOUS DISEASES

Disease	Agent	Transmission	Symptoms	Diagnosis	Treatment	Comments	Patient Education
Acquired immunodeficiency syndrome (AIDS)	Human immunodeficiency virus (HIV)	• Bloodborne • Sexual contact • Intrauterine • Lactation	Opportunistic infections, **lymphadenopathy,** fatigue, malaise, fever	CD4 percentage level less than 14%	Palliative care and treatment for **opportunistic infections,** antiviral drugs	World Health Organization (WHO) estimates 36 million people infected with HIV	1. Careful infection control and **asepsis** to reduce contact with pathogens that cause opportunistic infections 2. Use of latex condoms in conjunction with effective spermicide 3. Support groups/education
Hepatitis B	Hepatitis B virus (HBV)	• Bloodborne • Sexual contact • Intrauterine • Human bites	Fatigue, malaise, **anorexia,** headache, liver tenderness and enlargement, fever, jaundice	Serum antibody tests; liver function studies elevated	Immunization of all those at risk for exposure; palliative therapy, monitor bilirubin levels, bed rest, frequent low-fat, high-carbohydrate diet for those infected	May lead to liver cancer or cirrhosis; 100 times more infectious than AIDS; report to public health authorities	1. Follow-up required to monitor liver function studies 2. Close personal contacts of patient should receive HB vaccine or HBIG (HB immunoglobulin) 3. Teach infection control to patient to prevent spread to close contacts 4. Avoid alcohol, sedatives, or aspirin during acute phase
Hepatitis C	Hepatitis C virus (HCV)	• Tattooing • Body piercing • Sexual contact • Blood and body fluids • Needle exchange	Few or none for years or decades; progresses to chronic liver disease	Blood test for HCV; liver enzymes; liver biopsy	Medication combination of peginterferon with ribavirin; liver transplant	Most serious type of hepatitis; 5 million cases in the United States; may surpass mortality rate of AIDS if not contained; unknown to general public; progresses to cirrhosis or cancer; no vaccine	1. Ultimate defense is knowledge and awareness 2. Use protection during sexual contact 3. Be aware that ink used for tattooing can be contaminated with the virus 4. Do not use other people's toothbrush or razor 5. Do not donate blood 6. Zero alcohol consumption because of liver stress 7. Get hepatitis A and B vaccines 8. Testing is important
Tuberculosis (TB)	Mycobacterium tuberculosis bacillus	• Inhalation of contaminated airborne mucous droplets • Possibly ingestion	Productive cough, fatigue, fever, weight loss (older adults: behavior changes, anorexia, weight loss), night sweats	Sputum culture for M. tuberculosis, Mantoux skin test (PPD), chest X-ray, pleural needle biopsy	Antituberculosis agents, airborne transmission-based precautions, until drug agents started	Increase in incidence of TB, especially among persons with AIDS and the homeless; may be drug resistant; health care professionals should have annual skin testing; report outbreaks	1. Encourage hand washing and proper sputum tissue disposal 2. Promote compliance with medications 3. Encourage close contacts to have skin tests 4. Well-balanced diet

(continues)

TABLE 10-4 EXAMPLES OF SOME COMMON INFECTIOUS DISEASES (continued)

Disease	Agent	Transmission	Symptoms	Diagnosis	Treatment	Comments	Patient Education
	Bacteria or viruses (i.e., staphylococci, clostridium, botulinum, E. coli, shigella)	• Ingestion of contaminated food or water	Nausea, intestinal cramps, vomiting, diarrhea, dehydration, respiratory failure, death	Culture of feces, vomitus, or suspected food or water	Fluid balance restoration, medications, emergency treatment as required	Report outbreaks to local authorities; especially dangerous in children and older adults	1. Teach proper food handling 2. Carefully washing hands before handling all food 3. Report to physician all signs of dehydration 4. Gastroenteritis usually communicable via feces for up to seven weeks after exposure
	Influenze viruses A, B, or C, haemophilus (bacteria)	• Inhalation • Aerosolized • Mucous droplets	Acute upper/lower respiratory infection, severe cough, fever, malaise, sore throat, **coryza**	Tissue culture of nasal or pharyngeal secretions	Palliative therapy, active immunization (annual vaccine recommended for persons at risk [older adults, heart patients] for complications from infection)	Report cases to local health authority; may be fatal in older adults and children; may cause meningitis; may easily become epidemic	1. Bed rest for two to three days after fever decline 2. Force fluids 3. Report signs of secondary infections (pneumonia, otitis media) 4. Vaccine available
	Varicella-zoster virus	• Direct and indirect contact with respiratory droplets	Sudden-onset fever, malaise, **maculo-papular-vesicular** skin rash	Vesicular fluid tissue culture during first three days after eruption; serology: increased antibodies two weeks after rash; **lesion** appearance characteristic of varicella	**Acyclovir** helpful to reduce severity of disease; zoster immunoglobulin (ZIG) for high-risk persons only within 96 hours of exposure; palliative therapy	Vaccine (varicella virus vaccine live) available in United States for children older than 12 months	1. Communicable one to two days before rash until lesions crust 2. Avoid scratching lesions to prevent secondary infection and scarring 3. Benadryl and calamine lotion for itch 4. Acetaminophen for fever
	Virus	• Infected mosquito	Central nervous system; fever, headache, coma, convulsions, paralysis; 80% of people infected show no signs or symptoms	West Nile Virus IgM Capture ELIZA	None; supportive only	Potentially serious illness	1. Use insect repellent with DEET 2. Wear long sleeves and pants when outside, especially at dawn and dusk 3. Get rid of mosquito breeding sites by emptying standing water in flowerpots, buckets, and barrels 4. Keep children's pools empty and on their sides when not in use

(continues)

TABLE 10-4 EXAMPLES OF SOME COMMON INFECTIOUS DISEASES (continued)

Disease	Agent	Transmission	Symptoms	Diagnosis	Treatment	Comments	Patient Education
Severe acute respiratory syndrome (SARS)	Virus	• Close person-to-person contact • Kissing • Sharing eating or drinking utensils • Perhaps respiratory droplets	High fever, headache, cough, shortness of breath, diarrhea	SARS serum antibodies validated by Centers for Disease Control and Prevention	None; supportive only; may treat pneumonia with antibiotics but will not cure patient	Potentially serious illness; currently no known SARS transmissions; last transmission was in China, April 2004; because no one knows if SARS will recur, early recognition of cases and appropriate infection control are essential to control outbreaks; Transmission-Based Precautions (Isolation); airborne and direct contact	1. Travel to a previously SARS-affected area (China, Hong Kong, or Taiwan) or close contact with an ill person who has such a travel history 2. A diagnosis of pneumonia raises the suspicion of exposure to SARS 3. Avoid close contact such as kissing, hugging, sharing of eating or drinking utensils

People who know they are infected with HCV should not donate blood; share razors, toothbrushes, or other articles of personal use; and should cover wounds (cuts and sores) on their skin with a dressing. Health care providers caring for infected individuals should recommend that latex condoms be used during intercourse, and that sexual partners be tested for the virus.

HCV can be transmitted to the infant of an infected mother. This occurs in about 5% of cases. There is no prevention strategy for this occurrence.

The virus is not spread by contaminated food or water, sneezing, coughing, breast-feeding (unless blood is present), or by hugging or casual contact.

Once individuals with HCV have been diagnosed, they must see their physicians regularly, not consume any alcohol (causes further liver damage), and get the vaccines for HAV and HBV. Because there is no vaccine for HCV, antiviral drugs, such as peginterferon and ribavirin are used for treatment. The treatment is usually effective in only 20% to 30% of patients undergoing treatment.

Symptoms of HBV. HBV is considered a serious **biohazard** for health care providers. The American Medical Association has said that loss of health care workers to HBV overshadows the risk for AIDS and is almost entirely preventable.

HBV is easier to contract than HIV. Symptoms of HBV include loss of appetite, fatigue, nausea, headache, fever, and **jaundice,** a yellow discoloration of the skin. The liver function is impaired and, in severe cases, may even be lost. Notably, in some individuals, HBV may be asymptomatic and can still damage the liver and possibly lead to cancer of the liver. Usually, once patients become infected, they remain so for life and are capable of transmitting the virus to others. This is a chronic disease.

HBV and HCV represent the greatest risk to health care providers. There is a vaccine to help prevent HBV, but none exists for HCV. It is important to practice Standard Precautions (hand washing, infection control, personal protective equipment) to stem the transmission of these diseases.

Transmission of HIV, HBV, and HCV

HIV, HBV, and HCV are transmitted essentially through the same means. Contracting any of these diseases requires direct contact with the virus living in infected blood and body fluids. The viruses are transmitted primarily through the following means:

- Sexual contact with multiple partners or any infected person (heterosexual, homosexual, or bisexual). The virus enters the bloodstream through small tears in the mucous membrane of the vagina, rectum, penis, or mouth (less risk for HCV)
- Sharing needles for intravenous (IV) drug use with an infected person
- Using unsterilized tattoo and body piercing tools after their use on an infected person
- Receiving blood or blood products from an infected person. (All blood collected for transfusions is routinely checked for HIV, HBV, and HCV; therefore, risk from this is now rare.)
- Intrauterine infection of the fetus by a pregnant infected woman
- Human bite of an infected person

Despite the similarities among HIV, HBV, and HCV, the risk for contracting HBV and HCV is greater than contracting HIV. See Figure 10-2 and Table 10-5.

Medical assistants and all other health care providers must understand the importance of protecting themselves from the viruses that cause AIDS, HBV, and other pathogenic microorganisms. Through strict adherence to safety precautions and routine infectious disease control measures such as those found in **medical asepsis,** the risk for contracting an infectious disease is minimized.

Standard Precautions

The CDC spent several years researching, improving, and developing recommendations to protect health care

Latex Sensitivity

Health care providers should be aware that some people, including professionals and patients, can be allergic to latex products. Some personal protective equipment (PPE) is made from latex; medical and surgical products also are often made from this product.

The allergic reaction can be a localized one such as dermatitis or a more severe systemic reaction such as anaphylaxis (see Chapter 9), a form of shock marked by vascular collapse, respiratory failure, hypotension, arrhythmia, and laryngeal edema. Vinyl gloves can be worn in place of latex for hypersensitive individuals. Any person with an allergy to latex should wear a bracelet or other form of identification indicating this fact because, in any emergency, medical personnel wear latex gloves (see Chapter 9).

BLOODBORNE FACTS

WHAT IS HBV?

Hepatitis B virus (HBV) is a potentially life-threatening bloodborne pathogen. Centers for Disease Control estimates there are approximately 280,000 HBV infections each year in the United States.

Approximately 8,700 health care workers each year contract hepatitis B, and about 200 will die as a result. In addition, some who contract HBV will become carriers, passing the disease on to others. Carriers also face a significantly higher risk for other liver ailments which can be fatal, including cirrhosis of the liver and primary liver cancer.

HBV infection is transmitted through exposure to blood and other infectious body fluids and tissues. Anyone with occupational exposure to blood is at risk of contracting the infection.

Employers must provide engineering controls; workers must use work practices and protective clothing and equipment to prevent exposure to potentially infectious materials. However, the best defense against hepatitis B is vaccination.

WHO NEEDS VACCINATION?

The new OSHA standard covering bloodborne pathogens requires employers to offer the three-injection vaccination series free to all employees who are exposed to blood or other potentially infectious materials as part of their job duties. This includes health care workers, emergency responders, morticians, first-aid personnel, law enforcement officers, correctional facilities staff, launderers, as well as others.

The vaccination must be offered within 10 days of initial assignment to a job where exposure to blood or other potentially infectious materials can be "reasonably anticipated." The requirements for vaccinations of those already on the job took effect July 6, 1992.

WHAT DOES VACCINATION INVOLVE?

The hepatitis B vaccination is a noninfectious, yeast-based vaccine given in three injections in the arm. It is prepared from recombinant yeast cultures, rather than human blood or plasma. Thus, there is no risk of contamination from other bloodborne pathogens nor is there any chance of developing HBV from the vaccine.

The second injection should be given one month after the first, and the third injection six months after the initial dose. More than 90 percent of those vaccinated will develop immunity to the hepatitis B virus. To ensure immunity, it is important for individuals to receive all three injections. At this point it is unclear how long the immunity lasts, so booster shots may be required at some point in the future.

The vaccine causes no harm to those who are already immune or to those who may be HBV carriers. Although employees may opt to have their blood tested for antibodies to determine need for the vaccine, employers may not make such screening a condition of receiving vaccination nor are employers required to provide prescreening.

Each employee should receive counseling from a health care professional when vaccination is offered. This discussion will help an employee determine whether inoculation is necessary.

WHAT IF I DECLINE VACCINATION?

Workers who decide to decline vaccination must complete a declination form. Employers must keep these forms on file so that they know the vaccination status of everyone who is exposed to blood. At any time after a worker initially declines to receive the vaccine, he or she may opt to take it.

WHAT IF I AM EXPOSED BUT HAVE NOT YET BEEN VACCINATED?

If a worker experiences an exposure incident, such as a needlestick or a blood splash in the eye, he or she must receive confidential medical evaluation from a licensed health care professional with appropriate follow-up. To the extent possible by law, the employer is to determine the source individual for HBV as well as human immunodeficiency virus (HIV) infectivity. The worker's blood will also be screened if he or she agrees.

The health care professional is to follow the guidelines of the U.S. Public Health Service in providing treatment. This would include hepatitis B vaccination. The health care professional must give a written opinion on whether or not vaccination is recommended and whether the employee received it. Only this information is reported to the employer. Employee medical records must remain confidential. HIV or HBV status must NOT be reported to the employer.

U.S. Department of Labor
Occupational Safety and Health Administration

Single copies of fact sheets are available from OSHA Publications, Room N3101, 200 Constitution Ave. N.W., Washington, D.C. 20210 and from OSHA regional offices.

Figure 10-2 *Bloodborne Facts,* published by the U.S. Department of Labor, Occupational Safety and Health Administration (OSHA). This publication includes facts about hepatitis B virus, declination, and steps to be taken by the employer should exposure to blood, body fluids, or other potentially infectious material occur.

TABLE 10-5 HEPATITIS VIRUSES A TO E

	A	B	C	D	E
Causative Agent	Hepatitis A virus (HAV)	Hepatitis B virus (HBV)	Hepatitis C virus (HCV)	Hepatitis D virus (HDV)	Hepatitis E virus (HEV)
Transmission	Fecal-oral; contaminated water or food; person to person	Blood; sexual contact; perinatal; breast milk; drug use (sharing needles); tattooing and body piercing	Blood or body fluids; intravenous drug use; mother to fetus; tattoo and body piercing	Only persons with hepatitis B can get hepatitis D; blood and blood products; needlesticks; seldom sexual; rarely perinatal	Oral-fecal route; contaminated water; person to person uncommon
Risk groups	Household/sexual contact with infected person; international travelers; men having sex with men; drug users	Injection drug users; sexual/household contact with infected person; infants born to infected mothers; health care workers; multiple sex partners	Recipients of blood transfusions or organ transplants before 1992; people sharing needles; people exposed to blood and blood products; HBV- and HIV-infected individuals	People sharing needles; health care workers	Travelers to countries where HEV is **endemic**
Incubation period	15–50 days	45–160 days	14–180 days	15–60 days	15–60 days
Infectious period	Usually less than two months	Before symptoms appear; lifetime if carrier	Before symptoms appear; lifetime if carrier	Not determined	Not determined
Diagnostic tests	IgM anti-HAV	HBsAG HBeAG	Anti-HCV; serum ALT increased 10x; HCVRNA	IgG anti-HDV	None available
Symptoms	Flulike; jaundice; dark yellow urine; light-colored stools; anorexia	Flulike; may have jaundice; dark yellow urine; light-colored stools	Many have no symptoms; flulike	Flulike; may have jaundice; dark yellow urine; light-colored stools	Abdominal pain, anorexia; dark yellow urine; jaundice; fever
Prevention	Hepatitis A vaccine (entire series); Standard Precautions; enteric precautions; good personal hygiene, sanitization; immunoglobulin (for short term)	Hepatitis B vaccine (entire series); Standard Precautions; reduce risk behaviors; good personal hygiene, sanitization; immunoglobulin (for short term)	Standard Precautions; reduce risk behaviors; no vaccine	Standard Precautions; reduce risk behaviors; hepatitis B vaccine; if client already has hepatitis B, no prevention for hepatitis D	Standard Precautions; be sure water is safe when traveling; no vaccine
Treatment	Immunoglobulin within two weeks of exposure	Immunoglobulin (HBIg); alpha-interferon	Alpha-interferon; ribavirin (Virazole)	Alpha-interferon	None given
Prognosis	Rarely fatal; not a carrier	No cure; may become a carrier; liver cancer may develop	85% or less have chronic infection; chronic liver disease or cancer develop in 70%	May lead to cirrhosis	Acute infection only

Source: Centers for Disease Control and Prevention and National Institute of Diabetes and Digestive and Kidney Diseases.

providers, patients, and their visitors from infectious diseases. This intensive period of research resulted in Standard Precautions, a set of infection control guidelines that are now used by all health care professionals for all patients.

According to the CDC, Standard Precautions are "designed to reduce the risk of transmission of microorganisms from both recognized and unrecognized sources of infection in hospitals." They apply to:

1. Blood
2. All body fluids, secretions, and excretions regardless of whether they contain visible blood
3. Nonintact skin
4. Mucous membranes

To be effective, Standard Precautions must be practiced conscientiously at all times. Although the Standard

STANDARD PRECAUTIONS
FOR INFECTION CONTROL

Wash Hands (Plain soap)
Wash after touching **blood, body fluids, secretions, excretions,** and **contaminated items.** Wash immediately **after gloves are removed** and **between patient contacts.** Avoid transfer of microorganisms to other patients or environments.

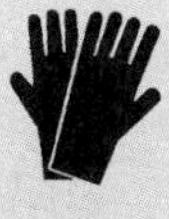

Wear Gloves
Wear when touching **blood, body fluids, secretions, excretions,** and **contaminated items.** Put on **clean** gloves just **before touching mucous membranes** and **nonintact skin.** Change gloves between tasks and procedures on the same patient after contact with material that may contain high concentrations of microorganisms. Remove gloves promptly after use, before touching noncontaminated items and environmental surfaces, and before going to another patient, and wash hands immediately to avoid transfer of microorganisms to other patients or environments.

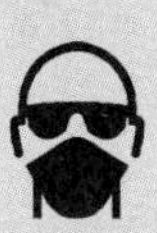

Wear Mask and Eye Protection or Face Shield
Protect mucous membranes of the eyes, nose, and mouth during procedures and patient-care activities that are likely to generate **splashes** or **sprays** of **blood, body fluids, secretions,** or **excretions.**

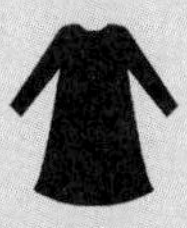

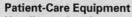

Wear Gown
Protect skin and prevent soiling of clothing during procedures that are likely to generate **splashes** or **sprays** of **blood, body fluids, secretions,** or **excretions.** Remove a soiled gown as promptly as possible and wash hands to avoid transfer of microorganisms to other patients or environments.

Patient-Care Equipment
Handle used patient-care equipment soiled with **blood, body fluids, secretions,** or **excretions** in a manner that prevents skin and mucous membrane exposures, contamination of clothing, and transfer of microorganisms to other patients and environments. Ensure that reusable equipment is not used for the care of another patient until it has been appropriately cleaned and reprocessed and single use items are properly discarded.

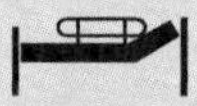

Environmental Control
Follow hospital procedures for routine care, cleaning, and disinfection of environmental surfaces, beds, bedrails, bedside equipment, and other frequently touched surfaces.

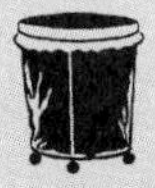

Linen
Handle, transport, and process used linen soiled with **blood, body fluids, secretions,** or **excretions** in a manner that prevents exposures and contamination of clothing, and avoids transfer of microorganisms to other patients and environments.

Occupational Health and Bloodborne Pathogens
Prevent injuries when using needles, scalpels, and other sharp instruments or devices; when handling sharp instruments after procedures; when cleaning used instruments; and when disposing of used needles.

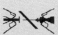

Never recap used needles using both hands or any other technique that involves directing the point of a needle towards any part of the body; rather, use either a one-handed "scoop" technique or a mechanical device designed for holding the needle sheath.

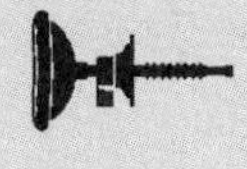

Do not remove used needles from disposable syringes by hand, and do not bend, break, or otherwise manipulate used needles by hand. Place used disposable syringes and needles, scalpel blades, and other sharp items in puncture-resistant sharps containers located as close as practical to the area in which the items were used, and place reusable syringes and needles in a puncture-resistant container for transport to the reprocessing area.

Use **resuscitation devices** as an alternative to mouth-to-mouth resuscitation.

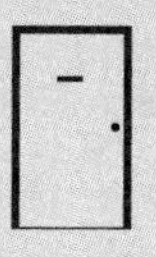

Patient Placement
Use a **private room** for a patient who contaminates the environment or who does not (or cannot be expected to) assist in maintaining appropriate hygiene or environmental control. Consult Infection Control if a private room is not available.

Figure 10-3 Standard Precautions for Infection Control issued by the Centers for Disease Control and Prevention in 1997. (Courtesy Brevis Corp.)

Precautions include many criteria specific to inpatient settings such as hospitals and skilled nursing facilities, they are absolutely applicable to any medical facility, including ambulatory care settings where medical assistants are more likely to work.

Figure 10-3 provides a comprehensive review of Standard Precautions.

Transmission-Based Precautions

When the CDC was in the process of developing a new guideline for isolation precautions in hospitals, the agency arrived at what it terms two tiers of precautions. The first tier is called the Standard Precautions, discussed earlier, designed for all patients regardless of their diagnosis or presumed infection status. The second tier of precautions is intended for patients diagnosed with or suspected of having specific highly transmissible diseases. These are known as Transmission-Based Precautions.

Transmission-Based Precautions reduce the risk for **airborne, droplet,** and **contact transmission** of pathogens and are always to be used *in addition to* Standard Precautions.

These airborne, contact, and droplet precautions also list specific syndromes that can appear in adult and pediatric patients who are highly suspicious for infection. They identify the appropriate Transmission-Based Precautions to be used until a diagnosis can be made. See Figures 10-4, 10-5, and 10-6 for specific information on these three Transmission-Based Precautions. Remember that these precautions are for specific categories of patients and are to be used in addition to Standard Precautions, which are used for all patients.

Some medical assistants' externship experiences take place in a hospital setting. For example, the electrocardiography and clinical laboratory departments of the hospital are areas some students rotate through during their externships. It is important for medical assistants to know and understand how to protect themselves from infectious diseases. Transmission-Based Precautions (isolation) reduce the risk for airborne, droplet, and contact transmission of pathogens. Procedure 10-3 describes the use of barriers (gown, mask, goggles, gloves, and cap) that are used when entering an isolation room to perform an electrocardiogram or phlebotomy on a patient with an infectious disease such as tuberculosis (airborne contact), meningitis (respiratory droplets contact), and wound drainage (direct contact).

Blood and Body Fluids

In all infection control efforts, it is important to understand what is meant by blood and body fluids. Specifically, they are described as the blood, secretions, and excretions of a patient. Examples of blood and body fluids and

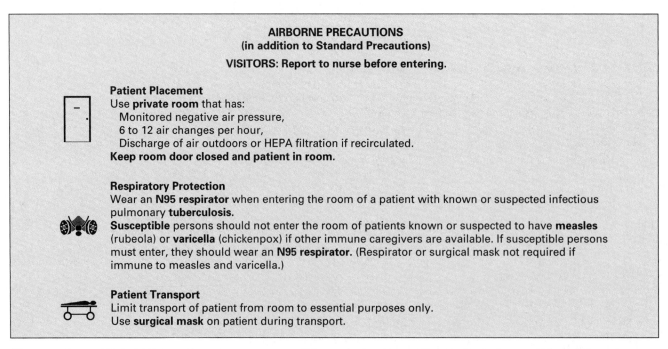

AIRBORNE PRECAUTIONS
(in addition to Standard Precautions)

VISITORS: Report to nurse before entering.

Patient Placement
Use **private room** that has:
Monitored negative air pressure,
6 to 12 air changes per hour,
Discharge of air outdoors or HEPA filtration if recirculated.
Keep room door closed and patient in room.

Respiratory Protection
Wear an **N95 respirator** when entering the room of a patient with known or suspected infectious pulmonary **tuberculosis.**
Susceptible persons should not enter the room of patients known or suspected to have **measles** (rubeola) or **varicella** (chickenpox) if other immune caregivers are available. If susceptible persons must enter, they should wear an **N95 respirator.** (Respirator or surgical mask not required if immune to measles and varicella.)

Patient Transport
Limit transport of patient from room to essential purposes only.
Use **surgical mask** on patient during transport.

Figure 10-4 Airborne Precautions, one category of Transmission-Based Precautions, for use in hospital settings. (Courtesy of Brevis Corp.)

CONTACT PRECAUTIONS
(in addition to Standard Precautions)

VISITORS: Report to nurse before entering.

Patient Placement
Private room, if possible. Cohort if private room is not available.

Gloves
Wear gloves when entering patient room.
Change gloves after having contact with infective material that may contain high concentrations of microorganisms (**fecal** material and **wound drainage**).
Remove gloves before leaving patient room.

Wash
Wash hands with an **antimicrobial** agent immediately after glove removal. After glove removal and handwashing, ensure that hands do not touch potentially contaminated environmental surfaces or items in the patient's room to avoid transfer of microorganisms to other patients or environments.

Gown
Wear gown when entering patient room if you anticipate that your clothing will have a substantial contact with the patient, environmental surfaces, or items in the patient's room, or if the patient is **incontinent,** or has **diarrhea,** an **ileostomy,** a **colostomy,** or **wound drainage** not contained by a dressing. **Remove** gown before leaving the patient's environment and ensure that clothing does not contact potentially contaminated environmental surfaces to avoid transfer of microorganisms to other patients or environments.

Patient Transport
Limit transport of patient to essential purposes only. During transport, ensure that precautions are maintained to minimize the risk of transmission of microorganisms to other patients and contamination of environmental surfaces and equipment.

Patient-Care Equipment
Dedicate the use of noncritical patient-care equipment to a single patient. If common equipment is used, clean and disinfect between patients.

Figure 10-5 Contact Precautions, one category of Transmission-Based Precautions, for use in hospital settings. (Courtesy of Brevis Corp.)

DROPLET PRECAUTIONS
(in addition to Standard Precautions)

VISITORS: Report to nurse before entering.

Patient Placement
Private room, if possible. Cohort or maintain spatial separation of **3 feet** from other patients or visitors if private room is not available.

Mask
Wear mask when working within **3 feet** of patient (or upon entering room).

Patient Transport
Limit transport of patient from room to essential purposes only.
Use **surgical mask** on patient during transport.

Figure 10-6 Droplet Precautions, one category of Transmission-Based Precautions, for use in hospital settings. (Courtesy of Brevis Corp.)

some of the areas in which medical assistants may become exposed to them are:

Blood:

- Specimens drawn during venipuncture
- Open wounds or lesions of any kind
- **Epistaxis,** or nosebleeds
- Vaginal bleeding, including **menses** (menstruation), **lochia** (discharge after childbirth), and hemorrhage
- Feces and vomit or other body fluids with or without visible blood

Vaginal secretions:

- Physiologic **leukorrhea** (normal vaginal discharge)
- Vaginitis with discharge

Cerebrospinal fluid:

- Fluid **aspirated,** or withdrawn, during a **lumbar puncture** (spinal tap)
- Leakage of fluid due to trauma to the brain or spinal cord (through ear, nose)

Synovial fluid:

- Fluid aspirated during arthroscopic procedures

Pleural fluid:

- Fluid aspirated during **thoracentesis,** a surgical puncture of the thoracic cavity
- Fluid leakage caused by chest trauma

Pericardial fluid:

- Fluid around the heart exposed during cardiac surgery or caused by cardiac trauma

Peritoneal fluid:

- Fluid exposed during abdominal surgery (least likely fluid with which medical assistant will come into contact), but exposure can occur during a **paracentesis**

Semen:

- Seminal fluid as a laboratory specimen for sperm count in examination for fertility level

Amniotic fluid:

- Fluid aspirated during **amniocentesis,** a surgical puncture of the amniotic sac
- Vaginal leakage during pregnancy, labor, and delivery

Breast milk (possibility exists)

Sputum:

- Material coughed up and **expectorated** from the respiratory tract

Saliva:

- Oral mucous gland fluid in mouth during oral/dental procedures

Any other body fluid visibly contaminated with blood

Thus far, only blood and blood products, semen, vaginal secretions, and possibly breast milk have been directly linked to transmission of HIV; the virus is not spread casually or through close family contacts. There is not yet a vaccine to protect individuals from HIV.

HBV has been found in blood and blood products, vaginal secretions, semen, and saliva. Infection can spread through close family contacts, kissing, sexual contacts, intrauterinely, and during delivery. An infant may become a chronic **carrier,** one who has no symptoms but can transmit disease. If there has been an exposure to the virus, a prompt injection of immunoglobulin, an antibody, will help provide protection from the virus. HBV vaccine is available, and the series of three injections usually immunizes an individual from an attack of hepatitis B for approximately 18 years.

Some states require health care providers and allied health students to be immunized before employment and before admission into a health program in an educational institution. Also, many states require infants to be routinely immunized with HBV vaccine.

Personal Protective Equipment

Standard and Transmission-Based Precautions all make use of barriers or personal protective equipment (PPE). The barriers consist of gloves, mask, gown, and goggles/face shield. Gloves reduce the risk for contamination to hands but do not prevent needles or other sharp instruments from penetrating the skin. Masks and protective eyewear reduce the contamination risk to mucous membranes of the eyes, nose, and mouth. Gowns protect clothing from contamination. Barriers or PPE are used in various combinations depending on the procedure or treatment being performed on patients. As a medical assistant, you may be exposed to infected blood and body fluids and must wear PPE (Figure 10-7).

Needlestick

One reason for exposure to blood is caused by accidentally sticking oneself with a dirty (used) needle after performing invasive procedures such as injections and

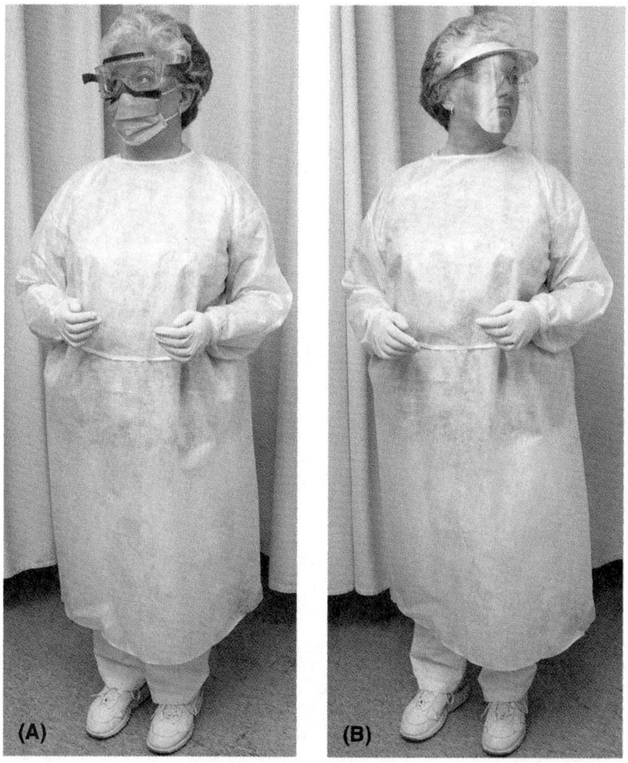

Figure 10-7 Medical assistant wearing personal protective equipment: (A) goggles, mask, gown, latex gloves; (B) full-face shield, gown, latex gloves.

venipuncture. In the past, needlesticks were common because of the practice of needle recapping. Contaminated (used) needles should never be recapped, broken off, removed from syringes, or manipulated by hand in any way. They are disposed of in the approved puncture-proof container designated for **sharps** (Figure 10-8A). The disposal container for sharps must be in the closest proximity as practical to the area where sharps are used. If a needle is used and an appropriate disposal container is not nearby ("point-of-use disposal"), the **scoop technique** of recapping may be used: the cap may be "scooped up" with the needle, using one hand, and then carried to the sharps container. The cap is not, under any circumstances, pushed into place over the needle (see Figure 10-9A–C). The risk to a health care provider of HIV infection caused by a needlestick is slight; however, the risk for HBV or HCV infection caused by a needlestick can be significantly greater.

Occupational Safety and Health Administration (OSHA) mandates that (1) employers select the safest needle device available, (2) employers must involve employees in identifying these devices, and (3) employers maintain a log of injuries caused by contaminated sharps ([66FR5325] OSHA 1910.1030). See Figure 10-10.

Desirable characteristics of safety devices include:

- The device is **jet injection.**
- The safety feature is built into the device.
- The device works passively (i.e., requires no activation by the user). If user activation is necessary, the safety feature can be engaged with a single-handed technique, allowing the worker's hands to remain behind the exposed sharp.
- The user can easily tell whether the safety feature has been activated. Some safety features have a sound, such as a click, indicating that the feature is engaged.
- The safety feature cannot be deactivated and remains protective through disposal.
- If the device uses needles, it performs reliably with all needle sizes.
- The device is easy to use and practical.
- The device is safe and effective in patient care.

Additional information regarding specific procedures to follow should an accidental needlestick occur, as well as other safety procedures included in the OSHA and CLIA rules and regulations will be found later in this chapter and in Chapter 26.

Disposal of Infectious Waste

Infectious waste (contaminated items) is described as any item that has come in contact with patient blood or body fluids. These items must be handled with gloves and disposed of by placing them in the appropriate biohazard containers that are provided by an agency with which your employer has contracted (see Figure 10-8B). Infectious waste is either **incinerated** (burned) or subjected to sterilization by autoclave to render it harmless before it is disposed of in a sanitary landfill. For your local rules and regulations of how to dispose of sharps and biohazard/infectious waste, contact your local Department of Health. Their staff can refer you to companies who specialize in the proper disposal of infectious waste and sharps. These companies follow strict state and federal regulations and can provide your clinic with containers, labels, and instructions. They will often work out a schedule for pickups, such as daily, weekly, monthly or "on-call." Charges will usually be based on the amount of infectious waste that requires disposal.

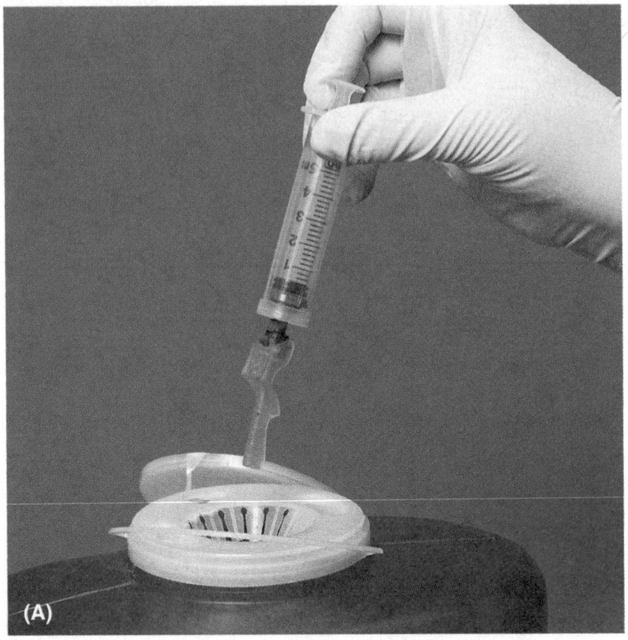

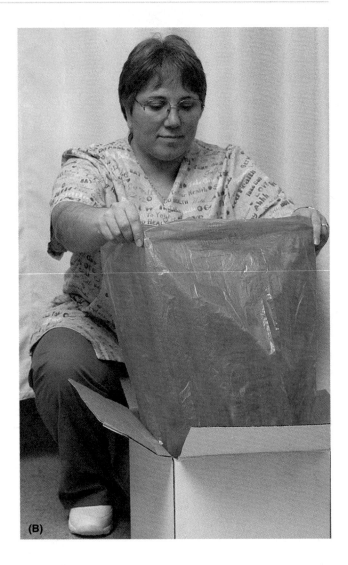

Figure 10-8 (A) Discard the entire disposable safety syringe and needle into the biohazard puncture-proof Sharps container. (B) The medical assistant is placing a sturdy disposable plastic bag marked with the biohazard waste symbol into a durable cardboard box for collection of infectious waste material. When full, these boxes are picked up by an agency for incineration or for autoclaving before disposal in a public landfill.

Federal Organizations and Infection Control

The CDC is responsible for studying pathogens and diseases in an effort to prevent their spread. A division of the U.S. Public Health Department, the CDC has issued a number of guidelines over the last 25 years that have enabled health care professionals to practice responsible infection control. As diseases evolve, and as new diseases are introduced into our society, the CDC revises and updates existing guidelines or issues new control measures to contain the spread of infection.

In 1970, the CDC developed a system of seven **isolation categories** for patients with known infectious diseases. This category system included strict **isolation,** respiratory isolation, protective isolation, enteric precautions, wound and skin precautions, discharge precautions, and blood precautions.

In 1985, the agency released a set of guidelines known as Universal Blood and Body Fluid Precautions, or simply **Universal Precautions.** These infection control practices were written in response to an increase in AIDS and HBV, both bloodborne diseases, and other infectious diseases as well.

Beginning in 1991, the CDC infection control guidelines were reviewed and subsequently revised. In 1996, a new set of guidelines was released. Standard Precautions

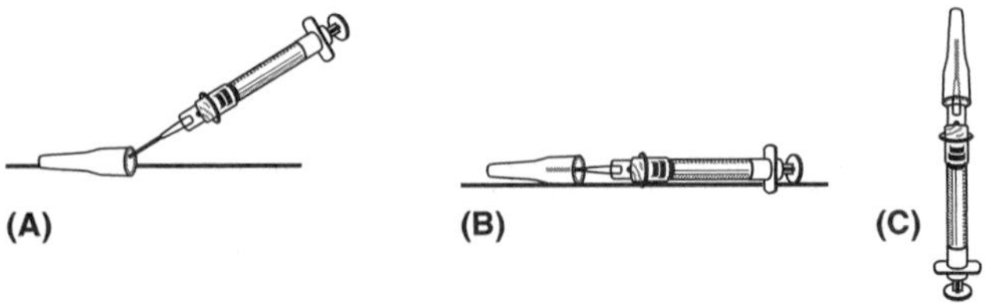

Figure 10-9 (A) Scoop into cap using one hand. Do not touch the cap with the other hand. (B) Slide needle into cap resting on table. (C) Holding the barrel of the syringe in one hand, carry to the sharps container. Do not push the cap into the syringe.

reflect improved recommendations intended to protect all health care providers, patients, and their visitors from a wide range of **communicable** diseases. At the same time that the CDC issued the new Standard Precautions, they also released a second tier of precautions called Transmission-Based Precautions. These are intended to be used in addition to Standard Precautions when caring for patients with known specific infectious diseases.

To understand the intent of these various CDC infection control guidelines, Standard Precautions and Transmission-Based Precautions are examined here in more detail.

OSHA REGULATIONS

OSHA regulations are intended to ensure that employers have a safe and healthful work environment for their employees. They represent requirements that employers must follow to ensure employee safety and health.

There are two standards that comprise the regulations: *The Occupational Exposure to Hazardous Chemicals in the Laboratory*, an amended version of the original standard *The Hazard Communication Standard*, and *The Bloodborne Pathogen Standard*.

EXAMPLES OF SAFETY DEVICES

Type of Device	Safety Features
Syringes and Injection Equipment	**Needleless or jet injection** – the medication/immunization is injected under the skin without a needle, using the force of the liquid under pressure to pierce the skin.
	Retractable needle – the needle (usually fused to the syringe) is spring-loaded and retracts into the barrel of the syringe when the plunger is completely depressed after the injection is given.
	Protective sheath – after giving an injection, the worker slides a plastic barrel over the needle and locks it in place.
	Hinged re-cap – after the injection, the worker, using the index finger, flips a hinged protective cap over the needle, which locks into place. This safety feature may be fused to the syringe or come separate and detachable from the syringe.
IV Access – Insertion Equipment	**Retractable** – the spring-loaded needle retracts into the needle holder upon pressing a button after use or the needle withdraws into the holder when withdrawn from the patient's arm.
	Passive – a metal safety clip unfolds over the needle as it is withdrawn.
	Shielded IV catheters (midline and peripheral) – a protective shield slides over the exposed needle.
	Hemodialysis safety fistula sets (butterfly) – a protective shield slides over the needle as it is withdrawn.

(continued)

Figure 10-10 Examples of Safety Devices published by the U.S. Department of Labor. This publication includes information about various types of safety devises and their features.

EXAMPLES OF SAFETY DEVICES (continued)

Type of Device	Safety Features
Blood-Collection and Phlebotomy	**Retractable needle** – the spring-loaded needle is pulled into the vacuum tube holder after use.
	Shielded butterfly needle – a protective shield slides over the needle after use.
	Self-blunting needle – after use, the needle is blunted while still in the patient.
	Plastic blood collection tubes – used to replace glass tubes.
Suture Needles	**Blunt suture needles** – used for sewing internal fascia.
Lancets	**Retracting lancet** – following skin puncture, the sharp automatically retracts back into the device.
Surgical Scalpels	**Retracting scalpel** – after use, the blade is withdrawn back into the body of the scalpel.
	Quick-release scalpel blade handles – a lever is activated that allows for a "touchless" attachment of the blade to the handle and releases it after use.

Figure 10-10 (continued)

The Bloodborne Pathogen Standard

The Bloodborne Pathogen Standard became effective in March 1992. It came about principally in the hope of reducing the occupational-related cases of HIV and HBV infections among health care workers. Figure 10-24 outlines *The Bloodborne Pathogen Standard*.

It covers all employees who can be "reasonably anticipated" to come into contact, as a result of performing their job duties, with blood and other potentially infectious materials. *The Bloodborne Pathogen Standard* seeks to limit exposure to bloodborne pathogens. The law covers:

- Exposure determination
- Methods of control of exposure, especially Standard Precautions
- HBV vaccine
- Postexposure follow-up
- Disposal of biohazardous waste
- Labeling
- Housekeeping and laundry functions
- Training for employee safety and documentation

See Figure 10-23 for an overview and summary of the OSHA *Bloodborne Pathogen Standard*.

Blood and Other Potentially Infectious Material. Blood and other potentially infectious material are defined by the CDC and OSHA as the same human fluids listed previously as well as the following:

- Unfixed human tissue (alive or dead); e.g., breast tissue from a frozen section biopsy
- Any tissue culture, cells, or fluid known to be HIV-, HBV-, or HCV-infected

When the origin of a specimen is unknown, it must be handled as if it were infectious.

Critical Thinking

Give eight examples of body fluids considered to be biohazardous substances. Explain how medical assistants could become exposed to blood and body fluids.

Bloodborne Pathogens. Disease-producing microorganisms are called pathogens; **bloodborne** refers to the manner in which the microorganisms can be transmitted—via blood or other potentially infectious material. Three pathogens of particular importance to health care professionals are HBV, HCV, and HIV.

Exposure Determination. Exposure determination requires an employer to list all the job classifications and employees in those job classifications that are exposed to blood and other potentially infectious material in the course of performing their jobs (Figure 10-11). Existing job descriptions can be used by the employer to identify the job categories that are considered high risk for exposure to blood and/or other potentially infectious material (Figure 10-12). It is important to note that exposure determination is made without regard to the use of PPE.

Plan to Control Exposure. Every employer who has an employee(s) who is identified and determined to be at risk for potential exposure must have a written exposure control plan (Figures 10-13 through 10-15). The plan must consist of methods of compliance for prevention of exposure, HBV vaccination and postexposure evaluation, communication of hazards to employee(s), documentation of the bloodborne standard, and a procedure for the determination of the events surrounding an exposure occurrence. The written plan must be employee accessible, updated regularly (at least annually), and modified when necessary and appropriate, especially to reflect changes in employee positions.

Methods of Compliance to Prevent Exposure. There are seven major strategies mandated by OSHA for the prevention of exposure to bloodborne pathogens and other potentially infectious material.

1. *Standard Precautions*. Adherence to the CDC's Standard Precautions is required. Hand washing is stressed and employers must provide hand washing facilities and must ascertain that employees use them frequently and especially following exposure to blood or other potentially infectious material.
2. *Engineering Controls and Work Practice Controls*. Engineering controls and **work practice controls**

SAMPLE

Exposure Activity Form for Category 2 Employees
Tasks Involving Occupation Exposure to Blood and Body Fluids

Employee at Risk and Job Title	Task Involving Risk and PPE	Risk Rating

Figure 10-11 Sample Exposure Activity Form for Category 2 Employees (no exposure to blood or body fluids), including tasks and risk rating. (Courtesy of POL Consultants, 2 Russ Farm Way, Delanco, NJ 08075, 856-824-0800.)

SAMPLE

Exposure Classification Record of Employee

The following employee was classified according to work task exposure to certain body fluids as required by the current OSHA infection control standard on (Date) ____________ as follows:

Employee Name: ______________ SS# __________

____ Category 1. "All procedures or other job related tasks that involve an inherent potential for mucous membrane or skin contact with blood, body fluids, or tissues, or a potential for spill or splashes of (blood or body fluids)."

____ Category 2. Tasks in which "The normal work routine involves no exposure to blood, body fluids, or tissues, but exposure or potential exposure may be required as a condition of employment." For example, receptionists, accounting, or insurance staff or others who may, as a part of their duties, be asked to help in clean up, instrument recirculation, laboratory, or other similar procedures where exposure may result.

____ Category 3. Tasks in which "The normal work routine involves no exposure to blood, body fluids, or tissues. Persons who perform these duties are not called upon as part of their employment to perform or assist in emergency medical care or first aid or to be potentially exposed in some other way."

Employer Signature ____________________

Because of a change of job assignment, the above employee was reclassified according to tasks exposure on (Date) _________ as follows:

_______ Category 1

_______ Category 2

_______ Category 3

Employer's Signature ______________________

Because of a change of assignment, the above employee was reclassified according to task exposure on (Date) __________ as follows:

_______ Category 1

_______ Category 2

_______ Category 3

Employer's Signature ______________________

NOTE: This record should be retained for length of employment plus thirty years.

Figure 10-12 Sample Exposure Classification Record of employee shows exposure categories into which employee's tasks fall. This record is kept for 30 years. (Courtesy of POL Consultants, 2 Russ Farm Way, Delanco, NJ 08075, 856-824-0800.)

OFFICE WORK PRACTICE EXPOSURE CONTROL PLAN

Effective Date: ____________

Office of ________________________________

As of the above date the office will follow the rules below to reduce exposure and contamination:

Observe Standard Precautions.

Wear gloves when drawing blood and performing procedures/tests.

Wash hands after removing gloves.

Change gloves frequently during the day and between patients.

Do not answer phone, handle papers, or word process while wearing gloves.

Do not cap or break needles.

Dispose of all needles in sharps containers.

Do not allow sharps containers to fill beyond ⅔ full.

Wear lab coats when performing tests.

Leave lab coats in laboratory/work area.

Dispose of all contaminated material in infectious waste container. (Biohazard)

Disinfect the laboratory work surfaces frequently.

Disinfect the examining room surfaces, daily and as needed.

Sterilize nondisposable examination and testing equipment.

Monitor sterilization procedure.

Do not eat or drink in work area.

Place gauze over tops of blood tubes when removing caps or use safety caps.

Clean up all specimen and chemical spills properly and immediately.

Label all chemicals according to OSHA regulations.

Label refrigerator that blood is stored in.

Centrifuges will have lids or specimens will be capped when spun.

Centrifuges will be disinfected regularly.

Hepatitis B vaccines will be offered to all employees.

Employees will take a safety training program.

Figure 10-13 Office Work Practice Exposure Control Plan indicates a sample list of precautions to take to minimize employee risk exposure. (Courtesy of POL Consultants, 2 Russ Farm Way, Delanco, NJ 08075, 856-824-0800.)

SAMPLE

Office Procedures Safety Form

PROCEDURE: ______________________

Type of hazard: ______________________

Person performing procedure: ______________________

Person assisting procedure: ______________________

Personal protective equipment used: ______________________

____

Proper techniques for safety:

____

____

____

What is done with used materials and soiled instruments?

____

____

____

What chemical products are involved?

____

____

____

What are the specific risks of procedure?

____

____

____

Additional comments:

____

____

____

____

Prepared By: ______________ Date: __________

Figure 10-14 Sample Office Procedures Safety Form lists procedures, type of hazard, employee performing procedure, employee assisting with procedure, and personal protective equipment. (Courtesy of POL Consultants, 2 Russ Farm Way, Delanco, NJ 08075, 856-824-0800.)

SAMPLE

Safety/Work Practice Controls for Office Procedures

Each office has special safety procedures that are unique to that particular practice. These are also known as work practice controls. The fundamental work practice control is using Standard Precautions. Work practice controls reduce the likelihood of exposure to hazards. Many times the risks can be eliminated by changing the way a procedure is performed. Make copies of the PROCEDURES SAFETY FORM. Fill in the information for any procedure that involves exposure to potentially infectious body fluids. File these procedures in the office operation section of your manual. Do not limit this section to only body fluid exposures. General safety for other hazards such as chemicals and X-ray should be listed as well. Common examples are listed below. Check the ones you do and add to this list.

____ Patient exams
____ Aspirations
____ Inoculations
____ Taking blood samples
____ Lab testing
____ Lesion excisions
____ Wound care
____ Dressing changes
____ Colposcopies
____ Surgical procedures
____ X-rays
____ Arthroscopies
____ Vaginal exams
____ PAP smears/IUDs
____ OB care
____ Norplants
____ Vasectomies
____ Biopsies
____ Sigmoidoscopies
____ ____________
____ ____________
____ ____________

Figure 10-15 Sample Safety/Work Practice Controls for Office Procedures lists procedures that involve exposure to blood, body fluids, and other potentially infectious material. (Courtesy of POL Consultants, 2 Russ Farm Way, Delanco, NJ 08075, 856-824-0800.)

consist of the physical equipment and mechanical devices an employer provides in an attempt to safeguard and minimize employee exposure. A common example of an engineering control is sharps disposal containers (Figure 10-16). Others are mechanical pipettes, fume hoods, splash guards, and eye wash stations (Figure 10-17). If and when occupational exposure continues after the engineering controls are in place, PPE must be used. Hand washing facilities or appropriate antiseptic hand cleanser (when hand washing facilities are unavailable) must be readily available.

3. *Personal Protective Equipment* (*PPE*). The employer must be certain that PPE is available and accessible and provide an alternative type of glove if an employee is allergic to those originally provided.

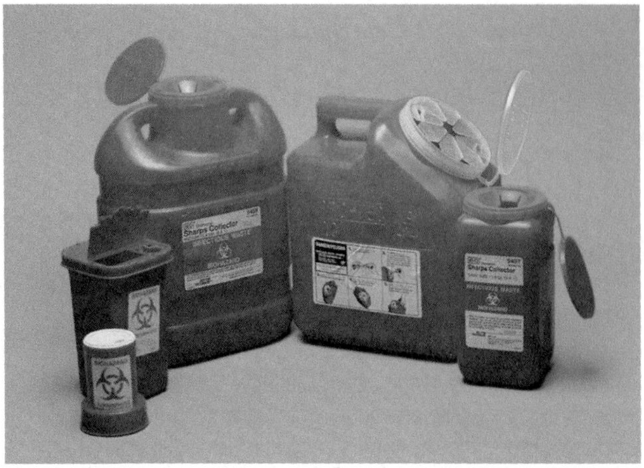

Figure 10-16 Various sizes of puncture-proof sharps containers. These and other biohazard waste containers are autoclaved when full and sent out to a biohazard agency for safe disposal.

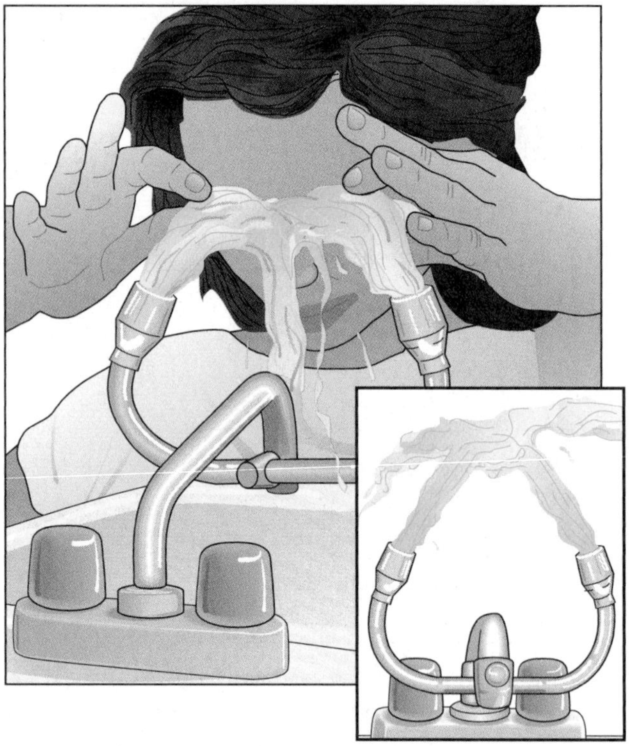

Figure 10-17 Emergency eyewash station: two streams of water or saline wash both eyes simultaneously and continuously.

(See Latex Sensitivity box earlier in chapter.) Cleaning and laundering and disposal of PPE is the responsibility of the employer, and the employee does not incur any expense for such.

All PPE must be removed before the employee leaves the work site and placed in an appropriate container that is supplied by the employer (Figure 10-18).

4. *Cleanliness of Work Areas*. The employer must maintain a work site that is clean and sanitary and have a written schedule for cleaning and decontaminating the work area after contact with blood and other potentially infectious material. **Spill kits** must be readily accessible (Figure 10-19).

   Broken glass is placed in a sharps container after using cardboard or a dust pan and brush to remove it.

   Laundry that is contaminated is handled with gloves and placed in a labeled container. If the laundry is damp or wet, gloves and other appropriate PPE must be worn, and the damp/wet laundry must be placed in a plastic bag(s) to prevent blood or other potentially infectious material from leaking through it. PPE cannot be laundered at home. All other Standard Precautions must be adhered to.

5. *Hepatitis B Vaccine*. HBV vaccine must be made available free of charge to every employee, full-time, part-time, or temporary, within 10 days of work assignment (Figure 10-20). This refers to employees who have the potential for occupational exposure, and who can "reasonably" be expected to have skin, eye, mucous membrane, or **parenteral** contact with blood or other potentially infectious material. The vaccine is given in three doses over a six-month period and is used to protect the employee from infection with HBV. It is an intramuscular injection with an approximate 96% rate of effectiveness.

   An employee has the right to decline taking the vaccine, but must sign a **declination form.** There is the option to reconsider receiving the vaccine at a later time.

6. *Follow-Up After Exposure*. An accidental exposure is broadly defined as one in which blood, blood-contaminated body fluids, or body fluids or tissues to which Standard Precautions apply are introduced onto a mucous surface, onto nonintact skin, or to the conjunctiva via a needlestick, skin cut, or direct splash. If an incident exposes an employee to any of these, the employer must make available a confidential medical evaluation in which is documented:

   - The circumstances surrounding the event
   - The route or routes of exposure
   - The identification of the person who was the source of the exposure

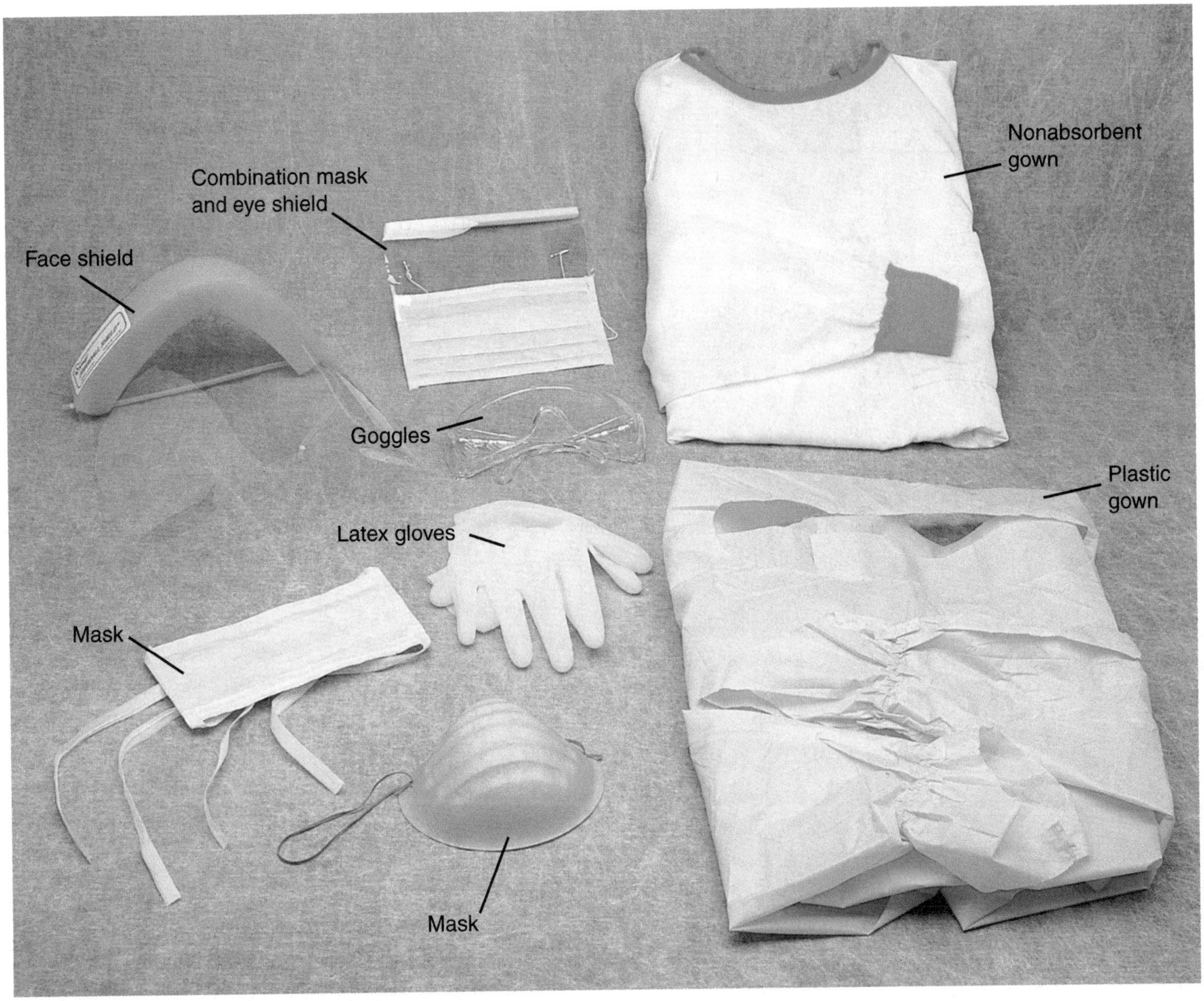

Figure 10-18 Personal protective equipment.

The following procedure describes the steps to take following an exposure incident:

- Immediately wash exposed area with soap and warm water.
- If mouth area is exposed, rinse with water or mouthwash.
- If eyes are exposed, flush with large amounts of warm water.
- Report incident to a supervisor immediately for **documentation** (Figure 10-21).

In addition, OSHA requires the following information:

- The exposed employee must be tested for HBV and HIV only if consent is given. An employee may refuse or may have blood drawn and stored for 90 days at which time the choice can be made whether to have the blood tested.
- The source individual's blood, if permission is granted, is tested for HBV and HIV, and the employee shall know the results (unless protected by the law).
- The employee is offered prophylaxis, gamma globulin, or HB vaccine after the exposure according to the current recommendation of the U.S. Public Health Service.
- The employee is counseled regarding precautions to take to avoid possible transmission and is provided information on potential illnesses for which to be alert.
- An OSHA 200 form must be filed.

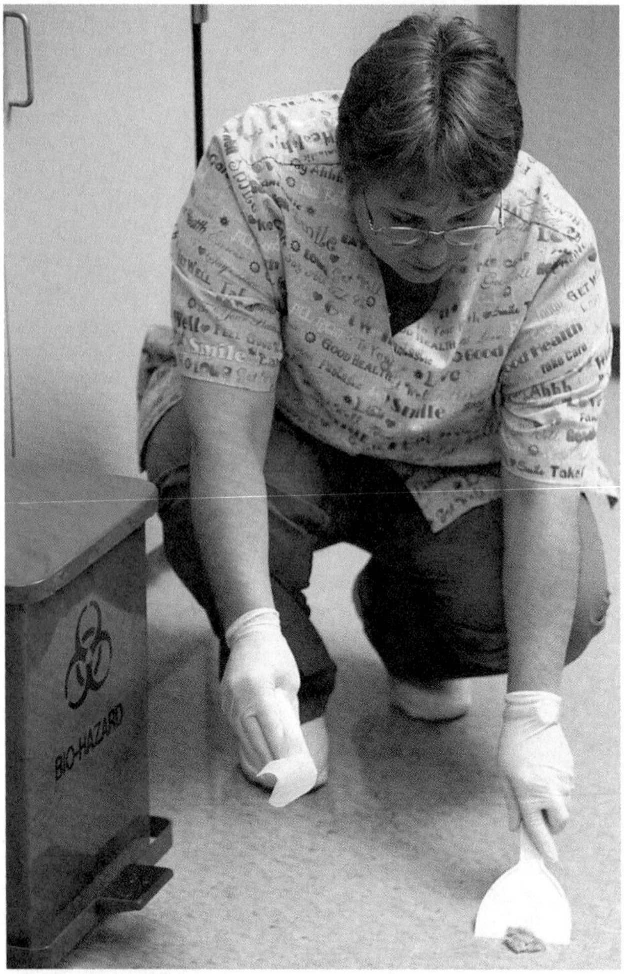

Figure 10-19 Medical assistant is wearing latex gloves to clean up a specimen spill. The biohazard waste bag is used to dispose of contaminated materials. The spill area is then cleaned with a 10% bleach solution.

7. *Medical Records*. Medical records of an employee who has suffered an occupational exposure must be kept for the length of employment plus 30 years and confidentiality must be guaranteed.

   The following information is to be included in the employee's record: name and Social Security number, HB vaccination status with dates, results of any examinations or tests, a copy of the health care provider's written opinion, and a copy of the information that was provided to the health care provider.

   The records must be available to the employee, to OSHA, and anyone with the written consent of the employee, but *not* the employer.

Hazard Communication for Blood. The employer is required to label containers of **regulated waste,** refrigerators, freezers, and other containers that are used to

SAMPLE

Hepatitis B Employee Vaccination Form

MEMO: To all employees with occupational exposure to blood or other infectious materials on an average of one or more times per month.

OSHA and the CDC have identified the potential exposure of health care workers to hepatitis B virus (HBV) in the course of performing their duties in this office. For the protection of our employees, we are offering prescreening testing and the HBV vaccination with follow-up evaluation to all employees who are exposed to blood or other potentially infectious materials on an average of one or more times per month. *In accordance with recommended OSHA guidelines, this vaccine and testing will be offered at no cost to the employee.* You have the ability to decide whether or not you want the testing and/or vaccine.

At the bottom of this memo, you may indicate your choice. Please return this memo with your signature and date to your immediate supervisor.

[ ] I want to receive the prescreening (optional)

[ ] I want to receive the vaccine and follow-up evaluation testing

[ ] I *do not* want the vaccine and testing and have read the following statement:

I understand that due to my occupational exposure to blood or other potentially infectious materials I may be at risk of acquiring hepatitis B virus (HBV) infection. I have been given the opportunity to be vaccinated with hepatitis B vaccine at no charge to myself. However, I decline hepatitis B vaccination at this time. I understand that by declining this vaccine I continue to be at risk of acquiring hepatitis B, a serious disease. If in the future I continue to have occupational exposure to blood or other potentially infectious materials and I want to be vaccinated with hepatitis B vaccine, I can receive the vaccination series at no charge to me.

____________________ ________________

NAME DATE

____________________ ________________

SIGNATURE SS#

PRESCREENING DATE ________ RESULTS _______

DATE OF VACCINATIONS ____________________

DATE OF FOLLOW-UP EVALUATION ____________

RESULTS _____________________________

NOTES:

Figure 10-20 Sample Hepatitis B Employee Vaccination Form provides employee information regarding hepatitis B vaccine and space to sign indicating whether employee declines vaccine. (Courtesy of POL Consultants, 2 Russ Farm Way, Delanco, NJ 08075, 856-824-0800.)

SAMPLE

Post-Exposure Management Record

The following employee was the subject of an infectious exposure incident on (date) _______ and was examined and treated as follows:

Employee Name: ______________ SS# ____________

Type of Incident (describe) ______________________

____

Route of Exposure: ___________________________

Source Patient Information:

____ Source patient could not be identified.

____ Source patient was identified but refused to contribute blood.

____ Source patient was identified and blood was secured from such patient. Results of blood testing of source patient's blood are attached to this form.

Employee hereby grants permission for tests for antibodies of human immunodeficiency virus (HIV-1) and/or hepatitis B virus and acknowledges that the employee has been counseled concerning such tests.

Employee Signature _______________ Date ________

The following test(s) were administered under supervision of a qualified physician:

____ Human Immunodeficiency Virus (HIV-1) Antibodies

____ Hepatitis B Virus Antibodies

Date(s) of Tests(s): ______________ Results of Test(s)—See attached Physician's or Laboratory statement/report.

Employee hereby acknowledges that the employee was counseled and a written copy(ies) of the results of the above test(s) were furnished to such employee on (date): _________

Employee Signature _______________ Date ________

____ Additional follow-up was performed as indicated by attached reports.

NOTE: This record should be retained for length of employment PLUS thirty years.

Figure 10-21 Sample Post-Exposure Management Record can be used to document employee exposure to blood, body fluids, or other potentially infectious material; tests performed on the employee by a qualified physician, and their results. (Courtesy of POL Consultants, 2 Russ Farm Way, Delanco, NJ 08075, 856-824-0800.)

BIOHAZARD LABELS

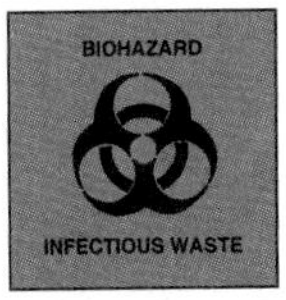

Containers that hold biohazardous materials must be properly labeled. Biohazardous materials include blood and body fluids as well as garments, gloves, masks, needles, gauze, wipes, aprons, and so on that may be contaminated with blood or other potentially contaminated body fluids. Labels shall be used to identify the presence of an actual or potential biological hazard.

CONSIDERATIONS:

- Labels shall be fluorescent orange or orange-red, with lettering or symbols in a contrasting color.
- Labels should be affixed onto or as close as feasible to the container by adhesive, string, wire, or other method.
- Red bags or red containers may be substituted for labels.
- If blood or control serum is stored in a refrigerator, the refrigerator shall be marked with a biohazard label.
- If blood is stored in a refrigerator for transport or same-day shipment, it does not need to be labeled but should be put in containment bags.

Figure 10-22 Biohazard labels alert employees to biohazardous materials such as blood, body fluids, and other potentially infectious material.

keep or transport blood or other potentially infectious material with warning labels that are orange or orange-red and have the biohazard symbol affixed to them. Red bags may be used in place of labels. The labeling serves to warn employees of the hazard possibility of container contents (Figure 10-22).

Information and Training for Employees. Employers must ascertain that employees take part in training sessions during working hours at no cost to employees. The initial session must be provided when occupational exposure may occur and annually thereafter. If employee tasks and job description change, training must take place at that time.

Training components are listed in Figure 10-23. Documentation of training sessions must be available and kept for three years.

OSHA REGULATIONS AND STUDENTS

With the passage of the OSHA law, all students with potential exposure to chemicals and bloodborne pathogens should follow all safety procedures as outlined by

Scope and Application

- The Standard applies to all occupational exposure to blood and other potentially infectious materials (OPIM), and includes part-time employees, designated first aiders, and mental health workers as well as exposed medical personnel.
- OPIM includes saliva in dental procedures, cerebrospinal fluid, unfixed tissue, semen, vaginal secretions, and body fluids visibly contaminated with blood.

Methods of Compliance

- General—standard precautions.
- Engineering and work practice controls.
- Personal protective equipment.
- Housekeeping.

Standard Precautions

- *All* human blood and OPIM are considered to be infectious.
- The *same* precautions must be taken with *all* blood and OPIM.

Engineering Controls

- Whenever feasible, **engineering controls** (devices that isolate or remove health hazards from the workplace) must be the primary method used to control exposure.
- Examples include needleless IVs, self-sheathing needles, sharps disposal containers, covered centrifuge buckets, aerosol-free tubes, and leak-proof containers.
- Engineering controls must be evaluated and documented on a regular basis.

Sharps Containers

- Readily accessible and as close as practical to work area.
- Puncture-resistant.
- Labeled or color-coded.
- Leak-proof.
- Closeable.
- *Routinely replaced* so there is no overflow.

Work Practice Controls

- Hand washing following glove removal.
- No recapping, breaking, or bending of needles.
- No eating, drinking, smoking, and so on in work area.
- No storage of food or drink where blood or OPIM are stored.
- Minimize splashing, splattering of blood, and OPIM.
- No mouth pipetting.
- Specimens must be transported in leak-proof, labeled containers. They must be placed in a secondary container if outside contamination of primary container occurs.
- Equipment must be decontaminated prior to servicing or shipping. Areas that cannot be decontaminated must be labeled.

Personal Protective Equipment (PPE)

- Includes eye protection, gloves, protective clothing, resuscitation equipment.
- Must be readily accessible and employers must require their use.
- Must be stored at work site.

Eye Protection

- Is required whenever there is potential for splashing, spraying, or splattering to the eyes or mucous membranes.
- If necessary, use eye protection in conjunction with a mask or use a chin-length face shield.
- Prescription glasses may be fitted with solid sideshields.
- Decontamination procedures must be developed.

Gloves

- Must be worn whenever hand contact with blood, OPIM, mucous membranes, nonintact skin, contaminated surfaces/items, or when performing vascular access procedures (phlebotomy).
- Type required—Vinyl or latex for general use.
  —Alternatives must be available if employee has allergic reactions (i.e., powderless).
  —Utility gloves for surface disinfection.
  —Puncture-resistant when handling sharps (i.e., Central Supply).

Protective Clothing

- Must be worn whenever splashing or splattering to skin or clothing may occur.
- Type required depends on exposure. Prevention of contamination of skin and clothes is the key.
- Examples—Low-level exposure lab coats.
  —Moderate-level exposure fluid-resistant gown.
  —High-level exposure fluid-proof apron, head and foot covering.
- *Note:* If PPE is considered protective clothing, then the *employer must* launder it.

Housekeeping

- There must be a written schedule for cleaning and disinfection.
- Contaminated equipment and surfaces must be cleaned as soon as feasible for obvious contamination or at end of work shift if no contamination has occurred.
- Protective coverings may be used over equipment.

(*continues*)

Figure 10-23 Overview of *The Bloodborne Pathogen Standard*. (Courtesy of the Occupational Safety and Health Administration, U.S. Department of Labor.)

Regulated Waste Containers (non-sharp)

- Closeable.
- Leak-proof.
- Labeled or color-coded.
- Placed in secondary container if outside of container is contaminated.

Laundry

- Handled as little as possible.
- Bagged at location of use.
- Labeled or color-coded.
- Transported in bags that prevent soak-through or leakage.

Laundry Facility

- Two options:
  1. Standard precautions for all laundry (alternative color coding allowed if recognized).
  2. Precautions only for contaminated laundry (must be red bags or biohazard labels).
- Laundry personnel must use PPE and have a sharps container accessible.

Hepatitis B Vaccination

- Made available within ten days to all employees with occupational exposure.
- At no cost to employees.
- May be required for student to be admitted to college health program as well as for externship.
- Given in accordance with United States Public Health Service guidelines.
- Employee must first be evaluated by health care professional.
- Health care professional gives a written opinion.
- If the vaccine is refused, the employee signs a declination form.
- Vaccine must be available at a future date if initially refused.

Post-Exposure Follow-Up

- Document exposure incident.
- Identify source individual (if possible).
- Attempt to test source if consent obtained.
- Provide results to exposed employee.

Labels

- Biohazard symbol and word *Biohazard* must be visible.
- Fluorescent orange/orange-red with contrasting letters may also be used.
- Red bags/containers may be substituted for labels.
- Labels required on —Regulated waste.
  —Refrigerators/freezers with blood of OPIM.
  —Transport/storage containers.
  —Contaminated equipment.

Information and Training

- Required for all employees with occupational exposure.
- Training required initially, annually, and if there are new procedures.
- Training material must be appropriate for literacy and education level of employee.
- Training must be interactive and allow for questions and answers.

Training Components

- Explanation of bloodborne standard.
- Epidemiology and symptoms of bloodborne disease.
- Modes of HIV/HBV transmission.
- Explanation of exposure control plan.
- Explanation of engineering, work practice controls.
- How to select the proper PPE.
- How to decontaminate equipment, surfaces, and so on.
- Information about hepatitis B vaccine.
- Post-exposure follow-up procedures.
- Label/color code system.

Medical Records

Records must be kept for each employee with occupational exposure and include:

- A copy of employee's vaccination status and date.
- A copy of post-exposure follow-up evaluation procedures.
- Health care professional's written opinions.
- Confidentiality must be maintained.
- Records must be maintained for thirty years plus the duration of employment.

Training Records

Records are kept for three years from date of training and include:

- Date of training.
- Summary of contents of training program.
- Name and qualifications of trainer.
- Name and job title of all persons attending.

Exposure Control Plan Components

- A written plan for each workplace with occupational exposure.

(*continues*)

Figure 10-23 (continued)

- Written policies/procedures for complying with the standard.
- A cohesive document or a guiding document referencing existing policies/procedures.

Exposure Control Plan

- A list of job classifications where occupational exposure control occurs (e.g., medical assistant, clinical laboratory scientist, dental hygienist).
- A list of tasks where exposure occurs (e.g., medical assistant who performs venipuncture).
- Methods/policies/procedures for compliance.
- Procedures for sharps disposal.
- Disinfection policies/procedures.
- Procedures for selection of PPE.
- Regulated waste disposal procedures.
- Laundry procedures.
- Hepatitis B vaccination procedures.
- Post-exposure follow-up procedures.
- Training procedures.
- Plan must be accessible to employees and be updated annually.

Employee Responsibilities

- Go through training and cooperate.
- Obey policies.
- Use universal precaution techniques.
- Use PPE.
- Use safe work practices.
- Use engineering controls.
- Report unsafe work conditions to employer.
- Maintain clean work areas.

Cooperation between employer and employees regarding *The Bloodborne Pathogen Standard* will facilitate understanding of the law, thereby benefiting all persons who are exposed to HIV, HBV, and OPIM by minimizing the risk of exposure to the pathogens.

Meeting the OSHA standard is not optional and failure to comply can result in a fine that may total $10,000 for each employee.

To obtain copies of *The Bloodborne Pathogen Standard,* contact OSHA at 800-321-6742 or www.osha.gov.

Figure 10-23 (continued)

OSHA. Because students are not considered employees of a health care facility and are attending an educational institution, they do not fall under the OSHA guidelines. They should, however, take precautions to avoid contact with potentially infectious materials and toxic chemicals wherever learning is taking place.

Avoiding Exposure to Bloodborne Pathogens

Students can come into contact with blood and other potentially infectious material during laboratory practices and externships. The potential for exposure and contact increases whenever **invasive procedures** are being performed. Some examples of invasive procedures are:

- **Phlebotomy,** the process of withdrawing blood
- Administering an injection
- Performing or assisting with medical/surgical procedures such as suturing of wounds or removal of sutures; assisting with certain procedures such as Pap smears, arthroscopies, amniocentesis, thoracentesis, or lumbar puncture; dressing changes, colposcopies, vaginal exams, obstetrical care, vasectomies,

Student Precautions

Gloves must be worn:
- During phlebotomy
- When giving injections
- When performing or assisting with invasive procedures
- When processing blood specimens

Eye protection with side projections must be worn:
- Whenever there is the potential for chemical exposure or the possibility of spray, splash, or splatter from blood or body fluids

Face shields or masks must be worn:
- When there is a chance of spray, splash, or splatter from blood or body fluids

Gowns or **aprons** must be worn:
- Where there exists any potential for exposure to contaminated materials

Lab coats must be worn and buttoned:
- When performing laboratory procedures

biopsies, and sigmoidoscopies are other examples in which students can contact blood and other potentially infectious material.

Students must be aware of and think about the procedures they are involved in and be certain that they use essential safety equipment (PPE) and procedures when necessary. Students should adhere to the same responsibilities that employees do.

PPE should be available in the student laboratory and used as necessary. Standard precautions must be strictly adhered to.

Students should always be on guard and make safety a priority by taking all precautions to avoid injuries. Some of the precautions are:

- Needles and other sharps (such as microscope slides and coverslips, sharp surgical instruments, and glass containers) should be handled with the same strict guidelines as outlined in the OSHA *Bloodborne Pathogen Standards* and the CDC's Standard Precautions.
- Obey all safety rules and know where the spill kits are located and how to clean up biohazard spills.
- Know where the eyewash stations are and know how to operate them.

Be familiar with all the information about solutions and chemicals used in the laboratory as outlined in the Material Safety Data Sheet (MSDS).

An exposure to blood or other potentially infectious material experienced by a student must be immediately reported to the instructor if the accident occurs at the college or to the supervisor of the clinical agency and the externship coordinator if the student is exposed during externship. OSHA procedures as outlined earlier in this chapter should be followed with the exception of the filing of the OSHA 200 form.

Many colleges require students studying the health professions to obtain the hepatitis B vaccine because it is approximately 96% effective against HBV. Because the vaccine is given in three doses over a period of six months, students should plan to have the injections in a timely fashion to be prepared for college laboratory courses and the externship period.

PRINCIPLES OF INFECTION CONTROL

By understanding the dependent nature of the chain of infection which holds that each link in the process must occur for infectious disease to occur, medical assistants may apply principles of infection control to eliminate or reduce the transmission of infectious microorganisms in the health care setting. Conscious and continual reliance on infection control is a professional standard and protects employees, patients, families, and the public from contracting infectious diseases. There are two general types of infection control: medical asepsis and surgical asepsis. Each is indicated in specific circumstances and each is achieved by the various techniques that are described in this chapter and in Chapter 19.

MEDICAL ASEPSIS

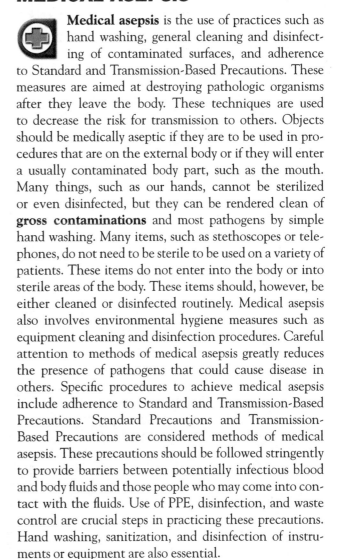

Medical asepsis is the use of practices such as hand washing, general cleaning and disinfecting of contaminated surfaces, and adherence to Standard and Transmission-Based Precautions. These measures are aimed at destroying pathologic organisms after they leave the body. These techniques are used to decrease the risk for transmission to others. Objects should be medically aseptic if they are to be used in procedures that are on the external body or if they will enter a usually contaminated body part, such as the mouth. Many things, such as our hands, cannot be sterilized or even disinfected, but they can be rendered clean of **gross contaminations** and most pathogens by simple hand washing. Many items, such as stethoscopes or telephones, do not need to be sterile to be used on a variety of patients. These items do not enter into the body or into sterile areas of the body. These items should, however, be either cleaned or disinfected routinely. Medical asepsis also involves environmental hygiene measures such as equipment cleaning and disinfection procedures. Careful attention to methods of medical asepsis greatly reduces the presence of pathogens that could cause disease in others. Specific procedures to achieve medical asepsis include adherence to Standard and Transmission-Based Precautions. Standard Precautions and Transmission-Based Precautions are considered methods of medical asepsis. These precautions should be followed stringently to provide barriers between potentially infectious blood and body fluids and those people who may come into contact with the fluids. Use of PPE, disinfection, and waste control are crucial steps in practicing these precautions. Hand washing, sanitization, and disinfection of instruments or equipment are also essential.

Some specific examples of appropriate use of medical asepsis include:

- Wash hands before and after handling equipment and supplies, on arrival and before leaving, and before and after working with each patient even if gloves were worn.

- Handle all specimens as if they were contaminated.
- Use disposable equipment whenever possible and dispose of it properly in a biohazard waste container. All equipment is contaminated after patient use.
- Use PPE as outlined in Standard Precautions and wash hands after removal of any PPE, including gloves.
- Keep contaminated equipment and supplies away from clothing to prevent transmission of pathogens to self and others.
- Place dressing materials, gauze, cotton balls, and any other damp or wet contaminated absorbable material in a waterproof bag before disposal in the biohazard waste container.
- Any break in the medical assistant's skin should be covered with a sterile dressing.
- Items that fall to the floor are contaminated. Either discard or sanitize then disinfect, or sterilize before using.
- If uncertain whether equipment or supplies are clean or sterile, clean or sterilize them before use.

Hand Washing

Hand washing is the most important aspect of all infectious control procedures. Proper hand washing removes gross contamination and reduces pathogens that could be transmitted by direct or indirect contact to others. Because hand washing is frequently required, the use of a good lotion is advised to reduce the possibility of skin breaks caused by dryness. The use of antibacterial soaps has not proven to increase the effectiveness of hand washing, can actually cause irritation of skin, and may even cause bacteria resistance through adaptation. Although these soaps are not recommended on a regular basis, they can be effective tools for use when soap and water are not readily available.

Procedure 10-1 outlines the steps of a medical asepsis hand wash.

Sanitization

Sanitization (washing) of instruments and equipment rids them of gross contamination and blood, body fluids, tissue, and other contaminated **debris.** Enzymatic detergent especially designed for medical instruments and a soft scrub brush are used to remove all contaminates from surfaces, crevices, hinges, and serrations. Use of enzymatic detergents will help break down the proteins found in body fluids and tissues. Water temperature should be warm but not hot. Heat coagulates protein, making it more difficult to remove. A critical component to promoting effective sanitization is to complete the procedure as soon as possible after contamination, so tissue or body fluids do not have the opportunity to dry on the instruments. Dried debris is more difficult to remove and may require much scrubbing. Instruments may be left to soak in disinfectant solution or water with a **solvent** if sanitization cannot be performed immediately after use (see Fig. 10-34).

To avoid the risk for punctures or cuts from sharp instruments during sanitization, heavy-duty gloves should be worn. Some facilities use an **ultrasonic cleaner.** It uses high-frequency sound waves and agitates the instruments (sanitizes them) before sterilizing them. Goggles are worn to protect eyes from splashing of contaminated debris during the scrubbing procedure. A plastic apron provides protection from splashing of clothing (see Chapter 19). Hot water may be used for rinsing to remove all residue and aid in the drying process. Drying thoroughly will prevent damage from rust or water spots.

Larger items such as instrument trays or Mayo stands, stools, chairs, examination tables, and lamps should also have a decontaminating sanitization process with thorough washing, rinsing, and drying.

See Procedure 10-4 for instrument sanitization. Gloves contaminated with blood and body fluids should be removed carefully to contain the contamination. Procedure 10-2 describes how to remove contaminated gloves thereby preventing further exposure to biohazard substances.

Disinfection

Disinfection, a third procedure used in medical asepsis practices, consists of various chemicals that can be used to destroy many pathogenic microorganisms but not necessarily their spores. Disinfection chemicals are used on inanimate objects. Because of their **caustic** nature, these chemicals can irritate the skin and mucous membranes. Chemicals can be used to disinfect items or equipment made from materials that could be damaged by heat or that are too large to fit into an autoclave such as stethoscopes, percussion hammers, examination tables, and Mayo trays and stands. These and other items that are chemically disinfected are used during *external* physical examination or procedures.

Boiling water (temperature 212°F) is considered a form of disinfection because it will kill some forms of microorganisms. It is important to note that this method *cannot* be considered a sterilization technique because the temperature is not high enough to kill the hepatitis virus, tuberculosis bacteria, or microbial spores. Articles such as nasal and ear specula can be disinfected by vigorous boiling for at least 15 minutes, or soaked in a disinfectant according to manufacturer's instructions. The only reasonable use for boiling as a means of disinfection in today's medical setting is for items that:

1. Will *not* be used in invasive procedures
2. Will *not* be inserted into body orifices nor be used in a sterile procedure

Before either chemical disinfection or disinfection by boiling, articles must first be thoroughly sanitized and dried. Of special note are stainless steel gynecologic and proctologic examination instruments. These instruments are not sanitized with other instruments because of the risk for transmission of sexually transmitted diseases (STDs). They are sterilized in the autoclave after sanitization to eliminate transmission of microorganisms.

Chemical disinfectant solutions must be carefully prepared and used according to the manufacturer's instructions to ensure effective disinfectant properties. Medical offices should use the disinfectant solution that best meets the needs of the ambulatory care setting as to the quantity of instruments to be disinfected, cost, preparation requirements, storage needs, and handling procedures. When choosing a chemical disinfectant solution, pay close attention to the manufacturer's report of the chemical disinfectant properties of the product. Some solutions are effective against a wide spectrum of microorganisms, whereas other solutions may be selective for certain common microorganisms. When chemically disinfecting, as with chemical sterilization, items must be thoroughly sanitized and dried. Any debris or water left on the item being chemically treated will dilute the chemical solution, thereby decreasing its effectiveness and compromising the disinfecting (or sterilization) process.

For surfaces such as countertops, the least expensive and most readily available chemical is a 1:10 solution of ordinary household bleach **(sodium hypochlorite).** However, besides the obvious disadvantage of bleaching clothing, bleach is not easily rinsed, and it is only effective if the solution is mixed fresh daily. Nevertheless, its effectiveness is so highly respected that many medical laboratories depend almost entirely on bleach to chemically kill pathogens on countertops.

In summary, medical asepsis includes procedures for which all medical assistants must be responsible and qualified to incorporate into daily work practices. The responsibility for maintaining medical asepsis is the combined goal of the office staff and physicians.

SURGICAL ASEPSIS AND STERILIZATION

Surgical asepsis means all microbial life (pathogens and nonpathogens) are destroyed before an invasive procedure is performed. Therefore, all equipment used is sterile. The terms *surgical asepsis* and *sterile technique* often are used interchangeably (see Chapter 19).

The main purpose of surgical asepsis is to prevent organisms from entering the patient's body during an invasive procedure. An invasive procedure refers to an opening in the skin such as a surgical incision, laceration, or an injection; or exposing a sterile inner surface to possible invasions of microorganisms such as when a urinary catheter is inserted through the urethra and into the sterile urinary bladder.

Because microorganisms are on virtually every surface such as the skin, instruments, surgical instrument trays, clothing, and even in the air, it is necessary to destroy as many of them as possible before doing any surgical (sterile) procedure. Any item that will come into

Maximum Process	Stethoscope	Chair	Ear Speculum	Vaginal Speculum	Fiberoptic Endoscope	Surgical Instrument	Skin
Sanitization	X	X	X	X	X	X	X
Chemical disinfection by wiping	X	X	X				
Chemical disinfection by soaking			X				
Chemical sterilization					X	X	
Antiseptic solution (surgical scrub)							X
Boiling			X				
Autoclave sterilization				X		X	
Use sterile barrier							X

contact with the sterile field (the area in which the sterile procedure will be performed or where sterile supplies will be maintained during the procedure) must be sterilized using physical or chemical agents. Once the surfaces are sterilized, every precaution must be taken to prevent contamination of the sterile areas either from a nonsterile surface or from airborne contamination. In this context, to **contaminate** is to make impure; for example, by the introduction of microorganisms or infectious material.

Before items can be sterilized, they must first be thoroughly sanitized and dried. The contaminated instruments are taken to a work area designated for that purpose. See Procedure 10-4 regarding sanitization of instruments. Care must be taken to prevent contamination of self. Heavy-duty gloves, goggles, and a plastic apron are worn for protection. This is a good time to check instruments for their working condition. Check ratchets, serrations and alignment, and ensure that they open and close readily. Check edges for nicks or roughness. Separate improperly working instruments. Instruments are now ready to be wrapped for sterilization.

As stated earlier, living tissue surfaces such as skin cannot be sterilized but can be rendered as free of pathogens as possible before the use of a sterile covering. One example of this concept is preparing the patient's skin with a surgical scrub solution before applying sterile drapes around the intended surgical site (see Chapter 19). Another example is the use of surgical hand washing technique before applying sterile gloves. The differences between hand washing for medical asepsis as discussed in this chapter (Procedure 10-1) and hand washing for surgical asepsis are addressed in Chapter 19.

There are four methods of sterilization:

1. Gas sterilization
2. Dry heat
3. Chemical sterilization
4. Steam sterilization (autoclave)

Gas Sterilization

Gas sterilization is accomplished in a gas oven large enough for wheelchairs and beds and takes hours for the extremely toxic gases to permeate and dissipate. These features make the gas oven useful in a large hospital setting but much too costly for the office.

Dry Heat Sterilization

Dry heat sterilization requires higher temperatures than steam sterilization and requires longer exposure times as well (at least one hour at 320°F). This method can be used for instruments that easily corrode such as sharp cutting instruments. Powders, oils, ointments, rubber goods, and plastic tubing may be sterilized using the dry heat method. Procedures for wrapping are the same as when wrapping for steam sterilization (see Procedure 10-6). Dry heat is seldom used in today's medical office or clinic.

Chemical Sterilization

Chemical sterilization, or cold sterilization, may use the same chemical agents used to chemically disinfect instruments or fomites. However, the exposure time for sterilization is achieved through prolonged immersion. The handling of instruments after chemical sterilization differs from handling procedures for instruments that are steam sterilized in that instruments must be handled with sterile gloves, rinsed with sterile water, and dried with a sterile towel before placement on a sterile surface.

Chemical sterilization is an effective method used in many medical offices when the object being sterilized is too large or too heat sensitive for autoclaving (see following section for information on autoclaving). Fiber-optic endoscopes are one of the most common items sterilized with the use of chemicals. These items are delicate and unable to withstand the high heat of an autoclave. The necessary equipment for chemical sterilization is a container or basin of adequate size for the intended item (and should be maintained for that purpose only) with a well-fitting lid and the chemical of choice. A vent hood is required for safety. Two of the most popular brands of chemicals available through medical supply sources are Wavecide and Cidex. Both have advantages and disadvantages. Offices must make individual choices based on convenience, expense, and other personnel preferences.

The effectiveness of any of these products depends greatly on the strength of the solution. If the strength is a 1:1 ratio of water to chemical, effectiveness will be lost if the solution is not mixed according to that dilution. Any attempt to cut cost by mixing a weaker solution will greatly compromise the effectiveness. Sometimes solutions are weakened unintentionally by placing wet items into them, thereby adding more water than is intended. For this reason, wet items must be carefully dried before chemical sterilization. A well-fitting lid is essential to avoid evaporation, which also interferes with the strength of the solution. The lid also lessens the chance of dust and airborne microbes from falling into the solution.

Another factor influencing the effectiveness of the sterilizing chemicals is exposure time. The manufacturer will provide specific time charts for each purpose. Manufacturer's directions will also include a time frame for replacing the solution. The ability of the solution to kill pathogens will be directly related to its freshness or shelf life. Regardless of the chemical used for sterilization, ventilation is important.

When using commercial chemicals, make certain the lid is placed on the soak basin at all times except when placing or removing items. Care must be taken to avoid contact with skin, eyes, and mucous membranes. Wear protective gloves, goggles, and apron if splashing is anticipated. The effects on skin can range from slight irritation to serious caustic burns.

Before any chemically sterilized items are used for patient contact, the chemicals must be thoroughly rinsed off using either sterile gloves or sterile transfer forceps to remove the item from the container. To maintain sterility, sterile water must be used for the rinsing process. Then dry with a sterile towel, and place onto a sterile field. This process is performed just before use of the item. (See Procedure 10-5.)

Steam Sterilization (Autoclave)

Steam sterilization is the most widely used method of sterilization in the medical office. An autoclave, basically a pressure cooker, is used to achieve sterilization. The autoclave uses steam under pressure to obtain higher temperatures than can be achieved with boiling (Figure 10-24). Water reaches a maximum temperature of 212°F through boiling. When under pressure, water is converted to steam and is then able to reach a temperature of 250–254°F. Exposing items to this extremely high heat and at least 15 pounds of pressure for a specific amount of time assures that all microorganisms and their spores are killed. The autoclave is actually an inner sterilizing chamber surrounded by a metal jacket. This creates a middle steam chamber between the inner sterilizing chamber and the jacket. Inside the jacket is a reservoir for water. When water is poured into the reservoir, the autoclave door closed and secured, and the autoclave turned on, several processes occur. The water in the reservoir heats until vapor is produced. The vapor enters the middle steam chamber inside the jacket. The air in the steam chamber is pushed out and replaced with steam. Because the air has been pushed out, the pressure increases. The increase of pressure causes the steam to then enter the inner sterilizing chamber (this is where the surgical instruments are placed), which pushes out the air. With the air being displaced with steam, the pressure increases in the inner chamber. The steam under pressure is able to reach a much higher temperature than boiling water. When the steam is able to reach all surfaces of the items placed in the autoclave and exposure is maintained for adequate amounts of time, sterility of those items is assured.

The recommended temperature for effective sterilization in an autoclave is 250–254°F. Unwrapped items should be sterilized for 20 minutes, loosely wrapped items for 30 minutes, and tightly packed items for at least 40 minutes. When uncertain about the proper amount of time necessary, the medical assistant should refer to the manufacturer's recommendations. The overall effectiveness of the autoclave in sterilizing contents is totally dependent on the medical assistant following proper operating procedure.

Only distilled water should be used to prevent mineral buildup in the machine. Before every use, check the

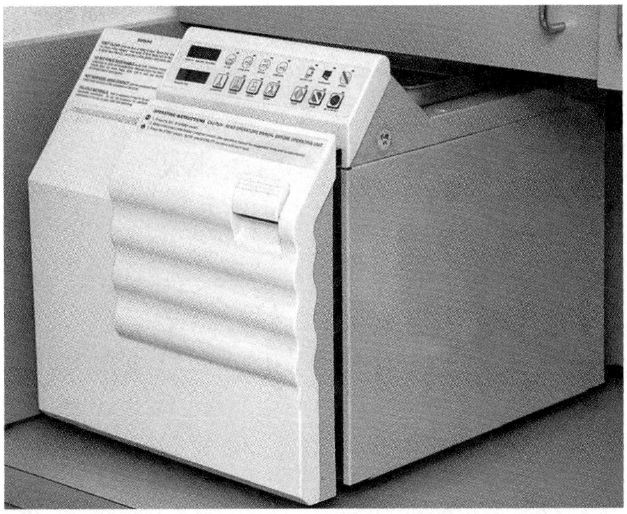

Figure 10-24 Commonly found in physician's offices, autoclaves are used for sterilization by steam pressure, usually at 250–254°F (121°C) for a specified length of time.

General rules to ensure proper sterilization using an autoclave:

- Articles placed into the autoclave must have been sanitized and dried.
- The articles are wrapped and placed to allow adequate exposure of all surfaces (see Figure 10-25). Instruments inside packages should have hinges open and serrations exposed.
- To avoid trapped air pockets, containers should be placed on their sides with lids loosely in place.
- Any wrapping material used must be approved for autoclave use.
- Timing should not start until the gauges reach 15 pounds of pressure and 254°F.
- When the cycle is complete, the door must be opened slightly to allow steam to escape. The sterile wrapped articles will be hot and damp and should be left in the autoclave to cool and dry. Microorganisms can contaminate the sterile articles through the damp wrapping if the door is opened too wide or if articles are handled while damp.

water level and add to fill line if necessary. Distilled water is inexpensive and readily available.

How to Load Packages. It is of extreme importance that instruments and materials be positioned properly in the autoclave for the steam to circulate through and between packs and penetrate them. Do not overload the autoclave. Place items as loosely as possible inside the chamber. Leave a 1- to 3-inch space between packs and the walls of the autoclave. Correct positioning and spacing allows sterilization to take place provided the medical assistant adheres to proper temperature, pressure, and time requirements (Figure 10-25).

Autoclave Maintenance and Cleaning. The autoclave, like any piece of equipment in the medical office, needs regular cleaning and maintenance. Frequency of cleaning the autoclave will depend somewhat on its usage. If the autoclave is used everyday, the inner chamber should be washed with a mild detergent and cloth, rinsed, and dried on a daily basis. The outer jacket should be wiped clean of dust and soil. Follow the manufacturer's instructions and recommendations for cleansers. Omni® cleanser is a well-known brand of autoclave cleanser.

At least once a week or following the manufacturer's instructions, the autoclave should be drained of water and cleaned thoroughly. Cleaning the autoclave requires that it be drained, filled with cleaning solution, run through a 20-minute heated cycle, drained of solution, filled with distilled rinse water, run through another 20-minute heated cycle, drained of rinse solution, and filled with distilled water again. Then the inner shelves are removed and scrubbed, and the inner chamber is wiped clean. Because this process is fairly time-consuming and will certainly put the autoclave out of use for a while, consideration should be given to scheduling the weekly cleaning at a time when personnel can devote the time and when the autoclave is not in demand for sterilization processes.

During the cleaning process, attention should be given to inspecting the rubber seal for cracks or wear. An extra replacement rubber seal should always be kept on hand. The seals are available through medical supply sources. Refer to the manufacturer's instructions for regularly scheduled replacement of the rubber seal and other recommended maintenance procedures.

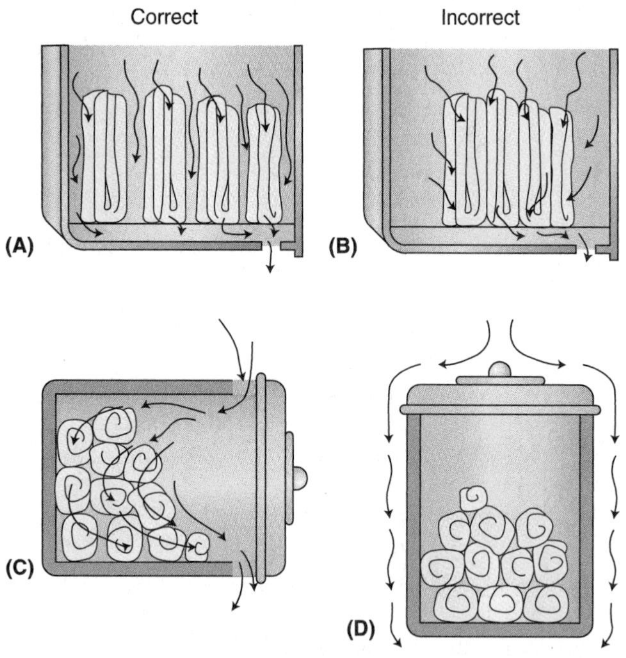

Figure 10-25 (A) Proper placement of packages in the autoclave allows steam to circulate and penetrate from all sides. (B) Packages incorrectly loaded in autoclave. (C) When placed correctly, the jar should lay on its side with the cover loosely in place to allow steam to freely circulate through the jar and properly sterilize the dressings. (D) Incorrect method. (Courtesy of Steris Corporation, Mentor, OH.)

Quality Control and Assurance for Autoclave. Quality control when using an autoclave consists of proper maintenance, proper operation, and observation of the temperature and pressure gauges. Equally important is the regular use of sterilization indicators and culture tests. Several types of sterilization indicators and culture methods are available:

- *Sterilization strips.* Contain a **thermolabile** dye that darkens when exposed to steam at the proper temperature and pressure for the proper amount of time. These indicators are placed in the center of the wrapped article (Figure 10-26).

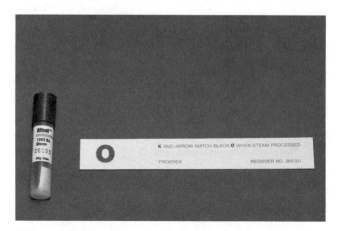

Figure 10-26 Types of sterilization indicators.

- *Culture tests*. Available as a culture strip containing heat-resistant spores. The strip is placed in the center of a wrapped article and placed in a fully loaded autoclave. After processing is complete, the article is unwrapped and the strip is placed into a culture medium. If the autoclave is functioning properly and the medical assistant has followed proper operating procedure, no growth should occur. Also available through Becton-Dickinson Microbiology Systems is an ampule called the Kilit Ampule. These biological indicators are ampules that contain spores of the thermophile "Bacillus stearothermophilus." After being processed through the autoclave, the Kilit Ampule is sent to a cooperating laboratory for week-long observation for survival of the bacilli spores. A written report of the results is generated by the laboratory and sent to the office for its records.

Autoclave Wrapping Material and Packaging Supplies. Wrapping or otherwise packaging surgical instruments and other surgical and medical articles before placing them in the autoclave will extend their shelf life up to six months. Before these articles are wrapped, they must first be sanitized, rinsed, and dried. Several materials are available for wrapping. Cost, convenience, visibility, time, space, and ease of use will help determine which to use. Many offices will use a combination of materials.

- Muslin is a cloth wrap available in several sizes and colors. Even with the cost of the initial purchasing, occasional replacements, autoclave tape, and laundering, muslin is still an economical option. Besides these cost-effective advantages, many surgical instruments may be wrapped together in muslin, making up a convenient surgery/procedure set. One of the main disadvantages of muslin is the inability to view the contents. Another disadvantage is the need for constant examination for holes, tears, and wearing out of the cloth. Patching is not a reasonable option because iron-on patches impede penetration of steam and sewn-on patches create their own set of perforations. A defective muslin cloth should be discarded. Wrapping space and training of personnel are necessary when using cloth. Special autoclave tape is required to seal the package.
- Paper sterilization wrapping squares are available in many different sizes and types. This disposable type of material requires that a new paper be used each time items are sterilized, but it eliminates the need for laundering. Similar to cloth wrapping, paper wraps also lend themselves to larger sets of articles being wrapped together for surgery or procedural packs. As with muslin cloth, wrapping space and some personnel training are necessary. Paper wraps are opaque, making viewing of the contents impossible. Autoclave tape is required to seal the package.
- Sterilization pouches or bags may be either plastic or paper or a combination (Figure 10-27). They are fairly inexpensive and very easy to use. Because no wrapping is involved, additional work space is not required. Another advantage of bags is the visibility of the items inside. Some pouches are packaged on a continuous roll and are available in a variety of widths. This allows the medical assistant to cut the bag to fit the article. Because both ends need to be taped closed, it is difficult to remove the article while maintaining its sterility. Probably the best bag-type option is individual bags with the top end open for instrument placement and the bottom end factory closed with a peel-apart seal. The article is inserted into the top opening, the bag is taped closed, and the package is sterilized (Figure 10-28). When needed, the sterile article is removed through the factory-sealed bottom end in a peel-apart sterile fashion. These bags need to be purchased in several individual sizes and are expensive but have the advantages of ease of use and item visibility and are probably the preferred method for most medical offices today.

Autoclave Tape. Autoclave tape is chemically treated to become "striped" when exposed to heat. The striped pattern indicates exposure to high temperature but does

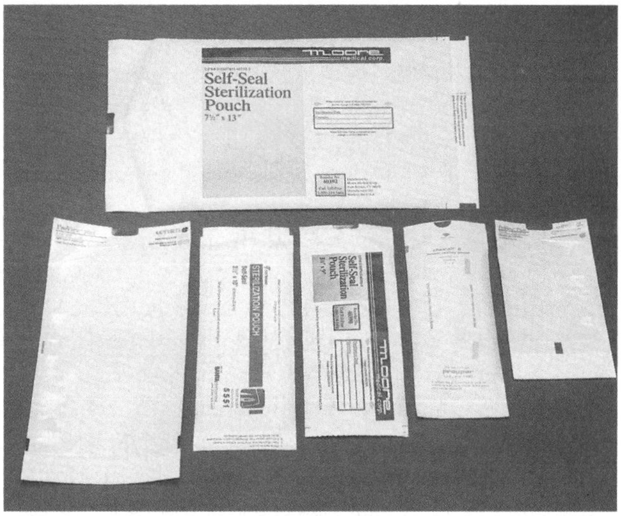

Figure 10-27 Various types and sizes of self-sealing bags for sterilization.

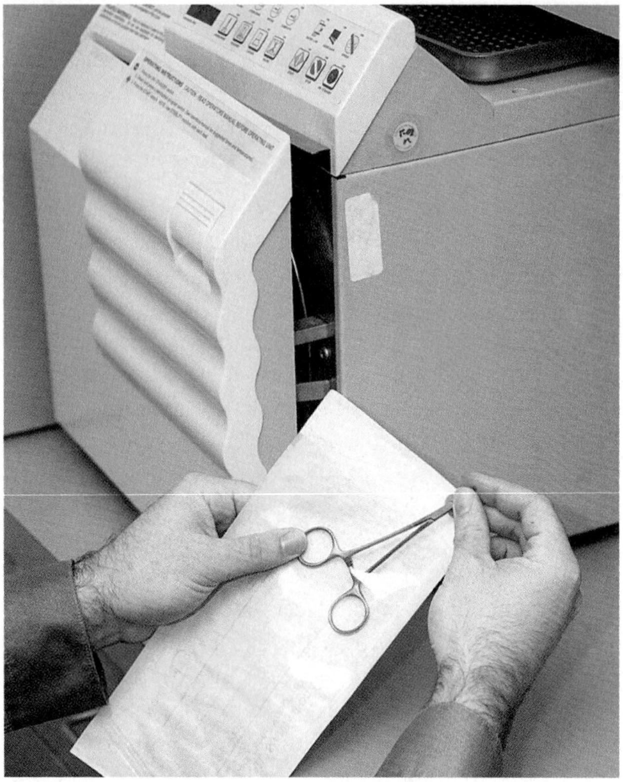

Figure 10-28 The medical assistant is placing a sanitized instrument into a sterilization bag for autoclaving by inserting the tips of the instrument in first.

not measure pounds of pressure or duration of exposure. Because of these limitations, autoclave tape does not assure that the wrapped package is sterile, only that it has been in a heated autoclave. Because it is placed on the outside of the package, it does not assure that steam has penetrated to the inner article but does help to determine if a package has been processed (Figure 10-29).

Labeling Packages for Autoclave. Surgical packages should be labeled clearly. Clear bags usually have a designated place for labeling, and muslin- or paper-wrapped packages may be labeled across the autoclave tape. Proper labeling should include the names of the articles in the pack, the date of sterilization, and the initials of the medical assistant responsible for the wrapping. The name of the instrument or article should be as specific as possible, especially when using the opaque cloth or paper wraps. If many instruments have been wrapped together for a specific surgery or for a specific physician, the label should clearly state which surgery or surgeon. For example, a "laceration repair set" could contain all the necessary instruments for repairing a laceration. "Dr. Peterson's vasectomy set" would contain all the instruments Dr. Peterson needs to perform a vasectomy, including, perhaps, personal preference instruments. The date of sterilization will help determine the expiration of sterility and determine a "pull date" for resterilizing. Initialing the package allows for accountability if necessary. Labels should always be written with a permanent marker. Ballpoint pen should never be used because the ink will smear when wet. Caution should be taken to avoid puncturing through the package during labeling.

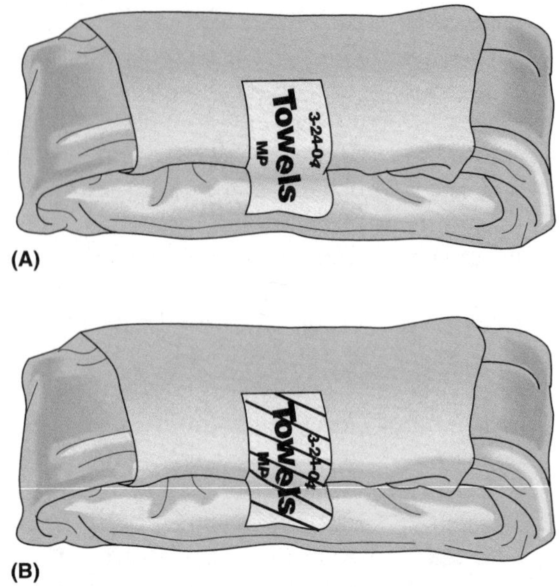

Figure 10-29 Package of towels (A) before and (B) after autoclaving. Note that the autoclave tape has a striped pattern indicating that the package was exposed to a high temperature. This does not assure sterility, however.

Critical Thinking

What is the purpose of OSHA's standards for bloodborne pathogens and whom does it cover?

Wrapping Techniques. Articles must be wrapped in a specific way to ensure they remain sterile when opened. Wrapped surgical instruments need to be double wrapped. Some methods advocate placing both layers of wrapping material together and double wrapping the pack in one process. A much more useful method is the "wrapping twice" technique (see Procedure 10-6). The wrapping twice technique allows for additional options at the time of opening. Wrapping twice allows for a completely wrapped inner sterile package to be applied to the surgical tray. This wrapping twice technique eliminates struggling to control multiple instruments during the unwrapping process; and, if the inner package becomes contaminated during the unwrapping, the medical assistant has the additional option of unwrapping the inner package using the same technique without having to start over. All packs should be neatly and securely wrapped; firm enough to prevent the instruments from movement, but loose enough to permit adequate steam penetration. See Procedures 10-6 and 10-7.

Procedure 10-1 Medical Asepsis Hand Wash

STANDARD PRECAUTIONS:

PURPOSE:

To reduce pathogens on the hands and wrists, thereby decreasing direct and indirect transmission of infectious microorganisms. Average duration is 2 minutes before beginning to work with patients, 30 seconds following each patient contact.

EQUIPMENT/SUPPLIES:

Sink (preferably with foot-operated controls)
Soap (preferably liquid soap in foot-operated container; bar soap discouraged)
Water-based antibacterial lotion
Disposable paper towels
Nail stick or brush

PROCEDURE STEPS:

1. Remove all jewelry (plain wedding band is only acceptable jewelry). Push watch up on arm or remove. RATIONALE: Jewelry harbors microorganisms on the hands.
2. Prepare disposable paper towel (if using pull-down dispenser, prepare the amount of paper towel necessary for drying hands after wash; if using folded towels, have accessible). RATIONALE: After the hand washing, you may not touch any contaminated surface, such as the handle on a paper-towel dispenser or the water faucets.
3. Never allow your clothing to touch the sink; never touch the inside of the sink with your hands. RATIONALE: The sink is considered contaminated at all times (Note: Sinks must be sanitized and disinfected at the end of each day).
4. Turn on the faucet with a dry paper towel (Figure 10-30A). Discard paper towel. Adjust water temperature to lukewarm. RATIONALE: Lukewarm water is best for hand washing because excessively hot water may overdry the skin.
5. Wet hands and apply soap using a circular motion and friction; rub into a lather (Figure 10-30B). RATIONALE: This initial hand wash is to remove visible soil and some microorganisms. Interlace fingers to clean between them (Figure 10-30C).
6. Use an orange stick or brush at the first hand washing of each day (Figures 10-30D and E). RATIONALE: Nails harbor excessive numbers of microorganisms. Even with trimmed nails, this step must be performed on a daily basis.
7. Rinse hands with hands pointed down and lower than elbows (Figure 10-30F). RATIONALE: When hands are held lower than elbows, pathogens and contaminated water run off the hands and not up on the forearms.
8. Repeat soap application and lather; interlace fingers well; wash with vigorous, circular motions all parts of hands including wrists; wash for at least one minute or longer depending on degree of contamination. RATIONALE: Appropriate length of hand washing is required to provide enough friction to remove soil and microorganisms.
9. Rinse well, keeping hands pointed downward. RATIONALE: Rinsing removes microorganisms, contaminated water, and soap from the hands.
10. Repeat hand washing for the first hand washing of the day or if necessary for contaminated or visibly soiled hands. Lather wrists using a circular motion and friction. Rinse arms and hands. RATIONALE: When the hands are excessively

(continues)

Procedure 10-1 (continued)

contaminated or soiled, two hand washings may be necessary to remove microorganisms from the hands.

11. Dry hands and wrists with disposable paper towel; do not touch towel dispenser after hand washing; blot instead of rubbing with towel; if sink is not foot operated, use a clean disposable towel to turn off water faucet. RATIONALE: Touching the towel dispenser contaminates the hands. Blotting the hands dry reduces drying of the skin. Turning faucet off with paper towel prevents recontamination from dirty faucet.

12. Discard paper towel in waste container. Do not leave contaminated towels for repeated use. NOTE: Repeat hand washing procedure before and after each patient contact, procedure, or meal. RATIONALE: Hand washing must be performed on a regular and frequent basis to ensure the reduction of microorganisms transmitted by hands.

Water-based antibacterial lotion can be applied to prevent chapped, **excoriated** skin. If skin is excoriated, the medical assistant may not be able to work because of breaks in the skin or may have to wear gloves during any patient contact.

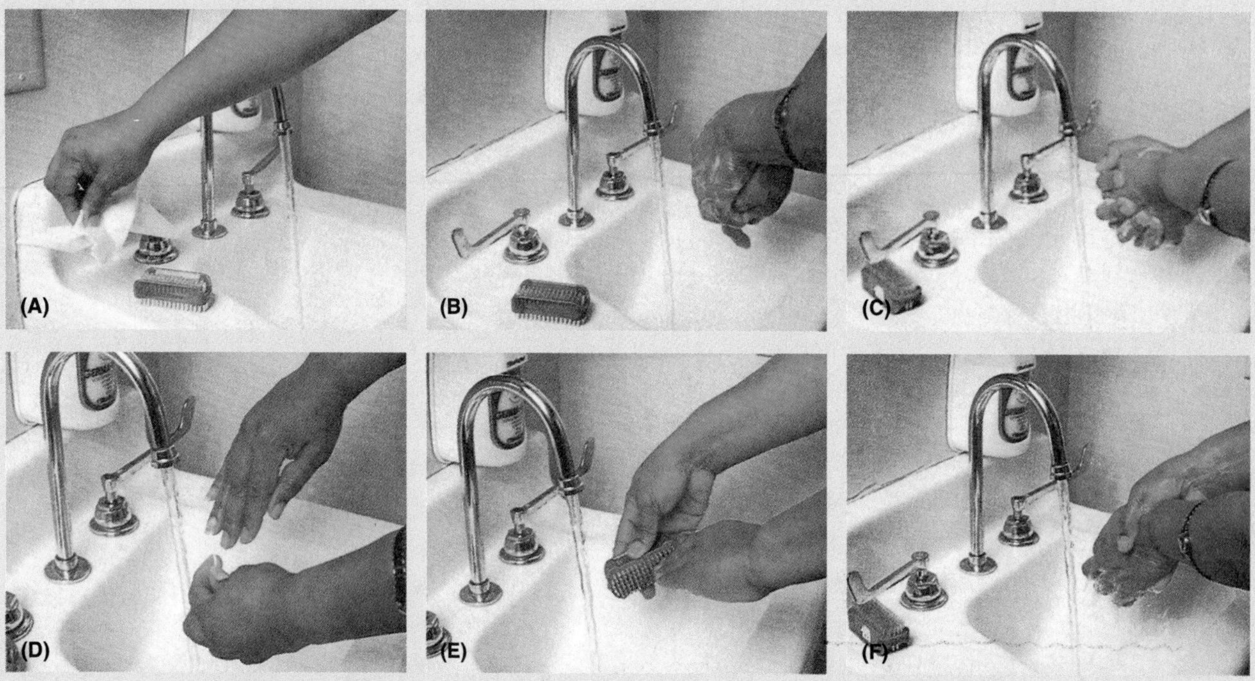

Figure 10-30 (A) Prepare towels for use. Turn on the faucet and adjust water to a lukewarm temperature. (B) Wet hands. Let water flow downward off hands and fingertips. (C) Use a circular motion to create friction and wash the palms and backs of hands. Interlace the fingers to clean between them. (D) Use an orange stick to clean under fingernails. (E) A hand brush may also be used to clean under fingernails. (F) Rinse hands thoroughly, letting the water flow downward off your hands and fingertips.

Procedure 10-2 Removing Contaminated Gloves

STANDARD PRECAUTIONS:

PURPOSE:

To carefully remove and dispose of contaminated gloves to contain exposure.

EQUIPMENT/SUPPLIES:

Biohazard waste container

PROCEDURE STEPS:

1. Grasp the palm of the used left glove with the right hand to begin removing the first glove. Notice hands are held away from the body and pointed downward (Figure 10-31A and B). RATIONALE: Holding the hands away from the body will further prevent exposure to biological contaminants.
2. Turn the used left glove inside out and hold it in the right gloved hand. Be careful not to touch your bare left hand on the contaminated right glove (Figure 10-31C–E). RATIONALE: Turning the glove inside out helps isolate the biological contaminants.
3. Holding the glove that has been removed with the hand that still has the glove on, the medical assistant inserts two fingers of the ungloved hand between her arm and the inside of the dirty glove (Figure 10-31F).

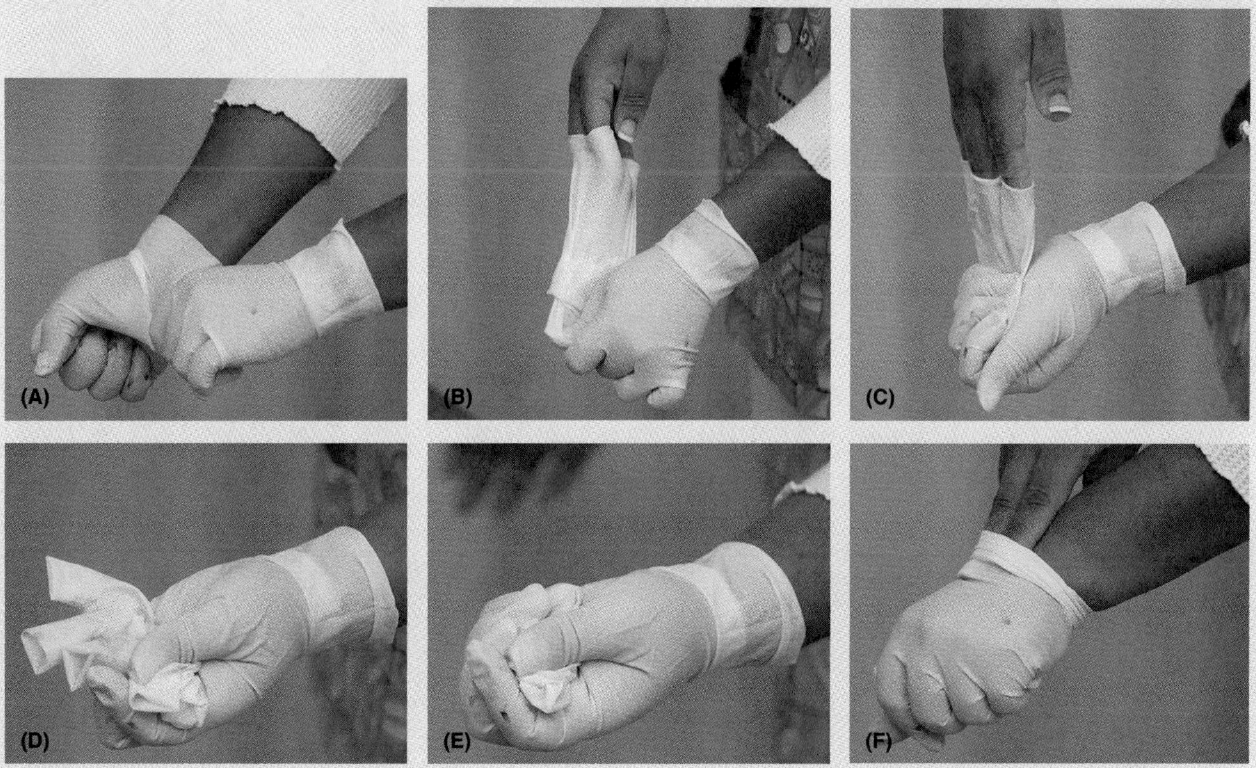

Figure 10-31 (A) Grasp the palm of the used glove with the right hand. (B) Begin removing the first glove. (C) Glove is turned inside out as it is being removed. Take care to not touch bare skin on the contaminated glove. (D) Inverted glove is completely removed into the contaminated glove. (E) Contain the inverted glove completely in the gloved hand. (F) Insert two fingers of the ungloved hand inside the back of the contaminated glove and turn it inside out over the other.

(continues)

Procedure 10-2 (continued)

4. Turn the right dirty glove inside out over the other. One glove is inside the other and the medical assistant can handle the gloves because the dirty, contaminated area is inside the gloves (Figure 10-31G and H). RATIONALE: Both gloves are inverted with the biological contaminates isolated.
5. Dispose of the inverted gloves into a biological waste receptacle (Figure 10-31I). RATIONALE: All biological waste should be placed into a red biohazard bag.
6. Wash hands thoroughly. RATIONALE: Immediate washing of hands is an additional precaution.

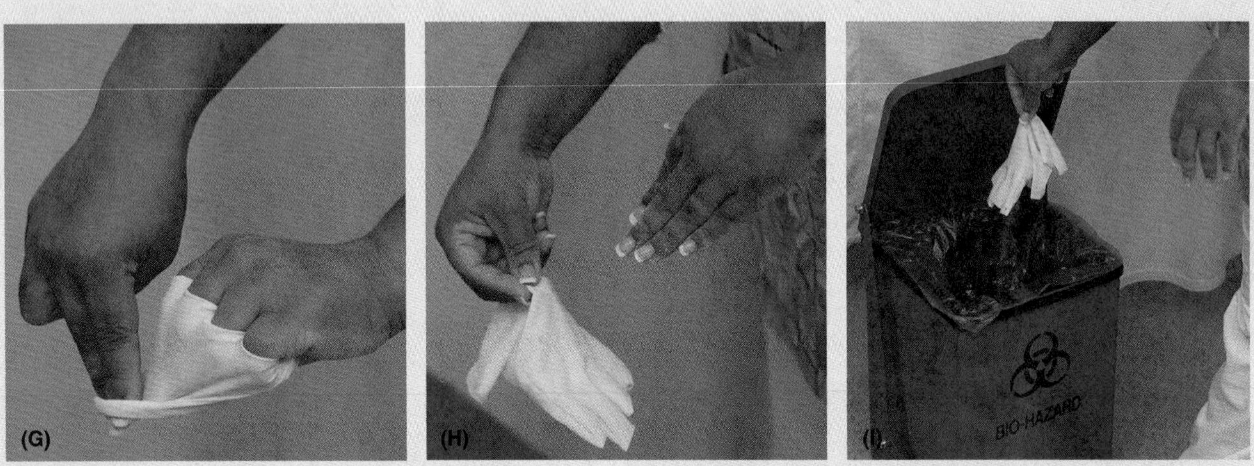

Figure 10-31 *(continued)* (G) Invert the second glove over the first. (H) One glove is now inside the other. (I) Dispose of gloves in biohazard container.

Procedure 10-3 Transmission-Based Precautions: Donning a Gown, Mask, Gloves, and Cap (Isolation Technique)

STANDARD PRECAUTIONS:

PURPOSE:

To provide barriers for medical assistant to be protected from airborne, contact, or droplet infectious diseases.

EQUIPMENT/SUPPLIES:

Disposable gowns
Disposable caps
Disposable masks
Gloves (nonsterile and sterile)
Room with sink and running water
Paper towels
Other supplies relative to client's condition

PROCEDURE STEPS:

1. Review physician orders and agency protocols relative to the type of isolation precautions. RATIONALE: Provides for patient comfort and decreases the spread of microorganisms.

(continues)

Procedure 10-3 (continued)

Limits the number of personnel coming into the patient's room and the patient's exposure to microorganisms.

2. Place appropriate isolation supplies outside the patient's room and note type of isolation sign on the door (e.g., airborne, droplet, or contact). RATIONALE: Ensures staff follows isolation protocol and alerts visitors to check with the nurses' station before entering the room.
3. Remove jewelry, laboratory coat, and other items not necessary in providing patient care. RATIONALE: Decreases the spread of microorganisms.
4. Wash hands and don disposable clothing:
   a. Apply cap to cover hair and ears completely.
   b. Apply gown to cover outer garments completely. Hold gown in front of body and place arms through sleeves (Figure 10-32A). Pull sleeves down to wrist. Tie gown securely at neck and waist (Figure 10-32B and C).
   c. Don nonsterile gloves and pull gloves over the cuff to cover completely.

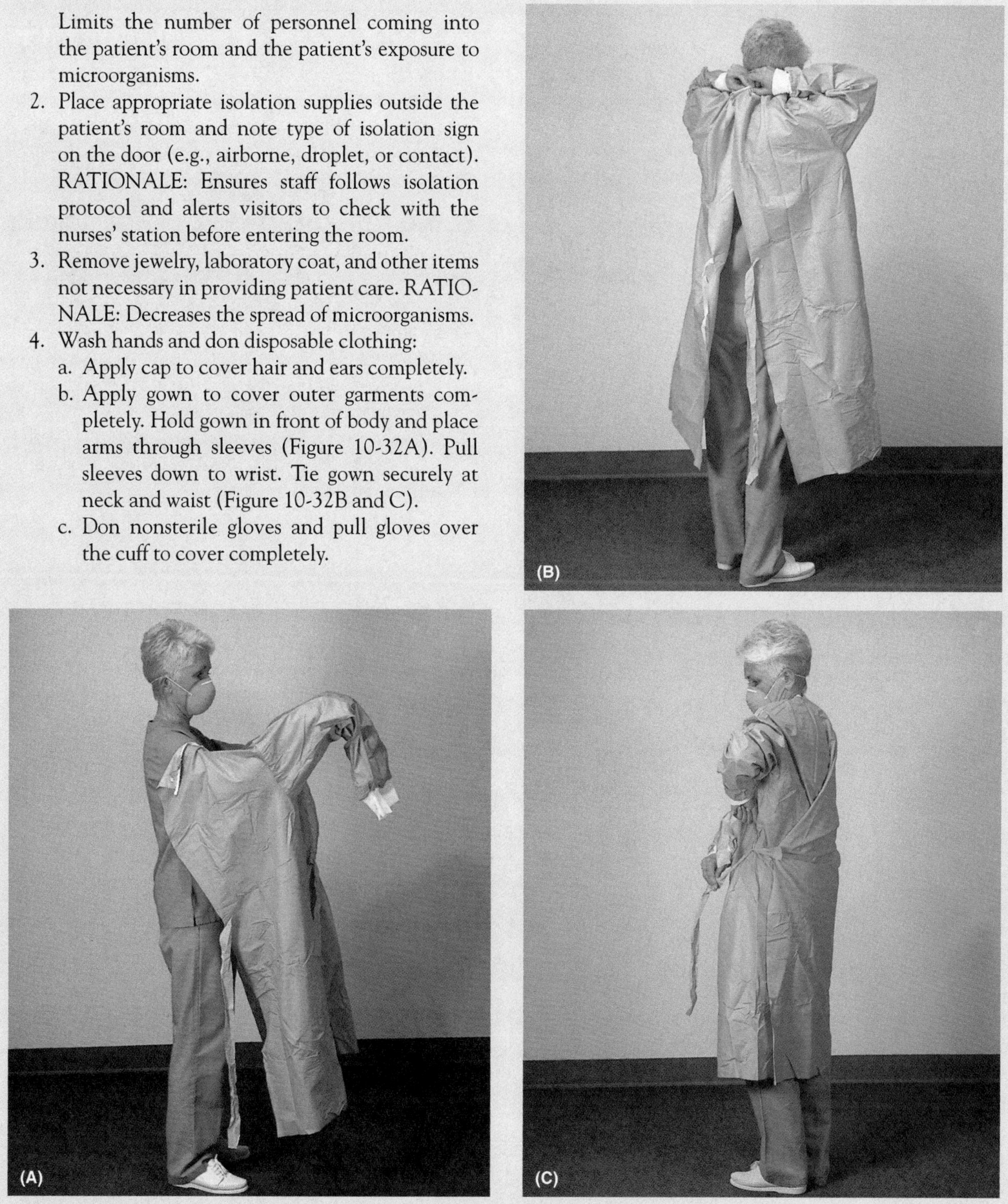

Figure 10-32 (A) Medical assistant has put on a mask and is donning the gown, pulling on the sleeves. (B) The neck of the gown is tied first, and (C) the back of the gown, last.

(continues)

Procedure 10-3 (continued)

d. Apply mask by placing the top of the mask over the bridge of your nose (top part of mask has a metal strip) and pinch the metal strip to fit snugly against the skin of the nose.

RATIONALE: Disposable garments act as a barrier in preventing the transmission of microorganisms from medical assistant to patient and protect the medical assistant from contact with pathogens.

5. Enter patient's room with all gathered supplies. RATIONALE: Prevents trips into and out of the patient's room and keeps supplies clean.
6. Assess vital signs and perform other functions (ECG, phlebotomy) of care to meet the needs of the patient. Record assessment data on a piece of paper, avoiding contact with any articles in the patient room. RATIONALE: Allows for data collection and the performance of patient care.
7. Dispose of soiled articles in the impermeable biohazard bags, which should be labeled correctly according to contents. If soiled, reusable equipment is removed from the room, label bag accordingly. RATIONALE: Impermeable biohazard bags prevent the leakage of contaminated materials, thereby preventing the transmission of infection. Labeling is a warning to other personnel that the contents are infectious.

EXITING THE ISOLATION ROOM: REMOVING GOWN, GLOVES, MASK, AND CAP

1. Remove contaminated gloves (see Procedure 10-2). Wash hands and then untie waist tie of gown (Figure 10-33A).
2. Remove mask by untying top ties first, then bottom ties (Figure 10-33B). Holding mask by ties, place in contaminated waste.
3. Untie neckties of gown (Figure 10-33C). Wash hands. RATIONALE: Removes microorganisms from hands before proceeding.

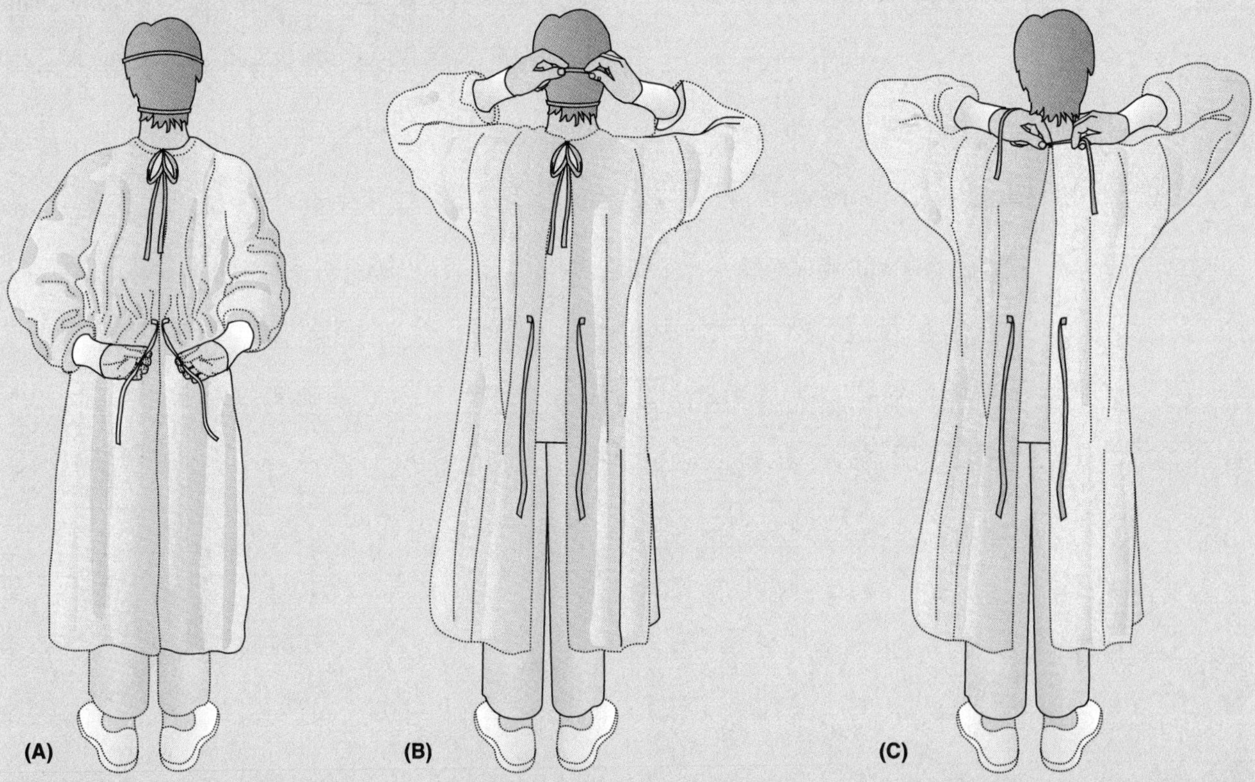

Figure 10-33 (A) When finished in the isolation room, the medical assistant removes the contaminated gloves (see Procedure 10-2), washes hands (see Procedure 10-1), and then unties waist tie of gown. Remove mask by untying top ties first, then bottom ties. (B) Holding mask by ties, place in biohazard container. (C) Untie neck ties of gown. Wash hands. RATIONALE: Hands are contaminated from touching the outside of the mask and gown and must be washed to remove microorganisms before proceeding to remove the gown.

(continues)

Procedure 10-3 (continued)

4. Slip fingers of one hand inside cuff (Figure 10-33D) of the other hand. Pull the gown over the hand, being careful not to touch the outside of the gown.
5. Using the hand covered by the gown, pull down the gown over the other hand (Figure 10-33E).
6. Pull gown off your arms. Hold gown away from yourself and roll into a ball with the contaminated side inside (Figure 10-33F). RATIONALE: The gown is removed and folded, touching only the inside of the gown to prevent transmission of microorganisms to yourself.
7. Dispose of gown in biohazard container.
8. Wash hands thoroughly.

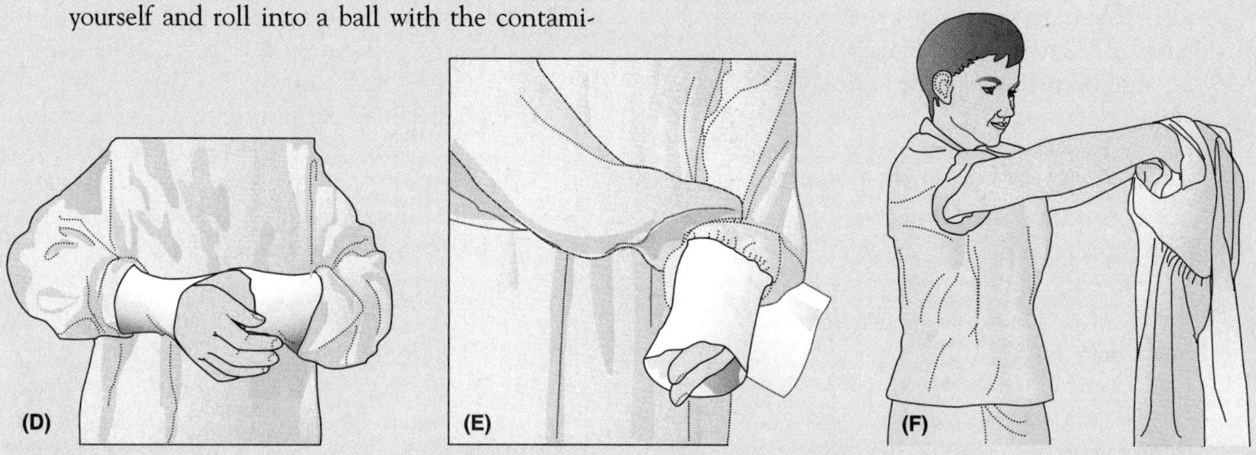

Figure 10-33 *(continued)* (D) Slip fingers of one hand inside cuff of the other hand. Pull gown over the hand, being careful not to touch the outside of the gown. RATIONALE: Outside of gown is contaminated. (E) Using the hand covered by the gown, pull down the gown over the other hand. (F) Pull gown off arms and hold away from body and clothing. Roll into a ball with the contaminated side of gown on the inside. RATIONALE: Gown is removed and folded, touching only the inside of the gown to prevent transmission of microorganisms. The outside is contaminated. Wash hands thoroughly.

Procedure 10-4 Sanitization of Instruments

STANDARD PRECAUTIONS:

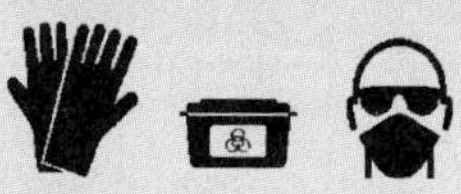

PURPOSE:

To properly clean contaminated instruments to remove tissue and debris.

EQUIPMENT/SUPPLIES:

Sink (or ultrasonic cleaner: follow manufacturer's instructions)
Sanitizing agent (low-sudsing detergent, approved chemical disinfectant, or blood solvent)
Brush
Disposable paper towels
Plastic apron
Disposable gloves, heavy-duty if cleaning sharps
Goggles
Biohazard waste container

(continues)

Procedure 10-4 (continued)

PROCEDURE STEPS:

1. Wear disposable gloves, goggles, and apron. RATIONALE: Contaminated instruments pose a blood and body fluid precaution as indicated by OSHA standards. Disposable gloves must always be worn to sanitize instruments. Wear heavy-duty gloves if cleaning sharp instruments. Goggles are worn to protect eyes from splashing of contaminated debris during scrubbing procedure. A plastic apron provides protection from splashing of clothing.
2. As soon as possible after a procedure in which an instrument is contaminated, rinse the instrument in water and disinfectant solution; rinse again under running water. RATIONALE: Rinsing contaminated instruments as soon as possible after use removes debris and tissue that could quickly dry onto the instrument, making sanitization more difficult.
3. If contaminated instrument must be carried from one place to another for sanitization, place the instrument in a basin labeled "Biohazard." RATIONALE: Do not carry contaminated instruments in your hands. Biohazard basins must be sanitized and disinfected daily according to procedures for Standard Precautions.
4. Scrub each instrument well with detergent and water; scrub under running water, and be sure to scrub inside any edges and all surfaces (Figure 10-34). RATIONALE: Thorough scrubbing removes tissue and debris from all areas of the contaminated instrument. If all tissue is not removed with scrubbing, the instrument may not be sterilized during sterilization procedures.
5. Rinse well with hot water. RATIONALE: Tissue and debris, as well as detergent, must be completely removed. Hot water will help remove all residue and aid in the drying process while rust and water spots will be eliminated.
6. After they are rinsed, place instruments on muslin or disposable paper towel until all instruments have been scrubbed and rinsed. RATIONALE: Often more than one instrument is sanitized; do not place sanitized instrument in the bottom of the sink or on a countertop without a disposable paper towel or muslin towel.
7. Dry instruments with muslin or disposable paper towels. RATIONALE: Wet instruments may rust or corrode. When preparing instruments for the sterilization procedures, they should be dry. Check instruments for working condition.
8. Remove gloves, wash hands.

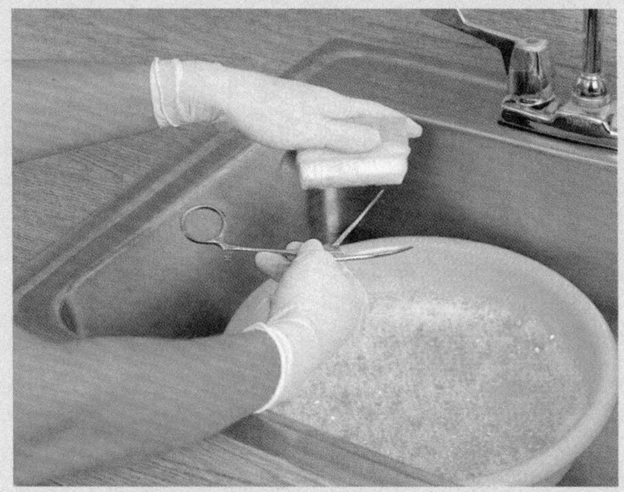

Figure 10-34 Medical assistant is using a scrub brush, plastic basin, and protein solvent enzymatic detergent to sanitize surgical instruments. Note the medical assistant also is wearing gloves.

Procedure 10-5 Chemical "Cold" Sterilization of Endoscopes

STANDARD PRECAUTIONS:

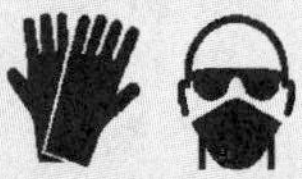

PURPOSE:

To sterilize heat-sensitive items such as fiber-optic endoscopes and delicate cutting instruments using appropriate chemical solution.

EQUIPMENT/SUPPLIES:

Chemical solution such as Cidex	Timer
Steris System®	Sterile water
(Percacetic acid)	Gloves (heavy-duty)
	Sterile towel
Airtight container	Plastic-lined sterile drapes

PROCEDURE STEPS:

1. Sanitize items that require chemical sterilization. Rinse and dry. RATIONALE: Recall that debris and body proteins must be scrubbed from items before sterilization.
2. Read manufactuer's instructions on original container of chemical sterilization solution. RATIONALE: Each brand of chemical sterilization solution has specific preparation instructions and germicidal properties; choose the solution that best fits the needs of the ambulatory care setting. Keep the solution in its original container to reduce chances of accidental poisoning.
3. Put on gloves. RATIONALE: Heavy-duty gloves help protect from sharp items puncturing the skin. Chemicals are harsh on the skin.
4. Prepare solution as indicated by manufacturer; place the date of opening or preparation on the container and initial it. RATIONALE: Following manufacturer's instructions ensures sterility. Note the expiration date of solution.
5. Pour solution into a container with an airtight lid, avoid splashing (Figure 10-35). RATIONALE: Chemicals should not be left exposed to open air to prevent evaporation and loss of potency, exposure to environmetal contaminants, accidental inhalation, or poisoning. Splashing may cause skin or mucous membrane contact and result in injury.
6. Place sanitized and dried items into the solution, completely submersing item(s). Avoid splashing when placing items into airtight container. RATIONALE: Total immersion is necessary for sterility to be achieved.

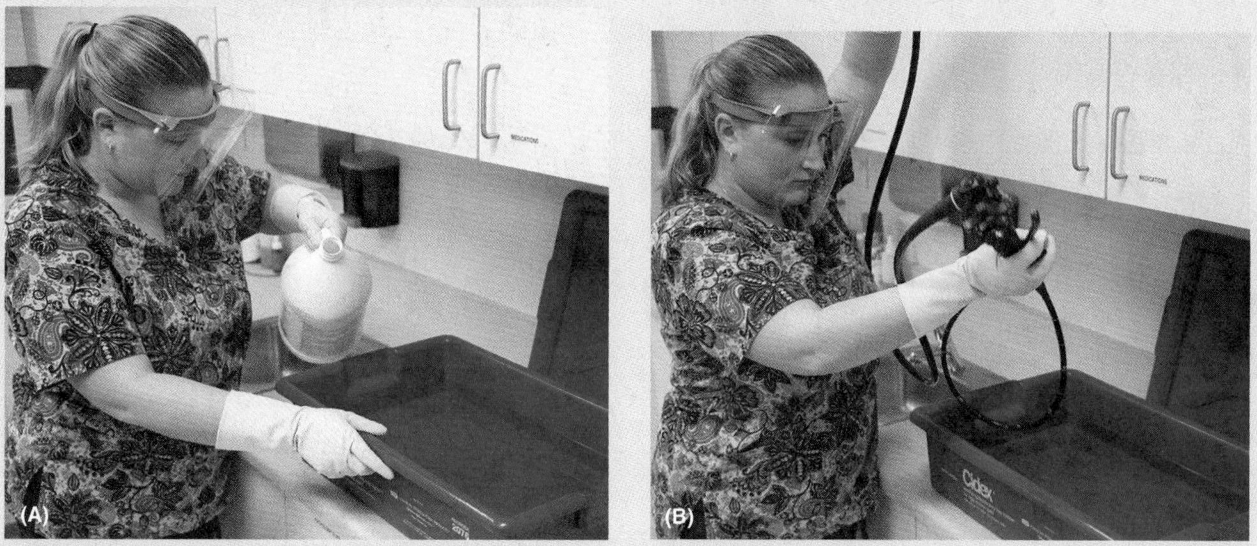

Figure 10-35 (A) Medical assistant pours chemical sterilization solution into a large soaking container. Note the use of heavy-duty gloves and face shield. (B) Medical assistant adds the endoscope to the chemical sterilization solution in the container.

(continues)

Procedure 10-5 (continued)

7. Close lid of container, label with name of solution, date, and time required per manufacturer, and initial (Figure 10-35C). RATIONALE: Exposure time is the required time indicated by the manufacturer to achieve sterility. Initialing work ensures accountability and responsibility.
8. Do not open lid or add additional items during the processing time. RATIONALE: Adding to the container interrupts the sterilization process and limits the effectiveness of the chemical.
9. Following the recommended processing time, lift item(s) from the container using sterile gloved hands or sterile transfer forceps. Carefully hold item above sterile basin and pour copious amounts of sterile water over it and through it (endoscopes) until adequately rinsed of chemical solution. RATIONALE: Item(s) once processed are sterile and must be handled appropriately. Using sterile gloved hands or sterile transfer forceps ensures sterile-to-sterile contact and no contamination of the item(s). Sterile water is poured through the inner channels of endoscopes to rinse chemicals from the inside, as well as the outside.
10. Hold item(s) upright for a few seconds to allow excess sterile water to drip off.
11. Place the sterile item on a sterile towel (which has been placed on a sterile field) and dry it with another sterile towel. The towel used for drying is removed from sterile field. The use of sterile drapes that have a plastic polylined barrier layer between two layers of paper is recommended for the sterile field. RATIONALE: Plastic-lined sterile drapes create a barrier to prevent moisture from drawing contaminants from the metal surgical instrument tray or countertop up into the sterile area.

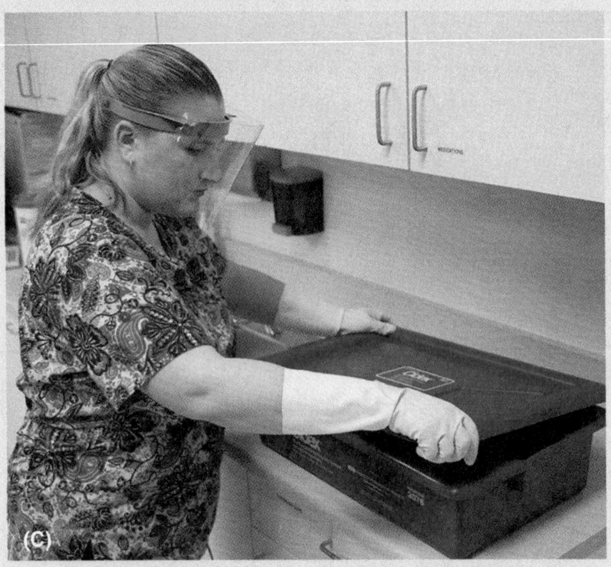

Figure 10-35 *(continued)* (C) Medical assistant secures lid tightly, then records the date, time of day, and her initials.

Procedure 10-6 Wrapping Instruments for Sterilization in Autoclave

PURPOSE:

To properly wrap sanitized instruments for sterilization in an autoclave.

EQUIPMENT/SUPPLIES:

Sanitized instruments
Wrapping material (muslin or disposable wrapping paper)
Sterilization indicator
2 × 2 gauze or cotton balls (if instrument has hinges)
Autoclave wrapping tape
Permanent marker or felt-tip pen (Figure 10-36A)

PROCEDURE STEPS:

1. Prepare a clean, dry, flat surface of adequate size to lay the wrapping material. RATIONALE: A clean area reduces risk for contamination. Adequate space is required for proper wrapping.
2. Select two wraps of adequate size in which to wrap instruments.
3. Place one square of wrapping material at an angle in front of you on the dry surface with one corner pointed directly toward you.
4. Place the sanitized instrument or articles to be placed in the autoclave just below the center of the wrap. Open instruments with hinges as wide as possible and place a 2 × 2 gauze or cotton ball in the opening (Figure 10-36B). RATIONALE: Instruments with hinged parts that are not spread open before autoclaving may not be properly sterilized.
5. Place one sterilization indicator with the instrument. RATIONALE: Sterilization indicators inside packages ascertain sterilization of each individual package. Indicators change colors when the required temperature has been reached, documenting the effectiveness of the sterilization. NOTE: Quality control for autoclave operation can be evaluated with sterilization indicators.
6. Bring the corner of the wrap closest to you up and over the article toward the center. Bring the tip of the same corner back toward you until it reaches the folded edge, creating a fan-fold effect. Smooth the edges of the fold. The article should remain completely covered (Figure 10-36C).
7. Fold one side edge toward the center line; fan-fold back to side, and crease (Figure 10-36D).
8. Repeat step 7 for the other side edge (Figure 10-36E).
9. Fold the package up from the bottom (Figure 10-36F).
10. Fold the top edge down and over the entire package (Figure 10-36G). RATIONALE: Final

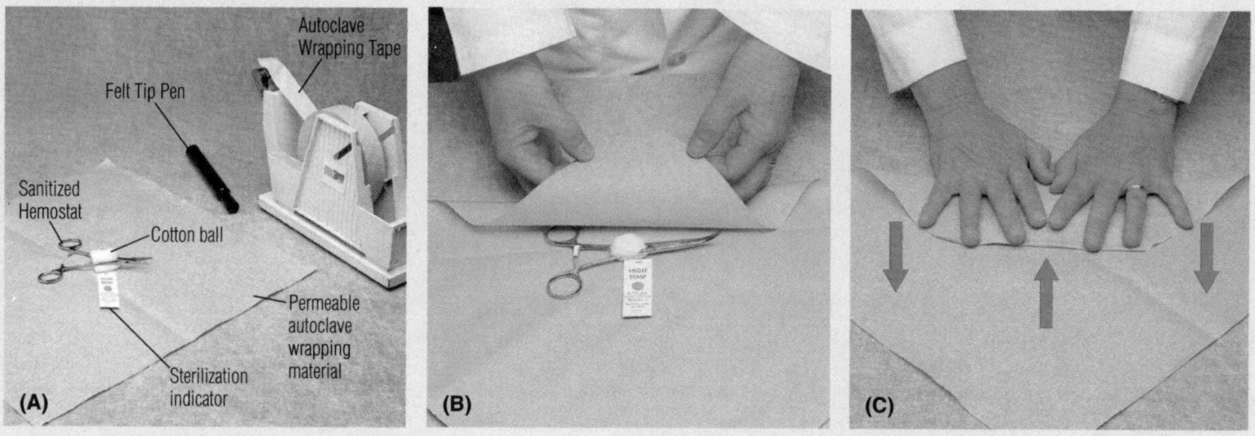

Figure 10-36 (A) Equipment needed to wrap surgical instruments or equipment for sterilization in an autoclave. (B) Place a cotton ball between the hinge joints of instruments to keep them open. Do not ratchet instruments closed. Pad the tips of sharp instruments. Put a sterilization indicator in with the instruments to be wrapped. (C) The wrapping paper is folded toward center. A small corner is turned back on itself.

(continues)

Procedure 10-6 (continued)

edge should wrap entire package for assurance of adequate coverage and protection once contents are sterilized. If wrap does not cover adequately, unwrap and start over with larger wrapping material.

11. To "wrap twice," place this package into the center of a second wrap (Figure 10-36H). Repeat Steps 7 through 10. RATIONALE: Double wrapping allows more control of multiple instruments when setting up a surgical tray.
12. Tape with autoclave tape across the point left exposed. RATIONALE: Autoclave tape indicates whether the package has been through the autoclave; it is not a form of sterilization indicator or quality control.
13. Label the tape with the name of the instrument or type of pack (i.e., laceration repair pack), date of sterilization, and your initials (Figure 10-36I). RATIONALE: Proper instrument labeling is required to identify wrapped sterilized instruments. Instruments wrapped and sterilized in paper or cloth wrappers are considered sterile for four weeks from the date of sterilization. Initialing packages ensures accountability and responsibility.
14. Place wrapped instruments in autoclave. RATIONALE: If wrapped instruments are not to be immediately autoclaved, do NOT date the package. Leave the package on a clean, dry surface and date the package just before autoclaving.

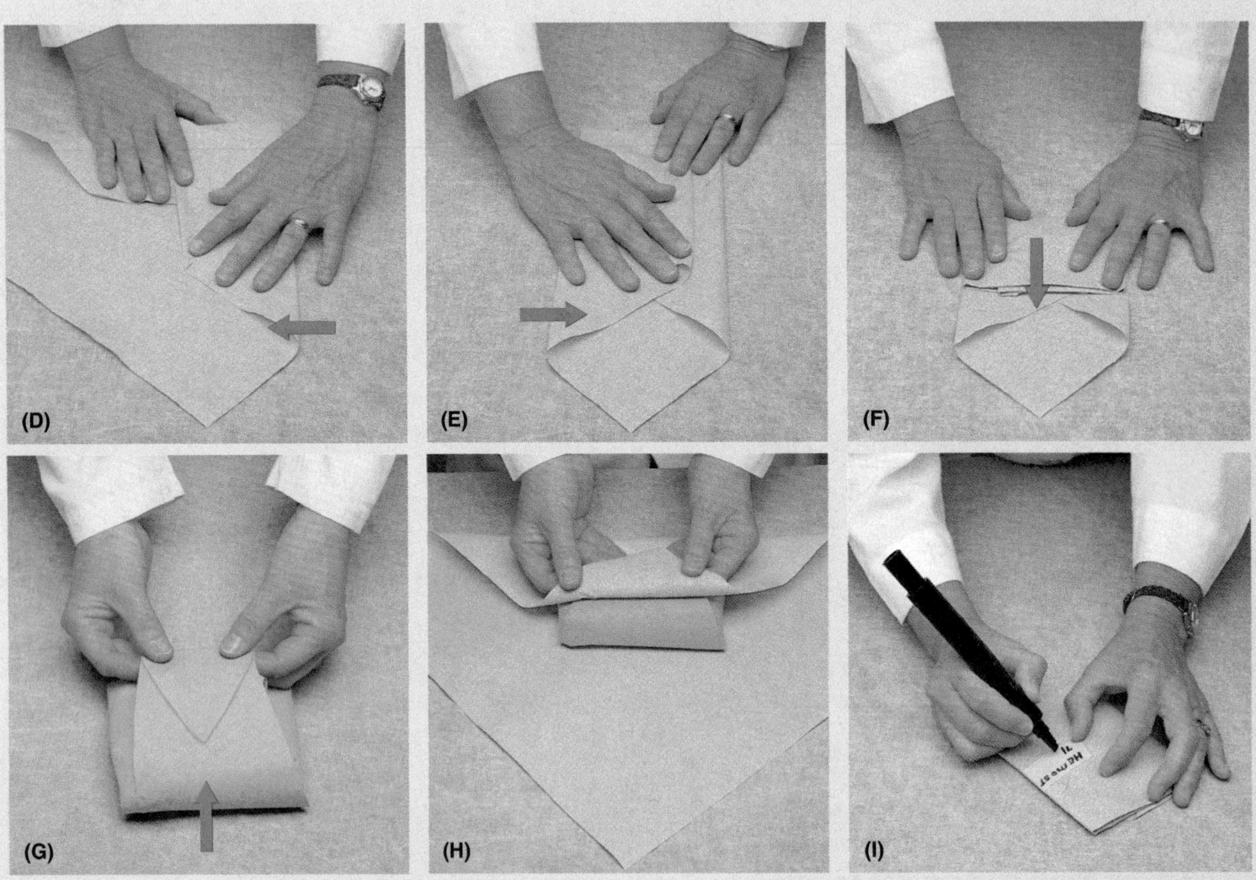

Figure 10-36 *(continued)* (D) Fold one side toward center leaving small corner turned back on itself. (E) Fold other side toward center leaving small corner turned back on itself. (F) The package is folded up from the bottom and secured. (G) Fold corner back on itself. (H) Wrap first package in another wrap. Double wrapping allows more control of multiple instruments when setting up a surgical tray. (I) Wrapped package is secured with heat-sensitive autoclave tape and labeled with the date, contents, and medical assistant's initials.

Procedure 10-7 Sterilization of Instruments (Autoclave)

PURPOSE:

To rid items of all forms of microbial (microorganisms) life for use in invasive procedures.

EQUIPMENT/SUPPLIES:

Steam sterilizer (autoclave)
Autoclave manufacturer instructions
Wrapped sanitized instrument package(s) with sterilization indicators placed inside package (or unwrapped item if removed with sterile transfer forceps)

PROCEDURE STEPS:

1. Check water level in the autoclave reservoir and add distilled water to fill line if necessary. RATIONALE: Not enough or too much water will impair the efficiency of the autoclave. Distilled water will not leave deposits (tap water leaves deposits) inside the autoclave. Deposits can impair the efficiency of the autoclave.
2. Depending on your autoclave, turn the knob to "fill" line and allow water into the chamber until it reaches the "fill" line. Turn the knob to the next position. This stops water from continuing to enter the chamber.
3. Load packages into autoclave tray; allow room for steam to circulate (Figure 10-37). RATIONALE: Steam circulates in predictable patterns in an autoclave. When packages are loaded too closely or improperly, proper sterilization will not occur in individual packages.
   a. Load jars of dressings or cups on their sides, with tops ajar or loosely in place. RATIONALE: Steam is trapped within a jar when it is right side up; containers and goods will not be sterilized if loaded sitting up vertically.
   b. Load unwrapped instruments flat with handles opened, exposing all surfaces. RATIONALE: Steam must reach all surfaces.

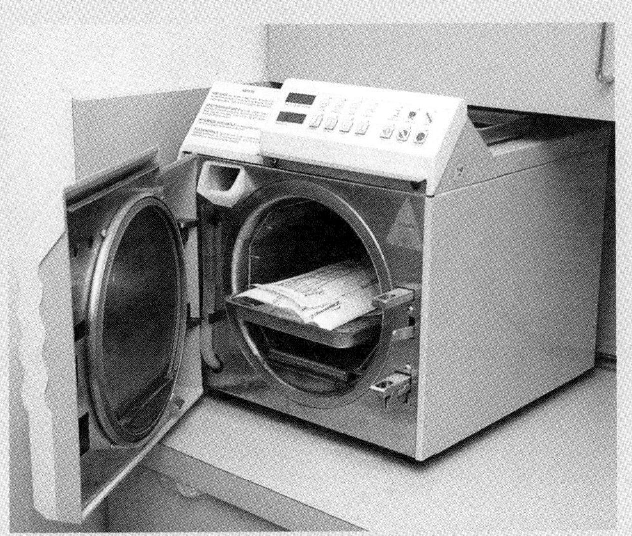

Figure 10-37 Load packages into the autoclave so steam is able to reach all surfaces, allowing for proper sterilization.

4. Close autoclave door and seal. RATIONALE: Pressure cannot be achieved without a proper seal.
5. Turn on autoclave. When the temperature dial indicates 250–254°F (121°C) and 15 pounds of pressure has been achieved inside the autoclave, begin necessary exposure time by setting timer. RATIONALE: Proper heat, pressure levels, and exposure time must be achieved to kill all microorganisms within the autoclave. Careful note should be given to setting exposure time only after the proper temperature and pressure settings have been achieved.

Item	Required exposure time
Wrapped instrument packages or trays	30 minutes
Unwrapped items	15 minutes
Unwrapped items covered with cloth	20 minutes

6. After completion of the autoclave cycle, vent exhaust steam pressure from the autoclave by following the manufacturer's instructions. RATIONALE: Following the manufacturer's instructions carefully will assure safe and proper use of the autoclave.
7. Open the door approximately 1 inch after the pressure gauge indicates zero (0) pressure and the temperature gauge indicates a decrease to at least 212°F. RATIONALE: You will not be able to open the door until the pressure is zero. Be

(continues)

Procedure 10-7 (continued)

aware that steam burns can occur when opening the door. Use caution.

8. Allow the contents to completely dry, approximately 30 to 45 minutes; do NOT touch contents until completely dry. RATIONALE: If packages are still wet or damp, microorganisms can enter a wrapped package, rendering it contaminated. Liquids travel along paper or cloth by capillary action and will be contaminated by microorganisms on countertops or from hands.
9. Remove wrapped contents with dry, clean hands and store in clean, dry closed cupboard or drawer. RATIONALE: Sterilized wrapped packages can be held with clean hands, because only the interior contents require maintenance of sterility. If the outer wrapper is required to remain sterile, remove with sterile transfer forceps and place on a sterile field or in sterile storage areas.
10. Remove unwrapped contents with sterile transfer forceps; resanitize and resterilize the transfer forceps following use. RATIONALE: Sterile transfer forceps must have been sterilized immediately prior to or along with the unwrapped item if they are to be used immediately in a sterile procedure. Place onto sterile surface.
11. Perform quality control on a regular basis, based on usage. RATIONALE: Quality control and maintenance of an autoclave is critical to assurance of proper operation. Accountability and responsibility to monitor quality control should be the responsibility of the medical assistant(s) most often responsible for sterilization.
    a. Monitor sterilization indicators with each use of sterilized instruments.
    b. Weekly perform quality control by documenting sterilization indicator outcome on a log; date and initialize quality-control log entries.
12. Clean and service the autoclave regularly according to the manufacturer's guidelines. When sterilization is not being achieved, take equipment out of service and contact a service agency for repair. RATIONALE: It is the responsibility of the medical assistant to take out of service any equipment that is not operating properly as a component of risk management.
13. Keep a log of cleaning, services, and quality-control measures performed.

Case Study 10-1

Your physician employer asks you to help develop an exposure control plan. Include the measures the employer must take to eliminate or lessen an employee's risk for exposure to blood or other potentially infectious materials. How often will the plan be reviewed?

Case Study 10-2

Considering the growth requirements for pathogens, describe how to discourage bacterial growth in the clinical area of the ambulatory care setting.

SUMMARY

Effective infection control measures are the first defense against the transmission of infectious diseases in the ambulatory care setting. Reliance on Standard and Transmission-Based Precautions, protective barriers, and basic principles of disinfection and sterilization promotes professional and responsible clinical care for patients. When the processes of infection control are applied to all clinical procedures, the chain of infection may be broken by many varied means. Remember that an infectious disease will not spread to another person if the chain is sufficiently broken at any stage.

Infectious diseases spread and accidents occur through lack of education and carelessness. Medical assistants must understand the importance of the regulations and guidelines set forth by the federal government and follow through by helping employers and fellow employees implement them. In doing so, the health and safety of patients and health care workers can be protected, the spread of infectious diseases can be kept under control, and the risk for contracting a serious infectious disease such as HIV, HBV, or HCV will be greatly minimized.

Every medical office and ambulatory care setting must, by law, have clearly written and readily available manuals containing information about Standard Precautions and OSHA for the safe handling, storage, and disposal of blood, body fluids, and chemicals.

Through consistent use of Standard Precautions and adherence to OSHA laws, health care providers can acquire the behaviors and techniques needed to safeguard themselves and their patients.

Because of frequent changes in the laws, it is necessary for medical assistants and all other health care providers to keep abreast of the government mandates.

STUDY FOR SUCCESS

To reinforce your knowledge and skills of information presented in this chapter:

- ❑ Review the Key Terms
- ❑ Practice any Procedures
- ❑ Consider the Case Studies and discuss your conclusions
- ❑ Answer the Review Questions
  - ❑ Multiple Choice
  - ❑ Critical Thinking
- ❑ Navigate the Internet and complete the Web Activities
- ❑ Practice the StudyWARE activities on the textbook CD
- ❑ Apply your knowledge in the Student Workbook activities
- ❑ Complete the Web Tutor sections
- ❑ View and discuss the DVD situations

REVIEW QUESTIONS

Multiple Choice

1. Standard Precautions are issued by:
   a. Health and Human Services
   b. Centers for Disease Control and Prevention
   c. Food & Drug Administration
   d. Occupational Safety and Health Administration
2. *The Bloodborne Pathogen Standard* is primarily concerned with:
   a. reducing the transmission of HIV, HBV, and HCV infections
   b. protecting the employer from lawsuits
   c. regulating the use of personal protective equipment
   d. taking blood samples from patients
3. In the chain of infection, the location of the infectious agent is known as the:
   a. reservoir
   b. portal of exit
   c. portal of entry
   d. means of transmission

4. The stage in infectious disease in which symptoms are vague and undifferentiated is called the:
   a. incubation stage
   b. prodromal stage
   c. acute stage
   d. onset of disease stage
5. An autoclave is an instrument used during:
   a. chemical sterilization
   b. steam sterilization
   c. dry heat sterilization
   d. gas sterilization

Critical Thinking

1. Analyze the importance of infection control and give five examples of how a medical assistant would practice responsible infection control in the ambulatory care setting.
2. Your patient has a draining wound. After you change the dressing, explain how to prevent the transmission of the microorganisms from the wound and dressing to you or another patient.
3. Give an example of how the proper disposal of contaminated objects can break a link in the chain of infection.
4. You notice a coworker sanitizing surgical instruments in preparation for sterilization. He or she did not scrub the serrations on the instruments well. What will be the result of his or her improper sanitization technique? Explain your answer.
5. You notice a tear in the wrapping of a sterilized pack. What actions do you take and why?
6. Describe eight procedures/techniques that you could be performing on a patient that could expose you to bloodborne pathogens.
7. What becomes of the biohazard containers once they are full?
8. What alternative do you have if you do not have access to soap and water after performing a procedure on a patient?
9. Explain the differences among sanitization, disinfection, and sterilization.

WEB ACTIVITIES

1. The U.S. Department of Labor Occupational Safety and Health Administration (OSHA) Web site (http://www.osha.gov) provides you with significant amounts of information about OSHA—the federal agency that seeks to protect health care workers from bloodborne pathogens. Visit the site to determine when the most recent changes have been made to *The Bloodborne Pathogen Standard*. What are they?
2. The HIV and Hepatitis.com Web site (http://hivandhepatitis.com/hep_b.html) gives information about simultaneous infections of HIV, HBV, and HBC. What are the statistics for persons who are infected with HIV and HBV, or HIV and HBC?
3. The Center for Disease Control and Prevention National Center for Infectious Diseases Web site (http://www.cdc.gov) provides a tremendous amount of information regarding infectious diseases and hepatitis in particular. Information also is available about HIV and AIDS. Are there other hepatitis viruses in addition to A, B, and C? Look on this site for the treatment of choice for all hepatitis viruses you find, and describe what the most common side effects are of treatment.
4. Health information from WebMD Healthwise, Inc. P.O. Box 1989, Boise, ID 83701 (http://www.medscape.com) provides information on current recommendations for adult immunization in the United States. Check this site and determine if you, your adult relatives, and adult friends are current and up to date with the recommendations.
5. The Medical College of Wisconsin Web site (http://www.intmed.mcw.edu/drug/InfectionRx.html) provides an antibiotic guide and treatment recommendations for common infections. Visit this site to discover the likely antibiotic treatment for (1) pneumonia (community acquired), (2) pharyngitis (exudative), and (3) gonorrhea.

THE DVD HOOK-UP

DVD Series
Skills Based Series

Program Number
4

Chapter/Scene Reference
- *Watch entire program*

In this chapter, you learned about proper infection control guidelines.

During one of the scenes, Mr. Breech became very ill and vomited. The vomit sprayed on the medical assisting extern and on and around the sink area. The extern turned around and quietly told the medical assistant that there was blood in the vomit.

1. Do you think that the extern should have said something in front of the patient about the blood in the vomit? What might have been a more tactful way of letting the medical assistant know about the blood in the vomit?
2. During the aseptic hand cleansing scene, the extern did not clean under her nails because it was not the first hand wash of the day. Do you think that the medical assistant should have instituted a nail cleansing anyway, because of the particular circumstances? Why?

DVD Journal Summary

Write a paragraph that summarizes what you learned from watching today's DVD program. In one of the scenes, Sandy accidentally stuck herself on a used needle. She was quite frightened when she spoke with her supervisor. She wrestled with the idea of starting prophylactic treatment. Do you think that Sandy was overreacting? What do you think you would do if you accidentally stuck yourself with a contaminated needle? Would you start prophylactic treatment right away?

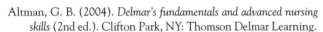

REFERENCES/BIBLIOGRAPHY

Altman, G. B. (2004). *Delmar's fundamentals and advanced nursing skills* (2nd ed.). Clifton Park, NY: Thomson Delmar Learning.

Delaune, S. C., & Ladner, P. K. (2002). *Fundamentals of nursing standards and practice* (2nd ed.). Clifton Park, NY: Thomson Delmar Learning.

Josephson, D. L. (2004). *Intravenous infusion therapy for nurses principles and practices* (2nd ed.). Clifton Park, NY: Thomson Delmar Learning.

Occupational Safety and Health Administration Bloodborne Pathogens-1910.1030 (Regulations [Standards-29CFR]). Retrieved from http://osha.gov. Accessed January 19, 2005.

Taber's cyclopedic medical dictionary (21st ed.). (2002). Philadelphia: FA Davis.

U.S. Department of Health and Human Services, Centers for Disease Control and Prevention. (2001). (Federal Register). Washington DC: U.S. Government Printing Office. Retrieved from http://cdc.gov/ncidod/hip/isolat/isoapp_a.html. Accessed January 19, 2005.

CHAPTER 11

Taking a Medical History, the Patient's Chart, and Methods of Documentation

KEY TERMS

Allergy
Chief Complaint
Clinical Diagnosis
Objective
Problem-Oriented Medical Record (POMR)
SOAP
Source-Oriented Medical Record (SOMR)
Subjective

OUTLINE

Preparing for the Patient
The Function of the Medical History
The Cross-Cultural Model
Patient Information Forms
- Administrative or Demographic Data Forms
- Medical Forms

Computerized Health History
The First Office Contact
- Telephone Contact
- Personal Visit
- Emergency Visit

Completing the Medical History Forms
- Interacting with the Patient
- Displaying Cultural Awareness
- Being Sensitive to Patient Needs
- Dealing with Sensitive Topics

Communication across the Life Span
The Medical Health History
- Chief Complaint
- Present Illness
- Medical History
- Adult Immunizations
- Family History
- Social History
- Review of Systems

The Patient's Record and Its Importance
- HIPAA Compliance
- Contents of Medical Records
- Continuity of Care Record
- Rules of Charting

Methods of Charting/Documentation
- Source-Oriented Medical Records
- Problem-Oriented Medical Records
- Computer-Modified Records
- SOAP Method of Charting
- Abbreviations Used in Charting
- Correcting an Error
- Chart Organization

FEATURED COMPETENCIES

CAAHEP—ENTRY-LEVEL COMPETENCIES

Patient Care

- Obtain and record patient history

General Competencies

- Recognize and respond to verbal communication

Legal Concepts

- Document appropriately

ABHES—ENTRY-LEVEL COMPETENCIES

Professionalism

- Maintain confidentiality at all times
- Evidence a responsible attitude
- Be courteous and diplomatic

Communication

- Be impartial and show empathy when dealing with patients
- Adapt what is said to the recipient's level of comprehension

Clinical Duties

- Interview and record patient history

Legal Concepts

- Determine needs for documentation and reporting
- Document accurately

OBJECTIVES

The student should strive to meet the following performance objectives and demonstrate an understanding of the facts and principles presented in this chapter through written and oral communication.

1. Define the key terms as presented in the glossary.
2. Understand the necessity and function of the medical history in patient treatment.
3. Define the parts of the medical history.
4. Identify and use effective methods of interacting with a patient.
5. Obtain a medical history from the patient.
6. Explain the different methods of charting/documentation.
7. Define the meaning and function of SOAP and problem-oriented medical records.
8. Explain some issues of cultural sensitivity in taking a medical history.
9. Describe the contents of a medical record.
10. State five reasons why the medical record is important.
11. Identify three areas of concern regarding HIPAA compliance and the patient's chart.
12. Discuss the continuity of care record.
13. Document accurately.

SCENARIO

When clinical medical assistant Audrey Jones, CMA, of Drs. Lewis and King takes a patient history, she typically uses a form custom designed for the office. Audrey uses the form as a guideline to be sure she gathers all pertinent information. However, she has learned that she must tailor her questions to the patient and sometimes will rearrange the order of the questions if necessary. Although Audrey is adept at gathering specific and necessary patient information, she also is aware of patient concerns and sensitivities and adapts her approach to accomplish the task while making the patient feel at ease.

INTRODUCTION

To treat a patient effectively, the physician must know the patient's medical history. If the patient is already established in the ambulatory care setting, the physician can work from the existing chart (record) with additional information obtained at the time of the office or clinic visit.

For a new patient, however, or for an established patient who has not been in for some time, an updated medical history form is of vital importance. Information contained in this history includes past medical problems, current medications and medication allergies, as well as other factors contributing to the patient's health.

Often, the family practice clinic will have a broad questionnaire for patients to complete, or the physician may tailor the medical history form to a particular specialty. These questionnaires, whether practice specific or general forms, can be created on the computer by the administrative medical assistant, if desired. A specialist physician will often mail the form to the patient before the appointment so that the patient can answer the questions in a quiet environment and have access to some of the information requested, such as names and addresses of other physicians that they have seen. When the office calls new patients the day before the appointment, they can be reminded to bring the completed questionnaire with them.

The role of the medical assistant in taking the patient history is to be as thorough as possible while being as sensitive as possible. Respect for the patient's privacy must be balanced with the need for the kind of complete information that results in informed medical treatment and care.

The patient chart or medical record is a legal document that is a collection of confidential patient information. Should a patient's medical record be introduced in court, it becomes a legal record of care given. It is important that charting in the record be accurate, clear, concise, and complete.

Spotlight on Certification

RMA Content Outline
- Oral and written communications
- Charts
- Problem oriented records

CMA Content Outline
- Recognizing and responding to verbal and nonverbal communication
- Professional communication and behavior
- Evaluating and understanding communication
- Interviewing techniques
- Medical records
- Documentation/reporting
- Performing telephone and in-person screening
- Patient history interview

CMAS Exam Outline
- Basic Health History Interview
- Basic Charting

PREPARING FOR THE PATIENT

Before the patient's visit and obtaining the medical history, make preparations while keeping the patient's comfort in mind. For example,

1. Make certain the examination room is clean, tidy, and in readiness for the patient.
2. Check to see that all necessary supplies are available.
3. Review the patient's chart before bringing the patient into the examination room. Note the age, any possible need for assistance, and identified reason for appointment.

When everything is ready, go to the reception area for the patient. It is preferable to call the patient by title and last name (Mr. Nichols) unless the patient previously requested the use of the first name. Speak clearly and plainly, making certain that your patient will be able to hear. When the patient stands, quickly determine if assistance is necessary. (The physical assessment has begun.) If assistance is warranted, make that offer and accompany the patient to the examination room, remembering later to note in the chart the kind of assistance provided. A friendly greeting is appreciated and helpful; a greeting such as, "How are you today?" may not be appropriate. If patients are in the physician's office, they generally are not feeling well and take that question seriously. Also, the reception area is not the most appropriate place for the patient to begin sharing his or her medical issues. The following comments may be acceptable: "Did you have any trouble finding parking?" or "I really like the colors in the shirt you are wearing. They remind me of summer."

Once in the examination room, seat the patient comfortably and sit face-to-face with the patient to begin the interview. The room should have good light, and the door should be closed for privacy. Build rapport with the patient. Use the patient's name often and make certain you pronounce it correctly. Finally, think globally. Ask about factors in the patient's life that might influence health. These topics might be sports, travel, pets, family, and hobbies. Not only does this provide vital information for the health history, it usually eases and relaxes the patient for the more difficult questions in the interview.

THE FUNCTION OF THE MEDICAL HISTORY

The medical history is the basis for all treatment rendered by the physician, any on-call physician, and any specialist consulted to treat the patient. During the history-taking process, the physician often will discover information that helps guide treatment for the patient. The medical history in the chart, or record, makes it easier for the physician to recall previous treatment. Notes and laboratory results in the chart quickly show the progress of the treatment.

In addition, the charts give a base for statistical analysis: for the physician's own research, for insurance records, and for the health department, especially for infectious diseases. The health history and chart notes also become a legal record of the treatment rendered to the patient. This is especially important if the patient is making an injury claim against another party or if the patient makes a malpractice claim against the physician. If the records in the chart are precise and correct, the chart becomes a good defense; however, if the charting or documentation is sloppy or incomplete, the entire record may be questioned as an insufficient or incorrect record of treatment. The best procedure is to document everything concerning a patient including all treatment rendered, telephone calls, missed appointments, and discussions with other specialists regarding the patient's treatment.

THE CROSS-CULTURAL MODEL

It is important for the medical assistant to understand that every patient interview is a cross-cultural one. Physicians and patients view the gathering of the patient history and the personal visit differently. Health and illness are inseparable from social and cultural beliefs. Who patients are—their background, their belief system, their family orientation, and their cultural heritage—influences their choices in health care. Physicians and patients have different concerns and anticipations, and the medical assistant conducting the interview who is aware of these perspectives will keep the following in mind:

- *Patient's chief concern:* The illness. The personal and social significance and the problems created by a perceived illness are important to the patient.
- *Physician's chief concern:* Disease. The physician is concerned with the malfunctioning and maladaptation of biological and psychological processes.

Critical Thinking

With another student in the classroom, discuss the chief concerns and treatment successes of both physicians and patients. Is it difficult to put yourself in the physician's place? Can you think of other questions that might help patients and physicians cross the cultural barrier?

- *Patient's idea of treatment success:* Being able to successfully manage an illness and its problems is often more important to the patient than the curing of the disease.
- *Physician's idea of treatment success:* Treatments, medications, and procedures that control disease problems and evaluating outcomes in these terms.

The medical assistant may find it helpful to ask certain questions of patients to help them move across cultures; for example:

1. What do you think caused your problem?
2. When do you think it started?
3. What affect does it have on you?
4. What do you fear from this problem?
5. What kind of treatment do you expect?

These questions involve and respect the patient's perception while providing helpful information to the physician.

PATIENT INFORMATION FORMS

There are two sets of information forms in the medical office.

Administrative or Demographic Data Forms

The first set of forms includes the patient demographic data form and the financial information form. The demographic data form (Figure 11-1) registers the patient's full name, address, mailing address if different, home and work telephone numbers, date of birth, Social Security number and all insurance information, person to be contacted in case of emergency, and a release of information signature. Some medical offices include a second form, the financial information form (Figure 11-2), to be signed regarding the financial policy of the practice including billing, insurance billing, co-payment billing, and any finance charges added

CODE | **PATIENT INFORMATION** | ACCOUNT

PLEASE PRINT

PATIENT Mr. Mrs. Miss/Ms. Last	First	MI	HOME PHONE: ( )	
Patient's Home Address	Street	City	State	Zip
Patient's Billing Address	Street	City	State	Zip
Social Security #	Date of Birth	Age	Sex	Driver's License #
Patient's Employer	Work Address		Work Phone:	
Spouse's Name	Spouse's Employer (Name & Address)		Work Phone:	
Emergency Contact: (Local Relative or Friend) Name	Address		Phone:	

REFERRED TO THIS OFFICE BY: ______

WHO IS YOUR PRIMARY PHYSICIAN? ______

INSURANCE PLEASE LIST ALL HEALTH CARE INSURANCE COMPANIES WHICH COVER THIS PATIENT:

PRIMARY: Name ______ Policy # ______ Subscriber ______

Insurance Address ______

SECONDARY: Name ______ Policy# ______ Subscriber ______

Insurance Address ______

MEDICARE # ______ (Please Include Letter)

MEDICAID # ______
(MEDI-CAL)

RESPONSIBLE PARTY Mr. Mrs. Miss/Ms. Last	First	Middle
Address		Phone
Occupation	Employers Name & Address	Bus. Phone:

Please remember that insurance is considered a method of reimbursing the patient for fees paid to the doctor and is not a substitute for payment. Some companies pay fixed allowances for certain procedures, and others pay a percentage of the charge. It is your responsibility to pay any deductible amount, co-insurance, or any other balance not paid for by your insurance.

METHOD OF PAYMENT: CASH ______ CHECK ______ CREDIT CARD ______

PLEASE READ & SIGN THE FOLLOWING:
I directly assign all medical / surgical benefits to ______
and understand that I am financially responsible for all charges whether or not paid by insurance. I hereby authorize the doctor to release all information necessary to secure the payment of benefits. I further agree that a photocopy of this agreement shall be as valid as the original.

SIGN HERE ______ DATE: ______

FORM # 58-8421-01 • BIBBERO SYSTEMS, INC. • PETALUMA, CALIFORNIA © 10/85 (REV. 8/93) TO REORDER CALL TOLL FREE: 800-BIBBERO (800 242-2376) OR FAX: (800) 242-9330

Figure 11-1 Sample patient information form. (Courtesy of Bibbero Systems, Inc., Petaluma, CA (800) 242-2376; www.bibbero.com.)

FINANCIAL POLICY

In order to reduce confusion and misunderstanding between our patients and the clinic, we have adopted the following financial policy. If you have any questions about this policy, please discuss them with our Billing Manager. We are dedicated to providing the best possible care and service to you and we regard your complete understanding of your financial responsibilities as an essential element of your care and treatment.

Unless other arrangements have been made in advance by yourself or your health coverage carrier, payment is due at time of service. For your convenience, we accept Visa, MasterCard, or we can arrange a payment schedule.

YOUR INSURANCE:

We accept assignment of benefit from Medicare. We also have direct billing agreements with many insurance companies. We will bill those plans for whom we have an agreement and will only require that you pay the copayment at the time of service.

If your medical plan determines a service is "not covered," you will be responsible for the entire charge. Payment is due upon receipt of statement from this office.

MINOR PATIENTS:

The adult accompanying the patient and the parent or guardian with custody will be billed for all services rendered to minor patients.

MISSED APPOINTMENTS:

In order to provide the best service and availability to our patients, we ask you to notify us 24 hours in advance if you know that you will be unable to keep the appointment. We reserve the right to charge for missed appointments.

I have read the financial policy and I understand it and agree to be bound by its terms.

______________________ Date ______________

Figure 11-2 Sample financial information form.

to monthly billings. The information from these forms provides the foundation for the patient's database.

Medical Forms

The second set of forms is the medical health history form, which can be as short as one page ($8^1/_2'' \times 11''$) or as long and detailed as six to eight pages. This form includes information on:

1. Present health history, including why the patient is being seen
2. Health history, personal and family
3. Social history including marital status, sexual orientation, and occupation
4. Body systems review/questionnaire
5. Medications currently being taken; includes over-the-counter and prescription medications
6. Physician's review of systems (ROS) (completed by the physician)

The best form is neither too long nor too complicated. Patients may feel overwhelmed with a long form and may not finish it or will give up, stating they cannot remember all the information. The form that is simple and brief can provide the most information. Some patients find a history form too intimidating. It is often easier for these patients to talk directly with the medical assistant or the physician about social history, feeling a one-to-one exchange is more personal and private.

A sample of a history form is included in Figure 11-3. This form asks the reason for the visit (chief complaint); symptoms the patient may be experiencing; medical history including allergies to medications, past medical problems and surgeries; current medications; family history; and social history. Depending on the ambulatory care setting, this form can be tailored to include vaccines and immunizations, usage of recreational drugs, exercise and diet regimens, accident information (especially if patient was hurt on the job), and any other information suited to the physician's specialty.

COMPUTERIZED HEALTH HISTORY

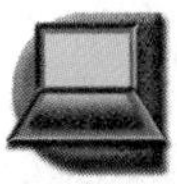

Some health care facilities use computerized health histories. These can be of two types: patient-generated and health care provider-generated. In patient-generated health histories, the patient responds on the computer to various questions, and then reviews information with the medical assistant for completeness. When using a health care provider-generated health history, the medical assistant completes the information on the screen during or after the patient interview. The medical assistant should remember to interact with the patient by looking up from the computer from time to time during the entry of information. It is easy to forget to look at patients as you ask them questions and enter the information. This habit can make the patient feel disconnected to the process. Frequently, these programs are user-friendly and save time for both the patient and medical assistant. Some patients may not want to use a computer, however, and should be given the option of answering questions face to face.

Andrus/Clini-Rec®
General Health History Questionnaire & Physical Examination Male or Female

CONFIDENTIAL

INSTRUCTIONS TO MY PATIENT

One of the most important parts of the medical record your doctor keeps for you is a health history concerning your past and present health problems, and any personal information which might affect the state of your health.

Your answers will be treated confidentially as are all parts of your visit. Please return this questionnaire to your doctor or to the doctor's nurse or assistant after you complete it.

Take all the time you need to complete this questionnaire. Answer each question as best you can by filling in the information asked for or by putting an "X" in the appropriate space. Choose the answer to each question which in your mind comes closest to applying to you.

If there is any question you have difficulty answering, just circle the question. You can discuss it with the doctor when you return the questionnaire.

If you have completed this questionnaire at home, be sure to bring it with you so that you and the doctor can go over your answers during your appointment within a confidential setting.

If this is a RE-EXAMINATION and you have previously filled out one of these "Patient Administered Comprehensive Health History Questionnaires", fill in PART A - Present Health History, sections I & II. *You do not* have to redo sections III & IV, or PART B - Past History.

Any changes which have occurred since you last filled out the questionnaire should be noted.

BIBBERO SYSTEMS, INC.

Created and Developed by "Medical Economics" Professional Systems

BIBBERO SYSTEMS, INC.
1300 N. McDOWELL BLVD.
PETALUMA, CA 94954

STOCK NO. 19-742-4 8/95

Figure 11-3 General health history questionnaire and physical examination, male or female. (Courtesy of Bibbero Systems, Inc., Petaluma, CA (800) 242-2376; www.bibbero.com.)

THE FIRST OFFICE CONTACT

Telephone Contact

The first contact with a medical assistant in the ambulatory care setting is usually a telephone call. The patient or a relative of the patient calls to get information about the physician and the practice. When this occurs, primary administrative information is obtained including the patient's full name, telephone number, medical problem, insurance company, and sometimes the address as well. At the same time, the patients learn about the practice's hours, location, financial policies, and answers to other questions they might have. The base of the patient information form has been obtained and can be completed on the patient's arrival at the office. The patient demographic information form and the financial information form are most likely completed and signed at the first visit, before the interview for the patient history. Occasionally, these forms may be mailed to the patient to be completed before the office visit.

Personal Visit

At times a patient may be referred to your office by another physician. When this happens, the patient may come to your office in person to bring records, X-ray films, or a referral and to make an appointment. If the patient is a member of a health maintenance organization, a referral from the primary care physician is usually mandatory. When the patient has a referral, the information forms are given to the patient to fill out in the office or to take home to complete in a quiet, undisturbed environment where the patient has access to records of past medical care.

Emergency Visit

When an acutely ill patient is referred by another physician to be seen immediately, or if your office or urgent care center accepts new patient emergency visits, the medical assistant has little advanced notice. To facilitate the history-taking process, the medical assistant may take the patient directly to an examination room where the atmosphere is quiet and private. This helps put the patient at ease, which helps in completing the forms. Depending on the nature of the emergency, the medical assistant can help by asking the questions on the forms and writing down the patient's responses.

COMPLETING THE MEDICAL HISTORY FORMS

Interacting with the Patient

When the medical assistant is taking the medical history, the first responsibility is to put the patient at ease. A comfort level must be developed between medical assistant and patient. The medical assistant must guide the conversation, keeping it on track to obtain the most information for the physician. Allowing conversation to wander, talking about other people, or letting the patient tell anecdotes does not help to complete the history. Explaining a term or concept that the patient does not understand is helpful to the patient. The medical assistant must remain professional and not be embarrassed or made uncomfortable by the patient's answers, whether regarding illness, actions, or personal choices. Refer to Table 11-1.

If the patient is already an established patient but has not seen the physician for several months or longer, update the medical history by asking if any illnesses have occurred in the months elapsed, if any new allergies to any medications or other substances have occurred, and the reaction to each. The chief complaint for the current visit should always be documented. The chief complaint is the problem that brings the patient to the physician this particular visit. Sometimes when patients know they are going to be seen, they save several problems to discuss. Depending on the appointment schedule for the day, this may be difficult to accomplish. If there is time in the schedule, every effort should be made to accommodate

TABLE 11-1 GENERAL APPROACH TO THE HISTORY

1. Ensure an appropriate environment that is lit well, at a comfortable temperature, quiet, private, and free of distractions.
2. Sit facing the patient at eye level; the patient also should be seated. Ensure that the patient is as comfortable as possible, because obtaining the health history can be a lengthy process. Figure 11-4 illustrates an appropriate setting.
3. Avoid the use of medical jargon. Use terms the patient can understand.
4. Reserve asking intimate and personal questions until rapport is established.
5. Remain flexible in obtaining the health history. It does not need to be obtained in the exact order it is presented in this chapter or on the form.
6. Remind the patient that all information will be treated confidentially.
7. Ask the patient if he or she has any questions.

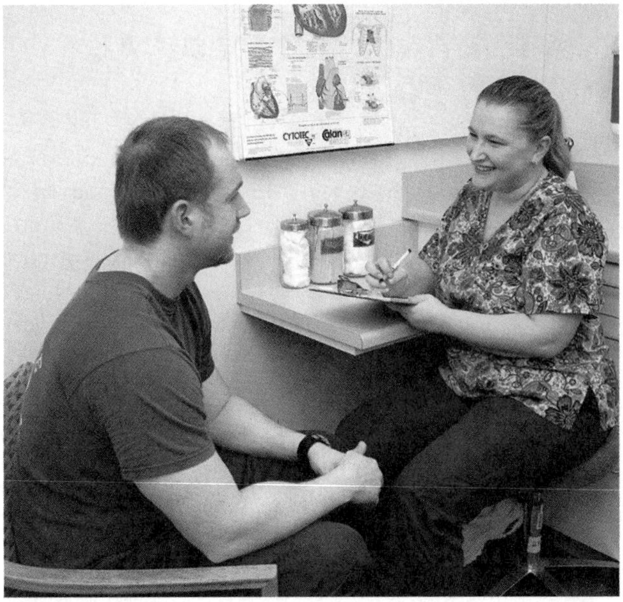

Figure 11-4 Show concern for the patient's well-being to put the patient at ease while the medical assistant takes the medical history.

Patient Education

In some cultures (e.g., Chinese, some Native Americans), it is disrespectful to speak of the dead. Thus, the patient may be reluctant to provide detailed information on the family health history of dead relatives. In these cases, you can ask the patient if there has been any history of specific diseases in the family and not focus on the specific individual if that person is deceased. The patient may be willing to share in which previous generation and which side of the family the condition existed. If these approaches are unsuccessful, explain to the patient the importance of this information, because it may provide clues to the patient's current health conditions.

the patient's needs. The medical assistant should always note the chief complaint before the physician sees the patient to assure the main problem is addressed.

Displaying Cultural Awareness

As the medical assistant begins the encounter with the patient, awareness of cultural differences and other problems that may inhibit communication is important. Any number of situations may arise that the medical assistant must be prepared to address. The medical assistant will overcome major obstacles if it is known that the patient does not speak English as a first language or needs an interpreter, if the patient is deaf and needs an interpreter, if the patient is from a culture in which the female patient does not disrobe for a male physician, or if the patient has a mental disorder making communication difficult.

If there is a language difficulty, the medical assistant may be required to arrange for an interpreter. There are language interpreters in most areas; especially in large urban areas, an interpreter might be found for nearly any language. If the patient is receiving medical care through Medicaid, special arrangements can be made for an interpreter through the state agency administering the program. Often the patient will bring a family member to interpret; however, if the matter is personal, the patient may not want to reveal personal matters with the family member present and may prefer an outside, objective interpreter. If the interpreter comes to the clinic as a contractor, a business associate contract should be completed to comply with Health Insurance Portability and Accountability Act (HIPAA) regulations. The contract is not necessary for a family member, a volunteer, or a clinic employee serving as an interpreter.

The medical assistant should be accessible and should listen to the patient. Sometimes the patient will be uneasy talking to the physician but may be more comfortable telling the medical assistant about the problem. Medical assistants can play an important part in the medical practice by listening and communicating both with the patient and with the physician.

Being Sensitive to Patient Needs

Some patients are frightened, hostile, or depressed. It is important to be open to nonverbal and verbal communication in answer to questions. Some patients react positively to a hand placed gently on the forearm; it calms and reassures them. Other patients have a negative response, pulling away from any such contact. Maintaining a professional boundary with the patient is essential. Boundaries respect the patient's needs for privacy, nurturing, validation, and separation. See Chapter 4 for additional information.

Patient Education

Some Asian cultures calculate age from conception, not from the actual birth date. For example, a newborn infant is considered to be 1 year old. The medical assistant needs to clarify the chronologic age with the patient or caregiver. This is particularly important for pediatric patients because of the link between age and developmental milestones.

Critical Thinking

With two others in your class, role-play a scenario where one person is the patient, another the medical assistant, and the third is an observer. A social history is being taken. Ask the patient about the use of any recreational drugs or chemicals. The patient responds, "Yes." What additional questions will you ask the patient? What will you include in the medical record?

The medical assistant needs to know when to touch the patient appropriately, always with permission either expressed or implied. (If the medical assistant tells the patient a blood pressure reading is next and reaches for the patient's arm and the patient extends an arm, permission to take the reading is implied. If, however, the patient pulls away and states no blood pressure is to be taken, permission is not given, and the reading must not be done at that time.) This is charted as "patient refused."

Trying to get information from a reluctant patient can be difficult and requires patience and understanding. If the patient is hesitant to discuss a problem with the medical assistant, it is better not to press for information. Pressing for information may make the patient become defensive or angry and can impair communication altogether.

A patient may come to the office upset and crying. This patient must be made to feel more in control, that no one is going to rush care being given. Sometimes just taking a few moments to sit with such patients until they feel more settled is enough to calm them and enable the history-taking interview to proceed.

Uncommunicative patients may require some special questioning techniques. The medical assistant may have to supply a sample of problems to get these patients to acknowledge the health concerns they have. Or they may shrug their shoulders at every question and be unresponsive. Some patients may simply say, "I don't know. I just don't feel well." If a relative has accompanied the patient to the appointment, it may be appropriate initially to have the relative present with the patient. In this way the patient has a familiar face in the unfamiliar, often frightening, physician's office. It is always the patient's decision if anyone else is to be in the room.

Some patients may have particular needs which they often will state to the medical assistant. Meeting these needs is usually a minor matter and makes patients feel more comfortable. For example, "Can you help me undress and get into the gown?"

Dealing with Sensitive Topics

Some of the most sensitive topics addressed in the health history include the use of alcohol, recreational drugs or chemicals, smoking, dietary habits, obesity, and sexual practices. An honest reporting on these topics, however, can be important to the patient's well-being and the physician's treatment. Some considerations in dealing with these sensitive topics include:

- Ask these questions in the later stages of the interview after rapport has been established.
- Use casual, direct eye contact without staring; this demonstrates the importance of the topic to the patient and your lack of embarrassment.

Patient Education

Some patients may seem reluctant to answer your questions regarding birthplace or Social Security number. Noncitizens may fear deportation if they are identified in the health care system, especially if they are seriously ill. Remind these patients that you are there solely to assist them with their health care needs and encourage them to provide accurate information to assist you in appropriate diagnosis and treatment, because many diseases are specific to geographic locations.

- Pose questions in a matter-of-fact tone.
- Adopt a nonjudgmental demeanor.
- Use the communication technique of "normalizing" when appropriate (e.g., "Some high school students drink alcohol/use drugs/engage in sexual relationships on a regular basis. Does this happen at your school? With you?").

If the medical assistant can enhance communication with the patient, communication between physician and patient will be more effective.

COMMUNICATION ACROSS THE LIFE SPAN

Keep in mind your patient's age when communicating and seeking information for the medical history. A parent or caregiver often accompanies a child. An infant will want to feel your physical support, your warmth, and a smile. As the child grows, time will be spent communicating with the child, as well as the parent. During this time, you may be dealing with two patients, discussing with the parent the problem the child has and assisting the parent in understanding procedures, treatment, and so on. There can come a time, also, when a child may do much better without a parent present. This can be a sensitive issue for parents. Sometimes a couple of simple statements might help; for example, "The physician will want to establish some rapport with your son for a few minutes. Please come with me while I get the literature that the physician wants you to have. Often these visits can be harder on parents than the children."

Teenagers are old enough to make the decision about being seen alone or with a parent present. Some are comfortable; others are not. Teenagers who have had the same primary care physician since early childhood and have already established a relationship are more likely to feel comfortable without parents. You may want to review a teenager's right to consent in Chapter 7.

Older adults may be accompanied by another adult and may request that individual be present during the interview. Others may prefer to be alone. Adults who have difficulty hearing, who are memory impaired, who are visually impaired, or whose language may not be understood are likely to be accompanied by another person. Keep in mind, however, that family members may not be the best person to be present. Some older adults find it difficult to answer questions in front of one of their children or even a spouse. Although it is not necessary for relatives, it is a good idea to have a HIPAA waiver signed by the patient, so long as they understand what is being signed. Remember that the intent of HIPAA is *not* to make communication more difficult or cumbersome; it is intended to protect a patient's privacy.

Chapter 15, which discusses pediatrics, and Chapter 17, which discusses gerontology have helpful suggestions for communications with children and older adults.

THE MEDICAL HEALTH HISTORY

The patient's medical health history will contain the following components:

- Personal data from the demographic or administrative form
- Chief complaint as noted at each visit by the medical assistant
- Present illness
  - Medications
  - Allergies
  - Other physicians or alternative therapy practitioners being seen
- Medical history
- Family history
- Social and occupational history
- Review of systems by physician

Chief Complaint

The **chief complaint** (usually abbreviated CC) is the specific reason that brought the patient to see the physician. It should be noted in as few words as possible but be very specific. It can be a direct quote from the patient.

A good example of a chief complaint notation might be: "I've had nausea and vomiting for three days." This is a **subjective** complaint in that it is known by the patient but cannot be seen or measured by the physician. It is specific, however, in relating the patient's condition. Another example is: "I hurt my ankle yesterday when I tripped over a curb." Again this is subjective but specific about cause, time of onset, and complaint. The ankle is visibly swollen and painful to touch. The swelling is an **objective** sign, a manifestation that can be seen, heard, or measured by any observer.

In contrast, a poor example of a chief complaint is "has not been feeling well." This notation tells the physician nothing about what symptoms or problems the patient has been experiencing. It gives no specific clue as to what the problem is from the patient's perspective. The medical assistant should try to pinpoint a complaint to a body system, to a time frame, to pain in a specific area. The patient usually will respond to questions that offer several options.

Certain characteristics of each chief complaint should be ascertained for a complete history. These characteristics are:

- Location
- Radiation
- Quality
- Severity
- Associated symptoms
- Aggravating factors
- Alleviating factors
- Setting and timing

Present Illness

The present illness is usually reflected in the chief complaint. The chief complaint is expanded on to give more information and detail. *Location* will describe the place where the symptom is located. Ask the patient to be as specific as possible. For instance, "I have pain on the inner thigh of my left leg" is more helpful than "my leg hurts." *Radiation* helps describe the symptom more by identifying how large an area the symptom covers. The patient might describe a "tingling sensation" all over my left leg, for instance. *Quality* addresses the characteristic of the symptom. The description might be "tingling and buzzing," or the pain described as "a dull ache" or "throbbing" or "stabbing." *Severity* of symptoms will include such descriptions as "keeps me awake at night," or "causes me to put little or no pressure on the leg." When the symptom is pain, patients may be asked to identify the pain on a scale of 1 to 10 with 10 being the most severe. *Associated symptoms* allows the patient to describe what other minor symptoms accompany the chief complaint. "Because I am limping and putting more weight on my right leg, my right hip aches much of the time." *Aggravating factors* and *alleviating factors* get at what makes the symptoms worse and what makes the symptoms decrease. "Walking fast or bending forward really hurts. Sitting down with my feet up on a stool makes it all feel better." You will also want to know what the patient has done to treat the problem and if any medications have been taken for the symptoms. The *setting* and *timing* have to do with when the symptoms started and what the patient was doing at symptom onset.

In the preceding example of nausea and vomiting, the patient may indicate inability to eat or take fluids. This would alert the physician to possible dehydration. Often the present illness is based on a prior health problem. For instance, a history of congestive heart failure gives a patient's symptoms of fluid retention, wheezing, and shortness of breath more importance because these are common complications. Without this knowledge of the patient's medical history, these symptoms could be confused with bronchitis, asthma, or pneumonia.

Some practitioners will want the medical assistant to address other topics in the present illness. Other practitioners will include these questions in the medical history. The topics include the following:

- Are there any other problems you are experiencing at this time? This question allows patients to indicate if there is something other than the chief complaint about which they have concerns.
- What medications are you taking? Even though the patient's chart will indicate some of this information, this is not the case for a new patient. Most patients do not include any over-the-counter medications or alternative therapies they may be using. Some facilities will ask the patients to bring every medication they are currently taking with them to the first visit. Be certain to ask about over-the-counter items such as vitamins, pain medications, herbal remedies, and so on.
- Are you allergic to anything? Again, the medical chart may note any allergies, but this question assists in alerting the staff to any potential problems, as well as updating the chart. It is a safety measure important to both the patient and the physician.

Medical History

The medical history includes all health problems, major illnesses, and surgeries that the patient has had. If not included under present illness, all current medications are noted, including dosages and reasons for taking them, as well as all allergies to any medications and the specific allergic reaction to each. These are important to the medical history, because many health problems can overlap and affect the patient in several areas. A patient with a long history of diabetes mellitus may present with an ulcer on his foot. Whereas the same ulcer in an otherwise healthy patient will heal with little intervention, the diabetic patient may require major treatment and attention including debridement (removal of dead or damaged tissue or foreign debris), antibiotics, and close monitoring.

Medications have side effects and contraindications that can affect patients. **Allergies** to medications can be serious and need to be noted in a readily visible part of the chart. Usually a red sticker is placed in a conspicuous area on the inside cover of the chart noting medication allergies. The information needs to be updated at least annually. Also document herbal, vitamin, and mineral supplements the patient is taking.

Adult Immunizations

If possible, update immunizations for adults at this time. Childhood immunizations are regularly checked in pediatric examinations. Not all adults recall their records, but some questions can help the physician determine if any immunizations are to be given. The Advisory Committee on Immunization Practices recommends the following immunization schedule for adults by age groups:

- *Tetanus and diphtheria* (Td) booster is given once every 10 years.
- *Influenza* vaccination is given to persons aged 19 to 49 years with medical or exposure indications and to all persons 50 years and older once yearly.
- *Pneumococcal polysaccharide* vaccination is given to persons aged 19 to 64 years with medical or exposure indications and to all persons 65 years and older.
- Three doses of *hepatitis B* vaccination during adulthood for persons with medical or exposure indications. Increasingly, physicians are giving hepatitis B and A vaccines to everyone.
- Two doses of *hepatitis A* vaccination to adults with medical or exposure indications.
- One dose of *measles, mumps, rubella (MMR)* if vaccination history is unreliable; two doses for persons with occupational or other indications.
- Two doses of *varicella vaccine* for persons who are susceptible.
- One dose of *meningococcal (polysaccharide)* vaccine for persons with medical or exposure indications.

AUTHORIZATION TO RELEASE HEALTH CARE INFORMATION

Patient ____________ Date of Birth ____________
SSN ____________ Previous Name ____________
I request and authorize ______________________ to release the health care information of the patient named above to:
Name ______________________
Address ______________________
This request and authorization applies to:
(Please initial the appropriate box)
__ Health care information relating to the following treatment, condition, or dates of treatment:
____
__ All health care information **EXCLUDING** specific information relating to sexually transmitted diseases (including HIV/AIDS), alcohol or drug use, or visits related to psychiatric disorders or mental health.
__ All health care information **INCLUDING** specific information relating to sexually transmitted diseases (including HIV/AIDS), alcohol or drug use, or visits related to psychiatric disorders or mental health.
__ Other: ______________________
I understand that my express consent is required to release any health care information relating to testing, diagnosis, and/or treatment of HIV (AIDS virus), sexually transmitted disease, psychiatric disorders/mental health, or drug and/or alcohol use. If I have been tested, diagnosed, or treated for HIV (AIDS virus), sexually transmitted disease, psychiatric disorders/mental health, or drug and/or alcohol use, you are specifically authorized to release all health care information relating to such diagnosis, testing, or treatment.

______________________ / ____________
Signature of patient or patient's authorized representative / Relationship to patient

____
Date

Figure 11-5 Sample Release of Information form.

To review these recommendations further and note contraindications, see the first Web Activity at the end of this chapter.

New patients may be asked to complete a Release of Information form (Figure 11-5) that is often created in the office. This form is sent to their former physicians to obtain past medical records and can be used to allow sharing of information with family members at the request of the patient.

If the patient has several physicians, the examining physician will encourage the patient to choose one physician to manage primary medical care so that all medical care and records are concentrated in one office. Under most managed care insurance policies, patients have one primary care physician (women may also have an obstetrician/gynecologist) who coordinates the patient's health care.

Family History

The family history can provide clues to the patient's present condition. By asking open-ended questions about medical problems of siblings, parents, and grandparents, the physician will be alerted to hereditary and familial diseases and disorders such as coronary artery disease, hypertension, breast cancer, and so forth. Present ages of siblings, parents, and grandparents, or cause of their death and age at time of death are noted. For instance, a family history of diabetes together with the patient's symptoms of frequent urination and thirst may make a diagnosis of diabetes mellitus a possibility.

Social History

The social history of patients includes their marital status, sexual habits, occupation, hobbies, and use of alcohol, tobacco, and recreational drugs or other chemical substances. This part of the history includes those lifestyles and behaviors that may put the patient at greater risk for injury or disease than would normally be found from factors in the family history and medical history. If the patient's usage of alcohol exceeds an average amount and a hobby the patient pursues is auto racing, the physician will counsel the patient about the danger of the combination of these two behaviors.

Be aware that patients may not want to answer questions pertaining to sexual history; attempt to return to these questions later. Ask the patient if a medical assistant of a different sex would make the patient more comfortable in discussing sexual practice.

For instance, the adolescent patient may refuse to answer questions of a sexual matter or provide false answers if the parent or caregiver is present. It may be best to ask the caregiver to leave the room at the completion of the health history so you can ask the patient if there is anything else to note in the sexual history.

Be alert for cues that demonstrate the patient's desire for knowledge on sexual matters, such as questions or requests for written information. Answer the patient's questions, provide educational materials, and refer the patient to a specialist when indicated.

It may be necessary to inquire about the patient's home environment. You need to be attentive for clues that signal the necessity of performing an in-depth home environment assessment. Some clues include, but are not limited to, poor hygiene, frequent infections, smoke inhalation, burns, malnutrition, and falls (especially in older adults).

Review of Systems

Once the medical history has been taken, it is time to prepare the patient for the physician's examination. Note on the forms for the physician any questions for which you were unable to get a complete answer from the patient or any areas where you have concerns. Thank the patient for their time and information during the interview. In clear terms and not speaking too rapidly, explain to the patient the need to disrobe, put on a gown, and be seated on the examination table. Note in Chapter 21 how to transfer a patient in a wheelchair to the examination table. *Always* ask if the patient needs assistance in disrobing. It is also wise to let the patient know that you can return in a few minutes to assist them onto the examination table if they need help. This allows you to see that the patient is comfortably settled and to give him or her an estimate of how long it will be before the physician is coming in for the examination.

The ROS is performed by the physician during the physical examination. This is an orderly and systematic check of each part of the body and is recorded. The physician asks questions concerning each organ and system of the body during the examination of the patient. The ROS, in conjunction with the physical examination, helps elicit information that is essential to the diagnosis of disease. The physician usually begins with an overall assessment and proceeds to check each body system in an organized manner. The order in which this is done may vary from one physician to another, but all will check the cardiovascular, respiratory, gastrointestinal, genitourinary, and neurological systems, as well as the extremities, the musculoskeletal system, and the skin.

Both positive and pertinent negative findings are documented in the ROS. When a response is positive, the physician asks the patient to describe it as completely as possible. Table 11-2 lists the symptoms and diseases that can be ascertained during the ROS. Many ambulatory care settings have preprinted ROS sheets. These are convenient, as positive findings can be circled and noted. Negative responses are not circled. In the electronic medical record, the same is available as point and click.

By the completion of this portion of the history, the physician usually has an idea about the patient's condition.

To complete the examination, the physician usually orders laboratory tests depending on the findings and the probable diagnosis. These results, together with the history, examination, and patient symptoms, help to lead to a **clinical diagnosis.**

All of the components of the patient's medical history document integral parts of the patient's health. If any part is lacking, the current understanding of the patient's health is not complete. By using all the components, the physician can evaluate the patient's health completely and more easily.

See Procedure 11-1 for steps in taking a medical history.

TABLE 11-2 REVIEW OF SYSTEMS

General

Patient's perception of general state of health at the present time; difference from usual state; vitality and energy levels

Neurological

Headache, change in balance, incoordination, loss of movement, change in sensory perception/feeling in an extremity, change in speech, change in smell, fainting, loss of memory, tremors, involuntary movement, loss of consciousness, seizures, weakness, head injury

Psychological

Irritability, nervousness, tension, increased stress, difficulty concentrating, mood changes, suicidal thoughts, depression

Skin

Rashes, itching, changes in skin pigmentation, black and blue marks, change in color or size of mole, sores, lumps, change in skin texture, odors, excessive sweating, acne, loss of hair, excessive growth of hair or growth of hair in unusual locations, change in nails, amount of time spent in the sun

Eyes

Blurry vision, visual acuity, glasses, contacts, sensitivity to light, excessive tearing, night blindness, double vision, drainage, bloodshot, pain, blind spots, flashing lights, halos around objects, glaucoma, cataracts

Ears

Hearing deficits, hearing aid, pain, discharge, lightheadedness, ringing in the ears, earaches, infection

Nose and Sinuses

Frequent colds, discharge, itching, hay fever, postnasal drip, stuffiness, sinus pain, polyps, obstruction, nosebleed, change in sense of smell

Mouth

Toothache, tooth abscess, dentures, bleeding/swollen gums, difficulty chewing, sore tongue, change in taste, lesions, change in salivation, bad breath

Throat/Neck

Hoarseness, change in voice, frequent sore throats, difficulty swallowing, pain/stiffness, enlarged thyroid

Respiratory

Shortness of breath, shortness of breath on exertion, phlegm, cough, sneezing, wheezing, coughing up blood, frequent upper respiratory tract infections, pneumonia, emphysema, asthma, tuberculosis

Cardiovascular

Shortness of breath that wakes you up in the night, chest pain, heart murmur, palpitations, fainting, sleep on pillows to breathe better, swelling, cold hands/feet, leg cramps, myocardial infarction, hypertension, valvular disease, pain in calf with walking, varicose veins, inflammation of a vein, blood clot in leg, anemia

Breasts

Pain, tenderness, discharge, lumps, change in size, dimpling

Gastrointestinal

Change in appetite, nausea, vomiting, diarrhea, constipation, usual bowel habits, black and tarry stools, vomiting blood, change in stool color, excessive gas, belching, regurgitation or heartburn, difficulty swallowing, abdominal pain, jaundice, hemorrhoids, hepatitis, peptic ulcers, gallstones

Urinary

Change in urine color, voiding habits, painful urination, hesitancy, urgency, frequency, excessive urination at night, increased urine volume, dribbling, loss in force of stream, bed-wetting, change in urine volume, incontinence, pain in lower abdomen, kidney stones, urinary tract infections

Musculoskeletal

Joint stiffness, muscle pain, back pain, limitation of movement, redness, swelling, weakness, bony deformity, broken bones, dislocations, sprains, gout, arthritis, osteoporosis, herniated disc

Female Reproductive

Vaginal discharge, change in libido, infertility, sterility, pain during intercourse, menses (last menstrual period, age period started, regularity, duration, amount of bleeding, premenstrual symptoms, intermenstrual bleeding, painful periods), menopause (age of onset, duration, symptoms, bleeding), obstetrical (number of pregnancies, number of miscarriages/abortions, number of children, type of delivery, complications), type of birth control, estrogen therapy

Male Reproductive

Change in libido, infertility, sterility, impotence, pain during intercourse, age at onset of puberty, testicular pain, penile discharge, erections, emissions, hernias, enlarged prostate, type of birth control

Nutrition

Present weight, usual weight, food intolerances, food likes, food dislikes, where meals are eaten

Endocrine

Bulging eyes, fatigue, change in size of head, hands, or feet, weight change, heat/cold intolerances, excessive sweating, increased thirst, increased hunger, change in body hair distribution, swelling in the anterior neck, diabetes mellitus

Lymph Nodes

Enlarged, tenderness

Hematological

Easy bruising/bleeding, anemia, sickle cell anemia, blood type

THE PATIENT'S RECORD AND ITS IMPORTANCE

The patient's chart or record is a collection of confidential information that concerns the patient, care given to the patient, patient progress, and laboratory and other diagnostic test results that have been completed. This information is arranged in a file folder or a binder, or is held together by other suitable means. It is used for a variety of purposes, but primarily it is used to provide a foundation for planning patient care and making decisions about patient care. Other purposes for a medical record include using it as a basis for communication among caregivers, for statistical analysis in research, and for reporting infectious diseases to the health department. It is also a legal document and belongs to the physician or the agency in which the physician is employed. See Chapter 7 regarding legal guidelines and medical records. Because it is a legal document, the medical record can be used to determine if patient care has been given according to the standards of care that the law recognizes; therefore, it must be complete, concise, accurate, and legible. Many important items of information must be written in the patient record and the medical assistant will be one of the professionals making chart entries.

HIPAA Compliance

HIPAA regulations focus on three vulnerable areas with respect to medical records and the patient's chart. These three areas include:

- Paper record storage and computer/server areas
- Fax machines
- Workstations

The patient's chart must be stored in locked areas, usually a locking file cabinet. It is important that only those persons with need for access to charts have a key. Locks should be changed periodically to ensure security. Sprinkler and fire detection systems should be installed and tested annually to protect paper records. Patients will respect and appreciate all procedures and policies to keep their history and medical records confidential and protected from harm.

Faxing is a growing vulnerability to the threat of unintended disclosure of patient confidential information. Unintentional human, software, and telecommunication carrier code errors contribute to the security problem. Faxes are easily misdirected or intercepted by individuals for whom access was neither intended nor authorized. Only authorized personnel should have access to the fax machine area, and patient information should be faxed only with assurance that the same security is afforded where the fax is being sent.

Further protection of the patient's medical information means that computer workstation terminals should have directional screen filters if they are located in areas where unauthorized individuals may view the screen. Automated screen time-out features should be installed to protect information from passersby. If the office connects to the Internet, telecommuters, or hospital networks, a commercial-grade network firewall should be installed, tested, and maintained to ensure security. Antivirus software should be in place and updated regularly.

Contents of Medical Records

Each patient has his or her own medical record. All patients' records hold standard information. In addition to the patient information forms previously mentioned, other important components of the record include:

- Informed consent forms
- Physical examination outcomes
- Laboratory and diagnostic test results
- The physician's diagnosis and plan of treatment
- Surgical reports
- Progress reports
- Follow-up care
- Telephone calls
- Discharge summary
- Other communications (from other physicians, laboratories, or agencies)
- Patient records from other physicians
- Medication history

Continuity of Care Record

The Continuity of Care Record (CCR) is being developed by a number of medical groups including the American Academy of Family Physicians and the American Academy of Pediatrics. It is being developed to make it easier and more effective to transport patient medical information between physicians. The CCR is intended to improve the continuity of patient care, reduce errors, and assure a minimum standard of information that is to be shared with another health care provider. The CCR will include patient and provider information, insurance data, patient's health status, recent care given, recommendations for future care, and the reason for referral or transfer. The patient's health status should include allergies, medications, immunizations, vital signs, pertinent laboratory results and recent procedures, and diagnoses. An expanded CCR also would likely include any advanced directives the patient might have. In a time when much referral takes place, especially in managed care, or when patients are transferred from a hospital setting to an assisted living environment where care is likely provided by someone other than the current primary care physician, such a record is most beneficial to patient and physician alike.

The CCR is likely to be completed by physicians, nurses, medical assistants, and ancillary providers such as social workers, physical therapists, among others. It can include outpatient, community-based, and inpatient services. It should be machine readable, as well as human readable, and can be transferred through a number of electronic formats. At all times, however, the CCR is to be protected and designed to enhance patient confidentiality.

Rules of Charting

Charting is required for each medication, treatment/procedure, or medical assistant action. Accounts of the patient's condition and activities must be charted in a clear and meaningful way. What is charted in the patient's record must be accurate, clear, complete, timely, and written properly. There is a saying, "If it is not charted, it was not done." Some basic rules to follow are:

- Entries on the patient's chart should always be written in blue or black ink.
- After charting, sign with your first initial, last name, and title.
- Do not leave empty space between your chart entry and your initial/signature. Draw a line through the center of an empty line or part of a line, if necessary. This prevents charting by someone else in an area signed by you.
- Ditto marks may not be used.
- Do not erase or obliterate any entry. Erasures provide reason for question if the chart is used in court. If a mistake is discovered immediately, a single line is drawn through the mistake. Charting then continues in a normal manner. If a mistake is discovered and corrected at a later date, a single line is drawn through the error and the correct information is written directly above it. Some policies require that "Correction" or "Corr" be placed by the entry and that it is dated and initialed. Follow your office protocol. Red pen may be used for the correction and notation.
- Leave no blank lines in the chart. Enter your data in the next available line.
- Use standard abbreviations only. Be alert to abbreviations that have been determined to be too easily misinterpreted, and do not use them. See "Abbreviations Used in Charting" section later in this chapter.
- Avoid medical terminology unless absolutely certain of spelling and definition. If you are unsure of the spelling of a word, use the dictionary to make certain.
- Confirm the patient's name is on every page.
- Use present tense. Never use future tense, such as "patient to be given a tetanus shot"; instead, wait until the injection is given, then chart the event.
- Never chart for another person; chart only what you know, not what someone else has told you.
- Describe events and behaviors; do not label them. "Patient was really angry" does not describe the event as well as "Patient yelled and threw the pencil on the counter."
- Be as specific as you can. Charting "Patient complained of shoulder pain" is not as clear as "Patient complains of right shoulder pain when reaching overhead."

METHODS OF CHARTING/DOCUMENTATION

There are three primary ways to maintain chart notes. They are:

- Source-oriented medical records
- Problem-oriented medical records
- Computer-generated/modified records.

Source-Oriented Medical Records

The traditional or conventional method of charting, **source-oriented medical record (SOMR),** consists of a chronologic set of notes for each visit beginning with the patient's first visit (Figure 11-6). This form of charting makes it difficult to follow or track a specific patient problem. The caregiver must search through the record to locate information about a particular patient problem. Source-oriented notes may be typed by the medical transcriptionist from dictation after the physician has seen the patient.

The example of handwritten chart notes shows the complete history taken at the time of examination including the present illness (if any), the medical history, allergies, family history, habits (social history), and ROS. The physical examination follows with each area noted. Impressions and changes in medications and plan finish the examination notes.

Problem-Oriented Medical Records

A more efficient way of keeping chart notes is the **problem-oriented medical record (POMR).** This method is used extensively today, especially by clinics or any medical practice where more than one physician

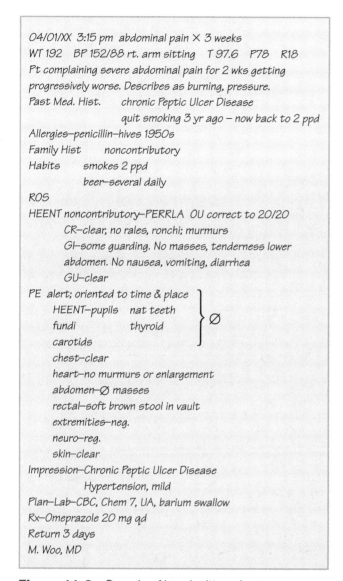

04/01/XX 3:15 pm abdominal pain × 3 weeks
WT 192 BP 152/88 rt. arm sitting T 97.6 P78 R18
Pt complaining severe abdominal pain for 2 wks getting progressively worse. Describes as burning, pressure.
Past Med. Hist. chronic Peptic Ulcer Disease
quit smoking 3 yr ago – now back to 2 ppd
Allergies–penicillin–hives 1950s
Family Hist noncontributory
Habits smokes 2 ppd
beer–several daily
ROS
HEENT noncontributory–PERRLA OU correct to 20/20
CR–clear, no rales, ronchi; murmurs
GI–some guarding. No masses, tenderness lower abdomen. No nausea, vomiting, diarrhea
GU–clear
PE alert; oriented to time & place
HEENT–pupils nat teeth } Ø
fundi thyroid
carotids
chest–clear
heart–no murmurs or enlargement
abdomen–Ø masses
rectal–soft brown stool in vault
extremities–neg.
neuro–reg.
skin–clear
Impression–Chronic Peptic Ulcer Disease
Hypertension, mild
Plan–Lab–CBC, Chem 7, UA, barium swallow
Rx–Omeprazole 20 mg qd
Return 3 days
M. Woo, MD

Figure 11-6 Sample of handwritten chart note.

may see the patient. This method calls for a list of problems to be made, dated, and numbers assigned to them. When a patient is seen, the problems are identified by number throughout the record. This system makes it easier for the physician to follow the patient's progress.

The POMR has four major components:

- *The database:* The patient's medical history, results from laboratory and other diagnostic tests, and results of physical examination are the core of the record.
- *The problem list:* Each problem is listed individually and assigned a number and dated.
- *The diagnostic and treatment plan:* This component addresses the laboratory and other diagnostic tests completed and the physician's plan for treating the patient.
- *Progress notes:* These notes are entered on every problem initially recorded. Documentation is done chronologically and includes patient's complaints, problems, condition, treatment, and responses to treatment and care given.

Leo McKay
Date of Birth 01/22/49
Office visit 04/01/XX

This 57-year-old patient is seen after a several year absence because of abdominal pain which began approximately 2 weeks ago with progressively worsening abdominal pain. He has stopped eating to see if pain would improve, which it did not. Finally yesterday he stopped taking fluids as well. Until this episode, he was drinking several beers daily and smoking approximately 2 ppd.

Weight is 192. BP 152/88 rt. arm sitting P 78 R 18 T 97.6. He is a well-developed, moderately obese male in moderate distress. Abdomen is tense with some guarding at RUQ.

Abdominal pain - pt needs barium swallow, CBC, Chem 7 and UA. To restrict diet to clear liquids until seen in 2 days, omeprazole 20 mg qd.

JW/tlm

Figure 11-7 Example of dictated and transcribed chart note.

Physicians may dictate their notes to be typed by a medical transcriptionist, and then filed in the chart (Figure 11-7). These notes may follow the form seen in the handwritten chart note or as in Figure 11-7.

Computer-Modified Records

The final example (Figure 11-8) shows a computer chart note that ties both methods together: the problems are stated, but the record grows in chronologic order. Note that the past health problems are shown at the top of each entry and all current medications are shown on each entry.

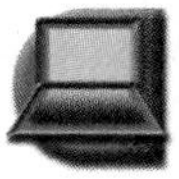

Computer-modified records are advantageous if an agency has computer terminals in a network connected to a main computer. Records can be brought up on a terminal by a physician and reviewed, updated, and saved whenever the physician wants to do so. Records are available 24 hours a day and therefore can be accessed by the physician on a home computer.

Protecting patient's confidentiality must always be a priority when medical records are computerized.

Patient: Leo McKay
Date of Birth: 01/22/49
Visit Date: 04/01/XX

Chief Complaint: Abdominal pain
History: Has been ill over the last 2 weeks with progressively worsening abdominal pain.
Review of Symptoms: Patient denies the following:
- Chest pain, Chest pressure, Chest heaviness, Circulation problems, Palpitations, Rapid heartbeat, Irregular heartbeat, Ankle swelling
- Cough, Phlegm, Coughing up blood, Shortness of breath, Wheeze, Change in exercise tolerance
- Burning or pain on urination, Difficulty starting or stopping urination, Dribbling after urination, Incontinence of urine, Blood in urine, Cloudiness of urine
- Change in appetite, Unexpected weight loss, Nausea, Vomiting, Difficulty Swallowing, Belly pains, Gas pains, Change in bowel habit: change in frequency, shape, color, consistency, size of stool; Blood, Mucus, or Slime, Rectal pain or discomfort, Hemorrhoids
- Skin rash, New or changing moles, Excess bruising or bleeding
- Mouth sores, Denture problems, Sinus drainage or stuffiness, Facial pain
- Panic attacks, Anxiety, Depression, Sadness, Seizures, Problems with concentration or memory, Disturbance of sleep, Insomnia, Early wakefulness
- Dizziness, Fainting, Lightheadedness on standing, Headaches, Vision problems, Hearing problems, Numbness or tingling in arms or legs, Weakness in arms or legs

Medications, including Herbal, Vitamin, and Mineral Supplements

Drug	Dose	Freq.	Started
none			

Medical Problem List

Problem	When Dx'd	Active?
Peptic Ulcer	1985	no

List of Surgeries

Surgical Procedure	When
none	

Family History: Parents deceased, father died of heart attack, mother of breast cancer.
Social History: Divorced, no children
Habits: Smokes 2 ppd, Several beers daily
Allergies: Penicillin

Physical Examination

GENERAL: Well developed and well nourished gentleman in no distress. No jaundice, cyanosis, clubbing, or edema.
VITALS: Weight = 192, Temp = 97.6, Pulse = 78, R = 18, BP = 152/88
HEENT: Normocephalic and without evidence of trauma, tympanic membranes and external auditory canals are normal. Pharynx and mouth are normal.
NECK: supple, no masses or thyromegaly.
NODES: No cervical nodes palpable. No axillary or inguinal adenopathy.
CARDIOVASCULAR SYSTEM: Heart sounds: no murmurs, rubs or gallops, carotids with good upstrokes, no bruits heard. Peripheral pulses including radials, brachials, and femorals intact. Posterior tibial, and dorsalis pedis pulses intact.
RESPIRATORY SYSTEM: resps 18/min, trachea central, expansion, fremitus, resonance, and breath sounds normal.
ABDOMEN: soft, no masses, organomegaly, or tenderness. No loin or costo-vertebral angle tenderness. Inguinal canals are intact without herniae. Bowel sounds active.
GENITOURINARY: Penis without lesions or discharge, scrotum, testicles, epididymis and cords all normal
RECTAL: no masses, tenderness, or hemorrhoids. Soft brown stool in vault. Prostate normal in size, and shape without nodules or tenderness.
MUSCULOSKELETAL SYSTEM: Joints with full ROM, no joint tenderness or swelling. Muscle bulk symmetric and normal.
SKIN: without masses, skin tags, rash, blisters or ulcerations. Nails are normal without splinter hemorrhages.
NEUROLOGICAL SYSTEM: Alert and oriented to place, person, and time. Communicates with good word recognition and appropriate word usage. Cranial nerves and spinal nerves grossly intact.

Assessment and Plan

Problem	Plan/Status
Abdominal pain	Reports about two weeks of epigastric and retrosternal chest pain radiating up and to the left. Episodes of pain occur usually during the day and last for 3-4 hours. No associated dyspnea, palpitations, sweats, dizziness. No nausea, vomiting or diarrhea. No blood in the stool. To get barium swallow, CBC, Chem 7 and UA. Begin omeprazole 20 m qd.

Follow-up appointment: 3 days
Mark Woo MD

Figure 11-8 Sample of computer-generated medical history and physical examination.

SOAP Method of Charting

Charting under SOMR and POMR techniques for follow-up visits is accomplished most efficiently using a method with the acronym **SOAP.** In this method, the *subjective* complaint (patient's symptoms) is listed. This is the patient's description of the current problems. These problems are not discernible to an observer. The *objective* findings are those made by the physician during the physical examination, vital signs, and laboratory and other test results. These findings can be seen, felt, or measured, and the findings are observable. *Assessment* of the problem is next. The physician weighs the objective findings with the subjective information the patient has given and forms a diagnosis. The physician then formulates a *plan*. The plan includes further laboratory tests, radiographs, medications, and instructions to the patient. Usually there is a follow-up appointment made for a few days or two to three weeks for a new problem, followed by a several month follow-up for the problem once it has been brought under control.

Examples of the transcribed and the computer-generated follow-up visit notes are shown in Figures 11-9 and 11-10, respectively.

Abbreviations Used in Charting

Abbreviations are used extensively in charting to document information. Some are used as a short-hand to save time and space, whereas other abbreviations are used to give an exact meaning to a finding. For instance, the abbreviation N&V indicates "nausea and vomiting" without having to write out the entire expression. See Table 11-3 for commonly used abbreviations.

Although the use of abbreviations in medical charts is common, it should be remembered that there is an increasing expectation that the medical chart should be understandable to any person reading it, especially if it is required in any legal matter. Therefore, keep abbreviations to a minimum and use only standard abbreviations. Be prepared to provide any attorney a list of commonly used and accepted abbreviations in your medical practice. The Joint Commission on Accreditation of Healthcare Organizations has posted a listing of prohibited abbreviations on their Web site (http://jcaho.com) to further satisfy their goal of patient safety.

Correcting an Error

When an error has been made in the chart and it needs to be corrected, the proper procedure is to draw a line through the error, note "Corr." and the correct information just above the line. Sign your initials and the date (Figure 11-11). Do not erase, obliterate, or otherwise try to change the error because that will invalidate the legal and medical value of the patient's chart. As a medical assistant, you will be responsible for

Leo McKay
Date of Birth 01/22/49
Visit Date: 04/04/XX

S: Patient returns after undergoing barium swallow. He is not in as much discomfort as last visit. States he has been taking clear liquids only and is hungry.
O: Lab results are back. Chem 7 shows slightly elevated glucose at 133. CBC and UA normal. Barium swallow shows two small areas of ulceration.
A: Gastric ulcer.
P: Reduce omeprazole to 10 mg qd. Recheck glucose at return visit in 4 weeks. MW/tlm

Figure 11-9 Sample of a dictated and transcribed SOAP follow-up visit note.

Leo McKay
Visit Date: 04/04/XX

Symptoms: Feeling somewhat better.
Abdominal pain is less on the Omeprazole.
Exam: Weight = 185 BP = 150/84
Patient had barium swallow showing two areas of ulceration. Lab tests show normal findings for CBC and UA. Chem 7 shows slightly elevated glucose at 133.

Assessment	Plan
Gastric ulcer	Omeprazole 10 mg qd. Recheck glucose at return visit.

Follow-up appointment: 4 weeks.

Mark Woo, MD

Figure 11-10 Sample of computer-generated follow-up visit note.

TABLE 11-3 ABBREVIATIONS COMMON TO MEDICAL CHARTING

BP or B/P	blood pressure
c̄	with
CBC	complete blood count
CC	chief complaint
CPE	complete physical examination
D&C	dilation and curettage
dx	diagnosis
ECG, EKG	electrocardiogram
EEG	electroencephalogram
ER	emergency room
GI	gastrointestinal
GU	genitourinary
GYN	gynecology
HEENT	head, eyes, ears, nose, and throat
I&D	incision and drainage
MI	myocardial infarction
N&V	nausea and vomiting
NVD	nausea, vomiting, and diarrhea
OPD	outpatient department
OR	operating room
P	pulse
PERRLA	pupils equal, round, reactive to light and accommodation
PT	physical therapy
R	respiration
ROM	range of motion
ROS	review of systems
s̄	without
SOAP	subjective, objective, assessment, plan
SOB	short of breath
T	temperature
T&A	tonsillectomy and adenoidectomy
UCHD	usual childhood diseases
URI	upper respiratory infection
UTI	urinary tract infection
WNL	within normal limits
XR	X ray
>	greater than
<	less than
↑	increase
↓	decrease
Δ	change

16 *corr. D. Warden 12/18/XX*

12/~~15~~/XX Leona McKay called to say, "Pain meds and PT are really working; was able to comb and brush her hair this morning." D. Warden

Figure 11-11 Correcting a charting error.

entering information in a patient's record and keeping it confidential. Remember that a patient's medical record is a legal document and it may be necessary to use it as evidence in a court of law.

Chart Organization

The chart notes are kept in chronologic order for the primary physician. The laboratory tests, hospital notes, consultations by other physicians, and any correspondence should be kept in an orderly fashion.

The chart order presents current medications on the left side of the chart with the laboratory reports and pathology reports underneath, each in chronologic order. In the POMR system, often the list of medical problems is found above the current medications.

On the right side of the chart, the physician's notes are in chronologic order with the most recent on top. The radiographs and EKGs follow, including MRIs, mammograms, CT scans, exercise tolerance tests (ETTs), echocardiograms, and other similar tests. Following these are the hospital notes, including the history and physical, hospital consultations, and discharge summary. Consultations by other physicians are grouped next, again in chronologic order.

The miscellaneous section may include anything from referrals for insurance companies to orders and updates from nursing homes or home health services. Finally, the correspondence section includes letters, insurance claim forms, and requests for prior medical records.

If a chart is kept in a specific order, information needed is easily gleaned by the medical assistant, the physician, or the front-office administrative assistant.

Procedure 11-1 Taking a Medical History

PURPOSE:

To obtain a medical history from a patient new to the ambulatory care setting.

EQUIPMENT/SUPPLIES:

Patient history forms
Clipboard
Pens

PROCEDURE STEPS:

1. Introduce yourself to the new patient. Confirm identity of the patient and escort to the examination room or private area.
2. Make eye contact and use positive body language to put patient at ease.
3. Explain the purpose and importance of obtaining the patient information. Ask the questions on the form, trying to get as much information as possible without letting the patient wander from the subject.
4. Ask each question clearly. Be sure patient understands all questions. Ask about allergies.
5. Repeat patient answers when needed to confirm. Be specific when documenting answers. Do not just write "yes" for tobacco use. List "2 packs per day." Be specific.
6. Write legibly using dark ink (blue or black).
7. Recheck the medical history form to be sure all parts are complete. Note any additional information provided by patient. Make sure numbers, dates, spelling, and other information are accurate and legible.
8. Prepare the patient for the review of systems and physical examination if this is indicated.
9. Document the procedure.

Case Study 11-1

Maria Jover, a patient of Dr. Elizabeth King at Drs. Lewis and King, has finally convinced her teenage son to make an appointment for a physical. Adam Jover is 17 years old, outgoing, fun loving, and apparently healthy. But Maria is concerned that he may be engaging in harmful social activities and hopes that by seeing Dr. Winston Lewis, Adam may discover ways to protect himself and his health. Adam agreed to the appointment but is adamant that his mother not accompany him. At the ambulatory care setting, it is decided that Adam might be more forthcoming with a male medical assistant, so Joe Guerrero is scheduled to take Adam's medical history before Dr. Winston does a ROS.

CASE STUDY REVIEW

1. When Joe Guerrero first sits down with Adam to take the history, he notices that Adam is ill at ease and nervous. What can Joe do to reassure Adam that his privacy will be protected?
2. When Joe attempts to take the social history, Adam seems evasive about answering Joe's questions and finally admits that he doesn't want his mother, Maria, to know about his social activities. What is Joe's response?
3. By the end of the interview, it becomes apparent that Adam may be engaging in some behaviors that put him at high risk for contracting the human immunodeficiency virus. How can Joe provide Adam with guidance without alienating him?

Case Study 11-2

Harvey DiAntonio is a 52-year-old patient who lives at 45 W. Smith Avenue, Baltimore, Maryland, 21208. His date of birth is July 8, 1954. His phone number is 667-1870. He is a Baltimore City fire fighter and has been for 21 years. He has union medical insurance, and Blue Cross/Blue Shield (BC/BS) is his carrier. His number is 211-67-87-56. He also carries major medical and his policy is Diagnostic #4. He has been referred by the fire department physician, Dr. Alan Byers. Mr. DiAntonio's complaint is severe "gripping" pain in the anterior mid-chest sometimes radiating to the abdomen, neck, and both arms. Pain seems to occur with strenuous exercise and when walking uphill. Pain usually lasts 20 minutes with each episode. Pain does "ease up" when he ceases activity. Mr. DiAntonio states his episodes have occurred while he was shaving, climbing stairs at work, after a heavy meal, and during sexual intercourse. One episode last week was accompanied with dizziness, nausea, and fatigue. The episodes have been going on now once or twice a month for five months. Mr. DiAntonio's history is essentially noncontributory. It is questionable whether this is due to good health or the fact that the patient has not had a physical examination for eight years. Surgeries include tonsillectomy and adenoidectomy, T&A, 1958, and appendectomy in 1964. Fractured rib, left side, in 1984 due to fire fighting incident. Usual childhood diseases. Hospitalized for observation, 1962, Sinai Hospital, for an unusually long episode of bronchitis. Social history shows that the patient is a pump operator on the job with much heavy exertion. Smokes 1½ to 2 packs of cigarettes per day and is a moderate drinker. He has a weight problem off and on and tends to eat too much while on duty. Lives in a one-story home. Hobbies include carpentry and music. Some family problems and tension exist as both of his children are in adolescence. Patient describes himself as "fun loving" with a "quick temper" and worries about meeting financial needs of the family. Is in a position to retire from active duty but states he could not tolerate the boredom.

Family history shows both parents deceased—mother of heart attack, age 59, and father of unknown cause at age 49. Has two siblings, one brother with history of hypertension and one sister living and in good health. Has two children both living and well. Family history otherwise negative.

Physical examination revealed a well-nourished, well-developed male in no acute distress at this time. Patient does seem a bit anxious about this examination. T. 98.6 - P. 94 - R. 24 - BP 175/104. Ht. 69", Wt. 198 pounds. HEAD, EYES, EARS, NOSE, THROAT—normal. NECK—supple. Trachea in midline. CHEST—normal in contour. Calcium deposit on left sixth rib probably due to history fracture. HEART—after careful examination with the patient recumbent and the scope placed lightly on the chest wall near the apex, a left atrial sound was heard (presystolic gallop). ABDOMEN—negative. EXTREMITIES—negative. GENITALIA—negative. SKIN—negative. NEUROLOGICAL—negative. Laboratory tests performed show a hemoglobin of 11.0 Gms. Awaiting results of serum cholesterol, calcium, phosphorus, and blood urea nitrogen. Chest radiograph essentially negative. EKG report showed atrial sounds occurring presystolically with long P-R intervals. DIAGNOSIS: 1) angina pectoris; 2) anemia; 3) hypertension. TREATMENT: Nitroglycerin tabs, sublingually as needed. To return to office in two weeks to follow medication effects. In consultation with patient, the patient was advised to control physical activity and quantity of food intake. Avoid extreme cold, eight hours of sleep/night. Avoid emotional upsets. Attempt four meals/day. Low-fat 1,600-calorie diet. No smoking, moderate alcohol intake.

CASE STUDY REVIEW

1. Identify the following parts of the case study above and extract from the case study the portion that matches the appropriate medical history component.
   - Personal data
   - Chief complaint
   - Present illness
   - Medical history
   - Family history
   - Social history
   - Review of systems
2. Using appropriate terminology and abbreviations, make a charting entry for Mr. DiAntonio by using the SOAP method of charting.

SUMMARY

The patient's medical history and the information that appears in the medical chart form the base for any and all treatment given to a patient. An efficient and effective medical chart tells the patient's story. It is critical that all information be accurate, documented appropriately, and complete in every way. Taking the medical history, maintaining the patient's chart, and documenting information is a major task for medical assistants.

STUDY FOR SUCCESS

To reinforce your knowledge and skills of information presented in this chapter:

- ❑ Review the Key Terms
- ❑ Practice any Procedures
- ❑ Consider the Case Studies and discuss your conclusions
- ❑ Answer the Review Questions
  - ❑ Multiple Choice
  - ❑ Critical Thinking
- ❑ Navigate the Internet and complete the Web Activities
- ❑ Practice the StudyWARE activities on the textbook CD
- ❑ Apply your knowledge in the Student Workbook activities
- ❑ Complete the Web Tutor sections
- ❑ View and discuss the DVD situations

REVIEW QUESTIONS

Multiple Choice

1. If the patient has difficulty with English, the medical assistant should:
   a. make the appointment for the patient and obtain the services of an interpreter to be present
   b. set the appointment after contact is made with the interpreter
   c. speak more loudly so the patient will understand
   d. suggest that the patient find a physician who speaks his or her first language
2. A helpful question to ask the returning patient is:
   a. Are you feeling bad today?
   b. Didn't you get better with the treatment prescribed last visit?
   c. Have you noticed any changes in your condition since your last visit?
   d. Do you realize you have gained six pounds since your visit last week?
3. When the patient reports not feeling well, the medical assistant should:
   a. mark the chief complaint as "patient not feeling well"
   b. ask helpful questions to help the patient express specific problems or symptoms
   c. pin down the symptoms by guessing what the problem could be
   d. let the physician work with the patient
4. Source-oriented medical records:
   a. are chronologic notes beginning with the patient's first visit
   b. have four major components
   c. are the best for finding information quickly
   d. are best when many physicians see the patient
5. Name, address, telephone numbers, birth date, Social Security number, insurance information, and person to contact in an emergency is information referred to as:
   a. administrative or demographic data
   b. CCR of patient information
   c. social history
   d. none of the above
6. The chief complaint:
   a. often is referred to as the CC in the chart
   b. is a statement of objective findings made by the staff
   c. is subjective data as expressed by the patient
   d. a and c

7. Interviewing patients for their medical history requires:
   a. special credentials such as Certified Medical Assistant (CMA) or Registered Medical Assistant (RMA)
   b. cross-cultural interviewing and communication skills
   c. computer skills in medical note taking
   d. a major portion of the receptionist's time and energy
8. The CCR is being developed:
   a. by the Academies for Family Practice and Pediatric physicians
   b. to reduce errors and assure certain information is shared among providers
   c. for input from all health care providers, nurses, and medical assistants
   d. all the above
9. Progress notes include:
   a. medical history and results of laboratory tests
   b. the physician's plan for treating the patient
   c. the CC, problems, conditions, treatment, and responses to care
   d. a and c
10. Subjective, objective, assessment, and plan charting is sometimes referred to as:
    a. SOAP
    b. POMR
    c. SOMR
    d. CCRP

Critical Thinking

1. Describe the ideal setting that you as a patient would like to have when a complete history is taken. For what reasons did you make your choices?
2. Compare and contrast the patient's chief concern with the physician's chief concern in the cross-cultural model. How can those concerns be brought together into one focus?
3. A male patient you are interviewing denies that he smokes, but his fingers are darkened with tobacco stain and he reeks of the tobacco odor. What questions might you ask to clarify his response?
4. The health and well-being of family members contributes what kind of information to a patient's medical history? When that information is essentially unknown for one reason or another, how is that information addressed in the chart?
5. There are two major "patient examples" of histories in this chapter: Mr. Leo McKay and Mr. Harvey DiAntonio. From the social and family history, identify how that information may or may not relate to the presenting problem.

WEB ACTIVITIES

1. Search the Web site for the Recommended Adult Immunization Schedule in the United States to determine if any changes have been made to the text information. Identify when or if any of the immunizations can be given to a woman who is pregnant or to a person who is severely immunosuppressed or has HIV infection.
2. Search the Web site for information on the electronic POMR. Are you able to see samples? Discuss the advantages and disadvantages of the electronic record and the POMR.

THE DVD HOOK-UP

DVD Series
Skills Based Series

Program Number
6

Chapter/Scene Reference

- *Introduction to Taking a Patient History*
- *Preparing an Exam Room*
- *Patient Assessment and Measurement*

In this chapter, you learned about the proper method for obtaining a patient's medical history and the proper technique for recording in a patient's chart.

In today's designated scenes, you observed Anita going over Mrs. O'Neil's patient history form. Anita first gathered information about the patient's personal history, and then the patient's familial history. Once Anita finished going over the history form, she asked Mrs. O'Neil what brought her into the office today?

1. Why did Anita need to ask the patient what brought her into the office today? After all, she just obtained the patient's entire medical history.
2. What do you think of Anita's personality? Do you think that she was a bit solemn?
3. Why must you also include over-the-counter medications when posting current medications being taken by the patient?

DVD Journal Summary

Write a paragraph that summarizes what you learned from watching today's DVD program. How do you feel about asking patients questions regarding sensitive subject matters such as sexual health and emotional stability?

REFERENCES/BIBLIOGRAPHY

U.S. Department of Health and Human Services, Centers for Disease Control and Prevention. *Recommended adult immunization schedule by age group and medical conditions, United States, 2003–2004*. Summary published by the Advisory Committee on Immunization Practices. Retrieved from www.cdc.gov. Accessed June 9, 2005.

CHAPTER 12

Vital Signs and Measurements

OUTLINE

OBJECTIVES

The student should strive to meet the following performance objectives and demonstrate an understanding of the facts and principles presented in this chapter through written and oral communication.

1. Define the key terms as presented in the glossary.
2. Discuss normal and abnormal temperatures, including factors affecting temperature.
3. Identify and explain the procedures for using, caring for, and storing of the various types of thermometers.

(continues)

KEY TERMS

Afebrile
Apical
Apnea
Arrhythmia
Baseline
Bradycardia
Bradypnea
Cheyne–Stokes
Diastole
Dyspnea
Emphysema
Eupnea
Febrile
Frenulum
Gallium
Hyperpnea
Hypertension
Hyperventilation
Hypotension
Hypoventilation
Increment
Lumen
Manometer
Orthopnea
Pyrexia
Rales
Stertorous
Stridor
Systole
Tachycardia
Tachypnea
Wheezes

FEATURED COMPETENCIES

CAAHEP—ENTRY-LEVEL COMPETENCIES

Fundamental Procedures

- Dispose of biohazardous materials
- Practice Standard Precautions

Patient Care

- Obtain vital signs

Legal Concepts

- Identify and respond to issues of confidentiality
- Document appropriately

ABHES—ENTRY-LEVEL COMPETENCIES

Professionalism

- Maintain confidentiality at all times

Clinical Duties

- Apply principles of aseptic techniques and infection control
- Take vital signs
- Use quality control
- Dispose of biohazardous materials
- Practice Standard Precautions

Legal Concepts

- Document accurately

OBJECTIVES (continued)

4. Discuss the Environmental Protection Agency's initiative to phase out mercury thermometers and other mercury-containing equipment.
5. Describe the locations and procedure for obtaining pulse rate.
6. Explain the procedure for obtaining respiration rates.
7. Identify and describe normal and abnormal pulse and respiratory rates and the factors affecting each.
8. Describe the appropriate equipment and procedure for obtaining a blood pressure measurement.
9. Identify normal and abnormal blood pressure, including factors affecting blood pressure.
10. Describe the procedures for obtaining height, weight, and chest measurements of adults.
11. Accurately record measurements on the patient chart.
12. Explain two reasons why a professional individual shows responsibility by learning about the dangers of mercury.

SCENARIO

At Drs. Lewis and King, clinical medical assistant Joe Guerrero, CMA, assists both physicians in taking patients' vital signs. One of his favorite patients is Abigail Johnson, a friendly woman in her 70s who always has a kind disposition despite her financial and medical difficulties. Abigail is overweight and has hypertension, thus her blood pressure is monitored on a regular basis to be certain that it is under control. In reviewing Abigail's chart, Joe notices that her blood pressure has been quite stable for the last few visits. He also checks her weight and notices that Abigail is slowly losing weight. Abigail's chart, with its history of blood pressure and other measurements, informs Joe's perspective and is a helpful record when evaluating the progress Abigail has made since she became a patient three years ago.

INTRODUCTION

One of the most important and commonly performed tasks of a medical assistant is obtaining and recording patient vital signs and body measurements. Vital signs, also sometimes referred to as cardinal signs, include temperature, pulse, respiration, and blood pressure, abbreviated TPR B/P. They are indicative of the general health and well-being of a patient, and with regular monitoring, may measure patient response to treatment. Vital signs, in total or in part, are an important component of each patient visit. Height and weight measurements, although not considered vital signs, are often a routine part of a patient visit.

Patients will exhibit vital sign readings that are uniquely their own. As a result, baseline assessments of vital signs are usually obtained during the patient's initial visit. These baseline results are used as a reference point for future readings, differentiating between what is normal and abnormal for the patient.

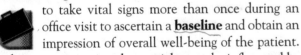

Two important habits must be developed by the medical assistant before taking a patient's vital signs: aseptic technique in the form of hand washing and recognition and correction of factors that may influence results of vital signs. Proper hand washing before taking vital signs will assist in preventing cross contamination of patients. Refer to the discussion on standard precautions and medical asepsis in Chapter 10. Also, emotional factors of patients must be recognized and addressed. Explaining procedures and allowing the patient the opportunity to relax will ease apprehension that may affect vital sign readings.

THE IMPORTANCE OF ACCURACY

Vital signs may be altered by many factors. Medical assistants must recognize and correct factors that may produce inaccurate results. For example, patients may exhibit anxiety over potential test results or findings of the physician. They may be angry or may have rushed into the office. A patient may have had something to eat or drink before the visit or may have had a long wait in the reception area. Patient apprehension and mood must always be considered by the medical assistant, because these factors can affect vital signs. The medical assistant may be required to take vital signs more than once during an office visit to ascertain a **baseline** and obtain an impression of overall well-being of the patient. Body measurements such as weight may be influenced by what the patient is wearing; height may be influenced by the patient's shoes and how his or her posture is while being measured.

Accuracy in taking vital signs is necessary because treatment plans are developed according to the measurement of the vital signs. Variations can indicate a new disease process or the patient's response to treatment. They may also indicate the patient's compliance with a treatment plan. Although taking vital signs is a task commonly performed by the medical assistant, it is never to be taken casually or lightly, and it should never be rushed or incompletely performed. Concentration and attention to proper procedure will help assure accurate measurements and quality care of the patient. The following text discusses procedures used to measure the vital signs of children and adults. Procedures used for infant examinations are discussed in Chapter 15.

Spotlight on Certification

RMA Exam Outline
- Vital signs

CMA Content Outline
- Principles of operation
- Vital signs

CMAS Exam Outline
- Vital Signs and Measurements

TEMPERATURE

Body temperature is maintained and regulated by two processes functioning in conjunction with one another: heat production and heat loss.

Body heat is produced by the actions of voluntary and involuntary muscles. As the muscles move, they use energy which, in response, produces heat. Cellular metabolic activities, such as the process of breaking food-sugars down to simpler components (catabolism), are another source of heat.

The body loses heat by a combination of five processes:

1. *Convection*. The process by which heat is lost through the skin by being transferred from the skin by air currents flowing across it; such as a fan used on a hot day for cooling purposes.
2. *Conduction*. The transfer of heat from within the body to the surface of the skin, and then to surrounding cooler objects touching the skin, such as clothing.
3. *Radiation*. Body heat lost from the surface of the skin to a cooler environment, much like a cool room becoming warm when occupied by many people.
4. *Evaporation*. A heat loss mechanism that uses heat absorption through vaporization of perspiration.
5. *Elimination*. Heat that is lost through the normal functioning of the intestinal, urinary, and respiratory tracts.

The delicate balance between heat production and heat loss is maintained by the hypothalamus in the brain. The hypothalamus monitors blood temperature and will trigger either the heat loss or heat production mechanism with as little as 0.04°F change in blood temperature.

Body temperature is measured in degrees and is influenced by several factors, including:

- An increase in temperature may result from a bacterial infection, increased physical activity or food intake, exposure to heat, pregnancy, drugs that increase metabolism, stress and severe emotional reactions, and age. Age becomes a factor in that infants have an average body temperature that is one to two degrees higher than adults.

- Decrease in temperature may result from viral infections, decreased muscular activity, fasting, a depressed emotional state, exposure to cold, drugs that decrease metabolic activities, and age. Age in this instance refers to older adults, in that older adults have decreased metabolic activity resulting in a decrease in body temperature.
- Another factor that can increase or decrease body temperature is time of day. During sleep and early morning, the temperature is at its lowest, whereas later in the day with muscular and metabolic activity the temperature increases.

Because of the many factors influencing body temperature and the uniqueness of individuals, there is no "normal" temperature. The medical assistant must think of temperatures in terms of the "average," which for an adult is 98.6°F, or 37.0°C.

Terms Used to Describe Body Temperature

The following terms are used to describe body temperature:

- **afebrile:** absence of fever
- **febrile:** fever is present
- *fever:* body temperature increased beyond normal range; **pyrexia** is another term for fever
- *onset:* time when fever begins
- *lysis:* body temperature gradually returns to normal after a period of fever
- *crisis:* body temperature decreases suddenly to normal levels; the patient may perspire profusely (diaphoresis)
- *intermittent:* a fluctuating fever that returns to or below baseline, then increases again
- *remittent:* a fluctuating fever that does not return to the baseline temperature; it fluctuates, but remains increased
- *continuous:* a fever that remains above the baseline; it does not fluctuate, but remains fairly constant

Figure 12-1 depicts types of fever.

Phase Out of Mercury Thermometers and Other Mercury-Containing Equipment

Glass mercury thermometers have been used for decades and have been common in health care agencies, as well as the home. In recent years, concerns have arisen about mercury toxicity when mercury thermometers or other equipment containing mercury breaks and spills mercury into the environment.

This can create a mercury vapor in the indoor air, which is a serious problem. The mercury also can cause environmental damage if it enters the lakes and rivers where it can contaminate fish, which are part of the food chain. Even small amounts of mercury can do great harm. The fetus is at risk because its developing nervous system is susceptible to mercury toxicity if a pregnant woman eats fish contaminated with mercury. When thermometers break or are disposed of improperly, the mercury can enter the atmosphere, especially if the mercury waste is burned in an incinerator.

If spilled mercury is not cleaned up (perhaps the individual using the thermometer is unaware that it is broken, and the mercury has seeped into a carpet or crevice), the mercury will evaporate and can reach dangerous levels in indoor air. There is medical literature that illustrates some cases of serious illnesses and even death from exposure to mercury from broken thermometers. Most cases involved young children. According to the Environmental Protection Agency (EPA), a 32-month-old child who was exposed to mercury became ill with hypertension, tachycardia, apathy, pulmonary edema, and coma. The mercury from a broken thermometer had not been cleaned up.

Even small mercury spills should be cleaned up as soon as possible. Becton-Dickinson, a thermometer manufacturer, makes the following recommendations for cleaning up a broken thermometer:

- Pick up the mercury with an eyedropper or scoop up the beads of mercury with a piece of heavy paper (cardboard, index card, or playing card).
- Place mercury, the dropper, heavy paper, and any broken glass in a plastic resealable bag. Place this bag into two more resealable bags, zipping each within the other, finishing up with the contents bagged three times. Place this into a wide-mouth, sealable plastic container.
- Call the local health department for the nearest mercury disposal location. If no disposal location is available, dispose of the container according to local and state regulations. The health department can refer you regarding how to obtain the information.
- Leave windows open for about two days to assure complete ventilation.

Do not do the following:

- Do not use household cleaning products. Combinations of some cleansers with mercury can release toxic gases.

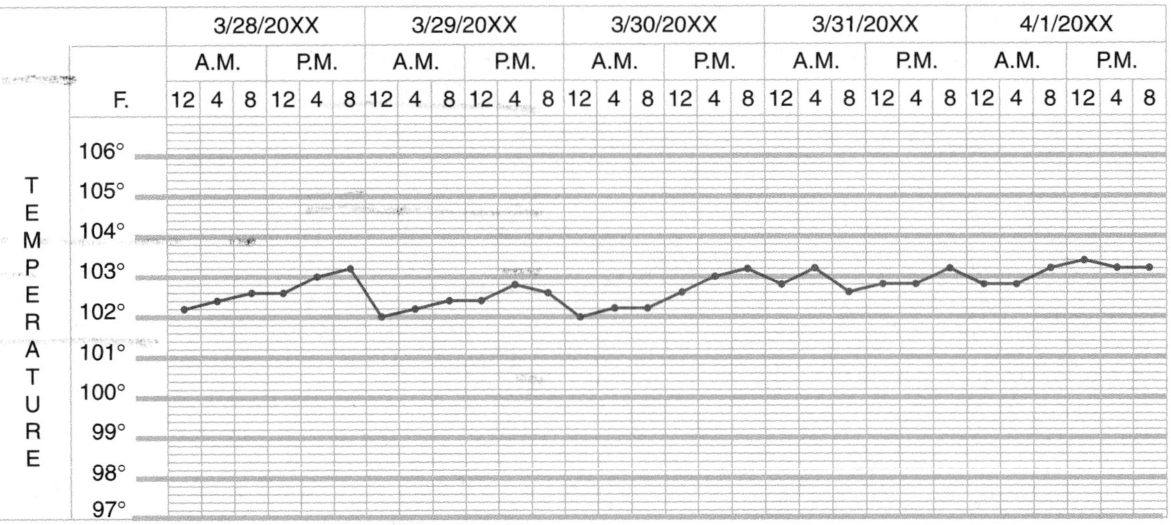

(A) Continuous

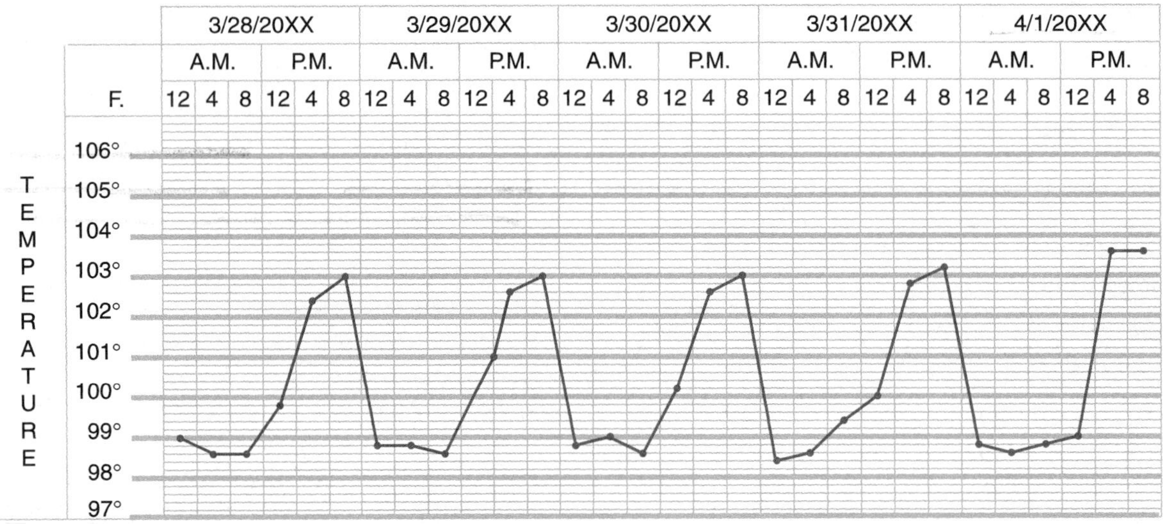

(B) Intermittent

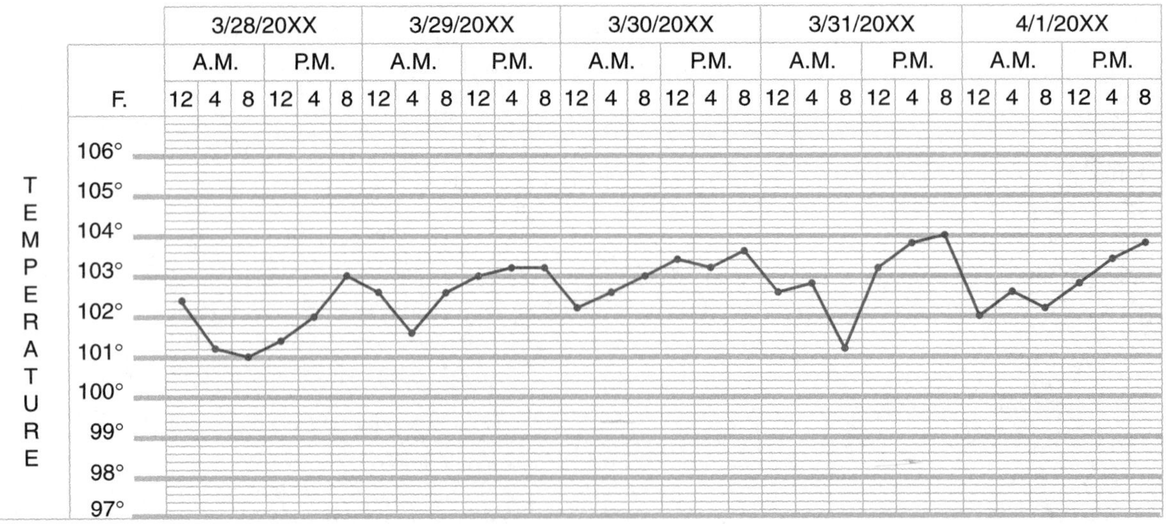

(C) Remittent

Figure 12-1 Types of fevers. (A) Continuous—remains above baseline. Does not fluctuate. (B) Intermittent—a fluctuating fever. Returns to or below baseline, then rises again. (C) Remittent—a fluctuating fever but does not return to baseline temperature. Remains elevated, but fluctuates.

- Do not use a broom or brush to clean up mercury; they only spread it around.
- Do not use a vacuum cleaner or shop vacuum. The mercury vapor escapes into the air and increases exposure by individuals in the area.

In 1998, the American Hospital Association signed an agreement with the EPA to eliminate mercury from their hospitals' waste systems. Hospitals and other health care agencies are therefore phasing out the use of mercury thermometers and other medical equipment that contain mercury such as sphygmomanometers, among others. Many states have recalled mercury thermometers and replaced them with digital ones.

The best alternative is to use nonmercury thermometers such as digital, electronic, alcohol, or glass **gallium** (Galinstan) or alcohol-filled thermometers adopted by the U.S. Food and Drug Administration (FDA) in the 1990s. All of these can be used orally, rectally, or axillary. Also available are tympanic (ear canal) and flexible, disposable, forehead, or oral thermometers (less accurate). There are no known risks with any of the above thermometers.

Types of Thermometers

The following are types of thermometers available for use in the ambulatory care setting:

- disposable
- digital
- electronic
- tympanic
- glass Galinstan (gallium or alcohol)
- temporal artery

Disposable Thermometers. Disposable thermometers are individually wrapped strips with heat-sensitive dots that change color to indicate temperature. They are used once, and then discarded. There are strips for use on the forehead and others for oral use. Although strips are easy to use and prevent patient cross contamination, accuracy is questionable.

Electronic Thermometers. Electronic thermometers are widely used, handheld, battery-operated or plug-in units that have easy-to-read electronic display screens to indicate results (Figure 12-2). Electronic thermometers are available in Fahrenheit or Celsius scales. Probes are attached and are color-coded blue for oral and red for rectal. The probes have disposable plastic covers. The plastic cover acts as a barrier to prevent contamination of the probe and is replaced for each patient to prevent cross contamination of the patient. An accurate result can be obtained in approximately 10 seconds.

Inexpensive digital thermometers are widely available for home use. They are quick, easy to use, and accurate. Encourage your patients to switch to these from the mercury glass thermometers. These lightweight thermometers do not require recharging; their small imbedded batteries last for years but are not replaceable.

Suggest patients watch for "Turn in Your Mercury Thermometer Days." Some communities, in conjunction with local pharmacies, will set aside a day or two each year for residents to take mercury thermometers to their local pharmacy. In exchange for the mercury thermometers, free digital thermometers are given as replacements.

Tympanic Thermometers. The use of tympanic thermometers is becoming more popular because they are fast, provide no discomfort to the patient, can be used on infants, as well as adults, and are usually accurate. They consist of a handheld unit with a probe tip that is inserted into the ear securely to make a seal. Disposable tips are used to prevent cross contamination. Accurate results are obtained in less than two seconds. With the tympanic method of measuring body temperature, the procedure is complete in a few seconds. It is comfortable for the patient, nonthreatening to infants and children, and may be used when other methods are inappropriate. It is the thermometer of choice for pediatric patients older than 2 years. However, physicians have found that inaccurate readings can result if patients have impacted cerumen in the ear of which they may be unaware. Also, if the patient has otitis media, a middle ear infection, the reading tends to be inaccurate and the procedure is painful.

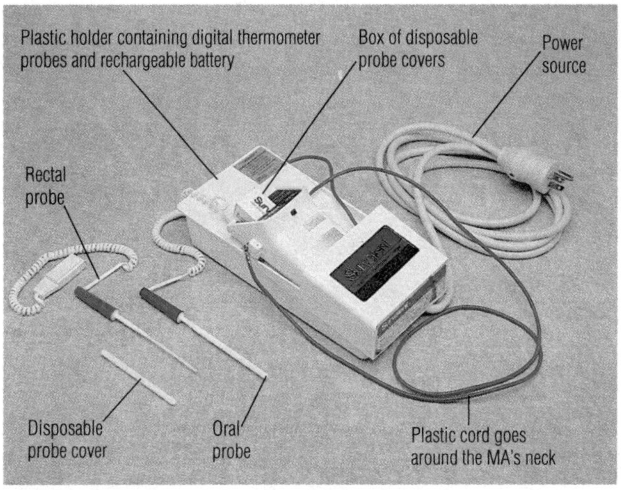

Figure 12-2 Electronic thermometers have interchangeable oral and rectal probes attached to a battery-operated portable unit.

Glass Thermometers. Glass Galinstan thermometers, although approved by the FDA, are expensive and not in wide distribution. Alcohol-filled thermometers, another type of glass thermometer, are not used widely either.

The most commonly used thermometers are the digital, electronic, disposable, and tympanic thermometers.

Temporal Artery Thermometers. A new, non-invasive thermometer has been developed and is currently in use. It is known as a temporal artery thermometer, or "TA" thermometer. Studies done by Harvard Medical School and the Hospital for Sick Children found the TA thermometer to be more accurate than the aural (tympanic) and rectal thermometers. It is used on adults and children.

The temporal artery is a major blood vessel in the head. The thermometer measures the temperature of the skin surface over the temporal artery.

A probe that contains a sensor is used and by sliding the TA thermometer straight across the forehead (midline forehead), the infrared heat from the artery is picked up by the sensor. Software accurately determines and displays the temperature. The TA thermometer can also be used behind the ear lobe (if the forehead is wet with perspiration). This painless, non-invasive method used for taking a temperature is very fast, accurate, and convenient.

Recording Temperature

Temperature may be taken on each visit to the physician's office to obtain a baseline for the patient. When recording the temperature, the scale used for the results must be designated F for Fahrenheit and C for Celsius. The route used must be labeled as well; methods other than oral must be labeled according to the route used because there is a difference in the measurement. Use R for rectal, and Ax for axillary, and Tym for tympanic.

> **Patient Education**
>
> Teach patients the importance of replacing mercury thermometers with an alternative such as digital, disposable, or aural (tympanic) thermometers. The risk for mercury poisoning is great if a mercury thermometer (or other mercury-containing item) is broken and the mercury escapes into the environment.

Temperatures will be recorded as shown:

Oral	T 98.6°F
Rectal	T 99.6°(R) F
Axillary	T 97.6°(Ax) F
Tympanic	T 98.6°(Tym) F
Temporal artery	T 99.4°(TA) F

When a facility uses a tympanic thermometer exclusively, the route is known and therefore does not have to be labeled.

The medical assistant must read all manufacturer's instructions before using any digital or tympanic thermometer. Each may have a slight difference in operating procedure.

Procedures 12-1 through 12-5 detail steps involved in taking temperature by various routes.

Measuring Temperature

To convert °F to °C:
Subtract 32 from F temperature, then multiply by 5/9.

Example:

$$97°F = 97 - 32 = 65 \quad 65 \times \frac{5}{9} = 9\overline{)325.0} = 36.1°C$$

36.1
27
55
54
10

To convert °C to °F:
Multiply C temperature by 9/5, then add 32.

Example:

$$36.1°C \times 9 = \frac{36.1}{1} \times \frac{9}{5} = 36.1 \times \frac{9}{5} = 5\overline{)324.90}$$

64.98
30
24
20
49
45
40

$= 64.98 + 32.00 = 96.98$ or 97°F

Oral Temperatures. To read a glass alcohol thermometer, hold the thermometer at eye level and move it slightly until the column can be seen. Note where the column is in relation to the numbers and lines on the thermometer. The longer lines on a Fahrenheit scale are calibrated by one full degree, whereas the smaller lines are calibrated by 0.2 degree (Figure 12-3). On a Celsius thermometer, each long line represents a degree. They are numbered consecutively, with nine lines between numbers, each line representing 0.1 degree.

To use an oral strip for taking a temperature, make certain that the package is not damaged, then peel it back to reveal the strip. The strip is then inserted into

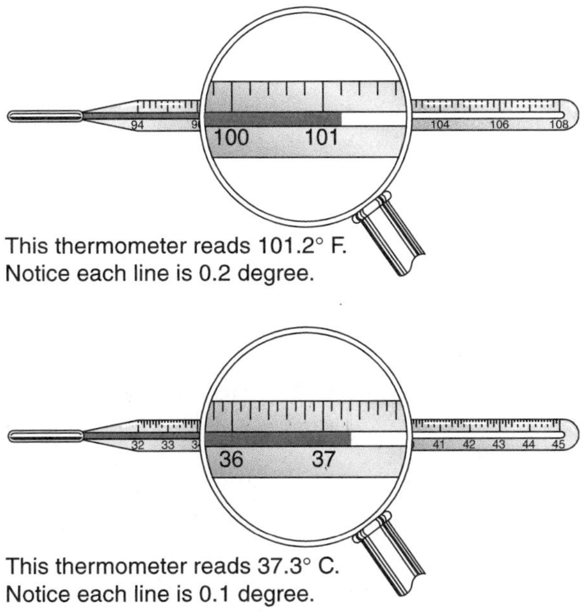

Figure 12-3 (A) Fahrenheit thermometer. (B) Celsius thermometer.

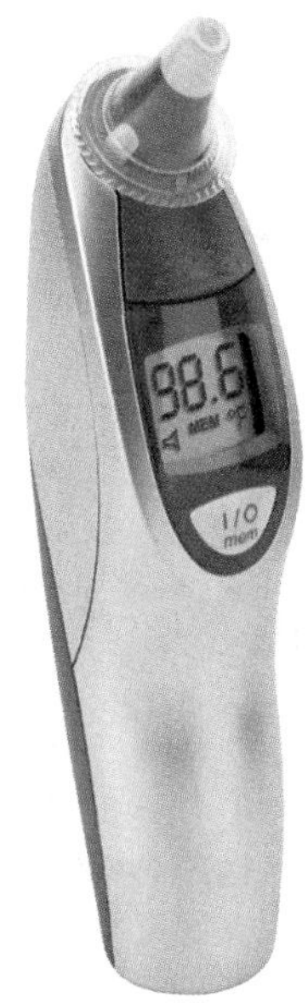

Figure 12-4 Thermo-scan tympanic thermometer. (Courtesy of Welch-Allyn.)

the patient's mouth. After the appropriate time interval has elapsed, the thermometer is removed, and the dots that have changed color are read using the scale located on the strip. Although convenient to use, accuracy is not always assured with the strips, and therefore they may not be the best choice for clinical use. See Procedure 12-5 to take an oral temperature using a disposable oral strip.

The procedure for obtaining an oral temperature with an electronic thermometer (see Procedure 12-1) follows the same steps as when using a glass thermometer. Some electronic thermometers are stored on a recharging base. When removed from the base, they are turned on and ready for use. A disposable cover is placed over the probe, and the probe is placed in the patient's mouth. When the temperature has been obtained, the thermometer will beep and the temperature will be displayed on the screen. The probe cover is ejected into a biohazard container without touching it, and the unit is returned to the base. The temperature is then recorded in the patient's chart. Always read and follow the manufacturer's directions for use and care of a digital unit.

Aural Temperature. Taking a temperature with a tympanic thermometer is a fast, safe method for obtaining a patient's temperature (Figure 12-4). It is common in ambulatory care settings. Tympanic temperature can be obtained without discomfort for the patient whether older, an infant, or reluctant.

The tympanic thermometer measures the patient's temperature by measuring the infrared waves produced by the tympanic membrane and recording the temperature in less than two to three seconds on a digital screen. The tympanic membrane and the hypothalamus of the brain share the same blood supply, thus an accurate measurement of the body temperature can be obtained.

The greatest benefits of the tympanic thermometer are that it gives nearly instant results; does not come into contact with mucous membranes, thereby minimizing cross contamination; uses a site that is readily accessible; is not affected by the patient smoking or drinking hot or cold liquids; does not require that the patient be conscious; and is an easy instrument to use. The unit is battery operated and uses a disposable probe cover or ear speculum.

Drawbacks to the tympanic thermometer have been demonstrated in pediatric patients with ear conditions such as otitis media. An inaccurate recording can result because the fluid buildup in the inner ear limits infrared wave transmission.

The tympanic thermometer is a handheld unit that is inserted into the outer third of the ear canal. See Procedure 12-2 to obtain an aural temperature using a tympanic thermometer.

Rectal Temperature. The rectal method of obtaining a temperature is used on infants and young children and patients who are unable or incapable of cooperating with the oral method of temperature taking. Pediatric procedures are covered in Chapter 15. Patients experiencing breathing difficulties, such as an upper respiratory infection, asthma, or emphysema, or those who are unable to follow instructions, as seen with dementia, mental retardation, unconsciousness, or Alzheimer's disease, in most cases will require a rectal temperature method. Rectal temperatures will have a reading that is approximately one degree higher than oral temperatures because the rectum is a closed body cavity. Rectal thermometers are rarely used in an office or ambulatory care setting because tympanic and axillary methods are available.

Axillary Temperature. An axillary temperature may be used when the patient is an infant or for other reasons is unable to have an oral or rectal temperature taken. This method may be used for patients who display breathing difficulties or who are unable to follow directions as a result of mental incapacity. This is the least accurate method of obtaining a patient's temperature and should be used when other routes are unavailable or inappropriate. An axillary temperature is approximately one degree lower than an oral temperature because the axilla is an open body cavity. See Procedure 12-4.

Cleaning and Storage of Thermometers

Oral and rectal digital thermometers must always be separated. Axillary thermometers may be cleaned with the oral thermometers. Storage will depend on the policy of the facility.

Digital, electronic, and tympanic thermometers are cleaned according to the manufacturer's directions. The covers protect the probes from contamination. Each type of thermometer has a storage case or a wall-mounted base made specially for storing the unit. Disinfect these types of thermometers by wiping with a mild disinfectant as instructed by the manufacturer.

PULSE

The pulse rate consists of two phases of the heart action and can be felt when compressing an artery. As the heart contracts it increases pressure on the arterial walls. The increased pressure passes through the arteries in a wave-like movement resulting in a slight expansion in the arterial wall. When the heart relaxes, the pressure is decreased in the arteries, resulting in the wall returning to its previous position. One contraction and relaxation of the heart is equal to one heart cycle or heart beat. The pulse and heartbeat rate should be the same.

Pulse Sites

The pulse can be felt in those areas of the body where an artery is close to the surface and an underlying solid structure such as a bone. The common pulse sites include the radial, carotid, temporal, brachial, femoral, popliteal, and dorsalis pedis arteries (Figure 12-5). An apical pulse, located at the apex of the heart, may also be taken. Although the radial, brachial, and carotid arteries are the most frequently used sites for pulse rates, it is important to recognize pulse beats because circulation may be monitored by palpating the other sites. Pulse sites are also used when necessary as pressure points for controlling severe bleeding.

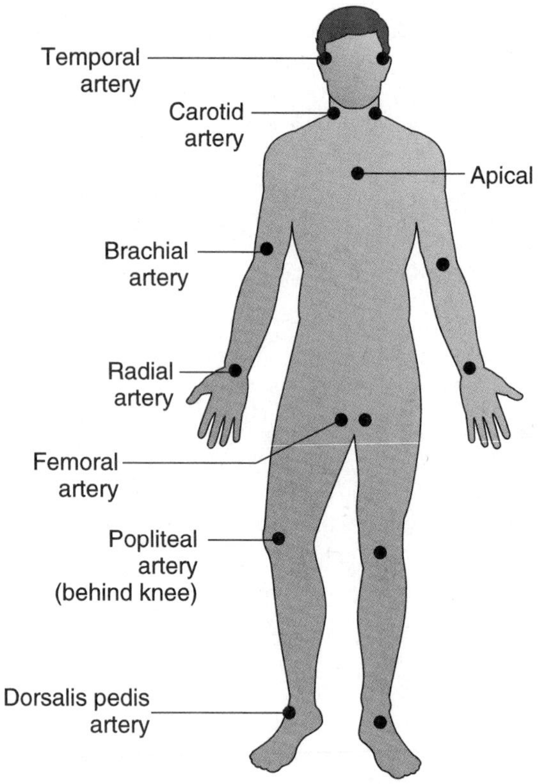

Figure 12-5 Pulse sites in the body.

- The *radial* pulse is located at the thumb side of the wrist approximately 1 inch above the base of the thumb. This is the most commonly used site for obtaining a pulse rate.
- The *carotid* pulse, used during emergency situations and when performing cardiopulmonary resuscitation (CPR), is found between the larynx and sternocleidomastoid muscle in the front side of the neck on either side of the trachea. When measuring the pulse at the carotid site, compress only one side at a time.
- The *brachial* pulse is found in the inner aspect of the elbow called the antecubital space. This pulse site is the most commonly used site to obtain blood pressure measurements.
- The *temporal* pulse is located at the temple area of the head. It is rarely used to obtain a pulse rate but may be used to monitor circulation or control bleeding from the head and scalp.

- Posterial tibial - medial side of ankle

- The *femoral* pulse is located in the groin area. It is a deep artery and must be compressed firmly to be felt.
- The *popliteal* pulse is located at the back of the knee. The patient must be in a supine position with the knee flexed for it to be felt because the artery is deep within the knee. This artery is the one used for leg blood pressure measurements and to monitor circulation.
- The *dorsalis pedis* pulse is felt on the top of the foot slightly to the side of midline next to the extensor ligament of the great toe, between the first and second metatarsal bones. It is commonly used to monitor lower limb circulation.
- ***Apical*** *pulse* is found at the apex of the heart, located at the fifth intercostal space left side, midclavicular line. That is, between the fifth and sixth ribs perpendicular to the middle of the clavicle, left of the sternum. A stethoscope is required to obtain an apical pulse. Apical pulse is used on cardiac patients and to obtain infant pulse rates because they are difficult to obtain by the usual methods.

Measuring and Evaluating a Pulse

When measuring a pulse rate, other characteristics besides the rate are noted. These characteristics include rhythm, volume of pulse, and condition of the arterial wall.

The rate is the number of pulsations or beats felt for one minute. The pulse is counted for 30 seconds, then the number is doubled. Pulse rates may vary according to age, activities, general health, sex, emotions, pain, and medications. The rate is lower when sleeping and higher when active or exercising. Rates for infants and children are greater than for adults. Well-conditioned athletes will have a lower than average resting rate because their cardiovascular system has been developed to function more efficiently.

Rhythm of the pulse refers to the time between pulsations and regularity of the beat. Normal rhythm occurs when the beats are felt at regular intervals. Abnormal rhythms, **arrhythmias,** are those rhythms in which the interval between pulsations is altered by either an increased or decreased time span. Arrhythmias must be noted and reported because they may indicate heart disease.

The volume of the pulse refers to the strength of the beat that is felt. The pulsations may feel full, strong, hard, soft, thready, or weak. A pulse may have a regular rate and yet have a variation in intensity or volume. Volume should be noted and reported.

Condition of the arterial wall can be felt as the pulse is taken. The normal artery feels soft and elastic. The abnormal artery may feel hard, knotty, wiry, or a combination of these. These should be noted and reported because they may indicate cardiac disease.

Normal Pulse Rates

Average pulse rates vary from birth to adulthood. At birth, the pulse rate is much higher; as we age, it generally decreases. Average rate by age group is as follows:

Birth	130–160 beats per minute
Infants	110–130 beats per minute
Children between 1 and 7 years old	80–120 beats per minute
Children older than 7 years	80–90 beats per minute
Adults	60–80 beats per minute

Pulse Abnormalities

Abnormalities may be in the rate, rhythm, and feel of the arterial wall. Common pulse rate abnormalities include **bradycardia,** a pulse rate less than 60 beats per minute, and **tachycardia,** a pulse rate greater than 100 beats per minute. Common arrhythmias would include a pulsation felt before expected, which is called a premature ventricular contraction (PVC), and sinus arrhythmia. An occasional premature contraction can occur in response to stress, caffeine, nicotine, alcohol, or lack of sleep. Sinus arrhythmia is a variation of rhythm during respiration and may be found in children and young adults. The rate increases with inspiration and decreases with expiration. This usually does not require treatment.

When any pulse rate abnormalities or arrhythmias are felt, take the pulse for one full minute, note the frequency of the abnormality, record the abnormality, and alert the physician.

Recording Pulse Rates

Pulse rates are normally recorded after the temperature; for example: T 98.6°F P 72 regular. Any unusual findings should be recorded and reported to the physician; for example: P 72 irregular × 2 minutes.

Procedure 12-6 describes measuring a radial pulse; Procedure 12-7 describes measuring an apical pulse.

RESPIRATION

The function of respiration (breathing) is the exchange of gases: oxygen and carbon dioxide. External respiration occurs when oxygen is drawn into the lungs and carbon dioxide is expelled from the lungs. Internal respiration occurs when oxygen is used by the cells for cellular function. Carbon dioxide is a by-product of cellular function and is expelled as a waste product. Respiration is an involuntary act controlled by the medulla oblongata of the brain. The medulla oblongata measures blood levels of carbon dioxide and triggers a respiration when the level of carbon dioxide increases. Although it is an involuntary act, respiration may be altered by holding the breath or when hyperventilation occurs. One inspiration (inhalation) drawing in of air and one expiration (exhalation) expelling air together equals one respiration.

Abnormalities in the characteristics of respiration such as rate, rhythm, and depth are noted when measuring respiration.

Respiratory rate is the number of respirations per minute. The normal respiratory rate, **eupnea,** varies with age, activities, illness, emotions, and drugs. The average respiration rate to pulse rate is 1:4, one respiration to four pulse beats.

Respiratory rhythm refers to the pattern of breathing. This can vary with age, with adults having a regular pattern, whereas infants have an irregular pattern. Rhythm may be altered by laughing and sighing.

Normal respiratory rates

Infants	30–60 respirations per minute
Children (1–7 years)	18–30 respirations per minute
Adults	12–20 respirations per minute

Depth of respiration is the amount of air that is inspired and expired with each respiration. In the resting state, the amount should be consistent. Depth is noted by watching the degree of rise and fall of the chest wall when measuring respiration rate.

Respiration Rate

Respiratory rate is measured by counting breaths for 30 seconds and doubling the amount. This will give the number of respirations per minute. It is important that patients not be aware you are measuring their respirations. Procedure 12-8 describes steps involved in measuring respiration rate.

Abnormalities

Abnormalities of the respiration rate may be found in the rate, depth, rhythm, and sounds of respiration. Rate abnormalities include apnea, tachypnea, bradypnea, and Cheyne–Stokes.

Apnea is the temporary complete absence of breathing. This may be a result of a reduction in stimuli to the respiratory center of the brain. Apnea will occur when the breath is voluntarily held and in Cheyne-Stokes respiration. It can be a serious symptom of other conditions of the cardiovascular and renal systems. It also can result from a head injury such as a concussion.

Sleep Apnea. Airflow during respiration that stops for more than 10 seconds is considered to be sleep apnea. The periods of apnea cause carbon dioxide to accumulate in the blood and oxygen to be depleted. For these reasons, sleep apnea can be dangerous. Oxygen depletion to the brain can cause memory impairment, cognitive changes, and daytime sleepiness. If the condition goes untreated, sleep apnea can result in cardiac arrhythmias, congestive heart failure, cerebral vascular accident (CVA), hypertension, and death.

Sleep apnea is associated with airway obstruction. The soft palate (especially in males who are overweight and who snore) can collapse while the patient is asleep. The result is apnea. The patient usually awakens from sleep enough to resume breathing.

Sleep apnea is diagnosed by sleep laboratory studies when apnea is observed while the patient is sleeping.

Treatment of sleep apnea consists of weight loss and continuous positive airway pressure (CPAP), a device that puts pressure on the airway while the patient sleeps. A mask is placed over the patient's face to keep the airway open. This prevents sleep apnea. A surgical procedure can be performed to remove parts of the soft palate and uvula.

Narcolepsy. Narcolepsy is another type of sleep disorder that causes patients to have daytime sleeping while driving, eating, or sitting in a movie theater. The patient can become paralyzed from the sleep, being unable to move, but can still breathe. The cause may be genetic.

The diagnosis is made by ruling out sleep apnea (through sleep studies) and by the history of repeated episodes of daytime sleeping for a few seconds to a half an hour. The disorder is not under the patient's control.

Tachypnea is a respiratory rate greater than 40 respirations per minute. It may be caused by hysteria or be transient in the newborn. Excessive loss of carbon dioxide may occur if tachypnea is prolonged; there is a potential for this to lead to more serious problems.

Bradypnea is a decrease in the number of respirations and is commonly seen during sleep or because of certain diseases.

Cheyne–Stokes is a regular pattern of irregular breathing rate. The cycle starts with a period of apnea lasting 10 to 60 seconds followed by increasing depth and rate of respiration, which is then followed by a decrease in rate with apnea starting the cycle once again. This cycle may be normal for children but may indicate brain dysfunction.

Orthopnea is a respiratory condition of severe **dyspnea** (labored breathing). Breathing is difficult in any position *other* than sitting erect or standing. This may be seen in patients with heart failure, angina pectoris, asthma, pulmonary edema, emphysema, pneumonia, and spasmodic coughing. Patients who experience orthopnea must be examined in a sitting position. Other positions will cause discomfort and may not be possible.

Abnormalities in the depth of respiration may be divided into shallow abnormalities, such as hypoventilation, and deep abnormalities, such as hyperpnea and hyperventilation.

Hypoventilation occurs when respiration is decreased in rate and shallow in depth; it may result from a depression of nervous stimuli of the respiratory center in the brain.

Hyperpnea is respiration that is increased both in depth and rate. This is commonly seen with activities such as physical exercise. It can also be associated with pain, respiratory diseases, cardiac diseases, hysteria, and some drugs.

Hyperventilation is a type of breathing in which the amounts of oxygen drawn in during inspiration are greatly increased; this results in a decrease in the amount of blood carbon dioxide. Hyperventilation may be associated with asthma, pulmonary embolism or edema, and acute anxiety. The patient may be treated by reducing the amount of oxygen inhaled during an inspiration. The patient may be instructed to hold one nostril closed while breathing, or may be instructed to breathe into a paper bag. Either procedure will reduce the amount of inspired oxygen and bring the oxygen and carbon dioxide blood levels back to within normal range.

Breath Sounds. The presence or absence of breath sounds can be indicative of respiratory problems. Sounds should be listened for and noted when taking the patient's respiratory rate.

Rales (pronounced "rawles") are rattling sounds heard during inspiration and expiration when the lung passageways contain secretions. The physician uses a stethoscope to auscultate or listen for rales, which are associated with some lung diseases. Rhonchi are sounds similar to snoring, usually produced by a rattle in the throat. These are also heard by auscultation.

Wheezes are high-pitched musical sounds heard on expiration. They can be the result of an obstruction in the bronchi and bronchioles of the lungs. Wheezes are commonly associated with asthma and **emphysema,** a chronic pulmonary disease characterized by dilated and damaged alveoli.

Stridor is a crowing sound heard on inspiration as a result of an obstruction of the upper airway. It is associated with laryngitis, a foreign body obstruction, and croup in children.

Stertorous respiration is described as a snoring sound with labored breathing. The sound is created by obstruction of air passages in the head. It may be heard in a patient with a brain injury.

BLOOD PRESSURE

Blood pressure measures cardiovascular function by measuring the force of blood exerted on peripheral arteries during the cardiac cycle or heartbeat. The measurement consists of two components. The first is the force exerted on the arterial walls during cardiac contraction and is called **systole.** The second is the force exerted during cardiac relaxation and is called **diastole.** They represent the highest (systole) and lowest (diastole) amount of pressure exerted during the cardiac cycle. Blood pressure is recorded as a fraction, with the systolic measurement written, followed by a slash, and then the diastolic measurement.

Example: systole/diastole or 120/80

Blood pressure may be affected by many factors including blood volume, peripheral resistance, vessel elasticity, condition of the muscle of the heart, genetics, diet and weight, activity, and emotional state.

- Blood volume is the amount of blood in the arteries. Increased volume increases blood pressure, whereas a decrease in volume will decrease blood pressure as in the case of a hemorrhage or severe dehydration.
- Peripheral resistance is the resistance to blood flow in the arteries. The resistance is in direct relation to the **lumen** of the arteries. The smaller the lumen, the more pressure needed to push blood through, whereas the reverse is also true: the larger the lumen, the less resistance and less pressure needed to push the blood through. The size of the lumen can become smaller from deposits of fatty cholesterol (plaque), resulting in an increase in blood pressure.
- Vessel elasticity refers to the ability of arteries to expand and contract to provide a steady flow of blood. As a person ages, elasticity of the vessels is reduced. Atherosclerosis can cause an increase in arterial wall resistance, resulting in an increase in blood pressure.

- The condition of the heart muscle is extremely important to blood flow and blood pressure. A strong heart muscle provides a forceful pump resulting in efficient blood flow and normal blood pressure. A weak heart muscle results in an inefficient pumping action of the heart leading to a decrease in blood pressure and blood flow. See Chapter 25, Electrocardiography.

The viscosity of the blood also is a factor in blood pressure. Viscosity refers to how sticky a substance is, in this case, the blood. If the blood is sticky, it acts thicker. Imagine holding a bottle of thin syrup upside down over your pancakes. The thin syrup comes out of the bottle quite readily. Now imagine holding a bottle of thick molasses over the pancakes. Being very viscous, the molasses is thicker and much more difficult to pour. So it is with viscous blood; it is thicker and requires a lot more work for the heart muscle to move it through the vessels, thus increasing the pressure inside the walls of the arteries. In fact, it may be so viscous that it might not be able to reach the tiniest capillaries of the kidney, eyes, and other areas without substantial increase in blood pressure. The viscosity of the blood and the resulting increased blood pressure helps explain why uncontrolled diabetes can adversely affect the kidneys and the small capillaries of the eyes and other organs.

Equipment for Measuring Blood Pressure

Blood pressure is measured by the auscultatory (listening) method using a sphygmomanometer and a stethoscope (Figure 12-6). There are three types of sphygmomanometers commonly used in the ambulatory care setting: mercury, digital, and aneroid manometers (Figures 12-7 to 12-9).

Mercury sphygmomanometers are being phased out with other mercury-containing medical equipment, such as mercury thermometers. Aneroid and electronic blood pressure measuring devices are more commonly used. Many medical facilities continue to use mercury sphygmomanometers while phasing them out in agreement with the EPA, but the process has been slower than the phasing out of mercury thermometers; therefore, information about the mercury sphygmomanometers is provided in this chapter.

The mercury **manometer** consists of a cuff containing a rubber bladder attached by rubber tubing to a glass column of mercury. The blood pressure is read at the meniscus of the mercury as it descends the column. Mercury manometers are the most accurate method of blood pressure measurement and are considered the standard because blood pressure is measured in millimeters of mercury. Although the most accurate, mercury manometers do have disadvantages: they are not as portable as aneroid manometers, and there is always the danger of a mercury spill should the glass column break and cause health and environmental problems. Mercury manometers need to be cleaned and checked regularly for accuracy by a professional technician. Care in handling and storage is important to prevent air bubbles and dirt from forming in the column or breaking the glass containing the mercury.

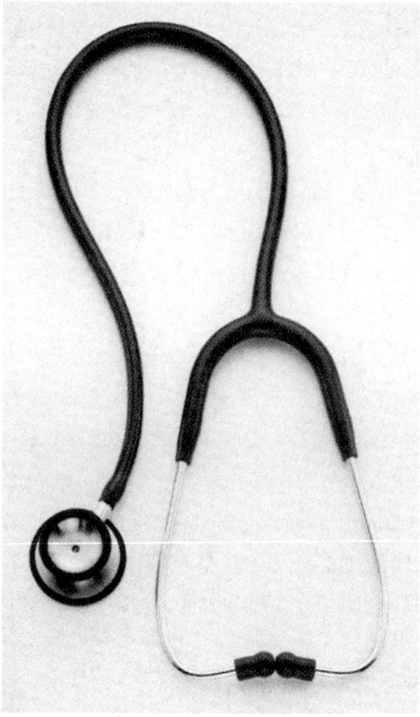

Figure 12-6 Adult stethoscope used with a sphygmomanometer to measure blood pressure. (Courtesy of Welch-Allyn.)

The aneroid manometer is a cuff containing a rubber bladder attached to a dial. The blood pressure is read at the point of the needle descending the dial. Aneroid manometers need to be calibrated regularly because they do not maintain calibration easily. Care in handling and storage will decrease the loss of calibration. Although not as accurate as a mercury manometer, aneroid manometers are easily portable and there is no danger of a mercury spill.

Cuff sizes in both mercury and aneroid manometers range from the smallest pediatric cuff to the largest obese and thigh cuff (Figure 12-10). The appropriate cuff size is necessary to obtain an accurate blood pressure measurement. A cuff that is too small will give an artificially high blood pressure reading, whereas a cuff that is too large will give an artificially low reading. The selection of the cuff size depends on the size of the arm, not the age of the patient. Due to the size of the arm, it may be necessary

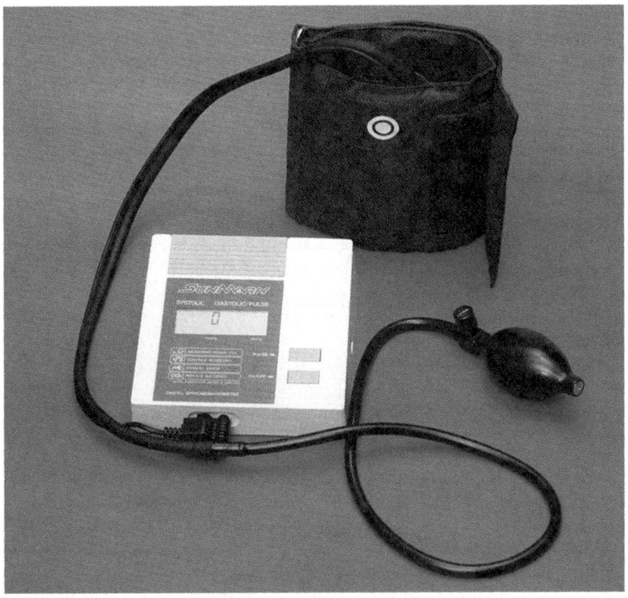

Figure 12-7 Digital sphygmomanometer.

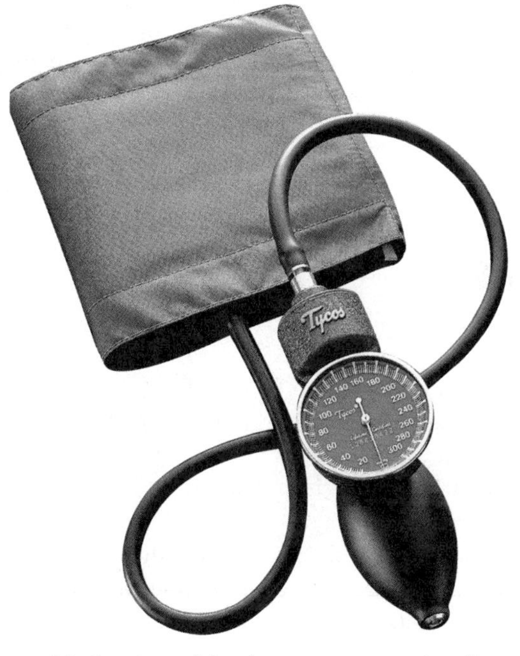

Figure 12-8 Aneroid sphygmomanometer. (Courtesy of Welch-Allyn.)

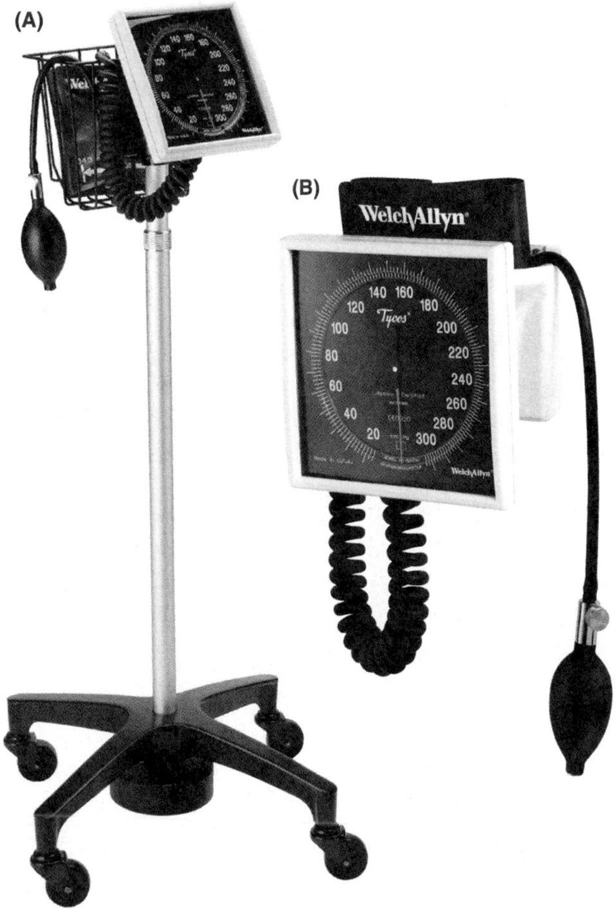

Figure 12-9 (A) Mobile aneroid sphygmomanometer. (B) Wall-mounted aneroid sphygmomanometer. (Courtesy of Welch-Allyn.)

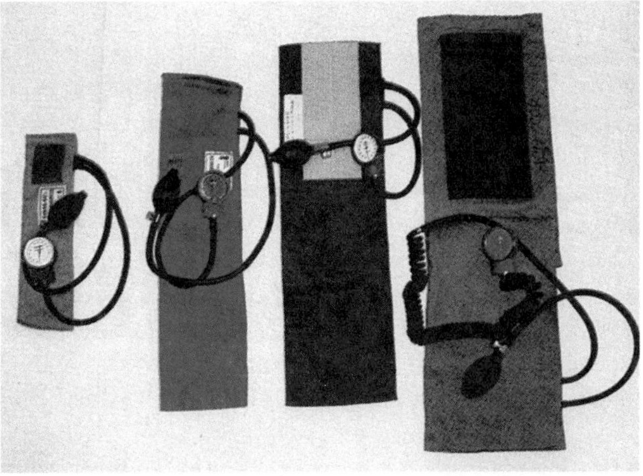

Figure 12-10 Blood pressure cuffs in sizes to fit the arm of a small child to an adult thigh. It is important to have the correct size to obtain an accurate reading.

to use an adult-size cuff on a child or a pediatric-size cuff on an adult. Adult cuffs should have a width that covers one-third to one-half the circumference of the arm. The length of the bladder should cover approximately 80% of the arm (about twice the size of the width). The cuff for a child should cover two thirds of the upper arm.

Measuring Blood Pressure

The sounds heard during blood pressure measurement are named the Korotkoff sounds. The cause of the sounds is not known. They may be a result of distention of the vessels or the sound of the blood passing through the vessels. In either case, Korotkoff sounds have five distinct phases. Not all phases are heard easily, especially for beginners.

- *Phase I*. Begins with the first sound heard when deflating the cuff. It is a sharp tapping sound. Note this first sound as this will be the *systolic reading* of the blood pressure.
- *Phase II*. This sound is the result of more blood passing through the vessels as the cuff is deflated. The sound is that of a soft swishing sound.
- *Phase III*. More blood continues to pass through the vessels as the cuff is deflated. The sound is a rhythmic tapping sound. If blood pressure measurements are not carefully followed and Phases I and II are missed, Phase III may erroneously be reported as the systolic pressure.
- *Phase IV*. Blood is now passing through the vessels fairly easily as the cuff is deflated. The sounds heard will be a muffling and fading of the tapping sounds. This phase may be used to record the diastolic pressure in children and in those patients where a tapping sound is heard to zero.
- *Phase V*. Blood is flowing freely at this time, consequently all sounds disappear. The disappearance of sounds is noted and recorded as the *diastolic pressure*.

When measuring blood pressure, keep two things in mind: patient comfort and accuracy.

Auscultatory gap is heard in some patients. It is a time, usually between Phases I and II or III, when all sounds disappear. Within 20 to 30 mm Hg, or 20 to 30 **increments** on the aneroid, the sounds reappear. If the procedures are not followed carefully, the auscultatory gap is easily missed, and the blood pressure measurement is incorrect in that systolic and diastolic readings may be in error according to the length of the gap. See Table 12-1.

Pulse pressure is the difference between the systolic and diastolic measurements. The normal range for pulse pressure is 30 to 50 mm Hg. The difference should be no more than one third of the systolic reading.

TABLE 12-1 ERRORS IN BLOOD PRESSURE MEASUREMENT PROCEDURES

Errors in measuring blood pressure must be avoided. Common errors include:

1. Improper cuff size.
2. The arm is not at heart level. Do not hold the arm up or let the patient hold up the arm. Pressure is increased when this is done.
3. Cuff is not completely deflated before use or after palpatory method, resulting in a higher pressure measurement.
4. Deflation of the cuff is faster than 2 to 4 mm Hg per heartbeat or 20–30 increments on the aneroid. Sounds are missed if this happens.
5. Reinflating the cuff during the procedure without allowing the arm to rest for one to two minutes.
6. Patient is not relaxed and comfortable. An anxious, apprehensive patient will have a reading that is higher than the actual blood pressure.
7. Improper cuff placement. Cuff is too loose, too tight, or not positioned correctly over the brachial artery.
8. Defective equipment in which there are air leaks in the bladder or valve, the mercury column is dirty, or air bubbles are present. Mercury and aneroid sphygmomanometers are not calibrated at zero.
9. Taking blood pressure measurements over clothing.

All of these errors are easily corrected by following careful procedure and by having the manometers calibrated and cleaned according to a regular maintenance schedule.

Recording Blood Pressure Measurement

The blood pressure is recorded on the patient chart in a fraction format. The position of the patient (sitting or lying down) may be noted. The arm used is also noted, particularly if the blood pressure has been taken in both arms.

Example: 120/80, rt. arm, supine

For children and those patients whose blood pressure can still be heard to zero, the beginning of Korotkoff Phase IV and zero are both recorded.

Example: 120/70/0

Procedure 12-9 outlines the procedure for measuring blood pressure.

Normal Blood Pressure Readings

Normal blood pressure is low at birth and gradually increases with age until adulthood, at which point it should remain fairly constant.

Newborn	50–52/25–30
Child 6 years	95/62
Child 10 years	100/65
Adolescent 16 years	118/75
Adult	Systolic less than 120 Diastolic less than 80
Prehypertension	120–139/80–89
High blood pressure	Above 140/90

Blood Pressure Abnormalities

There are only two possible blood pressure abnormalities: hypertension, blood pressure that is consistently above normal; and hypotension, blood pressure that is consistently below normal in which the patient is unable to function.

Hypertension. There are four types of **hypertension:** primary or essential, secondary, benign, and malignant.

- The most commonly seen form of hypertension is primary or essential. It is hypertension with no apparent cause or cure but is treatable. Treatment is designed to control hypertension and is a lifelong process. It will not be cured, just controlled. The American Heart Association (AHA) suggests that to diagnose hypertension, the diagnosis is based on the average of two or more readings at each of the two or more visits to the physician's office after the initial baseline screening. According to the AHA, normal blood pressure for adults 18 years and older is less than 120/80, prehypertension is 120–139/80–89, hypertension stage 1 is 140–159/90–99, and hypertension stage 2 is ≥160/≥100.
- Secondary hypertension is the result of some underlying problem such as renal disease, pregnancy, endocrine imbalances, obesity, arteriosclerosis, or atherosclerosis. Once the underlying problem has been removed, the blood pressure returns to normal or near normal. Secondary hypertension can be successfully treated.
- Hypertension that has a slow progression but may progress to the same end point as in malignant hypertension is referred to as benign hypertension.
- Malignant hypertension progresses rapidly with severe damage to the cardiovascular system, possibly to the point of death.

Hypotension. **Hypotension** is blood pressure persistently less than normal, usually less than 90/60, although this may be normal for some healthy adults. Hypotension is defined as a blood pressure so low that the patient is unable to function normally. It is usually a result of various shocklike conditions such as hemorrhage, traumatic or emotional shock, central nervous system disorders, or chronic wasting diseases. With successful treatment of the underlying problems, the blood pressure usually will be in the range of normal readings.

Orthostatic hypotension, sometimes called postural hypotension, occurs when a person rapidly changes position from supine to standing, when standing in one position for too long, or as a side effect of certain medications. In this instance, the blood pressure has momentarily decreased, and the person will experience vertigo (dizziness) and may have blurred vision. These symptoms usually last only a few seconds, just long enough for the blood pressure to return to normal. Care should

Patient Education

Hypertension is at epidemic proportions in the United States, and many patients are not treated because they do not know that they have the problem. It is known as the "silent epidemic" because most people do not experience any symptoms over a span of years. However, untreated or poorly treated hypertension over time can damage the heart, cause myocardial infarction, cause a stroke (cerebral vascular accident), or lead to kidney failure.

There are several nondrug ways to reduce blood pressure, even for people who have inherited hypertensive tendencies. Steps to take include: eating plenty of produce, grains, and low-fat dairy foods; cutting back on salt; stopping smoking; exercising regularly; maintaining a healthy weight; limiting alcohol intake; and reducing stress. It is easy to see that these recommendations all are lifestyle changes. They can significantly reduce blood pressure if practiced daily.

Critical Thinking

Discuss the normal vital signs differences expected between an infant and an adult.

be taken when helping patients to an upright position from a supine position because orthostatic hypotension can lead to syncope (fainting) and injury from falling.

HEIGHT AND WEIGHT

Although not considered a vital sign, height and weight are routinely measured if warranted by the age and the physical condition of the patient. Many physicians prefer that height and weight be measured as part of a yearly physical examination and otherwise may vary the frequency of patient height and weight measurements. Height and weight are normally measured simultaneously.

For children, height and weight are typically measured during each physician visit. The height of adults may be obtained on the initial visit only and weight taken on all visits. An adolescent or young adult may have height measured more frequently to plot body changes. Because older adult patients tend to lose the cushioning between vertebrae through osteoporosis as part of aging, they may need to have their height measured more frequently to check the stage of any degeneration.

Older adult patients require special attention by the medical assistant when measuring height and weight. It is especially important to assist older adult patients both on and off the scale, for the scale platform is movable, and older adult patients may lose their balance and fall if unassisted. A stand-alone walker can be placed over the scale platform to aid in stabilizing the patient.

Height

To measure a patient's height, a scale with a measuring bar is necessary (Figure 12-11). A paper towel is placed on the scale because the patient's shoes should be removed for accurate measuring. The patient is asked to step on the scale and face away from the measuring bar. Assist patient onto the scale; the scale platform is movable and the patient could fall.

There are two reasons for having the patient's back to the scale. When the measuring bar is lifted, it could cause face or eye injuries if the patient were facing the bar. Lifting the measuring bar prior to the patient stepping on the scale can also lead to eye and face injuries in that the patient could inadvertently walk into the bar. Another reason to have the patient's back to the scale is if the patient does not look straight ahead, the head is not level, which could result in a less than accurate measurement.

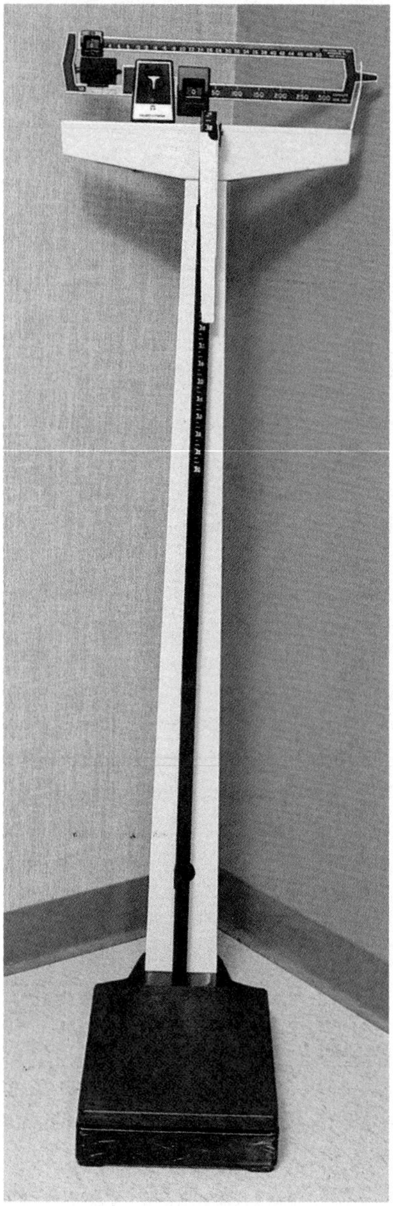

Figure 12-11 Traditional beam balance scale with measuring bar.

After the patient is on the platform, the measuring bar is placed firmly on the patient's head, and the line between where the solid bar and sliding bar meet is read. The bars are measured in quarter inches (Figure 12-12). Children's heights may be recorded in inches, whereas adults will be recorded in feet and inches. Conversion from inches to feet is accomplished by taking the num-

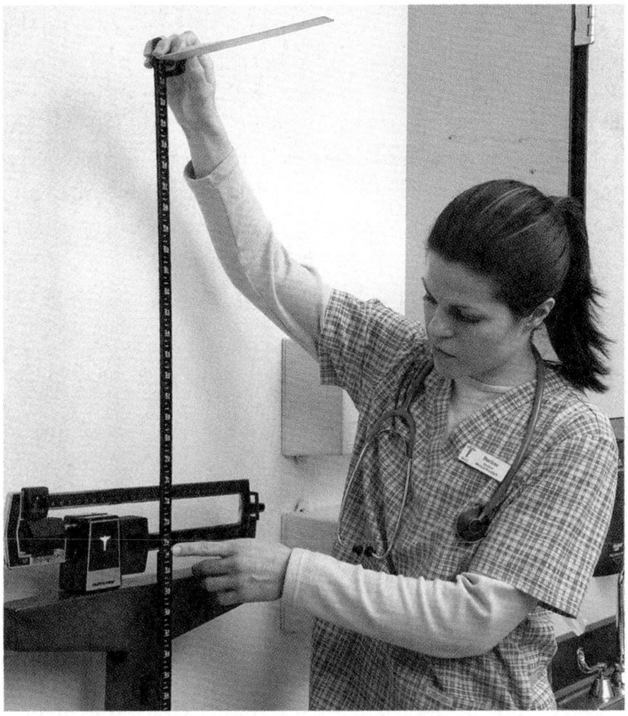

Figure 12-12 Read the height at the movable point of the ruler. The bars are measured in quarter inches.

ber of inches and dividing by 12. See Procedure 12-10 to measure height.

Weight

Physician preference and patient health will dictate the frequency of measuring an adult's weight. Some physicians require the patient's weight measured on each visit, whereas others do not if there are no health problems that require weight monitoring. Some health conditions that do require weight monitoring include obesity, eating disorders, hormone disorders such as diabetes and thyroid malfunction, hypertension, pregnancy, cancer, and some digestive disorders.

When measuring the weight of a patient, the medical assistant must maintain the patient's privacy. Most people are conscious of their weight and may become embarrassed if the measurement is taken where others may see and hear. Privacy is important and often overlooked. The medical assistant must also be careful of comments regarding a patient's weight particularly with the obese patient and with those being treated for eating disorders (see Chapter 22). Encouragement for weight loss for the dieting patient is beneficial but must be done in privacy. Other comments are inappropriate.

Occasionally a patient will be instructed by the physician to monitor weight at home. It is important for the patient to understand the necessity of weighing at the same time each day because weight may vary significantly throughout the day. A normal routine is to measure weight before breakfast.

Before an accurate weight can be obtained, the scale must be calibrated. The point of the balance beam must be floating in the center when no weight is applied to the scale. Some scales are equipped with a screw at the end that can be turned slightly until the beam is in the correct floating position. Once it is centered, it is calibrated and ready for use.

An eye-level digital scale with measuring bar measures height in the same way on the measuring bar of the digital scale as it is on the balance beam measuring bar. Weight measurement is quicker, easier, and usually safer taken on the digital scale. The scale platform is stationary, and the patient is assisted as needed onto the scale; the digital reading is ready in a few seconds.

The patient will wear normal indoor clothing, rather than disrobing, for weight measurement. Heavy coats or other outerwear should be removed. Heavy objects and purses should not be held during the procedure. A chair or counter should be provided to place these objects on while the procedure is being performed. Shoes should be removed. See Procedure 12-11 for measuring adult weight.

Occasionally, as in the case of medication dosage, the medical assistant may be required to convert pound weight into kilogram weight.

1 kilogram = 2.2 pounds

To convert pounds to kilograms:

Take the number of pounds and divide by 2.2

Example: 130 pounds divided by 2.2 = 59.09 kg

To convert from kilograms to pounds:

Take the number of kilograms and multiply by 2.2

Example: 40 kilograms multiplied by 2.2 = 88 lb.

Significance of Weight

The careful monitoring of a patient's weight may provide an insight into metabolic, nutritional, and emotional problems.

Critical Thinking

Discuss the methods the medical assistant may use to obtain patient cooperation when taking vital signs. Describe and demonstrate the appropriate charting procedure for normal vital sign results.

MEASURING CHEST CIRCUMFERENCE

Occasionally, the medical assistant may be instructed to measure the chest of an adult. This procedure is done on patients with emphysema and as a requirement for insurance and truck driver licenses. Two measurements will be taken, one on the deepest inspiration and one on the deepest expiration. A comparison is then made to ascertain chest capacity. To perform the procedure, ask the patient to disrobe from the waist up. Place a tape measure around the chest at nipple level. Instruct the patient to inhale deeply while you measure, then ask the patient to exhale completely while you take the second measurement. Record the results as inspiration number and expiration number. The physician performs any necessary comparison (see Chapter 18, Examinations and Procedures of Body Systems).

Procedure 12-1 Measuring an Oral Temperature Using an Electronic Thermometer

STANDARD PRECAUTIONS:

PURPOSE:

To obtain an oral temperature.

EQUIPMENT/SUPPLIES:

Electronic thermometer
Probe covers
Biohazard waste container

PROCEDURE STEPS:

1. Wash hands and follow standard precautions.
2. Assemble equipment.
3. Identify patient.
4. Position the patient in a comfortable position.
5. Determine if the patient has ingested hot or cold drinks or food or has been smoking within the previous half hour. RATIONALE: Ingesting hot or cold substances or smoking can result in an arbitrary increase or decrease in temperature results.
6. Explain the procedure. RATIONALE: To obtain patient cooperation and consent.
7. Select blue (oral) probe.
8. Cover with probe cover (Figure 12-13). RATIONALE: To prevent microorganism cross contamination.
9. Insert under the tongue to either side of the mouth (Figure 12-14). RATIONALE: Under

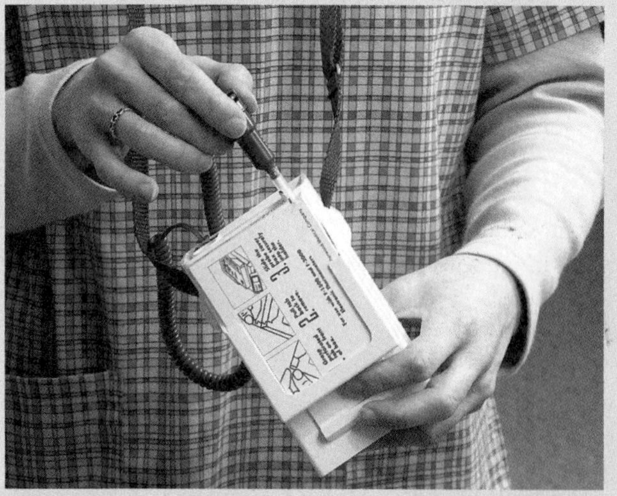

Figure 12-13 Slide the probe into the disposable cover, adjusting if necessary.

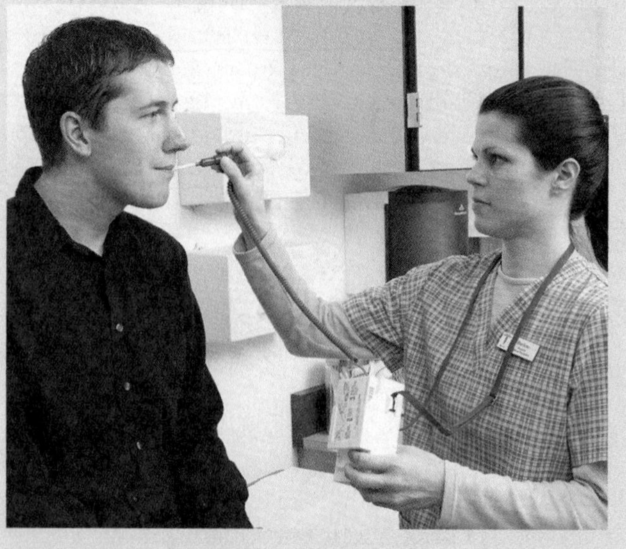

Figure 12-14 Insert the thermometer under tongue to either side of mouth.

(continues)

Procedure 12-1 (continued)

the center of the tongue is the **frenulum**, which impedes placement in this area.

10. Instruct patient to close mouth without placing teeth on thermometer. RATIONALE: To prevent air leakage.
11. Leave in place until the beep is heard.
12. Remove thermometer after appropriate time has elapsed.
13. Read the results on the digital display window.
14. Discard probe cover in biohazard waste container (Figure 12-15).
15. Replace electronic thermometer in the base holder, if required for recharging.
16. Wash hands.
17. Record temperature.
18. Document the procedure.

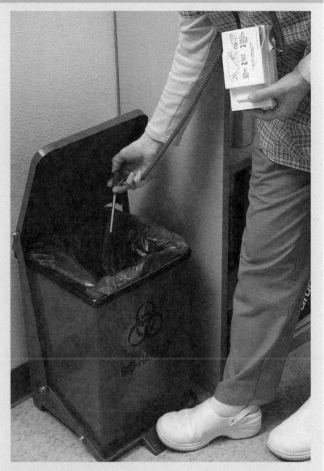

Figure 12-15 Discard probe cover in biohazard waste container.

DOCUMENTATION

5/26/20XX 11:00 AM T 99.2°F, P 96, R 14. C. McInnis, RMA

Procedure 12-2 Measuring an Aural Temperature Using a Tympanic Thermometer

STANDARD PRECAUTIONS:

PURPOSE:
To obtain an aural temperature using a tympanic thermometer.

EQUIPMENT/SUPPLIES:
Tympanic thermometer (Figure 12-16)
Covers or ear speculum
Waste container

PROCEDURE STEPS:
1. Wash hands following Standard Precautions.
2. Assemble equipment.
3. Identify the patient.
4. Explain procedure. RATIONALE: This will help gain patient's cooperation and consent.
5. Place cover on thermometer (Figure 12-17).
6. Set thermometer to start.
7. Gently straighten ear canal up and back for adults and place probe into ear canal to seal the area and activate the system (Figure 12-18). RATIONALE: Air leaks will occur if the ear canal is not sealed.
8. Wait until the temperature is displayed on the screen.
9. Remove from the ear.
10. Discard cover into waste container by pressing the release button.
11. Wash hands.
12. Replace thermometer.
13. Record temperature in patient chart.

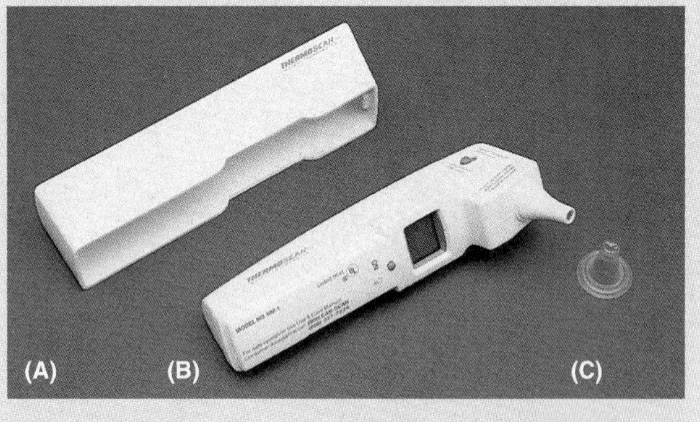

Figure 12-16 Tympanic thermometer: (A) holder, (B) tympanic thermometer, and (C) disposable speculum or cover.

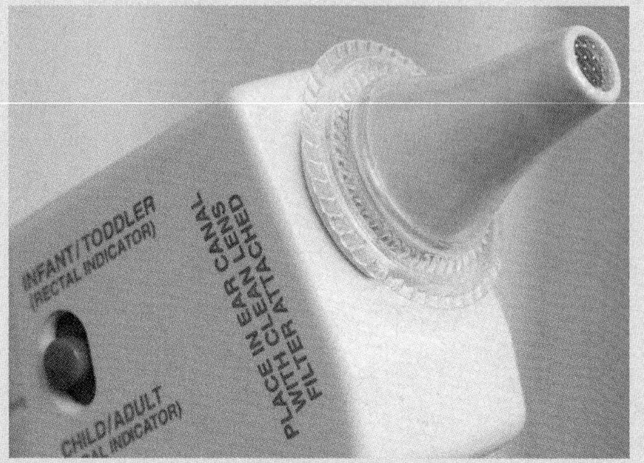

Figure 12-17 Attach the disposable speculum or cover to the tympanic thermometer to prevent spread of microorganisms between patients.

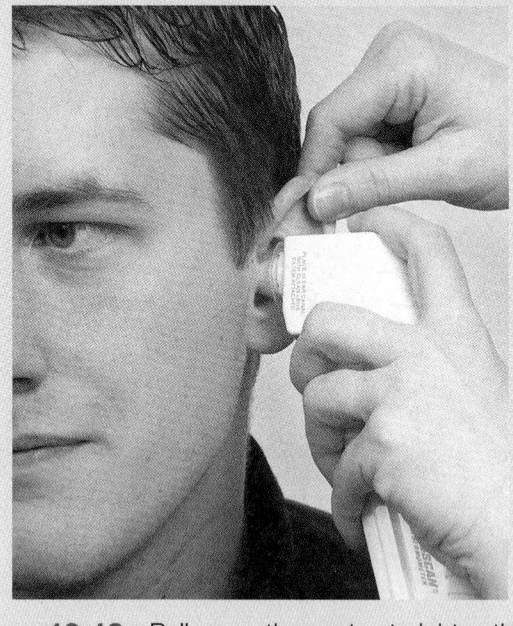

Figure 12-18 Pull up on the ear to straighten the auditory canal for an accurate reading.

DOCUMENTATION
5/26/20XX 4:00 PM T 99.6° (Tym) F, P 100, R 20. C. McInnis, RMA

Procedure 12-3 Measuring a Rectal Temperature Using a Digital Thermometer

STANDARD PRECAUTIONS:

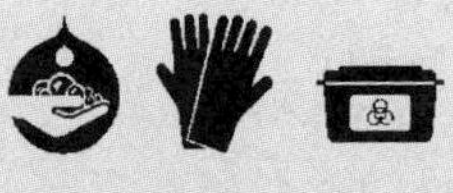

PURPOSE:

To obtain a rectal temperature using a digital thermometer.

EQUIPMENT/SUPPLIES:

Digital thermometer with red probe (rectal)
Probe cover
Lubricating jelly
Gloves
Biohazard waste container

PROCEDURE STEPS:

1. Wash hands and glove following Standard Precautions.
2. Assemble equipment.
3. Identify patient.
4. Explain procedure to patient. RATIONALE: Ensures understanding and gains patient cooperation and consent.
5. Remove clothing from the waist down, drape as necessary. RATIONALE: Maintains patient modesty, privacy, and warmth.
6. Position patient in Sims' position.
7. Place probe cover on red probe (rectal). RATIONALE: To prevent microorganism cross contamination. Red probe indicates rectal thermometer.
8. Lubricate with lubricating jelly. RATIONALE: Easier insertion of thermometer and safety for patient.
9. Spread buttocks, gently insert thermometer into the rectum past the sphincter (1½ inches) for adult.
10. Hold buttocks together while holding the thermometer. Do not let go of thermometer. RATIONALE: Holding buttocks together prevents air leaks and inaccurate recording. Holding onto thermometer ensures patient safety.
11. Hold in place until the beep is heard.
12. Read results on digital display window.
13. Remove from rectum.
14. Discard probe cover into biohazard waste container by pushing the release button.
15. Replace thermometer on holder base.
16. Remove gloves, discard in biohazard waste container, and wash hands.
17. Offer tissue to patient to wipe anus. Assist patient in dressing and position as necessary.
18. Record on the patient chart labeled with (R), indicating a rectal temperature.

DOCUMENTATION

5/28/20XX 8:00 AM T 99.6° (R) F, P 104, R 20. C. McInnis, RMA

Procedure 12-4 Measuring an Axillary Temperature

STANDARD PRECAUTIONS:

PURPOSE:

To obtain an axillary temperature using a glass or digital thermometer.

EQUIPMENT/SUPPLIES:

Glass or digital thermometer
Sheath
Towelettes
Paper towels

PROCEDURE STEPS:

1. Wash hands following Standard Precautions.
2. Assemble equipment; place sheath on thermometer.
3. Identify patient.
4. Explain procedure. RATIONALE: This elicits patient cooperation and consent.
5. Ask patient to remove clothing to provide access to axilla.
6. Cover patient with gown as necessary to maintain patient modesty and warmth.
7. Wipe axillary area with dry towel or towelette to remove moisture. RATIONALE: Moisture in the axilla will cause inaccurate reading.
8. Place thermometer in axilla.
9. Ask patient to fold arm against chest or abdomen (Figure 12-19).
10. Leave in place for appropriate time according to manufacturer's instructions, usually 10 minutes.
11. Carefully remove.
12. Remove sheath and discard.
13. Read thermometer.
14. Sanitize thermometer. Place on clean paper towel.
15. Wash hands.
16. Place clean thermometer in alcohol for 30 minutes.
17. Document temperature in patient's record, indicating axillary temperature.

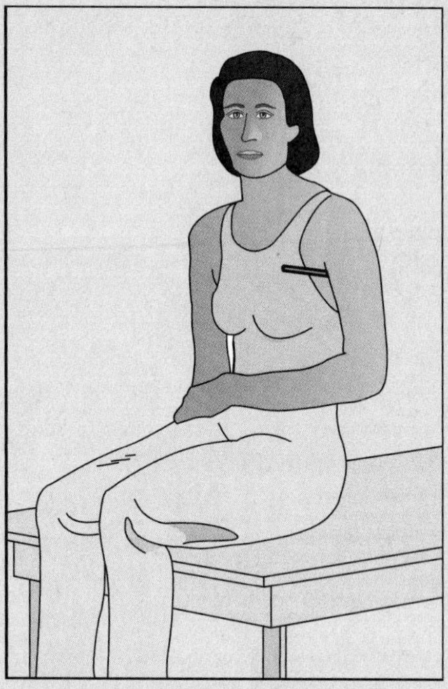

Figure 12-19 After placing thermometer in axilla, ask patient to fold arm against chest or abdomen.

DOCUMENTATION

4/30/20XX 2:00 PM T 97° (A) F, P 64, R 12. J. Guerra, CMA

Procedure 12-5 Measuring an Oral Temperature Using a Disposable Oral Strip Thermometer

STANDARD PRECAUTIONS:

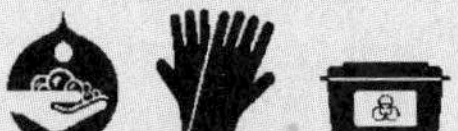

PURPOSE:

To obtain an oral temperature.

EQUIPMENT/SUPPLIES:

Oral strip thermometer (Figure 12-20)
Gloves
Biohazard waste container

PROCEDURE STEPS:

1. Wash hands following Standard Precautions.
2. Assemble equipment.
3. Identify patient.
4. Position the patient in a comfortable position.
5. Determine if the patient has ingested hot or cold drinks or food or has been smoking within the previous half hour. RATIONALE: Ingesting hot or cold substance or smoking can result in an arbitrary increase or decrease in temperature results.
6. Explain the procedure. RATIONALE: To obtain patient cooperation and consent.
7. Apply gloves.
8. Insert disposable oral strip thermometer under the tongue to the side of the mouth. RATIONALE: Under the center of the tongue is the frenulum, the fold of mucus membrane that attaches the tongue to the floor of the mouth, which impedes placement in this area.
9. Instruct patient to close mouth tightly. RATIONALE: To prevent air leakage.
10. Leave in place for 60 seconds.
11. Remove thermometer after appropriate time has elapsed.
12. Wait 10 seconds to read the dots.
13. Read temperature by locating the last dot that has changed color (Figure 12-21).
14. Discard strip in biohazard waste container.
15. Remove gloves and discard in biohazard waste container.
16. Wash hands.
17. Record temperature.
18. Document the procedure.

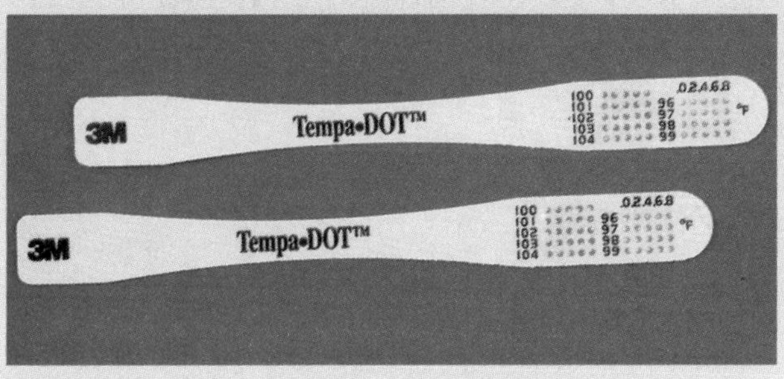

Figure 12-20 Disposable oral strip thermometer.

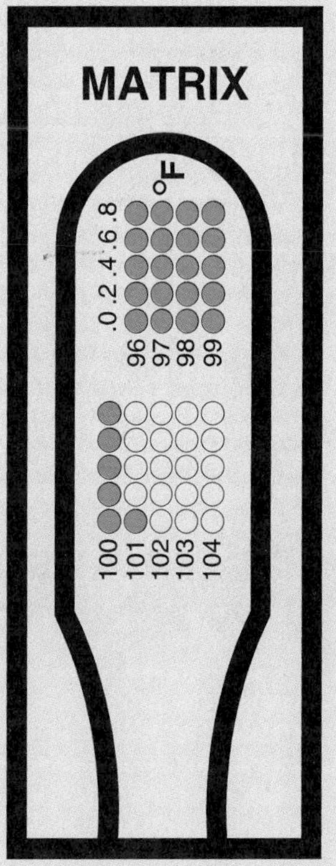

Figure 12-21 The reading on this disposable oral thermometer is 101°F.

DOCUMENTATION

4/16/20XX 3:15 PM T 101°F, P 100, R 22 (disposable oral thermometer reading)
J. Guerra, CMA

Procedure 12-6 Measuring a Radial Pulse

STANDARD PRECAUTIONS:

PURPOSE:
To obtain a pulse rate.

EQUIPMENT/SUPPLIES:
Watch with a second hand

PROCEDURE STEPS:

1. Wash hands.
2. Identify patient.
3. Explain procedure. RATIONALE: Ensures patient cooperation and consent.
4. Position patient with the wrist resting either on a table or on lap (Figure 12-22).
5. Locate the radial pulse with the pads of your first three fingers. Do not use thumb; it has its own pulse.
6. Gently compress the radial artery enough to feel the pulse.
7. Count the pulsations for one full minute.
8. Note any irregularities in rhythm, volume, and condition of artery.
9. Wash hands.
10. Record the pulse in the patient chart after the temperature, noting any irregularities.

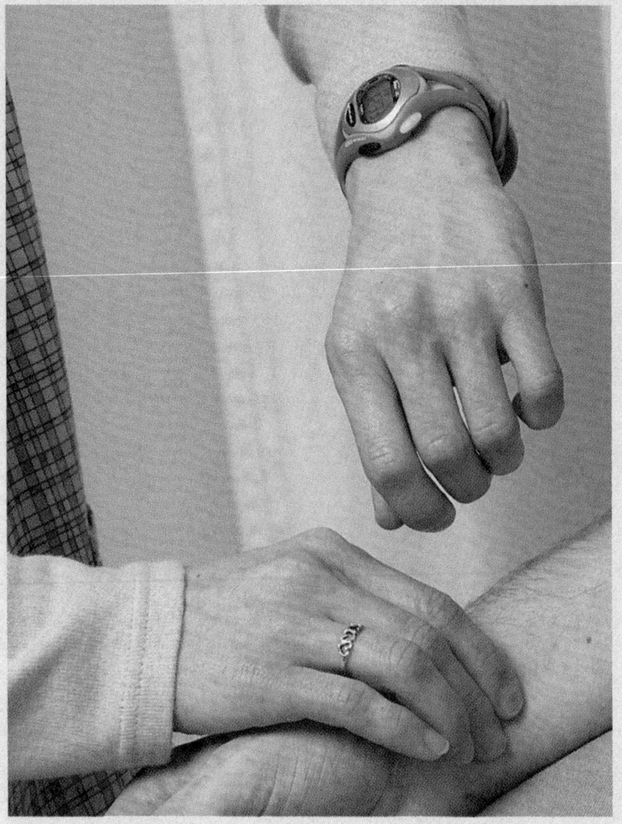

Figure 12-22 Position patient with wrist resting on table or lap.

DOCUMENTATION

2/10/20XX 3:00 PM P 80, regular and strong. D. Kolter, RMA

Procedure 12-7 Taking an Apical Pulse

STANDARD PRECAUTIONS:

PURPOSE:
To obtain an apical pulse rate.

EQUIPMENT/SUPPLIES:
Stethoscope
Watch with second hand
Alcohol wipes

PROCEDURE STEPS:
1. Wash hands.
2. Assemble equipment.
3. Wipe earpiece with alcohol wipes.
4. Identify patient.
5. Explain procedure. RATIONALE: Ensures patient cooperation and consent.
6. Assist patient in disrobing, removing clothing from the waist up.
7. Provide a gown or drape for patient modesty and warmth.
8. Position the patient in a supine position. RATIONALE: Easier access to apex of heart.
9. Locate the fifth intercostal space, midclavicular, left of sternum (Figure 12-23). RATIONALE: Location of apex of heart.
10. Place stethoscope on the site and listen for the lub-dup sound of the heart.
11. Count the pulse for one minute; each lub-dup equals one pulse.
12. Assist the patient to sit up and dress.
13. Wash hands.
14. Wipe earpieces, diaphragm, and tubing of stethoscope.
15. Record the pulse in the patient chart with the designation of (AP) to denote method of obtaining the pulse and note any arrythmias.

NOTE: Apical pulse and radial pulse are frequently taken simultaneously, with the radial pulse taken by another individual (Figure 12-24). Both pulse rates should be identical. A discrepancy may indicate a cardiac problem.

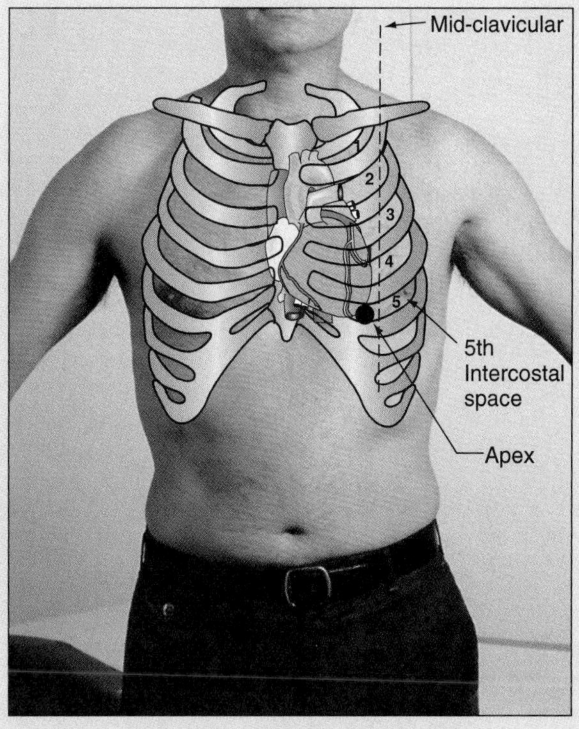

Figure 12-23 Locate the apical pulse by counting intercostal spaces. Locate the fifth intercostal space.

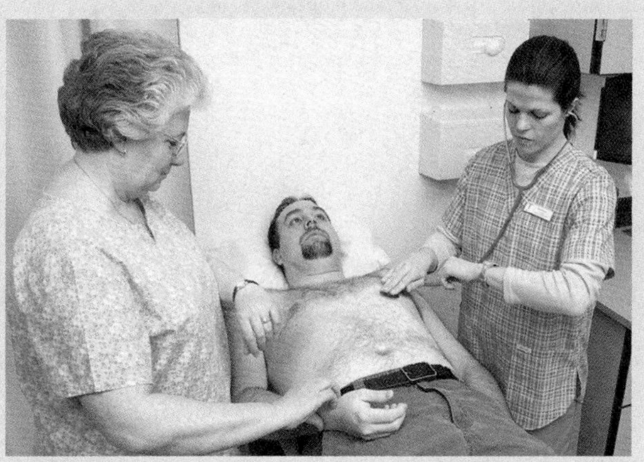

Figure 12-24 Sometimes apical and radial pulses are taken simultaneously.

DOCUMENTATION
7/8/20XX 12 PM T 98.6°F, P (apical) 96 reg. (radial) 100 slightly irregular. Dr. King notified. D. Kolter, RMA

Procedure 12-8 Measuring the Respiration Rate

STANDARD PRECAUTIONS:

NOTE: The respiration rate is normally taken immediately before or after the pulse rate. It should be taken without patient knowledge, because respiration can voluntarily be altered. While counting respirations, it is best to continue grasping the wrist as if still taking the pulse. This procedure will assist in preventing alteration of breathing by the patient.

PURPOSE:
To obtain an accurate respiratory rate.

EQUIPMENT/SUPPLIES:
Watch with second hand

PROCEDURE STEPS:

1. Wash hands.
2. Identify the patient.
3. Position patient in a comfortable position.
4. Watch the rise and fall of the chest wall for one minute, or while holding the patient's arm, place it across the chest and feel for the rise and fall of chest wall. Alternatively, place a hand on the patient's shoulder and feel and watch for the rise and fall of the chest wall.
5. Note depth, rhythm, and breath sounds while counting.
6. Wash hands.
7. Record respiration rate in patient chart, noting any irregularities and sounds.

DOCUMENTATION

8/7/20XX 2:00 PM T 98.6°F, P 84. Rate and rhythm regular. J. Guerra, CMA

Procedure 12-9 Measuring Blood Pressure

STANDARD PRECAUTIONS:

PURPOSE:
To measure blood pressure.

EQUIPMENT/SUPPLIES:
Stethoscope
Sphygmomanometer
Alcohol wipes

PROCEDURE STEPS:

1. Wash hands.
2. Assemble equipment, making sure that cuff size is correct. RATIONALE: Inappropriate cuff size will result in inaccurate measurement.
3. Clean earpieces of stethoscope with alcohol wipe.
4. Identify patient.
5. Explain procedure. RATIONALE: May be the first instance where blood pressure is measured; to allay anxiety and ensure cooperation and consent.
6. Position patient comfortably; if sitting, feet flat on the floor, arm resting at heart level on the lap or a table. RATIONALE: Legs crossed may arbitrarily increase blood pressure; arm above heart level may result in inaccurate reading.
7. Bare the upper arm. If clothing is restricting, have patient remove it. RATIONALE: Tight clothing on the arm can produce inaccurate results.

(continues)

Procedure 12-9 (continued)

8. Palpate brachial artery.
9. Securely center the bladder of the cuff over the brachial artery above the bend of the elbow. RATIONALE: Cuff should be high enough so stethoscope does not touch it. Extraneous sounds may be heard.
10. Palpate the radial pulse and smoothly inflate cuff until the pulse is no longer felt; note the number.
11. Quickly deflate the cuff and allow arm to rest for about one minute. Calculate peak inflation level. RATIONALE: This ensures that an auscultatory gap is not missed.
12. Make sure cuff is completely deflated.
13. Position stethoscope over the brachial artery and hold in position with the fingers only.
14. Inflate cuff smoothly and quickly to the peak inflation level (Figure 12-25).
15. Deflate the cuff at a rate of 2 to 4 mm Hg per heartbeat. RATIONALE: No matter how experienced you become, accurate blood pressure readings cannot be obtained if the cuff deflation is greater than 2 to 4 mm Hg per heartbeat.
16. Listen for Korotkoff Phase I; note when it appears.
17. Continue deflation, noting the Korotkoff phases.
18. Note when all sounds disappear, Korotkoff Phase V.
19. Continue deflating the cuff at the same rate for at least another 10 mm Hg after sounds have disappeared. RATIONALE: To hear an auscultatory gap should one be present.
20. The cuff may then be deflated quickly.
21. Remove the cuff.
22. Clean earpieces and diaphragm of stethoscope with alcohol wipes.
23. Wash hands.
24. Record the measurement in patient's chart.

NOTE: On a patient's initial visit and in patients with hypertension, the physician may want the blood pressure taken in both arms. There is normally a slight variation in pressure between the arms. If it is necessary to repeat the procedure, wait approximately five minutes before doing so.

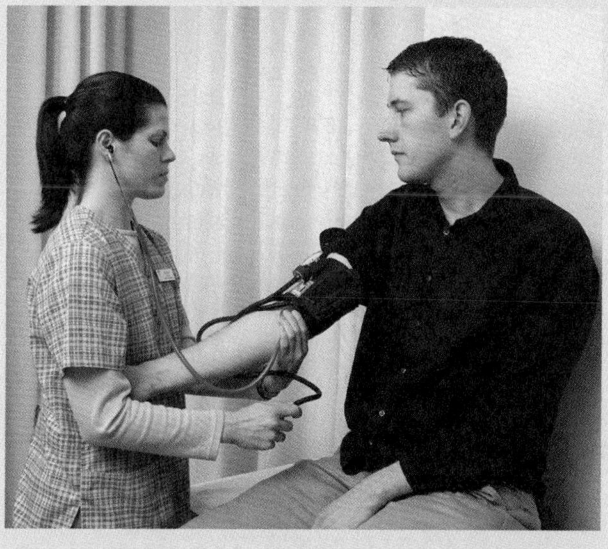

Figure 12-25 Inflate cuff smoothly and quickly.

DOCUMENTATION

2/16/20XX 3:00 PM BP 146/90 in right arm. BP 150/92 in left arm. D. Swingle, CMA

Procedure 12-10 Measuring Height

STANDARD PRECAUTIONS:

PURPOSE:
To obtain the height of a patient.

EQUIPMENT/SUPPLIES:
Scale with measuring bar
Paper towel

PROCEDURE STEPS:

1. Wash hands.
2. Identify patient.
3. Explain the procedure to patient to ensure understanding, cooperation, and consent.
4. Instruct patient to remove shoes and stand on paper towel on scale with back against scale, looking straight ahead. RATIONALE: Back against scale aids patient safety.
5. Assist patient onto scale. RATIONALE: Scale platform is movable, and patient may become unsteady and lose balance and fall.
6. Lower measuring bar until firmly resting on top of head (Figure 12-26).
7. Assist patient to step off of the scale. Allow patient to sit and help with shoes if necessary.
8. Read line where measurement falls.
9. Lower measuring bar to its original position.
10. Wash hands.
11. Record height in patient chart.

Example: Ht. 5′ 6″

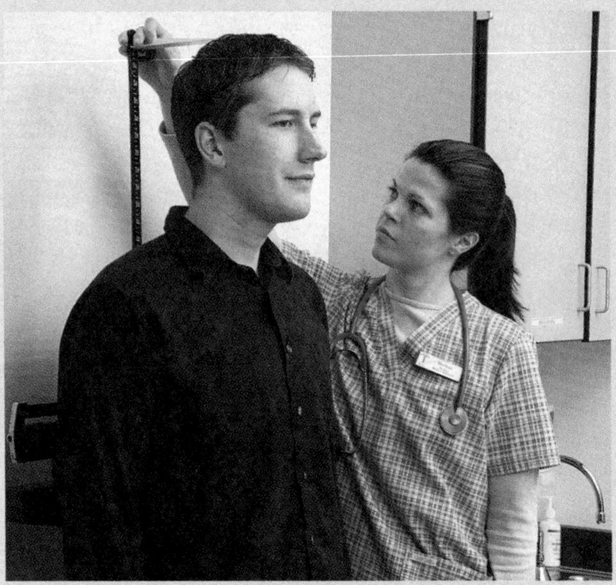

Figure 12-26 To measure height, have the patient stand with back against scale and keep head level.

DOCUMENTATION

3/4/20XX 2:00 PM Ht. 5′ 6″. B. Abbott, RMA

Procedure 12-11 Measuring Adult Weight

STANDARD PRECAUTIONS:

PURPOSE:
To obtain the weight of the patient.

EQUIPMENT/SUPPLIES:
Balance beam or digital scale
Paper towels

PROCEDURE STEPS:

1. Wash hands.
2. Identify patient.
3. Explain the procedure to patient to ensure understanding and cooperation.
4. Place a paper towel on scale. RATIONALE: Paper towel protects patient's feet from microorganisms.
5. Instruct the patient to place heavy objects on the area provided, including heavy objects that may be in their pockets.
6. Instruct the patient to remove shoes, jackets, and heavy sweaters and step on the scale. Assist patient to the center of the scale. RATIONALE: The scale platform is movable, and the patient may become unsteady, lose balance, and fall. The platform on the digital scale is stationary, but assist the patient onto the scale platform and read the digital reading. If using a balance beam scale, continue with Steps 7 through14 (Figure 12-27).
7. Move the lower weight bar (measured in 50-pound increments) to the estimated number (the patient may be asked for approximate weight).
8. Slowly slide the upper bar until the balance beam point is centered (see Figure 12-27).
9. Read the weight by adding the upper bar measurement to the lower bar measurement.
10. Assist the patient to step off of the scale.
11. Provide a chair for the patient to sit to put on shoes. Return objects to the patient.
12. Return the weights to zero.
13. Wash hands.
14. Record measurement in the patient chart.

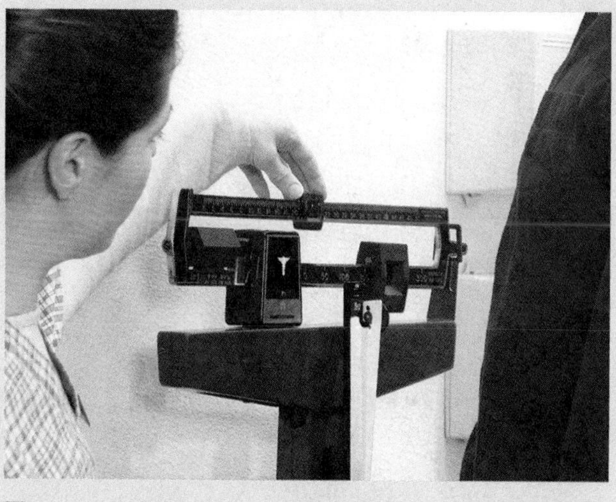

Figure 12-27 When weighing the patient, slide the upper bar until the balance beam point is centered.

DOCUMENTATION

5/2/20XX 3:00 PM Wt. 142 lbs. B. Abbott, RMA

Case Study 12-1

Herb Fowler, a regular patient of Dr. Lewis at Drs. Lewis and King, is a black man in his 50s. He has smoked for many years and only recently has thought about quitting smoking because of a chronic cough. Herb is also significantly overweight but has a hard time making the decision to give up smoking *and* change his diet. Although his blood pressure has been stable for the last few years, Audrey Jones, CMA, is concerned when she takes Herb's vital signs during his most recent checkup. His weight is slightly up and his blood pressure has jumped from 140/90 to 156/100.

CASE STUDY REVIEW

1. Is a blood pressure reading of 156/100 a cause for concern? Should Audrey take a second reading?
2. In addition to alerting the physician to the change in Mr. Fowler's blood pressure and weight, Audrey feels she may be able to provide advice to the patient (with physician's permission). How can Audrey use her communication and medical assisting knowledge to counsel Herb Fowler on lifestyle changes?
3. To follow up, Audrey reviews her knowledge of hypertension and discusses the four types with the physician. What are the four kinds of hypertension and what are their characteristics?

SUMMARY

Throughout life, a patient will undergo various measurements to ascertain growth, development, and general health and well-being. The normal range for each of these measurements will vary according to the stage of life of the patient at the time of examination. The medical assistant must be aware of what to expect when measuring a patient in each life stage. Awareness of normal expectations for each stage of life will help the medical assistant to perform the procedures in a more effective and efficient manner and aid in observing any abnormal signs and measurements.

Together with differences seen with age, the medical assistant will see differences in patients because each patient has unique medical problems.

The medical assistant has a great responsibility when performing patient measurements and must ensure accuracy, patient safety, comfort, and confidentiality while obtaining accurate results.

STUDY FOR SUCCESS

- ❑ Review the Key Terms
- ❑ Practice the Procedures
- ❑ Consider the Case Study and discuss your conclusions
- ❑ Answer the Review Questions
  - ❑ Multiple Choice
  - ❑ Critical Thinking
- ❑ Navigate the Internet by completing the Web Activities
- ❑ Practice the StudyWARE activities on your student CD
- ❑ Apply your knowledge in the Student Workbook activities
- ❑ Complete the Web Tutor section
- ❑ View and discuss the DVD situations

REVIEW QUESTIONS

Multiple Choice

1. The most dependable and accurate route for taking a temperature is:
   a. oral
   b. aural (tympanic)
   c. rectal
   d. axillary
2. The artery commonly used for taking a patient's pulse is:
   a. carotid
   b. brachial
   c. radial
   d. popliteal
3. A blood pressure cuff that is too small for the patient's arm will:
   a. have no effect on the results
   b. give an arbitrarily low result
   c. give an arbitrarily high result
   d. have an effect on certain patients only
4. The term used to indicate a pulse rate significantly above the average is:
   a. bradycardia
   b. tachycardia
   c. arrhythmia
   d. sinus rhythm

Critical Thinking

1. Discuss the responsibilities of the medical assistant when measuring vital signs.
2. Describe the care and use for each of the various types of thermometers.
3. Discuss the reasons that a professional must be aware that mercury thermometers and other mercury-containing equipment are being phased out of use.
4. Describe the procedure for converting temperatures from Fahrenheit to Celsius and vice versa and calculate the following conversions:
   a. 98.6°F = ____________________ °C
   b. 39.1°C = ____________________ °F
5. Discuss the rationale for not using the thumb for taking the pulse rate of a patient.
6. Discuss the reasons for taking the respiratory rate of a patient without the patient's knowledge.
7. Discuss the importance of using the appropriate blood pressure cuff size when measuring a patient's blood pressure.
8. Describe the following:
   a. hypertension
   b. tachycardia
   c. apnea
   d. remittent fever

WEB ACTIVITIES

1. Using a search engine, access information on the Internet from the American Heart Association regarding essential hypertension and answer the following:
   a. What population of people in the United States is at greatest risk for essential hypertension?
   b. List four patient education tips for reducing blood pressure without the aid of medication.
   c. Check the list of normal blood pressure readings in this chapter and compare it with what the American Heart Association says are normal blood pressure measurements at various ages.
2. Access information on the Internet from the National Research Council and list its recommendations for weight of the following women:

Height	Age	Weight in Pounds
5′ 2″	19–34 years	?
5′ 4″	19–34 years	?
5′ 6″	19–34 years	?

THE DVD HOOK-UP

DVD Series
Skills Based Series

Program Number
5

Chapter/Scene Reference
- *Watch entire program*

This chapter discusses the proper techniques for obtaining the patient's vital signs and steps for measuring and weighing the patient.

This program illustrated many techniques for obtaining various vital signs. In the taking a radial pulse scene, the medical assistant noticed a problem with the patient's rhythm and decided to take an apical pulse as well. The chapter states that you should place the patient in a supine position and locate the apex of the heart when taking an apical pulse. The DVD program illustrated the medical assistant taking an apical pulse with the patient sitting in an upright position. It also had a more complicated technique for finding the apex of the heart.

1. How do you think you should manage a patient with an arrhythmia? How can you keep the patient from becoming concerned?
2. Which method do you think would work better for measuring an apical pulse: the method listed in the book or in the DVD program? Why?

DVD Journal Summary

Write a paragraph that summarizes what you learned from watching today's DVD program. At the end of the blood pressure scene, the medical assistant told the patient that her blood pressure was 158/100, which is quite elevated. Do you think it was wise of the medical assistant to tell the patient her reading? Do you think it is acceptable to tell patients their blood pressure when it is normal? Why or why not?

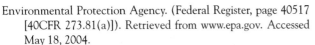

REFERENCES/BIBLIOGRAPHY

Environmental Protection Agency. (Federal Register, page 40517 [40CFR 273.81(a)]). Retrieved from www.epa.gov. Accessed May 18, 2004.

Michigan State University. *Mercury containment initiative*. Retrieved from www.aware.msu.edu. Accessed March 22, 2004.

National Library of Medicine, National Institute of Health. http://cerhr.niehs.nih.gov/genpub/topics/mercury.html. Accessed April 28, 2005.

Taber's cyclopedic medical dictionary. (22nd ed.). (2003). Philadelphia: FA Davis.

CHAPTER 13

The Physical Examination

OUTLINE

KEY TERMS

- Ataxia
- Bruits
- Catheterization
- Cyanosis
- Fenestrated Drape
- Jaundice
- Labyrinthitis
- Pallor
- Pyorrhea
- Scleroderma
- Symmetry
- Tinnitus
- Vertigo
- Vitiligo

OBJECTIVES

The student should strive to meet the following performance objectives and demonstrate an understanding of the facts and principles presented in this chapter through written and oral communication.

1. Define the key terms as presented in the glossary.
2. Describe the six methods used in physical examinations.
3. Name and describe eight positions used for physical examinations.
4. Discuss the purpose of draping and demonstrate the appropriate draping procedure for each type of position.
5. Identify at least 10 instruments and supplies used for examination of various parts of the body.
6. Identify eight basic components of a physical examination.
7. Describe the sequence followed during a routine physical examination.
8. Recall method of examination, instrument used, and position for examination of at least eight body parts.

FEATURED COMPETENCIES

CAAHEP—ENTRY-LEVEL COMPETENCIES

Patient Care

- Prepare and maintain examination and treatment areas
- Prepare patient for and assist with routine and specialty examinations

ABHES—ENTRY-LEVEL COMPETENCIES

Clinical Duties

- Prepare patients for procedures
- Prepare and maintain examination and treatment area
- Assist physician with examinations and treatments

SCENARIO

At the multiphysician Inner City Health Care facility, five physicians are employed on a rotating basis, with two or three working at any one time. Clinical medical assistants Wanda Slawson, CMA, and Bruce Goldman, CMA, have developed a clear understanding of what each physician prefers in both room and patient preparation. Wanda and Bruce also coordinate with each other and with office managers Jane O'Hara and Walter Seals, both CMAs, to ensure patient comfort. Depending on the patient and the type of examination, Wanda will often assist with patient preparation when the patient is female and Walter will assist when the patient is a male.

INTRODUCTION

Physical examinations are performed to obtain a picture of the health and well-being of the patient. An initial examination will provide a baseline reference for future examinations. The examination follows a standard routine, usually starting at the head and following through the entire body, including all major organs and body systems. Although the sequence of events for the physical examination is relatively standard, variations will occur according to physician preference, type of practice, and patient's chief complaint. Diagnostic procedures such as laboratory tests and X-rays may be ordered or performed in the facility or sent to an outside laboratory. At the conclusion of the physical examination, the physician will have an impression of the patient's general health, a diagnosis if possible, and treatment plans. The physician uses information from three major sources to aid in making a diagnosis: the health history, the physical examination, and laboratory tests and diagnostic procedures.

The role of the medical assistant throughout the physical examination will greatly depend on the physician. Some physicians will delegate many duties to the medical assistant, whereas others will require little assistance. Commonly performed clinical medical assisting duties related to physical examinations can be divided into two categories: patient preparation and room preparation. Patient preparation includes patient explanation and preparation, positioning, draping, vital signs, specimen collection such as urine and blood, and electrocardiogram (ECG). Room preparation includes assembling the appropriate instruments and equipment for the physician and assuring patient privacy and comfort.

Additional medical assisting duties include supporting the patient, handing the physician instruments and equipment as required, and taking notes dictated by the physician. Throughout and after the examination, the medical assistant will adhere to the principles of medical asepsis and standard precautions as required by Occupational Safety and Health Administration (OSHA). The effective medical assistant will establish an efficient but flexible routine providing for the needs of both the patient and physician.

Spotlight on Certification

RMA Content Outline
- Physical examinations

CMA Content Outline
- Preparing/maintaining treatment areas
- Examinations
- Procedures
- Explanation and instructions
- Instruments, supplies and equipment

CMAS Content Outline
- Examination Preparation

METHODS OF EXAMINATION

There are six methods used by the physician to examine the body. They include observation or inspection, palpation, percussion, auscultation, mensuration, and manipulation. The physician will use all in total or in part depending on the type of examination being performed.

Observation or Inspection

Observation or inspection is the process of observing the patient. The general health, posture, body movements, skin, mannerisms, and care in grooming are all noted. Closer observation will be focused on body **symmetry** (correspondence in shape and size of body parts located on opposite sides of the body) and contour. Deformities and skin rashes will be observed. Skin color is also noted (Figure 13-1).

Palpation

Palpation is an examination of the body using touch and may be used to help verify observations. A body part or organ may be felt for size and condition. Abdominal masses may be felt through the abdominal wall. Skin texture, moisture, and temperature can be felt. The contour of limbs and rigidity and position of bones and joints may be felt. Palpation may be performed with the use of fingertips, one or both hands, or the palm of the hand (Figure 13-2).

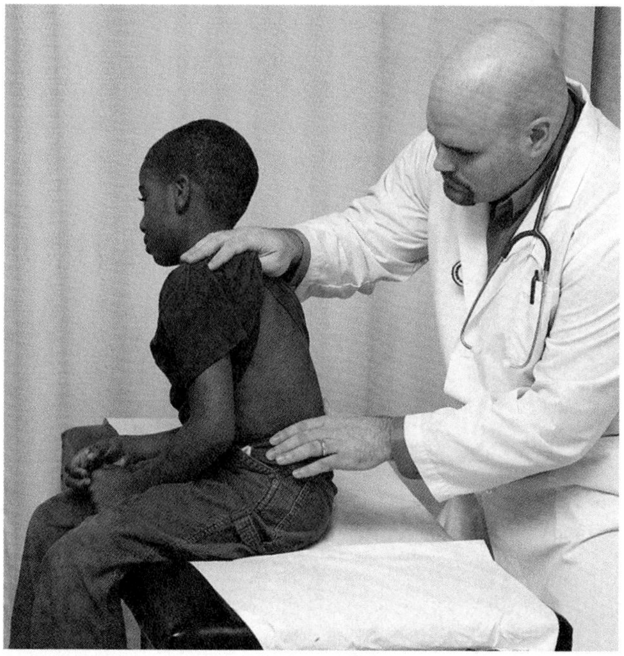

Figure 13-1 The physician observes the patient for signs of disease. This method of examination is known as observation or inspection.

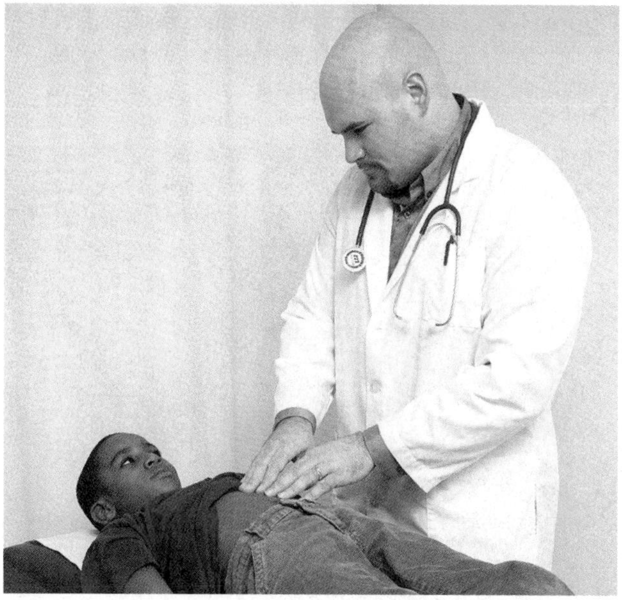

Figure 13-2 The physician palpates the abdomen during the physical examination to feel for abnormalities.

Percussion

Percussion is the process of eliciting sounds from the body by tapping with either a percussion hammer or fingers. The vibrations and sounds from underlying organs and cavities can be felt and heard. Using this method can determine the presence of air or solid material in the organ or cavity being checked. Healthy structures that are dense, such as the liver, produce a dull sound. Hollow structures such as the lungs should produce a more hollow sound. There are two methods used to perform percussion. The direct method is by tapping directly on the surface of the skin. The indirect method is performed by placing a finger or hand on the surface of the skin and tapping the hand (Figure 13-3).

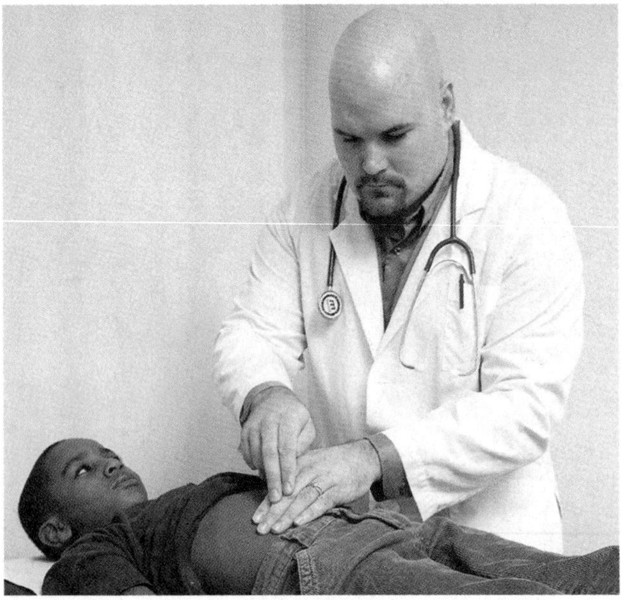

Figure 13-3 The physician uses percussion during the physical examination to tap the body to produce sounds that may indicate disease.

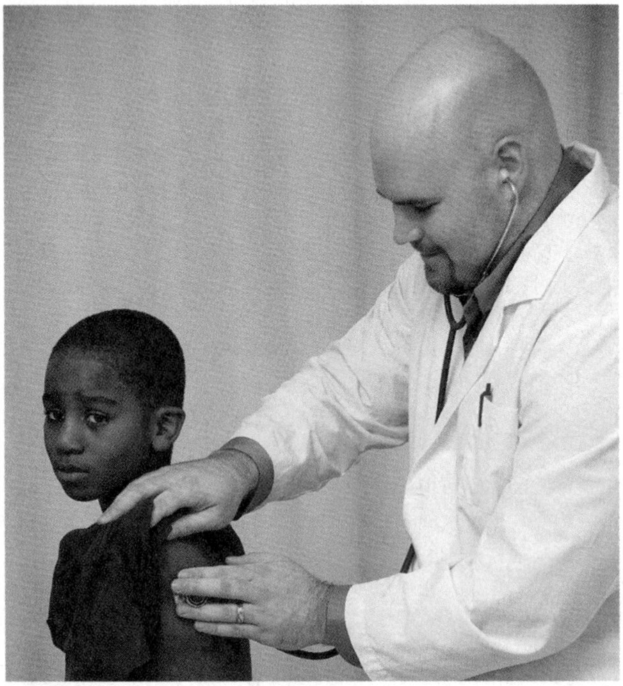

Figure 13-4 The physician uses a stethoscope to listen to sounds from the patient's body. This method of physical examination is known as auscultation.

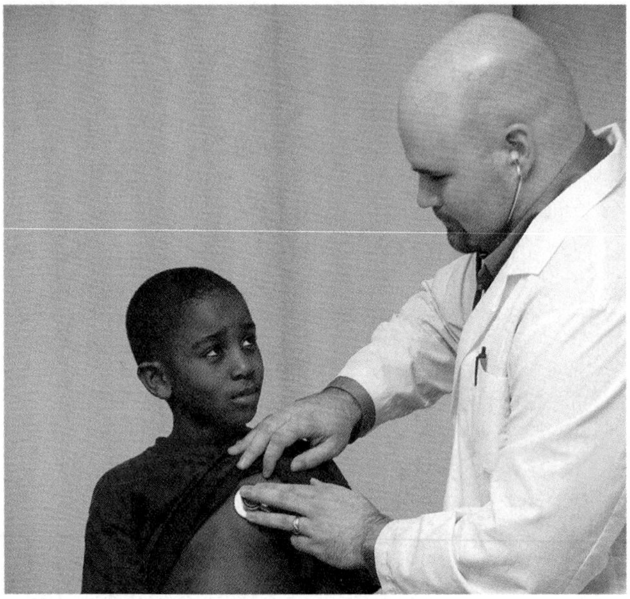

Figure 13-5 Auscultation is performed on the anterior and posterior portion of the body.

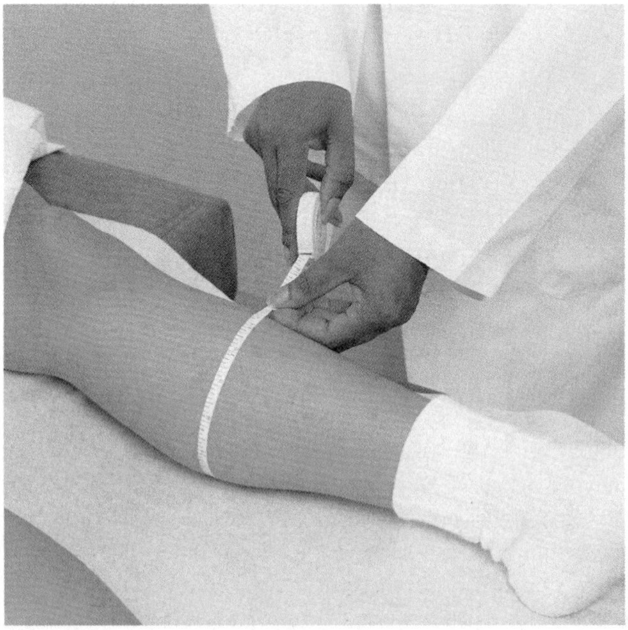

Figure 13-6 A tape measure may be used to measure the circumference of the calf of the patient's leg or other body part. This method of physical examination is known as mensuration.

Auscultation

Auscultation is the process of listening directly to body sounds, normally with a stethoscope. The physician listens for lung and heart sounds such as murmurs, rales, or **bruits,** which generally are abnormal sounds heard on auscultation of an organ or vessel such as a vein or an artery. The abdomen will be examined for bowel sounds that include the clicks and gurgles of normal bowel activity, the sounds that occur with peristalsis (Figures 13-4 and 13-5).

Mensuration

The mensuration method of examination uses the process of measuring. The measurement of height and weight, the length of a limb, and the amount of flexion and extension of an extremity are all forms of mensuration. Measurement of chest and infant head circumference are also forms of mensuration. In most instances, a tape measure is used to perform mensuration of an infant's head or circumference of a body part (Figure 13-6).

Manipulation

Manipulation checks the amount of flexion and extension of a joint by applying forceful passive movement on the joint. Range of motion of some joints may be checked using this method.

POSITIONING AND DRAPING

Physical examinations may require the patient to be placed in various positions. Each position is designed to make examination of a particular area of the body easier and more efficient. The medical assistant may assist the patient in undressing and will provide the appropriate drape and gown. The medical assistant also instructs the patient about the appropriate position required for the examination and may assist the patient into position by providing support and guidance. Always provide for patient safety.

Proper draping to protect modesty and prevent embarrassment and comfort from chills is essential. If patients are capable of helping themselves, the medical assistant should leave the room while the patient undresses and puts on a gown. If the patient is disoriented or extremely ill, the medical assistant must stay in the room; patient privacy can be provided by discreetly removing clothing and covering the patient as quickly as possible. When the patient is a child, the medical assistant should note the comfort level of the child while the child undresses. Children develop modesty at an early age and may be embarrassed by sitting on the examination table wearing only underwear. Respect a child's right to privacy by offering a gown or drape. Older adults will need assistance with undressing and draping. Care must be taken to provide as much modesty and privacy as possible as you assist patients of all ages.

Never turn your back on seriously ill or disoriented patients or young children. Ensure patient safety at all times.

Examination Positions

There are a number of positions that may be required of the patient during the physical examination. The position used will depend on the type of examination. Seven common positions are outlined in Procedures 13-1 through 13-7. These include:

1. Supine (horizontal recumbent) (see Procedure 13-1)
2. Dorsal recumbent (see Procedure 13-2)
3. Lithotomy (see Procedure 13-3)
4. Fowler's (see Procedure 13-4)
5. Knee-Chest (see Procedure 13-5)
6. Prone (see Procedure 13-6)
7. Sims' (see Procedure 13-7)

Supine (Horizontal Recumbent). The supine position is assumed when lying flat facing up (Figure 13-7). It is used for examination of the anterior surface of the body from head to toe. When the physician is performing a physical examination on a female patient that includes a breast examination, she should be provided with a gown and instructed to wear it with the opening in the front. A drape is then placed over the lap or from the waist down.

Dorsal Recumbent. The patient lies on his or her back (dorsal) face up, legs separated, knees flexed with feet flat on the table (Figure 13-8). This is the most

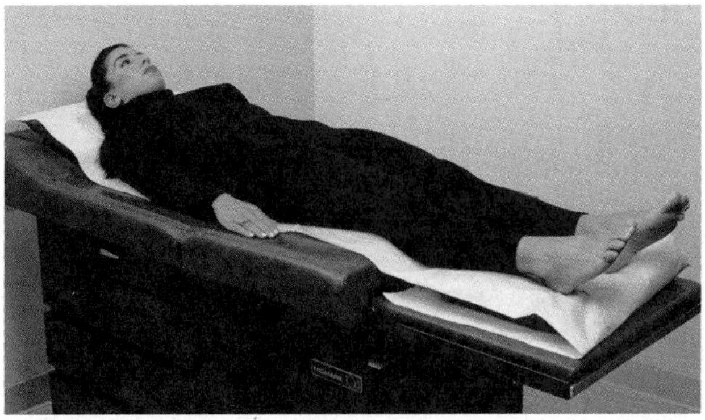

Figure 13-7 Supine or horizontal recumbent position.

comfortable position for patients with back and abdominal problems. Examinations performed in this position include rectal, genital, head, neck, and chest, as well as abdominal palpation. It can also be used for urinary **catheterization.** Preteen and early teen girls requiring a pelvic examination may be placed in this position and will require careful instructions and procedure explanations. The patient is covered with a drape that is diamond shaped. One edge of the diamond can be lifted to examine the genitalia without exposing the rest of the body.

Lithotomy. The patient is assisted to lie on her back similar to the dorsal recumbent position except the buttocks should be as close to the bottom edge of the table as possible, and feet are placed in stirrups attached to the foot of the table (Figure 13-9). The lithotomy position is used for genital and pelvic examinations. It can also be used for urinary catheterization. At the conclusion of the examination, the patient should slide toward the head of the table before getting up from this position. Patients with special needs, such as older adults and those physically challenged as with severe arthritis, may not be able to assume this position. If this is the case, assist patient into Sims' position or modified Dorsal position (see Procedure 13-7) and the sigmoidoscopy, proctoscopy, or pelvic exam can be done in this position for these patients.

A modification of the dorsal recumbent position is often used for female external genitalia examinations, especially female urologic examinations, some gynecologic examinations, and examinations during pregnancy. This position consists of the patient lying on the examination table on her back, with her knees bent. The feet are together with the heels pulled up toward the buttocks. During the examination, the knees are relaxed apart. The physician may stand to the side of the patient during the examination. This position has many advantages over the lithotomy position, if a full pelvic examination is not required.

Fowler's. The patient sits in a position with the back of the examination table raised to either 45 degrees (Semi-Fowler's; Figure 13-10) or 90 degrees (High-Fowler's; Figure 13-11). Legs rest flat on the table. A pillow may be placed under the knees. This position is used for patients having cardiovascular or respiratory problems to facilitate

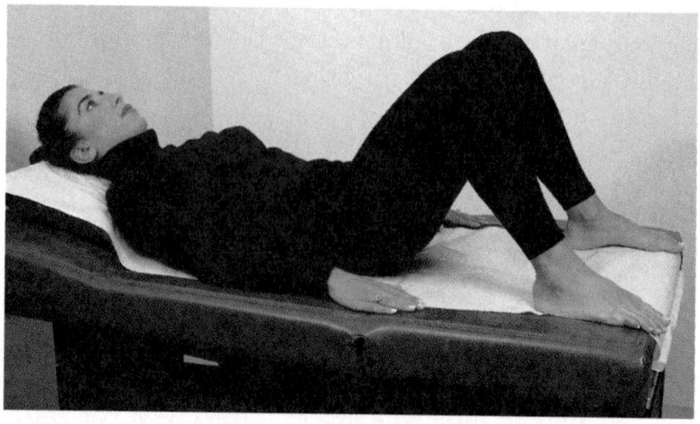

Figure 13-8 Dorsal recumbent position.

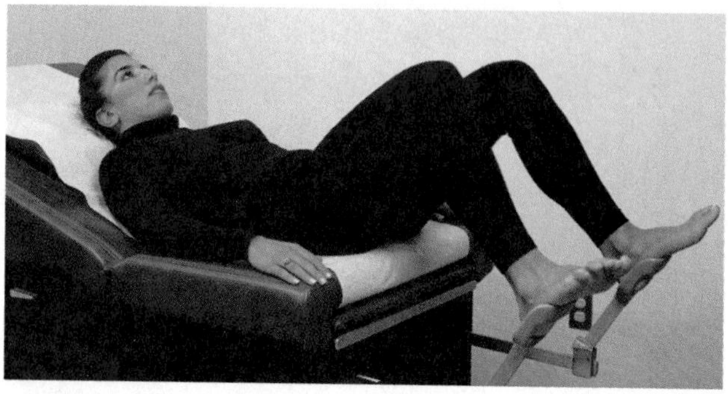

Figure 13-9 Lithotomy position.

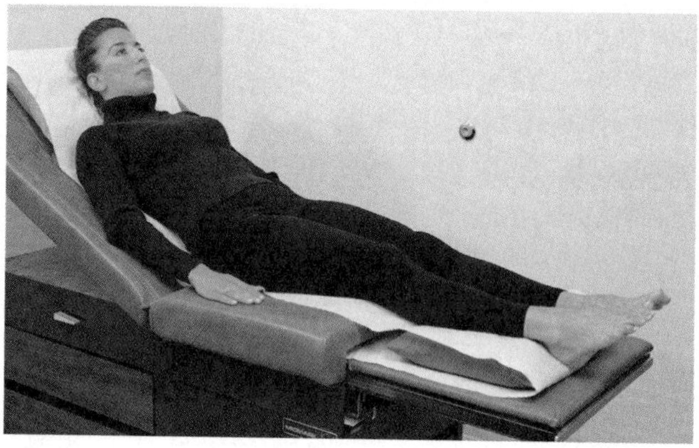

Figure 13-10 Semi-Fowler's position (45-degree angle).

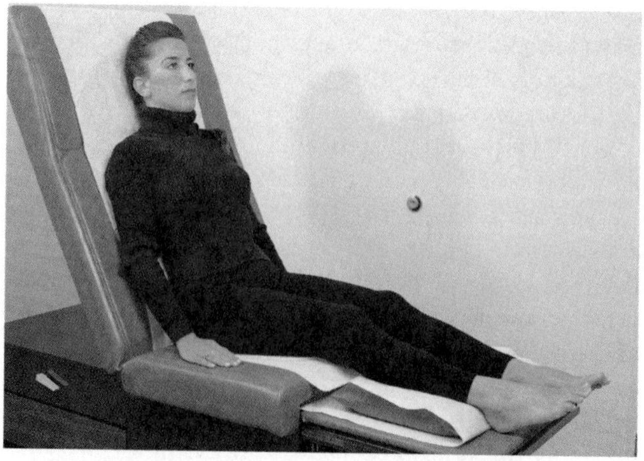

Figure 13-11 High Fowler's position (90-degree angle).

their breathing, and for examination of the upper body and head.

Knee-Chest. The knee-chest position puts the weight of the body on the knees and chest (Figure 13-12). The patient is instructed to kneel on the table and spread the knees shoulder width apart. The buttocks should be elevated, back straight with the chest resting on the table. The head is positioned to one side, with arms flexed on the side of the head and hands under the head. This is not a comfortable position, and the patient may need assistance. If the position is too uncomfortable or difficult, have the patient rest on the elbows. The knee-chest position is unnecessary if the clinic has a proctologic table (Figure 13-13). This position is used primarily for proctologic examinations, sigmoidoscopy procedures, and in some instances vaginal examinations. Draping will require a large drape to cover the entire body. It may be necessary to use two smaller drapes, holding them together with towel clamps. A diamond- or triangle-shaped drape allows for one edge to be lifted to expose only the rectal area. Do not place the patient in knee-chest position until the physician is ready to begin the procedure.

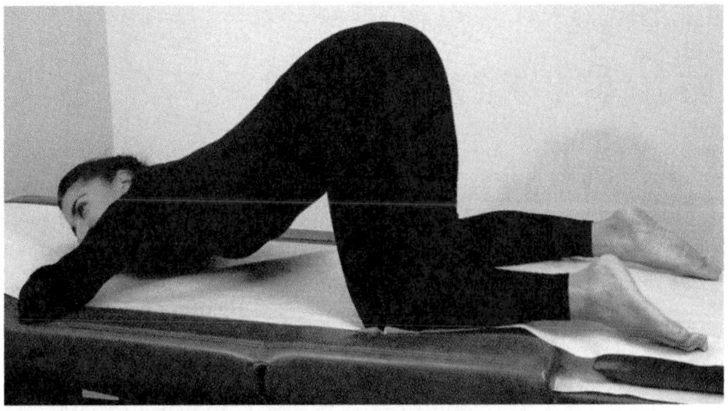

Figure 13-12 Knee-chest position.

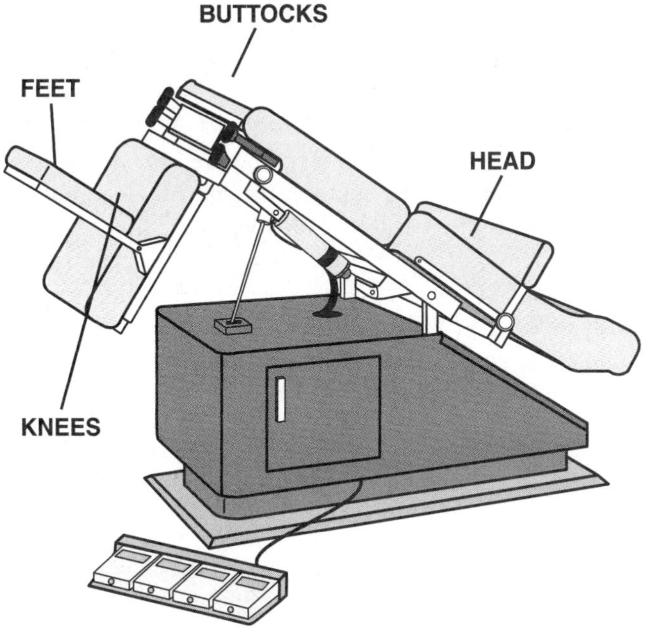

Figure 13-13 Proctologic table.

Proctologic. This position requires the use of a specialized table known as a proctologic examination table (Figure 13-13). The patient is instructed to undress from the waist down and to kneel on the knee board of the table. The patient then bends at the hips and rests the chest on the table. The head is supported by a head board. The table is then turned to elevate the buttocks. A triangular, diamond-shaped, or **fenestrated drape** will cover the patient from the shoulders to the knees. This position is used for proctologic examinations.

Prone. The patient is instructed to lie face down on the table with head turned to side, arms may be placed above head or along side of body (Figure 13-14). The drape must cover from the mid-chest area to the legs. This position may be used for examining the posterior aspect of the body, including the back or spine.

Sims' (lateral). The patient is instructed to lie on the left side; the left arm and shoulder may be drawn back behind the body (Figure 13-15). The left knee is

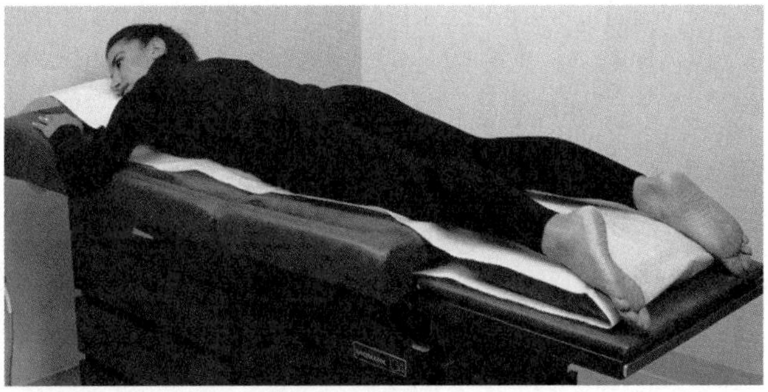

Figure 13-14 Prone position.

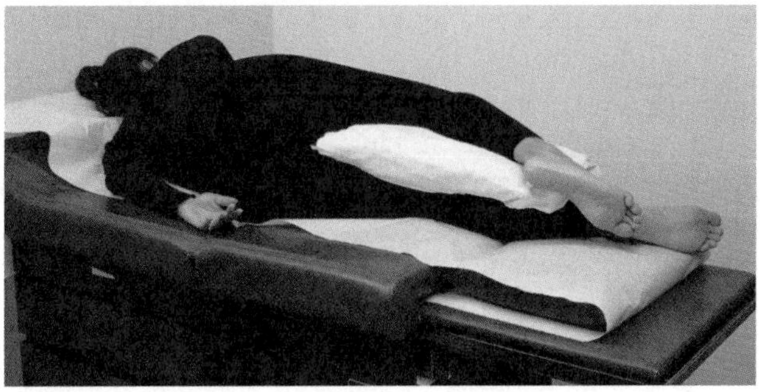

Figure 13-15 Sims' or lateral position.

Critical Thinking

Describe a type of examination that may be performed while the patient is placed in each of the following positions: (1) lithotomy, (2) Sims', (3) knee-chest, and (4) supine.

slightly flexed to support the body, and the right knee is flexed sharply. A small pillow is provided for under the patient's head and a pillow may also be placed between the patient's legs if it does not interfere with the examination being performed. The drape should be large enough to cover the patient from the shoulders to the knees (triangle or diamond shape to expose rectum). This position may be used for vaginal or rectal examination, for rectal temperatures, sigmoidoscopy, or for enemas.

Trendelenburg. Trendelenburg position can be used for two reasons. The first is to aid a person who is in shock. By lowering the head and elevating the legs, blood flow from the major vessels in the lower extremities will, by gravity, flow upward toward the brain and major organs. This may help to increase blood pressure enough to sustain the patient until taken to the emergency department. (See Chapter 9, Emergency Procedures and First Aid.) The other reason for Trendelenburg position is to elevate and incline the legs so that the abdomen and pelvic organs are pushed up toward the chest by gravity, making visibility and maneuverability easier for the physician doing either abdominal or pelvic surgery. In this case, the legs are elevated and inclined. (See Chapter 19, Assisting with Office/Ambulatory Surgery.)

EQUIPMENT AND SUPPLIES FOR THE PHYSICAL EXAMINATION

Equipment and supplies used for physical examinations should be properly cleaned and ready for the physician's use. Refer to Chapters 10 and 19 for proper cleaning and care of instruments. The list of instruments and supplies in Table 13-1 includes those that may be used in the physical examination. However, this is a limited list. Actual equipment and supplies needed will vary with the physician and with the type of examination. Figure 13-16 shows some common instruments that may be used in the physical examination. See Chapter 18, Examinations and Procedures of Body Systems, for instruments used in specialty examinations.

TABLE 13-1 INSTRUMENTS AND SUPPLIES NEEDED FOR A PHYSICAL EXAMINATION

Balance beam or digital scale	Tongue depressors
Patient gown	Laryngeal/pharyngeal mirror
Drape	Percussion hammer
Thermometer	Tape measure
Stethoscope	Cotton balls
Sphygmomanometer	Gloves
Alcohol wipes	Tissues
Examination lights	Emesis basin
Otoscope	Gauze sponges
Tuning fork	Tonometer
Ophthalmoscope	Specimen bottles/slides—request forms
Penlight	Biohazard and regular waste containers
Nasal speculum	

BASIC COMPONENTS OF A ROUTINE PHYSICAL EXAMINATION

The physical examination of the patient begins as soon as the patient enters the office. Although the physical examination is performed by the physician, it is important for the medical assistant to be aware of the various examination components and the significance of each as an indicator of patient well-being.

Patient Appearance

General appearance and actions are noted as the patient is received by the medical assistant and during the patient history (see Chapter 11). Skin color is checked, general grooming, ease of conversation, and answers to questions are noted. Be aware of cultural differences while assisting with a physical examination. Some patients of other cultures may appear to you to be unclean in their appearance, have an unpleasant body order, have poor hygiene, or otherwise appear to be different from your culture. In some cultures, a daily bath is considered unnecessary, and body odor is not considered offensive. Regard your patient in a nonjudgmental way, taking into account the other's cultural beliefs. The medical assistant should be alert to a patient with abnormal skin color, confusion or disorientation, or difficulty in movement. Such a patient may have a serious problem and should be placed in an examination room and the physician contacted immediately.

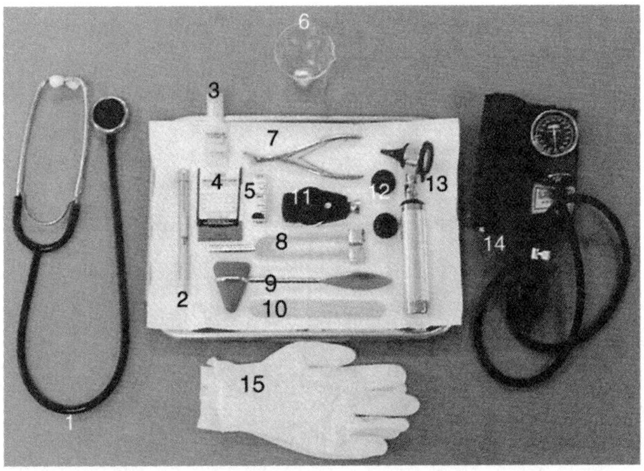

Figure 13-16 Instruments and supplies used in the physical examination: (1) Stethoscope. (2) Penlight. (3) Guaiac/occult blood test developer. (4) Guaiac/occult blood test. (5) Flexible tape measure. (6) Urine specimen container. (7) Metal nasal speculum. (8) Tuning fork. (9) Percussion hammer. (10) Tongue depressor. (11) Ophthalmoscope (head). (12) Ear/nose-speculum. (13) Otoscope head attached to base handle. (14) Sphygmomanometer. (15) Latex gloves.

The following aspects of the patient's health are evaluated by the physician through the method of physical examination known as observation.

Gait

Gait pertains to the manner or style of walking. The patient may have a limp, walk with feet wide apart, appear to be dragging one leg, or have difficulty maintaining balance. The physician will observe the patient's gait by instructing the patient to walk on a designated straight line. Abnormal gait can include **ataxia,** uncoordinated wide-based walk; steppage, in which the leg stepping forward is raised high enough to raise the toes off the ground; drag-to, in which the feet are dragged forward rather than lifted and moved; and spastic, in which the legs are held stiffly together and the feet are slightly dragged forward. Each of these gaits can indicate a disease process or health problem associated with neurologic functioning.

Stature

The height of the patient is measured. The physician will look for height, trunk, and limb proportion.

Posture

Because normal posture is erect with the head held up, a patient in pain may exhibit postural differences. The spine might be in a fixed position, or there may be limited motion in an extremity. The physician will observe spine movement and alignment as the patient performs prescribed movements. Abnormalities can include kyphosis (humpback), which may be seen in older adult patients, particularly women with osteoporosis; lordosis, abnormal curvature of the lumbar area; and scoliosis, curvature of the upper spine.

Body Movements

Body movements may be either voluntary or involuntary. Voluntary body movements describe those movements intended to be made by the patient. Involuntary body movements are movements not controlled by the patient. Tremors are a form of involuntary movement that may be seen in the mouth, fingers, hands, arms, and legs of a patient. Tremors can indicate a neurologic health problem. Involuntary body movements are usually easily observed.

Speech

The patient's speech may indicate abnormal conditions. Abnormalities include aphonia, loss of voice usually because of laryngitis, but which may have other causes; aphasia, the inability to express oneself through speech or writing, which may indicate brain injury or disease; and dysphasia, an inability to use appropriate speech patterns, such as using words in the wrong order. This may indicate a brain lesion or disorder.

Breath Odors

Breath odors may be detected when speaking with the patient or when obtaining vital signs. A sweet fruity odor may indicate acidosis. This may result from diabetes mellitus, starvation, or renal disease. A musty odor may indicate liver disease, and an ammonia odor may indicate uremia.

Poor oral hygiene results in gingivitis (gum disease), caries (cavities), tooth loss, and foul breath odors. Gum disease and caries encourage the growth of microorganisms in the mouth and throat. Because of the vascularity of the oral cavity, microorganisms can enter into the circulatory system and travel to the heart, causing endocarditis. The importance of good oral health is necessary for general health and well-being. Regular dental checkups, cleaning, and flossing daily promote good health.

Nutrition

There are various published charts containing guidelines for normal weight established by height and age. Overweight and underweight are defined as being above or below the published charts. Obesity and underweight are mentioned in Chapters 12 and 22. Edema is a condition that causes weight gain and is an excessive accumulation of fluids in the body tissues. To test for edema, the physician will press a finger against the skin of the patient in an area over a bony prominence such as the ankle. If edema is present, pitting will be evident when the finger is removed. Fat tissue will not leave an indentation when pressed.

Skin and Appendages

Skin problems include abnormal skin color such as redness, **pallor, cyanosis, jaundice,** and **vitiligo.** Pallor is defined as lack of color or paleness; cyanosis is a slightly blue or gray discoloration of the skin, often seen in patients with severe anemia; jaundice is a yellowing of the skin, often caused by obstructed bile ducts or liver disease; and vitiligo is characterized by white patches on the skin, observed against normal pigmentation. Other skin conditions are lesions, ulcers, and bruises. Texture may be smooth, rough, and scaly and have loss of elasticity. These findings may indicate health problems or excessive exposure to the sun. The nails can also indicate some forms of health problems. Infections, either local or systemic, may be observed in nails that are brittle, grooved, or lined. The appearance of the fingertips can be indicators of disorders as seen in clubbing, which may indicate congenital heart disease, and spooning, which may be seen in severe iron deficiency anemias. Abnormal hair distribution, as in facial hair on a female patient, may indicate hormonal changes.

When patients arrive for their appointments, the medical assistant will consider confidentiality of the utmost importance. From the time the patient arrives until the patient leaves, there are multiple occasions to protect patient confidentiality. The medical history and personal finances and insurance matters must be handled privately, out of the hearing range of others. Pertinent personal information that you may elicit from the patient that will be helpful to the physician during his or her examination also must be kept private. When the patient is having testing performed such as electrocardiology that requires the patient to undress in preparation for the examination, care must be taken to avoid violating the patient's right to privacy. Respecting the dignity of all patients by protecting their privacy and confidentiality is a sign of a professional who is aware of patient rights.

The Physical Examination Sequence

There is a sequence followed for a physical examination, although physician preference and the patient's chief complaint can produce a variation to this sequence.

The physical examination begins with the medical assistant taking and recording the patient's vital signs, height, weight, and visual acuity, as well as auditory ability when appropriate. Additional laboratory procedures, such as urinalysis and blood analysis or electrocardiography, may be performed as directed by the physician before the physical examination. Before the examination, a patient will be instructed to empty the bladder saving a urine specimen for analysis. The patient is then told about the examination and what to expect during the examination. Any questions the patient might have should be answered by the medical assistant or referred to the physician. The patient should be instructed about undressing (a private area should be provided for undressing). The medical assistant should be explicit as to what clothing is to be removed and what can be left on. If a complete physical examination is required, all clothing should be removed. A gown and drape are provided for the patient. The medical assistant may leave the room while the patient undresses unless the patient asks for help or is unable to manage alone. It is appropriate to knock before reentering the room.

It is customary for the medical assistant to remain in the room when the physician is examining a patient for patient comfort, to assist the physician, and as a deterrent to potential lawsuits.

The medical assistant will place the instruments for the examination on the counter or Mayo stand, according to physician preference, but usually in order of use. When lamps are used for the examination, the medical assistant may turn them on and have them ready for the physician. Make sure that the light is not directed into the patient's eyes. Inform the physician that the patient is ready when the patient is comfortably positioned on the examination table. Normally the physical examination will start at the head and proceed downward. See Table 13-2 for a detailed review of the components of the physical examination.

TABLE 13-2 COMPONENTS OF THE PHYSICAL EXAMINATION

Body Part	Position	Instrument Used	Method of Exam	Physician's Findings: Normal	Physician's Findings: Abnormal
General appearance	Standing	—	Inspection	Patient is cooperative, good hygiene, good skin color, ease of gait	Uncooperative, behavior inappropriate, unkempt appearance
Skin	Supine and Prone	Flashlight	Inspection Palpation	Good color, warm to touch; no lesion such as warts, moles, abscesses, rashes	Jaundice, cyanosis, pallor, redness, flakiness of skin, lesions, rashes
Head and neck	Supine or Semi-Fowler's or sitting on edge of table	Light source	Inspection Palpation	Symmetry of head; hair not dry or oily and distributed evenly; scalp free of lesions and not dry; no lymph node enlargement	Asymmetry of head; alopecia, dry, flaky scalp; swelling, lumps or pain in head or neck
Eyes	Supine or Semi-Fowler's or sitting on edge of table	Flashlight Ophthalmoscope	Inspection Mensuration	Snellen test shows accurate visual acuity; able to identify color plates; no tearing; pupillary reaction to light equal; retina pink and blood vessels healthy; tonometer measurement of intraocular pressure within normal limits; no bulging of eyeballs	Poor visual and color ability; dull-appearing eyes; drainage; unequal pupils; clouded lens; unequal pupillary reaction; intraocular pressure increased; torturous, unhealthy retinal blood vessels; bulging eyeballs
Ears	Supine or Semi-Fowler's or sitting on edge of table	Otoscope Flashlight Tuning fork and audiometer	Inspection Percussion	Cerumen not impacted on tympanic membrane; tympanic membrane gray and intact; no discharge or pain; able to hear tuning fork or audiometer	Impacted cerumen; red, bulging tympanic membrane; discharge (pus or blood); inability to hear sound from tuning fork; poor auditory ability when checked with audiometer
Nose	Supine or Semi-Fowler's or sitting on edge of table	Nasal speculum Flashlight Aromatic substance	Inspection	Mucous membranes moist and pink; able to detect specific odors; septum straight; nostrils equal in size; no abnormal discharge; no lesions	Dry, red, swollen mucous membranes; unable to detect odors; deviated septum; nostrils flaring; discharge, polyps noted
Mouth and throat	Supine or Semi-Fowler's or sitting on edge of table	Flashlight Tongue depressors Laryngeal and pharyngeal mirrors	Inspection	Gag reflex present; mucous membranes moist and pink; teeth intact, pink tongue; tonsils nonswollen, pink	No gag reflex; tongue rough; pallor of mucous membranes; dental caries; swollen tonsils
Arms and hands	Supine or Semi-Fowler's or sitting on edge of table	Percussion hammer	Inspection Palpation Percussion	Good muscle tone; normal range of motion; nails pink, smooth; ability to squeeze doctor's hands with equal strength; normal reflexes	Poor muscle tone; poor range of motion; nails cyanotic; brittle, ridged nails; abnormal reflexes
Chest and lungs	Supine or Semi-Fowler's or sitting on edge of table	Stethoscope Tape measure	Inspection Palpation Auscultation Mensuration Percussion	Axillary lymph nodes not palpable; lungs clear; no cough; ribs nontender; symmetrical chest wall; respirations and heart rate normal; normal chest sounds	Enlarged axillary lymph nodes; asymmetry of chest wall; respiration and heart rate abnormal; abnormal chest sounds
Heart	Supine or Semi-Fowler's or sitting on edge of table	Stethoscope Electrocardiogram (ECG)	Auscultation Palpation Mensuration	Normal heart function per ECG; regular rhythm, rate of heart sounds; no murmurs; blood pressure normal range; pulse points good quality	Abnormal heart function per ECG. Irregularity of rhythm, rate; murmurs; blood pressure outside normal ranges; poor pulse quality

(continues)

TABLE 13-2 COMPONENTS OF THE PHYSICAL EXAMINATION (continued)

Body Part	Position	Instrument Used	Method of Exam	Physician's Findings: Normal	Physician's Findings: Abnormal
Breasts	Supine	—	Inspection Palpation	No lumps, tenderness, swelling, or thickening; no sores or lesions; no bleeding or discharge from nipples; no lymph node swelling in axilla; no dimpling or "orange peel" appearance	Lumps, tenderness, swelling, thickening; sores or lesions; bleeding or discharge from nipple; lymph node enlargement in axilla; "orange peel" appearance to breast tissue; dimpling of skin
Abdomen	Supine	Stethoscope Measuring tape	Inspection Palpation Auscultation Mensuration Percussion	Liver, spleen not palpable; symmetry to abdomen; no abnormal bowel sounds; no abnormal sounds from organs in abdomen; abdomen soft; no abdominal or inguinal hernias	Liver, spleen enlarged; asymmetric abdomen; increased or decreased bowel sounds; unusual sounds elicited from percussion of abdominal organs; abdominal distention; ascites; presence of abdominal, umbilical, or inguinal hernia
Female genitalia and rectum	Lithotomy or dorsal recumbent or Sims'	Vaginal speculum Light source	Inspection Palpation	External genitalia without lesions, sores, ulcerations; vaginal mucosa pink and without discharge; nontender ovaries; cervix smooth, noneroded, noninflamed; good muscle tone in perineal floor and rectum; negative stool for occult blood; nonpalpable lymph nodes in groin	Lesions, sores, ulcerations; discharge from vagina, cervix; painful ovaries; cervix ulcerated, inflamed; poor muscle tone in perineal and rectum floor; prolapse of uterus or bladder into vagina; hemorrhoids; positive hemoccult; enlarged inguinal lymph nodes
Male genitalia and rectum	Supine Standing	—	Inspection Palpation	Penis pink, no discharge; no lesions, sores, ulcers; testicles firm, nontender, and movable; rectal musculature intact; nonpalpable prostate; nonpalpable lymph nodes in groin	Discharge from penis; ulcers, sores, other types of lesions; testicles tender, swollen; relaxed anal sphincter; hemorrhoids; positive hemoccult slide; enlarged prostate; enlarged lymph nodes in groin
Legs and feet	Supine Prone	Tape measure	Inspection Mensuration Palpation	Normal muscle tone and range of motion; no edema; pulses normal; no varicosities; toenails smooth; no signs of fungus or other infection; calves equal in size	Muscle weakness; poor range of motion; edema; diminished pulse; varicose veins; toenails ridged, infected; unequal calf measurements
Neurological examination	Supine	Percussion hammer Safety pin Cotton ball	Percussion Inspection	Normal reflexes; oriented to time and place; appropriate responses; normal responses to sensation; alert; steady gait; no vertigo or syncope	All reflexes disoriented; inappropriate responses; dulled response to pain and sensation; lethargic; unsteady gait; poor coordination; vertigo; syncope

Head. The patient will be in a sitting position for this examination. The face will be checked for puffiness especially around the eyes. Facial skin will be checked for **scleroderma,** a tight and atrophied skin. The older adult patient may have fatty patches that appear raised and yellowish on the eyelids. The hair and scalp are checked. The head and neck are palpated for lumps and swelling.

Eyes. The appearance of the eyes is examined. The pupils of the eyes will then be checked for light and accommodation. When a penlight or flashlight is placed in front of the pupil, the pupil will constrict. The other pupil should constrict equally. The physician will note that pupils are equal and react to light and accommodation. (This is abbreviated PERLA.) If they do not constrict and return to normal equally, it may indicate a problem in the brain. A tonometer may be used to measure the intraocular eye pressure of patients older than 35 years. Normal eye pressure is 13 to 22 mm Hg. An increase above normal will be found in glaucoma. The physician will use an ophthalmoscope to view the blood vessels of the retina. This is done by turning out the lights in the room allowing pupils to dilate. The patient is instructed to look straight ahead while the physician looks into the eye. Retinal changes indicate disease such as hypertension. The sclera are checked for jaundice.

Ears. An otoscope is used by the physician to examine the ears. The external ear is checked for redness in the ear canal and buildup of cerumen. A healthy tympanic membrane has a pearly gray appearance. A red appearance to the tympanic membrane may indicate infection in the middle ear, known as otitis media. **Vertigo** may indicate that the patient has an inner ear infection or **labyrinthitis. Tinnitus** or ringing in the ears may indicate inner ear problems. Other symptoms of ear problems include pain, discharge, and deafness. The tuning fork is used in testing the sensations of hearing, including bone conduction and air conduction.

Nose. The nasal cavity will be visualized by the physician with the use of a nasal speculum. Discharge from the nose may indicate a postnasal drip in which the sinuses may be draining into the nose and throat. Other abnormalities may include obstruction because of a deviated septum. Polyps and ulcerations may be found in the nasal cavity. Epistaxis or nosebleed may be seen when the capillaries rupture on the surface of the nasal mucosa.

Mouth and Throat. The physician will use a tongue blade or depressor and a light source. The teeth and gums will be checked for dental hygiene such as caries and the gums will be checked for signs of **pyorrhea** (discharge of pus from the gums around the teeth). If the tonsils are present, they will be checked for signs of infection such as redness or white pockets of pus. The larynx and pharynx are examined in the same manner, using laryngeal and pharyngeal mirrors to look for abnormal redness and patches indicating a disease. The floor of the mouth is examined both visually and by palpation for indications of swollen glands and ulcerations.

Neck. The physician palpates the neck looking for swollen lymph nodes. The thyroid gland is palpated anteriorly and posteriorly for size, symmetry, and texture. The patient will be asked to swallow several times while the physician feels the thyroid gland. A small glass of water may be given to the patient to aid in swallowing. Range of motion will be checked by having the patient turn the head in each direction. Care must be taken with older adult patients. The patient should be instructed to move the head slowly.

Chest. The symmetry of the chest is observed, both anteriorly and posteriorly. Chest measurement may have been performed before the examination. The chest of a patient with emphysema will appear barrel-like in shape. While the patient is sitting, the physician will listen to the lungs with a stethoscope. The patient may be instructed to take several deep breaths during this process.

Carefully monitor the patient, particularly older adult patients, because deep breathing may cause dizziness. The physician will be listening for abnormal lung sounds previously discussed. The physician may examine the lungs by percussion. Heart sounds will be auscultated both anteriorly and posteriorly. In cases of heart disease, the medical assistant may be instructed to obtain an electrocardiogram.

Breast. The patient will be placed in a supine position and instructed to place the hand behind the head on the side on which the examination is taking place. The physician will examine the breast for masses by using a circular motion starting at the outer edge of the breast and working toward the center. The nipple will then be gently squeezed to see if there is any discharge. The patient is then instructed to change arm positions so that the other breast may be examined. With the patient in a sitting position, the physician will observe the breasts for symmetry. Female patients should be instructed on the procedure to follow for performing monthly breast self-examination. This may be an embarrassing procedure for the female patient. Maintain as much modesty as possible by carefully draping and giving emotional support. See Chapter 14 for more detailed information on breast examination and breast self-examination.

Abdomen. The patient is placed in a dorsal recumbent or supine position with the arms at the sides for examination of the abdomen. The drape is lowered to just above the pubic hair. The female patient will wear a gown open in the front that can be pulled to the sides while still covering the breast. The physician will normally stand on the right side of the patient while performing this part of the examination. The abdomen will be examined by palpation, percussion, and auscultation. Following the quadrants of the abdomen, the physician will gently palpate the organs in each quadrant working from side to side. The physician will feel for organ size and location, as well as the presence of masses, percuss the abdomen listening for sounds from abdominal organs, use the stethoscope to listen for presence of abdominal sounds, and visually inspect the abdominal area for changes in skin color, scars, or other abnormalities. The contour of the abdomen may be flat or slightly convex. The presence of hernias will be checked both in the supine and standing positions. Patients with abdominal disorders may give a history of dyspepsia, dysphagia or excessive flatulence, nausea, vomiting, bloating, and pain.

Genitalia. Also refer to Chapters 14 (Obstetrics and Gynecology) and 16 (Male Reproductive System) for more detailed information in genitalia examinations.

Female Genitalia. The patient is placed in the lithotomy position. The physician will examine both the external genitalia and reproductive organs. The rectum may be examined and a hemoccult test done at the conclusion of the pelvic examination. See Chapters 18 and 32 for information regarding the hemoccult slide test. After the examination, the patient is instructed to slide toward the head of the table and may be allowed to sit up slowly. Sitting up quickly may cause orthostatic hypotension and dizziness.

Male Genitalia. Care must be taken to protect patient modesty and privacy. The physician will begin the examination by inspecting and retracting the foreskin of the penis if the patient is uncircumcised. The glans penis will be inspected for discharge and redness. The penis and scrotum will then be palpated for possible tenderness and masses. Because of the seriousness of testicular cancer, the patient will be instructed, usually by the physician, in the procedure to perform monthly testicular examinations. See Chapter 16, Male Reproductive System, for detailed information.

Rectal Examinations. The physician may examine the rectum as a part of the male genitalia examination. The patient may be placed in either the Sims' or knee-chest position. The physician will perform a manual examination. The prostate gland is then examined by digital rectal palpation. The physician inserts the gloved index finger into the rectum and palpates the prostate gland for any masses or swelling (see Chapter 16, Male Reproductive System, for more information). A lubricated rectal speculum may then be inserted for visual examination. Because this is uncomfortable for the patient, emotional support is important. The physician can visualize the rectum for bleeding, fissures, polyps, or other lesions.

Reflexes. The patient's reflexes are observed by the physician in both the supine and sitting positions. A percussion hammer is used. While sitting with the arm flexed, the elbow will be lightly tapped to elicit movement from the biceps. The patellar or knee-jerk reflex is tested by tapping the area just below the patella at the knee. The Achilles reflex or ankle-jerk is tested by tapping the Achilles tendon. The Babinski reflex is tested on the sole of a relaxed foot (the great toe will flex) with the patient in a supine position. Reflexes determine the integrity of the neurologic system.

Procedure 13-8 outlines the steps in assisting with the physical examination.

Once the examination has been completed, the patient will be instructed to dress. The patient should be given privacy while dressing. Assist the patient as needed. Do not remain in the room to clean it while the patient is dressing. Remain in the room if the patient requires assistance. Further instructions regarding other testing procedures and treatment plans will be provided by the physician. Be specific with instructions to patients regarding what they should do after they are completely dressed.

Patient Education

Throughout the physical examination, from the time the patient arrives and until the patient leaves, there are many opportunities for patient education. Written instructions should be given when necessary, and physician information should be clarified if needed.

Opportunities for teaching the patient how to adopt a healthy lifestyle are abundant. Regular exercise, no smoking, weight control, limiting alcohol consumption, and using stress reduction techniques, such as meditation, yoga, massage therapy, and so forth, all help to decrease blood pressure and reduce risk for heart attack, stroke, and other illnesses.

Critical Thinking

List and describe the various components of a physical examination.

Procedure 13-1 Positioning Patient in the Supine Position

STANDARD PRECAUTIONS:

PURPOSE:
To safely and properly assist patient into supine position for examination of anterior surface of the body from head to toe.

EQUIPMENT/SUPPLIES:
Drape
Gown

PROCEDURE STEPS:
1. Wash hands and follow Standard Precautions.
2. Assemble supplies.
3. Assist patient to sit on end of table.
4. Assist patient to lie back on table as you pull out the table extension. Support patient's back while extending foot of table.
5. Cover patient with drape from shoulders to ankles.
6. Place small pillow under patient's head.
7. On completion of a procedure, assist patient to sitting position. RATIONALE: Allowing the patient to remain seated helps to prevent dizziness caused by orthostatic hypotension.
8. Push table extension back into place while supporting patient's feet.
9. Once patient is stable (check color of skin, pulse), give further instructions as required.

Procedure 13-2 Positioning Patient in the Dorsal Recumbent Position

STANDARD PRECAUTIONS:

PURPOSE:
To safely and properly assist patient to dorsal recumbent position for catheterization or pelvic examination, head, neck, chest, abdominal, or lower limb examination.

EQUIPMENT/SUPPLIES:
Drape
Gown

PROCEDURE STEPS:
1. Wash hands and follow Standard Precautions.
2. Assist patient to sit on end of table.
3. Assist patient to lie back on table; extend the foot of the table while you support the patient's back.
4. Assist patient to bend knees and place feet flat on the surface of the table. Push in foot extension.
5. Cover patient with drape (diamond shape) from shoulders to ankles.
6. Place small pillow under patient's head.
7. On completion of procedure, assist patient to sitting position while you push table extension back into place and support patient's feet.
8. Have patient sit at end of table for a few minutes. RATIONALE: This helps prevent dizziness and possible fall from low blood pressure caused by orthostatic hypotension.
9. Once patient is stable (check color of skin, pulse), give further instructions as required.

Procedure 13-3 Positioning Patient in the Lithotomy Position

STANDARD PRECAUTIONS:

PURPOSE:
To safely and properly assist patient in lithotomy position for genital or pelvic examination or for urinary catheterization.

EQUIPMENT/SUPPLIES:
Drape
Gown

PROCEDURE STEPS:
1. Wash hands and follow Standard Precautions.
2. Have patient disrobe from waist down and put on gown.
3. Assist patient to sit on end of table. Cover patient's lap and legs with drape.
4. Assist patient to lie back on table as you support patient's back while extending foot of table.
5. Position stirrups level with the table and approximately one foot from edge of table. Lock stirrups into position. RATIONALE: Facilitates patient examination and ensures patient safety.
6. Have patient slide down on table. Have patient move as close to edge of examination table as possible.
7. Assist patient to bend knees and assist her in placing feet in stirrups. Move drape to diamond shape to ensure privacy.
8. Place small pillow under the patient's head.
9. On completion of procedure, extend foot extension of table.
10. Place feet on foot extension and assist patient to slide toward head of table.
11. Assist patient to sitting position while replacing foot extension.
12. Have patient sit at end of table for a few minutes. RATIONALE: This helps prevent dizziness and possible fall from low blood pressure caused by orthostatic hypotension.
13. Once patient is stable (check color of skin, pulse), give further instructions as required.

Procedure 13-4 Positioning Patient in the Fowler's Position

STANDARD PRECAUTIONS:

PURPOSE:
To safely and properly assist patient into the Fowler's position for examination of upper body and head; often used for patients with cardiovascular or respiratory problems.

EQUIPMENT/SUPPLIES:
Drape
Gown

PROCEDURE STEPS:
1. Wash hands and follow Standard Precautions.
2. Provide gown and assist to disrobe if necessary.
3. Assist patient to sit on end of table. Cover lap and legs with drape.

(continues)

Procedure 13-4 (continued)

4. Assist patient to slide back on table leaning against the back rest, which has been raised slightly.
5. Support patient's feet while extending foot of table.
6. Position head of table at a 90-degree angle (45-degree for Semi-Fowler's).
7. Place pillow under the patient's knees for comfort.
8. Cover patient with drape from shoulders to ankles.
9. On completion of procedure, replace foot extension.
10. Have patient sit at end of table for a few minutes. RATIONALE: This helps prevent dizziness and possible fall from low blood pressure caused by orthostatic hypotension.
11. Once patient is stable (check color of skin, pulse), give further instructions as required.

Procedure 13-5 Positioning Patient in the Knee-Chest Position

STANDARD PRECAUTIONS:

PURPOSE:

To safely and properly assist patient in knee-chest position for examination of the rectum, sigmoid colon, and, in some instances, the vagina.

EQUIPMENT/SUPPLIES:

Drape
Gown

PROCEDURE STEPS:

1. Wash hands and follow Standard Precautions.
2. Have patient completely undress. Provide gown.
3. Instruct patient to sit on end of table with drape over lap and legs.
4. Instruct patient to lie back on table while you support the patient's back and extend foot of table.
5. Assist patient to turn onto abdomen by turning toward you, being careful to stay in center of table to avoid a fall. Support patient by placing your left hand on the patient's back and guide the patient toward you. Adjust drape.
6. Assist patient to rise to knees while bending at hips to place chest on table, keeping covered with drape.
7. Arms are bent to side of head with hands under head.
8. If this position is uncomfortable, have patient rest on elbows. Adjust drape from shoulders to ankles, creating a triangle or diamond shape.
9. On completion of procedure, assist patient to lie flat on abdomen, then turn onto the back toward you, and then return to sitting position.
10. Have patient sit at end of table for a few minutes. RATIONALE: This helps prevent dizziness and possible fall from low blood pressure caused by orthostatic hypotension.
11. Once patient is stable (check color of skin, pulse), give further instructions as required.

NOTE: Because this can be an embarrassing and uncomfortable position, it is best that the patient not be placed into this position until the physician is ready for the examination.

Procedure 13-6 Positioning Patient in the Prone Position

STANDARD PRECAUTIONS:

PURPOSE:

To safely and properly assist patient into the prone position for examination of posterior aspect of the body including the back, spine, or legs.

EQUIPMENT/SUPPLIES:

Drape
Gown

PROCEDURE STEPS:

1. Wash hands and follow Standard Precautions.
2. Have patient undress. Provide gown.
3. Assist patient to sit on end of table. Place drape over lap and legs.
4. Assist patient to lie back on table while you support the patient's back and extend foot of table.
5. Assist patient to turn toward you, then onto abdomen, being careful to stay in center of table to avoid a fall. Place pillow under feet and head.
6. Adjust patient drape from shoulders to ankles.
7. On completion of procedure, assist patient to turn toward you, then assist to sitting position.
8. Have patient sit at end of table for a few minutes. RATIONALE: This helps prevent dizziness and possible fall from low blood pressure caused by orthostatic hypotension.
9. Once patient is stable (check color of skin, pulse), give further instructions as required.

Procedure 13-7 Positioning Patient in the Sims' Position

STANDARD PRECAUTIONS:

PURPOSE:

To safely and properly assist patient into Sims' position for rectal examination, rectal temperature, proctoscopy, sigmoidoscopy, an enema, and, in some instances, for vaginal examination.

EQUIPMENT/SUPPLIES:

Drape
Gown

PROCEDURE STEPS:

1. Wash hands and follow Standard Precautions.
2. Have patient undress. Provide gown.
3. Assist patient to sit on end of table. Place drape over lap and legs.
4. Assist patient to lie back on table while you support the patient's back and extend foot of table.
5. Assist patient to turn toward you onto the left side with left arm behind body, placing body weight on chest. Adjust drape.
6. Assist patient to slightly flex left knee and flex right knee to a 90-degree angle for support.
7. Right arm is bent in front of body with hand toward head at an angle to provide support.
8. Adjust drape from shoulders to ankles creating triangle or diamond shape.
9. On completion of procedure, instruct patient to turn toward you, then onto back, and then to sitting position.
10. Have patient sit at end of table for a few minutes. RATIONALE: This helps prevent dizziness and possible fall from low blood pressure caused by orthostatic hypotension.
11. Once patient is stable (check color of skin, pulse), give further instructions as required.

Procedure 13-8 Assisting with a Complete Physical Examination

STANDARD PRECAUTIONS:

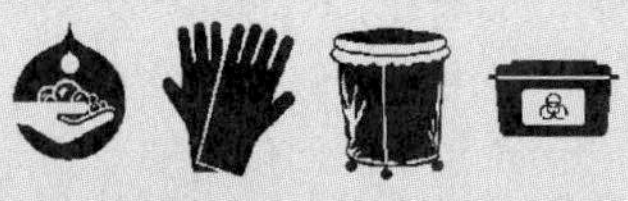

PURPOSE:

To assist physician in a complete physical examination.

EQUIPMENT/SUPPLIES:

Balance beam or digital scale	Tongue depressor
Patient gown	Percussion hammer
Drape	Tape measure
Thermometer	Cotton balls
Stethoscope	Safety pin
Sphygmomanometer	Gloves
Alcohol wipes	Tissues
Examination lights	Lubricant
Otoscope	Emesis basin
Tuning fork	Gauze sponges
Ophthalmoscope	Specimen bottles/slides—request forms
Penlight	Biohazard and regular waste container
Nasal speculum	

PROCEDURE STEPS:

1. Wash hands. Adhere to Standard Precautions.
2. Assemble equipment.
3. Place instruments in easily accessible sequence for physician use. RATIONALE: Efficient use of time and space.
4. Greet and identify patient.
5. Explain procedure to patient. RATIONALE: To obtain patient cooperation and allay apprehension.
6. Review medical history with patient. Refer to Chapter 11 for obtaining patient history. RATIONALE: To assure complete history has been obtained and is current.
7. Take and record patient vital signs, visual acuity, and hearing test results.
8. Obtain a urine specimen. Refer to Chapter 30 for urine collection procedures.
9. Obtain all required blood samples. Refer to Chapters 28 and 29 for blood specimen collection procedures.
10. Perform electrocardiogram (ECG) if directed by physician. Refer to Chapter 25 for ECG procedure.
11. Provide patient with appropriate gown and drape.
12. Assist patient to disrobe completely; explain where the opening for the gown is to be placed. RATIONALE: To assist patient in maintaining modesty, privacy, and warmth.
13. Assist patient in sitting at the end of the table; drape patient across lap and legs. RATIONALE: Always drape patient to maintain modesty.
14. Inform physician when patient is ready.
15. When the physician arrives, remain by the patient ready to assist the patient and physician.
16. Position patient in a sitting or supine position for the head, throat, eye, ear, and neck examination.
17. Lights may be turned off to allow pupils to dilate for retinal examination.
18. Hand the physician instruments as required (some physicians will not require the medical assistant to hand the instruments).
19. The sitting position will be maintained for auscultation of the chest and heart.
20. Assist the patient into a supine position and drape for examination of the chest. Breast examination is discussed in Chapter 14.
21. Maintain a quiet atmosphere to enhance the ability of the physician in hearing heart and lung sounds. RATIONALE: Quiet is necessary to hear heart and chest sounds accurately.
22. Position patient in supine position and drape for abdominal examinations and examination of extremities.
23. Gynecologic examination may then be performed. Refer to Chapter 14. Assist patient into lithotomy position for gynecological examination. Male genitalia examined.
24. If rectal examination is necessary, assist patient into Sims' position.
25. Place patient in prone position for examination of posterior aspect of body.

(continues)

Procedure 13-8 (continued)

26. On completion of the examination, assist patient to sitting position and allow to sit at end of table for a few minutes. RATIONALE: Allows patients to recover from potential dizziness.
27. Assure patient stability (check color of skin, pulse) before allowing patient to stand up. RATIONALE: Prevents the possibility of a patient fainting from orthostatic hypotension.
28. Assist patient in dressing; provide privacy.
29. Chart any notes or patient instructions per physician orders.
30. Escort patient to physician's office for discussion of examination results.
31. Put on disposable gloves.
32. Dispose of gown and drape in biohazard waste container. RATIONALE: Prevent microorganism cross contamination; gown and drape may have body secretions on them.
33. Dispose of contaminated materials in biohazard container. RATIONALE: Prevent microorganism cross contamination of bloodborne pathogens and other potentially infectious materials (OPIM).
34. Remove table paper and dispose in biohazard waste container. RATIONALE: Prevent microorganism cross contamination.
35. Disinfect counters and examination table with a solution of 10% bleach. RATIONALE: Prevent microorganism cross contamination by blood and OPIM.
36. Clean, disinfect, or sterilize reusable instruments as appropriate (refer to Chapters 10 and 19). RATIONALE: Prevent microorganism cross contamination.
37. Remove gloves and discard in biohazard waste container. RATIONALE: Prevent microorganism cross contamination by blood and OPIM.
38. Wash hands.
39. Replace table paper and equipment in preparation for the next patient.
40. Document the procedure.

DOCUMENTATION

11/8/20XX T 98.2, P 84, R 16 Complete physical examination performed by Dr. Woo. Urinalysis negative, hemoccult slide negative. Venipuncture performed and specimens sent to laboratory for complete blood count and electrolytes. Electrocardiogram completed. Patient given written instructions and appointment made for a colonoscopy. Says she understands the preparation for the colonoscopy. W. Slawson, CMA

Case Study 13-1

At Inner City Health Care, clinical medical assistant Wanda Slawson is helping Liz Corbin, a part-time administrative/clinical medical assistant, learn to prepare the examination room and patients for the physical examination. In addition to alerting Liz to physician preferences, Wanda wants to be sure that Liz has a solid understanding of the methods of examination, positions and draping, and the components of the physical examination.

CASE STUDY REVIEW

1. In reviewing with Liz the methods of examination used by physicians, what six primary methods would Wanda have Liz describe?
2. What patient positions would Liz need to know?
3. Wanda asks Liz to recall the various examination components and their significance. How should Liz respond?

Case Study 13-2

Mrs. Mason, a 72-year-old somewhat frail woman with arthritis and hypertensive heart disease has an appointment today for a complete physical examination. It will include a basic physical examination and an examination of the pelvis because she has had bright red vaginal spotting.

CASE STUDY REVIEW

1. Discuss positions and draping for the physical examination including pelvic examination for this patient.
2. Discuss any special safety needs for Mrs. Mason.
3. What additional supplies and equipment should be available for the physician?

SUMMARY

A complete physical examination should be performed on the initial visit of the patient. Findings at this examination, both normal and abnormal, provide a baseline for future examinations.

The role of the medical assistant throughout the examination is twofold. The assistant assembles the necessary instruments and may hand them to the physician when requested. The medical assistant will also prepare specimens as required by the examination and physician. Responsibilities to the patient include explanations and careful positioning, protecting modesty by careful draping and, most important, providing comfort, emotional support, and safety. By performing these duties, the medical assistant can assure patient compliance and physician efficiency.

STUDY FOR SUCCESS

To reinforce your knowledge and skills of information presented in this chapter:

- ❑ Review the Key Terms
- ❑ Practice the Procedures
- ❑ Consider the Case Studies and discuss your conclusions
- ❑ Answer the Review Questions
  - ❑ Multiple Choice
  - ❑ Critical Thinking
- ❑ Navigate the Internet by completing the Web Activities
- ❑ Practice the StudyWARE activities on your student CD
- ❑ Apply your knowledge in the Student Workbook activities
- ❑ Complete the Web Tutor sections
- ❑ View and discuss the DVD situations

REVIEW QUESTIONS

Multiple Choice

1. The method of examination that is the process of listening directly to body sounds is called:
   a. percussion
   b. auditory
   c. auscultation
   d. the direct method
2. The supine position is also known as:
   a. horizontal recumbent
   b. dorsal recumbent
   c. knee-chest
   d. Sims'
3. During the physical examination, ataxia might be observed, which relates to:
   a. stature
   b. posture
   c. body movement
   d. speech
4. When the patient asks a question of the medical assistant, the medical assistant should:
   a. refer all questions to the physician
   b. try to answer all questions, even if uncertain
   c. answer questions to the extent of knowledge; refer others to the physician
   d. ask the patient to please hold all questions until the examination is complete
5. When the abdomen is being examined, the patient is typically in a:
   a. supine position
   b. prone position
   c. Fowler's position
   d. Sims' position

Critical Thinking

1. Discuss the responsibilities of the medical assistant during a physical examination.
2. Review the six methods used in the physical examination.
3. Evelyn Williams has a physical examination scheduled for today. She is recuperating from back surgery and still has pain when she moves to raise her legs. What position is most comfortable for her? Which body parts can be examined with her in this position?

4. Explain the sequence of a physical examination.
5. List the instruments and supplies needed for examining the following body areas:
   a. head
   b. reflexes
   c. chest
   d. abdomen
6. Describe the cleaning process that the following instruments will need after their use in an examination:
   a. nasal speculum
   b. tuning fork
   c. percussion hammer
   d. reusable otoscope speculum
7. List and describe the three sources of information the physician uses to aid in making a diagnosis.
8. List two procedures or tests the medical assistant might perform as part of the patient's physical examination.

WEB ACTIVITIES

1. Using one of the "gateways" for general health and medical information and its links to other sites, gather information about the U.S. government's guidelines for average adult height and weight measurements. According to the government tables, what is considered an appropriate weight for your height?
2. Explore the Web for information about the following conditions and their possible causes:
   - changes in retinal blood vessels
   - enlarged liver
   - ascites
   - varicose veins
   - vertigo

REFERENCES/BIBLIOGRAPHY

Hegner, B. R., Acello, B., & Caldwell, E. (2004). *Nursing assistant: A nursing process approach* (9th ed.). Clifton Park, NY: Thomson Delmar Learning.

Taber's cyclopedic medical dictionary (22nd ed.). (2003). Philadelphia: FA Davis.

Thibodeau, G., & Patton, K. (1996). *The human body in health & disease* (2nd ed.). St. Louis: Mosby Year-Book.

THE DVD HOOK-UP

DVD Series: **Skills Based Series** | Program Number: **6**

Chapter/Scene Reference
- *Positioning the Patient*

This chapter discusses the proper techniques for positioning patients and various methods that physicians use to examine the patient.

In the designated scene, the medical assistant is seen placing the patient in various positions. You probably noticed that many of the positions were awkward for the patient. It should be noted that the position that the DVD lists as the Trendelenberg position is not the true Trendelenberg position. The position illustrated in the DVD starts off by having the patient lying in a supine position. The medical assistant then carefully lifts the patient's legs and feet straight up in into the air. This is actually a maneuver that can be used in place of the Trendelenberg position when you do not have access to a tilt table.

1. What types of physical concerns do you need to be aware of when using this alternative maneuver to the Trendelenberg position?
2. What is the purpose of lifting the legs straight up into the air instead of just propping them up on some pillows?

DVD Journal Summary

Write a paragraph that summarizes what you learned from watching the scenes in today's DVD program. When positioning patients, you are going to see parts of the body that the patient may not be able to see. What would you do if you saw some fecal matter on the back part of the patient's upper leg?

UNIT 5

Assisting with Specialty Examinations and Procedures

CHAPTER 14

Obstetrics and Gynecology

OUTLINE

OBJECTIVES

The student should strive to meet the following performance objectives and demonstrate an understanding of the facts and principles presented in this chapter through written and oral communication.

1. Explain the importance of prenatal care, and discuss what examinations will be performed as part of the initial visit.
2. Explain why the initial prenatal visit is important.
3. Describe what laboratory tests and procedures are performed during the initial prenatal visit.
4. List 12 conditions or diseases that can cause a pregnant woman and her fetus to be at greater risk for problems during the pregnancy.
5. List signs and symptoms and their possible corresponding conditions that the physician searches for during the prenatal history and physical examination.
6. Calculate an expected date of confinement (EDC) or expected date of birth (EDB) using Nägele's Rule.
7. Calculate an EDC (EDB) using a gestation wheel.
8. Explain the purpose of ultrasonography and amniocentesis.

(continues)

KEY TERMS

Abortion
Amniocentesis
Amniotomy
Bartholin Gland
Bimanual Examination
Braxton–Hicks
Candidiasis
Carcinoma in situ
Cervical Punch Biopsy
Cesarean Section
Chlamydia
Colposcopy
Condylomata
Congenital Anomalies
Coupling Agent
Cryosurgery
Diethylstilbestrol (DES)
Dilation
Dysmenorrhea
Dyspareunia
Dysplasia
Eclampsia
Ectopic
Effacement
Endometriosis
Erosion
Exfoliated
Formalin
Fulgarated
Genitalia
Gestation
Gestational Diabetes
Gravidity
Human Chorionic Gonadotropin
Hyperemesis Gravidarum
Hypoxia
Hysterosalpingogram
Intraepithelium
Involution
Lamaze

(continues)

KEY TERMS (continued)

Lochia
Meconium
Metrorrhagia
Multigravida
Nägele's Rule
Neonatal
Nullipara
Oxytoxin
Parity
Parturition
Patent
Pelvic Inflammatory Disease
Placenta Abruptio
Placenta Previa
Polycystic
Preeclampsia
Prenatal
Primigravida
Prostaglandin
Puerperium
Sickle Cell Anemia
Stigma
Tay–Sachs
Thalassemia
Titer
Trichomoniasis
Trimester
Ultrasonography
Vesicle
Viable
Wet Mount

FEATURED COMPETENCIES

CAAHEP—ENTRY-LEVEL COMPETENCIES

Fundamental Procedures

- Practice Standard Precautions

Specimen Collection

- Obtain specimens for microbiological testing

Patient Care

- Prepare and maintain examination and treatment areas
- Prepare patient for and assist with routine and specialty examinations

(continues)

OBJECTIVES (continued)

9. List and describe six types of abortion.
10. Explain what occurs in each of the three stages of labor.
11. Describe what takes place during the postpartum examination.
12. List and describe the diseases and disorders that can affect the female patient.
13. Describe the laboratory tests and procedures that can help diagnose the diseases and disorders that can affect the female patient.
14. Describe seven sexually transmitted diseases.
15. Explain the medical assistant's responsibilities with a gynecologic examination.
16. Describe breast self-examination and method of teaching patient breast self-examination.
17. Discuss menopause.
18. Describe the findings and concerns surrounding hormone replacement therapy.
19. Describe several methods of contraception.
20. Explain reasons for impaired fertility.
21. Describe three therapies that assist in reproduction.

SCENARIO

In the obstetrics department at Inner City Health Care, Wanda Slawson and Bruce Goldman, both certified medical assistants, are preparing for the day's appointments. Both take responsibility for being certain all rooms have appropriate equipment and supplies needed for today's patients. There are three ultrasonograms in addition to the pelvic examinations, Pap smear, and breast examinations scheduled for the afternoon. Wanda is responsible for assisting the physician with each of them. She is careful to follow all safety precautions before, during, and after assisting with examinations and procedures. She is careful to explain procedures to the patients and to direct any questions to the physician.

K-4
46
4

FEATURED COMPETENCIES (continued)

- Prepare patient for and assist with procedures, treatments, and minor office surgeries
- Screen and follow-up test results

Patient Instruction

- Instruct individuals according to their needs

ABHES—ENTRY-LEVEL COMPETENCIES

Communication

- Serve as a liaison between physician and others

Clinical Duties

- Prepare patients for procedures
- Prepare and maintain examination and treatment area
- Assist physician with examinations and treatments
- Collect and process specimens
- Screen and follow up patient test results
- Practice standard precautions

Legal Concepts

- Perform risk management procedures

Spotlight on Certification

RMA Content Outline

- Anatomy and physiology
- Medical terminology
- Patient education
- Physical examinations
- Laboratory procedures

CMA Content Outline

- Medical terminology
- Anatomy and physiology
- Patient instruction
- Patient education
- Examinations
- Procedures
- Collecting and processing specimens; diagnostic testing

CMAS Content Outline

- Medical terminology
- Anatomy and Physiology
- Examination preparation

INTRODUCTION

Obstetrics is the medical specialty in which the physician treats the female patient from the prenatal period through labor, delivery, and during the six-week postpartum period. Gynecology is the specialty that treats the medical and surgical disorders and diseases of the female reproductive tract. Both specialties are usually combined, and the physician who practices them is known as an obstetrician/gynecologist, or simply, an OB/GYN physician. Knowledge of the female anatomy, the laboratory tests and procedures for both specialties, the diseases and disorders that affect the female patient during her nonpregnant and pregnant states, and patient education are essential for the medical assistant who will care for these patients. The goal of the OB/GYN specialty is to promote the health and well-being of the woman and her baby.

OBSTETRICS

Obstetrics is the branch of medicine that provides care to the mother and fetus during pregnancy, labor, delivery, and the postpartum period known as the **puerperium.** Pregnancy is a period of approximately 40 weeks from the day conception takes place (Figure 14-1). The puerperium is the period of six weeks after delivery when the mother's body is returning to its prepregnant state. Visits to the physician for prenatal and postnatal care are the initial **prenatal** visit, return visits, and the six-week postpartum checkup.

Initial Prenatal Visit

The initial prenatal visit is of utmost importance and usually occurs after a woman has missed a second menstrual period or after an at-home pregnancy test result is positive. It is a time of health promotion for the expectant

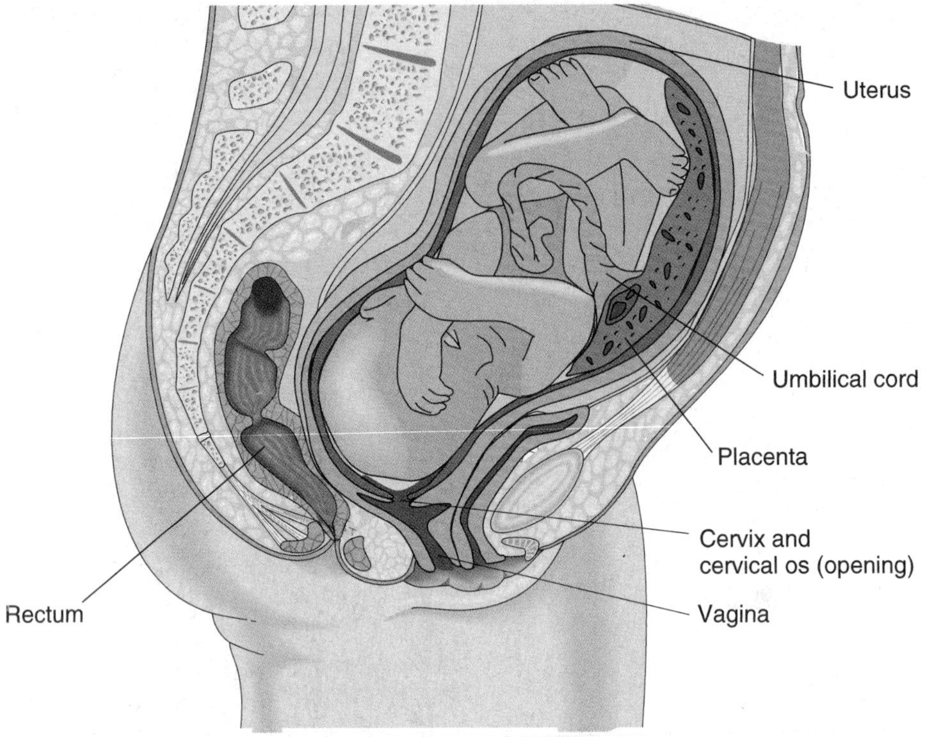

Figure 14-1 Normal uterine pregnancy.

mother and her baby. It is also the time for diagnosis and treatment of maternal disorders that may have been present before the pregnancy or that may have developed during the course of the pregnancy. Growth and development of the fetus are followed and identification of problems that may impede a normal labor are sought. There is ongoing assessment of the expectant mother and the fetus. Any abnormalities can indicate a problem or complication necessitating further testing and assessment. Early detection and management of conditions such as **gestational diabetes,** urinary tract infections, anemia, and **preeclampsia** can prevent serious complications.

The initial visit requires more time than subsequent visits because a thorough history and physical examination are done, including breast, abdominal, pelvic, and vaginal examinations. Pelvic measurements are taken to help ascertain if the pelvis is adequate for a fetus to be delivered vaginally.

The initial visit is followed by monthly visits and then weekly visits beginning about the 28th week. The routine visits consist of checking weight, blood pressure, testing blood and urine; education about nutrition, activity, and rest; and preparing for childbirth.

Many groups of women do not receive prenatal care. Lack of financial resources, lack of transportation, and poor communication by health care providers are some of the reasons that some women do not participate in prenatal care. Modesty may deter some women from seeking prenatal care. Exposing the body to a man is viewed as a major violation of modesty in some cultures. This is why protecting the privacy of all patients is critical.

Certain cultures expect their women to observe practices believed to ensure a favorable pregnancy. Mexican women are advised not to watch an eclipse of the moon; the belief is that the baby will be born with congenital anomalies. Some Spanish women in the United States wear a braided cord around the midsection to ward off nausea and to ensure safe birth. Medals and beads, often worn by

Cultural differences are another reason to keep the Health Insurance Portability and Accountability Act (HIPAA) regulation in mind. During pregnancy, some women's cultures demand modesty, and protecting their privacy is critical. Infertility is a **stigma** in some cultures. Maintaining confidentiality is a requirement of HIPAA for all patients.

The patient's partner may be unaware of the patient's obstetrical history such as previous pregnancies, abortion, or sexually transmitted diseases. Confidentiality is of utmost importance, and it is best to be alone with the patient when obtaining this type of medical information.

TABLE 14-1 LABORATORY TESTS AT THE INITIAL PRENATAL VISIT

Laboratory Test	Disease or Condition
Complete blood count (CBC), hemoglobin, and hematocrit	To detect anemia or infection
Urinalysis with microscopic examination (pH, specific gravity, color, glucose, albumin, proteins, white and red blood cell counts, casts, ocetone, **human chorionic gonadotropin** [HCG])	To screen for diabetes mellitus, renal disease, infection, hypertensive disease, pregnancy
Blood type, Rh factor	To detect Rh incompatibility
Rubella **titer**	To determine immunity to rubella
Renal function	Renal impairment evaluation in women with history of diabetes mellitus, hypertension, or kidney disease
Tuberculin skin test	Screens for tuberculosis
Venereal disease research lab (VDRL) and rapid plasma reagin (RPR)	To detect syphilis
Human immunodeficiency virus (HIV) with patient permission	Screens for HIV antibodies
Hepatitis B and C virus	Screens for hepatitis B and C viruses
Blood glucose	Screens for gestational diabetes
Cardiac evaluation electrocardiogram (ECG), chest radiograph, or echocardiogram	Evaluates cardiac function in women with history of heart disease or hypertension
Pap smear	To check for cervical dysplasia, herpes simplex virus 2
Vaginal, cervical, or rectal smear or culture	To check for gonorrhea, chlamydia, human papilloma virus (HPV)

women, are believed to ward off evil spirits. Other cultures believe that inactivity during pregnancy will safeguard the mother and baby. There are also many dietary influences within different cultures. (See Chapter 22 for more information about culture and diet and food choices.) Respect for all cultures is of great importance, and judgments should not be made that some women are ignorant or lazy. Incorporating customs and beliefs demonstrates that you value cultural diversity and women's self-esteem.

All women should be fully involved in their care. Women with physical or emotional disabilities must have their particular needs addressed. When necessary, make adaptations whenever possible for women who are mentally challenged, blind, deaf, or physically incapacitated.

Laboratory Tests. The laboratory tests that may be part of the initial prenatal visit are described in Table 14-1.

Patient Education. Patient education includes such topics as nutrition, dental care, rest, and exercise, as well as discussion about over-the-counter (OTC), prescription medications, and herbal products. Alcohol and tobacco and their dangers and potential harm to fetus and mother should also be discussed. Medications, alcohol, cigarettes,

Patient Education

Whatever the pregnant woman ingests or inhales affects the fetus. Smoking during pregnancy poses serious risks to mother and fetus. Low birth weight, placenta abruptio, and deliveries before term are some of the possible effects to the fetus. Lung cancer, emphysema, and cardiovascular disease can affect the mother. Other kinds of substance abuse such as alcohol, cocaine, and other recreational drugs are commonly seen in pregnant women who are abused such as in a domestic abuse situation; however, women do not have to be in an abusive situation to abuse drugs or alcohol. Ask the patient if she is in immediate danger. If so, a referral can be made to a community resource (e.g., women's shelter, hotline phone number, district attorney's office) or the physician can help devise a safety plan until the community resource steps in to help. (See Chapters 7 and 23 for more information about domestic violence and drug abuse.)

and mind-altering substances taken by the mother have harmful effects on the fetus and should not be used.

Before the birth, the expectant couple is encouraged to choose a method of feeding the infant. During the initial prenatal visit, benefits of breast-feeding the newborn are discussed. If the mother is HIV negative, breast-feeding is encouraged because it offers many nutritional, psychological, and immunologic benefits. Because the immune system of newborns is not fully developed, the high level of immunoglobulins in breast milk gives them protection against some pathogenic diseases of the respiratory and gastrointestinal tracts. Close contact between mother and newborn is certain with breast-feeding, and bonding can readily take place. Breast-fed infants seem to have fewer allergic reactions. For the mother, one benefit of breast-feeding is that the uterus **involutes,** or returns more quickly to the non-pregnant state. Breast-feeding is the optimal way to feed a newborn. The services of a lactation consultant (available in most women's hospitals and some pediatric offices) can be helpful especially during the initial phase of breast-feeding. The consultant can provide hands-on instructions to the patient to optimize the experience for the mother and baby.

Formal childbirth education classes given in various languages teach the fundamentals of labor, delivery, and newborn care and feeding.

Prenatal History. The prenatal history will be comprehensive and include much of the same information that is obtained during the taking of a regular medical history. However, emphasis will be on identification of the high-risk patient. Particular attention is given to women who have a history of one or more of the following situations or conditions because they may place women at greater risk during pregnancy:

- Use of legal drugs (OTC, prescription, tobacco, caffeine, alcohol), illegal drugs (marijuana, cocaine), and herbal products
- Age under 16 and over 35 years
- Rh-negative blood
- A history of repeated premature labors and deliveries, abortions, or stillbirths
- Genetic diseases in the family
- Previous **Cesarean section**
- Diabetes
- Hypothyroidism or hyperthyroidism
- Sexually transmitted disease
- Hypertension
- Nutritional deficiencies
- Cardiac problems
- Kidney conditions
- Epilepsy
- Headaches

Any of these conditions or diseases can place the woman and fetus at risk for serious complications.

During the initial prenatal visit, an obstetrical history is taken, which includes the **gravidity,** or total number of pregnancies, including the present pregnancy, regardless of duration. The history also includes the **parity,** the number of pregnancies carried to the point of viability regardless of whether the baby was born alive or dead. Multiple births, twins, and triplets count as one pregnancy (gravida) and one delivery (para). For example, a woman pregnant for the first time is referred to as Gravida 1, Para 0. After this woman delivers, regardless if the baby is born alive or dead, if it reached the age of **viability,** the history of the woman is Gravida 1, Para 1. Viability is the ability to grow and develop after birth. The term **multigravida** refers to a woman who has been pregnant more than once. **Nullipara** describes a woman who has not carried a pregnancy to viability.

Para sometimes has four letters that can be used to give more information about past deliveries. It does *not* include the present pregnancy. The four letters are FPAL:

F—number of full-term deliveries (37–40 weeks gestation)

P—number of preterm or premature deliveries (20–36 weeks gestation)

A—number of abortions (induced or spontaneous terminations before 20 weeks gestation)

L—number of living children born to the patient who are still alive at the time of history data collection

For example, a woman has had four term pregnancies, delivered four live infants, but lost a child to leukemia at 7 years of age. This women is considered to be 4-0-0-3.

The present prenatal history includes information about the present pregnancy. The physician searches for problems indicative of high-risk factors. Identifying high-risk patients helps to limit maternal and newborn deaths and diseases. Some factors that indicate that a patient is at high risk are inadequate nutrition; use of drugs such as alcohol, tobacco, or cocaine; existing medical conditions such as high blood pressure or diabetes; sexually transmitted disease; and poverty. The physician watches for signs and symptoms that indicate a potentially serious condition. Examples are listed in Table 14-2.

TABLE 14-2 SIGNS AND SYMPTOMS OF POTENTIALLY SERIOUS CONDITIONS

Signs and Symptoms	Possible Condition
Rapid weight gain	Preeclampsia
Headaches	Preeclampsia
Hypertension	Preeclampsia
Vision changes	Preeclampsia
Severe nausea and vomiting	Hyperemesis gravidarum/ dehydration
Bleeding, discharge, abdominal pain/cramping	Threatened abortion, placenta previa, placenta abruptio
Edema	Preeclampsia
One-sided pelvic or abdominal pain	**Ectopic** pregnancy (Figure 14-2)
Chills, fever	Vaginal infection, sexually transmitted disease, other infections

Subsequent or Return Prenatal Visits

Subsequent visits include weight, blood pressure, urinalysis, complete blood count with hemoglobin and hematocrit, measurement of the height of the uterine fundus (a tape measure is used by placing it on the anterior symphysis pubis and the crest of the uterus) (see Figure 14-7A and B), and fetal heart measurements (see Figure 14-8A and B). Generally, it is not possible to determine with accuracy the exact date of conception. Many formulas have been used for calculating the EDB (expected date of birth) or EDC (expected date of confinement). Although none is foolproof, **Nägele's rule** is the usual method used because it is reasonably accurate. Nägele's rule is to add seven days to the first day of the last menstrual period (LMP), subtract three months, and add one year. An example is:

the first day of LMP = July 10, 2005
add 7 days = July 17
subtract 3 months = April 17
add one year = April 17, 2006

Another method to calculate EDB or EDC is to add seven days to LMP and count forward nine months. Most women give birth seven days before or after the EDB or EDC.

Pregnancy wheels help determine the EDC. Line up the arrow of the first day of the LMP, then read off the date that corresponds to the 40-week designation (Figure 14-3).

Vaginal examinations are only done periodically up to two to three weeks before the EDB or EDC. Patients are encouraged to attend classes in the **Lamaze** method of childbirth, as well as classes in the care of the newborn (Figures 14-4 through 14-9).

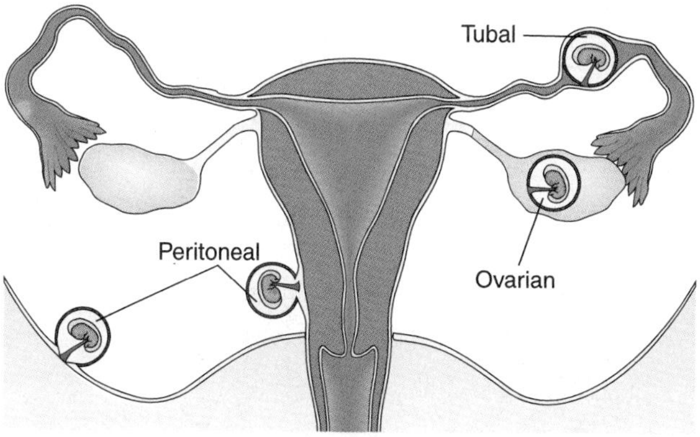

Figure 14-2 Sites of ectopic pregnancy.

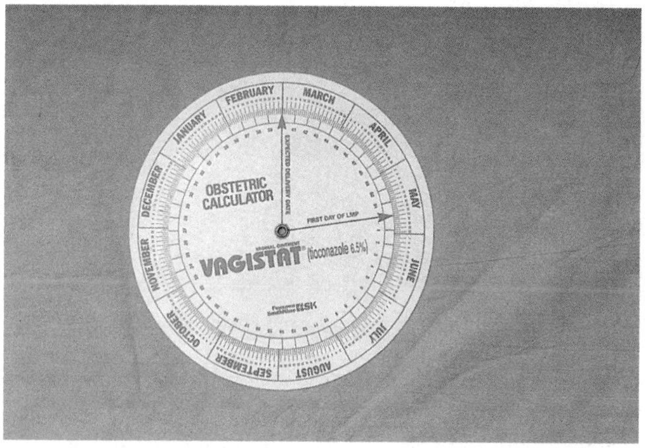

Figure 14-3 Gestation wheel. Place arrow labeled "first day of LMP" on date of last menstrual period (LMP). Read date at arrow labeled "expected delivery date."

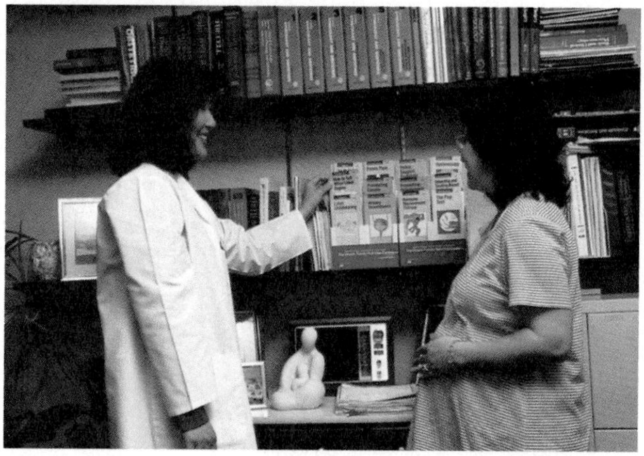

Figure 14-4 Supplying patients with information on a healthy pregnancy and potential risks and danger signs is an important responsibility of the medical assistant.

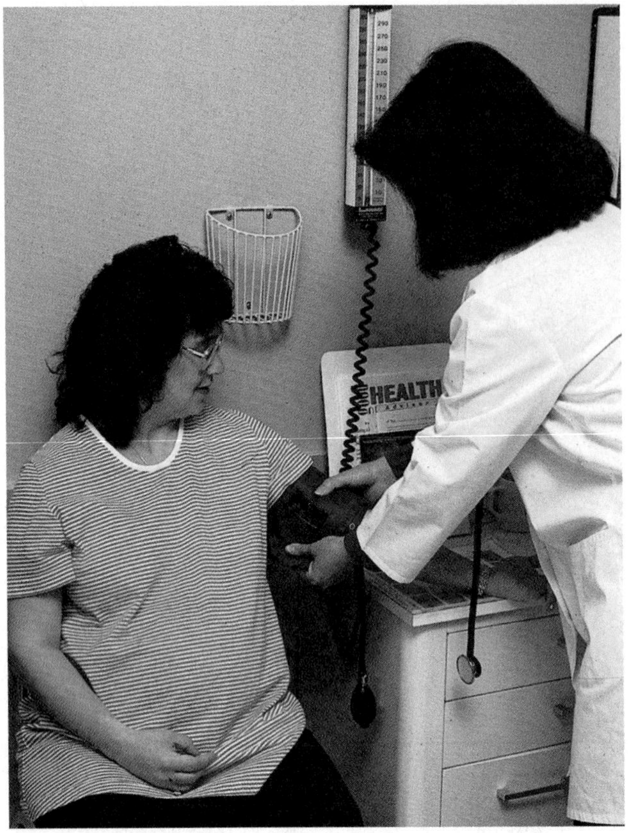

Figure 14-5 Blood pressure is measured at each prenatal visit.

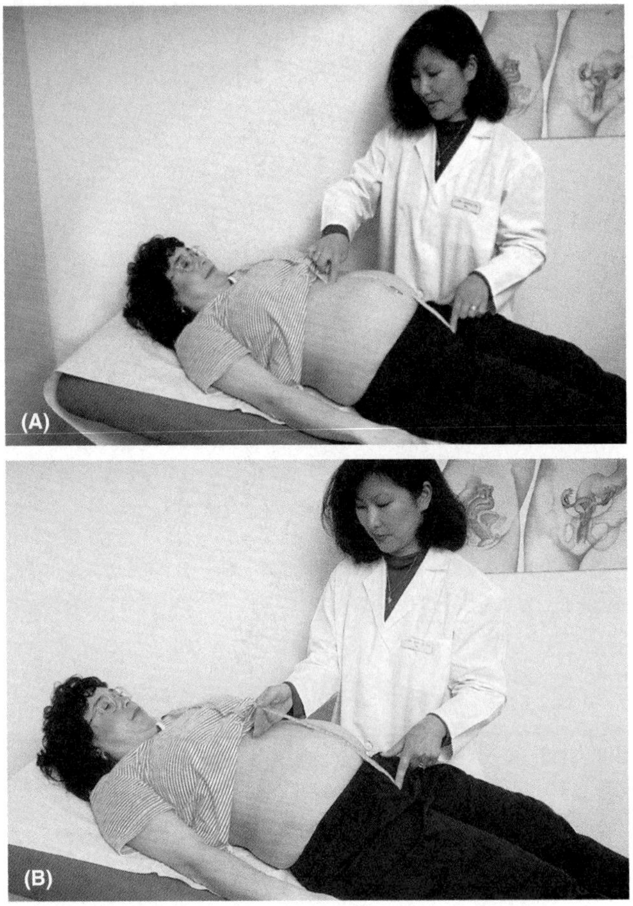

Figure 14-7 Fundal height is measured by placing the end of the tape at the symphysis pubis and extending it in either a (A) curved or (B) straight pattern to the fundus.

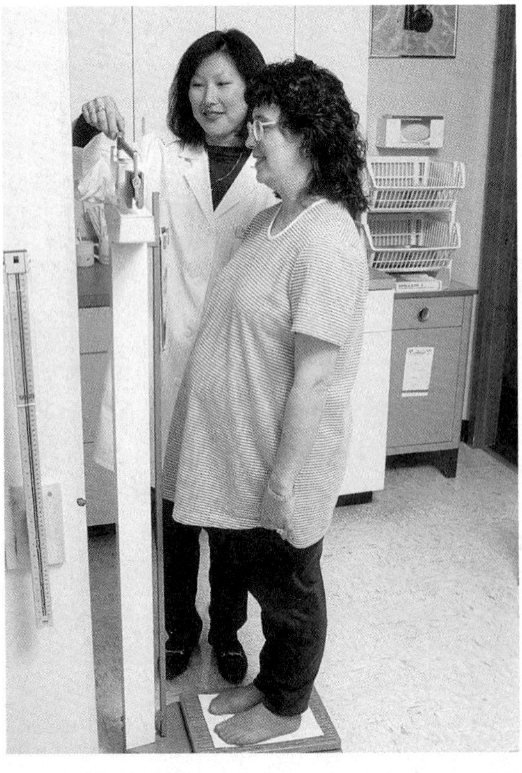

Figure 14-6 Weight gain is tracked throughout the pregnancy.

Tests and Procedures

Alpha Fetal Protein. Another test that may be done during a subsequent visit is a blood test known as alpha fetal protein (AFP) blood test. It is done about the 16th week of pregnancy. It is a screening test only, done to rule out neural tube defects, abdominal wall defects, and chromosomal problems such as Down syndrome. If the test is positive, additional testing such as an **amniocentesis** or an ultrasound will be used to help make a diagnosis.

Chorionic Villi Sampling (CVS). Chorionic villi sampling (CVS) is a test performed on women who are older than 35 years, have a history of chromosomal abnormalities, and are known carriers of a genetic disorder such as **thalassemia, sickle cell anemia,** or **Tay–Sachs.** The test is done at about 8 to 10 weeks **gestation** and has an advantage over amniocentesis because the latter cannot be done before the 14th week. In one method of the CVS test, a sample of tissue that surrounds the fetus is taken through a catheter by means of suction: The

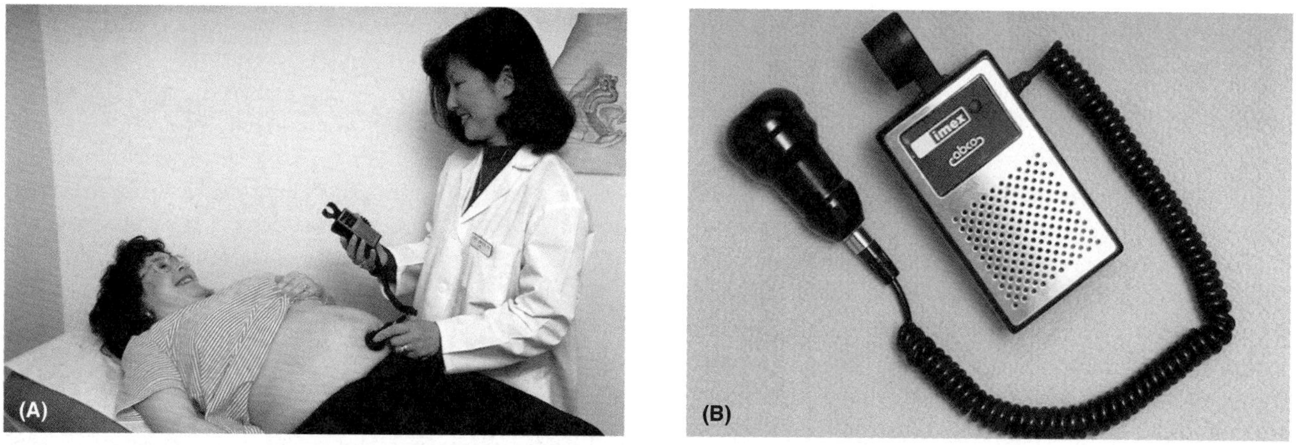

Figure 14-8 (A) Fetal heart tones are measured with a handheld Doppler. (B) Handheld Doppler.

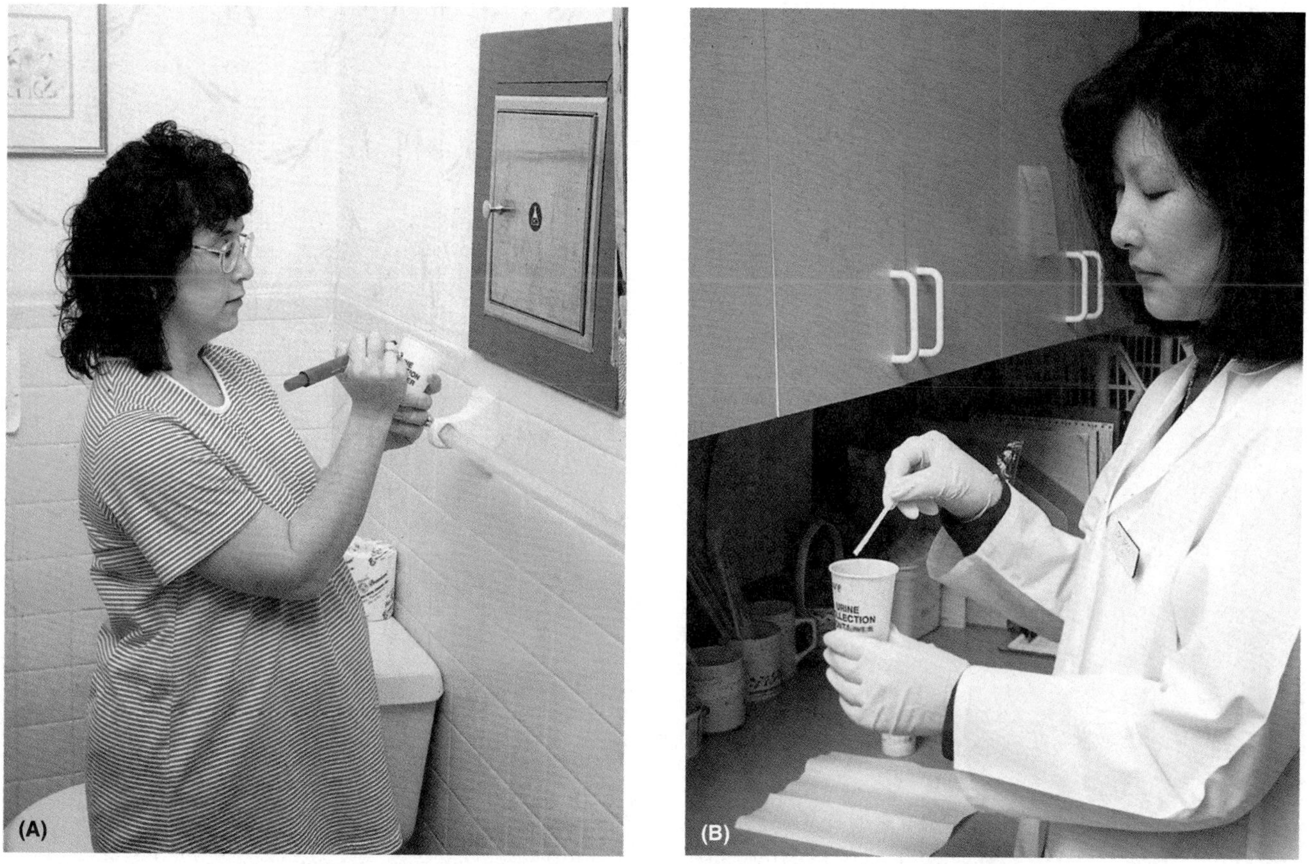

Figure 14-9 Urine is tested at each visit for glucose and protein. (A) Client provides a urine sample. (B) Medical assistant uses dipstick to check for glucose and protein.

sample is analyzed in the laboratory for genetic abnormalities. An ultrasonogram is done simultaneously with an amniocentesis to avoid possible injury to the fetus or placenta.

Ultrasonography/Amniocentesis. Two tests can be done that can supply vital information: **ultrasonography,** or ultrasound, and amniocentesis. Ultrasound can be performed in the first, second, or third **trimester.** It uses high-frequency sound waves to produce an image of the fetus. A **coupling agent** is spread onto the mother's abdomen to enhance penetration of sound waves through the tissue, and the scanning mechanism is moved over the abdomen. An image of the fetus can be viewed on a screen similar to a television screen. Photos are taken during the examination. The technique usually takes about a half hour. There are no known side effects to the fetus or mother, and ultrasound uses no X-rays. There is no pain involved, but slight discomfort can occur due to a full bladder. (A quart of fluid should be consumed one hour before the test and finished within 15 or 20 minutes.) A full bladder is essential to a good-quality ultrasound because it supports the uterus in position for good imaging. This procedure may be used to identify the number of fetuses, check the age of the fetus (number of weeks gestation), and detect some fetal abnormalities (e.g., Down syndrome; Figure 14-10).

A high-resolution ultrasonographic test is used more and more frequently to check for Down syndrome. The test is useful because it can detect chromosomal abnormalities. It can be done sooner in a pregnancy than blood testing and could minimize the need for CVS or amniocentesis, both of which are not without risks to the mother and fetus.

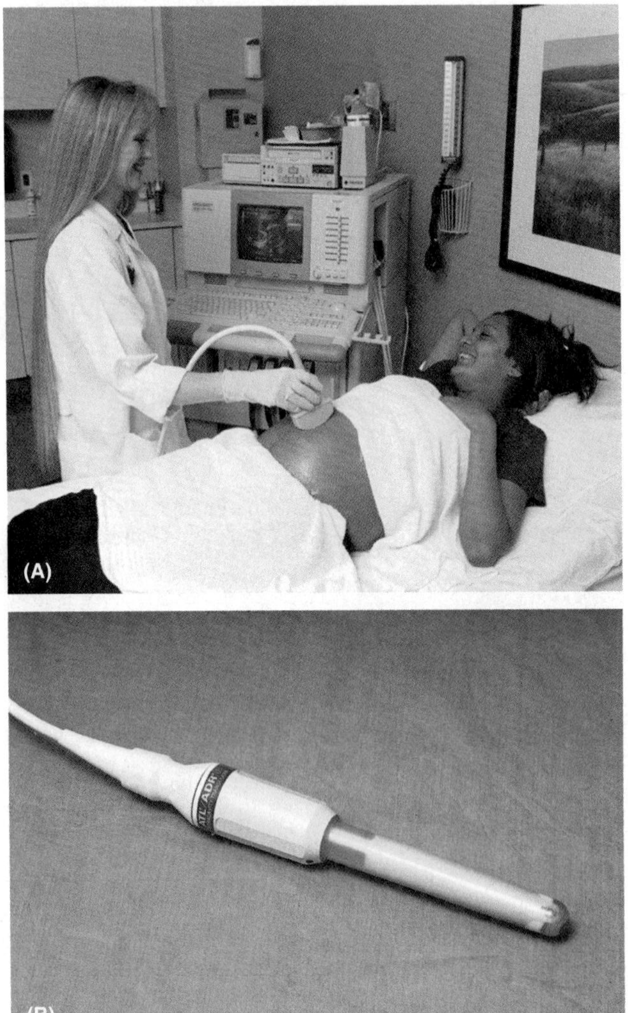

Figure 14-10 (A) Abdominal ultrasound. (B) Transducer for transvaginal ultrasound.

An amniocentesis is the surgical puncturing, with a long, thin needle, of the amniotic sac through the woman's abdomen. The purpose of this test is to obtain, by aspiration, a sample of amniotic fluid that contains fetal cells. The procedure can be done as early as 14 weeks and helps to diagnose genetic mishaps, **congenital anomalies** (present at birth), and chromosomal defects. It also can be used to determine the lung capacity of the fetus (Figure 14-11).

Ultrasonography is performed while the physician is doing the amniocentesis to identify the position of the fetus and placenta, thereby avoiding injury to either.

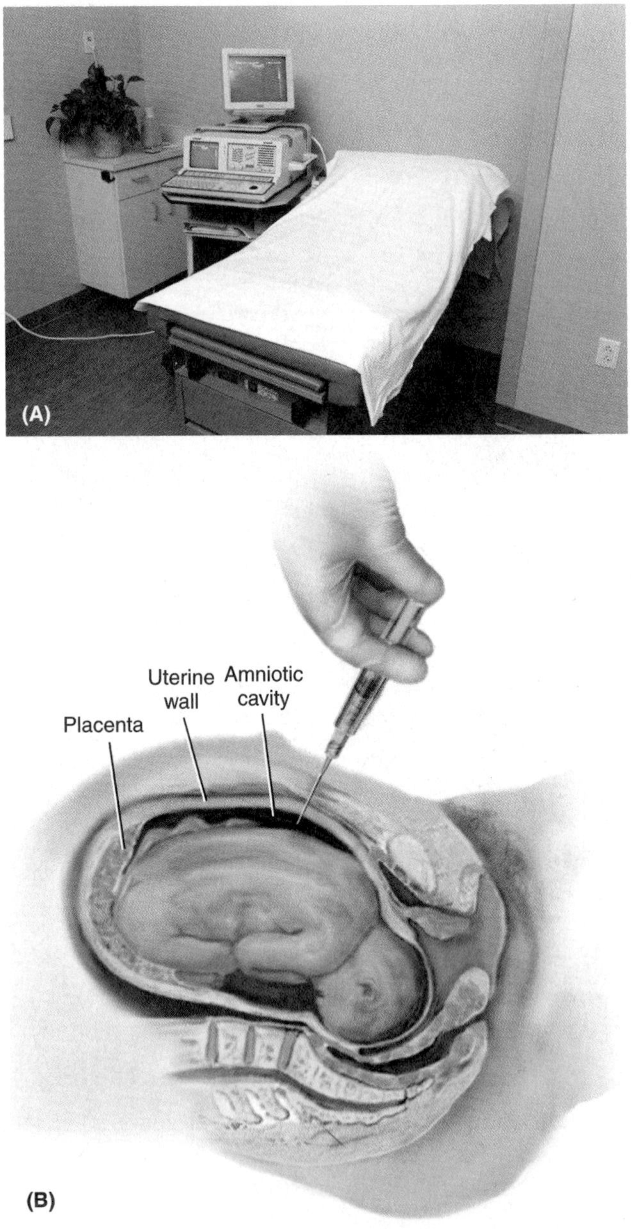

Figure 14-11 (A) An amniocentesis setup. (B) During amniocentesis, a sample of amniotic fluid is aspirated for evaluation.

The procedure is not without risk and is not universally accepted. There can be bleeding, leaking of amniotic fluid, and infection.

Fetal heart rate is another test. Monitoring can be done in one of two ways: a nonstress test monitors the fetus's heart rate while it is moving spontaneously or a stress test monitors the fetal heart rate while the mother is stimulated with medication to have mild uterine contractions. Normally, the fetal heart rate will accelerate to a certain safe limit while it is being stressed.

Complications of Pregnancy

Abortion/Interruption of Pregnancy. The interruption of pregnancy before the fetus is viable is known as **abortion.** Six types of abortion are listed here:

1. *Spontaneous:* unknown etiology (miscarriage)
2. *Complete:* expulsion of all products of conception, fetus, and placenta with no surgical intervention
3. *Missed:* Fetus dies in the uterus and must be removed; usually a dilation and curettage (D&C) is the surgical procedure performed
4. *Incomplete:* Only parts of the fetus and placenta are expelled. Tissue remains in the uterus and a D&C usually must be performed.
5. *Threatened:* Bleeding from the uterus, but there are no contractions or dilation of cervix. Pregnancy continues.
6. *Induced:* Evacuation of the fetus and placenta from the uterus at the mother's request or because mother's health is in jeopardy.

Eclampsia. **Eclampsia** syndrome, also known as pregnancy-induced hypertension, can occur in pregnancy and result in convulsions unrelated to epilepsy or other brain conditions. It is a potentially life-threatening disorder characterized by hypertension, generalized edema, and proteinuria. It can put the woman and her fetus in grave danger and can be fatal if not treated. Preeclampsia is less severe. The symptoms are the same, except there are no convulsions. This is why weight is measured, blood pressure checked, and a urinalysis (including a check for protein) are routinely performed. Sudden significant weight gain, increase in blood pressure, and the presence of protein in the urine can indicate possible preeclampsia. The cause is unknown. Prophylaxis is of great importance. The problem is seen more often in women who have received inadequate prenatal care, especially poor nutrition, in **primigravida** (pregnant for the first time) younger than 18 years, in women with preexisting cardiovascular and renal conditions, as well as in women who are diabetic.

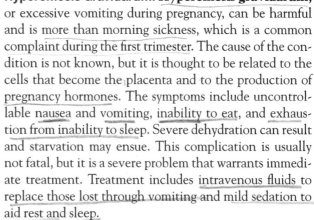

Critical Thinking

A 17-year-old girl has missed her period and has called the clinic describing sharp right quadrant pain. What tests/procedures will help the physician make a diagnosis?

Gestational Diabetes. Gestational diabetes first appears during the second or third trimester of the pregnancy and usually disappears after the woman has delivered her baby or when the pregnancy terminates for any other reason. This type of diabetes is usually a milder form of the disease. Prompt detection (through blood and urine glucose testing) and therapy are essential to avoid fetal and **neonatal** (newborn) illness and death.

Hyperemesis Gravidarum. **Hyperemesis gravidarum,** or excessive vomiting during pregnancy, can be harmful and is more than morning sickness, which is a common complaint during the first trimester. The cause of the condition is not known, but it is thought to be related to the cells that become the placenta and to the production of pregnancy hormones. The symptoms include uncontrollable nausea and vomiting, inability to eat, and exhaustion from inability to sleep. Severe dehydration can result and starvation may ensue. This complication is usually not fatal, but it is a severe problem that warrants immediate treatment. Treatment includes intravenous fluids to replace those lost through vomiting and mild sedation to aid rest and sleep.

Placenta Previa. **Placenta previa** occurs when the placenta implants low in the uterus and partially or completely covers the cervical os. It is an emergency. The cause is unknown. When labor ensues and the cervix begins to dilate, the placenta is pulled away from the wall of the uterus and causes bleeding. On occasion, the bleeding, which comes on suddenly and is painless, will stop spontaneously. If it continues, significant maternal blood is lost, and the fetus may suffer anoxia and die when the placenta separates from the blood supply (Figure 14-12B).

Ultrasonography will determine where the placenta is attached at which time the diagnosis can be made and treatment begun. Treatment depends on the gestational age of the fetus and the percent of placenta that covers the cervical os. Cesarean section may be necessary to remove the placenta, control bleeding, and deliver the fetus safely.

Placenta Abruptio. **Placenta abruptio** occurs when the placenta prematurely and abruptly separates from the uterine lining (see Figure 14-12A). It can result in fetal

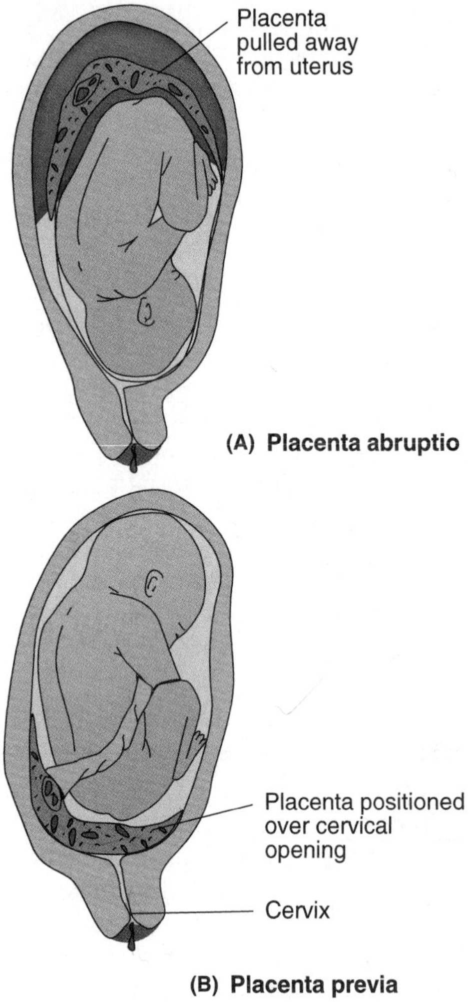

Figure 14-12 (A) Placenta abruptio. (B) Placenta previa.

distress and death, and maternal shock and death. It usually occurs late in pregnancy but can occur during labor.

Factors that contribute to this complication are multiple pregnancies, chronic hypertension, trauma to the uterus, and sudden release of amniotic fluid. Delivery as soon as possible either vaginally or by Cesarean section is indicated. The prognosis of the newborn depends on the extent of **hypoxia** suffered during labor and delivery.

Impaired Fertility. The inability to conceive and bear a child after a period of unprotected sex is known as impaired fertility. Some reasons for this problem can be that many couples delay pregnancy until later in life when fertility is naturally lower. The increase in the incidence of **pelvic inflammatory disease** (PID), endometriosis, the increase in substance abuse, and environmental conditions such as pesticides and lead all can contribute to impaired fertility.

Diagnosis and treatment of impaired fertility requires a physical, emotional, and financial investment over a long period. To diagnose impaired fertility in the female patient, a complete history and physical examination are performed. Endocrine system and anatomic and physiologic abnormalities are sought. Laboratory tests on urine and blood are performed. Proof of ovulation can be determined by retrieving an ovum from the uterine tube, performing an endometrial biopsy, assessing mucus characteristics, and taking the basal body temperature. Levels of estrogen, progesterone, follicle-stimulating hormone, and lutenizing hormone are also measured. A **hysterosalpingogram,** a radiograph of the uterus and tubes after the injection of dye, reveals defects in either the uterus or tubes.

Laparoscopy can be performed to visualize the internal pelvic structures. Tubal patency, **endometriosis,** pelvic adhesions, or **polycystic** ovaries can be seen. Endometrial biopsy is done to examine the tissue to determine whether the endometrium is capable of accepting a fertilized ovum for implantation. Ultrasonography, either abdominal or transvaginal, can assess pelvic organs for abnormalities.

Tests that can be performed on a male to diagnose impaired fertility are semen analysis, hormone analysis, and biopsy of a testicle. Once a diagnosis of impaired fertility has been made, a number of therapies are available to assist in reproduction. These include:

- In vitro fertilization (IVF), indicated for fallopian tube blockage and endometriosis: Eggs are retrieved from ovaries, fertilized with sperm in the laboratory, then transferred to her uterus.
- Gamete intrafallopian transfer (GIFT): Eggs are retrieved from ovaries. An egg and sperm are aspirated into a special catheter, then placed into the fallopian tube where fertilization can occur naturally.
- In vitro fertilization and gamete intrafallopian transfer (IVF + GIFT) with donor sperm: Eggs are retrieved from ovaries, fertilized with donor sperm in the laboratory, aspirated into a special catheter, then placed into the fallopian tube where fertilization can take place naturally.

New technology allows sperm to be retrieved from the testicles if ejaculation is impossible; sperm can be injected into the ovum, embryos can be frozen, and there can be surrogate pregnancies. With technology comes the ethical and legal questions of donor eggs and embryos, pregnancies in older adult women, how to define who the parents are, what to do with frozen embryos after death or divorce, and other such issues as disposal of unused (extra) embryos.

In some cultures, a woman is deemed the responsible party for impaired fertility, and the impairment is thought to be caused by her sins, evil spirits, or her own deficiencies. The virility of a male is questioned unless he is able to manifest his sexual potency by having a child.

Parturition

Parturition, or labor, is the process during which the uterus, through contractions, expels the fetus and placenta. There are three stages of labor:

- Stage I—Dilation: from onset of labor until complete **dilation** (expansion) and **effacement** (thinning and shortening) of cervix
- Stage II—Expulsion: from complete dilation and effacement through the birth of fetus (expulsion)
- Stage III—Placental: from birth of fetus through expulsion of the placenta

Labor is believed to be triggered by the release of **oxytoxin** and **prostaglandins** after the level of other hormones decreases. When the oxytoxin is released, it causes the muscles of the uterus to contract. **Braxton–Hicks** contractions, often referred to as false labor, can usually be differentiated from real labor because of their irregularity and tendency to disappear when the woman moves about and changes positions.

If fetal membranes do not spontaneously rupture during labor, an **amniotomy** (artificial rupture of the membranes) can be done. The procedure uses a sterile amniohook, and it may shorten the length of labor.

Signs and symptoms to watch for during labor that indicate complications are heavy vaginal bleeding, sudden increase and decrease in blood pressure, increased activity by the fetus, headache, extreme restlessness, and visual changes. **Meconium** in the vaginal discharge can indicate fetal distress.

Postpartum Period

The postpartum period is the time known as the puerperium during which the body returns to nonpregnant state. It is usually four to six weeks after delivery. The body undergoes changes during this time. The uterus involutes (returns to normal size) and healing of any injuries takes place.

A vaginal discharge, known as **lochia,** appears during the puerperium. It consists of tissue, blood, white blood cells, mucus, and bacteria. It can be described by its appearance. Lochia rubra is bright red and appears the first three days after delivery. Lochia serosa is pink or brown and is indicative of less blood. By about 10 days, the flow decreases, becomes whitish-yellow, and is known as lochia alba. Lochia usually disappears by the third week postpartum but may last for up to six weeks. Menstruation usually begins in a nursing mother three to six months after delivery, two months for nonnursing mothers. The mother is told to avoid heavy lifting, not to become fatigued, to eat a well-balanced diet, to continue to take her prenatal tablets, and to report any feelings of depression. An appointment in six weeks will evaluate the mother's general health, and the physician will discuss infant care, breast-feeding, the importance of exercise and good nutrition, and birth control. The medical assistant can stress the importance of yearly Pap smears and of monthly breast self-examinations because these are important aspects of patient education.

Contraception. Voluntary prevention of pregnancy is known as contraception. The opportune time to discuss contraception with the mother is soon after delivery and before discharge from the hospital. She should know what method of contraception she and her partner will use before resuming sexual activity. To discuss contraception at the six-week postpartum checkup can be too late. Sexually transmitted disease (STD) protection should also be reviewed before discharge.

Written instructions about methods of contraception are important and help the patient understand options that are available.

Some nonprescription kinds of contraception are the various barrier methods: latex condoms, male and female contraceptive foam, spermicide (nonoxynol-9) used with a condom to help prevent STDs, vaginal sponges that contain a spermicide, and abstinence.

Prescription methods of contraception include hormonal contraception in the form of oral birth control pills; Norplant®, a surgical implant of progestin in the upper arm, which provides up to five years of contraception; a diaphragm used with a spermicide; a cervical cap to fit over the cervix; an intrauterine device (a small device made of copper or progesterone-medicated plastic); and vaginal rings.

Sterilization is a surgical procedure that renders the individual infertile. The woman's uterine tubes are **fulgarated** (destroyed by means of an electric current) or bands and clips are placed around the tubes to block them (ligation). Both fulgaration and ligation are considered to be permanent methods. Female sterilization can be performed immediately after giving birth or any time afterward during any phase of the menstrual cycle. Laparoscopic surgery is the usual approach. Tubal ligation is the top contraceptive choice in the United States (Figure 14-13).

The surgical procedure performed on a male to render him sterile is a vasectomy. It can be performed on an outpatient basis under local anesthesia. Small incisions are made into the scrotum above and to the side of each testicle. Each vas deferens is identified, ligated twice, and then severed (Figure 14-14). It is important for the patient to realize that sterility is not immediate because some sperm remain in the sperm ducts after vasectomy. One week to several months may elapse before the ducts are sperm free. Some form of contraception is necessary until two consecutive sperm counts are zero.

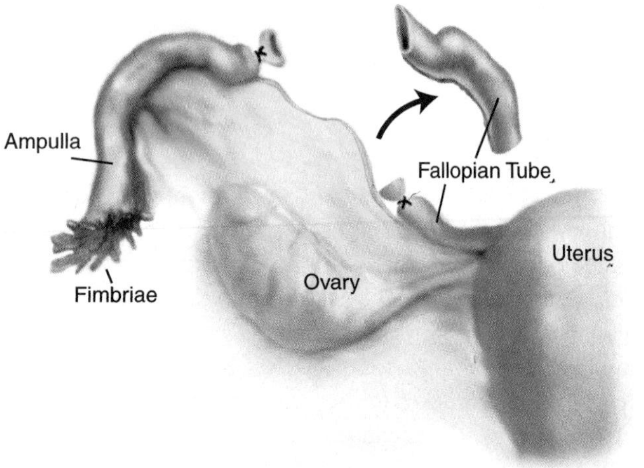

Figure 14-13 Tubal ligation.

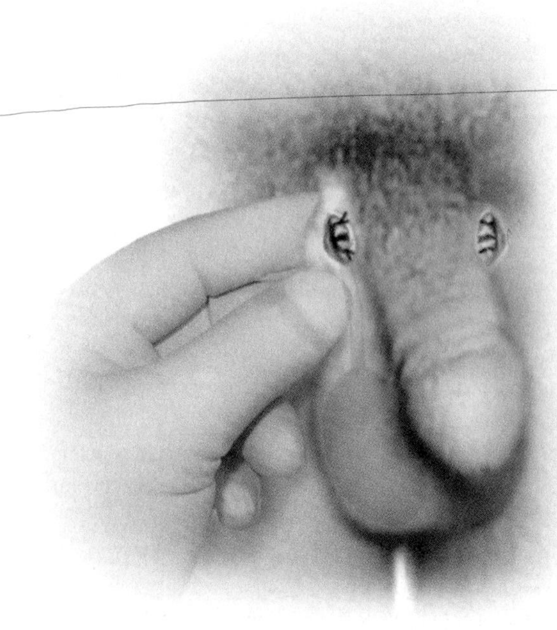

Figure 14-14 Vasectomy.

Another method of contraception approved by the Food and Drug Administration is a medication known as RU 486, an emergency contraceptive, which is used to cause or induce an abortion. Another method is a spring-like device called essure. It is inserted into the fallopian tubes where scar tissue forms and blocks the tubes. This also prevents pregancy. Injectable contraceptives are available. Depo-Provera® is given intramuscularly every three months. Lunelle® is given intramuscularly monthly. These injectables are best given within the first five days of the menstrual cycle to be certain the woman is not pregnant.

GYNECOLOGY

Gynecology is the specialty that studies diseases of the female reproductive tract and the breasts. The gynecologic examination is routinely performed in an office or clinic and usually includes abdominal, pelvic and breast examination, and a Pap smear. It can be done as part of the female's complete physical examination, or it can be a separate examination performed in the gynecologist's office or gynecology clinic. Early diagnosis and treatment of problems associated with the female reproductive organs helps the female to achieve optimum health of these organs and is the goal of the OB/GYN physician (Figure 14-15).

The Gynecologic Examination

It is recommended that a gynecologic pelvic examination and Pap smear be done annually on all women beginning when they become sexually active or by age 20 years. It is done to assess the female's health and to screen for cancer of the reproductive organs. It includes a breast examination by the physician and instructions for the patient about how to perform her own breast self-examination (BSE). It also includes a pelvic examination and Pap smear. Pap tests are done to detect cervical cancer. Women should be especially conscientious in scheduling annual Pap tests and mammograms if they have a family history of breast, uterine, or cervical cancer. Early detection of cervical and breast cancers and appropriate treatment can cure the disease. Any woman who has had a hysterectomy because of cancer should continue to be tested for pelvic cancer annually by having a Pap smear. Because the cervix has been removed, the specimen cells are taken from the inner vaginal vault instead. Even after hysterectomy, the woman still remains at risk for cancer cells to grow within the vaginal vault and she must be encouraged to continue with her regular pelvic examinations and Pap tests. Others feel that in healthy women a Pap test done every 1 to 3 years is sufficient. The American Cancer Society recommends that women have a Pap test at least every 3 years, beginning when they become sexually active, or at age 20 years, if there have been two initial negative Pap test results one year apart. Encourage patients to have regular Pap tests. Women at high risk should have a Pap test every six months and a mammogram yearly. If the patient is experiencing a vaginal discharge and there is a suspicion of a vaginal infection, smear(s) and cultures of discharge will be done to aid in diagnosis. See Chapter 31, Basic Microbiology, for more information.

Encourage your female patients to schedule their Pap smear and annual examination on a date that will be easy to remember, such as April Fool's Day, Flag Day, tax day, or first day of summer. Keep a tickler file to remind patients who "forget." Many patients think that because they have had a hysterectomy, they no longer need their annual examination and Pap smear. Every woman should have an annual (or regular) examination even if the Pap test is not included. A woman who has had a hysterectomy because of cancer should continue to have Pap smears on a regular basis. Many women are not aware of this and need to be educated (see Patient Education box).

Other gynecologic problems that may arise between annual gynecologic examinations may require that an appointment, in addition to the annual gynecologic checkup that is routinely done, be made and may include such symptoms and problems as severe **dysmenorrhea** (painful menses), lower abdominal pain, **metrorrhagia,** bleeding between menstrual periods, **dyspareunia** (painful intercourse), sexual dysfunction, infertility, and discomfort from menstrual symptoms. Women experiencing these problems should have a gynecologic examination, and the physician will determine a diagnosis based on the examination, the patient's history, symptoms, signs, and laboratory data.

It is important to realize that patients' health practices related to culture, values, and belief systems are deeply ingrained and not easily changed. Being aware of some of these practices and beliefs will benefit both you and your patients. You will have a better understanding of their cultural heritage and beliefs that are different from yours, and this will help patients to be more comfortable. At times, it might be necessary to modify care according to the patient's cultural background and practice.

Female circumcision is an ancient cultural custom that has been practiced worldwide for more than 2,000 years. Between 100 and 130 million women in 40 countries have had female circumcisions. Central Africa is one of the main areas where various forms of the procedure are performed.

There are four different types of female circumcision: (1) removal of the prepuce of the clitoris; (2) clitoridectomy, removal of prepuce and clitoris; (3) removal of prepuce, clitoris, upper labia minora, and some labia majora; and (4) infibulation, removal of all external genitalia (prepuce, clitoris, labia majora, labia minora). Some reasons given for this practice are that it is a right of passage, a sign of purity, marriage availability, sexual faithfulness, protection from rape and abortion, and for socialization into the role of a woman. Surgery is usually performed by a lay midwife, and a razor or broken glass is used; infections and hemorrhages are common. If an infibulation is performed, the two sides of the vulva are sewn together. Scar tissue forms over the vagina. A small opening for urination and menstruation is made by inserting a foreign object until the area heals. The most common reason given for this procedure is that it follows customs and tradition. During childbirth, the infibulation is cut to allow for delivery, then resutured after delivery.

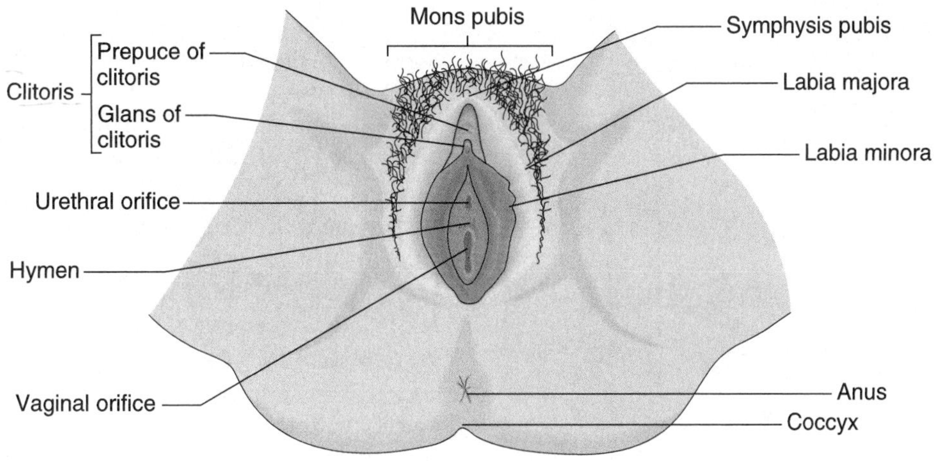

Figure 14-15 External genitalia of the female.

Critical Thinking

A 27-year-old woman wants to schedule an appointment because she has some bright red bleeding after sexual intercourse. What conditions or diseases might this woman have? Discuss your reasons for choosing the conditions or diseases. What equipment and supplies might the doctor require?

Always view patients as individuals whose cultural beliefs and practices may differ greatly from your own. Treat them as you do all patients, with respect and empathy.

Breast Examination. The physician performs a breast examination on the patient as part of a gynecologic examination. The physician looks for redness, dimpling, and puckering, and palpates each breast and axilla feeling for lumps or thickening. Part of the medi-

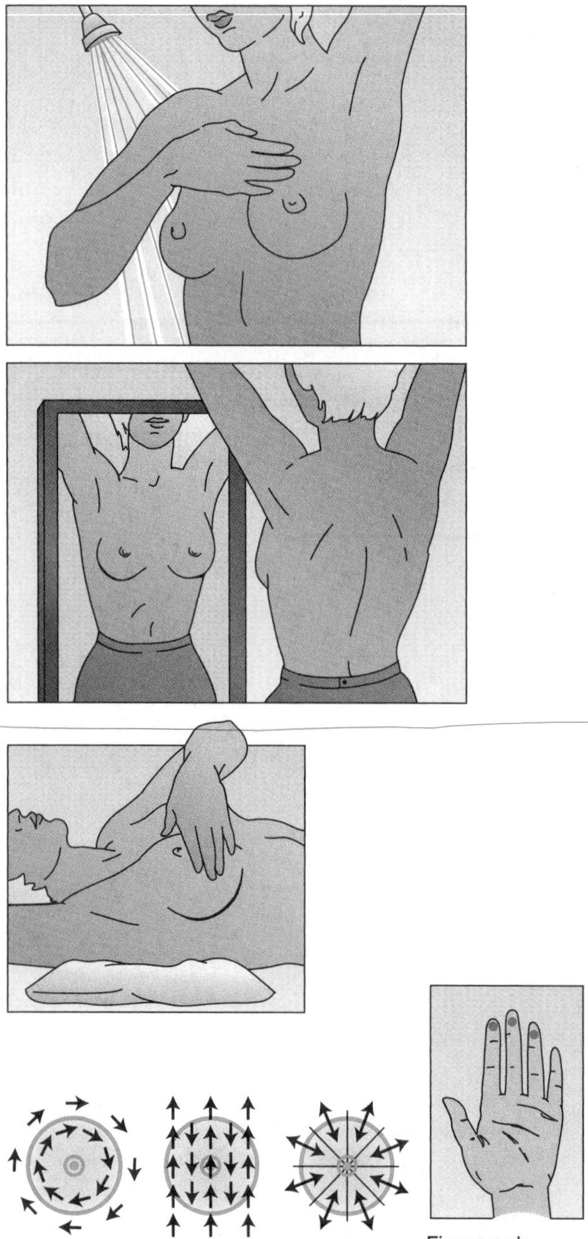

Figure 14-16 (A–D) Breast self-examination. (Courtesy of American Cancer Society.)

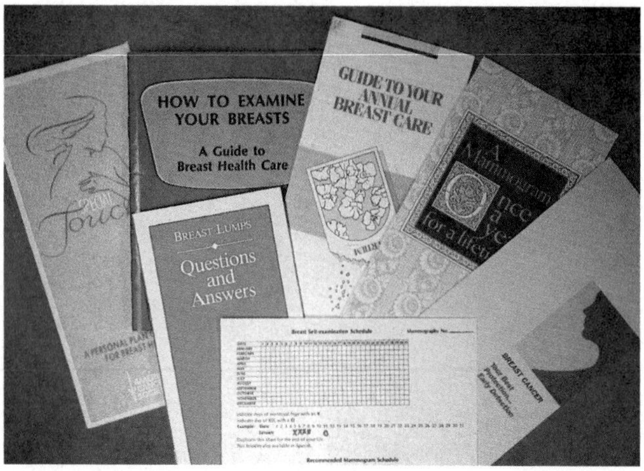

Figure 14-17A Informational pamphlets detailing the breast self-examination and its importance can be helpful to patients.

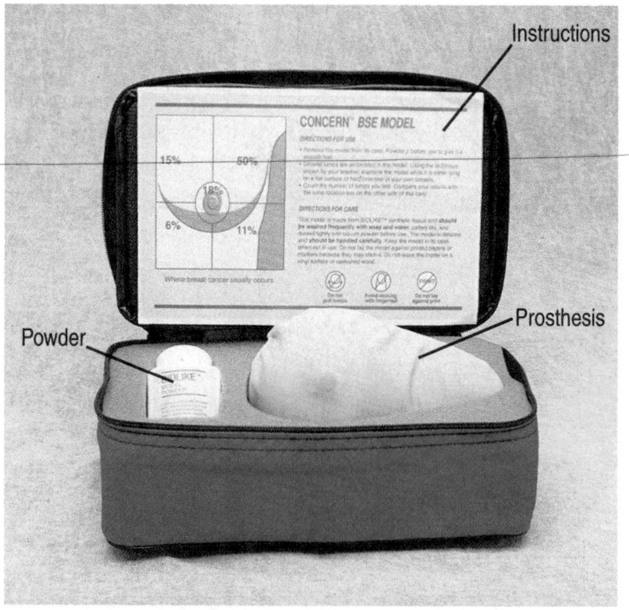

Figure 14-17B Breast self-examination model kit contains instructions for breast self-examination and powder to aid fingers in gliding over the breast prosthesis. The prosthesis contains lumps and thickened areas for identification and location.

Patient Education

Breast Self-Examination

1. Breast self-examination (BSE) should be done in three different positions.
   a. In a warm shower (soaping each breast) checking for lumps, thickening, or changes that differ from previous self-examination. Refer to Figure 14-16A.
   b. In front of a mirror, checking for changes in appearance. Refer to Figure 14-16B.
   c. Lying flat in a supine position helps breast tissue spread allowing better palpation of outer tissue. Refer to Figure 14-16C. Use pads of fingers.
   d. Examine the breasts in a circular motion starting at 12-o'clock position and moving around the breast clockwise. Use an up and down motion or an inward and outward motion from nipple outward or chest wall inward (Figure 14-16D).
2. Do the breast self-examination at the same time each month, 7 to 10 days after menses. Repeating the examination the same time each month provides familiarity with the contours of the body and allows for hormonal levels to return to premenstrual status. The breasts may be swollen, tender, and have thickening because of hormonal influence around the time of the menstrual cycle and for 7 to 10 days after menses.

Physician Breast Examination. The American Cancer Society recommends that:

a. Women aged 20 to 39 years have a breast physical examination by a physician every 3 years and women aged 40 years and older have one yearly.
b. Women without symptoms of breast cancer aged 40 to 49 years should have a mammogram every 1 to 2 years, and women aged 50 years and older, once a year (Figures 14-18 and 14-19). A tumor or mass can often be seen with a mammography up to 2 years before either the physician or patient notices or feels a tumor.

cal assistant's responsibility is to teach patients how to perform the BSE. Figure 14-16 provides illustrations for performing the BSE. The physician may also provide several pamphlets and a breast model with lumps and thickening for enhancing patient education and awareness about the importance of the examination (Figure 14-17A and B).

Assisting with a Gynecologic Examination. The gynecologic examination consists of four parts. These parts include:

1. Inspection of external **genitalia** (labia minora, labia majora, urinary meatus, clitoris, **Bartholin glands**, and vagina) for swelling, lesions, or ulcerations
2. Pelvic examination of cervix, uterus, tubes, and ovaries including a **bimanual examination;** this examination may or may not include a Pap test (Figure 14-20)
3. Rectal examination
4. Breast examination

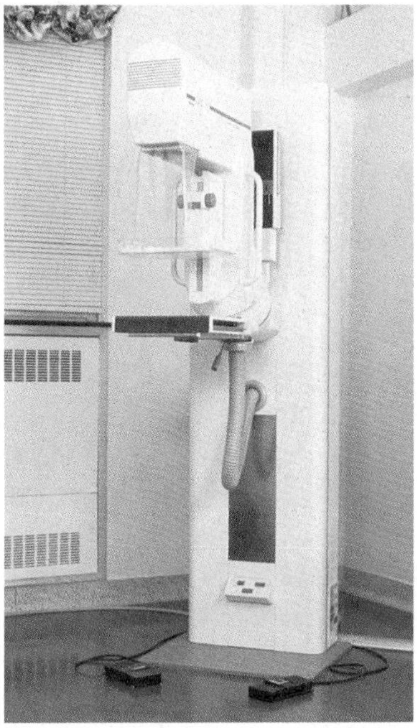

Figure 14-18 Breasts are compressed by the plates of mammographic X-ray unit.

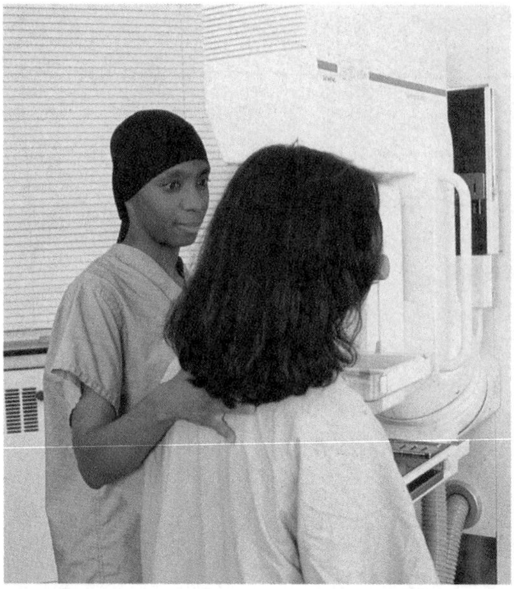

Figure 14-19 The technologist positions the patient for a mammography. The procedure requires the patient to move into various positions so different angles of the breast tissue may be X-rayed.

Patient Education

Many women think that if they have had a hysterectomy because of cancer they no longer need to have Pap smears performed. This is not true, and it is up to health care professionals to educate them. If the hysterectomy was performed because of cancer, the cancer cells can reappear in the vaginal vault after the surgery. During the pelvic examination, because the cervix has been removed, the physician will scrape the inner walls of the vaginal vault for cells to include in the Pap smear.

The medical assistant should prepare the patient, equipment, and room before the examination.

Gynecologic Examination with Pap Equipment. On a Mayo tray near the end of the examination table, place the instruments and supplies the physician needs to perform the gynecologic or pelvic examination with Pap test. Figures 14-21A and 21B show the equipment commonly needed for the examination. To aid in the inspection portion of the examination, you should place a gooseneck lamp at the foot of the table behind the stool on which the physician will sit. (See Procedure 14-3.)

In preparation for the annual examination, the patient is asked to avoid douching and sexual intercourse

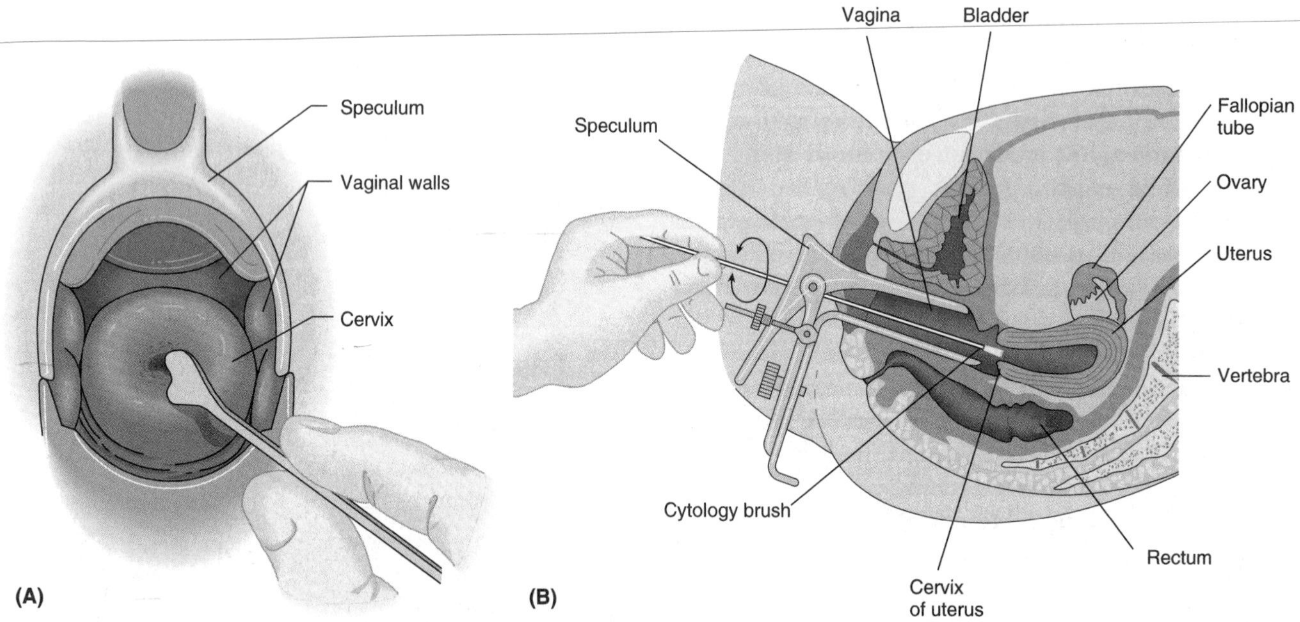

Figure 14-20 Use of speculum, cytology brush, and spatula to obtain a Pap smear. (A) The physician uses a spatula to obtain cells from the cervix. (B) The physician uses a cytology brush to obtain cells from the cervix.

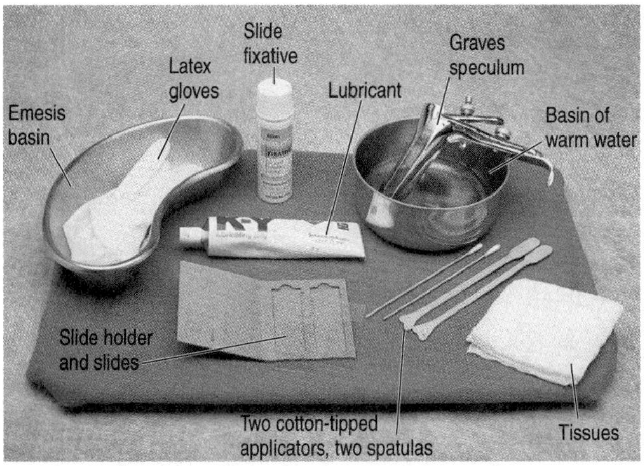

Figure 14-21A Setup for gynecologic examination including a conventional Pap smear.

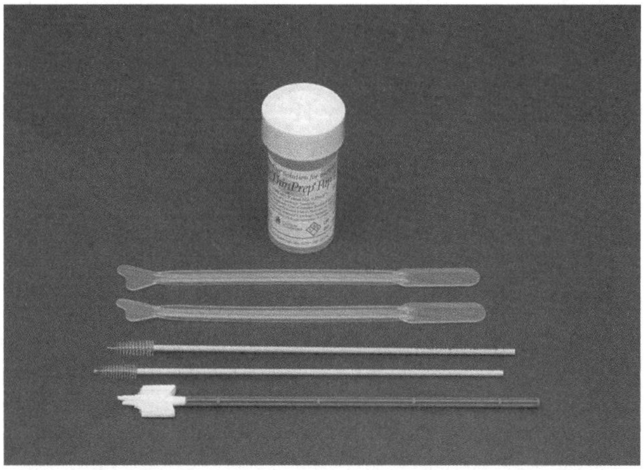

Figure 14-21B Thin Prep® Pap supplies: Transport medium container, spatula, cytology brush, and cytology broom.

for two days before a Pap test. Immediately before a pelvic examination, the patient is encouraged to empty her bladder. The urine may be collected for testing according to the clinic policy or the physician's preference and depending on any urinary tract complaints or symptoms the patient may have. If a Pap test is being performed, take a minute to interview the patient and gather the necessary medical and laboratory information. The data needed include:

- Last normal menstrual period. This question will bring up information about breakthrough bleeding (if patient is taking oral contraceptives), dysmenorrhea, metrorrhagia, postcoital bleeding, perimenopausal irregularities, and other idiosyncrasies of the menstrual patterns.
- Hormonal therapies, either oral contraceptives or hormone replacement therapy (HRT). These are excellent questions for birth control history, successes/failures, problems/solutions, and menopausal issues, concerns, and problems.
- Surgical history, especially related to the genitourinary tract. These questions will initiate discussions about bladder problems, hysterectomies, and so forth.
- Sexual history/habits. This will open discussions with the patient about disease prevention, birth control, hormonal problems, menopausal conditions, and so forth.
- Symptoms of diseases/disorders, such as pelvic or genital pain or discomfort; vaginal discharge, irritation, or itching; painful intercourse; dysuria; urinary frequency or incontinence; and breast pain or breast conditions/concerns.

All the information gathered during the patient interview should be shared with the doctor before the examination. Often a form is available that is specifically designed for this type of interview; the medical assistant simply fills in the blanks, makes appropriate check marks, and comments on the form. The doctor then uses the form and additional information gathered during his or her patient interaction to complete his or her report.

In preparation for the examination, have the patient undress and don a patient gown with the opening positioned in the front (for the breast examination) and a drape sheet. The patient is seated on the examination table. Provide the patient with privacy during the undressing. Ensure the patient's comfort by providing her with a blanket if she is cold and have her leave her socks on if her feet are cold. Assure her that the doctor will be in shortly.

During the breast and abdominal examinations, the patient will be placed into the supine or dorsal recumbent position. Provide her with a pillow for comfort. For the pelvic examination, the patient is placed into the lithotomy position. Assist the patient into this position, providing leg and back support as needed.

During the pelvic examination and the Pap smear, the medical assistant provides the doctor with assistance as needed. The tray of supplies should be at an appropriate height and position for the doctor to access it while seated. The vaginal speculum should be warmed to body temperature. Some examination tables are equipped with warming drawers for storing the specula so they are warm and ready for use. Or, the medical assistant may set up the pelvic exam/Pap smear supplies on a Mayo tray and position the gooseneck lamp so the warmth from the light bulb can warm the specula. Another method is for the physician to hold the speculum under warm running water just before use. Whichever method is used, the doctor will test the speculum to make sure it is not too hot before use. This is often done by touching the speculum on the patient's inner thigh to determine if the temperature is comfortable.

During the examination, the medical assistant will support the patient, hand the doctor supplies as needed, and adjust the light source as needed. When the doctor has obtained the appropriate cervical cells, he or she will hand the cytology broom or brush to the medical assistant. The medical assistant will uncap the ThinPrep container, swish the broom or brush vigorously in the ThinPrep solution until all the specimen has been deposited, dispose of the broom or brush in a biohazard container, reapply the cap, and complete the container label. If the patient is "status post hysterectomy," the physician will scrape cells (using the spatula) from the inner walls of the vaginal vault rather than from the cervix, which will no longer be present. Those cells are deposited into the ThinPrep solution in the same manner as a cervical specimen.

After the Pap test is performed, the physician will examine the internal organs. He or she will accomplish this bimanual (two-handed) examination by inserting two fingers into the vagina and, while pressing on the outside abdominal wall, manually feel the shape, consistency, movement, and positioning of the uterus and the ovaries. If any abnormalities are felt, further testing may be recommended. After the bimanual examination, a rectal examination is performed. This examination enables the doctor to assess the back side of the uterus, which is not felt during the bimanual examination.

When the pelvic examination is completed, the medical assistant will assist the patient off the table, offer tissue and the sink for her to clean up and wash her hands, and let her know you will be back in a few minutes. When you return, you may escort the patient to the physician's office for private discussion. Occasionally, the doctor will hold the discussion in the examination room after the patient has dressed.

Pap Smear. The conventional Pap smear is performed by scraping the patient's cervix with a spatula and cytology brush and smearing the cells onto a microscopic slide. The slide is then placed into a bottle of Pap fixative or sprayed with Pap fixative and sent to the regional laboratory for viewing. The ThinPrep® Pap Test differs in that the cells that are obtained on the collecting devices are swished vigorously into a vial of fluid transport medium rather than placed on a slide. The vial is sent to the regional laboratory for processing. Using the conventional method, approximately 80% of the specimen remains on the collecting device with only about 20% being submitted on the slide. With the ThinPrep® Pap Test, virtually 100% of the collected cells are rinsed off the collecting device and submitted in the vial. The conventional Pap slide preparation results in an inconsistently distributed specimen containing blood cells, mucus, and other debris that can interfere with the viewing. The ThinPrep® Pap Test uses a ThinPrep processor to suspend the cervical cells, to eliminate the blood cells, mucus, and other debris; and to distribute a thin and even layer of cells onto a slide for analyzing. The ThinPrep® Pap Test slide is of better quality, is much clearer and easier to read, and increases accuracy for both the manual assessment and the computerized assessment.

Although the conventional Pap smear has undoubtedly saved countless lives by detecting cervical cancer, the ThinPrep® Pap Test is significantly more effective. Another advantage of the ThinPrep® Pap Test is that the same specimen may be used to determine the presence of human papillomavirus (HPV) or chlamydia/gonorrhea if needed.

The federal government regulates laboratories that perform testing on Pap smears. There are requirements placed on the individuals who view or access the specimens for malignant cells, and they include specialized training. Limits are placed on the number of slides that can be read in one day. Proficiency testing, mandated by the Clinical Laboratory Improvement Act of 1988 (CLIA '88) ensures accuracy and precision of test results and is a requirement for Pap smear examination. See Chapter 26 for more information about CLIA '88.

A computerized method, known as PAPNET, is used to retest Pap smears that have been analyzed by technologists. The method duplicates the process that the technologists perform.

Another test, known as Virapap, can be used to screen for HPV in a Pap smear. There is higher incidence of cervical cancer in women who have HPV, and the test can help identify these women who are at greater risk for cervical cancer. Vaginal cancer can also be detected by a Pap smear. There is an increased risk for both cervical and vaginal cancer in daughters of women who used **diethylstilbestrol (DES)** during pregnancy.

A system for cytologic reporting of a Pap smear is a descriptive report that tells the physician exactly

Critical Thinking

A 38-year-old woman has been diagnosed with HPV infection. What is the significance of this infection?

what cellular changes have taken place. The classification includes the grades of cervical **intraepithelial** neoplasia (CIN).

CIN 1 = mild **dysplasia** (abnormal tissue development)
CIN 2 = moderate dysplasia
CIN 3 = severe dysplasia or **carcinoma in situ**

Pap Smear Results. The Pap smear will usually be sent to a reference laboratory where a pathologist will examine it and record the results on the cytology report form. The form will be returned to the physician.

Gynecologic Diseases and Conditions

The female reproductive system is affected by many diseases and conditions caused by hormonal imbalance, cysts, infection, and tumors. Some of the more common disorders and diseases are covered here.

Infertility. Most women, with unprotected intercourse, will be able to conceive within a year. The inability to conceive can be caused by a problem with either the male or the female individual. Some common causes of infertility in a female patient are:

- Endometriosis
- Certain medications
- Blocked fallopian tubes
- Problems ovulating
- Chronic stress
- Scar tissue from surgery, infection, or ectopic pregnancy
- Tumors

A woman who is having difficulty conceiving and has a history of any of the above will have a physical examination by a physician who specializes in infertility. The specialist will decide what tests and procedures are necessary. Hormone levels may be measured to look for hypothyroidism and ovarian function determined through a surgical procedure, such as laparoscopy. A test for **patency** (openness) of the fallopian tubes can be performed by a hysterosalpingogram, a radiographic procedure done after injection of dye into the vagina, through the cervix, into the uterus, and out the fallopian tubes. The dye will pass through all of these organs if there is no blockage in any of them (see "Impaired Fertility" section earlier in this chapter).

Menopause. The period of time that marks permanent cessation of menstrual activity is known as menopause. It usually occurs between the ages of 35 and 58 years. There may be a gradual decline in monthly menstrual flow, or a woman may suddenly cease to menstruate. Natural menopause occurs when the ovaries produce less and less estrogen. This causes the ovaries to cease ovulation and, therefore, menstruation stops. Surgical menopause is caused by the surgical removal of both ovaries (bilateral oophorectomy). Symptoms occur soon after ovulation ceases with both natural and surgical menopause. Symptoms may last for a few months to several years and include mild to severe symptoms. Hot flashes, chills, nervousness, fatigue, apathy, mental depression, crying episodes, insomnia, palpitations, and headache are some common symptoms experienced by some women. A long-term effect of lower estrogen levels is osteoporosis. HRT was thought to prevent osteoporosis and heart disease. An HRT study, the Women's Health Initiative (WHI), which was slated to run for 15 years, stopped testing what had been the most widely prescribed estrogen and progestin combination in 2002. Safety concerns brought an early end (5.5 years) to a trial testing the long-term benefits and risks for combined estrogen and progestin therapy (HRT). The testing was halted earlier than it was intended because it was determined that HRT, specifically Prempro®, was more harmful than helpful. There were increased risks for breast cancer and cardiovascular incidents; therefore, researchers told the women in the study to stop taking the combination medication. This situation has left many women with few choices for treating menopausal symptoms such as night sweats, hot flashes, dyspareunia, mood swings, fatigue, and osteoporosis. Switching to something else is risky because no other hormones have been as well studied as estrogen and progestin in Prempro®. There are many safe options for prevention and treatment of osteoporosis.

Researchers continued to study the estrogen-only hormone after halting the estrogen–progesterone trial. Because progesterone was initially added to the estrogen to protect women from uterine cancer, the thinking was that healthy postmenopausal women who had a hysterectomy and were given the estrogen-only hormone would not be at risk. However, data showed an increase in stroke in postmenopausal women given estrogen only. As of February 2004, the estrogen-only arm of the WHI study was halted, and the recommendation is for only short-term use of the hormone for women with moderate-to-severe menopausal symptoms. The FDA has urged manufacturers to add warnings to their labels on the estrogen-only hormone about the increased risk for dementia, strokes, abnormal mammograms, and uterine cancer in women who have not had a hysterectomy.

Endometriosis. Endometriosis is a painful, common condition characterized by endometrial tissue adhering to tissue and organs outside of the uterus. It is primarily found in the pelvis, adhering to an ovary, fallopian tube, or pelvic peritoneum. It also can be found outside of the pelvis, even in the abdomen adhering to tissue and organs, such as the bowel. The cause is unknown. The abnormal and engorged endometrial tissue responds to hormonal stimulation (estrogen) and builds up along with the normal endometrium of the menstrual cycle. It sloughs off at time of menstruation and is painful. The blood has not had a way to leave the body and is discharged into the pelvic or abdominal cavities.

Endometriosis symptoms may respond to contraceptive medication because these pills suppress menstruation and no further treatment is necessary (see Figure 14-22). However, long-term hormonal treatment may help alleviate symptoms. Hysterectomy may be necessary if the woman does not respond to hormonal therapy.

Ovarian Cysts. Cysts that appear on the ovary are common. As part of the menstrual cycle, the ovarian follicles enlarge and become graafian follicles. Only one of these graafian follicles ruptures at the time of ovulation. The follicles that do not rupture, but remain, are filled with fluid. They may enlarge and become cysts (Figure 14-23).

Ultrasonography will aid in viewing the ovaries. Most ovarian cysts resolve without treatment. Laparoscopy can be done to either drain or remove the cyst. Contraceptive therapy many times is helpful in resolving the cyst without surgery.

Direct viewing of the ovaries and surgery may be necessary because cancer of the ovary must be ruled out.

Ovarian Cancer. Because the symptoms of ovarian cancer do not appear until the disease has had an opportunity to become established, it is difficult to make a diagnosis early in the disease process. Therefore, if a woman has any symptoms, the cancer has been present for some time. Symptoms may be pressure in the pelvis, lower abdominal discomfort, weight loss, and fluid in the abdomen. Diagnosis can be made by laparoscopic surgery and a biopsy. Hysterectomy and bilateral salpingo-oophorectomy are done, followed by radiation therapy or chemotherapy. The cause is not known.

Pelvic Inflammatory Disease (PID). PID involves some or all of the female reproductive tract and can be a mild to serious infection. The causative microorganism is usually a sexually transmitted pathogen. The microorganism enters through the vagina and ascends through the cervix into the body of the uterus. It can spread out through the fallopian tubes into the pelvic cavity. Culture and sensitivity of the vaginal discharge are performed, and appropriate antibiotics are prescribed. Early treatment helps to lessen damage caused by scar tissue that forms in the pelvis and organs. Delayed treatment can cause septic shock, which can be life-threatening. Infertility and ectopic pregnancy are long-range problems that can occur (see Tables 14-3, 14-4, and 14-5).

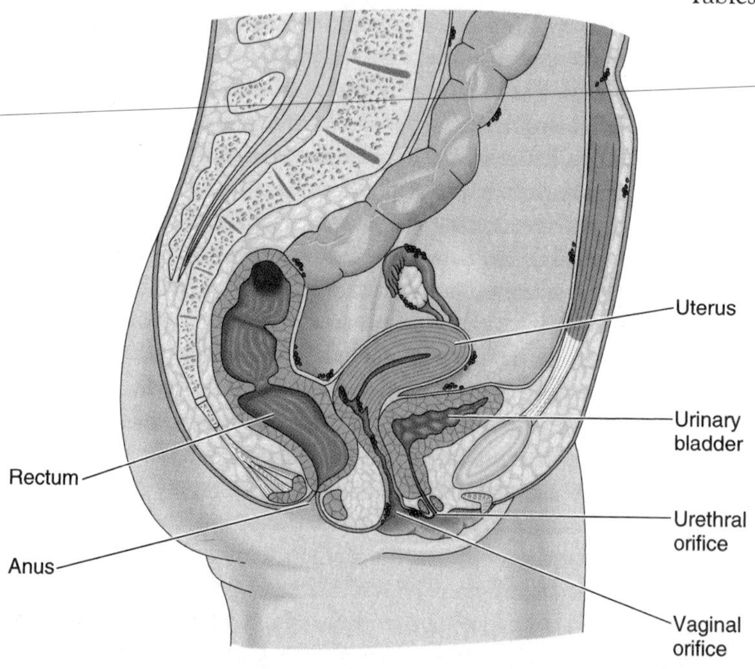

Figure 14-22 Endometriosis—common sites of endometrial implants.

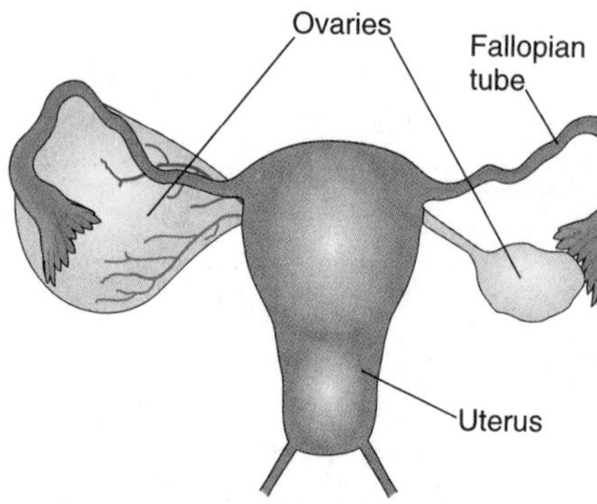

Figure 14-23 Ovarian cyst.

TABLE 14-3 FEMALE REPRODUCTIVE SYSTEM

Medical Tests or Procedures	Disease/ Disorder	Laboratory Diagnostic Tests: Blood	Laboratory Diagnostic Tests: Other	Radiography	Surgery
Pelvic examination	Bartholin Gland Infection		Exudate culture and sensitivity		Incision and drainage
Monthly breast self-examination	Breast Cancer	Breast cancer gene detection BRCA1, BRCA2		Mammography Ultrasonography	Biopsy of breast lesion Lumpectomy
Pelvic examination Colposcopy	Cervical Cancer		Pap smear		Cone biopsy Punch biopsy Dilation & curettage (D&C) Cryosurgery LEEP (loop electrosurgical excision procedure) Laser surgery Hysterectomy
Pelvic examination	Endometriosis		Urinalysis	Abdominal ultrasonography Chest radiograph	Laparoscopy Hysterectomy
Monthly breast self-examination	Fibrocystic Breasts			Mammography Ultrasonography	Biopsy
Pelvic examination	Pelvic Inflammatory Disease	Complete blood count and differential (CBC)	Urinalysis Culture and sensitivity of vaginal discharge	Pelvic ultrasonography	Laparoscopy
Sexually Transmitted Diseases					
Pelvic examination	• **Chlamydia**	Serology	Urinalysis Direct urethral or cervical smear using monoclonal antibodies ThinPrep® Pap Test		
Pelvic examination Pap smear	• **Condylomata**/HPV (genital warts)		ThinPrep® Pap Test	Excisional biopsy	
Pelvic examination	• Neisseria Gonorrhea	CBC	Urinalysis Direct smear of vaginal discharge, anal canal, and oropharynx Thayer-Martin culture ThinPrep® Pap Test	Pelvic ultrasonography	
	• Hepatitis B and C and HIV	Virology	Liver function	Abdominal ultrasonography	Liver biopsy
Vaginitis					
Pelvic examination	• **Candidiasis**	Blood glucose	Urinalysis **Wet mount:** direct vaginal smear with potassium hydroxide (1 drop)		
Pelvic examination	• **Trichomoniasis**		Urinalysis Wet mount: direct vaginal smear with isotonic saline (1 drop)		

TABLE 14-4 DESCRIPTION OF FEMALE REPRODUCTIVE SYSTEM DISORDERS AND CONDITIONS

- *Bartholin Gland Infection.* Infection of the mucous gland(s) that open near the vaginal opening.
- *Breast Cancer.* Most common site of cancer in females. A genetic cause has been identified for some breast cancers. Some symptoms are lump, thickening, swelling, dimpling, pain, and nipple discharge.
- *Cervical Cancer.* A carcinoma of the cervix of the uterus caused by a progressive cervical dysplasia. Most common in women aged 30 to 40 years. A significant risk factor is seen in women who become sexually active early in their lives and who have multiple sex partners. Presence of human papillomavirus (HPV) poses greater risk.
- *Endometriosis.* Presence of endometrium in sites other than inside the uterus. May be found on the ovaries, fallopian tubes, large bowel, lungs, and pleura. Causes pelvic pain, dysmenorrhea, and infertility.
- *Fibrocystic Breasts.* Benign cysts in breast tissue that increase or decrease in size during menses. Thought to be a normal variation in breast tissue due to monthly hormonal influence.
- *Pelvic Inflammatory Disease (PID).* Pelvic reproductive organs become inflamed and infected by bacteria, viruses, or parasites. An ascending infection can ensue involving the vagina, cervix of uterus, body of uterus, fallopian tubes, and ovaries. Symptoms include vaginal discharge, pain, fever. May cause infertility. Majority caused by sexually transmitted disease.
- *Premenstrual Syndrome (PMS).* Cluster of symptoms that occur monthly before the onset of menses thought to be caused by progesterone–estrogen imbalance. Symptoms include fluid retention, weight gain, irritability, and mood swings.
- *Sexually Transmitted Diseases (STDs).* Several diseases caused by bacteria, viruses, and protozoa that are transmitted through sexual intercourse (vaginal, anal, oral).
  - *Chlamydia.* An invasion by an intracellular parasite causing urethritis, cervicitis, PID, proctitis, infant pneumonia, and conjunctivitis.
  - *Condylomata (HPV).* Genital warts caused by a virus. Grow around the external genitalia, rectum, and cervix. Associated with abnormal Pap smears.
  - *Neisseria Gonorrhea.* An infection by a bacterium that can involve the cervix, urethra, fallopian tubes and ovaries, rectum, and mouth.
- *Vaginitis.* Inflammation of the vagina may be caused by bacteria, fungus, protozoa, chemical irritants, irritation from foreign bodies, vitamin deficiency, uncleanliness, and intestinal worms.
  - *Candidiasis.* A yeast (fungal) infection of the vagina caused by prolonged antibiotic therapy, pregnancy, or diabetes, which can change the normal vaginal flora leading to overgrowth of the fungus.
  - *Trichomoniasis.* An infection by a protozoan most commonly spread through sexual intercourse or may come from fecal contamination of the vagina.

TABLE 14-5 COMMON SEXUALLY TRANSMITTED DISEASES

Pathology	Symptoms	Test	Treatment
AIDS	Flulike, lymphadenopathy, infections, malignancies, pneumonia	HIV	Medication: antiretroviral medications such as zidovudine and didanosine
Chlamydia	Usually asymptomatic	Vaginal culture ThinPrep® Pap Test	Doxycyline, erythromycin
Condylomata	Warts on external and internal genitalia	Visual exam ThinPrep® Pap Test	Cryocautery or chemocautery preferred but electrocautery can be used Keratolytic agents used such as Podofilox
Gonorrhea	Usually asymptomatic; yellowish-green discharge with dysuria in advanced stages	Gram stain or Thayer-Martin culture ThinPrep® Pap Test	Penicillin, ceftriaxone
Herpes Simplex I & II	Itching and soreness followed by genital **vesicles,** which heal in 10 to 14 days	Visual exam with blood test for confirmation	Acyclovir®, Valtrex, Famvir
Syphilis	Stage I: papule develops into ulcer, which develops into chancre on vulva Stage II: fever, general malaise, dermal and mucosal lesions Stage III: degeneration of central nervous system, lesions of internal structures	Venereal Disease Research Laboratory, Fluorescent Antibody Test	Penicillin
Trichomonas	Milky white, frothy, malodorous discharge with genital burning and itching	Wet mount for microscopic examination	Oral Flagel®, partner(s) must also be treated

Other Diagnostic Tests and Treatments for Reproductive System Diseases

Colposcopy. **Colposcopy** is the examination of the vagina and cervix by means of a lighted instrument that has a three-dimensional magnifying lens called a colposcope. The examination is done to determine if areas in the vagina or the cervix contain precancerous cells or tissue. The procedure is performed after an abnormal Pap test. It can also be performed to evaluate a lesion noted during a pelvic examination and to follow up after treatment of cervical cancer. Because the instrument has the ability to magnify tissue, the cervix can be more readily examined and a biopsy taken.

The patient is placed in lithotomy position and is prepared as she would be for a gynecologic examination. A nonlubricated speculum is inserted into the vagina. The vagina is swabbed with a long cotton-tipped applicator that has been moistened with saline. (This provides better visualization of the cervical tissue.) The cervix is then swabbed with acetic acid to dissolve mucus and provide a good contrast between normal and abnormal tissue. A staining medium can be used as another means of identifying abnormal cells. If the physician finds an area of abnormal tissue, a biopsy can be performed using cervical punch biopsy forceps. The specimen is examined by a pathologist to determine whether malignant cells are present.

Endometrial Biopsy/Sampling. An endometrial biopsy/sampling is often performed when patients are experiencing postmenopausal bleeding. It is a fairly simple procedure. The sampling device is housed in a long strawlike tube that slides through the cervical os quite easily. Once the end of the tube is inside the uterus, a plunger is pulled back. The action of pulling the plunger suctions a sampling of the endometrial tissue. This is a sterile procedure and requires an application of a cleansing solution (such as Betadine) to the cervix before performing the biopsy. Endometrial biopsy/sampling is quick and almost painless for the patient. The patient might experience slight cramping.

Cervical Punch Biopsy. The **cervical punch biopsy** is usually done in conjunction with a colposcopy to obtain a sample of cervical tissue for pathologic examination. The specimen is examined for malignant cells and the biopsy usually follows an abnormal Pap smear report.

The procedure is performed with the patient in lithotomy position and with a vaginal speculum in place. The physician may stain the cervix to aid in identifying abnormal tissue. If the colposcope is being used, it illuminates and magnifies the cervical tissue and the physician will take several tissue samples using the cervical punch biopsy forceps. If bleeding ensues, it can be controlled with a vaginal packing, or the area can be cauterized to stop the bleeding. The specimen is placed in a container with **formalin,** a completed requisition form is attached to the container, and it is sent to the pathology laboratory for examination. The patient may expect a small amount of bleeding and should notify the physician if bleeding ensues that is greater than a menstrual period. A discharge that has a strong, foul odor is to be expected and can last for up to one month after the procedure.

Cervical Cone Biopsy. Another type of biopsy, known as a cone biopsy, can be performed. An inverted cone of tissue is excised after a local anesthetic. In this procedure, a larger sample of tissue is excised to rule out invasive cancer and to remove the lesion. It is the most comprehensive specimen to diagnose a premalignant or malignant lesion. The carbon dioxide laser scalpel or electrosurgery can be used in this procedure.

Cryosurgery. **Cryosurgery** is used to treat tissue by freezing temperatures. Chronic cervicitis and cervical **erosion** are two common problems treated in this manner. (Also refer to Chapter 19 for information on cryosurgery.) The freezing temperature causes cells to die; they are then cast off from the cervix and eventually replaced with healthy cells about a month after the procedure.

The procedure is performed with the patient in lithotomy position and the cervix is swabbed to remove mucous. The probe is placed against the affected area of the cervix and the machine is turned on. The liquid nitrogen flows over the area for about three minutes and freezes the tissue. The patient may have some pain similar to dysmenorrhea that may last for about a half hour.

Patient Education

Post Cervical Biopsy and Cervical Cone Biopsy

1. Rest for 24 hours after the procedure.
2. Do not lift heavy objects for two weeks.
3. Leave packing in place for 24 hours or as directed. Do not insert another tampon unless told to do so by the physician.
4. Report any bleeding greater than a normal menstrual period.

Patient Education

After Cryosurgery of Cervix

1. Expect a clear, watery, heavy discharge for up to one week, tapering off for up to four weeks.
2. Use only sanitary pads, not tampons. Change often, cleansing perineal area with each pad change.
3. Report signs of infection: fever, malodorous discharge, pain, nausea, or vomiting.
4. Do not engage in sexual intercourse, douche, or use tampons for four weeks (unless instructed otherwise by physician).
5. Expect a somewhat heavier than usual menstrual period the following month.
6. Report excessive bleeding.

There should be no strong, foul odor, but there can be a discharge for up to one month. Patients should report any malodorous discharges because this may indicate an infection. Healing usually takes four to six weeks.

Wet Prep/Wet Mount For Yeast, Bacteria, and Trichomonas. The wet prep or wet mount is an office procedure to determine the cause of vaginitis in women and urethritis in men. The doctor takes a sample of the discharge on a cotton-tipped applicator, the medical assistant rinses it vigorously in a test tube containing a few drops (about 0.5 ml) of normal saline, pressing the swab against the inside of the test tube to express all the specimen, places a drop of the solution onto a microscope slide, covers with a coverslip; then the physician views it microscopically for the following:

- If a yeast infection is present, budding yeast will be seen.
- If a bacterial infection is present, clue cells will be seen. Clue cells are vaginal epithelial cells that appear fuzzy with no clear cell edge. They appear this way because the outside edge is covered with bacteria.
- If trichomonas are present, they appear as motile single-cell protozoa. Movement will be noted. The trichomonas are sometimes identified in a microscopic portion of the urinalysis as well.

Potassium Hydroxide Prep For Fungus. After performing the previously mentioned test, a few drops of 10% potassium hydroxide (KOH) may be added to the remaining solution in the test tube and examined microscopically for fungi. The KOH destroys bacteria and vaginal epithelial cells, leaving only the cell walls of the fungus, which makes visualization easier. This slide is prepared in the same way as the wet prep: Place a drop of the solution onto a clean slide, cover with a coverslip. Dispose of all glass slides, coverslips, and test tubes into a sharps container.

Amplified DNA Probe Test for Chlamydia and Gonorrhea. The Amplified DNA Probe Test for Chlamydia and Gonorrhea is used as a screening tool for both men and women and on all pregnant women. It is not a culture. There are two types of kits available, the ProbeTec® blue kit for urethral specimens from the male patient (see Chapter 16) and the ProbeTec® pink kit for endocervical specimens from the female patient. The female kit contains preservative, swabs (one large swab and one small Mini-Tip Culturette Swab), and instructions. This test needs to be performed on the female patient before the digital/bimanual examination so there is not any lubricating jelly present. Using the large swab, the doctor will clean the cervix of any mucus, blood, and cellular debris and discard the swab. The Mini-Tip Culturette Swab is then inserted into the cervical canal and rotated for 15 to 30 seconds. Immediately it is placed into the transport tube. If the ProbeTec Wet Transport tube is used (Figure 14-24), the swab is broken off into the liquid before recapping. This test also may be used to test for chlamydia and gonorrhea in a urine specimen, following the manufacturer's instructions for collection and testing.

Laparoscopy. Laparoscopy is a procedure in which a lighted instrument is used to view the inside of the pelvic cavity. It can be helpful in diagnosing endometriosis and

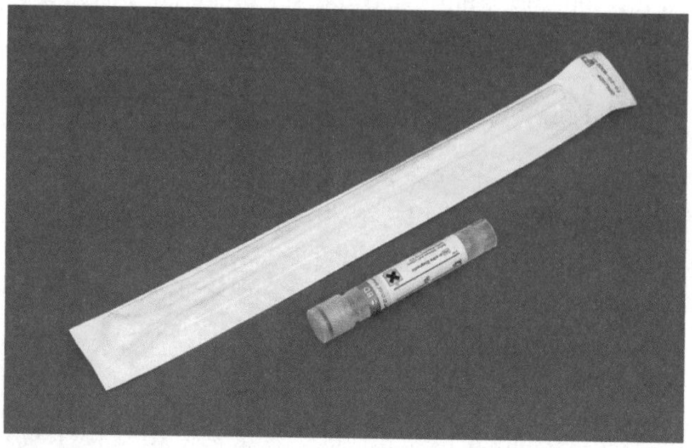

Figure 14-24 BD's ProbeTec Amplified DNA test kit for chlamydia and gonorrhea.

ovarian cysts or other abnormalities in the pelvic cavity. A tubal ligation, severing of the fallopian tubes, can be done laparoscopically. Laparoscopy can be done abdominally or vaginally (Figure 14-25).

Dilation and Curettage. Dilation and curettage (D&C) is a surgical procedure that involves the dilating and scraping the cervix of endometrial tissue. It is commonly performed to remove any remaining tissue after an incomplete abortion or to examine the tissue if the female patient has had abnormal uterine bleeding.

Complementary Therapy in Obstetrics and Gynecology

Most of the complementary therapy practiced today can be helpful in assisting women with easing the discomforts of pregnancy and labor. In our stress-filled world, emotional calm can be provided through the use of some of these therapies.

Neonatal intensive care unit infants benefit from a calm, warm touch, rocking, hugging, and singing softly.

Information about any form of complementary therapy (stress reduction, imagery, acupuncture, biofeedback, massage therapy, music therapy, among others) should be obtained from the obstetrics patient at each visit. Consultation with the provider concerning their safety during pregnancy is advisable.

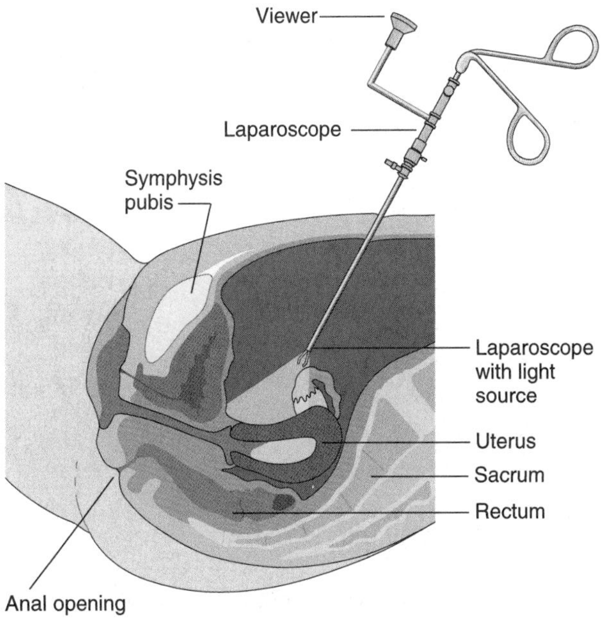

Figure 14-25 Laparoscopy.

Caution is advised when the use of herbal medicine is considered during the pregnancy. Because the herbal supplements are available over the counter and little is known about their effects on the fetus, women should be cautioned to avoid using any kind of herbal supplement during their first trimester. Women should ask their provider's advice about the use of the supplements after the first trimester.

Procedure 14-1 Assisting with Routine Prenatal Visits

STANDARD PRECAUTIONS:

PURPOSE:

To monitor the progress of the pregnancy.

EQUIPMENT/SUPPLIES:

Scale
Disposable gloves
Patient gown
Tape measure
Sphygmomanometer
Stethoscope
Doppler fetoscope and coupling agent
Urine specimen container
Urinalysis testing supplies
Biohazard waste container

PROCEDURE STEPS:

1. Wash hands.
2. Set up equipment.
3. Identify patient.
4. Obtain urine specimen. RATIONALE: A urine specimen for analysis is necessary. An empty bladder facilitates the examination and is more comfortable for the patient. The sample will be tested.
5. Weigh patient. RATIONALE: Assesses gain or loss of weight to help determine fetal development and maternal nutrition.
6. Measure blood pressure.
7. Have patient disrobe from waist down and put on a gown open in the front. RATIONALE: An open gown facilitates access to the abdomen for

(continues)

Procedure 14-1 (continued)

examination and measurement of the fundal height.

8. Test the urine specimen while waiting for the physician. RATIONALE: Urinalysis is done for detection of glucose and protein, which can indicate disease.
9. Assist patient onto examination table and drape her. RATIONALE: The patient may be off balance and unsteady on her feet because of the enlargement of the abdomen. Provide for her safety.
10. Assist the physician as the examination is performed.
    - Hand the physician the tape measure to measure height of fundus
    - Hand the physician the Doppler fetal pulse detector for measurement of fetal heart rate.

    The medical assistant may spread the coupling agent onto the patient's abdomen.
11. After the examination, assist patient to sit for a few moments. Assess her color, pulse. RATIONALE: Orthostatic hypotension can occur when a patient rises from a recumbent position. Give the patient time for the blood pressure to go back to normal so she will not experience dizziness from decreased blood pressure.
12. Provide any instruction or clarification of physician's orders.
13. Apply gloves. Discard disposable supplies per OSHA guidelines. Disinfect equipment used.
14. Remove gloves.
15. Wash hands.
16. Set up for the next patient.
17. Record all information in patient's record.

DOCUMENTATION

4/14/20XX 2:30 PM Wt. 148 3/4 lbs., T 98.8°F, P 82, R 16, BP 118/72[L] sitting. Urine dipstick negative for glucose and protein. Fundal height at 22 wks. FHR 120. Says she feels well and is sleeping and eating well. C. McInnis, CMA

Procedure 14-2 Instructing Patient in Breast Self-Examination

PURPOSE:

To properly instruct a woman in the procedure for performing a breast self-examination.

EQUIPMENT/SUPPLIES:

Breast model

Pamphlet on breast self-examination

PROCEDURE STEPS:

1. Using a patient information brochure (see Figure 14-16) and the knowledge you have gained from this unit, instruct the patient on the proper method to perform a breast self-examination. RATIONALE: Written information will be easier for her to follow, especially if there are instructional diagrams and pictures.
2. Discuss the ideal positioning, time of the month, frequency, methods, and the pattern to follow while examining the breasts. RATIONALE: Emphasizing the important points within the instructions will help her understand the procedure.
3. Help her determine a day each month that will be conducive for her to perform the examination. RATIONALE: If she is scheduled to perform a breast self-examination every month, she is more likely to follow through with the test.

(continues)

Procedure 14-2 (continued)

4. Answer any questions she has and give her your number to call if she needs further instruction. RATIONALE: Offering further support will give additional emphasis to the importance of this procedure and will let her know that you are available for assistance if she needs it.
5. Provide her with additional educational materials and resources that are approved by your physician–employer. RATIONALE: Educational materials in the form of brochures, videotapes, books/booklets, Web sites, and so on, are all good references for her. All education materials given to patients should first be approved by your physician–employer.
6. Have her report any abnormalities to you and/or the physician immediately. RATIONALE: The sooner any abnormalities are checked, the better the outcome. If the abnormality is benign, the patient can feel relief; if the abnormality is suspicious of malignancy, time is an important factor for cure.

Procedure 14-3 Assisting with Pelvic Examination and Pap Test (Conventional and ThinPrep® Methods)

STANDARD PRECAUTIONS:

PURPOSE:

To assist the physician in collecting cervical cells for laboratory analysis for early detection of malignant cells of the cervix and to assess the health of the reproductive organs to detect diseases leading to early diagnosis and treatment.

EQUIPMENT/SUPPLIES:

Nonsterile gloves (2–3 pair)
Vaginal speculum
Warm water or warming light
Light source
Drape sheet
Patient gown
Tissues
Vaginal lubricant
Lab requisition
Urine specimen container
Urine testing supplies
Biohazard specimen bag
Biohazard waste container
Adjustable stool for physician
Supplies for the Pap test according to the method used
For ThinPrep® Pap:

- Cervical spatula
- Brush and broom
- ThinPrep® container with solution

For Conventional Pap test:

- Microscope slides
- Fixative and/or specimen bottle
- Cervical spatula
- Cytology brush

PROCEDURE STEPS:

1. Wash hands and assemble necessary supplies near patient.
2. Request that patient empty her bladder. (Instruct patient to save urine specimen and provide specimen container if ordered by physician.) RATIONALE: An empty bladder facilitates examination of the uterus and a urine specimen is frequently used for a urinalysis.
3. Provide patient with gown and request her to completely undress.
4. Explain procedure to patient.
5. Instruct patient to sit at end of table when ready for pelvic examination. Drape patient for pri-

(continues)

Procedure 14-3 (continued)

vacy if performing conventional Pap test. Label the frosted end of the slide with a marking pencil. Include patient's name on slide. Indicate site from where specimen is collected: c = cervix, v = vagina, e = endocervical.

6. Assist patient into lithotomy position. Patient's knees should be relaxed and thighs rotated out as far as comfortable. Drape for privacy and warmth.
7. Encourage patient to breathe slowly and deeply through the mouth during examination. RATIONALE: Allows for relaxation of pelvic muscles and easier insertion of vaginal speculum.
8. Warm vaginal speculum with either warm water or under heat lamp or place on a heating pad. NOTE: Do not lubricate speculum. Lubricant obscures **exfoliated** cervical cells when Pap test is being performed.
9. Hand speculum and spatula, cytology brush, and broom to the physician as needed.
10. Apply gloves.
11. For conventional Pap test, hold slides for physician to apply smear of exfoliated cells, one for vaginal (v), one for cervical (c), and one for endocervical (e) in that order. If spraying Pap fixative, spray it over the slide within 10 seconds at a distance of about 6 inches. Allow to dry for at least 10 minutes. If using Pap fixative in a bottle, place slide directly into bottle. If using ThinPrep®, swish the cytology broom vigorously in the ThinPrep® solution until all the specimen has been deposited. Dispose of brush into biohazard container. RATIONALE: This maintains cell appearance and avoids contamination of cells. Avoid getting too close to slide with spray because this may destroy or damage cells. Slides must be fixed before they dry to protect the appearance of the cells.
12. For ThinPrep® Pap test, hand the speculum and cytology broom to the physician. Open the ThinPrep® solution container. When the cells have been obtained, take the broom and vigorously swish it into the container of solution until all the cells have been deposited. Replace the cap and label. Dispose of the broom into biohazard waste. RATIONALE: The ThinPrep® procedure requires that all cells obtained from the cervix be presented in the solution for complete testing.
13. Place lubricant on physician's gloved fingers without touching gloves, for bimanual and rectal examinations. The physician will insert the index and middle fingers into the vagina. The other hand is placed on the lower abdomen. The size, shape, and position of the uterus and ovaries are palpated.
14. The physician will insert one gloved finger into the rectum to check the ovaries and the tone of the rectal and pelvic muscles. Hemorrhoids, rectal fissures, or other lesions may be palpated.
15. Assist patient to wipe genitalia and rectum.
16. Help patient to a sitting position, allowing her to rest a while. Check her pulse and skin color. RATIONALE: Some patients, especially older adult patients, can experience orthostatic hypotension.
17. Discard disposable supplies per OSHA guidelines. If stainless steel speculum was used, soak in cool water. Sanitize and sterilize as soon as convenient.
18. Remove gloves and wash hands.
19. Assist patient down and off the table if necessary.
20. Instruct patient to dress. Inform patient of how and when test results will be reported to her.
21. Prepare laboratory requisition (cytology request) form. Include physician name and address, date, source of specimen, patient's name and address, date of LMP, and hormone therapy. Place slides in slide container. Place container into biohazard specimen bag. Place requisition into outer pocket of bag and send to laboratory.
22. Wash hands.
23. Document procedure in the patient's chart.

DOCUMENTATION

4/14/20XX 11:00 AM
Wt. 138 lbs., T 98°F, P 68, R 20, BP 138/72[L] sitting. Urine dipstick negative for protein and glucose. Pap smear performed by Dr. Woo. Slides of vaginal, cervical, endometrial cells sent to lab with requisition. Pelvic and rectal exams performed by Dr. Woo. Patient expressed no complaints of discomfort. BP 142/78 P 80. C. McInnis, RMA

Procedure 14-4 Wet Prep/Wet Mount and Potassium Hydroxide (KOH) Prep

STANDARD PRECAUTIONS:

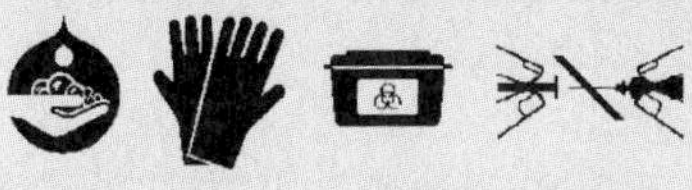

PURPOSE:

To test a vaginal specimen to determine the cause of vaginitis. The wet prep/wet mount tests for yeast, bacteria, and trichomonas; the KOH prep tests for yeast.

EQUIPMENT/SUPPLIES:

Cotton-tipped applicator
Small test tube
Normal saline (0.5 ml, or a few drops)
10% Potassium hydroxide (KOH; 0.5 ml, or a few drops)
Two microscope slides and cover slips
Microscope
Vaginal speculum
Patient drape
Gloves
Other equipment as necessary for a vaginal examination

PROCEDURE STEPS:

1. Prepare the patient for a pelvic examination as outlined in Procedure 14-3 (see Figure 14-26).
2. Place several drops of normal saline into a small test tube. RATIONALE: Preparing the test tube for the specimen.
3. Using the cotton-tipped applicator, the physician obtains a sampling of discharge from the vagina and hands it to the medical assistant. RATIONALE: The physician will complete the examination of the patient while the medical assistant prepares the sample for viewing.
4. Rinse the swab vigorously in the test tube containing saline, pressing the cotton tip against the inside of the test tube to express all the specimen. RATIONALE: It is important to get as much of the sample as possible for a more accurate diagnosis.
5. Dispose of the cotton-tipped applicator into a biohazard container. RATIONALE: All body fluid–contaminated supplies should be handled with care and disposed of according to Standard Precautions.
6. Apply a drop on a microscope slide and cover with a coverslip. Hand the slide to the physician

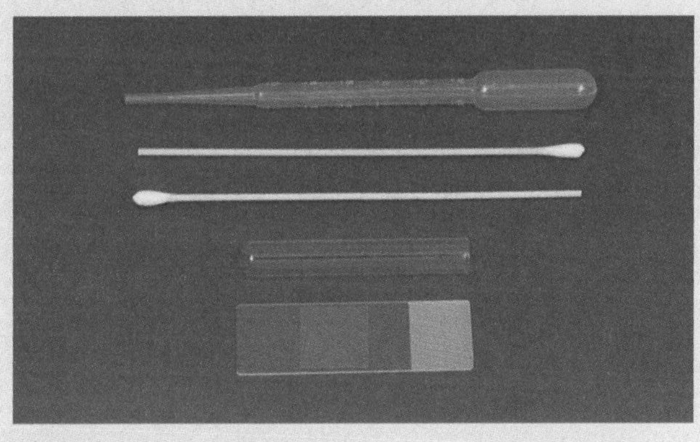

Figure 14-26 Supplies for wet mount and KOH prep: Pipette, cotton-tipped swabs, small test tube, and microscope slide with cover slip (not shown: Saline and KOH solution).

(continues)

Procedure 14-4 (continued)

for the microscopy examination. RATIONALE: Only a physician may perform the PPMP (Physician Performed Microscopy Procedure) for diagnosis, according to CLIA regulations.

7. Assist the patient back to a sitting position. Instruct her to dress and offer to assist if needed. RATIONALE: While the physician is viewing the slide, your responsibility is the safety and comfort of the patient.
8. In the laboratory, the physician will view the slide for yeast, bacteria, and trichomonas. RATIONALE: The physician will take the slide to the laboratory where the microscope is located.
9. After completion of the wet prep/wet mount, apply a few drops of KOH into the remaining solution in the test tube, place a drop on a fresh slide, and cover with a coverslip. RATIONALE: This is the second part of the microscopy test that can be performed on the vaginal secretion to diagnose the cause of vaginitis.
10. The physician will perform a microscopic examination for yeast. RATIONALE: This is a PPMP.
11. Dispose of all slides and the test tube into a sharps container. RATIONALE: As stated in Standard Precautions, all sharps must be disposed of in a sharps container.
12. Disinfect the laboratory area and equipment. RATIONALE: As stated in Standard Precautions, all biohazard contaminated surfaces must be disinfected after contamination.
13. Return to the patient and assist as needed. RATIONALE: The patient may need assistance and direction.
14. Chart the procedure and document the test as needed. RATIONALE: All patient testing must be documented. The physician may document the examination while the medical assistant documents the laboratory procedure. The physician must record the findings of the PPMP, or initial them if the medical assitant records the results under the physician's direction.

DOCUMENTATION

6/10/20XX 2:15 PM Wet mount and KOH prep done by Dr. Woo. Candidiasis diagnosed by Dr. Woo. Patient given prescription for Gyne-Lotrimin 3 Vaginal suppositories (200 mg) at bedtime for three consecutive nights. C. McInnis, RMA

Procedure 14-5 Amplified DNA ProbeTec Test for Chlamydia and Gonorrhea

STANDARD PRECAUTIONS:

PURPOSE:

To test a vaginal specimen for diagnosis of chlamydia and gonorrhea and as a screening tool for pregnant women.

EQUIPMENT/SUPPLIES:

Amplified DNA ProbeTec Kit (pink):

- Transport tube containing preservative
- Swabs (one large and one small Mini-Tip Culturette)

Vaginal speculum
Patient drape
Gloves
Other equipment as necessary for a vaginal examination

PROCEDURE STEPS:

1. Prepare the patient for a pelvic examination as outlined in Procedure 14-3.
2. Hand the large swab to the physician, who will use it to clean the cervix. RATIONALE: Mucus or blood on the cervix will interfer with the purity of the specimen.
3. Discard the large swab into the biohazard waste container. RATIONALE: According to Standard Precautions, all biohazard contaminated waste must be handled carefully and disposed of properly.
4. Hand the small Mini-tip Culturette Swab to the physician. He or she will insert the swab into the cervical os and rotate it for 15 to 20 seconds. RATIONALE: Accurate test results require obtaining adequate endocervical cells and secretions.
5. Immediately place the swab into the transport tube and recap. RATIONALE: The specimen needs to be placed in the tube with preservative immediately to preserve it.
6. If using the ProbeTec Wet Transport tube, break the tip of the swab off into the the liquid before recapping. RATIONALE: The tip of the swab is scored and will snap off easily. This allows the entire specimen to be transported in a small amount of preservative.
7. Attach requisition to specimen.
8. Document the procedure.

DOCUMENTATION

6/10/20XX 10:00 AM DNA ProbeTec test done by Dr. Woo. Entire specimen transported to laboratory. C. McInnis, RMA

Case Study 14-1

Maria Rodriguez has an appointment to see Dr. King today. It is her initial prenatal visit. She tells Liz Corbin, the medical assistant, as she is escorted from the reception area that she has been feeling "pretty good."

CASE STUDY REVIEW

1. Explain the importance of the initial prenatal visit. Discuss.
2. Name five specific diseases and conditions for which Dr. King will be on the alert during Maria's pregnancy.
3. What laboratory and other procedural tests may be performed at the initial visit?
4. Discuss areas of patient education and health promotion that Liz will discuss with Maria at the initial visit.

Case Study 14-2

Emily Harris is scheduled to have a cervical punch biopsy.

CASE STUDY REVIEW

1. What is the primary reason for a cervical punch biopsy?
2. Explain the post biopsy instructions she will need.

Case Study 14-3

Annette Sanderson has made an appointment with Dr. King because she has had symptoms of vaginitis. When she arrives at the clinic, you take her chief complaint and history. She tells you that she has a milky-white, frothy, vaginal discharge and that she itches in the genital area.

CASE STUDY REVIEW

1. What tests/procedures will you prepare for Dr. King in consideration of Annette's symptoms?
2. What is the most likely causative microorganism for these symptoms?
3. Describe the treatment that Dr. King may prescribe.

SUMMARY

Obstetrics and gynecology are two specialties that are usually practiced by the same physician. The OB/GYN physician will care for the health and well-being of the female patient in her pregnant and nonpregnant states. Knowledge of the numerous tests and procedures that are performed to diagnose and treat problems in the female patient are essential. Health promotion and patient education are of extreme importance whether the patient is an obstetric patient and scheduled for her initial prenatal visit or a gynecologic patient scheduled for yearly pelvic, Pap, and breast examinations.

STUDY FOR SUCCESS

To reinforce your knowledge and skills of information presented in this chapter:

- ❑ Review the Key Terms
- ❑ Practice any Procedures
- ❑ Consider the Case Studies and discuss your conclusions
- ❑ Answer the Review Questions
  - ❑ Multiple Choice
  - ❑ Critical Thinking
- ❑ Navigate the Internet and complete the Web Activities
- ❑ Practice the StudyWARE activities on the textbook CD
- ❑ Apply your knowledge in the Student Workbook activities
- ❑ Complete the Web Tutor sections
- ❑ View and discuss the DVD situations

REVIEW QUESTIONS

Multiple Choice

1. Which of the following conditions or diseases that an obstetrics patient experiences is considered to place her in the high-risk category?
   a. urinary tract infection
   b. 19 years of age
   c. both partners Rh negative
   d. poor nutritional habits
   e. poor hygiene
2. Using Nägele's Rule, calculate the expected date of birth of a patient whose last menstrual period was August 20, 2005.
   a. November 27, 2006
   b. December 13, 2006
   c. May 27, 2006
   d. April 20, 2006
3. The primary test performed at about the 16th week to check the fetus for neural tube defects is known as:
   a. alpha fetal protein analysis (AFP)
   b. amniocentesis
   c. chorionic villi sampling (CVS)
   d. rubella titer
   e. Rh factor
4. The release of which of the following hormones is thought to cause labor to begin?
   a. progesterone
   b. estrogen
   c. oxytoxin
   d. thyroxine
5. Ultrasonography is done to check for which of the following?
   a. gestational diabetes
   b. preeclampsia
   c. degree of effacement
   d. number of weeks of gestation
6. After a cervical punch biopsy, it is normal for the patient to experience which of the following?
   a. bleeding greater than a normal menstrual period
   b. no odor to vaginal discharge
   c. malodorous vaginal discharge
   d. severe abdominal cramps

7. To make the diagnosis of trichomoniasis, the medical assistant will need to prepare for which of the following?
   a. Pap smear
   b. ultrasonography
   c. wet mount
   d. culture and sensitivity
   e. blood glucose
8. To diagnose pelvic inflammatory disease (PID), the physician may order which of the following?
   a. wet mount
   b. Pap smear
   c. urinalysis
   d. rubella titer
   e. ultrasonography
9. Which of the following is/are primarily associated with abnormal Pap smears?
   a. endometriosis
   b. Bartholin cysts
   c. condylomata
   d. ovarian cysts
   e. PID
10. The primary purpose of colposcopy is to:
    a. treat advanced cancer of the vagina and cervix
    b. detect dysplastic cells of cervix after a positive Pap smear
    c. treat PID in the fallopian tube
    d. treat endometriosis of the pelvic cavity

Critical Thinking Questions

1. A pregnant woman who has had no prenatal care has not had a period for six months. She has called the OB/GYN clinic to schedule an appointment because she has had vaginal bleeding. She continues to feel fetal movement.
   a. What laboratory tests or procedures will the doctor order?
   b. What diagnosis is the physician most likely to make?
2. Lower abdominal and back pain that increases just before and during menses may be caused by what condition?

WEB ACTIVITIES

Obstetrics

Access a Web site for expectant parents to locate information about the following:

1. Obtain fact sheets about each trimester.
2. Compile a list of tests, complications, and postpartum recovery.
3. Visit the National Library of Medicine Web site.
   a. What are the time frames for the various stages of labor?
   b. What are the various breech presentations?
4. Find a Web site that gives information about the Lamaze method of childbirth. Is this something you might consider for yourself or your partner?
5. Search the Internet for a Web site that gives information about postpartum exercise routines. Also visit http://www.medscape.com for information.

Gynecology

Locate a Web site specific to cancer of the female reproductive tract to complete the following:

1. What treatment options are available for cancer of the endometrium?
2. What tests are available to help diagnose the cancer?
3. Print a list of local support groups for women with endometrial cancer.
4. Visit the American College of Obstetricians and Gynecologists Web site for information about managing pregnant patients with the following disorders or conditions:
   a. hypertension
   b. cardiovascular disease
   c. Rh factor incompatibility
5. Visit the American Cancer Society's Web site. Find information about diethylstilbestrol (DES) and male offspring malignancies.

THE DVD HOOK-UP

DVD Series: **Skills Based Series** | Program Number: **6**

Chapter/Scene Reference
- *Pap Examination*

In this chapter, you learned about the proper techniques for preparing a patient for a pap and pelvic examination as well as a prenatal examination.

The selected scene from today's program illustrates Anita preparing a tray for a Pap procedure. Anita places the speculum into some warm water.

1. What are two reasons to place the speculum in water?
2. Why did Anita stay positioned above the drape?
3. What was the purpose of the Hemoccult Card?

DVD Journal Summary

Write a paragraph that summarizes what you learned from watching today's selected DVD scene. Think of how you feel when you have to have a pelvic examination. Do you like having the assistant in the room when you are examined? Why is it considered good practice for a female medical assistant to stay in the room with a male physician during a pelvic examination? What kinds of things will you do to make your patient feel more comfortable during a Pap/pelvic procedure?

REFERENCES/BIBLIOGRAPHY

Consumer Reports on Health. (2004). "Estrogen therapy: not for prevention." *16*(5), 3.

Harvard Women's Health Watch. (2002). "Abbreviated hormone replacement therapy trial answers some questions, raises new ones." *10*(2), 2–4.

Littleton, L. Y., & Engebretson, J. C. (2002). *Maternal, neonatal, and women's health nursing*. Clifton Park, NY: Thomson Delmar Learning.

Spratto, G. R., & Woods, A. L. (2004). *2004 edition PDR, nurse's drug handbook*. Clifton Park, NY: Thomson Delmar Learning.

Taber's cyclopedic medical dictionary (21st ed.). (2002). Philadelphia: FA Davis.

Tamparo, C., & Lewis, M. (2000). *Diseases of the human body* (3rd ed.). Philadelphia: FA Davis.

CHAPTER 15

Pediatrics

OUTLINE

KEY TERMS

Cochlear Implantation
Exudate
Fontanel
Myringotomy
Phenylketonuria (PKU)
Sensorineural
Suppurative
Tympanostomy

OBJECTIVES

The student should strive to meet the following performance objectives and demonstrate an understanding of the facts and principles presented in this chapter through written and oral communication.

1. Define the key terms as presented in the glossary.
2. Describe the various theories of human development.
3. Describe pediatric care including measuring height, weight, head, chest circumference, and vital signs.
4. Explain the process of collecting a urine specimen.

(continues)

FEATURED COMPETENCIES

CAAHEP—ENTRY-LEVEL COMPETENCIES

Patient Care

- Obtain vital signs
- Prepare patient for and assist with routine and specialty examinations
- Maintain medication and immunization records

Legal Concepts

- Perform within legal and ethical boundaries
- Prepare and maintain medical records

Professionalism

- Treat all patients with compassion and empathy

Communication Skills

- Adapt communications to individual's ability to understand

ABHES—ENTRY-LEVEL COMPETENCIES

Professionalism

- Maintain confidentiality at all times
- Be cognizant of ethical boundaries

Communication

- Be attentive, listen and learn
- Be impartial and show empathy when dealing with patients
- Adapt what is said to recipient's level of comprehension
- Recognize and respond to verbal and non-verbal communication
- Adaptation for individualized needs

(continues)

OBJECTIVES (continued)

5. Explain the process of screening for hearing and visual impairments.
6. Describe common pediatric diseases and disorders.
7. Explain the importance of immunizations and scheduling of them.

SCENARIO

At Inner City Health Care, clinical assistant Bruce Goldman, CMA, is responsible for encouraging parents to keep track of their children's immunization records. Bruce teaches parents the importance of immunizations for long-term health protection and the importance of following recommended vaccination schedules for maximum benefit.

FEATURED COMPETENCIES (continued)

Clinical Duties

- Prepare patients for procedures
- Take vital signs
- Prepare and administer medications as directed by Physician
- Maintain medication records

Legal Concepts

- Document accurately

Instruction

- Instruct patients with special needs
- Teach patients methods of health promotion and disease prevention

Spotlight on Certification

RMA Content Outline

- Patient education
- Vital signs
- Physical examinations
- Clinical pharmacology

CMA Content Outline

- Adapting communication to an individual's ability to understand
- Vital signs
- Examinations
- Collecting and processing specimens; diagnostic testing
- Pharmacology
- Maintain medication and immunization records

CMAS Content Outline

- Vital signs and measurements
- Examination preparation
- Basic pharmacology

INTRODUCTION

New techniques and developments occur frequently in medicine, and medical assistants must refine existing skills and learn new ones to be knowledgeable and proficient and to provide the most current, up-to-date quality care to patients. The medical assistant who works in a pediatrician's office or a pediatric ambulatory care setting that treats infants and children will need additional skills when providing pediatric care to patients.

Knowledge of the developmental stages, knowledge of diseases of infants and children, and the ability to gain the child's confidence and trust and the caregivers' cooperation are all skills required to provide for the physiological, emotional, and psychological needs of the pediatric patient. This chapter covers the specialty examination and the appropriate clinical procedures in pediatrics.

WHAT IS PEDIATRICS?

Pediatrics is the branch of medicine that cares for newborns, infants, children, and adolescents. Pediatricians are physicians who diagnose and treat health problems and diseases specific to these age groups. This patient population has special needs, and medical assistants must be knowledgeable about the growth and development phases of life and diseases unique to pediatric patients. Children form judgments and have fears about health care providers. They need an atmosphere that is comfortable and one in which their physiological, emotional, and psychological needs are recognized and addressed.

Medical assistants must gain the confidence and trust of the child, allay fear, and help to promote positive relationships between the child and the physician and must themselves develop a positive relationship with the child. Children are likely to be cooperative when being examined or during a procedure if good rapport has been established. It is important to be honest with young patients and approach them at their level of understanding. Allow children to touch and hold a "safe" instrument, such as a stethoscope, and explain its purpose to them. Doing so can reduce anxiety and fear (Figure 15-1).

Taking a history of the child; assessing the child; measuring vital signs, height, weight, vision and hearing, laboratory work; administration of injections; observing the parent–child interactions; and noting the child's development level are all responsibilities in which a medical assistant takes part. It is important also for the medical assistant to recognize pediatric patients by their names no matter what their ages.

The first physical examination of a newborn is performed immediately after delivery. The pediatrician will assess the neonate's ability to exist outside of the mother's uterus. A scoring system is used to determine the neonate's physical condition at 1, 5, and 15 minutes after birth. It is known as the APGAR (appearance, pulse, grimace, activity, and respiration) score. Muscle tone, skin color, respiration, heart rate, and response to stimuli are given a score 0, 1, 2, and so on, with the highest score 10. Infants with low APGAR scores need immediate attention, such as stimulation, oxygen, medication, and so on. Their condition is monitored closely.

Tests are done to detect problems the neonate may have. **Phenylketonuria (PKU),** iron deficiency anemia, lead poisoning, and hypothyroidism are problems for which neonates are screened shortly after the APGAR scoring is done. Many patients seen in the pediatric setting are babies or children who are not ill. They are considered "well-baby" or "well-child" patients and are having routine checkups. Ill babies or children seen in the pediatrician's office or pediatric clinic are often called "sick-child" or "sick-baby" patients. Well-baby appointments are regularly scheduled appointments during which time the physician examines the child and evaluates the growth and development of the child. Most offices schedule well-baby appointments after birth according to the following time frame: 1, 2, 4, 6, 9, 12, 15, 18, 24 months, and yearly thereafter.

The goal of well-baby visits or checkups is prevention of health problems and diseases. Typically, immunizations are given during these appointments. The chart shown in Figure 15-2 includes immunization schedules from the National Immunization Program. The program urges that all children be immunized because the vaccines provide the best defense against many dangerous childhood diseases. Immunizations protect children against hepatitis A and B, polio, measles, mumps, rubella, pertussis, diphtheria, tetanus, haemophilus influenza type b, pneumococcal, chicken pox, and influenza. All of these need to be given before age 2 years to protect children during the period of their lives when they are more susceptible to infectious diseases (see Tables 15-1 and 15-2).

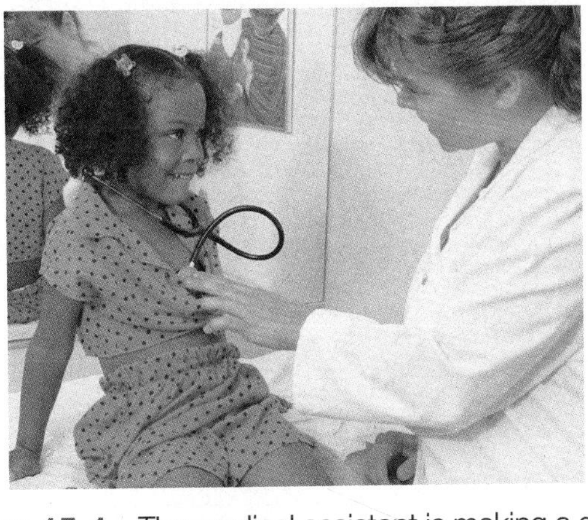

Figure 15-1 The medical assistant is making a game of a procedure to gain the child's cooperation.

Preparation of Vaccines for Administration

Careful attention to both proper storage of vaccines and thorough patient preparation for immunization will promote effective vaccination results. Access to vaccination should be available to all patients, especially to families with young infants and children. Most of the recommended vaccines are administered in the child's first 15 to 18 months of life. Access involves cost of vaccines, appointment requirements, and time required to receive vaccines. Some offices permit walk-in vaccination administration with free or low co-payment fee only.

Patient Education

Encourage parents to be aware of different vaccines and to keep track of vaccination schedules. By posting recommended schedules in visible locations in the ambulatory care setting, parents can be reminded.

Figure 15-2 illustrates the recommended vaccination schedule for children and adolescents, which is supported by the American Academy of Pediatrics, the Advisory Committee on Immunization Practices (ACIP), the Committee on Infectious Diseases (COID), the Commission of Public Health and Scientific Affairs (COPHSA), and the American Academy of Family Physicians (AAFP).

Vaccine	Birth	1 mo	2 mos	4 mos	6 mos	12 mos	15 mos	18 mos	24 mos	4–6 yrs	11–12 yrs	13–18 yrs
Hepatitis B[2]	HepB #1	only if mother HBsAg (-) / HepB #2			HepB #3				HepB series			
Diphtheria, tetanus, pertussis[3]			DTaP	DTaP	DTaP		DTaP			DTaP	Td	Td
Haemophilus influenzae type b[4]			Hib	Hib	Hib[4]	Hib						
Inactivated poliovirus			IPV	IPV	IPV					IPV		
Measles, mumps, rubella[5]						MMR #1				MMR #2	MMR #2	
Varicella[6]						Varicella			Varicella			
Pneumococcal[7]			PCV	PCV	PCV	PCV			PCV	PPV		
Influenza[8]					Influenza (yearly)				Influenza (yearly)			
- - - Vaccines below red line are for selected populations - - -												
Hepatitis A[9]									Hepatitis A series			

Range of recommended ages — Catch-up immunization — Preadolescent assessment

1. This schedule indicates the recommended ages for routine administration of currently licensed childhood vaccines, as of December 1, 2004, for children aged ≤18 years. Any dose not administered at the recommended age should be administered at any subsequent visit when indicated and feasible. ▭ Indicates age groups that warrant special effort to administer those vaccines not previously administered. Additional vaccines might be licensed and recommended during the year. Licensed combination vaccines may be used whenever any components of the combination are indicated and other components of the vaccine are not contraindicated. Providers should consult package inserts for detailed recommendations. Clinically significant adverse events that follow immunization should be reported to the Vaccine Adverse Event Reporting System; guidance is available at http://www.vaers.org or by telephone, 800-822-7967.

2. **Hepatitis B (HepB) vaccine.** All infants should receive the first dose of HepB vaccine soon after birth and before hospital discharge; the first dose may also be administered by age 2 months if the mother is hepatitis B surface antigen (HBsAg) negative. Only monovalent HepB may be used for the birth dose. Monovalent or combination vaccine containing HepB may be used to complete the series. Four doses of vaccine may be administered when a birth dose is administered. The second dose should be administered at least 4 weeks after the first dose, except for combination vaccines, which cannot be administered before age 6 weeks. The third dose should be administered at least 16 weeks after the first dose and at least 8 weeks after the second dose. The final dose in the vaccination series (third or fourth dose) should not be administered before age 24 weeks. ***Infants born to HBsAg-positive mothers*** should receive HepB and 0.5 mL of hepatitis B immune globulin (HBIG) at separate sites within 12 hours of birth. The second dose is recommended at age 1–2 months. The final dose in the immunization series should not be administered before age 24 weeks. These infants should be tested for HBsAg and antibody to HBsAg at age 9–15 months. ***Infants born to mothers whose HBsAg status is unknown*** should receive the first dose of the HepB series within 12 hours of birth. Maternal blood should be drawn as soon as possible to determine the mother's HBsAg status; if the HBsAg test is positive, the infant should receive HBIG as soon as possible (no later than age 1 week). The second dose is recommended at age 1–2 months. The last dose in the immunization series should not be administered before age 24 weeks.

3. **Diphtheria and tetanus toxoids and acellular pertussis (DTaP) vaccine.** The fourth dose of DTaP may be administered as early as age 12 months, provided 6 months have elapsed since the third dose and the child is unlikely to return at age 15–18 months. The final dose in the series should be administered at age ≥4 years. **Tetanus and diphtheria toxoids (Td)** is recommended at age 11–12 years if at least 5 years have elapsed since the last dose of tetanus and diphtheria toxoid-containing vaccine. Subsequent routine Td boosters are recommended every 10 years.

4. ***Haemophilus influenzae*** **type b (Hib) conjugate vaccine.** Three Hib conjugate vaccines are licensed for infant use. If PRP-OMP (PedvaxHIB® or ComVax® [Merck]) is administered at ages 2 and 4 months, a dose at age 6 months is not required. DTaP/Hib combination products should not be used for primary immunization in infants at ages 2, 4, or 6 months but can be used as boosters after any Hib vaccine. The final dose in the series should be administered at age ≥12 months.

5. **Measles, mumps, and rubella (MMR) vaccine.** The second dose of MMR is recommended routinely at age 4–6 years but may be administered during any visit, provided at least 4 weeks have elapsed since the first dose and both doses are administered beginning at or after age 12 months. Those who have not previously received the second dose should complete the schedule by age 11–12 years.

6. **Varicella vaccine.** Varicella vaccine is recommended at any visit at or after age 12 months for susceptible children (i.e., those who lack a reliable history of chickenpox). Susceptible persons aged ≥13 years should receive 2 doses administered at least 4 weeks apart.

7. **Pneumococcal vaccine.** The heptavalent **pneumococcal conjugate vaccine (PCV)** is recommended for all children aged 2–23 months and for certain children aged 24–59 months. The final dose in the series should be administered at age ≥12 months. **Pneumococcal polysaccharide vaccine (PPV)** is recommended in addition to PCV for certain groups at high risk. See *MMWR* 2000;49(No. RR-9).

8. **Influenza vaccine.** Influenza vaccine is recommended annually for children aged ≥6 months with certain risk factors (including, but not limited to, asthma, cardiac disease, sickle cell disease, human immunodeficiency virus [HIV], and diabetes), health-care workers, and other persons (including household members) in close contact with persons in groups at high risk (see *MMWR* 2004;53[No. RR-6]). In addition, healthy children aged 6–23 months and close contacts of healthy children aged 0–23 months are recommended to receive influenza vaccine because children in this age group are at substantially increased risk for influenza-related hospitalizations. For healthy persons aged 5–49 years, the intranasally administered, live, attenuated influenza vaccine (LAIV) is an acceptable alternative to the intramuscular trivalent inactivated influenza vaccine (TIV). See *MMWR* 2004;53(No. RR-6). Children receiving TIV should be administered a dosage appropriate for their age (0.25 mL if aged 6–35 months or 0.5 mL if aged ≥3 years). Children aged ≤8 years who are receiving influenza vaccine for the first time should receive 2 doses (separated by at least 4 weeks for TIV and at least 6 weeks for LAIV).

9. **Hepatitis A vaccine.** Hepatitis A vaccine is recommended for children and adolescents in selected states and regions and for certain groups at high risk; consult your local public health authority. Children and adolescents in these states, regions, and groups who have not been immunized against hepatitis A can begin the hepatitis A immunization series during any visit. The 2 doses in the series should be administered at least 6 months apart. See *MMWR* 1999;48(No. RR-12).

Approved by the **Advisory Committee on Immunization Practices** (http://www.cdc.gov/nip/acip), the **American Academy of Pediatrics** (http://www.aap.org), and the **American Academy of Family Physicians** (http://www.aafp.org). Additional information about vaccines, including precautions and contraindications for vaccination and vaccine shortages, is available at http://www.cdc.gov/nip or from the National Immunization Information Hotline, 800-232-2522 (English) or 800-232-0233 (Spanish).

Figure 15-2 Recommended childhood and adolescent immunization schedule—United States, 2005. MMWR 2005; 53 (Nos. 51 and 52): Q1–Q3. (National Immunization Program, Centers for Disease Control and Prevention.)

TABLE 15-1 VACCINE ADMINISTRATION GUIDELINES

Vaccine	Disease	About the Disease	Precautions and Contra-indications	Side Effects and Adverse Reactions	Vaccine Schedule
DTaP, DT, Td	Diphtheria, tetanus, pertussis	Diphtheria can cause breathing problems, paralysis, heart failure and death; tetanus causes paralysis of the jaw—cannot open mouth or swallow; Pertussis (whooping cough) causes severe coughing so infants have difficulty eating, drinking, or breathing or causes brain damage/death	Moderate to severe acute illness neurological disorder, allergic reaction to prior dose	Local reactions, fussiness, seizures, fever, allergic reaction	2 months, 4 months, 6 months, 15–18 months, 4–6 years; not given at 7 years or older
Inactive poliovirus (IPV)*	Poliomyelitis	Causes paralysis of skeletal muscles and diaphragm so infants cannot breathe on their own	Allergic reaction to prior dose or to neomycin, streptomycin, or polymixin B; moderate to severe acute illness; pregnancy	Local reactions, allergic reaction	2 months, 4 months, 16–18 months, 4–6 years (booster)
Haemophilus influenzae type B (Hib)	Meningitis, pneumonia, epiglottitis, pericarditis	Causes bacterial meningitis, pneumonia, epiglottitis, septicemia, death	Moderate to severe acute illness, allergic reaction to prior dose	Fever, swelling, redness and/or pain; allergic reaction	2 months, 4 months, 6 months, 12–15 months (booster); children younger than 6 weeks old should not get vaccine
Combination vaccines containing Hib			Moderate to severe acute illness	Local reaction, allergic reaction	Cannot be used at 2 months, 4 months, or 6 months; may be used as booster
• DTaP_Hib (TriHIBit)	Diphtheria, tetanus, pertussis, *Haemophilus influenzae*				
• Hepatitis B-Hib (-Comvax)	Hepatitis B and *Haemophilus influenzae*				2 months, 4 months, 12–15 months; not given to infants younger than 6 weeks old
Hepatitis B (HBV)	Hepatitis B	Anorexia, fatigue, diarrhea, vomiting, liver damage, cancer, death	Pregnancy, moderate to severe acute illness, allergic reaction to Baker's yeast	Mild systemic effects, soreness, fever, allergic reaction	Within 12 hrs of birth, 1–2 months, 6 months (3 doses needed)
Pediatrix, DTap, HepV, IPV	Diphtheria, tetanus, Pertussis, *Haemophilus influenzae,* hepatitis B, inactive poliovirus		Moderate to severe acute illness	Mild systemic effects, local reaction, allergic reaction	2 months, 4 months, and 6 months

(continues)

TABLE 15-1 VACCINE ADMINISTRATION GUIDELINES (continued)

Vaccine	Disease	About the Disease	Precautions and Contra-indications	Side Effects and Adverse Reactions	Vaccine Schedule
Td	Tetanus, diphtheria		Moderate to severe acute illness, severe allergic reaction to prior dose	Soreness; swelling; severe allergic reaction; deep, aching pain in muscles of upper arm(s)	7 years or older then every 10 years for life
MMR	Measles, mumps, rubella	Measles cause otitis media, pneumonia, seizures, brain damage, death; Mumps cause fever, swollen glands, deafness, meningitis, swelling of testicles or ovaries, death; Rubella can cause pregnant women to have miscarriages or babies born with severe anomalies	Do not give if allergic to gelatin or the antibiotic neomycin, moderate to severe acute illness, breast-feeding, pregnancy, immunosuppressed individuals	Fever, mild rash, swelling of glands in cheeks and neck, seizures, temporary pain in joints, severe allergic reaction	Two doses—12–15 months and 4–6 years (or any age if longer than 28 days from first dose)
Varicella	Chicken pox	Severe skin infection, pneumonia, brain damage, death; shingles (herpes zoster) may occur years later	Do not give if allergic to gelatin or the antibiotic neomycin, moderate to severe acute illness	Soreness and swelling at site, fever, mild rash, seizures, pneumonia	Between 12–18 months or any age if never had chicken pox
HAV	Hepatitis A	Liver disease with flu-like symptoms, jaundice, nausea and vomiting, abdominal pain	Allergic reaction to prior dose, tell doctor if pregnant (safety of vaccine during pregnancy has not been determined)	Soreness at site, headache, severe allergic reaction	1 month before traveling or when at risk for infection (two doses needed 6 months apart)
Influenza Inactivated (I.M.) Live, intranasal (I.N.) Ages 5–49	Influenza (flu)	Fever, cough, chills, aches, death	Pregnant women should not get, egg allergy, history of Guillain-Barré syndrome	Soreness, redness, fever, aches, allergic reaction	All children 6–23 months
Pneumococcal congugate	Pneumonia, bacterial meningitis	Meningitis, septicemia, otitis media, pneumonia, deafness, brain damage	Moderate to severe illness, allergic reaction to prior dose	Redness, swelling at site, fever, drowsiness	2 months, 4 months, 6 months, 12–15 months
Meningococcal	Meningitis	Infection of the brain and coverings of the spinal cord, septicemia, mental retardation, seizures, stroke, death	Severe allergic reaction to prior dose	Allergic reaction, redness or pain at site, fever	Not for children younger than 2 years (two doses needed 3 months apart)

*Oral polio vaccine no longer recommended

Routine well-infant examinations should be scheduled according to the recommended vaccination schedule to promote and facilitate maintenance of the schedule.

Vaccine storage should follow specific manufacturer's guidelines. Some vaccine preparations require refrigeration or protection from light.

Vaccines have trade names, and manufacturers have been tested for safety. The package insert of each vaccine describes the vaccine including its route of administration, purpose, contraindications, and possible side effects. Because some vaccines are grown in bird eggs weakened by addition of chemicals, or made from animals, it is

TABLE 15-2 ADMINISTERING VACCINES: DOSE, ROUTE, SITE, AND NEEDLE SIZE

Vaccines	Dose	Route	Site	Needle Size
Diphtheria, Tetanus, Pertussis (DTaP, DT, Td)	0.5 mL	IM	Vastus lateralis: for infants (& toddlers lacking adequate deltoid mass); Deltoid: for toddlers, children & adults	22–25g, 1–2"
Haemophilus influenzae type b (Hib)	0.5 mL	IM	Vastus lateralis: for infants (& toddlers lacking adequate deltoid mass); Deltoid: for toddlers & children	22–25g, 1–2"
Hepatitis A (HepA)	≤18 yrs.: 0.5 mL ≥19 yrs.: 1.0 mL	IM	Vastus lateralis: for infants (& toddlers lacking adequate deltoid mass); Deltoid: for toddlers, children & adults	22–25g, 1–2"
Hepatitis B (HepB)	≤19 yrs.: 0.5 mL* ≥20 yrs.: 1.0 mL	IM	Vastus lateralis: for infants (& toddlers lacking adequate deltoid mass); Deltoid: for toddlers, children & adults	22–25g, 1–2"
Influenza, live attenuated (LAIV)	0.5 mL	Intranasal spray	Administer 0.25 mL dose into each nostril while patient is in an upright position	NA
Influenza, trivalent inactivated (TIV)	6–25 mos: 0.25 mL ≥3 yrs.: 0.5 mL	IM	Vastus lateralis: for infants (& toddlers lacking adequate deltoid mass); Deltoid: for toddlers, children & adults	22–25g, 1–2"
Measles, mumps, rubella (MMR)	0.5 mL	SC	Anterolateral fat of thigh: for young children Posterolateral fat of upper arm: for children & adults	23–25g, 5/8"
Meningococcal (Men)	0.5 mL	SC	Anterolateral fat of thigh: for young children Posterolateral fat of upper arm: for children & adults	23–25g, 5/8"
Pneumococcal conjugate (PCV)	0.5 mL	IM	Vastus lateralis: for infants (& toddlers lacking adequate deltoid mass); Deltoid: for toddlers & children	22–25g, 1–2"
Pneumococcal polysaccharide (PPV)	0.5 mL	IM SC	Deltoid Anterolateral fat of thigh: for young children Posterolateral fat of upper arm: for children & adults	22–25g, 1–2" 23–25g, 5/8"
Polio, inactivated (IPV)	0.5 mL	IM	Vastus lateralis: for infants (& toddlers lacking adequate deltoid mass); Deltoid: for toddlers, children & adults	22–25g, 1–2"
		SC	Anterolateral fat of thigh: for infants & young children Posterolateral fat of upper arm: for children & adults	23–25g, 5/8"
Varicella (Var)	0.5 mL	SC	Anterolateral fat of thigh: for young children Posterolateral fat of upper arm: for children & adults	23–25g, 5/8"

*Persons 11 through 15 years of age may be given Recombivax HB® (Merck) 1.0 mL (adult formulation) on a 2-dose schedule.

Combination Vaccines

DTaP+HepB+IPV (Pediatrix™) DTaP+Hib (Trihibit™) Hib+HepB (Comvax™)	0.5 mL	IM	Vastus lateralis: for infants (& toddlers lacking adequate deltoid mass); Deltoid: for toddlers & children	22–25g, 1–2"
HepA+HepB (Twinrix®)	≥18 yrs.: 1.0 mL	IM	Deltoid	22–25g, 1–2"

Please note: Always refer to the package insert included with each biologic for complete vaccine administration information. The Advisory Committee on Immunization Practices (ACIP) statement for the particular vaccine should be reviewed as well.

(Immunization Action Coalition, 1573 Selby Avenue, St. Paul, MN 55104, (651) 647-9009, www.immunize.org/catg.d/rules1.pdf. Accessed Sept 19, 2004.)

essential to know what allergies a child has. For example, a child who is allergic to eggs cannot receive an MMR, varicella, or influenza vaccine because of the possibility of the child being allergic to the egg protein that is used in the manufacturing of the vaccine. Symptoms of side effects, contraindications, and allergies must be known by the medical assistant, who will be certain that the parents are informed and have given written consent before the vaccines are given. After administration of vaccines, the medical assistant is responsible for documentation of the types of vaccines, site of administration, manufacturer's lot number, and side effects, if any have been reported by the parents. The physician will report any clinically significant adverse reactions to the Vaccine Adverse Event Reporting System (VAERS) and will file a VAERS Events Form for the National Immunization Program. Every child must have a personal immunization record as part of their permanent medical record. It is mandated that the following information be included with each immunization:

- Month, day, and year of administration
- Vaccine given
- Manufacturer name
- Lot number and expiration date
- Site and route of administration
- Name, address, and title of health care provider giving the vaccine

See Procedure 15-1 for more information on maintaining immunization records.

Vaccines stimulate the immune system to produce antibodies against pathogens (see Chapter 10). Some patients may have conditions or preexisting conditions that would contraindicate vaccine administration. Safe vaccine administration requires assessment and recognition of conditions that would contraindicate vaccine administration at any specific time. Contraindications for each vaccine are presented in each package insesrt and in Table 15-1. When any vaccine is not given because of an existing contraindication, careful documentation and notification of the physician are required.

Recommended Vaccination Schedule

The recommended vaccination schedule for infants and children is based on the premise that repeated doses of several vaccines are required and vaccine manufacturers recommend administering only compatible vaccines at any one visit to avoid drug interactions. If no contraindications are present at the various ages, vaccines should be administered according to the schedule to ensure complete vaccination by the age of 15 to 18 months, with booster vaccines on school entry and again every 10 years throughout adult life. Should any vaccine be missed for any reason, vaccine schedules are available to ensure adequate vaccine administration.

Giving Injections to Pediatric Patients

Infants and toddlers who have injections must be held in such a way that they cannot move. This is done for two reasons: to protect the child from injury and to provide access to an injection site.

For an infant from birth to about 2 years of age, the vastus lateralis muscle is the preferred site. It is readily accessible when the infant is lying supine on the examination table. A parent or another staff member can hold down the upper half of the infant's body, and the medical assistant can use his or her nondominant elbow to hold down the right leg at the knee. With the infant immobilized, the injection can be given.

Children who are 2 to about 4 years old are not emotionally developed enough to understand the need for cooperation. You will need help from the parent or another staff member to hold the child securely, thus avoiding injury. The deltoid is the preferred site for this age group. One method used to restrict the child's movement is to seat the child on the parent's lap. The parent wraps his or her legs around the child's legs to limit movement. The parent or staff member holds down the noninjection arm. The injection can be given once the child is securely mobilized.

Keep the syringe and needle out of the patient's sight, because pediatric patients learn quickly that doctor office visits many times mean an injection, and with the injection is some degree of fear and pain.

Do not tell the child that the injection will not hurt; rather, explain that it will sting for a short while, but it will help to keep him or her strong and healthy. A cartoon character adhesive strip applied to the site after the injection helps direct the child's attention away from the discomfort.

Although the deltoid is the preferred site, occasionally other muscles (e.g., dorsogluteal and vetrogluteal muscles) can be used for pediatric injections (see Figure 15-3A–D).

Sick-baby or sick-child visits are those appointments that have been arranged for ill babies or children who will be examined by the pediatrician to determine a diagnosis and appropriate treatment for a particular problem.

Clinical responsibilities for medical assistants during either type of visit include the same or similar procedures as the adult examination. The instruments used for the pediatric physical examination are similar to those used for an adult physical examination. Vital signs are taken, visual acuity is measured, a urine specimen may be obtained, blood drawn and processed, height and weight measurements are taken, and head circumference is measured. To gain the child's confidence, begin the examination at the feet and work up to the head. These are some of the skills and procedures medical assistants will perform or with which they will assist during the pediatric office or clinic visit.

THEORIES OF GROWTH AND DEVELOPMENT

Before providing more indepth information about the various stages of growth and development in children, it is important to review the major theorists who contributed to understanding human growth and development.

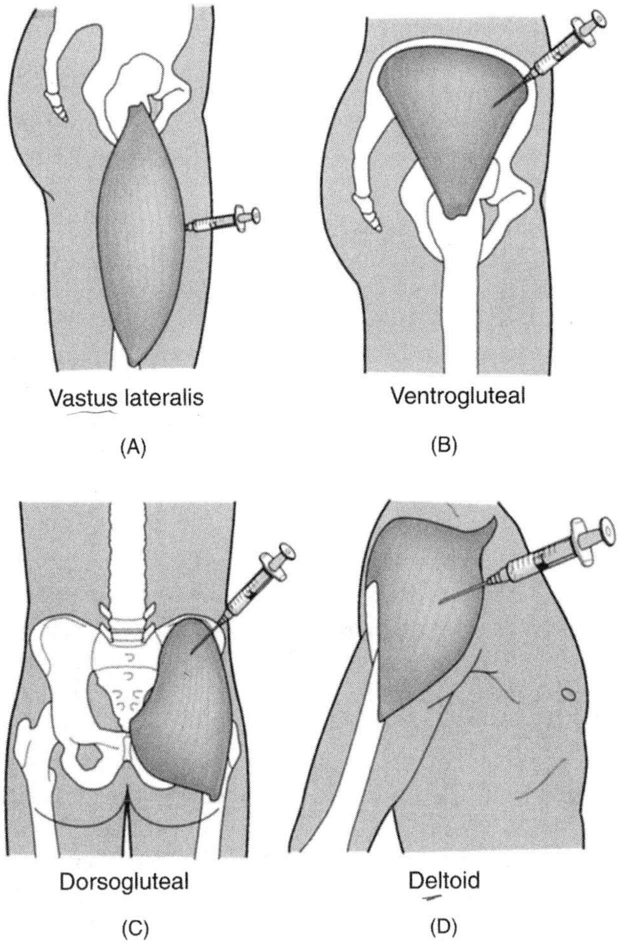

Figure 15-3 Intramuscular Injection Sites. (A) Vastus lateralis: Identify the greater trochanter. Place hand at the lateral femoral condyle. The injection site is in the middle third and anterior to the lateral aspect. (B) Ventrogluteal: Place palm of left hand on right greater trochanter so the index finger points toward the anterosuperior iliac spine. When middle finger is spread to form a V, the injection site is in the middle of the V. (C) Dorsogluteal: Place hand on iliac crest and locate the posterosuperior iliac spine. The injection site is the outer quadrant when an imaginary line is drawn between the trochanter and the iliac spine. (D) Deltoid: Locate the lateral side of the humerus. One finger width below the acromion process is the deltoid. (Potts, N.L., & Mandlero, B.L. (2002). *Pediatric nursing: Caring for children and their families*. Clifton Park, NY: Thomson Delmar Learning.)

There are at least eight or nine theories of human development put forth by Freud (psychosexual), Erickson (psychosocial), Sullivan (interpersonal), Piaget (cognitive), Kohlberg (moral), Bronfenbrenner (ecology), Pavlov, Skinner (behavioral), and Bandura (social learning). Each theory focuses on particular aspects of human development and its principles, strengths, and weaknesses.

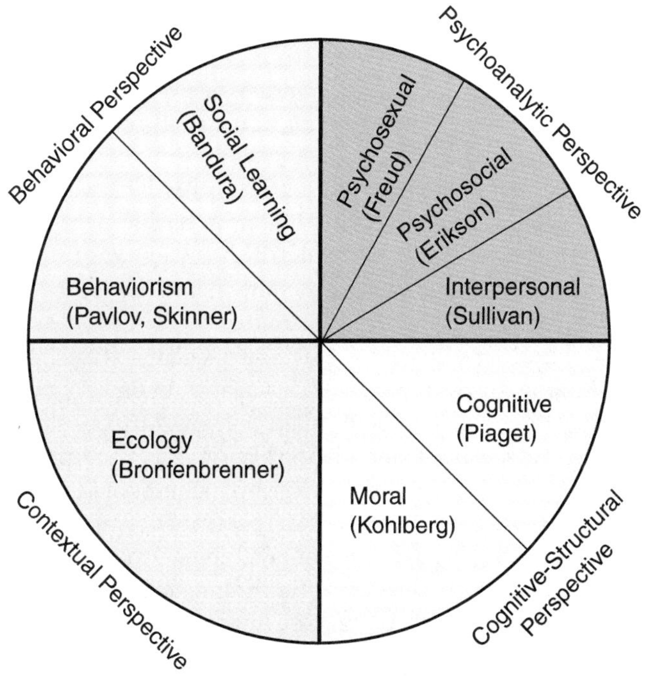

Figure 15-4 The eclectic nature of human development.

No single theory can explain human development. The medical assistant can apply the theory or theories with relevance and understanding to each individual child or adult. This will allow for an inclusive approach to human development that is appropriate for children and families (see Figure 15-4).

The following sections provide more information about growth and development at the various stages of a child's life.

Newborns

Even at a few days old, a newborn can imitate facial and manual gestures that adults make and can show a preference for certain colors (red, black, and white). The newborn can respond to auditory stimuli and is sensitive to being touched and handled. Respiratory rate is usually 30 to 60 breaths/min; breaths are somewhat irregular in depth and rhythm, shallow and abdominal. The heart rate ranges from 100 to 150 beats/min depending on whether the infant is awake or asleep. Urinary output is about 1 to 3 ml/hour or about 2 to 6 voidings a day.

Newborns can move and wiggle and can place themselves into dangerous or unsafe positions. One hand should always be kept on the newborn whenever she is on top of any object because he or she can easily roll off. The safest place is in a crib with the sides raised.

Infants

The infant stage is from one month to one year. Gross and fine motor skills develop starting at the head and moving toward the feet.

The infant usually doubles his or her birth weight during the first 6 months; by 12 months, birth weight has tripled. Height increases about 1 inch per month. By 12 months, the infant's height has slowed, and there can be a 50% increase from the birth length.

Head size changes quickly to accommodate fast brain growth. By 1 year old, the infant's brain is about 66% of the size of an adult brain, but growth does slow during the second six months of the first year. The **fontanels** (anterior and posterior) close by 2 months old (anterior) and 12 to 18 months old (posterior). The infant cannot control head movement until about 4 months old. This is known as "head lag," and the amount of head lag can be determined by pulling the infant by the arms from a supine to a sitting position. Because the infant cannot control the head, it will fall back until about 4 months old, at which time the infant has no head lag and can control the head while sitting.

Gross and fine motor development occurs quickly during the infant stage, but once developed, the infant can begin to walk, first with help, then alone. By 1 year old, in addition to being able to walk alone, the infant can feed himself or herself finger foods, grasp with his or her index finger and thumb, place and remove small objects from a container, and hold a crayon and make a mark with it.

The medical assistant can be helpful in relaying information to the infant's parents or caregivers regarding growth and development, nutrition, hygiene, safety, and vaccines.

Toddlers

The toddler period covers 2 years in the child's life from about 1 to 3 years of age. During the toddler period, there is rapid change. The child is becoming more independent, is able to move about quickly, and is verbal and inquisitive. Environmental dangers are of utmost concern because of the toddler's rapid development of motor skills and lack of judgment. This is a time for discipline and guidelines but also for encouraging independence and natural curiosity. Most injuries and deaths occur as a result of airway obstruction, poisoning, drowning, falls, burns, and auto accidents.

During the two years that the toddler is developing, his or her physical growth slows. Height averages about a 3-inch gain per year; weight gain is about 5 pounds per year. Most toddlers will walk by 12 to 15 months old and climb stairs by 18 months old.

Bladder and bowel control usually occur during this period. Vital signs move closer to adult norms, respiration (25–30 breaths/min awake) and pulse rates (70–110 heartbeats/min) slow, blood pressure increases to greater than 90/50 mm Hg. Serum lead levels are checked during this time.

It is during the toddler period that rapid onset of respiratory distress can occur, and there is an increase in tendency for airways to collapse. Otitis media, tonsillitis, and upper respiratory infections are common.

Often parents or caregivers are concerned their toddlers are eating little or they focus only on one particular food. Most toddlers will eat when they are hungry and caregivers worry unnecessarily. The toddler is less interested in food because of his or her slowdown in growth, thus fewer calories are needed.

Eating habits are established during the first two to three years of life, and good eating habits with children should start when they are toddlers. The early years are the time to teach lifelong healthy eating habits together with regular exercise. These two factors will significantly add years and quality of life because of disease prevention and maintenance of health. Many children in the United States are obese perhaps because their parents are. A 1998 study reported in *Annals of Human Biology* found that almost half of children who were overweight at 1 year old were obese by 21 years old. The earlier that one can prevent obesity, the healthier one's children will be. Parents are their children's role models.

Preschoolers

The preschool years include ages 3 to 6 years. The child now has control over bowel and bladder, can dress and feed himself or herself, and can interact with others. During this period, preschoolers gain about 2 pounds of weight per year and 3 inches in height per year. Visual acuity rates decrease slightly.

The Denver Developmental Screening Test can be used to determine motor skills development levels. Running, jumping, skipping, jumping rope, and bike riding with training wheels usually occurs in this time period. Preschoolers may begin to tie shoelaces.

Sexual curiosity is displayed, and questions about body parts, including genitalia, should be answered honestly. Children learn at this age that "private" body parts should not be touched by strangers.

Preschoolers learn through play and by imitating adult behaviors. It is now that children will play well with others and share. Preschoolers are creative and use their imaginations well.

During preschool years, a yearly physical examination should be done to note growth, vision, hearing, and blood pressure. Laboratory work includes a test for lead exposure, a tuberculosis test (once before beginning school), and a lipid profile. This age group suffers from otitis media, upper respiratory infections, and common stomach viruses. Teaching children the importance of good hand washing techniques and its significance in preventing illness is important.

Some preschoolers may refuse to eat for a few days or prefer one particular food everyday. Parents and caregivers should avoid issues over these matters. Instead, spend mealtimes in a pleasant way.

Regular physical activity is beneficial because it helps develop lifetime habits of exercise, leading to disease prevention and health promotion. Sports are an ideal way to get preschoolers active and to have fun. Noncompetitive activities such as dance, T-ball, karate, gymnastics, and bicycling also keep children active and healthy. Love of reading can be established now, especially when parents/caregivers read to their youngsters.

Playing near the road is an area of great concern for these children. They will listen to adults who set limits for their safety.

School-Aged Children

The years encompassed in the school-aged group are from 6 to 12 years of age. A steady progression in the children's rate of growth occurs during these years. Weight increases by about 5 pounds per year, and height increases about 2 inches per year. Muscle size increases, and the following motor skills continue to improve: climbing, running, jumping, throwing, catching, and balancing.

The circulatory and respiratory functions develop. The pulse and respiration rates slow. The pulse rate in this age group is about 90 beats/min; the average respiration rate is 20 breaths/min. Both rates are while the children are at rest.

This period shows relatively few infectious diseases because of the immunity the children developed to microorganisms during their preschool years.

The last years of the school-aged period are known as prepuberty. Breast development, axillary and pubic hair, and body odor may appear as early as 9 or 10 years of age.

Peers begin to play a major role now, and children will seek support from their peers to begin to gain independence from their parents and family. A sense of accomplishment happens when the children's energy is focused on sports, hobbies, and schoolwork and they see themselves succeed in these activities.

Language is the way to communicate, and children use their language skills to socialize with their family and peers.

Usually school-aged children experience excellent health, and when they do become ill, it is usually a minor illness. Routine physical examinations about every 2 years are suggested by the American Academy of Pediatrics at ages 5, 6, 8, 10, 11, and 12 years old. Height, weight, vital signs, physical examination, vision and hearing tests, review of nutrition, scoliosis screening and tuberculosis testing are checked. Use of recreational drugs, tobacco, and alcohol are addressed.

60

Booster immunizations of DPT (diphtheria, pertussis, tetanus) and MMR (measles, mumps, and rubella) are typically given between 4 and 6 years of age. Tetanus and diphtheria (Td) is usually repeated every 10 years.

Nutrition education is an ongoing process and children should be taught to eat breakfast daily and to make intelligent, healthy food choices. Good nutrition and physical activity are essential for their physical and emotional well-being and long-range health maintenance and disease prevention.

Accidents in this age group are the leading cause of death. The increased independence, need for their peer's approval, and increased involvement in physically challenging activities are some of the reasons. Most injuries are related to auto accidents and firearms. Violent crimes against children in this age group have increased dramatically in the last 20 years or so.

School-aged children comprehend rules related to safety regarding automobiles, bikes, swimming, and firearms, but they frequently resist these rules.

This group of children suffers from not looking the "same" as their peers, bullying, stress (peer pressure, divorce, drugs), both parents/caregivers work and are not home when child goes home after school (latchkey children).

Adolescents

The adolescent period of growth and development is noticeable for its wide range of physiological changes. It is the period between 11 and 21 years of age. During adolescence, there is a large growth spurt with gains in weight and height that occur rapidly. Boys can gain up to about 14 pounds and grow as much as 6 inches; girls gain up to about 10 pounds and grow up to 5 inches. Girls usually attain their adult height about one year before onset of menses; boys reach their adult height at about 13 years old, after axillary and pubic hair appear.

The average heart rate is about 60 to 70 beats/min; average blood pressure is 100/50 to 120/70 mm Hg. Girls have a slightly higher pulse and body temperature than boys; girls' systolic blood pressure is a bit less. Respiration rates in both sexes averages about 16 to 20 breaths/min.

Adolescents direct their energy to nonfamily relationships and career goals. It is a time of conflict because adolescents are trying to become independent from their parents and establish their own identities.

The Department of Adolescent Health of the American Medical Association urges annual health screenings that focus not only on the physiological and psychological health of the adolescent, but also on such matters as physical activity, birth control, recreational drugs, alcohol, depression, suicide ideation, injury prevention, and school accomplishments.

Laboratory tests include human immunodeficiency virus (HIV) and other sexually transmitted diseases (gonorrhea, syphilis, chlamydia, and hepatitis B and C if sexually active). Tuberculosis testing is also recommended. The physical examination is comprehensive and includes vital signs, height and weight, vision and hearing testing, urinalysis, and complete blood count (CBC). At this time, the provider will discuss issues of injury prevention (wearing seat belts, helmets for biking, no drinking and driving, contact sports, among others), violence prevention (gang memberships and anger management), nutrition (fast foods, high-sodium and fatty foods), how to avoid becoming overweight and obese, and regular physical activity. Motor vehicle accidents cause 50% of teenage deaths between ages 16 and

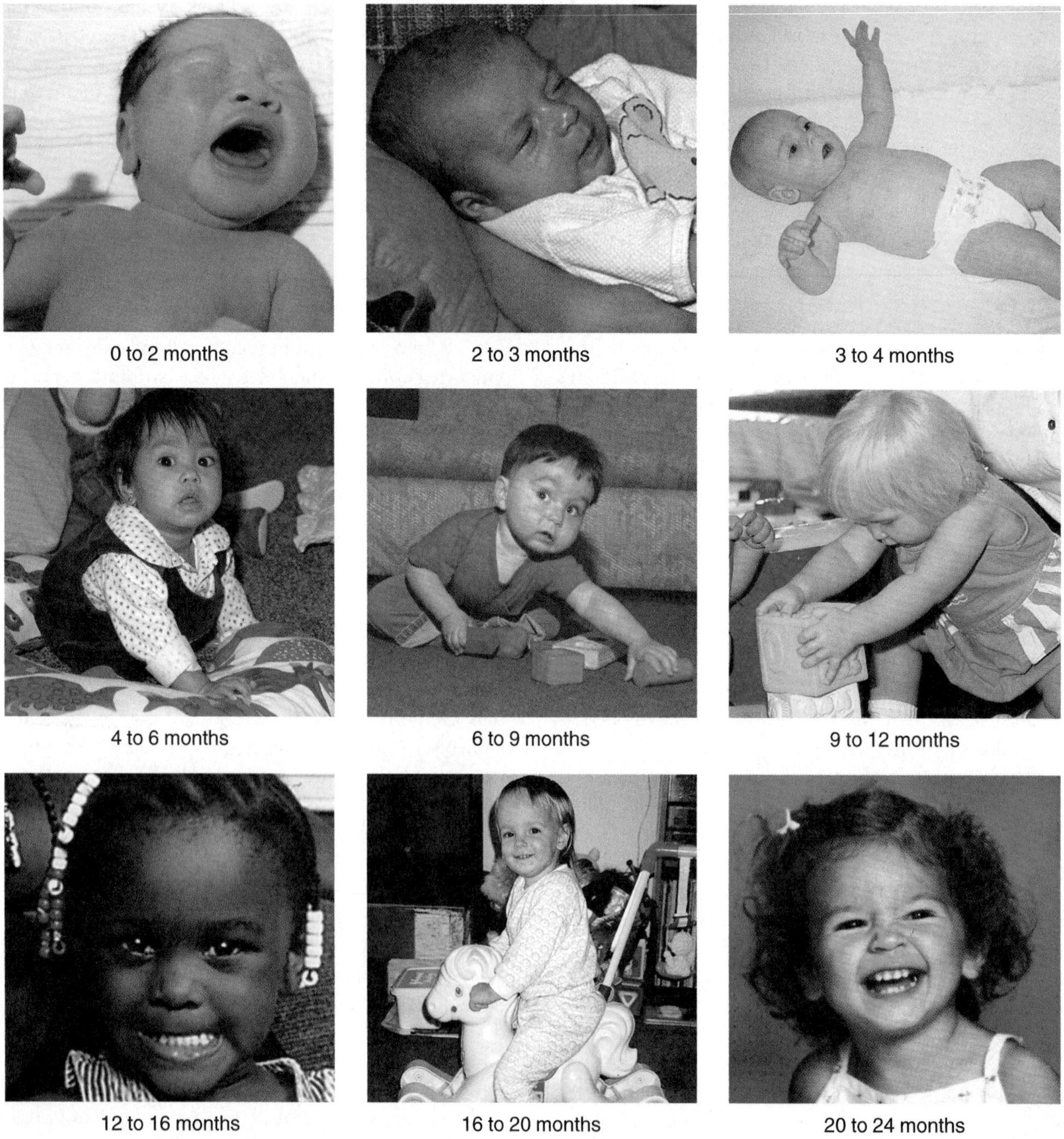

Figure 15-5 Growth and development stages of infants and toddlers.

19 years, and they are common in drivers who use alcohol or other drugs.

To be effective at all stages of growth and development, the medical assistant must understand the age and maturity level of pediatric patients, the psychological changes that occur, and the psychosocial aspects of the child at various ages.

Communication with pediatric patients needs to be individualized, accepting, showing of empathy, and encompassing honesty and openness. Confidentiality must be maintained regardless of age. Parents and caregivers are involved with the care of their youngsters; therefore, they have the legal right to know the medical matters that relate to their minor children. Adolescents may share information with the medical assistant that they do not want their parents or caregivers to know. It is important to stress that some matters may need to be shared with parents or caregivers, especially when adolescents are living at home (certain matters pertaining to birth control, abortion, pregnancy, and sexually transmitted diseases pose special problems). Some states allow minors to give their consent under these circumstances (see Chapter 7).

Medical assistants can teach parents and caregivers in various ways. Handouts, demonstrations, videos, and one-on-one instruction are helpful in keeping children safe and healthy.

The medical assistant must be caring, respectful, supportive, and nonjudgmental of all patients. The caregiver to pediatric patients must reflect these values. Family beliefs and values also must be taken into account. This will foster care for pediatric patients that is compliant and in the best interest of all (see Figure 15-5).

GROWTH PATTERNS

Growth patterns provide valuable information to the pediatrician regarding the infant's physical progress. They are also used to calculate pediatric doses of medication. Height and weight and head circumference are measured at each regularly scheduled appointment at the pediatric facility. The measurements are then plotted on a physical growth percentile chart that is part of the patient's permanent record (Figure 15-6).

MEASURING THE INFANT OR CHILD

Careful measuring of the infant or child and monitoring of growth patterns are essential and should be done in a consistent and accurate manner.

Length and Weight Measurements

To record or plot length and weight measurements, you must first locate one growth value, either length (highlighted yellow) or weight (highlighted red), in the vertical columns of the Physical Growth Percentile Chart in Figure 15-7. Find the child's age in months in the horizontal rows (highlighted green). Locate the area where the growth value lines intersect on the graph and plot the length and weight by marking with a dot. Connect dots from previous examination with a ruler to provide a neat and accurate graphic recording. The date, age, measurements, and comments should also be indicated at the bottom of the chart.

The curved lines printed across the growth charts show the normal range of growth of infants and children in the United States. The numbers on the right side of the chart, in the vertical boxes between age 34 and 35 months, show the percentiles of other children the same age. To determine into which percentile the infant falls in relation to other infants of the same age, follow the line (percentile) upward to the percentage values along the edge of the graph. The National Center for Health Statistics (NCHS) growth charts become a permanent record of the child's development. These give the physician a quick way to check the child's growth in relation to that of other children the same age. Growth charts aid in the diagnosis of growth abnormalities and nutritional disorders and disease. Hereditary factors also influence growth patterns; therefore, having the family's history is important.

Infant Holds and Positions

Lifting and carrying infants must be done safely. The medical assistant should be especially careful of the infant's neck. It should be supported whenever the infant is lifted or held. About the age of four months, an infant begins to be able to hold up its head without support. (Each infant's growth and development is unique; therefore, four months is an approximate age.)

There are two primary positions that the medical assistant uses when lifting or carrying an infant. The first is the upright position in which the anterior surface of the infant's body is held against the medical assistant's body with one hand, which supports the infant's buttocks. The other hand is placed behind the head and neck of the infant for support (Figure 15-8). This position can be used to carry the infant and to place him or her on the scale or examination table. The second position is called the cradle position; the medical assistant holds the infant under his back and neck with one arm, and the other arm supports the buttocks and legs (Figure 15-9). This position is commonly used by mothers when

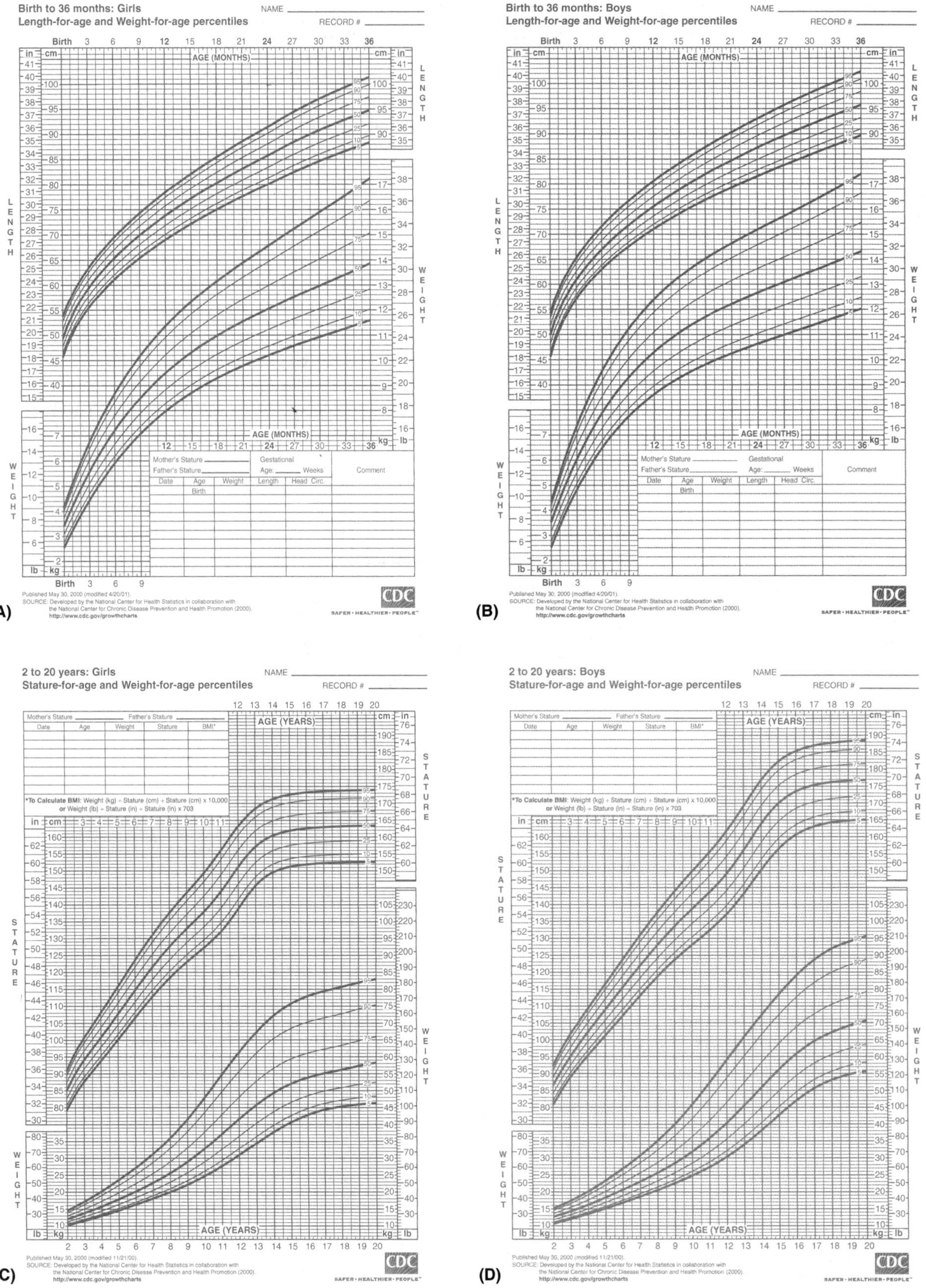

Figure 15-6 (A) Growth chart for girls' height and weight, age birth to 36 months. (B) Growth chart for boys' height and weight, age birth to 36 months. (C) Growth chart for girls' height and weight, age 2 to 18 years. (D) Growth chart for boys' height and weight, age 2 to 18 years. (Reprinted with permission of Ross Product Division, Abbott Laboratories, Inc.)

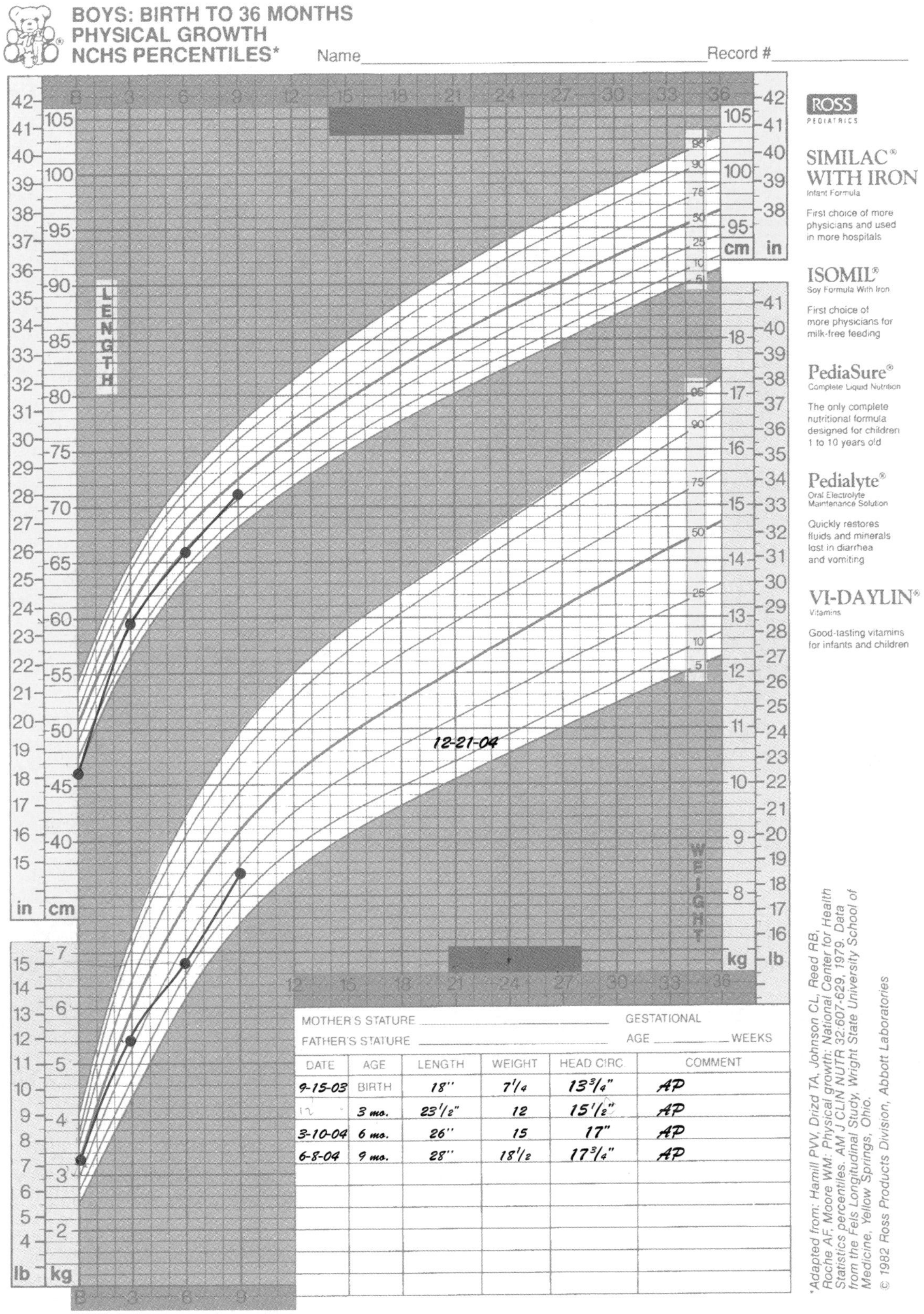

Figure 15-7 Sample growth chart with information plotted at birth, 3, 6, and 9 months. Sections in this figure have been highlighted to help you locate the values: length (yellow), weight (pink), age (green), and percentiles (white).
(Reprinted with permission of Ross Products Division, Abbott Laboratories, Inc.)

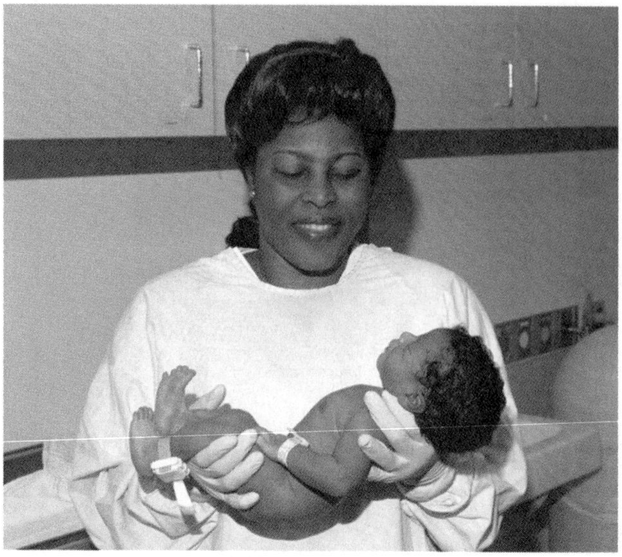

Figure 15-8 Infant carry—upright.

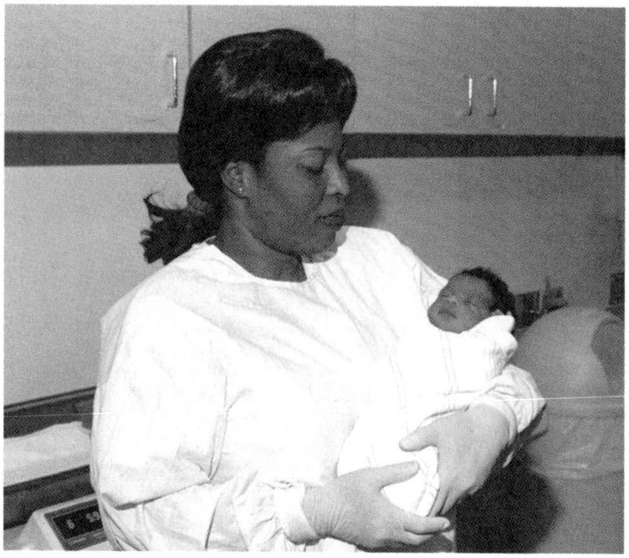

Figure 15-9 Infant carry—cradle.

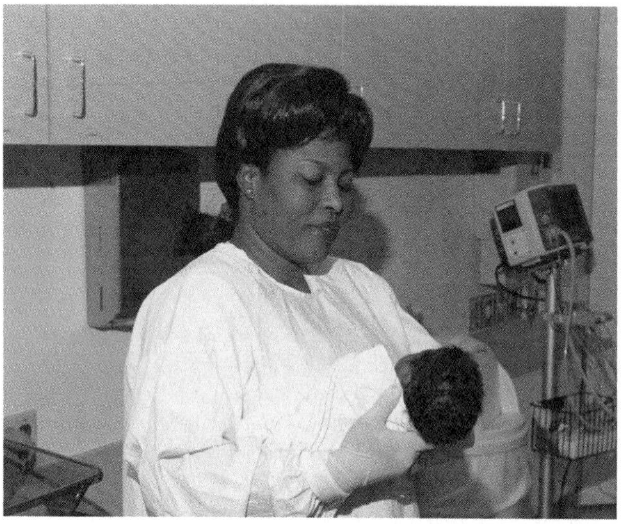

Figure 15-10 Infant carry—football.

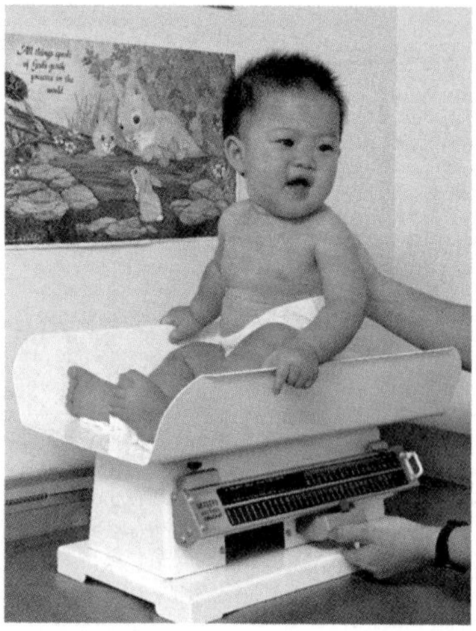

Figure 15-11 Infants who are able to sit and small children can be weighed on a platform scale.

feeding their babies. It is comforting to infants when they are able to see the parent or the familiar person. A third position that is used less often is known as the "football" carry or position. The posterior of the infant lays across the medical assistant's dominant outstretched arm and hand, and the infant's legs straddle the medical assistant's arm. The medical assistant supports the head, neck, and back of the infant with the dominant hand and arm and keeps the infant close to the body (Figure 15-10). If transporting the infant in this position, the medical assistant uses the nondominant hand to protect the back and top of the infant's head. When the medical assistant is stationary, the nondominant hand can be used if needed. When done properly, this position keeps the infant safe and secure.

Height and Weight Measuring Devices

Various devices are available for measuring height and weight in children. Infants and small children are weighed on an infant platform scale, which provides a measurement in pounds and ounces and kilograms and grams (Figure 15-11). The scale has a platform with curved sides in which the child may sit or lie. Weigh the infant or child in as few clothes as possible, removing the diaper and shoes or slippers. A small sheet, cloth diaper, or paper towel should be placed on the scale before weighing the infant or child, to avoid the transfer of microorganisms from bare skin.

Infant length can be measured using an infant measuring board, which consists of a rigid headboard and movable footboard. Place the measuring board on a table and position the infant on his or her back on the board, with the head touching the headboard. Move the footboard up until it touches the bottom of the infant's feet.

An infant can also be measured on a pad by placing a pin into the pad or making a pencil mark at the top of the head and a second pin or mark at the heel of the extended leg. The length is the distance between the two pins. A tape measure can also be used. Note: 1 inch = 2.54 cm.

A stature-measuring device may be used to measure height once the child is able to stand erect without support. The device consists of a movable headpiece attached to a rigid measuring bar and platform (Figure 15-12). A paper towel should be placed on the platform before use to avoid the potential transmission of microorganisms from bare feet.

Measuring Head Circumference

Head circumference measurement is routinely recorded on an infant's chart to alert the physician to any abnormal development. This procedure should be performed during routine visits until the child is 36 months old. Thereafter, it should be measured on a yearly basis until the age of 6 years. Head circumference measurement requires a flexible paper or metal measuring tape. A cloth tape may stretch and give a false measurement. Head circumference is plotted similarly to height and weight but on separate Growth Percentile Charts for head measurements (Figure 15-13). Generally, head and chest circumference are equal at about 1 to 2 years of age. Rapid growth above the normal percentile may indicate hydrocephalus, a disorder in which excessive fluid accumulates around the brain causing an increase in intracranial pressure and possible brain damage. This could lead to mental and physical problems. Conversely, the growth of the head that falls below the normal percentile may indicate microencephaly caused by a premature closure of the fontanels. In this instance, there is not enough room for the development of the brain, and mental retardation can result. Head circumference for a newborn should be between 12.5 to 14.5 inches or 31.75 to 36.83 cm.

Measuring Chest Circumference

Measuring the chest circumference of an infant is not normally performed during routine examinations. It may be performed and monitored when there is a suspicion of overdevelopment or underdevelopment of the heart or lungs or calcification of rib cartilage. To measure the chest of an infant, snugly wrap the measuring tape around the chest at nipple level. It is preferable to read the measurement during the resting phase between respirations.

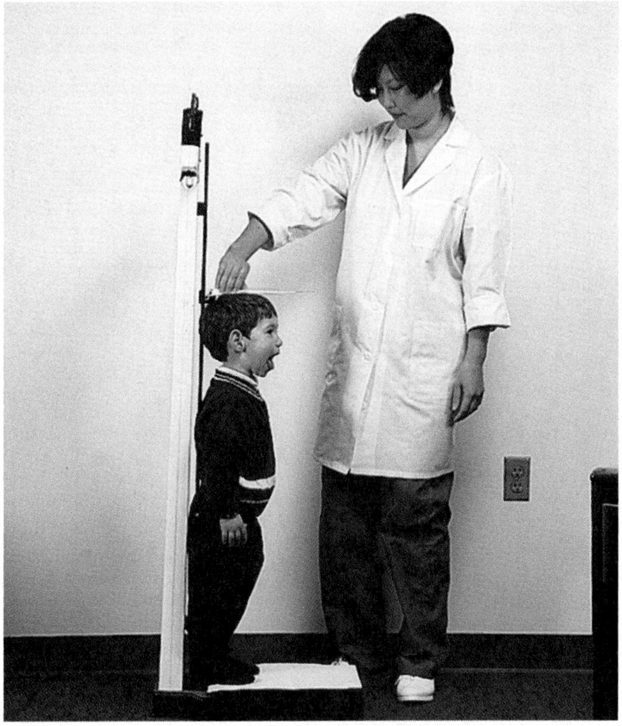

Figure 15-12 Measuring length and height in children.

Occasionally it may be necessary for the medical assistant to convert measurement results into inches or centimeters. To accomplish the task accurately, note that 1 inch equals 2.54 cm. (See Procedure 15-2 for measuring infant chest and head circumference and weight and height.)

To convert inches to centimeters, multiply the number of inches by 2.54:

$$\text{Inches} \times 2.54 = \text{Centimeters}$$

To convert centimeters to inches, divide the number of centimeters by 2.54:

$$\text{Centimeters} \div 2.54 = \text{Inches}$$

Infant/Child Failure to Thrive

The failure of an infant or a child to grow and thrive may have many organic and inorganic causes. There may be social and emotional causes. Many of the causes for an infant or a child failing to grow and thrive may be treated if found in time. The emotionally deprived infant needing affection will not grow, because there will be a lack of growth hormone production. Once this child is given physical and emotional warmth, the growth hormone is produced and the child will grow. Other reasons for an infant failing to thrive may be because the infant has a chronic disease; a diet that is inadequate especially in

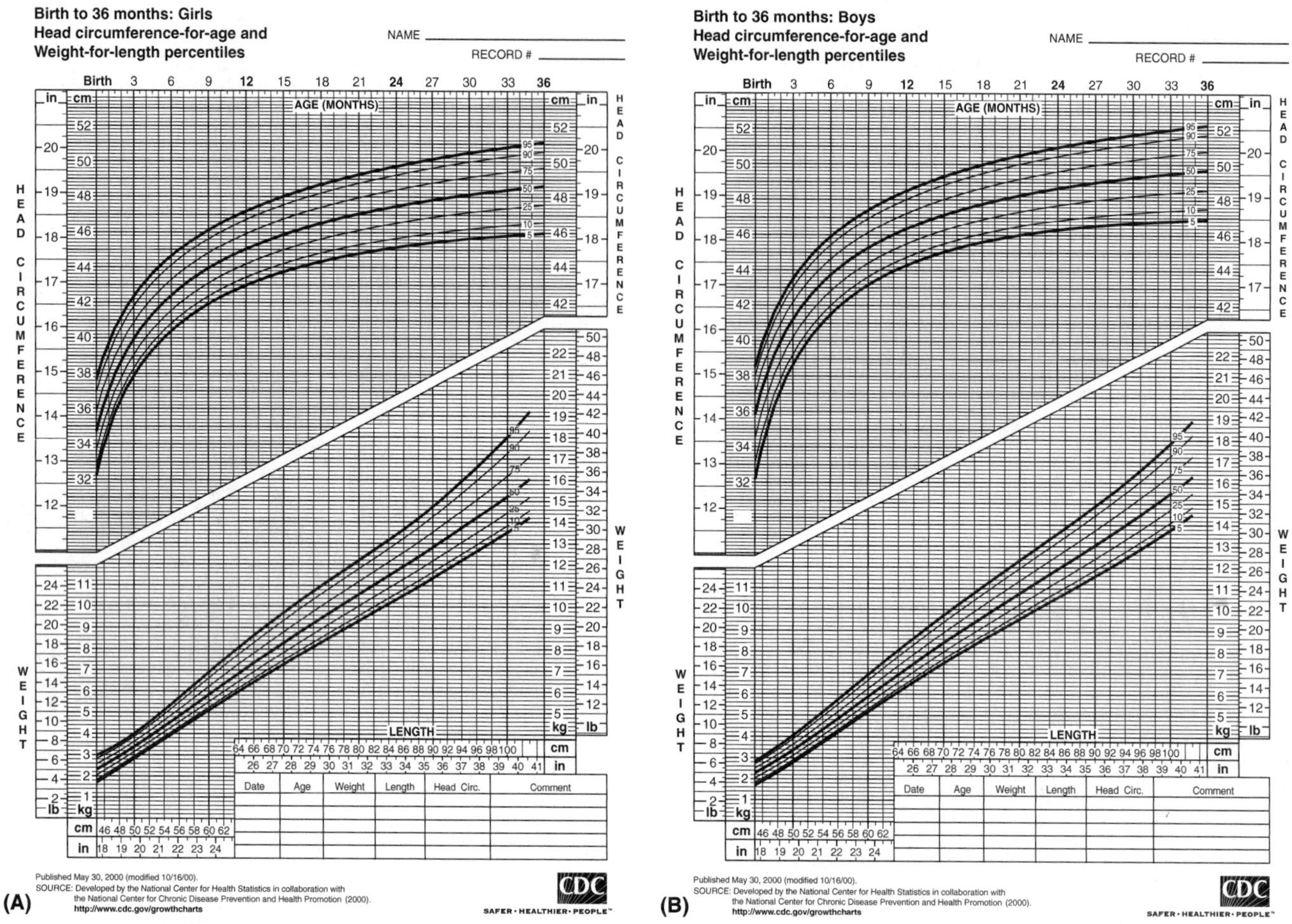

Figure 15-13 (A) Growth chart for girls' head circumference, birth to 36 months. (B) Growth chart for boys' head circumference, birth to 36 months. (Reprinted with permission of Ross Products Division, Abbott Laboratories, Inc.)

calories and proteins; a disorder of the heart, brain, or kidneys; or has been improperly fed.

PEDIATRIC VITAL SIGNS

As with older children and adults, pediatric vital signs are commonly taken by the medical assistant. The vital signs are more fully covered in Chapter 12 for adult patients; however, specific procedures for taking an infant's temperature, pulse, respiration, and blood pressure are explained here. These procedures are done differently for infants than for older children and adults.

Temperature

Body temperature may be measured in Fahrenheit (F) or Celsius (C) degrees through oral, rectal, axillary, or tympanic routes. Many types of thermometers are used. Mercury (glass) thermometers have been replaced in ambulatory care areas and offices by digital thermometers, electronic thermometers, and tympanic membrane sensors or aural, which provide accurate temperature readings in less time. Broken mercury thermometers release vapors into the air that are toxic when inhaled and lead to mercury poisoning. They should no longer be used. Proper disposal of the mercury is regulated by the health department and varies from state to state. Electronic and digital thermometers can display temperature within 15 to 60 seconds, depending on the model used. A reading can be obtained by infrared tympanic membrane sensor in as little as 2 seconds.

Oral Temperature. The oral route is used for children older than 5 years. Caution the child against biting down on the thermometer. Do not take an oral temperature if the child has a history of seizures.

Aural Temperature. The aural route uses the tympanic membrane thermometer. It is used on children older than 2 years because it is considered less accurate for children younger than 2 years. Otitis media and impacted cerumen are two other reasons why this route may not be selected. A reading can be obtained in a matter of seconds.

Rectal Temperature. Rectal temperatures may be taken with caution in infants and toddlers when other methods or routes are not advised. Place the child supine or prone, with the knees flexed. An infant can also lie prone on a parent's lap. Do not force the thermometer. Rectal temperatures are not indicated for children who have had rectal surgery or for those who have diarrhea. See Procedure 15-3.

Axillary Temperature. Axillary temperatures are often preferable to rectal or oral temperatures for toddlers and preschoolers because they are safe and nonintrusive to take. Place the probe of the digital thermometer in the axillary space and have the child hold the arm close to the trunk. Leave in place until beep is heard. This route is not used if accuracy is critical.

Pulse

The apical pulse is heard at the apex of the heart, located at the fifth intercostal space left side, midclavicular line. That is, between the fifth and sixth ribs in the middle of the clavicle (usually below the nipple), left of the sternum. A stethoscope is required to obtain an apical pulse. The apical pulse is generally preferred over other pulse locations for infants and small children (younger than 5 years). Each "lub-dub" sound is counted as one heartbeat. The pulse is counted for one full minute. See Procedure 15-4.

The normal pulse rate varies with age, decreasing as the child grows older (Table 15-3). The heart rate may also vary considerably among children of the same age and size. The heart rate increases in response to exercise, excitement, anxiety, and fever and decreases to a resting rate when the child is still.

Listen to the heart rate, noting whether the heart rhythm is regular or irregular. Children often have a normal cycle of irregular rhythm associated with respiration called sinus arrhythmia. In sinus arrhythmia, the child's heart rate is faster on inspiration and slower on expiration. Record whether the pulse is normal, bounding, or thready.

Respirations

In older children and adolescents, respiratory rate is counted in the same way as in an adult. In infants and young children (younger than 6 years), however, the respiratory rate is assessed by observing the rise and fall of the abdomen. Inspiration, when the chest or abdomen rises, and expiration, when the chest or abdomen falls, are counted as one respiration. Because these movements are often irregular, they should be counted for one full minute for accuracy. Normal respiratory rate varies with the child's age (Table 15-4). See Procedure 15-5.

TABLE 15-3 NORMAL HEART RATE RANGES FOR CHILDREN

Age	Heart Rate Range	Average Heart Rate
Infants to 2 years	100–160	110
2 to 6 years	70–120	100
6 to 10 years	70–110	90
10 to 16 years	60–100	85

Blood Pressure

The blood pressure of an infant is not normally taken unless requested by the physician. In children 3 years of age and older, blood pressure should be measured annually as part of a routine vital sign assessment.

Blood pressure may be measured using electronic or aneroid equipment and a pediatric cuff. The size of the blood pressure cuff is determined by the size of the child's arm or leg. A general rule of thumb is that the width of the inflatable bladder should be 40% of the circumference of the extremity used. If the cuff is too small, pressure will be falsely high; if too large, falsely low. Sometimes it is difficult to hear the blood pressure in an infant or small child. Use a pediatric stethoscope over pulse sites if possible.

If the pulse still cannot be auscultated, the blood pressure can be measured by touch. Palpate for the pulse. Keeping your fingers on the pulse, pump up the cuff until the pulse is no longer felt. Slowly open the air valve, watching the dial, and note the number where the pulse is again palpated. This is called the palpated systolic blood pressure (see Table 15-5).

TABLE 15-4 NORMAL RESPIRATORY RATE RANGES FOR CHILDREN

Age	Respiratory Rate per Minute
1 year	20–40
3 years	20–30
6 years	16–22
10 years	16–20
17 years	12–20

TABLE 15-5 NORMAL BLOOD PRESSURE RANGES

Age	Systolic (mm Hg)	Diastolic (mm Hg)
1 year	74–100	50–70
3 years	80–112	50–80
6 years	82–110	50–78
10 years	84–119	54–80
17 years	94–119	62–88

COLLECTING A URINE SPECIMEN FROM AN INFANT

Occasionally the medical assistant may be required to obtain a urine specimen from an infant for laboratory testing. Special procedures and equipment are required for this procedure. The collection bag is clear plastic with adhesive tabs for application to the perineum of the infant (Figure 15-14). See Procedure 15-6.

SCREENING INFANTS FOR HEARING IMPAIRMENT

In some hospitals, infants are screened for hearing impairment immediately after delivery. An automated system for checking hearing ability is used by some clinics. It is a more complex screening requiring the use of sensors. As the infant moves in response to sounds produced by the system, these responses are recorded by sensors attached to the infant. This procedure is a more definitive screening process. The medical assistant must maintain a quiet environment while these screening procedures are being performed because extraneous sounds may invalidate the results (Figure 15-15).

SCREENING INFANT AND CHILD VISUAL ACUITY

Measuring the visual acuity of an infant is difficult and is not usually performed unless visual impairment is suspected. Newborns will respond to light by tightly shutting their eyes, keeping them closed until the light is removed.

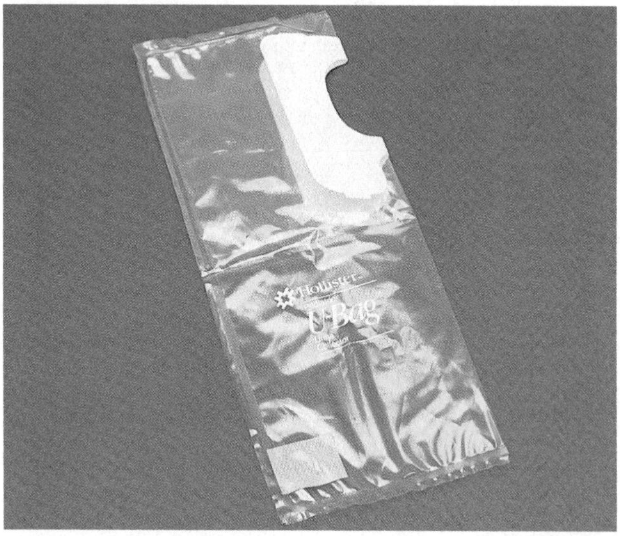

Figure 15-14 Pediatric urine collector. The collector is opened, and the paper backing is removed exposing the adhesive surface. The collector is firmly attached over the child's cleansed genitalia to prevent leakage.

Older infants will follow an object up and down when it is placed directly in front of the eyes. It is estimated that a newborn has the vision equivalent to 20/150, which will reach the adult level of 20/20 by the age of six months. The medical assistant will be required to maintain a nonstimulating environment while the physician is screening the infant, because any interference may invalidate results.

The kindergarten chart or Allen cards are used to test visual acuity in young children. It contains pictures in descending size, and the lines are labeled in the same manner as the Snellen Chart. The child is asked to identify the picture as the medical assistant points to it (Figure 15-16).

The E chart is a series of Es pointing in different directions in descending size. The size and labeling are the same as the Snellen chart. This chart is used for older children. The child will be asked to point in the direction of the *E* as the medical assistant points to it (Figure 15-17).

Make a game out of measuring young children's visual acuity because their attention span is very limited.

COMMON DISORDERS AND DISEASES

Young children grow and physically change very quickly. Their immune systems develop normally when they are healthy infants and children. Immunizations, together

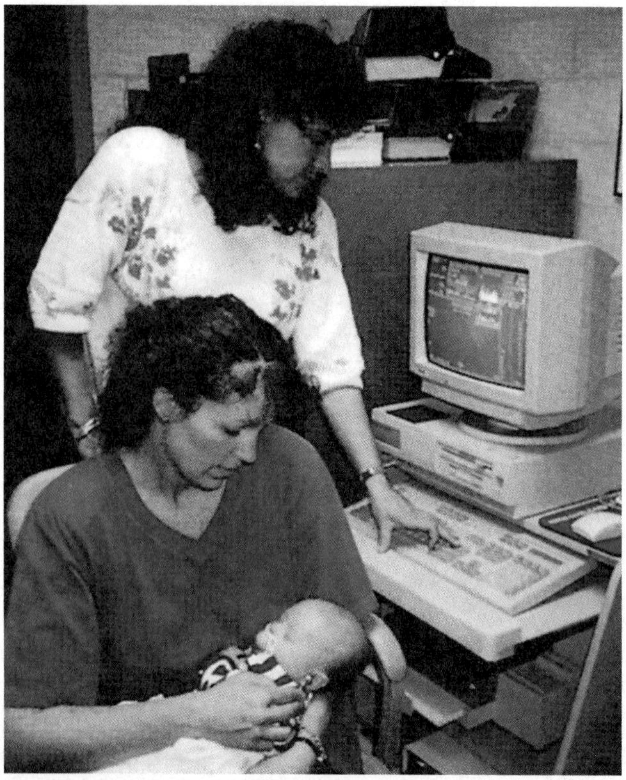

Figure 15-15 Infant getting hearing tested. (Courtesy of American Academy of Audiology.)

with their own developing immune system, give them protection from dangerous childhood diseases. Many life-threatening illnesses have been controlled because of scheduled immunization, the child's own developing immune system, and the wise use of antibiotics for infections.

Otitis Media

Otitis media is a commonly occurring disorder of infants and young children. It is characterized by inflammation of the middle ear. Fluid accumulates behind the tympanic membrane with a degree of temporary hearing loss. It is commonly known as a middle ear infection. Because of the infant and young child's eustachian tubes' connection to the nose and throat, bacteria that causes throat and respiratory infections can easily access the inner ear via the eustachian tube. The fluid in the middle ear can become infected by the bacteria present in the nose and throat. The fluid turns to pus and is known as **suppurative** otitis media. Pain and loss of hearing are common symptoms. Many young children have eustachian tubes that are horizontal and narrow, which predisposes them to otitis media. As children develop physically, they can outgrow otitis media.

The physician can diagnosis otitis media by visually examining the tympanic membrane with an otoscope. The membrane will be bulging and appear red and inflamed (Figure 15-18). If **exudate** or an oozing of pus is present, a culture and sensitivity can be done. The treatment for otitis media is antibiotics. To avoid antiobiotic overuse and pathogen resistance, physicians will attempt to prescribe antibiotic therapy only when necessary. Decongestants are helpful in some children. For chronic otitis media, a **myringotomy,** incision into the tympanic membrane, may be necessary to avoid the rupture of the tympanic membrane and the scarring that results. Scarring can cause permanently impaired hearing ability.

Tympanostomy is a surgical procedure in which pediatric ear tubes are placed through the tympanic

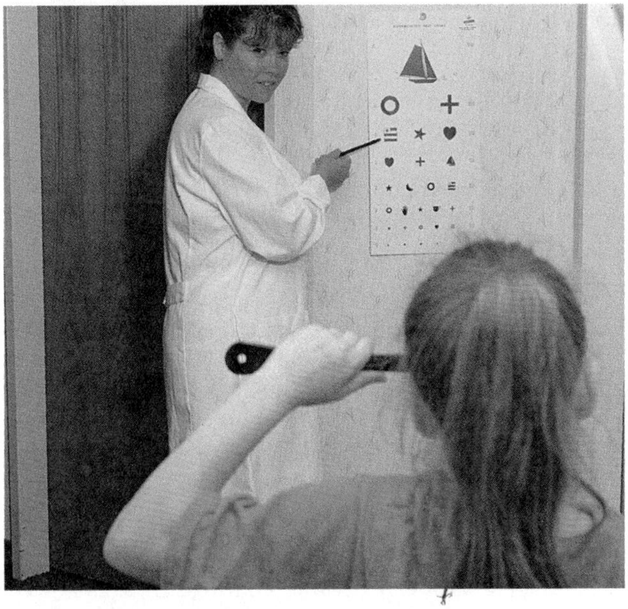

Figure 15-16 Measuring distance visual acuity of a child using a kindergarten vision screening chart.

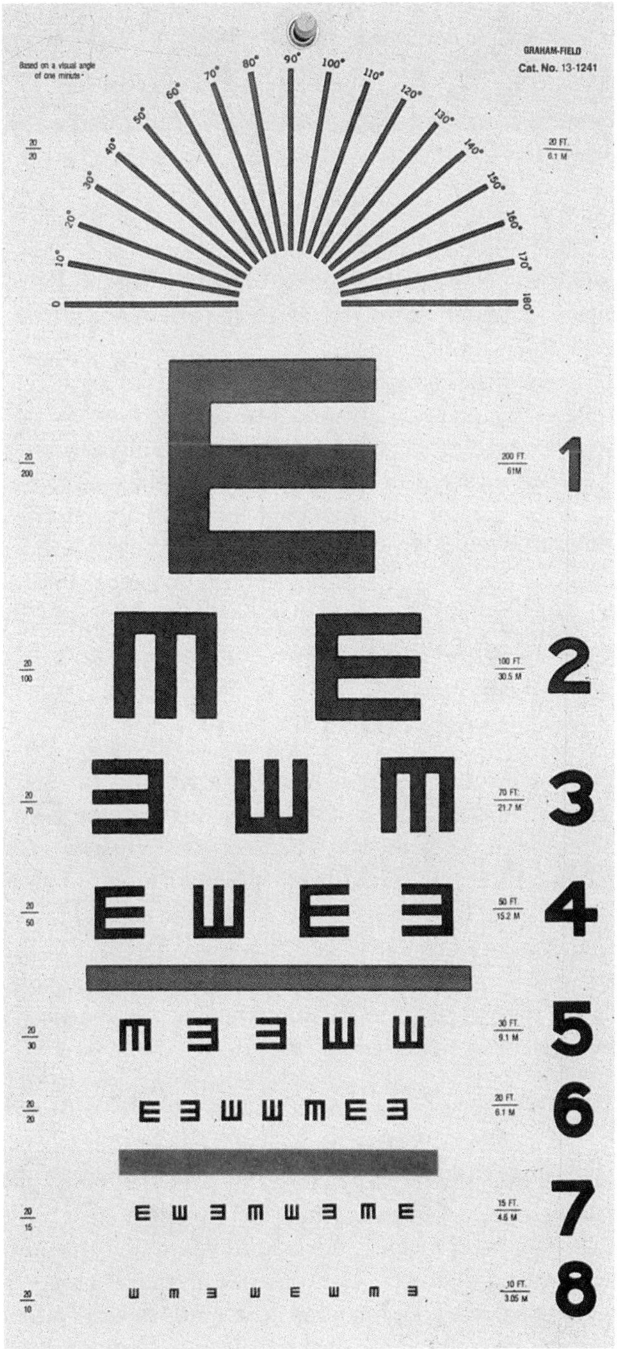

Figure 15-17 Snellen E or Big E chart for testing distance visual acuity of children.

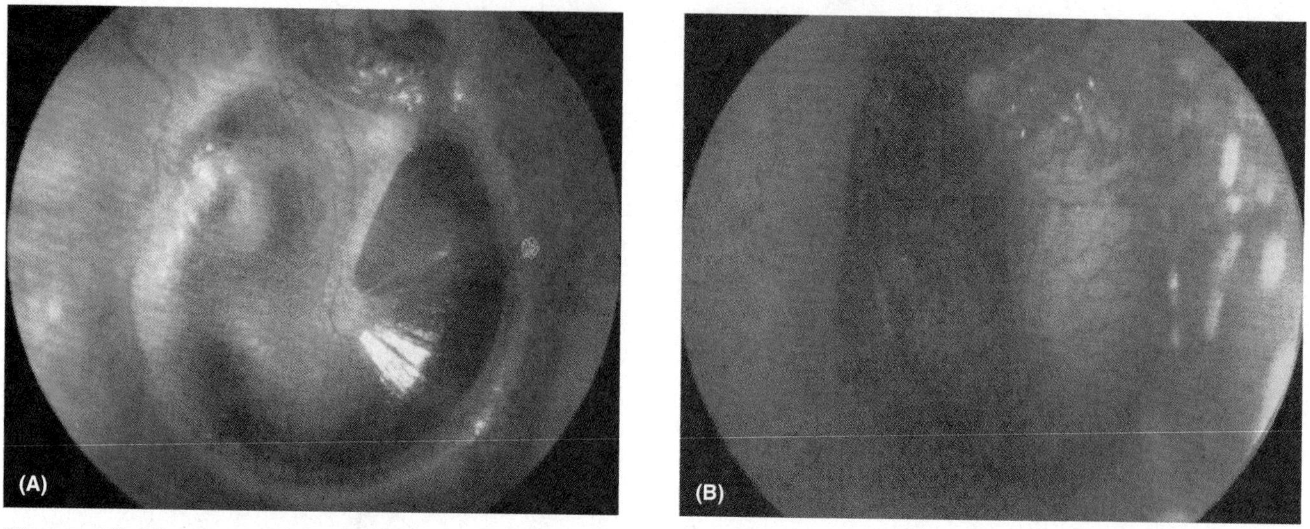

Figure 15-18 Comparison of (A) normal tympanic membrane and (B) acute otitis media.

membrane to promote ongoing drainage. Chronic otitis media that is left untreated can result in permanent hearing loss.

Hearing loss causes serious major problems in a child's development. Treatment of hearing loss depends on its cause. Hearing aids may be helpful to amplify sounds if the loss is caused by sounds not being conducted to the inner ear. Sensor neural hearing loss does not improve with hearing aids. **Cochlear implantation,** approved by the Food and Drug Administration (FDA) since 1990, is a relatively new procedure that can help children with bilateral **sesorineural** deafness.

The Common Cold

The common cold is aptly named because it is the most common and frequent disease that young children experience. Viruses are the usual microorganism that cause a cold, and they are spread by direct contact and droplets through the air when children cough and sneeze. Some symptoms are inflammation of the nasopharynx, coughing, nasal discharge, sneezing, and fever. Treatment consists of getting sufficient rest, forcing fluids, and eating a well-balanced diet.

Tonsillitis

The tonsils are located in the back of the nose and throat. They aid in protecting the respiratory tract from infection but frequently become inflamed and infected while doing their job. The cause most often is group A beta-hemolytic streptococcus or a virus. Fever, cough, sore throat, and red, swollen tonsils are common symptoms. Diagnosis can be made by doing a culture and sensitivity of tonsillar exudate. Antibiotics will rid the child of infection and must be taken as prescribed. Tonsillectomy is considered for older children who have chronic tonsillitis.

Pediculosis

Infestation with the head louse is known as pediculosis capitus and is common among school-aged children. The parasites suck blood from humans and are highly contagious. Diagnosis can be made by visual examination of the hair and scalp and observing the eggs (known as nits) on the hair. Special medications applied to the hair is an effective treatment. Care should be taken to launder bed linens and clothing everyday. The louse is not a vector for disease.

Asthma

Asthma has increased dramatically in the general population but especially in children. The cause of asthma is not known, but it can be brought on by environmental substances, such as pollen, chemicals, cigarette smoke, mold, and dog and cat hair. Its symptoms include wheezing, coughing, and shortness of breath. It is a serious chronic respiratory disease. Spasms of the bronchi trap air and mucus in the lungs. The child will complain of a tight chest and will have shallow respirations and a nonproductive cough. The asthma attack may become an emergency situation. The pediatrician may refer the child to an allergy specialist who will test the child for various allergies. Respiratory therapy is helpful for some children. Airways can become damaged over time as a result of chronic inflammation.

Croup

The common viral condition croup has symptoms of a croupy or "barking"-type cough, a high-pitched sound on inspiration (stridor) and respiratory distress. The condition is often associated with an upper respiratory infection that leads to inflammation of the larynx, trachea, and bronchi. Respiratory obstruction can occur if severe, but children with croup generally are not seriously ill.

Child Abuse

Child abuse has increased significantly in recent years. By law, health care professionals, including medical assistants, as well as others, must report suspected child abuse. The individual reporting the suspected abuse is protected against liability as a result of the reporting. If suspicion of abuse exists, the physician and health care professional should:

- Treat the child's injuries
- Send the child to hospital if necessary
- Inform parents of the diagnosis
- Inform parents that the incident will be reported to the public and social service agency
- Notify child protective agency
- Document all information
- Provide court testimony if requested

Some injuries commonly seen in child abuse include poor hygiene, bruises, welts, malnutrition, burns, fractures, head injuries, dislocated joints, and neglected well-baby appointments.

The cultural background of the family should be taken into consideration as should some folk medicine practices. Latin American and Russian cultures treat headaches or abdominal pain by the practice of placing a cup on the skin, creating a vacuum, and a small amount of burning material is placed on the skin. These children may present with burns. To treat minor ailments, Southeast Asians rub a coin or spoon in hot oil and rub it onto the child's neck, spine, and ribs, and a burn may occur.

Procedure 15-1 Maintaining Immunization Records

STANDARD PRECAUTIONS:

PURPOSE:
To establish and maintain a record of preventive immunizations against childhood diseases for the physician and parent or legal guardian.

EQUIPMENT/SUPPLIES:
Vaccine Administration Record
Vial of vaccine as ordered

PROCEDURE STEPS:

1. Give the parent or legal guardian the most recent copy of the Vaccine Information Statement (VIS). The statements explain risks and benefits of vaccines for each dose of vaccine given.
2. After the administration of a scheduled vaccine for the child, document in the patient's record and on the Vaccine Administration Record.
3. Using the medicine note and the vaccine vial, fill out the Vaccine Administration Record (Figure 15-19) according to which vaccine you administered. Note the headings, type of vaccine (use generic abbreviations, not the brand name), date given, month, day, year, dose, route, site, vaccine lot number and manufacturer, VIS; date on VIS, date given (VIS), and your initials as the individual who administered the vaccine.
4. The immunization record is kept by the physician and the parent or legal guardian. NOTE: Remind parent or legal guardian to keep immunization records safe and readily accessible for proof of immunization for daycare and school.
5. Document on child's record that vaccine was administered.

(continues)

Procedure 15-1 (continued)

Vaccine Administration Record

Record Number: ______________________

Patient Name: ______________________

Address: ______________________

Birth Date: ______________ Male ____ Female ____

Medicare Number: ______________________

Insurance Number: ______________________

Clinic Name and Address:	
Name(s) of Vaccine Administrator(s):	Initials
Use Reverse Side for Additional Names and Initials	

Vaccine administrator: Make sure to give the parent or legal representative the most recent copy of the Vaccine Information Statement (VIS) which explains risks and benefits of vaccine for **each** dose of vaccine given.

Vaccine	Type of Vaccine*	Date Given mo/day/yr	Dose	Route**	Site Given*** (RA,LA, RT, LT)	Vaccine lot #	Vaccine mfr.	Vaccine Information Statement Date on VIS	Vaccine Information Statement Date Given	Vaccine Admin Initials
Hepatitis B (e.g., HepB, HepB-Hib, DTaP-HepB-IPV)				IM						
				IM						
				IM						
Diphtheria, Tetanus, Pertussis (e.g., DTaP, DT, DTaP-Hib, DTaP-HepB-IPV, Td)				IM						
				IM						
				IM						
				IM						
				IM						
				IM						
				IM						
***Haemophilus influenzae* type b** (e.g., Hib, HepB-Hib, DTaP-Hib)				IM						
				IM						
				IM						
				IM						
Polio (e.g., IPV, DTaP-HepB-IPV)				IM•SC						
				IM•SC						
				IM•SC						
				IM•SC						
Pneumococcal Conjugate (PCV7)				IM						
				IM						
				IM						
				IM						
Measles, Mumps, Rubella (MMR)				SC						
				SC						
Varicella (Var)				SC						
				SC						
☐ Check box if this child has a physician-certified reliable history of chickenpox.**** Date box checked __/__/__										
Hepatitis A (HepA)				IM						
				IM						
Influenza Inactivated (Intramuscular) or Live (Intranasal)				IM•IN						
				IM•IN						
				IM•IN						
				IM•IN						
Pneumococcal Polysaccharide (PPV23)				IM•SC						
				IM•SC						
Other										
Other										

* Record the generic abbreviation for the type of vaccine given (e.g., DTaP), not the trade name. For combination vaccines, indicate the type (e.g.,DTaP-Hib) and all other information for each individual antigen (e.g., in the DTP and Hib sections) comprising the combination.

** Route: IM = Intramuscular, SC = Subcutaneous, IN = Intranasal, PO = Oral.

*** Site given: RA = Right Arm, LA = Left Arm, RT = Right Thigh, LT = Left Thigh.

****A reliable history of chickenpox is defined as: 1) physician interpretation of parent/guardian description of chickenpox; 2) physician diagnosis of chickenpox; or 3) laboratory proof of immunity.

Figure 15-19 Vaccination Administration Record.

DOCUMENTATION

5/2/20XX DTaP 0.5 mL (R) vastus lateralis. Recorded on vaccine administration record as well. Parent given vaccine information statement. W. Slawson CMA

Procedure 15-2 Measuring the Infant: Weight, Length, Head, and Chest Circumference

STANDARD PRECAUTIONS:

PURPOSE:

To obtain an accurate measurement of an infant's weight, length, head, and chest circumference for medical records and to screen for growth abnormalities.

EQUIPMENT/SUPPLIES:

Infant scale	Patient's chart
Paper protector	Pen
Flexible measuring tape	Ruler
Growth chart	Biohazard waste container

PROCEDURE STEPS:

Measuring infant weight:

1. Wash hands. Explain procedure to parent(s).
2. Undress infant (including the diaper).
3. Place all weights to left of scale to check balance.
4. Place a clean utility towel on scale, check balance scale for accuracy, being sure to compensate for the weight of the towel. RATIONALE: The protection that the paper utility towel affords helps to reduce transmission of microorganisms and will provide warmth because the scale will be cool.
5. Gently place infant on her back on the scale. Place your hand slightly above the infant's body to ensure safety (Figure 15-20). RATIONALE: This will safeguard the infant from falling.
6. Place the bottom weight to its highest measurement that will not cause the balance to drop to the bottom edge.
7. Slowly move upper weight until the balance bar rests in the center of the indicator. A balanced scale will provide an accurate weight. Read the infant's weight while he or she is lying still.
8. Return both weights to their resting position to the extreme left.
9. Gently remove infant and apply diaper. (Parent can help with diapering and holding infant.)

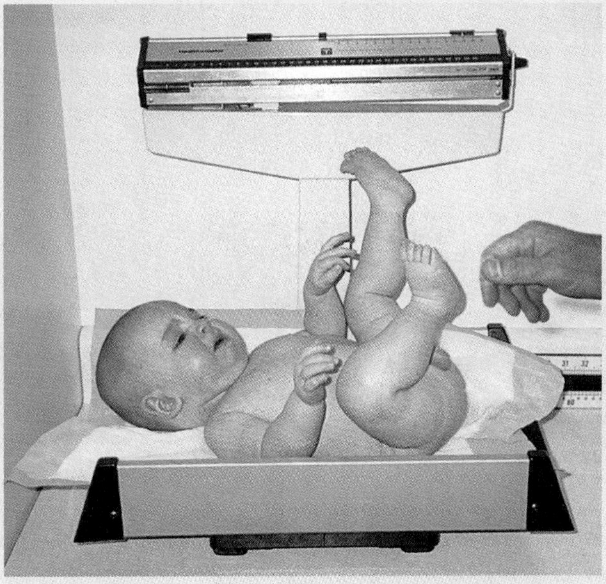

Figure 15-20 Infants who are unable to sit erect should be weighed on their back on a platform scale.

(continues)

DOCUMENTATION

3/10/20XX 4:00 PM 6 months of age, wt. 15 lbs. Recorded on growth chart. C. McInnis, RMA

Procedure 15-2 (continued)

10. Discard used protective paper towel per Occupational Safety and Health Administration (OSHA) guidelines.
11. Sanitize scale.
12. Wash hands.
13. Document results according to office policy (pounds and ounces or kilograms) on growth chart, patient's chart, and parent's booklet if available. Connect dot from previous examination with a ruler to complete graph.

Measuring infant length:

1. Wash hands. Explain procedure to parent(s).
2. Remove infant's shoes.
3. Gently place infant on his or her back on the examination table. If the pediatric table has a headboard, ask parent to hold infant's head against (end) headboard of table at zero mark of ruler while you place infant's heels against footboard. Gently straighten infant's back and legs to line up along ruler. If there is no footboard (to place infant's feet against), use your right hand as a guide (Figure 15-21). If necessary, gently place your left hand over the child's legs at the knees to secure the child in place and straighten the legs so you can read the recumbent length from the head to the heel. RATIONALE: Sometimes it is difficult to straighten the legs.
4. Read length on the measuring device in inches or centimeters.
5. Wash hands.
6. Document measurement on growth chart, patient's chart, and parent's booklet if available. Connect dot from previous examination with a ruler to complete graph.

Measuring Head Circumference:

1. Wash hands and explain procedure to parent(s).
2. Talk to infant to gain cooperation. Infant may be held by parent or lie on examination table for procedure. Older children of 2 or 3 years may stand or sit if they will remain still.
3. Place the measuring tape snugly around the head from the occipital protuberance to the supraorbital prominence. This is the largest part of the head (Figure 15-22).
4. Read the measurement, which will be in either inches (to nearest ½ inch) or centimeters (to nearest 0.01 cm).
5. Wash hands.
6. Document results according to office policy on growth chart, patient's chart, and parent's booklet if available. Connect dot from previous examination with a ruler to complete graph.

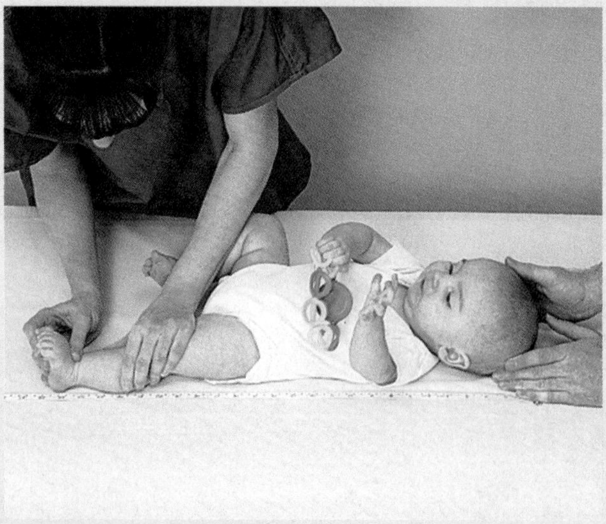

Figure 15-21 Measuring the recumbent length of an infant.

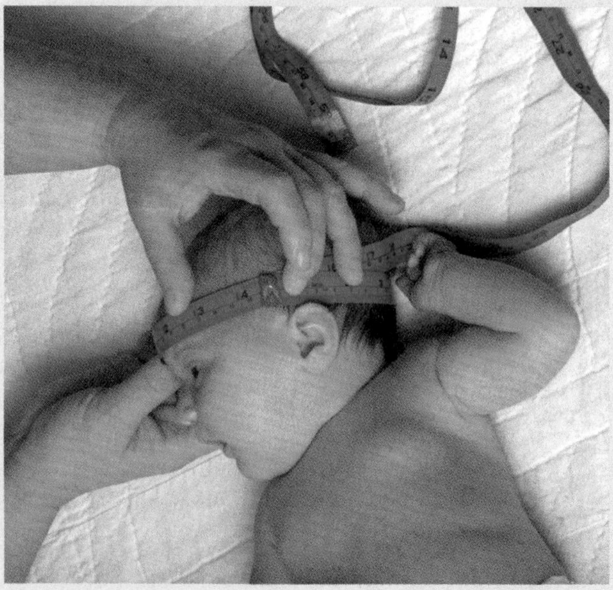

Figure 15-22 Measuring infant's head circumference.

(continues)

Procedure 15-2 (continued)

Measuring infant's chest circumference:

1. Wash hands and explain procedure to parent(s).
2. Use one thumb to hold tape measure with zero mark against the infant's chest at the midsternal area. With the other hand, bring the tape around/under the back to meet the zero mark of the tape in front. Take the measurement of the chest just above the nipples with the tape fitting around the child's chest under the axillary region. If you need assistance in holding the child still, ask the parent or another assistant. The measurement should be taken when the child is breathing normally and during the resting phase between respirations (Figure 15-23).
3. Read measurement to the nearest 0.01 cm.
4. Wash hands.
5. Document results in patient's chart.

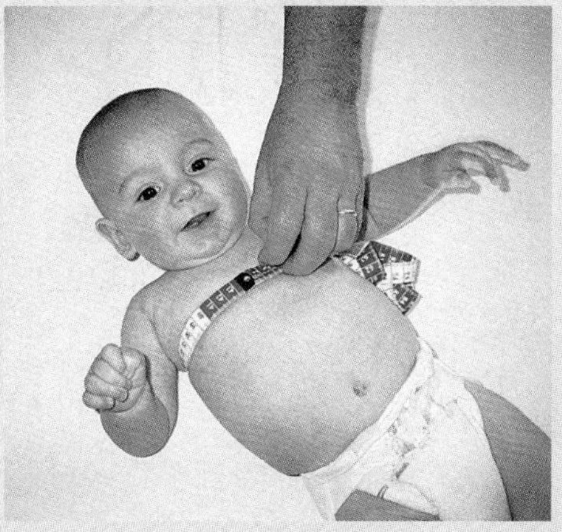

Figure 15-23 Measuring infant's chest circumference.

DOCUMENTATION

3/10/20XX 4:00 PM 6 months of age, length 26″ long. Recorded on growth chart. C. McInnis, RMA

DOCUMENTATION

3/10/20XX 4:00 PM 6 months of age, head circumference 43 centimeters. Recorded on growth chart. C. McInnis, RMA

DOCUMENTATION

3/10/20XX 4:00 PM 6 months of age, chest circumference 30 centimeters. Recorded on growth chart. C. McInnis, RMA

Procedure 15-3 Taking an Infant's Rectal Temperature with a Digital Thermometer

STANDARD PRECAUTIONS:

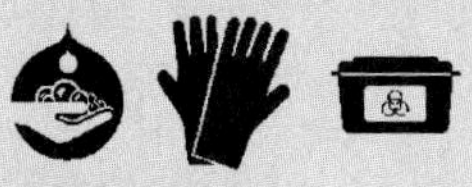

PURPOSE:

To obtain a rectal temperature using a digital thermometer.

EQUIPMENT/SUPPLIES:

Digital thermometer (red probe) and probe cover
Lubricating jelly
4 × 4 gauze sponges
Gloves
Biohazard waste container

PROCEDURE STEPS:

1. Wash hands.
2. Assemble equipment.
3. Identify patient.
4. Explain procedure to parent(s). RATIONALE: Gain cooperation and assistance in disrobing infant and positioning properly.
5. Remove infant's diaper.
6. Position infant in a prone (Figure 15-24A) or supine (Figure 15-24B) position having parent or another medical assistant safeguard infant.
7. Place sheath on thermometer. RATIONALE: Prevents microorganism cross contamination.
8. Lubricate with lubricating jelly. (Place lubricant on a 4 × 4 gauze sponge and place tip of thermometer in lubricant.) RATIONALE: Easier insertion of thermometer.
9. Apply gloves.
10. Spread buttocks, insert thermometer gently into the rectum past the sphincter; for an infant this is 0.5 inch (Figure 15-24).
11. Hold buttocks together while holding the thermometer. If necessary, restrain infant movement by placing your arm across infant's back. Parent can immobilize infant's legs. RATIONALE: Ensure infant's safety and comfort.
12. Hold in place until beep is heard. Do not let go of the thermometer. RATIONALE: Movement by infant can cause thermometer to move and injure the infant.
13. Remove from rectum. Have parent attend to infant.
14. Note temperature reading.
15. Remove probe cover by ejecting it into a biohazard container.
16. Remove gloves, discard in biohazard waste container.
17. Wash hands.
18. Wipe probe with antiseptic wipe. Replace thermometer on holder.
19. Assist parent in dressing infant if necessary.
20. Record on the patient chart labeled with (R); indicating a rectal temperature.

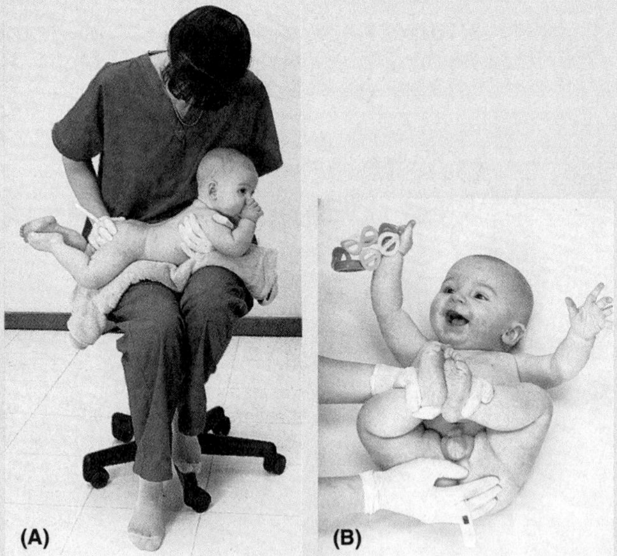

Figure 15-24 (A) Taking the rectal temperature of an infant in the prone position. (B) Infant in supine position having rectal temperature taken.

DOCUMENTATION

5/3/20XX 4:00 PM T 99.8 (R). M. Slawson, CMA

Procedure 15-4 Taking an Apical Pulse on an Infant

STANDARD PRECAUTIONS:

PURPOSE:
To obtain an apical pulse rate.

EQUIPMENT/SUPPLIES:
Stethoscope
Watch with second hand
Alcohol wipes

PROCEDURE STEPS:

1. Wash hands.
2. Assemble equipment.
3. Identify patient.
4. Explain procedure to parent.
5. Assist in disrobing infant if necessary.
6. Provide a drape for infant's warmth if necessary.
7. Position the infant in a supine position or sitting in the parent's lap. RATIONALE: The supine position may offer easier access to apex of heart if the child is calm.
8. Locate the fifth intercostal space, midclavicular line, left of sternum. RATIONALE: Location of apex of heart.
9. Place warmed stethoscope on the site and listen for the lub-dup sound of the heart.
10. Count the pulse for one minute; each lub-dup equals one heartbeat or pulse.
11. Wash hands.
12. Assist parent as needed.
13. Clean earpieces and diaphragm of stethoscope with alcohol wipes. RATIONALE: Prevents cross contamination of microbes between patients.
14. Record the pulse in the infant's chart with the designation of (AP) to denote method of obtaining the pulse. Note any arrhythmias.
15. Wash hands again.

Procedure 15-5 Measuring Infant's Respiration Rate

STANDARD PRECAUTIONS:

PURPOSE:
The respiration rate is normally taken immediately before or after the pulse rate to obtain an accurate respiratory rate.

EQUIPMENT/SUPPLIES:
Watch with second hand

PROCEDURE STEPS:

1. Wash hands.
2. Identify the patient and explain the procedure to the parent.
3. Position infant in a supine position.
4. Place hand on the chest to feel the rise and fall of the chest wall for one minute.
5. Note depth, rhythm, and breath sounds while counting.
6. Wash hands.
7. Record respiration rate in patient chart, noting any irregularities and sounds.

DOCUMENTATION

3/10/20XX 4:00 PM Respirations 22. Regular. W. Slawson, CMA

Procedure 15-6 Obtaining a Urine Specimen from an Infant or Young Child

STANDARD PRECAUTIONS:

PURPOSE:

To obtain a specimen of urine from an infant or young child.

EQUIPMENT/SUPPLIES:

Urine collection bag
Laboratory request form
Gloves
Washcloth
Soap
Water
Towel
Biohazard waste container

PROCEDURE STEPS:

1. Wash and glove hands following Standard Precautions.
2. Assemble equipment.
3. Identify patient and explain procedure to parent(s).
4. Instruct parent to remove diaper.
5. Wash and dry perineal area. RATIONALE: Cleaning area reduces microorganism level and provides better quality urine specimen.
6. Apply collection bag, secure with adhesive tabs.
   a. Girls: spread perineum, place bag over labia.
   b. Boys: place bag over penis and scrotum.
7. Replace diaper carefully.
8. Frequently check bag for urine.
9. Once specimen has been collected, remove bag carefully.
10. Prepare specimen as required. Send to laboratory in a specimen container with a requisition or process the specimen in the office laboratory.
11. Remove gloves and discard in biohazard waste container.
12. Wash hands.
13. Record collection in patient's chart.

DOCUMENTATION

3/10/20XX 4:00 PM Urine specimen collected via urine collection bag. Specimen sent to Bay Laboratory with requisition for routine urinalysis. J. Guerro, CMA

Case Study 15-1

After examining Joey Little, Dr. King confirms the diagnosis of otitis media.

CASE STUDY REVIEW

1. Explain otitis media, the most common reason for its occurrence, and its treatment.
2. How can parents and caregivers be educated to help prevent otitis media?

SUMMARY

Caring for the health and well-being of infants and children through their various developmental stages and into adolescence is the responsibility of the pediatric practice.

Careful observation of the parent or caregiver and the child is helpful to the treatment and care given to the child. The medical assistant is responsible for reporting to the physician any suspicion of child abuse.

Opportunities abound for educating parents about topics that will keep their children healthy throughout life and include nutrition, sleep, immunization, and exercise. Pamphlets, videos, and demonstrations are available to share with parents and caregivers.

Children need respect and should be treated with empathy, love, and honesty; in doing so, a positive relationship can be developed with the child.

STUDY FOR SUCCESS

To reinforce your knowledge and skills of information presented in this chapter:

- ❑ Review Key Terms
- ❑ Practice the Procedures
- ❑ Consider the Case Study and discuss your conclusions
- ❑ Answer the Review Questions
  - ❑ Multiple Choice
  - ❑ Critical Thinking
- ❑ Navigate the Internet by completing the Web Activities
- ❑ Practice the StudyWARE activities on your student CD
- ❑ Apply your knowledge in the Student Workbook activities
- ❑ Complete the Web Tutor sections
- ❑ View and discuss the DVD situations

REVIEW QUESTIONS

Multiple Choice

1. At what age should the first polio vaccine be given?
   a. birth
   b. one month
   c. two months
   d. three months
   e. six months

2. One procedure done to treat otitis media is:
   a. suppuration
   b. tympanostomy
   c. ear irrigation
   d. otoscopy
   e. myringectomy

3. The pathogen usually responsible for causing tonsillitis is:
   a. staphylococcus aureus
   b. meningococcus
   c. beta-hemolytic streptococcus group A
   d. beta-hemolytic streptococcus group B
4. Head circumference is measured on the child until what age?
   a. 1 year
   b. 2 years
   c. 4 years
   d. 6 years
5. An apical pulse is taken over which of the following sites?
   a. third intercostal space on the left side
   b. fourth intercostal space on the left side
   c. fifth intercostal space on the left side
   d. sixth intercostal space on the left side

Critical Thinking Questions

1. You notice when you undress a 2-year-old child to prepare for a physical examination that there are bruises on the buttocks and what appear to be burns on the feet. What course of action do you take?
2. Explain the importance of head circumference measurement.
3. Explain the importance of growth charts.
4. Describe the appropriate positions in which to place an infant for a rectal temperature.
5. Describe the appearance of the pediatric urine collector bag. What is the best way to make certain it will adhere to the child's body?
6. Explain the type of chart used to test visual acuity in young children.
7. When is it appropriate to use the tympanic thermometer while taking a child's temperature?
8. When taking an infant's rectal temperature, what precautions should be taken?
9. Chest circumference measurements on an infant are performed for what purpose?
10. What do the curved lines printed across growth charts indicate?

WEB ACTIVITIES

Search for the American Pediatric Academy on the World Wide Web (http://www.aap.org) to answer the following:

1. What information is available about immunization for hepatitis A, B, and C?
2. What is the most recent recommendation that the American Academy of Pediatrics has made regarding varicella influenza and pneumonia immunizations?
3. Visit the Zero to Three Web site (http://www.zerotothree.org). Search for "healthy development for 24- to 36-month-old toddlers." Describe four to five ways parents can encourage their 2- to 3-year old children to express themselves.
4. Visit the National Network for Child Care Web site (http://www.nncc.org). Search the site for information about fetal alcohol syndrome and birth defects. What specific problems can a newborn have if his or her mother consumed excessive alcohol during pregnancy?
5. Visit the American Academy of Family Physicians Web site (http://www.aafp.org). What information can you find about croup? List five symptoms that should alert parents to call their provider. What are pinworms? How do children get pinworms? How are pinworms detected? How are pinworms treated?

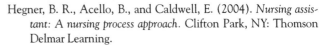

REFERENCES/BIBLIOGRAPHY

Hegner, B. R., Acello, B., and Caldwell, E. (2004). *Nursing assistant: A nursing process approach*. Clifton Park, NY: Thomson Delmar Learning.

Mandleco, B. L. (2004). *Growth and development handbook: Newborn through adolescent*. Clifton Park, NY: Thomson Delmar Learning.

Potts, N. L., Mandleco, B. L. (2002). *Pediatric nursing: Caring for children and their families*. Clifton Park, NY: Thomson Delmar Learning.

Taber's cyclopedic medical dictionary (22nd ed.). (2003). Philadelphia: FA Davis.

Tamparo, C., & Lewis, M. (2000). *Diseases of the human body* (3rd ed.). Philadelphia: FA Davis.

THE DVD HOOK-UP

DVD Series
Skills Based Series

Program Number
6

Chapter/Scene Reference
- *Infant Examination*

In this chapter, you learned about the proper techniques for assisting with pediatric examinations.

The designated scene from today's program illustrates the medical assistant assisting with an infant examination. In the first scene, the medical assistant asks the patient's mother to remove everything but the diaper. The mother tells the medical assistant that the diaper is pretty wet; therefore, the medical assistant instructs the mother to change the diaper before she weighs the infant.

1. Why would removing the diaper altogether as suggested in this chapter be a better method for weighing the infant?

The medical assistant measures the infant by placing a mark above the head and below the foot after straightening out the foot and leg. Spencer is quite playful, making it difficult for the medical assistant to get an accurate reading. The marking for the foot actually had two lines.

1. How does the medical assistant know which mark to use?
2. Is this an accurate reading?

DVD Journal Summary

Write a paragraph that summarizes what you learned from watching today's DVD selected scene. How do you feel about working in pediatrics? Do you have children of your own? How does having children affect your ability to work in pediatrics?

CHAPTER 16

Male Reproductive System

OUTLINE

Testicular Self-Examination
Disorders of the Male Reproductive System
- Testicular Cancer
- Epididymitis
- Prostatitis
- Prostate Cancer
- Benign Prostatic Hypertrophy
- Sexually Transmitted Diseases
- Balanitis
- Infertility
- Erectile Dysfunction

Assisting with the Male Reproductive Examination
Diagnostic Tests and Procedures
- Vasectomy
- Semen Analysis
- Urodynamic Studies

OBJECTIVES

The student should strive to meet the following performance objectives and demonstrate an understanding of the facts and principles presented in this chapter through written and oral communication.

1. Define key terms.
2. Describe common disorders and diseases of the male reproductive system.
3. Explain benign hyperplasia of the prostate.
4. Identify signs and symptoms of the various disorders and diseases of the male reproductive system.
5. Explain erectile dysfunction, its causes, and its treatments.
6. Describe the common diagnostic tests and procedures used in the male reproductive system.
7. Explain testicular self-examination to a male patient.
8. Show compassion and empathy.

KEY TERMS

Cryptorchidism
Intravenous Pyelogram
Libido
Metastasis
Nocturia
Orchidectomy
Residual Urine
Retention
Spermatogenesis
Transilluminator
Transurethral Resection

FEATURED COMPETENCIES

CAAHEP—ENTRY-LEVEL COMPETENCIES

Clinical

Patient Care

- Prepare patient for examinations, procedures, and treatments
- Assist with examinations, procedures and treatments

General

Professionalism

- Project a professional manner and image
- Adhere to ethical principles

Instruction

- Teach methods of health promotion and disease prevention

ABHES—ENTRY-LEVEL COMPETENCIES

Professionalism

- Be courteous and diplomatic

Clinical Duties

- Prepare patients for procedures

SCENARIO

Joe Guerro, CMA, finds many situations daily to educate patients because he knows how important it is. He keeps abreast of the latest techniques and procedures about diseases and problems of the male reproductive system. He attends lectures, workshops, and seminars when possible, and uses the World Wide Web to obtain the latest information from the American Cancer Society about prostate cancer and as a resource for people with prostate cancer. With Dr. Woo's permission, Joe shares that information with patients.

INTRODUCTION

The male reproductive system consists of a pair of testes suspended in the scrotum, in which sperm and hormones are produced. The scrotum can contract and relax to help regulate temperature of the testes for optimum ***spermatogenesis****.*

A system of tubes (the epididymis) transports the sperm to the outside of the body, and a penis transports the sperm into the female reproductive tract through the urethral opening. There are glands such as the prostate that secrete fluid that becomes part of the semen.

The male reproductive system is closely related to the male urinary system; thus, diseases and disorders of one system will naturally affect the other. Because the prostate gland encircles the male urinary urethra, any enlargement can cause urinary problems. The prostate gland is located directly next to the rectal wall. This location enables the physician to palpate the posterior of the prostate gland through the anterior rectal wall and, if need be, perform an ultrasound and biopsy of the prostate using the rectal route. It is recommended that men have their prostate gland routinely evaluated at 40 years old, and then annually after 50 years old. During the annual examination of the prostate gland, the physician can assess the gland for enlargement, nodules, and other abnormalities. When the prostate becomes inflamed or irritated in any way, it can release a protein into the bloodstream. This protein is an antigen called prostate-specific antigen, or PSA. Checking the PSA level can help the doctor determine if there is some pathology of the prostate gland. It is important that blood be drawn for the PSA test before the digital rectal examination of

Patient Education

1. Testicular cancer is one of the leading causes of death in men younger than 40 years.
2. Risk factors include an undescended testicle, cryptorchidism, childhood mumps, and history of chemotherapy.
3. Prognosis is good when found in the early stages.

the prostate, which can irritate the prostate gland, thus causing a slight increase of the PSA level.

Diseases, disorders, conditions, diagnostic tests, procedures, and treatments common to the male reproductive system are shown in Table 16-1.

Spotlight on Certification

RMA Content Outline
- Anatomy and physiology
- Medical terminology
- Patient education
- Physical examinations
- Laboratory procedures

CMA Content Outline
- Medical terminology
- Anatomy and physiology
- Patient instruction
- Patient education
- Examinations
- Procedures
- Collecting and processing specimens; diagnostic testing

CMAS Content Outline
- Medical terminology
- Anatomy and Physiology
- Examination preparation

TESTICULAR SELF-EXAMINATION

Early detection of testicular cancer relies heavily on the patient's willingness to perform self-examination of these body parts on a regular basis. Patient teaching is valuable when used to educate the patient about self-examination for detection of abnormalities such as lumps or thickenings. Figure 16-1 illustrates a testicular self-examination, and Procedure 16-1 outlines steps for instructions usually given to the patient by the medical assistant. The testicular self-examination is best performed in the shower because the warmth will cause the scrotum to relax, making the examination easier and more effective.

DISORDERS OF THE MALE REPRODUCTIVE SYSTEM

See Table 16-1 for a summary of male reproductive disorders.

Testicular Cancer

Testicular cancer is the most common kind of cancer in men between 20 and 35 years old; otherwise, it is rarely seen. Usually a painless lump is found in a testicle. An undescended testicle, cryptorchidism, and a history of mumps are predisposing factors. Diagnosis can be made by performing a biopsy after palpation of the testicle finds a mass. Surgery to excise the testicle, **orchidectomy,** followed by radiation and chemotherapy is the usual course of action. If caught early, there is a high cure rate. Monthly testicular examinations are recommended by the American Cancer Society for all men and are considered the best preventive measure for testicular cancer. See Figure 16-1 and Procedure 16-1.

Epididymitis

Epididymitis is an inflammation of the epididymis, which is a small oblong body resting on and beside the posterior surfaces of the testes. It consists of a convoluted tube 13 to 20 feet in length. It constitutes the first part of the secretory duct of each testis. The patient's symptoms are chills, fever, pain in the inguinal region, and a swollen epididymis that can be seen on an ultrasonogram. It is primarily caused by a sexually transmitted disease (STD) such as chlamydia, gonorrhea, or syphillis. Other causes are urinary tract infections, trauma, prostatectomy, and prolonged indwelling catheter. Treatment consists of antibiotics, scrotal support, and bed rest.

Prostatitis

Prostatitis, or inflammation of the prostate, occurs primarily in men older than 50 years. The prostate may enlarge and cause pain and discomfort, such as burning while urinating.

TABLE 16-1 MALE REPRODUCTIVE SYSTEM DISEASES AND DISORDERS

Disease/Disorder	Laboratory Diagnostics	Radiography and Technical Diagnostics	Medical/Surgical Diagnostics	Treatments
Prostatitis (inflammation of the prostate gland)	Complete blood count Urinalysis and culture Analysis of prostate secretion	Urodynamics (if not caused by a bacterium)	Digital rectal examination	Long-term treatment with antibiotics Increase fluid intake
Benign hyperplasia (hypertrophy/enlargement) of the prostate (BPH)	Prostatic-specific antigen (PSA) Urinalysis	Intravenous pyelogram (IVP) Pelvic ultrasound	Digital rectal examination Cystoscopy Ultrasound and biopsy	Medications Transurethral resection prostatectomy (TURP) is rare
Prostate cancer	PSA Urinalysis Acid phosphatase (blood)	IVP Pelvic ultrasound	Digital rectal examination Cystoscopy Ultrasound and biopsy	Prostatectomy Hormone manipulation Chemotherapy, radiation, or both
Epididymitis (inflammation of the tubes on the testis)	Complete blood count Urinalysis and culture and sensitivity Culture and sensitivity of urethra	IVP Pelvic ultrasound	Physical examination	Antibiotics, scrotal support
Testicular cancer		Testicular ultrasound	Physical examination (Palpation of testis) Biopsy	Excision of the testis Radiation therapy Chemotherapy
Erectile dysfunction (ED) (inability of male to achieve erection)	Complete blood count Fasting blood sugar Lipid profile Testosterone level Urinalysis	Angiogram, rarely Magnetic resonance imaging of the brain, rarely	Physical examination Neurological examination Psychological evaluation	Oral medications Localized injected medication Penile implant Penile pump
Balanitis (inflammation of the glans of the penis)	Culture, rarely		Physical examination Skin culture	Localized soaks and frequent cleansing Antibiotics
Sexually transmitted diseases (STDs):				
Nonspecific urethritis (NSU)	Rule out other STDs Culture and sensitivity of urethral discharge			Increase fluid intake Antibiotics Possibly test/treat partner
Chlamydia	Urinalysis Urethral smear			Patient education Antibiotics Test/treat partner
Genital herpes (type II herpes simplex)	Culture of lesion			Patient education Antiviral medications Test/treat partner
Gonorrhea	Urethral smear			Patient education Antibiotics Test/treat partner
Syphilis	Urinalysis with culture Venereal Disease Research Laboratory (VDRL) studies Culture of the lesion			Patient education Antibiotics Test/treat partner

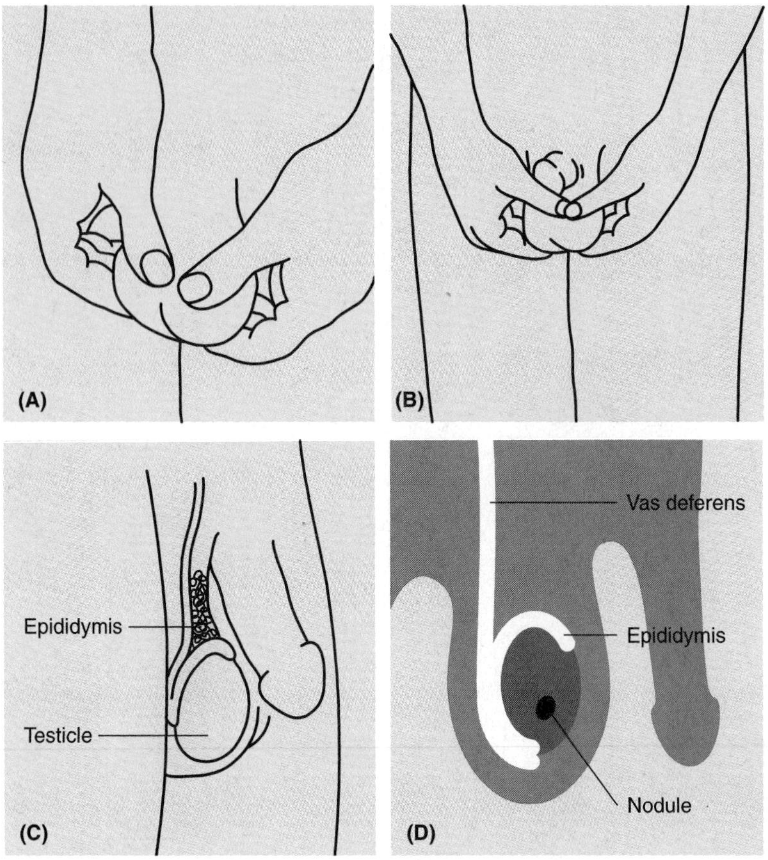

Figure 16-1 Testicular self-examination should be performed once a month after a warm bath or shower. The heat will relax the scrotum, making it easier to find abnormalities. (A) Stand in front of the mirror. Look for swelling on the skin of the scrotum. (B) Examine each testicle with both hands. Position your index and middle fingers under the testicle with the thumbs on top. Gently roll the testicle between your thumbs and fingers. (Having one testicle larger than the other is normal.) (C) Find the epididymis (the soft, tubelike structure and the back of the testicle). Do not mistake the epididymis for an abnormal lump. (D) If you find a lump, notify your doctor right away. Most lumps are found on the sides of the testicle, but some are located on the front. Testicular cancer is highly curable when detected early and treated promptly.

There can be pain in the back, muscle aches, and urinary frequency. The cause may be bacterial, such as from gonorrhea, or may be caused by another pathogen that produced a urinary tract infection. Urinalysis, urine culture, and digital rectal examination (to palpate the prostate) help in making a diagnosis. Treatment is usually medication, such as penicillin and pain medication, and the patient will be told to force fluids by increasing fluid intake significantly.

Prostate Cancer

Prostate cancer is the third leading cause of cancer death in men, after lung and colon cancer. **Metastasis** to the spine or pelvis is not unusual. The symptoms, if present, are similar to urinary obstruction, difficulty urinating, frequency of urination, and inability to urinate. It is of value to check the blood level of PSA, but a biopsy is necessary to be certain. An ultrasonogram and computed axial tomography (CAT) scan can help to determine if there has been any metastasis. Treatment may consist of prostatectomy, hormonal therapy, radiation, chemotherapy, and brachytherapy (internal radiation "seeds").

A prostatic ultrasound consists of a short probe inserted into the rectum. High-frequency sound waves are produced by the probe, and an image (either a photo or a video) of the prostate is recorded. A biopsy of the prostate can be done in conjunction with the ultrasound. The physician uses the ultrasound to guide a needle through the rectum into areas of the prostate that showed abnormalities on the ultrasound. The needle collects cells from the prostate through the rectum wall. The specimen is sent to the laboratory for analysis. Medical assistants are responsible for patient instruction and preparation and assisting with an ultrasound and biopsy of the patient.

A prostatectomy is major surgery done for prostate cancer and is performed through the abdomen or the perineum (the external region between the scrotum and the anus). Urinary incontinence, impotence, or both are possible complications.

If the cancer has metastasized, orchidectomy may be recommended because the surgery alters hormone production (loss of testosterone). Less testosterone can slow the metastasis but can lead to loss of muscle mass, osteoporosis, and sexual dysfunction.

An additional treatment consists of small pellets ("seeds") of a radioactive substance that are implanted in the prostate tissue through a small incision (brachytherapy). The seeds of radiation are concentrated in the prostate and will destroy the prostate without harming surrounding tissue as external beam radiation does. Various medications such as those that reduce or suppress the production of testosterone may be helpful when combined with radiation or surgery, but they have the same possible side effects as orchidectomy.

Patients who have been tested for prostate cancer are monitored for progression of the cancer, which includes PSA every 3 months to 1 year, CAT and bone scans, central venous catheter, and monitoring of the signs and symptoms that indicate cancer progression such as bowel and bladder function impairment, weight loss, pain, and fatigue.

Benign Prostatic Hypertrophy

Benign hypertrophy of the prostate gland or benign hypertrophic prostate gland, also known as benign prostatic hyperplasia (BPH), is common in men 50 years or older. Symptoms include **retention** (the inability to completely empty the bladder), a diminished flow of urine, and difficulty starting to urinate. Hesitancy and **nocturia** can occur. It is thought that the cause is aging and may be related to hormonal changes. The prostate enlarges and, because it surrounds the urethra, it causes constriction of the urethra and the associated symptoms. The physician can palpate the enlarged prostate gland when performing a rectal examination. This helps in making a diagnosis. Other tests may include a blood test known as PSA, a urinalysis, and an **intravenous pyelogram** (excretory urograph) (a radiograph of the kidneys, ureters, and bladder using a contrast medium). The enlarged prostate blocks urine flow and if **residual urine** stays in the bladder, infections can develop, and kidneys may cease functioning because they can't drain urine properly into the bladder when it is full (Figure 16-2). Catheterization may be necessary (see Procedure 18-3).

The PSA blood test is used to detect abnormally high levels of a protein substance that may indicate prostate cancer. The American Cancer Society recommends that men aged 50 years and older have an annual PSA blood test.

Ultrasound can be used to view the prostate, bladder, or kidneys. A biopsy of the prostate, done in conjunction with an ultrasound, can help diagnose either BPH or cancer.

Treatment of BPH, in some cases, consists of medication that can relax prostate muscles, hormones that block prostate growth, or bladder relaxants. **Transurethral resection** (TURP) of the prostate (removal of prostate tissue using a device inserted through the urethra) is the most common surgical treatment. Instruments are inserted through the penis and a laser or radio waves can be used to remove the excess tissue (Figure 16-3). Possible risks to the TURP procedure include impotence and urinary incontinence. BPH does not cause or lead to cancer.

Critical Thinking

How is benign prostatic hypertrophy treated?

Critical Thinking

List several sexually transmitted diseases that a male individual can contract.

Sexually Transmitted Diseases

STDs affect men and women; they can damage health and become life-threatening. Refer to Table 16-2. Also see information in Chapter 14 regarding STDs.

Balanitis

Balanitis is usually caused by poor hygiene in uncircumcised men. Bacteria, fungi, viruses, caustic soaps, and improper rinsing of soap while bathing also are causes. Some of the symptoms and signs that occur include redness of the foreskin or of the penis, rashes on the head of the penis, malodorous discharge, and pain in the penis and foreskin. Diagnosis of balanitis may be made by the physician through examination of the penis and foreskin, by a skin culture for microorganisms, or by both. If the cause is bacterial, then antibiotics can be used to treat balanitis. In severe cases, circumcision (surgical removal of prepuce of penis) may be necessary.

Infertility

When couples regularly have unprotected sexual intercourse, the majority of these couples usually conceive within one year. The inability or diminished ability to conceive is known as infertility.

An insufficient number or diminished motility of sperm can cause infertility. Other causes include an infection in the genitourinary tract or the presence of an STD, either of which can block the tract and prohibit sperm from being fully ejaculated. An injury to the blood or nerve supply in the area, radiation exposure, stress, and hormonal imbalances are other factors that can promote infertility.

A complete physical examination and medical history (including childhood illnesses such as parotitis [mumps]), semen analysis for count and motility, and tests for endocrine disorders can help determine the cause of infertility.

Treatment of a male patient with infertility depends on the cause; treatments include surgery to remove a blockage, antibiotics to treat an infection, use of artificial

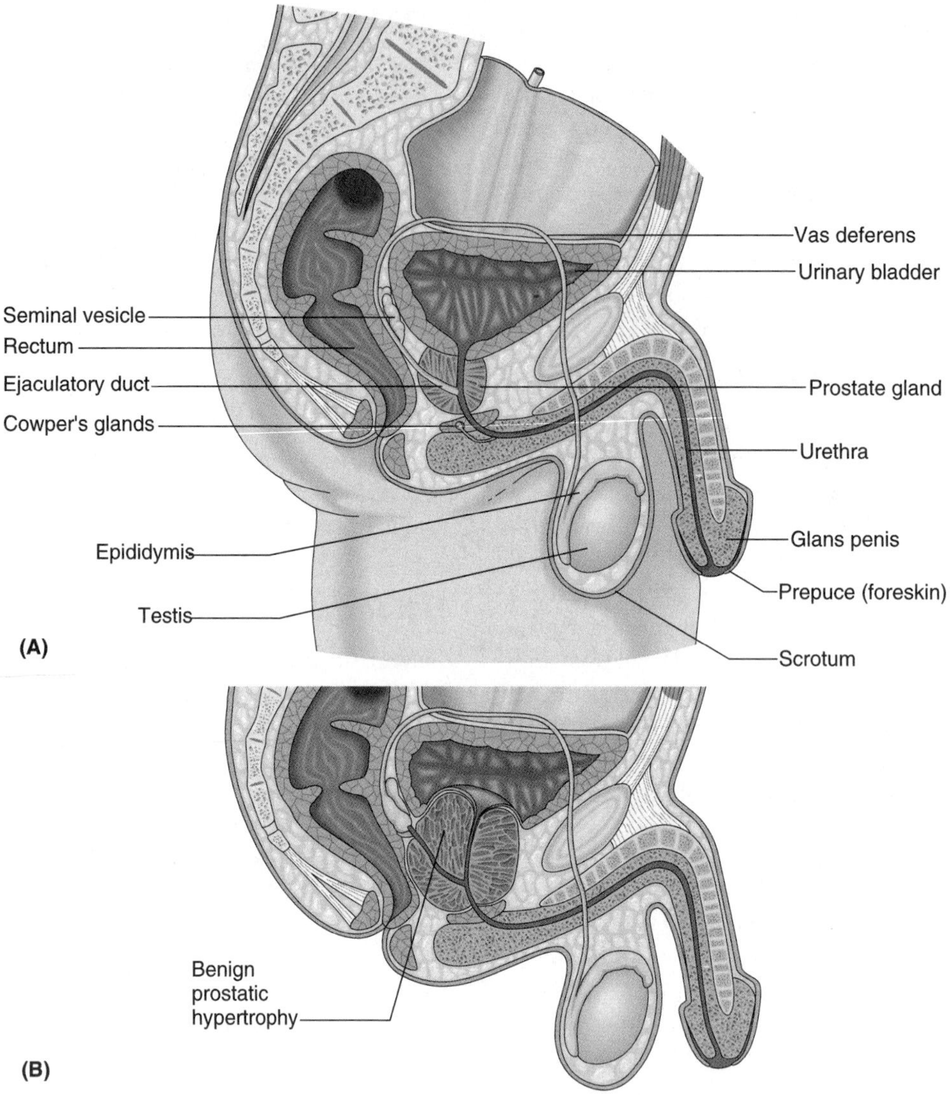

Figure 16-2 Normal and enlarged prostate: (A) normal; (B) enlarged.

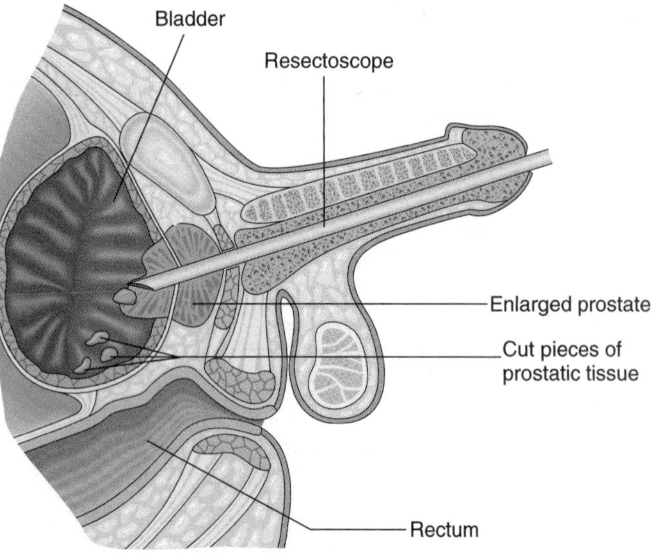

Figure 16-3 Transurethral resection of prostate.

TABLE 16-2 SEXUALLY TRANSMITTED DISEASES

- Chlamydial infection. Common in male and female individuals. A prevalent sexually transmitted disease that often coexists with gonorrhea.
- Genital herpes. Painful, viral disease that is dormant and recurs periodically. There is no cure. Characterized by blisters similar to chicken pox. Common in male and female individuals.
- Gonorrhea. Caused by a bacterium and the infection can spread producing a stricture of the urethra or the vas deferens. Sterility can result if both vas deferens become involved.
- Syphilis. Caused by a spirochete. Chancres develop. Can heal. If untreated, the disease progresses to stages two and three. Severe damage to the cardiovascular system and brain and vision and hearing loss occur. General paralysis and death can result. Highly contagious.
- Hepatitis B and C virus and HIV.

insemination, or the use of pharmaceuticals to treat the infertility.

Prevention of the factors that may cause infertility is preferable, because the percentage of couples treated for infertility who successfully become pregnant is relatively low.

Erectile Dysfunction

Also called impotence, erectile dysfunction (ED) occurs when a man is unable to achieve or to sustain an erection of the penis during sexual intercourse. This condition or dysfunction is not normal at any age and is different from other issues that impede sexual intercourse such as lack of **libido.**

Many men, at some point in their lives, can experience the inability to achieve an erection. This can happen on occasion from consuming too much alcohol or from extreme fatigue. This is not ED. The inability to achieve an erection more than 50% of the time is generally a reason for seeking treatment and is usually an indication of ED.

For an erection to occur, there must be certain physiologic conditions present. There must be a stimulus from the brain and adequate circulation and nerve supply to the penis. If any of these conditions is impeded, an erection cannot be achieved. Some reasons why ED occurs include conditions or diseases that impair circulation (artherosclerosis) and nerve stimulation (nerve diseases) and psychological factors such as stress and depression. Medications such as those used to treat certain conditions such as hypertension can cause ED. Diabetes, multiple sclerosis, cerebral vascular accident (stroke), surgery on the prostate or bladder, and brain and spinal cord injuries are some other causes of ED.

Treatment of the dysfunction is based on the cause. Referral to a urologist or psychologist, or both, is made if appropriate. Blood and urine tests will be done after the physician examines the individual for medical problems. Medications the patient may be taking will be addressed.

> Because of the very nature of erectile dysfunction, many men are embarrassed if they have the disorder, feeling that they are somehow less "manly" than other men. It is of extreme importance to be cautious and sensitive when caring for these patients. Confidentiality on the telephone and during conversations must be maintained. Protect your patient's privacy at all times. This is not only the law, but it is also an attribute of a professional medical assistant.

Some of the ways ED can be treated include oral medications (Viagra, Levitra, Cialis), penile injections (medication is injected into the penis), sex therapy, and surgery such as penile implants (a device surgically implanted to overcome impotence) and vacuum pumps. A vacuum pump device is a pump put over the penis and air is pumped out of the cylinder, creating a vacuum. This vacuum causes blood to fill the penis, making it erect. Once the penis is erect, the pump can be removed.

ASSISTING WITH THE MALE REPRODUCTIVE EXAMINATION

A female medical assistant may or may not be requested to assist the physician with the examination of the male reproductive system. The physician will examine the penis and the foreskin of the penis in an uncircumcised patient. The penis and testes are examined for swelling, masses, or discomfort. A **transilluminator** may be used by the physician to check the prostate gland. A lighted instrument used to inspect a cavity or organ, the transilluminator would be passed through the rectum to illuminate the prostate gland through the walls of the rectum. The physician will do a digital rectal examination to check the size of the prostate and will also check for an inguinal hernia.

DIAGNOSTIC TESTS AND PROCEDURES

Tests and procedures, in addition to those previously addressed, include vasectomy and a semen analysis.

Vasectomy

A vasectomy is performed to surgically sterilize the male individual. The vas deferens extends up into the abdomen where it connects to create the ejaculatory duct that opens into the urethra. By removing a portion of each vas deferens, sperm cannot travel to mix with semen, thereby causing the male to be sterile (Figure 16-4). See Chapter 19 for the vasectomy surgical procedure.

Semen Analysis

Semen testing is frequently performed in the physician's office or clinic to determine sperm cell counts before

> **Critical Thinking**
>
> Describe two reasons why the physician orders a semen analysis.

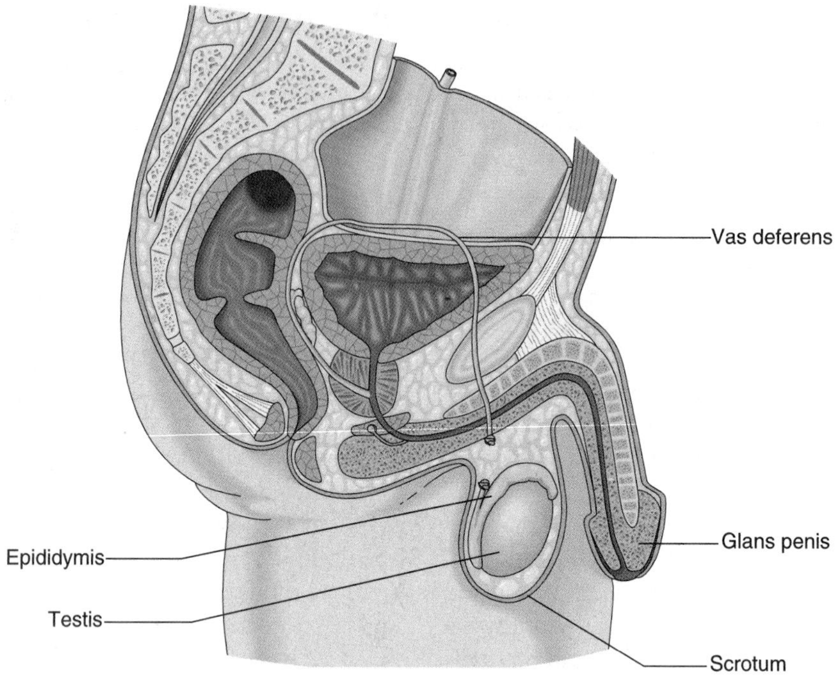

Figure 16-4 Vasectomy (one side).

referring patients to a specialist, such as a physician who treats infertility. It is also done as part of a complete fertility workup and to evaluate the effectiveness of a vasectomy. See Chapter 32 for extensive information about semen analysis.

Urodynamic Studies

Urodynamic studies are a way of testing the lower urinary tract. A catheter is used to instill water into the bladder and the information is fed into a computer via electrodes. Bladder capacity, strength of contraction, and the ability to retain urine in the bladder can be measured.

Procedure 16-1 Instructing Patient in Testicular Self-Examination

PURPOSE:
To provide a patient with information concerning testicular screening for the presence of a painless mass in the scrotum.

EQUIPMENT/SUPPLIES:
Testicular self-examination card
Anatomy illustration

PROCEDURE STEPS:

1. Identify yourself and explain the procedure.
2. Instruct patient to examine his testicles in a warm shower. RATIONALE: The warmth causes the scrotal skin to relax.
3. Examine each testicle separately with both hands.
4. Place the index and middle fingers underneath the testicle and the thumbs on top. Roll the testicle gently between the fingers.
5. Locate the epididymis. Provide a chart to the patient that illustrates the testes and epididymis. RATIONALE: A lump can be similar in size to the epididymis and needs to be distinguished from the epididymis.
6. Look for swelling or changes in the scrotal area.
7. Encourage the patient to report anything unusual to the physician.
8. Document the education provided.

DOCUMENTATION

11/4/20XX Patient instructed on how to perform testicular self-exam. Patient returned the demonstration and had no questions. Joe Guerro, CMA

Case Study 16-1

Adam Desmond has an appointment today in the clinic for a physical examination. His chief complaint is that he has been having trouble sitting through ball games or movies without having to go to the bathroom to urinate several times.

CASE STUDY REVIEW

1. How can Dr. Woo make a diagnosis of BPH?
2. What preliminary tests might Dr. Woo order for Mr. Desmond today?

Case Study 16-2

John Toomey called to say that he discovered "something hard in his right testicle, like a marble."

CASE STUDY REVIEW

1. What will Dr. King's examination consist of?

SUMMARY

A thorough knowledge of the diseases and disorders of the male reproductive system and the diagnostic tests and procedures that are performed for this specialty will enhance the quality of care given by the medical assistant.

STUDY FOR SUCCESS

To reinforce your knowledge and skills of information presented in this chapter:

- ❑ Review the Key Terms
- ❑ Practice the Procedures
- ❑ Consider the Case Studies and discuss your conclusions
- ❑ Answer the Review Questions
  - ❑ Multiple Choice
  - ❑ Critical Thinking
- ❑ Navigate the Internet by completing the Web Activities
- ❑ Practice the StudyWARE activities on your student CD
- ❑ Apply your knowledge in the Student Workbook activities
- ❑ Complete the Web Tutor sections

REVIEW QUESTIONS

Multiple Choice

1. Cancer of the prostate may be detected early by which of the following?
   a. prostate-specific antigen
   b. transurethral resection
   c. semen analysis
   d. urine culture
2. The best preventive measure for testicular cancer is which of the following?
   a. yearly physical examination
   b. yearly intravenous pyelogram
   c. monthly self-examination
   d. monthly urinalysis with cultures
3. Benign prostate hypertrophy (BPH) is thought to be caused by:
   a. excessive consumption of alcohol
   b. aging and hormonal changes
   c. recurrent epididymitis
   d. chronic chlamydia infections
4. Which of the following is a symptom of prostatitis?
   a. painful urination
   b. low sperm count
   c. eruptions on the scrotum
   d. high testosterone level
5. The most definitive way to diagnose cancer of the prostate is by which of the following?
   a. ultrasonography
   b. intravenous pyelogram
   c. biopsy of the prostate
   d. semen analysis

Critical Thinking

1. Describe how a self-testicular examination should be performed.
2. What is the purpose of severing the vas deferens?
3. List several symptoms of BPH and explain why the symptoms occur.
4. Describe the blood test that is helpful to diagnose prostate cancer.
5. Explain why BPH is more common in men aged 50 years and older.
6. What age group is afflicted by testicular cancer, and how can the patient take action to detect it?
7. How is a rectal examination on a patient useful to the physician in determining a diagnosis for a patient who has nocturia?

WEB ACTIVITIES

Navigate the Internet to find a medical Web site, then answer the following questions:

1. Describe two treatment choices for BPH.
2. Search for information about internal radiation or "seeds" as a treatment choice for cancer of the prostate. What did you find?
3. Find two other disorders or diseases of the male reproductive tract (other than those in the text) and (a) describe what they are, (b) how they are diagnosed, and (c) how they are treated.
4. Discover what contraindications exist for some men whose physician is considering prescribing Viagra or one of the other medications for ED treatment.

REFERENCES/BIBLIOGRAPHY

DeNoon, D. (2003). *Erectile dysfunction 2003: More choices*. Nazario, B., reviewer. (2003, December 17). Retrieved from WebMD Web Site: http://aolsvc.health.webmd.aol.com/content/article/78/95852.htm. Accessed November 17, 2004.

Gilbert, S. (2003). *Health, balanitis, prostate gland cancer*. Retrieved from http://www.allrefer.com. Accessed November 17, 2004.

Grayson, C. E., editor. (2003). *Ultrasound and prostate biopsy*. (2003, November). Retrieved from WebMD Web site: http://aolsvc.health.webmd.aol.com/content/article/45/1688_50829.htm. Accessed November 17, 2004.

Neighbors, M., & Tannehill-Jones, R. (2000). *Human diseases*. Clifton Park, NY: Thomson Delmar Learning.

Taber's cyclopedic medical dictionary (23rd ed.). (2003). Philadelphia: FA Davis.

Tamparo, C., & Lewis, M. (2000). *Diseases of the human body* (3rd ed.). Philadelphia: FA Davis.

CHAPTER 17

Gerontology

OUTLINE

Societal Bias
Facts about Aging
Physiologic Changes
- Senses
- Integumentary System
- Nervous System
- Musculoskeletal System
- Respiratory System
- Cardiovascular System
- Gastrointestinal System
- Urinary System
- Reproductive System

Prevention of Complications
Psychological Changes
The Medical Assistant and the Geriatric Patient
- Memory-Impaired Older Adults
- Visually-Impaired Older Adults
- Hearing-Impaired Older Adults
- Elder Abuse

Healthy and Successful Aging

OBJECTIVES

The student should strive to meet the following performance objectives and demonstrate an understanding of the facts and principles presented in this chapter through written and oral communication.

1. Define the key terms.
2. Identify expected physiologic changes that occur as part of the aging process.
3. List five common functional changes that can occur.
4. Describe prevention techniques for complications arising from age-related disorders.
5. Explain two myths about aging.
6. Explain the importance of communication with the older adults.
7. Identify several techniques or strategies to communicate with the visually and hearing impaired.
8. Describe aspects of healthy and successful aging.

KEY TERMS

Andropause
Arteriosclerosis
Cognitive Functioning
Cystitis
Dementia
Empathy
Geriatrics
Gerontology
Hyperthermia
Hypothermia
Incontinence
Macular Degeneration
Nevus
Pernicious Anemia
Presbycusis
Residual Urine
Senile
Transient Ischemic Attack

FEATURED COMPETENCIES

CAAHEP—ENTRY-LEVEL COMPETENCIES

Patient Instruction

- Instruct individuals according to their needs
- Provide instruction for health maintenance and disease prevention
- Identify community resources

ABHES—ENTRY-LEVEL COMPETENCIES

Professionalism

- Project a positive attitude
- Be courteous and diplomatic

Communication

- Be impartial and show empathy when dealing with patients
- Adapt what is said to recipient's level of comprehension
- Adaptation for individualized needs

Instruction

- Instruct patients with special needs
- Teach patients methods of health promotion and disease prevention

SCENARIO

Mrs. Johnson is an 82-year-old patient of Dr. King, and she is scheduled for an appointment in the cardiac clinic. She is being evaluated for congestive heart disease and has had hypertension for many years. Her condition was difficult to control, but now responds to medication. She has become a volunteer at the gift shop at St. Louis Hospital. She is an example of an older adult with chronic illnesses who has changed some long-time behaviors that were harmful to her health.

INTRODUCTION

Gerontology *is the scientific study of the problems associated with aging.* ***Geriatrics*** *is the branch of medicine that specializes in all aspects of aging: physiologic, pathologic, psychological, economic, and sociologic. The importance of studying gerontology is becoming more recognized because the expected life span is increasing. Thousands of people are living to be 100 years old or older. The aging population is growing rapidly, and according to the U.S. Census Bureau, by 2030, there will be 60 million people in the United States older than 65 years. The 80 and above age group is currently the fastest growing group. As a medical assistant, you will be experiencing the impact on the health care system of this growing population of people.*

Through knowledge of the physical and psychological changes that occur as an individual ages, as a medical assistant you will be better able to recognize the special needs of this group of people. You will draw on and use effective communication skills and provide quality health care to the geriatric patients.

Spotlight on Certification

RMA Content Outline

- Human relations
- Patient education

CMA Content Outline

- Developmental stages of the life cycle
- Hereditary, cultural and environmental influences on behavior
- Adapting communication to an individual's ability to understand
- Patient instruction
- Professional communication and behavior
- Evaluating and understanding communication

CMAS Content Outline

- Professionalism
- Basic health history interview

SOCIETAL BIAS

In our culture, there is a deeply ingrained bias about aging. Older adults are systematically stereotyped, and there is much discrimination because of age. Myths and stereotypes are common, and the medical assistant can be an advocate for older adults and can be sensitive to these myths and stereotypes. Accurate information and useful concepts about aging must be communicated to the general public. Older adults oftentimes are viewed as sick, frail, powerless, sexless, and burdensome. As a society, we are obsessed with the negative, rather than the positive, aspects of aging. The most popular myth is, "To be old is to be sick." Recent studies indicate that older adults in the United States are generally healthier than their counterparts of nearly a decade ago. Even in advanced old age, a majority of the older population has little functional disability. Years of research have debunked this myth. Because of better education about the practice of healthier lifestyles, to be old in the United States does not mean to be sick and frail. Thousands of people are living to be older than 100 years because of the recognition that healthy lifestyles are the most important factor in helping people to live long, healthy, productive lives. Such factors as good nutrition, regular exercise, stress reduction, yearly physical examinations, not smoking, and today's technology help forestall the aging process.

Critical Thinking

What is the most common myth about older adults? What are your thoughts about this myth?

FACTS ABOUT AGING

Following are general facts about aging:

- Aging is progressive and universal.
- There are no diseases specific to aging.
- As people age, not all functional changes are related to disease. Interest, personal, and financial resources, family structure, genetics, and attitude all play a part. The individual's lifestyle is also a factor. For example, smoking, misuse of chemicals such as alcohol or drugs, type of diet, and exercise all play a part in how people age.
- There is a wider range of what is considered "normal" function among older adults than among younger people. There is a greater variability among older people in their physical abilities, sizes, and characteristics than among younger groups (Figure 17-1).
- All old age is not alike. People in their 60s, 70s, 80s, and 90s are all different.

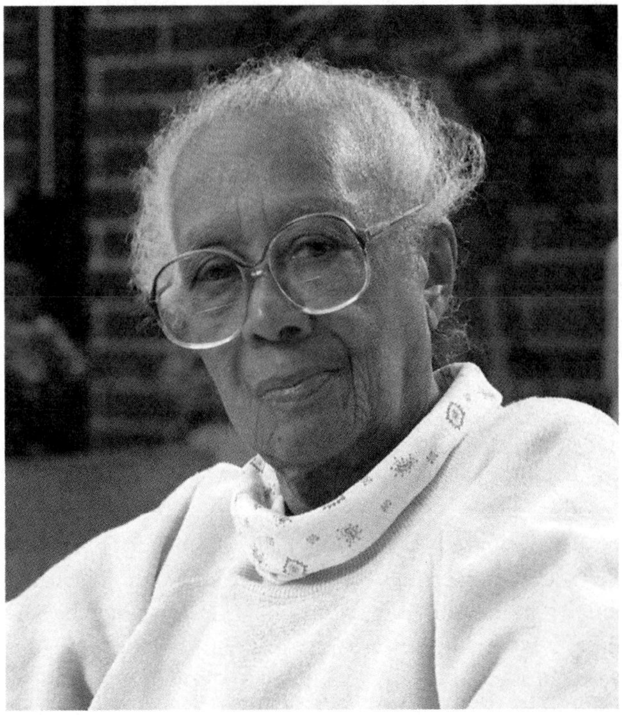

Figure 17-1 Note the many signs of aging.

PHYSIOLOGIC CHANGES

Although aging is a normal process, not all individuals age in the same way or at the same rate, because no two people have exactly the same genetic inheritance, personal lifestyle, or experiences in life. All of these factors strongly influence the ways in which we grow older. Some believe that the body endures wear and tear and stress during life and that because of this, eventually the body loses its ability to function as well as it had. Others believe that as people grow older, the body produces smaller and smaller amounts of various hormones and other chemicals that keep the body functioning. The fewer of these kinds of substances that are produced, the more susceptible an individual becomes to disease.

Every body system undergoes changes as we age. The changes are physiologic and psychological. As individuals move into their 60s and beyond, they will show physiologic changes that are part of the aging process. As people age, their body systems function less effectively, causing them to have difficulty performing their ordinary, everyday tasks of living. Also, as people grow older, they become more susceptible to disorders and diseases. When taking the medical history of an older patient, it is evident that many have one or several chronic illnesses. Heart disease, diabetes, arthritis, hypertension, and vision and auditory impairments are common.

Although it is important to be knowledgeable about the physiologic changes that occur as part of aging, it is important to realize that the majority of older adults are free of serious, chronic health problems.

Senses

Vision. Many changes occur in the eye's ability to function. Pupil size diminishes, limiting the amount of light that can go through it to reach the retina. There is a diminished production of tears so the eye may be dry, red, and irritated. The lens may become cloudy, and the cornea thickens. There is increased sensitivity to glare. Several problems can occur as a result of these changes. There is less ability to see clearly at any distance and to discern various shades of colors. Older people will need eyeglasses to help correct their vision loss, but reading small print can remain difficult. Glare can be minimized by incorporating a process known as polarization into corrective lenses.

Cataracts, **macular degeneration,** and glaucoma are common findings in older adults. Cataracts can be surgically excised if they are large. Glaucoma can be treated medically or surgically, but if left untreated can lead to blindness. Macular degeneration can lead to vision impairment. The macular of the retina is an important area in the visualization of fine details. Degeneration of it is the leading cause of visual impairment in adults older than 50 years, making it difficult to do fine work or such activities as threading a needle. Laser surgery may halt the progression of the degeneration.

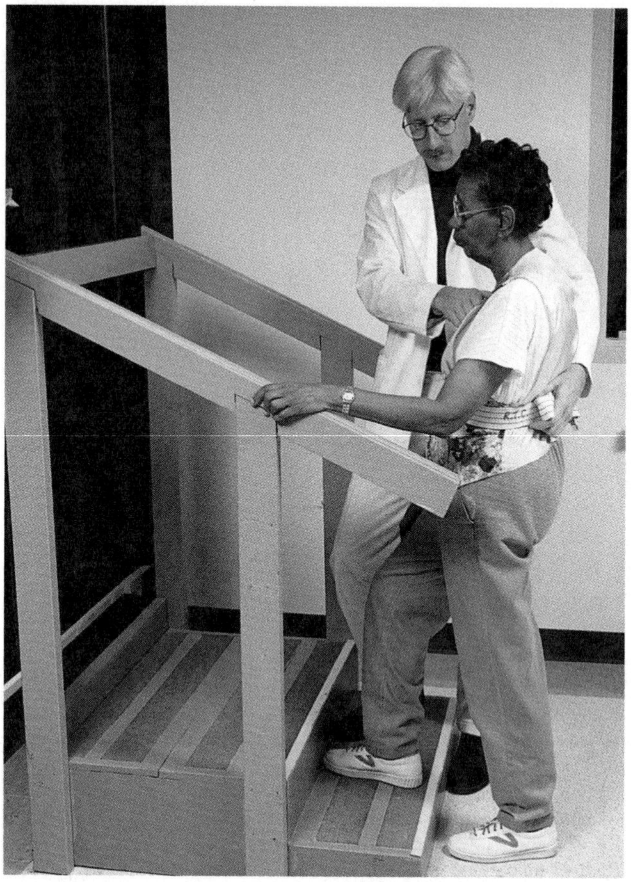

Figure 17-2 Learning to use handrails will help the older adult with poor balance or vision.

Because of failing vision and impaired balance and coordination, older adults should be cautioned to use handrails whenever possible (Figure 17-2).

Hearing. Loss of hearing in the aging process is not uncommon. It usually occurs over a period of years, and the older person may not be aware of the loss. Loss of hearing ability begins at about the third decade of life. Many times, individuals with hearing loss seem inattentive or confused and are thought to be mentally weak or **senile.** Presbyacusia or **presbycusis** is the progressive loss of hearing ability caused by the normal aging process.

Taste and Smell. Taste and smell diminish with age, making food less appealing because it no longer tastes as good as it once did (Figure 17-3). Taste buds decrease in size. Detecting odors becomes difficult and impaired and further lessens the desire for food. It is not unusual for older adults to lose weight and even to become malnour-

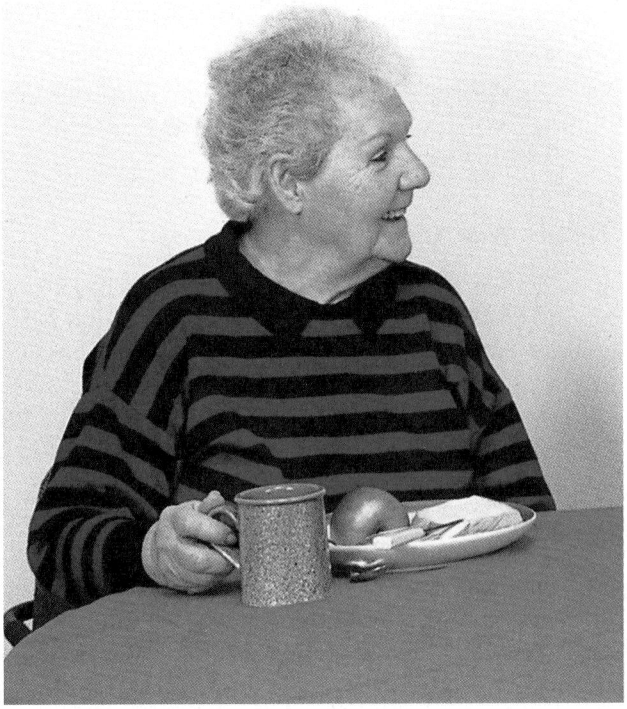

Figure 17-3 Older adults may tend to add more salt and sugar to their food to compensate for their diminished sense of taste.

ished because of the loss of the ability to taste and smell. Lacking the sense of smell can be dangerous because of the inability to smell smoke or gas and other dangerous fumes.

Integumentary System

Aging individuals' skin becomes more fragile with less subcutaneous and connective tissue. Exposure to sunlight is the major cause of wrinkled skin, liver spots, and leathery looking skin.

Sweat glands become smaller and the body becomes nonsensitive to heat and cold. **Hyperthermia,** an unusually high fever, and **hypothermia,** an unusually low body temperature, are serious problems, and exposure to excessive hot or cold temperatures should be avoided. See Chapter 21.

Hair loses color and becomes thinner. The skin dries and is less elastic. Fingernails and toenails thicken.

The development of skin cancer on the exposed skin surfaces is not uncommon in older adults. Basal and squamous cell carcinomas are the most common skin cancer types seen in this population. Both types of cancer can be serious if left untreated, but squamous cell cancer can metastasize. A complete skin assessment should be done on a yearly basis. Melanoma, a malignant tumor developing from a **nevus,** is the least common skin cancer, but it can be extremely serious because it metastasizes readily. It is caused by exposure to the sun. Many older adults live in the Sunbelt areas of the United States and should be cautioned to wear sunscreen of at least SPF 15. People of all ages should protect their skin daily with a sunscreen of at least SPF 15, regardless of where they reside.

Nervous System

The brain shrinks in size as an individual ages because brain cells do not continue to divide throughout life as other cells do. Some loss of memory or delay in memory can be expected in many, but not all, aging people. Mental competence is the rule rather than the exception for older adults. Sudden loss of memory accompanied by confusion and inability to do tasks once able to be performed could be an indication of an organic problem, such as **transient ischemic attack,** a temporary interference of the blood supply to the brain, or a brain lesion.

Problems with balance, temperature regulation, diminished pain sensation, and insomnia can occur as part of the physical changes of aging that affect the nervous system.

Chronic illnesses from which many older people suffer often require several different medications to keep under control. Side effects of medication (over-the-counter, prescription, and herbals) can cause decreased mental capacity, as can malnutrition and substance abuse.

Loss of balance can be a problem for some older adults. Their coordination of muscles for movement may need more time for processing than it does with younger individuals. Older adults need to be reminded to be sure of their balance before starting to walk and to do so slowly. There is a general unsteadiness and lack of coordination not only because of the aging process, but also possibly because of medications the older adult takes. Older adults may need to use a cane to help steady their gait (Figure 17-4).

Musculoskeletal System

The musculoskeletal system changes are evident because older adults have less muscle strength. This results in loss of mobility, and the activities of daily living become more difficult. There is less flexibility and joints can stiffen. Loss of height and a stooped appearance can result. Arthritis and osteoporosis are not unusual, and older adults can suffer fractured bones more easily. Poor nutrition, malnourishment, and lack of exercise all contribute to these conditions and prolong healing time as well. See Chapters 21 and 22.

Osteoporosis—a thinning of the long bones, pelvic bones, and vertebrae—is a fairly common problem in the aging population, with more women than men affected.

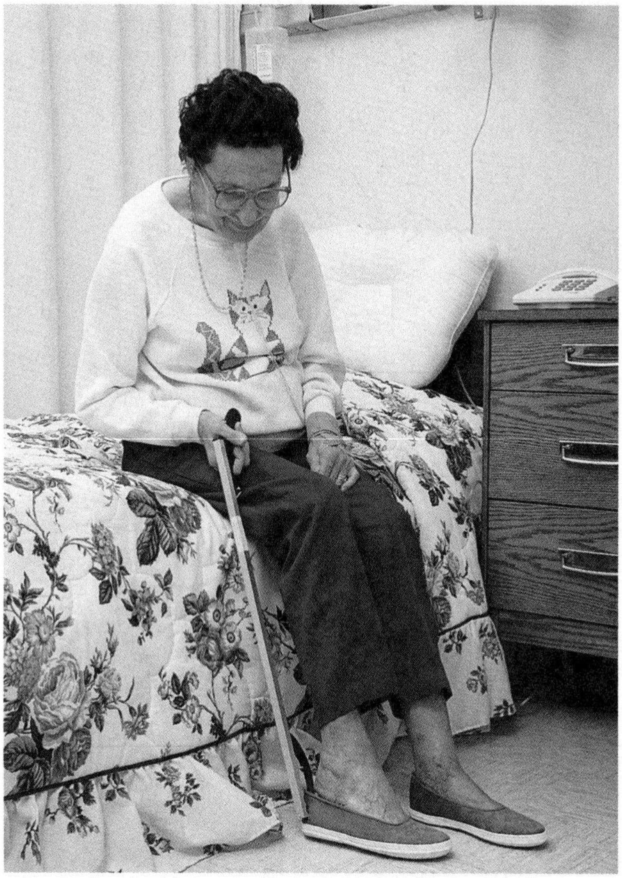

Figure 17-4 Older adults should be instructed to take their time when sitting, standing, and walking.

This thinning of bone makes these individuals more susceptible to pain and fractures in these and other bones. New medications (Fosamax, Evista) plus 1500 mg of calcium daily helps to slow the progress of osteoporosis. Vitamin D is essential for utilization of calcium. A deficiency of vitamin D in older adults occurs either because it is insufficient in their diets or because of insufficient exposure to sunlight. Vitamin D is added to milk.

Physical activity and a nutritional diet, including milk, can stall the development of bone and muscle loss; therefore, older adults should be encouraged to keep active by walking, gardening, swimming, bicycling, golfing, and so on. The pace of these activities should be suited to the individual's level of ability (Figure 17-5).

Respiratory System

Breathing capacity diminishes with age, and oxygen and carbon dioxide exchange is lessened. The rib and chest muscles become smaller and less efficient. Lungs lose their elasticity, and the older adult may be dyspneic, short of breath (SOB), and more prone to pneumonia.

As we age, there is a gradual decline in the muscle structure of the respiratory system, leading to a diminished ability to breathe; thus, development of cough and pneumonia is not uncommon. Regular exercise can help to maintain the ability to breathe and cough effectively. In people who have been active throughout their lives, there is greater lung capacity.

Cardiovascular System

Heart disease and blood vessel disorders are the major cause of death in the United States. Lifestyle has been implicated as the most significant cause of cardiovascular disease. Blood vessels lose their elasticity, become narrower, build up with plaque, and the arteries harden. This is known as **arteriosclerosis.** The myocardium loses some of its ability to pump effectively. This, together with narrowed and plaque-filled arteries, causes the heart to pump harder. Hypertension, or sustained high blood pressure, is a direct result of these factors. Hypertension can contribute to the accumulation of plaque in artery walls. Congestive heart failure is the inability of the heart to pump effectively to meet the body's demand for blood. Myocardial infarction, or heart attack, is another result of arteriosclerotic heart disease. Consistent, regular exercise is the most beneficial activity for older adults to maintain adequate cardiac output throughout their life span.

Gastrointestinal System

Stomach secretions and motility slow as part of aging. Peristalsis slows, and food moves through the gastrointestinal tract more slowly. **Pernicious anemia** is a disorder that can occur when cells of the stomach lining fail to secrete the intrinsic factor. Associated with the absence of hydrochloric acid, pernicious anemia affects the nervous system and red blood cell formation. Fewer calories are needed in the aging process because metabolism slows. Many overeat if they are lonely, gain weight, and may become obese. Eating is a social as well as a physiologic event, and if there is no one to eat with, many older adults will not prepare a meal or eat properly to have good nutrition. Loss of vigor and vitality occur. Malnourishment is not uncommon.

Poor eating habits, poor nutrition, overeating, or undereating can also lead to dental problems. Poor dental hygiene leads to gum disease and loss of teeth, many times making the chewing of food difficult and discouraging. Sometimes cardiac problems, such as endocarditis and myocardial infarction, occur from gum disease due to the invasion of pathogens and inflammation.

Urinary System

The kidneys decrease in size making urine production and output less with aging. With cardiovascular arteriosclero-

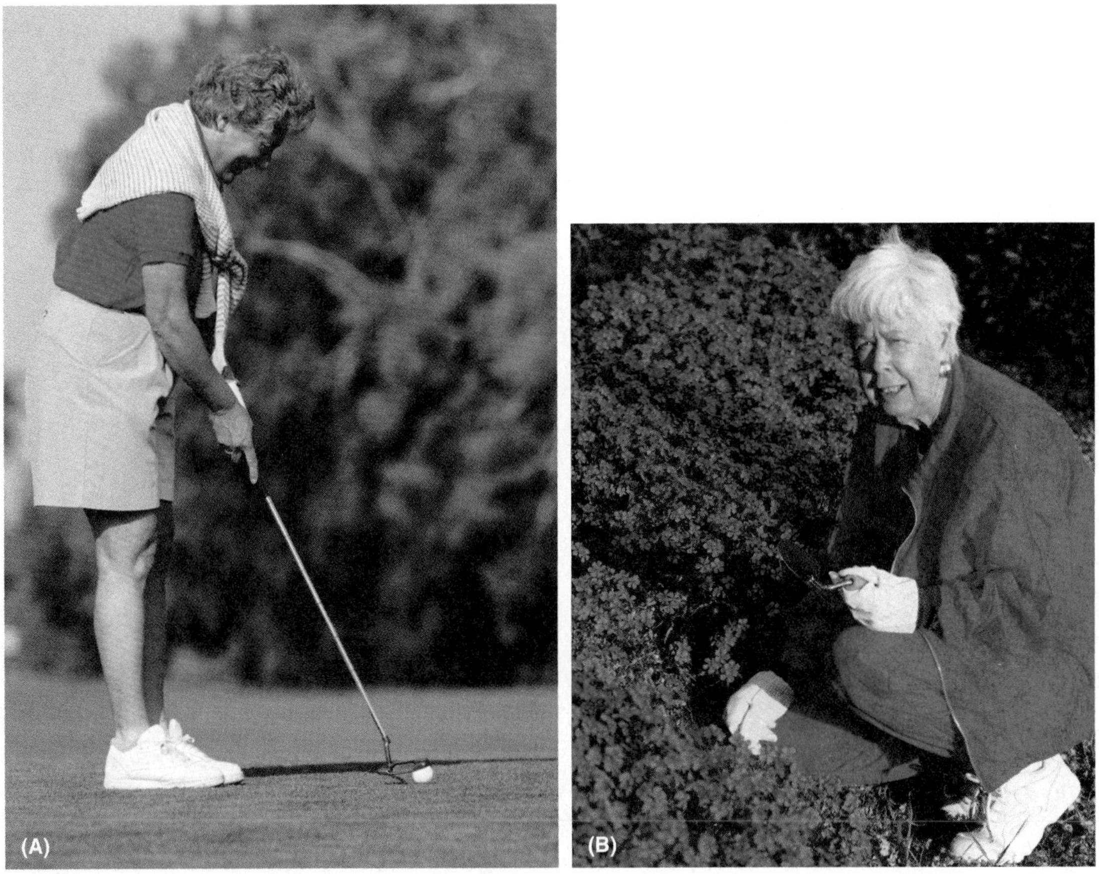

Figure 17-5 (A) A regular exercise program that helps promote successful aging. (B) Gardening is a beneficial form of exercise.

sis, blood flow to the kidney is less. Filtering waste products from the blood is impaired. Medications are not excreted as quickly as they are in a young, healthy person. Levels of medication may increase to a dangerous level with poor filtration. The bladder walls become more inelastic, and the ability to empty the bladder completely becomes difficult. **Residual urine** remains in the bladder, and microorganisms can cause an infection. **Cystitis** is infection and inflammation of the bladder. Urinary **incontinence,** the uncontrollable loss of urine, can be the result of many factors, such as relaxed muscles in the female pelvic floor, cystitis, hypertrophy of prostate gland, and diabetes.

Reproductive System

Women experience menopause at about 55 years old. Estrogen produced by the ovaries ceases, and changes in the female are noticeable with shrinking of vulva and genitalia. Hot flashes are not uncommon because of blood vessel dilation and contraction. Vaginal secretions diminish, the vagina becomes smaller, and infections are more likely. Estrogen replacement therapy helps to lessen symptoms but is used only for short-term therapy in women who experience severe menopausal symptoms. Long-term use of estrogen and progesterone has been proved to increase the risk for heart disease and breast cancer. (See Chapter 14 for information about hormone replacement therapy.)

Men continue to produce sperm well after 50 years of age; however, testosterone levels diminish and midlife changes occur in men. This is known as **andropause.** It is about this time that many men older than 50 years experience benign hypertrophy of the prostate (see Chapter 16). Medication may help in some cases; otherwise, surgery, a prostatectomy, may be performed.

Aging men and women maintain their sexual desires and many enjoy sexual intercourse more when there are no longer children in the home. There is more privacy and time to relax. Retirement centers, nursing homes, and assisted living centers are aware of sexual activity among their patients. Acceptance and privacy by the medical assistant is important as long as both adults are consenting and neither is cognitively impaired.

PREVENTION OF COMPLICATIONS

Older adults are at risk for complications as a result of changes in the structure and function of their body systems.

Accidents can happen because of impaired vision and the inability to see well or to hear a warning sound, such as a fire alarm.

Malnutrition and anemia can develop because of poor nutrition or poor absorption of food. This can be caused by lack of interest in food because of lack of sense of taste or smell.

Older adults may have diminished sensitivity and lack the ability to feel pain as well as a younger person does. Heat and cold applications can injure an aging person if not watched carefully. Also, simple fractured bones may go unnoticed for some time. Loss of balance, disorientation, and confusion may be signs of impaired nervous system function.

Because many older adults suffer from osteoporosis, bones are more easily fractured. Falls are more common because of a loss of vision and balance.

Respiratory tract infections are not unusual. Pneumonia is a serious complication in this group of people. Encourage fluid intake and activity to keep the lungs healthy.

Urinary infections are more common. Adequate fluid intake (eight 8-ounce glasses of liquid per day) help keep infections at bay. Incontinence occurs when pelvic floor muscles are relaxed after childbirth.

Circulatory problems because of cardiovascular disease can cause poor circulation to the extremities, especially the legs. Fluid retention with noticeable edema are a common complication, together with hypertension and congestive heart failure.

Vaginitis is more common because of vaginal dryness and irritation caused by lack of estrogen. The prostate gland enlarges, making urination difficult for men.

It is especially important for older adults to alert and consult with their physicians regarding consumption of an alternative substance, or when considering engaging in an alternative therapy. Many older adults take prescription drugs for a variety of health problems and there could be harmful and serious effects because of the interactions of the prescribed medications with the alternative substance. Tai chi, massage therapy, yoga, art therapy, music therapy, and meditation are examples of some alternative or complementary therapies in which an older adult patient can participate. Balance, mobility, strength, creativity, and stress reduction are some of the benefits for older adults who choose to add these alternatives to enhance their health and well-being.

PSYCHOLOGICAL CHANGES

There is a great deal of variation in the psychological functioning of older adults. Among the factors that contribute are the person's health, psychosocial history, race, sex, and environmental aspects, such as education, support system, and social class.

The level of decline in an older adult's intelligence is affected by social factors. People who maintain their intelligence tend to be in better health, have had more education, are in a high socioeconomic group, and are involved with others and in their community.

Dementia affects memory, personality, and **cognitive functioning** (awareness, reasoning, judgment, intuition). Alzheimer's disease is a common form of dementia. Some research has shown that there may be a genetic, as well as environmental, link to the cause of Alzheimer's disease. People who have had a stroke may suffer from dementia, impairing brain functioning.

Depression in the older adult can occur from loss of a spouse, chronic illness, or financial problems. Personality seems to help determine how individuals adapt to changes that they experience as they grow older.

THE MEDICAL ASSISTANT AND THE GERIATRIC PATIENT

Many older adults experience dementia, mental illness, depression, stress, boredom, fear of the unknown, loss of independence, feelings of rejection and worthlessness, low self-esteem, loneliness, dependence, failed expectations, and disappointments. All of these factors coupled with the physiologic changes that can occur offer a special challenge to the medical assistant caring for the health and needs of this group of patients. Allow patients time to ventilate and express their concerns, allow for private and confidential discussion, and **empathize** with their situation by being aware of their feelings, emotions, and behavior. Good communication is essential for quality care of older adults. Do not talk to older adults as if they were children. Speak

> Be cautious to limit access to patient health records only to those who need them to perform their jobs. Be sure to use passwords to safeguard databases and keep computer screens facing away from patients.
>
> Disclosure of suspected patient abuse is necessary to prevent serious threats or injuries to older adult patients and is required by law.

slowly and clearly. Face the individual while talking. Write instructions in addition to verbalizing them.

Memory-Impaired Older Adults

Geriatric care poses challenges when attempting to communicate with impaired older adults. The inability to communicate on a meaningful level can be frustrating and challenging, especially for the older person who is struggling to communicate but cannot find the right words. Following are some techniques that can be effective in improving verbal communication with older people experiencing memory impairment:

1. Talk to the person in a nondistracting place. It can be difficult for an older adult to concentrate or to sort things out when there are environmental distractions, such as other conversations, equipment noises, or people walking by.
2. Begin conversations with orientating information. Identify yourself, and call older adults by their preferred names. Explain the purpose of your visit.
3. Use short words and short, simple sentences with no pronouns.
4. Speak slowly and say individual words clearly.

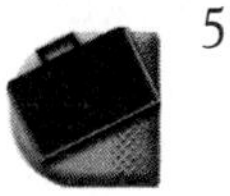

5. Never "talk down" or be condescending. This is demeaning. Speak in an adult manner as you would to a coworker or friend. Provide the dignity and respect you wish to receive yourself.
6. Lower the tone (pitch) of your voice. A raised pitch is a signal that one is upset. A lower pitch is also easier for people with hearing impairments to understand.
7. Talk to the person in a warm and pleasant manner. Use nonverbal cues, such as facial expression, tone of voice, or touch, to show your feelings of affection and concern. Smiling, taking the older person's hand, or touching the person on the arm can vividly communicate that you are interested and really care.
8. When giving instructions, allow plenty of time for the information to be absorbed.
9. Give clear and simple instructions.
10. Ask the person to do one task at a time.
11. Listen actively. If you do not understand, apologize to the person by saying that you did not understand exactly what was said. It is extremely important to phrase responses in a way that does not damage the self-esteem of the older adult.
12. Avoid asking direct questions that require the person to remember a fact.
13. Focus on well behavior or things that we know the patient can still do.
14. Use humor when appropriate. If expressed naturally, humor brings much needed laughter, a dimension that is often lost in the health care setting.
15. Let the person know when you leave and if you are returning.
16. When discussing a case with another staff member, do so in private to protect patient confidentiality.

Visually-Impaired Older Adults

Visually-impaired people need to know you are present, but do not approach the individual until you make your presence known. Help by explaining his or her location, and identify others who may also be present (Figure 17-6).

Hearing-Impaired Older Adults

For the hearing-impaired older adult to communicate and understand instructions, there are some techniques the medical assistant should keep in mind. These strategies will be beneficial and will facilitate communication and understanding. These techniques include:

1. Face the hearing-impaired person directly and on the same level when possible. (If he or she is standing, the medical assistant should stand; if the patient is seated, the medical assistant should be seated).
2. Keep your hands away from your face while talking.
3. Reduce background noises when talking. Move to a quieter room away from extraneous sounds and activities.
4. Hearing-impaired individuals hear and understand less when they are tired or sick.
5. Get the person's attention before beginning to speak and do not talk from another room.
6. Speak in a normal tone; do not shout.
7. Be sure that light is not shining in the eyes of the hearing-impaired individual.
8. If the hearing-impaired patient has trouble understanding, reword what you have said. Do not repeat the same words again and again.
9. Written instructions are useful, but the medical assistant must be certain that what is written is understood.

Critical Thinking

Describe strategies for communicating with hearing-impaired patients.

Making Contact

Introduce yourself. Ask the visually-impaired patient if he would like assistance. If he does, offer your arm by saying so and by touching your hand or forearm against his.

Grip

The patient grips your arm just above the elbow. The grip must be firm but not so tight that it becomes uncomfortable.

Stance

The patient stands next to you, slightly behind. His arm is bent and held close to his side. Relax your arm and let it hang naturally at your side.

Pace

The pace should be comfortable for both of you. If the patient tightens his grip or pulls on your arm, slow down; your pace may be too fast or he may be anxious. You should alert the patient to obstacles such as curbs, stairs, doors, and thresholds. Be specific, but do not confuse him with too much information.

Stairs

When approaching stairs, tell the patient. Let him know whether you are going to go up or down. Be sure you approach the stairs directly, not at an angle. Have the patient stand next to the handrail if there is one.

Pause at the top (or bottom) of the stairs and describe anything unusual about them. The patient will find the handrail and reach forward with his foot to locate the edge of the first step. Start down (or up) the stairs, keeping yourself one step ahead. Keep a steady pace.

When you reach a landing, stop immediately. (Do not take an extra step.) Doing so lets the patient know that there are no more steps, and he can then match his stride with yours.

The same procedure should be used when approaching curbs. Point out any changes in the terrain, even small ones.

Sitting

When guiding someone to a chair, walk up to it and place your hand on the back of the chair. Let the patient trail your arm down to its back. Tell him which way the chair is facing, and he can then seat himself.

If the chair lacks a back or is very large, bring the patient up to the chair so that his legs are against the front of it. He can then reach down to locate the arms and seat of it before he sits.

If the chair is at a table, describe the relationship of the chair, the table and the patient. Place one of his hands on the chair and the other hand on the table.

Doors

When approaching a closed door, tell the patient its position when open. For example, "The door opens away and to the left." Or say, "Take the door with your left hand." After you open the door and begin to walk through, the patient will have his hand ready to help hold it open as you walk through together. The patient will move his arm across the front of his body to find the door with the palm of his hand. He should close it behind you if it is not a self-closing door. Use the narrow passage technique in addition to this technique if the doorway is narrow.

Narrow Passage Technique

When coming to a narrow passage, tell the patient. Move your guiding arm to the center of your back. Slow your pace. He will move behind you and extend his arm, placing you in a single-file position. Once you pass through the narrow passage, bring your arm forward and return to the normal stance.

Figure 17-6 Sighted guide techniques.

Elder Abuse

What is elder abuse? Massachusetts law defines elder abuse as the committing or omitting of an act that results in serious physical or serious emotional injury to an older adult. All states have elder abuse laws. Abuse includes physical abuse, emotional abuse, and neglect. The law protects elders abused or neglected by caretakers.

All persons 60 years and older living in the community are protected under the law. Who must report elder abuse? Physicians, medical interns, dentists, medical assistants, nurses, family counselors, police officers, psychologists, homemakers, licensed home health care aides, and many others are required to report abuse. Agencies are also liable. Any person required to report abuse who fails to do so is subject to a fine. Anyone who has reasonable cause to believe an older adult has been abused may report it and has a moral obligation to protect older adults. In most states, the department responsible for elder affairs has established an elder abuse hotline to receive reports of abuse. Reports may also be made to the designated protective service agency in your community. Once reports are received by the elder protective services program, if appropriate, a caseworker will assess the situation to determine the nature and extent of the abuse. If abuse is confirmed, services will be provided to eliminate or alleviate abuse. Many social services are usually available. Mental health, legal, homemaker services, and alternative living arrangements may be provided. See Chapter 7.

Some signs and symptoms of mistreatment or abuse include:

Psychological Signs and Symptoms

- Increasing depression
- Anxiety
- Withdrawn/timid
- Hostile
- Unresponsive
- Confused
- New poverty
- Longing for death
- Vague health complaints
- Anxious to please

Physical Signs and Symptoms

- Lack of personal care
- Lack of supervision
- Bruises
- Welts
- Lack of food
- Beatings
- Neglect
- Unsatisfactory living conditions

There are many other signs and symptoms and not all of those listed by themselves indicate mistreatment, neglect, or abuse. If any seem to increase in number or severity, it may indicate a problem. By observing closely, you may be able to initiate corrective action or reduce or prevent the situation from deteriorating.

Usually the victim is frail (weak), physically or emotionally, and dependent on the abuser for basic survival needs. The victim may be afraid to speak out for fear of retaliation.

Where should one call for information? Contact elder protective services programs in the Yellow Pages of your phone book, or call the Eldercare Locator toll free at (800) 677-1116.

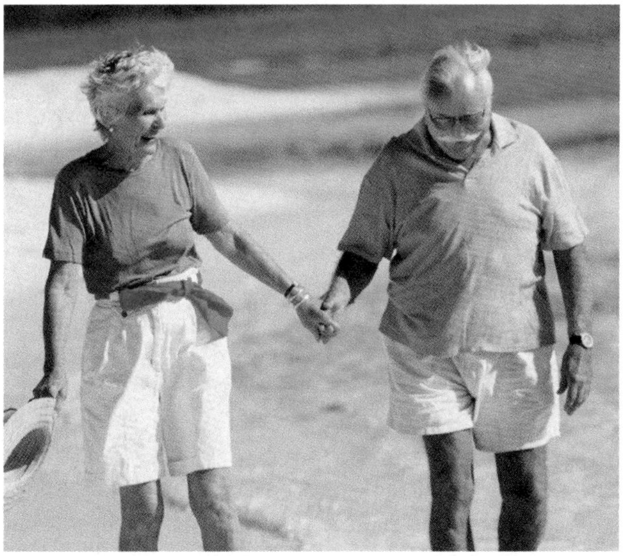

Figure 17-7 With improved geriatric care, older adults can look forward to longer, healthier lives.

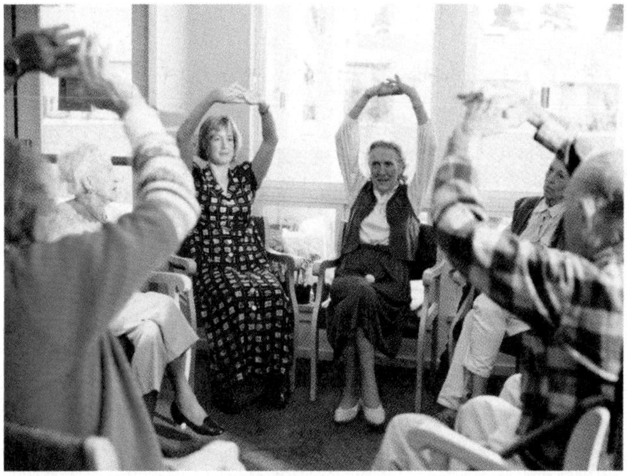

Figure 17-8 An exercise class in an assisted-living facility.

HEALTHY AND SUCCESSFUL AGING

Older adults are enjoying longer, healthier lives. Some of the reasons for healthy aging are the increase in the number of gerontologists (specialists who provide medical care only to older adult patients), more awareness and involvement of older adults with their health care, improved nutrition, regular exercise, new medications, and advancing medical technology (Figure 17-7).

Some tips for healthy aging according to the National Institute on Aging of the National Institutes of Health are:

1. Eat a balanced diet.
2. Exercise regularly.
3. Get regular checkups.
4. Don't smoke.
5. Wear a seatbelt when in the car.
6. Practice safety to avoid falls and fractures.
7. Keep in contact with family and friends and stay active through work, community, and recreation.
8. Avoid over exposure to the sun and cold.
9. Drink alcohol in moderation. Don't drink and drive.
10. Keep personal and financial records in order to simplify budgeting and investing. Plan for long-term financial needs and housing.
11. Keep a positive attitude toward life and engage in activities that make you happy.

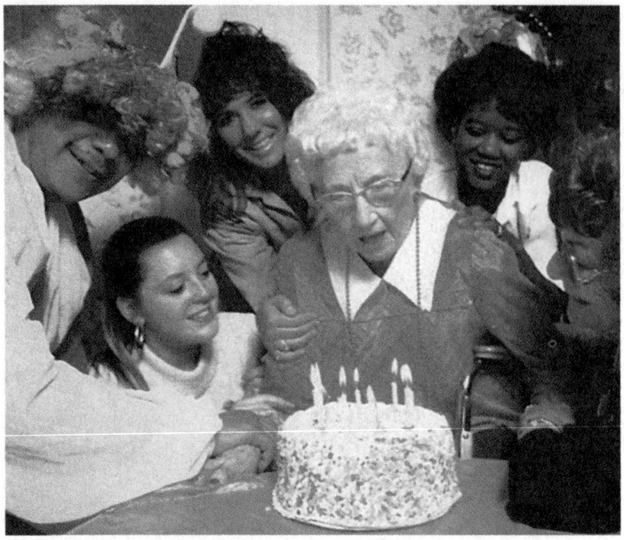

Figure 17-9 The woman is celebrating her 100th birthday and is surrounded by her family and friends.

Successful aging requires that healthy living and daily activities be combined. To age successfully, individuals need to be continually involved, must pursue what makes them happy, and make an effort to maintain a positive attitude. These actions of healthy habits should begin in childhood when they can be formed and encouraged. They become the responsibilities of each individual. Some activities that are important to successful aging are socialization with friends and family, intimacy, education, and employment (for income and social satisfaction). For successful aging to happen, the older person has to make a commitment to work at it. See Figures 17-8 and 17-9.

Critical Thinking

What are some strategies that older adults can do to keep mentally and physically stimulated?

Case Study 17-1

Adelaide Robinson, 83 years old, has an appointment Thursday morning for a recheck of her most recent complaint. She tells you that she is moving slower than she did just six months ago, and she has noticed less flexibility as well.

CASE STUDY REVIEW

1. What are the possible causes of Mrs. Robinson's complaints?
2. What effect will these problems have on Mrs. Robinson's daily routine?
3. What might Dr. King suggest Mrs. Robinson do to help alleviate symptoms?

Case Study 17-2

Sally Donovan, 92 years old, is in the gerontology clinic today. Her main concern, problem, and reason for appointment is that she "cannot taste or smell much anymore and food doesn't taste good." She wants suggestions from the physician about how to improve her taste and smell so she can enjoy food more freely.

CASE STUDY REVIEW

1. What are some reasons that older adults lose their sense of taste and smell?
2. Describe any dangers that can be associated with loss of taste and smell.

SUMMARY

Many aging people live well into their 80s, 90s, and even to 100 years of age. They remain physically and mentally stimulated. They learn a foreign language, learn to play a musical instrument, love to read, garden, and volunteer. Older people are more aware today than ever before of the importance of a healthy lifestyle and of its significant contribution to their long and healthy life span.

Other older adults, because of genetic inheritance, wear and tear, stress, and loss of chemicals and hormones, seem to age quickly but have little control over these factors.

Many others practice poor health habits, some by choice and others by circumstance. These habits contribute to chronic diseases, disability, and a shorter and unhealthy life span.

Above all, dispel myths about older adults. Be patient, kind, consistent, and thoughtful.

STUDY FOR SUCCESS

To reinforce your knowledge and skills of information presented in this chapter:

- ❑ Review Key Terms
- ❑ Consider the Case Studies and discuss your conclusions
- ❑ Answer the Review Questions
  - ❑ Multiple Choice
  - ❑ Critical Thinking
- ❑ Navigate the Internet by completing the Web Activities
- ❑ Practice the StudyWARE activities on your student CD
- ❑ Apply your knowledge in the Student Workbook activities
- ❑ Complete the Web Tutor sections

REVIEW QUESTIONS

Multiple Choice

1. The most chronic condition associated with older adults is:
   a. arteriosclerotic heart disease
   b. cystitis
   c. presbycusis
   d. pernicious anemia
2. An eye disease common to older adults that is characterized by fluid pressure buildup is:
   a. macular degeneration
   b. presbyopia
   c. cataract
   d. glaucoma
3. Joints in older adults become worn because:
   a. cartilage erodes in the joints
   b. osteoporosis makes bones brittle
   c. muscle fibers decrease
   d. vertebrae become thinner
4. Inability to cough deeply and raise mucous makes older adults more susceptible to which of the following?
   a. emphysema
   b. asthma
   c. pneumonia
   d. bronchitis
5. Residual urine refers to:
   a. catheterized urine for urinalysis
   b. first-voided specimen
   c. amount of urine left in bladder after voiding
   d. total amount of urine in the bladder when full

Critical Thinking

1. How can an older adult's food be made more appealing?
2. What are some ways that older adults can keep bones from becoming brittle?
3. Describe a vision problem that leaves older adults having difficulty seeing color intensity.
4. What are four causes of urinary incontinence?
5. Give three ways to enhance communication with older adults.

6. What is the best way to approach a visually-impaired person?
7. Older adults in the United States are generally healthier today than older adults of 10 years ago. What are some of the reasons for this?
8. How can you encourage older adults to choose a healthy lifestyle?

WEB ACTIVITIES

1. Visit the Institute on Aging Web site (http://www.umass.edu/aging) and determine why many older adults have cardiovascular disease.
2. The American Psychological Association Web site (http://www.apa.org) gives information about psychology. Find information that pertains to older adults and their psychological health. What are some resources for mental health issues that can be helpful for older adults?
3. The U.S. government has a Web site (http://www.aoa.dhhs.gov.aoa) for concerns and information about aging. What government agencies can an older adult contact for help with health insurance questions?
4. The National Osteoporosis Foundation Web site (http://www.nof.org) provides information about osteoporosis. Retrieve information about osteoporosis that is useful for all older adults.
5. Locate a Web site for older adults who have arthritis. Find some techniques for these patients to make their activities of daily living less difficult.

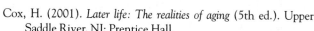

REFERENCES/BIBLIOGRAPHY

Cox, H. (2001). *Later life: The realities of aging* (5th ed.). Upper Saddle River, NJ: Prentice Hall.

Hegner, B. R., Accello, B., & Caldwell, E. (2004). *Nursing assistant: A nursing process approach* (9th ed.). Clifton Park, NY: Thomas Delmar Learning.

Hogstel, M. O. (2001). *Gerontology: Nursing care of the older adult*. Clifton Park, NY: Thomas Delmar Learning.

Markson, E., & Hollis-Sawyer, G. (2000). *Readings in social gerontology*. Los Angeles, CA: Roxbury Publishing Co.

Taber's cyclopedic medical dictionary (21st ed.). (2003). Philadelphia: FA Davis.

CHAPTER 18

Examinations and Procedures of Body Systems

OUTLINE

OBJECTIVES

The student should strive to meet the following performance objectives and demonstrate an understanding of the facts and principles presented in this chapter through written and oral communication.

1. Define the key terms as presented in the glossary.
2. Describe how to perform a urinary catheterization.
3. State the proper protocol when collecting urine for a drug screening.

(continues)

KEY TERMS

Alimentary Canal
Allergen
Alveoli
Amblyopia
Amsler Grid
Aphasia
Appendicular Skeleton
Aseptic
Auricle
Axial Skeleton
Biopsy
Bronchi
Bronchodilator
Calculi
Carbuncle
Catheterization
Closed Fracture
Colonoscopy
Comedone
Cystoscopy
Demyelination
Dislocation
Dysuria
Emaciation
Endoscopy
Equilibrium
Erosion
Erythema
External Respiration
Frequency
Furuncle
Gait
Hematemesis
Hematochezia
Hematuria
Hemoptysis
Hydronephrosis
Ingestion
Internal Respiration
Lesion

(continues)

KEY TERMS (continued)

Lithotripsy
Malabsorption
Malaise
Melena
Nebulizer
Nephrolithotomy
Nitrogenous
Nocturia
Nystagmus
Obturator
Occluder
Oliguria
Ophthalmoscope
Opticokinetic Drum Test
Otoscope
Paresthesia
Perforation
Peripheral Nerve
Peritonitis
Phacoemulsification
Polycystic
Polyp
Proteinuria
Pyuria
Rosacea
Salicylates
Spirometry
Strabismus
Stratum Corneum
Uremia
Urgency
Wheal

FEATURED COMPETENCIES

CAAHEP—ENTRY-LEVEL COMPETENCIES

Clinical Competencies

Fundamental Procedures

- Perform handwashing
- Perform sterilization techniques
- Dispose of biohazardous materials
- Practice Standard Precautions

Specimen Collection

- Obtain specimens for microbiological testing

(continues)

OBJECTIVES (continued)

4. Describe patient preparation for occult blood testing.
5. Differentiate between an instillation and an irrigation.
6. Discuss the different types of visual acuity charts and how to use them appropriately.
7. Explain the medical assistant's role when assisting with audiometry.
8. Describe the proper use of a metered dose nebulizer.
9. Briefly discuss the role of the medical assistant during spirometry.
10. Explain the medical assistant's role in cast application and cast removal and the guidelines for cast care.
11. List items required by a physician for a neurologic examination and explain the medical assistant's role in the examination.
12. Explain oxygen administration using a nasal cannula.
13. Explain the reasons for performing pulse oximetry.

SCENARIO

At Inner City Health Care, a number of specialty examinations are scheduled for Tuesday the 8th. Administrative medical assistant Jane O'Hara, who is office manager, is careful to schedule patients requiring specialty procedures so that times do not overlap; before she schedules, Jane makes certain examination rooms are available with an extra margin of time between patients. Clinical medical assistants Wanda Slawson, CMA, and Bruce Goldman, RMA, take responsibility to ensure that all supplies and equipment are assembled, that both physician and patient are comfortable with the physical environment, and that all safety precautions are followed before, during, and after the examination or procedure.

FEATURED COMPETENCIES (continued)

- Instruct patients in the collection of fecal specimens

Diagnostic Testing

- Perform respiratory testing

Patient Care

- Prepare and maintain examination and treatment areas
- Prepare patient for and assist with routine and specialty examinations
- Prepare patient for and assist with procedures, treatments, and minor office surgeries
- Apply pharmacology principles to prepare and administer oral and parenteral (excluding IV) medications

General Competencies

Legal Concepts

- Identify and respond to issues of confidentiality
- Perform within legal and ethical boundaries

Patient Instruction

- Instruct individuals according to their needs
- Provide instruction for health maintenance and disease prevention
- Identify community resources

Operational Functions

- Use methods of quality control

ABHES—ENTRY-LEVEL COMPETENCIES

Professionalism

- Conduct work within scope of education, training and ability

(continues)

INTRODUCTION

New techniques and developments occur frequently in medicine and medical assistants must refine existing skills and learn new ones to be knowledgeable and proficient and to provide the most current, up-to-date, quality care to patients. The medical assistant who works in a specialist's office or an ambulatory care setting that treats a variety of patient problems will need additional skills when providing specialty care to patients. Patients with conditions specific to a particular body system or body part need specialized care. The medical assistant will assist the physician with a multitude of clinical procedures that are an integral part of each specialty examination.

This chapter covers specialty and body system examinations and the appropriate clinical procedures in urology; endoscopy; and the sensory, respiratory, musculoskeletal, neurologic, circulatory, blood and lymph, and integumentary systems.

Each specialty description includes tables that contain information on diseases, disorders, and diagnostic tests and procedures used to confirm diagnoses. Other diseases and disorders and procedures related to each specialty are addressed in the body of the chapter.

Spotlight on Certification

RMA Content Outline

- Anatomy and physiology
- Terminology
- Asepsis
- Physical examinations
- Laboratory procedures

CMA Content Outline

- Medical terminology
- Anatomy and physiology
- Principles of infection control
- Treatment area
- Examinations
- Vision, hearing, respiratory testing

CMAS Content Outline

- Medical terminology
- Anatomy and Physiology
- Asepsis in the medical office
- Examination preparation

FEATURED COMPETENCIES (continued)

Communication

- Serve as a liaison between Physician and others

Clinical Duties

- Interview and take patient history
- Prepare patients for procedures
- Apply principles of aseptic techniques and infection control
- Prepare and maintain examination and treatment area
- Assist physician with examinations and treatments
- Use quality control
- Perform selected tests that assist with diagnosis and treatment
- Screen and follow up patient test results
- Prepare and administer medications as directed by Physician
- Maintain medication records
- Dispose of biohazardous materials
- Practice standard precautions
- Instruct patient in the collection of fecal specimen
- Perform respiratory testing

Legal Concepts

- Determine needs for documentation and reporting
- Document accurately

Instruction

- Teach patients methods of health promotion and disease prevention

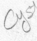

URINARY SYSTEM

The urinary system includes the kidneys, ureters, and bladder. The main function of the kidneys is to form and excrete urine, which contains waste products harmful to body tissues. The kidneys also regulate water balance in the body and help maintain the acid–base balance of body fluids.

Collecting and processing urine for laboratory analysis is covered in Chapter 30. Several other clinical and diagnostic procedures of the urinary system are covered in this section including urinary catheterization and an overview of performing a urine drug screen and a diagnostic X-ray known as an intravenous pyelogram (IVP) or excretory urography used to diagnose disorders of the urinary tract.

Diagnostic tests, procedures, disorders, and conditions common to the urinary system are shown in Tables 18-1 and 18-2.

Signs and Symptoms of Urinary Conditions and Disorders

Signs and symptoms of urinary tract diseases include any abnormality in urine or in the ability to urinate. Some common signs and symptoms are **dysuria** (painful urination), **proteinuria** (protein in the urine), **hematuria** (blood in the urine), **pyuria** (pus in the urine), **frequency, urgency, oliguria** (scanty urination), and **nocturia** (excessive urination at night). Patients may report flank or low back pain or experience fever, nausea, vomiting, general **malaise** (general discomfort), and fatigue.

Urinary tract infection (UTI) is the most common disorder of the urinary system, and it manifests itself with many of the above signs and symptoms. UTI is a broad diagnosis covering any infection of the urinary tract including the urethra, ureters, bladder, and kidneys. UTIs may be caused by virus or fungus, but by far the most common infection is caused by bacteria. The most common area is the bladder (cystitis).

Bacteria may reach the urinary tract through the blood (hematogenous infection) or by entering the tract through the urethra (ascending infection). Hematogenous infection is less common and is usually the result of septicemia. In this case, the urinary tract is a site of secondary infection. Primary infection of septicemia may begin in the respiratory or gastrointestinal tract and is carried to the urinary tract throughout the blood.

Diagnostic Tests

The most commonly performed test to diagnose urinary system disorders is a urinalysis. Many different disorders of the urinary system can be identified, making this test extremely valuable. A specimen of urine can be analyzed

TABLE 18-1 URINARY SYSTEM DISORDERS

Disease/ Disorder	Laboratory Diagnostic Tests: Blood	Laboratory Diagnostic Tests: Urine	Laboratory Diagnostic Tests: Radiography	Surgery	Medical Tests or Procedures	Treatment
Cancer of urinary bladder	• Complete blood count	• Urinalysis • Culture and sensitivity of urine	• Intravenous pyelogram • Pelvic ultrasound • Computed tomography scan	• Biopsy of bladder with endoscopy	• Cystoscopy	• Resection of cancer (transurethral resection of a bladder tumor [TURBT]) • Cystectomy • Radium implants • Chemotherapy
Cystitis	• Complete blood count	• Urinalysis including microscopic examination • Culture and sensitivity of urine	• Intravenous pyelogram		• Cystoscopy	• Appropriate antibiotic therapy
Glomerulo-nephritis	• Blood urea nitrogen • Creatinine • Blood culture • Sedimenta-tion rate • Electrolytes	• Urinalysis • Culture and sensitivity of urine	• Intravenous pyelogram • Ultrasound of kidneys • X-ray of kidneys, ureters, and bladder		• Biopsy of kidney(s)	• Diuretics • Antihypertensives • Dialysis (if necessary) • Kidney transplant
Polycystic kidneys	• Blood urea nitrogen • Creatinine • Electrolytes	• Urinalysis	• Intravenous pyelogram • Ultrasound of kidneys • Computerized tomography scan			• Dialysis • Kidney transplant
Pyelonephritis	• Blood urea nitrogen • Creatinine • Blood culture • Electrolytes	• Urinalysis	• Intravenous pyelogram • Ultrasound of kidneys			• Appropriate antibiotics
Renal calculi	• Complete blood count • Uric acid	• Urinalysis	• X-ray of kidneys, ureters, and bladder • Ultrasound of kidneys, ureters, and bladder • Intravenous pyelogram		• Cystoscopy	• **Lithotripsy** (crushing of a kidney stone) • Surgery **(nephrolithotomy)**
Urinary tract infection	• Complete blood count	• Urinalysis • Culture and sensitivity of urine			• Cystoscopy	• Appropriate antibiotics

for many components such as pH, specific gravity, protein, glucose, leukocytes, and blood. The specimen can be further analyzed by examination under the microscope to look for bacteria, white and red blood cells, crystals, and casts.

Urine culture and sensitivity can be performed and will indicate if a UTI is present so the appropriate antibiotic can be prescribed by the physician. To obtain a urine specimen for culture, there are two ways to collect the specimen: clean catch or by **catheterization** (insertion of sterile tube into urinary bladder). See Procedures 18-1 through 18-3 and Chapter 30, Urinalysis.

Blood tests can be done to determine whether waste products are being adequately filtered out of the circulatory system. A test for kidney function confirms the status of glomeruli function.

Two **nitrogenous** waste products normally filtered from the blood are urea and creatinine. A blood urea nitrogen (BUN) test will check for levels of these two wastes. High levels of waste products can result in **uremia** (waste products in the blood), a toxic condition of the blood that, if not reversed, leads to death. See Chapter 30, Urinalysis.

TABLE 18-2 DESCRIPTION OF URINARY DISORDERS AND CONDITIONS

- *Cancer of Urinary Bladder.* Linked to cigarette smoking, industrial chemicals, and ingested toxins. Microscopic hematuria one of the first symptoms.
- *Cystitis.* Inflammation of the urinary bladder. More common in female patients due to the short length of the urethra. *E.coli* may travel from the rectum to the bladder. Infectious organisms can invade the bladder during sexual intercourse. Frequency, burning, dysuria, and urgency are common symptoms.
- *Glomerulonephritis.* Seen in children and young adults after streptococcal infection; strep throat, scarlet fever. Causes degenerative inflammation of glomeruli. Chills, fever, weakness are common symptoms. Edema and albumin in urine are common. Hypertension occurs.
- *Polycystic Kidneys.* A congenital anomaly. Kidneys contain multiple cysts and greatly dilated tubules do not open into renal pelvis. Hypertension, kidney failure, and death can result.
- *Pyelonephritis.* Caused by pyogenic bacteria such as *E. coli*, streptococci, staphylococci, pregnancy, or calculi. May originate in the bladder and ascend to the kidneys. Pyuria, chills, fever, sudden back pain are symptoms. Dysuria is common. Tenderness in suprapubic area.
- *Renal Calculi.* May be present with or without symptoms. Cause intense pain when they lodge in the ureter(s). Formed by certain salts (perhaps calcium). Urinary urgency, nausea and vomiting, fever.

An intravenous pyelogram (IVP), a kidneys-ureters-bladder (KUB), and cystogram are radiologic examinations of the urinary tract.

Intravenous Pyelogram (Excretory Urography). An intravenous pyelogram (IVP) is used to examine the urinary tract (kidneys, ureters, and bladder) for blockage, narrowing, growths, and calculi. This urinary tract diagnostic radiograph is also used to diagnose disorders such as lesions, **hydronephrosis** (collection of urine in renal pelvis), and **polycystic** (many cysts) kidneys.

Patient Preparation for IVP. In studies of the urinary system, the IVP requires that the patient prepare with laxatives, enemas, and fasting (Table 18-3). The IVP consists of an intravenous injection of an iodine-based contrast medium that is used to define the structures of the urinary system. A retrograde pyelogram is a study of the urinary tract done by inserting a sterile catheter into the urinary meatus. Radiopaque contrast medium then flows upward into the kidneys. This diagnostic test is usually done in conjunction with cystoscopy. Patients should have iodine-sensitivity tests before the examination to determine the possibility of an allergic reaction. A voiding cystogram may be ordered in conjunction with an IVP. In this case, the contrast medium is instilled into the bladder by catheter and no special patient preparation is needed. See Chapter 20, Diagnostic Imaging.

Cystoscopy. **Cystoscopy** is a sterile procedure that uses a lighted scope (cytoscope) to view the urethra and bladder. Inflammation, bladder **calculi** (stones), **polyps,** and tumors can be seen using a cystoscope. A biopsy of the bladder can be done while performing a cystoscopy (Figure 18-1).

TABLE 18-3 INTRAVENOUS PYELOGRAM

Purpose	Patient Education	Precautions
To examine the urinary tract—kidneys ureters, bladder—for blockage, narrowing, growths, and calculi.	1. Light evening meal night before 2. Cathartic (laxative) 3. NPO after 9:00 PM 4. Cleansing enema(s) in AM	Contrast medium of iodine used for visualization (check with patient regarding seafood or iodine allergies) *Warn patients of possible warm flushed sensation when dye is injected and that they may experience a metallic taste.

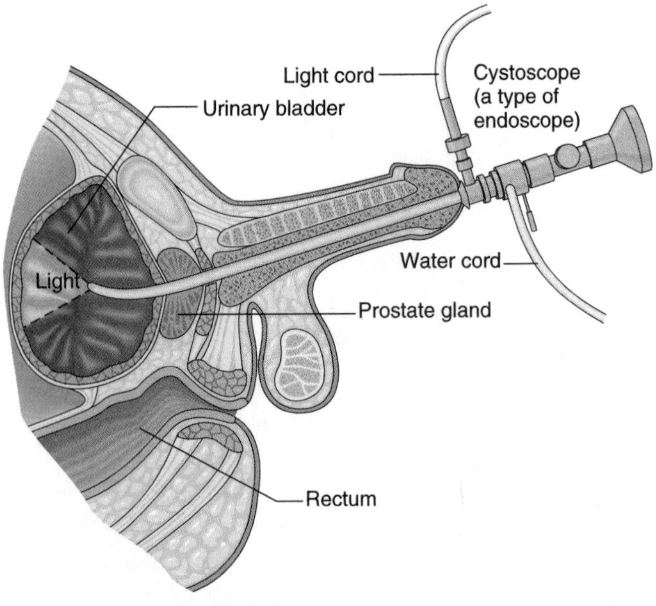

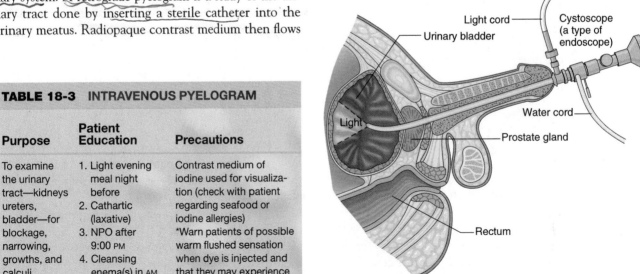

Figure 18-1 Cystoscopy.

Biopsy of the Kidney. Biopsies of the kidney will help confirm a diagnosis. Using radiology, a fine-gauge needle is inserted through the flank to remove a piece of kidney tissue for analysis and possible malignancy.

Urinary Drug Screening (Urine Toxicology Screening). There may be circumstances when it is necessary to check a patient's urine specimen for traces of drugs. At times, employees and athletes are required to have their urine tested to qualify for employment or sports activities.

It is legally necessary to have a signed consent form from patients for all drug screening tests performed. It may also be necessary to identify the patient or donor before a test is performed by requesting a photo identification that can be copied and filed with the consent form.

Depending on the drug collection kit used, the urine sample volume can vary from 1 to 40 ml. Some kits may also supply a bluing agent that the medical assistant will need to place in the toilet and toilet tank before the urine collection. The collector should wait immediately outside the collection area to receive the sample directly from the donor. See Procedure 18-1. When the urine drug screening is performed during the investigation of a crime, the patient is observed during urination and the sample is handled according to legal requirements. As in other drug screening tests, there must be a continuous record of who is handling the specimen at all times.

Critical Thinking

Why are the rules of evidence always followed during a drug screen?

Urinary Catheterization

The medical assistant may either perform or assist with the urinary bladder catheterization, which is the introduction of a sterile catheter (tube) through the urethra into the bladder for withdrawal of urine. See Figure 18-2

Patient Education

Urine Toxicology Screening

1. Inform the patient not to flush the toilet after voiding into the specimen container.
2. The urine sample should remain in full view of the donor until it is secured for transport to the laboratory.

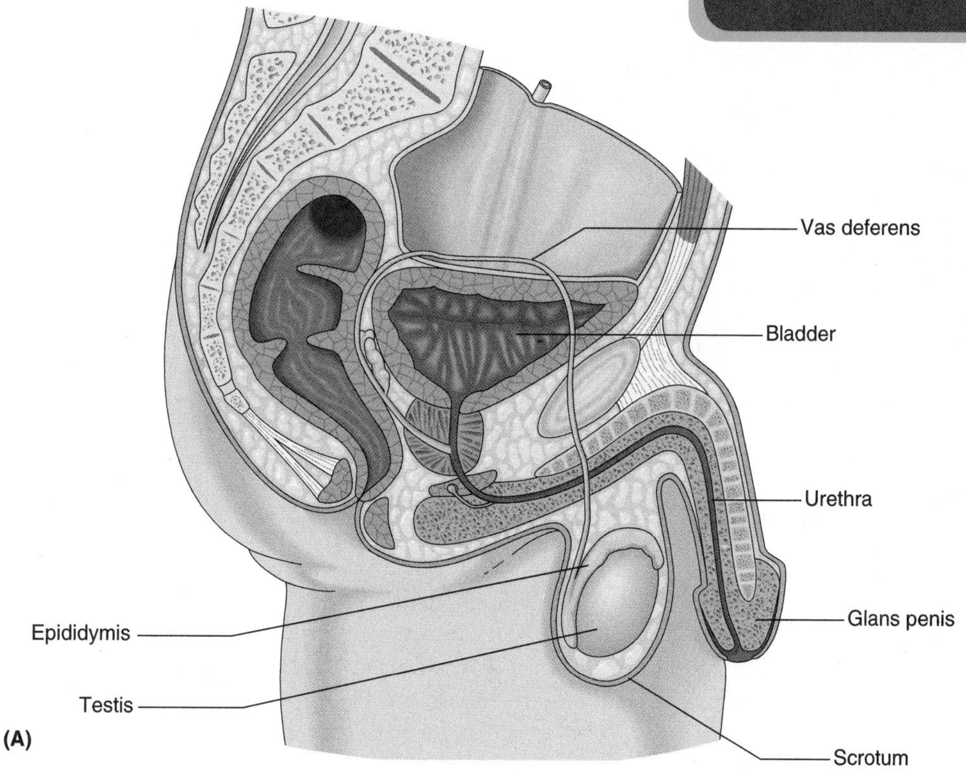

Figure 18-2 (A) Cross-sectional view of male anatomy showing urethra and bladder for catheterization. (continues)

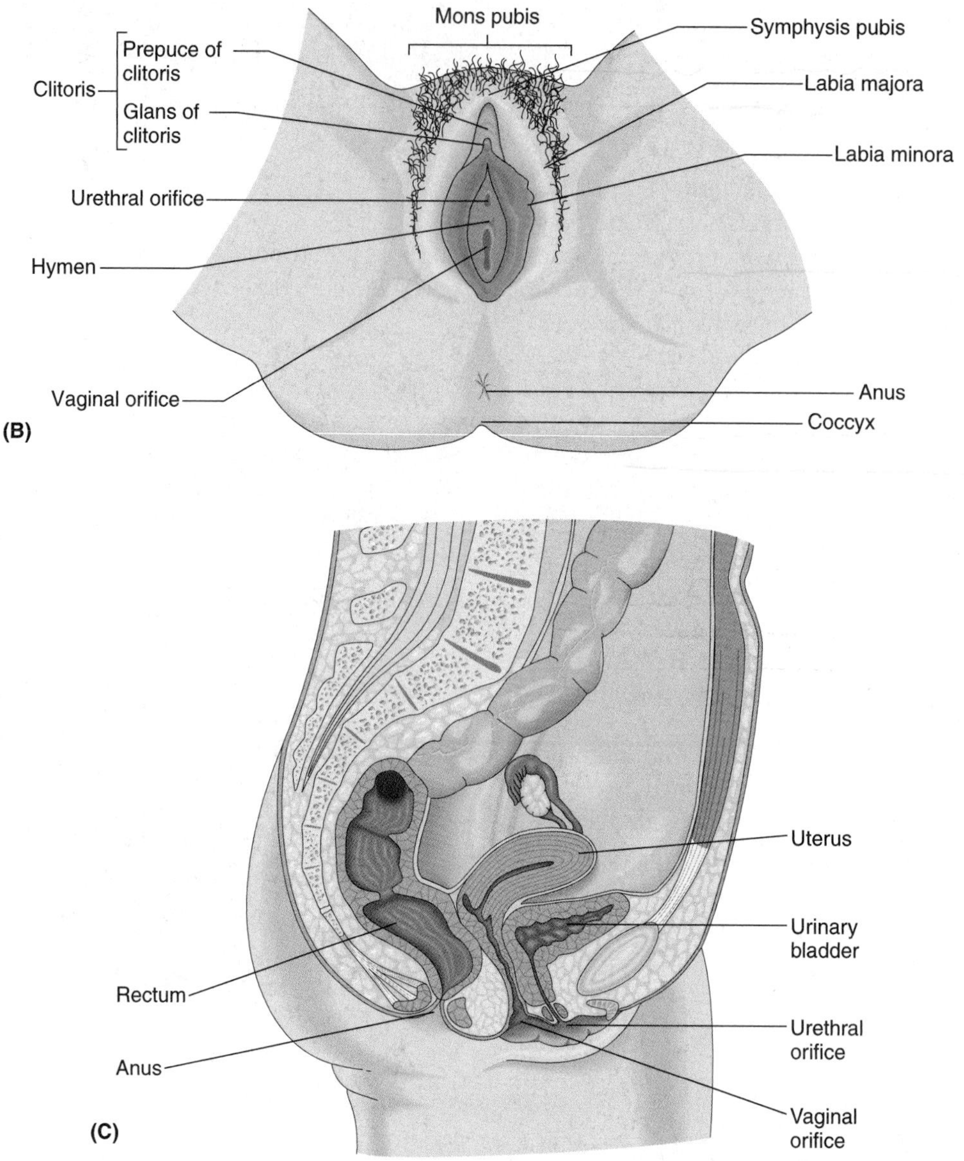

Figure 18-2 (continued) (B) External genitalia of the female. (C) Cross-sectional view of female anatomy showing urethra and bladder for catheterization.

for male and female anatomy for catheterization. There are basically four reasons for catheterizing patients:

1. To obtain a sterile urine specimen for analysis
2. For relief of urinary retention
3. To instill medication into the bladder, after the bladder is emptied
4. To measure post-void residual urine

In some cases, this procedure is done by a urologist; however, some physicians in obstetrics/gynecology and general and family practice may perform or have the medical assistant perform the catheterization. Catheterizing male patients is generally performed by the physician. The physician may order a culture and sensitivity of the urine obtained from catheterization if the patient is experiencing dysuria, frequency, hematura, and urgency. This is done to determine if microorganisms are present and, if so, what the causative microorganism is and which medication would irradicate it, in order to prescribe the appropriate antibiotics.

Sterile technique must be maintained throughout the catheterization. Contamination of any items during the procedure requires discarding the item and obtaining new sterile equipment before continuing the procedure (Figure 18-3).

See Procedure 18-2 to perform a urinary catheterization on a female patient and Procedure 18-3 for male catheterization.

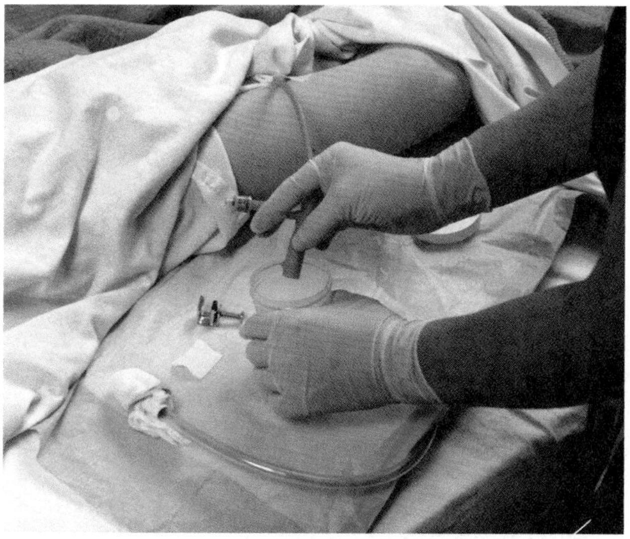

Figure 18-3 Urinary catheterization can be performed using a straight catheter, which is removed immediately after a urine specimen has been obtained, or it can be performed using a Foley catheter (an indwelling catheter). The indwelling catheter remains in the patient's bladder by means of a small inflated balloon at the bladder end of the catheter. A urine specimen can be obtained by disconnecting the tubing, being careful to make certain that sterility is maintained.

Catheterization Equipment. Urinary catheters are sized according to a system of French sizes. A common size catheter is Fr 12. The higher the number the larger the catheter. The physician will order the catheter size when ordering the catheterization procedure. Urethral catheters, sometimes called straight catheters, are used when the catheter is removed after the procedure. The Foley catheter is used when the catheter will remain in the urinary bladder (indwelling catheter). A suprapubic catheter (indwelling) is a surgical procedure. An incision is made in the suprapubic area. The bladder empties through the catheter. Sterile, disposable catheterization kits are available that contain all necessary items to perform the procedure. See Figure 18-4 for types of urinary catheterizations.

DIGESTIVE SYSTEM

The gastrointestinal system performs the following five functions:

1. **Ingestion** (taking in) of food and breaking it into smaller particles
2. Passage of food through the digestive system (peristalsis)
3. Digestion through secretions of digestive enzymes
4. Absorption of nutrients into the bloodstream
5. Defecation of the solid waste products of digestion

When any of these functions is hindered, the digestive system malfunctions.

The digestive process begins in the mouth and concludes at the anus. As food passes through the **alimentary canal** (gastrointestinal tract), or digestive tract, it is mixed with gastric juices and enzymes, allowing it to break down into smaller nutrients, which allows absorption through the walls of the small intestine. Contents that have not been absorbed travel through the large intestine and are excreted through the anus. See Tables 18-4 and 18-5 for the common tests, procedures, disorders, and conditions of the digestive system. Figure 18-5 shows the major organs of the digestive system.

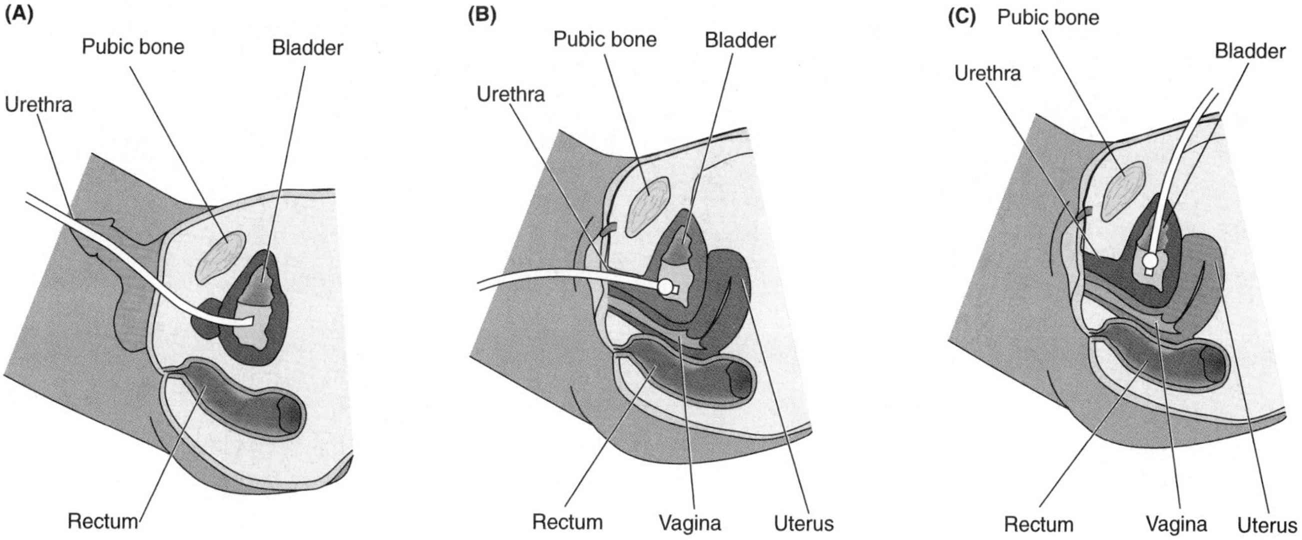

Figure 18-4 Types of urinary catheterizations: (A) straight catheter; (B) indwelling catheter; and (C) suprapubic catheter.

TABLE 18-4 DIGESTIVE SYSTEM DISORDERS

Disease/ Disorder	Laboratory Diagnostic Tests			Radiography	Surgery	Medical Tests or Procedures	Treatment
	Blood	Urine	Other				
Anorexia nervosa	• Complete blood count • Electrolytes • Blood glucose	• Urinalysis				• Electro-cardiography	• Replacement of fluids and electrolytes if needed • Psychiatric care
Appendicitis	• Complete blood count	• Urinalysis • Pregnancy test		• Abdominal ultrasound		• Rectal examination	• Appendectomy
Bulimia	• Complete blood count • Electrolytes	• Urinalysis				• Electro-cardiography	• Replacement of fluids and electrolytes if needed • Care of esophagus erosion • Psychiatric care
Cholecystitis	• Complete blood count • Serum bilirubin	• Urinalysis		• Cholecysto-gram (oral or intravenous) • Ultrasound of gall bladder			• Cholecystectomy
Cholelithiasis	• Complete blood count • Serum bilirubin			• Radioisotope scan • Ultrasound of gall bladder • Intravenous cholangiogram			• Cholecystectomy • Asymptomatic—no treatment other than diet modification (low-fat diet)
Colon cancer	• Complete blood count • Electrolytes			• Barium enema • Abdominal ultrasound • Computed tomography (CT) scan of abdomen	• Biopsy of colon	• Sigmoid-oscopy • Colonoscopy	• Colectomy • Resection of colon • Radiation • Chemotherapy
Crohn's disease	• Complete blood count • Electrolytes			• Abdominal ultrasound • Barium enema • Abdominal flat plate	• Biopsy of colon	• Sigmoid-oscopy • Colonoscopy • Stool culture	• Nutritional support • Medication (antibiotics, antiinflammatories) • Surgery of affected por-tion of colon (resection)
Diverticulitis	• Complete blood count • Erythrocyte sedimentation rate			• Barium enema • Abdominal flat plate		• Sigmoid-oscopy • Colonoscopy	• Antibiotics • Surgery if bowel perforates (colectomy)
Drug-induced ulcer	• Complete blood count • Electrolytes		• Guaiac test	• Upper gastrointestinal series	• Biopsy of stomach	• Gastroscopy	Cessation of: • Aspirin • Antiinflammatory drugs (Ibuprofen, Naproxen, etc.) • Corticosteroids • Iron • Methotrexate Treatments • Histamine H_2 blocking agents (Pepcid, Prilosec, Tagamet, Zantac)
Duodenal ulcer	• Complete blood count		• Breath test • H. pylori • Occult blood test	• Upper gastrointestinal series	• Biopsy duodenum	• Upper endoscopy	• Medication: gastric secretion–blocking agent antibiotics • Lifestyle changes • Small, frequent meals • Gastrectomy if perforation

(continues)

TABLE 18-4 DIGESTIVE SYSTEM DISORDERS (continued)

Disease/ Disorder	Laboratory Diagnostic Tests						
	Blood	Urine	Other	Radiography	Surgery	Medical Tests or Procedures	Treatment
Enterobiasis	• Complete blood count		• Stool sample for ova and parasites			• Perianal examination	
Gastric ulcer	• Complete blood count • Serum albumin • Transferrin		• Guaiac test • H. pylori • Culture stomach secretions • Breath test	• Upper gastrointestinal series • Abdominal radiographs	• Biopsy stomach lining	• Upper endoscopy	• Medication: gastric secretion–blocking agent antibiotics • Lifestyle changes • Small, frequent meals • Gastrectomy if perforation
Gastroenteritis	• Complete blood count • Electrolytes		• Stool culture	• Upper gastrointestinal series		• Upper endoscopy	• Usually self-limiting • Maintain electrolyte balance • Antibiotics if indicated • Infection control
Gastritis	• Complete blood count		• Samples of gastric content	• Upper gastrointestinal series	• Biopsy of stomach	• Gastroscopy	• Antacid medications (Prilosec, Tagamet, Zantac) • Antibiotics if needed
Gastroesophageal reflux disease				• Esophageal ultrasonography • Gastroscopy		• Esophageal manometry	• Medication • Diet modification • Weight loss
Hemorrhoids	• Complete blood count				• Hemorrhoidectomy	• Physical examination • Proctoscopy	• Hemorrhoidectomy • Ligation • Cryosurgery
Hepatitis	• Protein • Bilirubin • Liver functions • Alkaline phosphatase • Gammaglobulin	• Urinalysis		• Ultrasonography of liver	• Liver biopsy	• Liver scan	Hepatitis A • Immunoglobulin Hepatitis B • No specific treatment Hepatitis C • Medication (alpha-interferon; ribavirin)
Hiatal hernia			• pH studies of gastric secretions	• Upper gastrointestinal series • Chest radiograph	• Biopsy	• Gastroscopy	• Elevate head of bed for sleep • Antacids (Prilosec, Tagamet, Zantac) • Avoid foods that irritate stomach and esophagus • Avoid overeating (see Figure 18-6)
Pancreatitis	• Serum amylase • Complete blood count • Erythrocyte sedimentation rate			• Ultrasonography • Computerized axial tomography scan • Endoscopic retrograde cholangiopancreatography			• Analgesics • Diet modification
Pancreatic cancer	• Complete blood count			• Ultrasonography • Computerized axial tomography scan • Endoscopic retrograde cholangiopancreatography		• Percutaneous needle aspiration biopsy	• Surgical resection (if possible) • Radiation therapy • Chemotherapy

TABLE 18-5 DESCRIPTION OF DIGESTIVE DISORDERS AND CONDITIONS

- *Anorexia nervosa.* An eating disorder of psychological origin. The individual does not eat and becomes **emaciated** (extremely thin) and malnourished because of the need to avoid weight gain.
- *Appendicitis.* Acute inflammation of the appendix usually caused by infection or obstruction. Characterized by pain, nausea, vomiting, and fever.
- *Bulimia.* A syndrome in which an individual binges on food and then purges by inducing vomiting. Laxative abuse is common. The reason individuals engage in this behavior is to avoid weight gain; it is of psychological origin.
- *Cholecystitis.* Inflammation of the gallbladder. Usual cause is gall stones, but other causes may be bacteria or chemical irritants.
- *Colon cancer.* Common malignancy characterized by change in bowel habits, diarrhea or constipation, and abdominal discomfort as tumor grows.
- *Crohn's disease.* Chronic disease that exhibits inflammation of the ileum resulting in diarrhea, right lower quadrant pain, and attacks of diarrhea and frequent blood in the stools.
- *Diverticulitis.* Inflammation of diverticula usually caused by impacted feces or bacteria in the sacs. Pain, cramplike, usually in left side of abdomen. Obstruction can develop.
- *Diverticulosis.* Diverticula in colon without symptoms.
- *Drug-induced ulcers.* Ulcers of the stomach or duodenum caused by taking salicylates (aspirin), corticosteroids, antiinflammatory medications (ibuprofen, naproxen), iron, and Methotrexate.
- *Duodenal ulcer.* Lesion in the mucous membrane of the small intestine usually caused by hyperacidity or *Helicobacter pylori*.
- *Enterobiasis (pinworms).* Intestinal parasites causing intestinal and rectal infection. Pruritis of the anus is a symptom.
- *Gastric ulcer.* Caused by bacteria *H. pylori*, salicylates, smoking, and alcohol.
- *Gastroenteritis.* Inflammation of the stomach and intestinal tract. Causes nausea, vomiting, and diarrhea. May be caused by ingestion of pathogen.
- *Gastritis.* Inflammation of the stomach lining usually caused by an undefined irritant including alcohol, bacteria, or viruses. It can result in stomach discomfort, nausea, or vomiting.
- *Gastroesophageal reflux disease (GERD).* A small valve in the lower esophagus (between the stomach and esophagus) leaks causing stomach acid to back up from the stomach to the esophagus. There is frequent heartburn and discomfort behind the sternum.
- *Hepatitis.* Inflammation of the liver caused by infection from a virus resulting in hepatomegaly, anorexia, and jaundice.
  - *Hepatitis A.* Spread by fecal contamination of food or water.
  - *Hepatitis B.* Spread by blood and body fluids contamination through sexual contact, contaminated needles, perinatal fluids, semen.
  - *Hepatitis C.* Spread by blood (i.e., transfusion), contaminated needles, and sexual contact.

  Refer to Chapter 10 for more information about hepatitis.
- *Hiatal hernia.* Congenital or traumatic protrusion of stomach through the diaphragm into the chest cavity (Figure 18-6).
- *Pancreatitis (acute and chronic).* Inflammation of the pancreas. Acute: can be a life-threatening event; pancreatic enzymes begin to digest the pancreas causing necrosis and hemorrhage. Chronic: a slow, progressive destruction of the pancreas thought to be from enzymes digesting the pancreas as seen in acute pancreatitis. May be idiopathic or related to alcoholism. Diabetes can be a complication of pancreatitis.
- *Pancreatic cancer.* Cancer of the pancreas (usually the head). One of the leading causes of cancer deaths in the United States. Most commonly seen in the 60- to 70-year age group.

Signs and Symptoms of Digestive Conditions and Disorders

Common signs and symptoms of disorders and diseases of the digestive tract include nausea, vomiting, stomach cramping, diarrhea, heartburn, loss of appetite, weight loss, indigestion, fatigue, **hematemesis** (vomiting blood), **melena** (blood in feces), and **hematochezia** (bright red blood in feces).

There are many disorders and diseases of the digestive tract that can cause these signs and symptoms. Gastritis, a common ailment of the stomach, can be caused by caffeine, aspirin and other medication, spicy foods, and alcohol, and is characterized by epigastric pain, nausea, and vomiting of blood (hematemesis). Gastroenteritis, inflammation of the stomach and small intestine, another common ailment, is also known as food poisoning, intestinal flu, or traveler's diarrhea. It can be caused by infections from contaminated food or water, drug reactions, and allergic reactions to particular foods. Peptic ulcers found in the stomach are called gastric ulcers and can be caused by the action of pepsin, an enzyme. It is an **erosion** (eating away of tissue) of the mucous lining of the stomach. **Salicylates** (such as aspirin), alcohol, smoking, oversecretion of hydrochloric acid, and stress seem to be implicated in this disease. Some gastric ulcers may be caused by the bacteria *Helicobacter pylori* and require antibiotic treatment. Ulcers found in the duodenum are

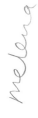

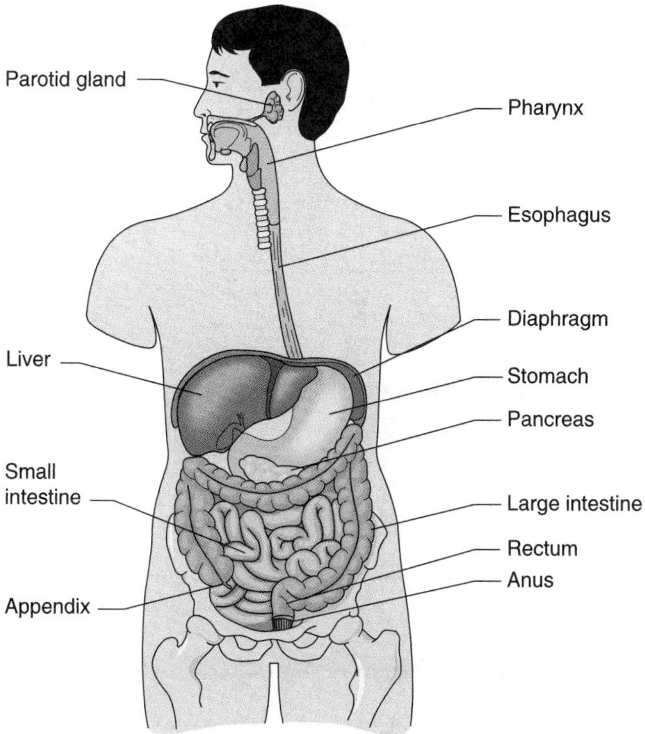

Figure 18-5 The digestive system.

called duodenal ulcers and are similar to gastric ulcers. A duodenal ulcer is an erosion of the mucous lining of the duodenum, a part of the small intestine. If determined that the ulcer is caused by the bacteria, antibiotics will be prescribed. Both types of ulcers seem to run a chronic

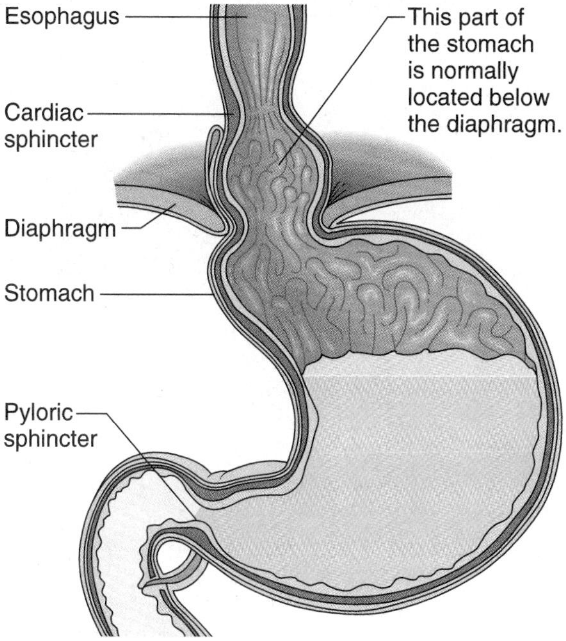

Figure 18-6 Hiatal hernia.

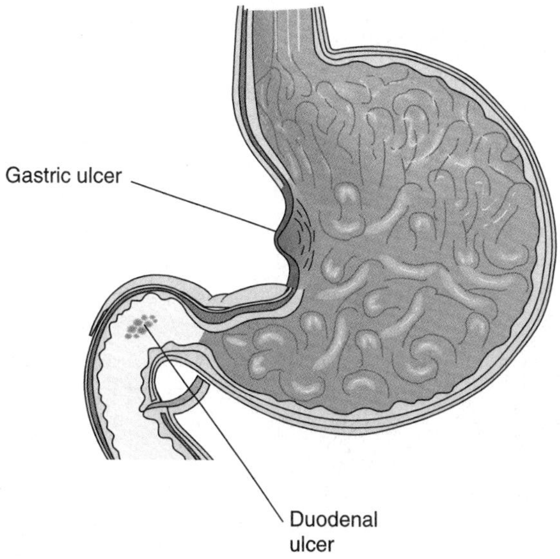

Figure 18-7 Peptic ulcers.

course, and if they are not controlled, the ulcerated area can **perforate** (a hole caused by ulceration) and hemorrhage ensues. Contents of the stomach or intestine can spill out into the abdominal cavity and cause a serious complication called **peritonitis** (infectious organisms enter the membrane covering the internal organs). See Figures 18-7 and 18-8.

Diarrhea is characterized by frequent liquid bowel movements. Diarrhea and vomiting may have many causes such as allergic reactions, infections from food or water, or from stress. Dehydration can become a problem if diarrhea continues for several days. Infants, children, and older adults are especially vulnerable to dehydration from vomiting and diarrhea.

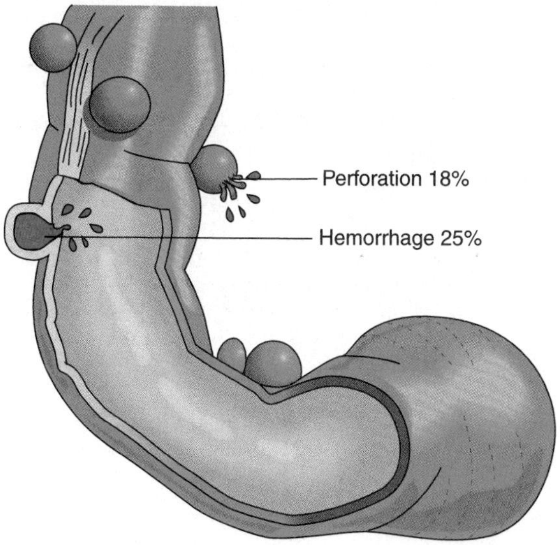

Figure 18-8 Diverticulosis.

Diagnostic Tests

Diagnostic tests for the digestive system commonly include radiography and **endoscopy** (viewing within the body with a lighted scope). An upper gastrointestinal (GI) series (barium swallow) is done to visualize the esophagus, stomach, and upper portion of the small intestine. A lower GI series (barium enema) will visualize the large intestine. See Figures 18-9 and 18-10, and Chapter 20.

Endoscopy allows the physician to look directly into the digestive organs with a lighted scope. Some examples of endoscopies used in the digestive tract are named by the organ being scoped:

stomach: gastroscopy
colon: colonoscopy
sigmoid colon: sigmoidoscopy
entire upper GI area: esophagogastroduodenoscopy (EGD; Figure 18-11)

Biopsies can be taken during an endoscopic procedure.

Sigmoidoscopy. Sigmoidoscopy is a diagnostic examination of the interior of the sigmoid colon. It is a useful aid in the diagnosis of cancer of the colon, ulcerations, polyps, tumors, bleeding, and other lower intestinal disorders. The sigmoidoscope is a metal or plastic (disposable) instrument with a light source and a magnifying lens, which permits the mucous membrane of the sigmoid colon to be seen.

The rigid metal and plastic types of scopes are used in some offices (Figure 18-12). An **obturator** (a tool used to obstruct a cavity) is inserted into the sigmoidoscope. The tip of the obturator and scope are lubricated and carefully inserted into the rectum. Then the obturator is

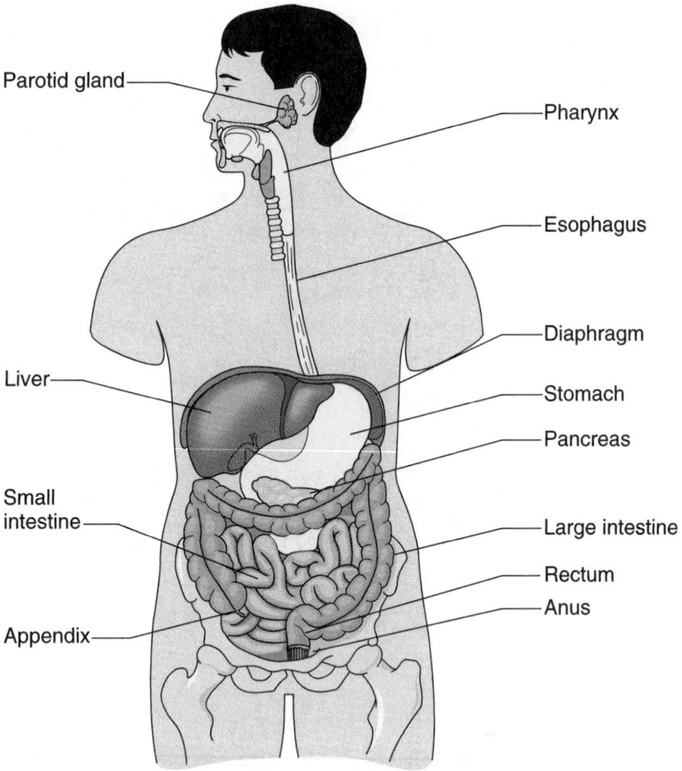

Figure 18-10 Upper gastrointestinal series; highlighted area is visualized.

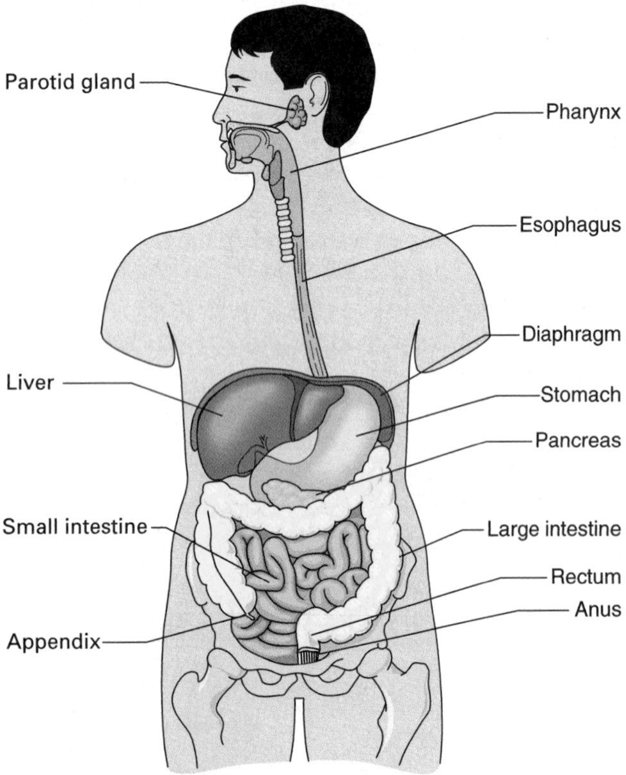

Figure 18-9 Lower gastrointestinal series; highlighted area is visualized.

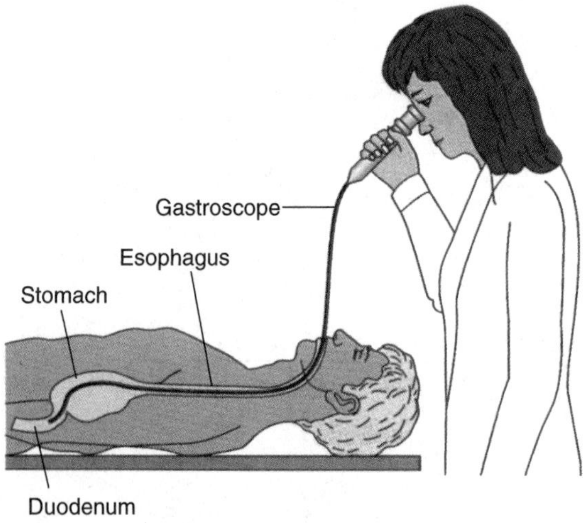

Figure 18-11 Esophagogastroduodenoscopy procedure.

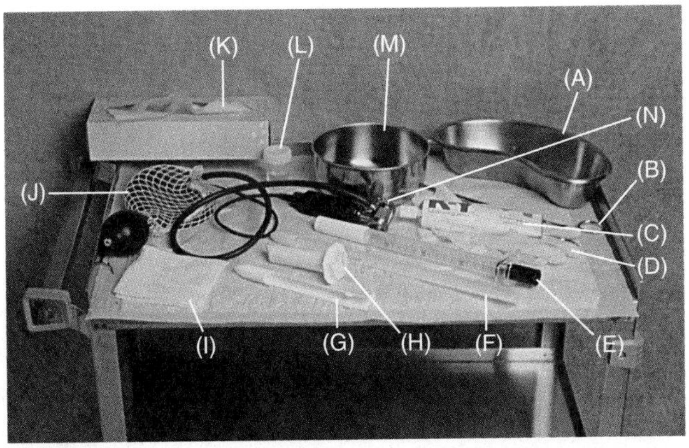

Figure 18-12 Setup for a proctosigmoidoscopy with a rigid sigmoidoscope and anoscope. (A) Kidney basin. (B) Sponge forceps. (C) Lubricant. (D) Gloves. (E) Disposable rigid sigmoidoscope. (F) Obturator for sigmoidoscope. (G) Obturator for anoscope. (H) Anoscope. (I) Gauze sponges. (J) Insufflator. (K) Tissues. (L) Biopsy container. (M) Basin of water. (N) Magnifying lens.

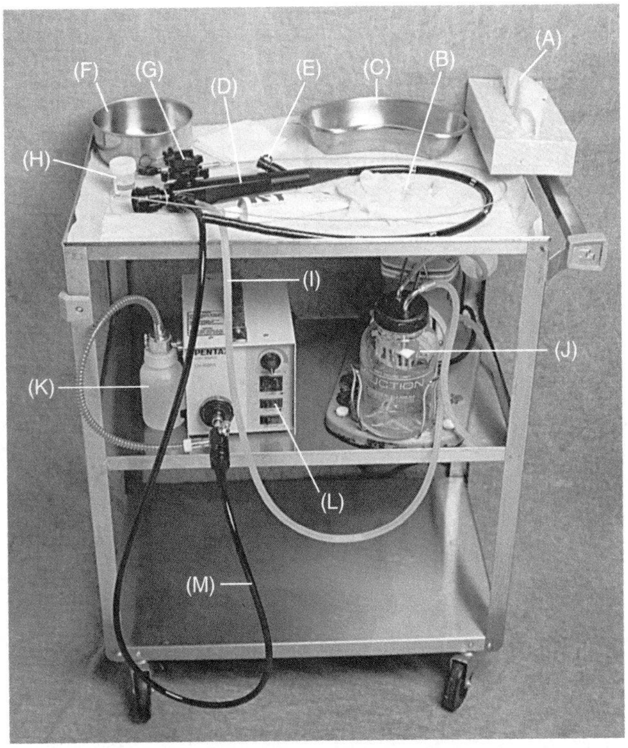

Figure 18-13 Setup for a proctosigmoidoscopy with a flexible sigmoidoscope. (A) Tissues. (B) Gloves. (C) Kidney basin. (D) Flexible sigmoidoscope. (E) Eye lens. (F) Basin for water. (G) Control head. (H) Biology container with formalin. (I) Suction tubing. (J) Suction apparatus. (K) Water bottle. (L) Light source control panel. (M) Power cord.

removed so that the sigmoid colon can be seen. Patients find this an unpleasant procedure. More commonly used now by physicians is the flexible sigmoidoscope, which is shown assembled with items necessary for the procedure. Because it is flexible, it can be inserted farther into the colon. This instrument makes it possible to view more of the mucous membranes of the intestines (Figure 18-13).

As with any examination of the pelvic or abdominal cavity, you should advise the patient to empty the bladder and evacuate the bowel before the procedure begins. This will make the examination easier for both patient and examiner. During the procedure the patient should be instructed to breathe through the mouth deeply and slowly to relax abdominal muscles. Patients may feel the urge to defecate during a colon examination because of the stretching of the intestinal wall from the instrument passing through and air being introduced with it. If patients use the breathing technique mentioned, this discomfort can be relieved. The procedure should last only a few minutes, especially if patients have followed preparation instructions.

Air is sometimes introduced into the sigmoid colon (by the examiner's use of the inflation bulb attached to the scope with tubing) to distend the wall of the colon for easier placement of the lumen of the endoscope. Patients find this to be uncomfortable and sometimes painful. The physician may need to use suction to remove mucus, blood, or fecal material that is obstructing the view of the sigmoid colon.

Handing necessary items to the physician and giving support to the patient are the medical assistant's roles during these examinations.

It will also most often be the medical assistant who teaches the patient how to prepare for the sigmoidoscopy and explains how the test is performed. For successful examination, proper preparation is essential. In addition to having patients restrict dairy products, raw fruits and vegetables, and grains and cereals from their diet, they should be encouraged to drink plenty of clear liquids and eat lightly the day before the scheduled appointment for the sigmoid colon examination. A plain commercial enema should be self-administered at home approximately two hours before the examination. Physicians may vary the instructions according to the patient's condition. If patients are not completely informed about preparations and the examination is attempted with unsatisfactory results, it will have to be repeated, which is both costly and inconvenient. Satisfactory results are obtained by giving patients both oral and written instructions.

There are occasions, during an appointment for which the patient was "worked in" to the schedules, when the physician believes that the patient's condition warrants the examination of the sigmoid colon. In this case, the physician will order an enema to be given to the patient in the office.

It is not a common procedure to administer an enema to a patient in the medical office or clinic, but it is sometimes necessary for the successful completion of a sigmoidoscopy or other rectal examination. Even though a patient may have received proper instructions and carried them out before the scheduled appointment, there is no guarantee that the patient achieved success. In the event that the patient comes in for the appointment and the colon is not sufficiently evacuated of feces for a sigmoidoscopy, the physician may order a cleansing enema so that the examination can be completed. It is generally best to proceed with the planned procedure, even with the delay of the enema. Usually this works out well for patient and staff, because rescheduling presents difficulties for everyone.

Often the patient did follow the list of instructions but was not able to retain the enema solution long enough to get satisfactory results. You will more likely be able to encourage the patient to retain the contents of the enema longer. You may want to explain that the longer the contents are retained, the more successful the results will be. Otherwise, it may have to be repeated, or the examination rescheduled. Be certain that you use an examination room that is close to the rest room for the patient's convenience when you administer an enema. Your patience and understanding are needed, because many patients are embarrassed to have an enema administered to them.

Some examinations, such as diagnostic sigmoidoscopy and X-rays, require the use of laxatives by the patient the day before or the morning of the examination. This may present a problem in the patient's personal or employment schedule if instructions are not made clear before the appointment is scheduled. Most patients are fearful of what the diagnostic examination will disclose. Helping them choose a convenient appointment time and explaining the reasons for the preparations they must undergo is usually appreciated.

Proper positioning of the patient during the sigmoidoscopy is important for both the physician's viewing of the rectum and sigmoid colon and the patient's comfort. Proctology tables are designed especially for this procedure (Figure 18-14). They provide support of the patient's chest and head with the arm resting against the headboard as the table is tilted to the knee-chest position. Those who cannot tolerate this position are assisted into Sims' position for the examination. Many physicians

Patient Education

With the physician's direction, you may discuss the following topics with your patients about their digestive health.

1. Remind them that laxatives and enemas should only be used by direction of the physician.
2. Constipation may be avoided/relieved by including fresh fruits and vegetables, cereals, and grains in the diet; drinking plenty of liquids (water); and getting regular exercise.
3. Instruct them that if they have any of the following symptoms persistently it could mean that a disease or an abnormal condition is present and consulting the physician is strongly advised: heartburn or indigestion, nausea or vomiting (especially if coffee grounds consistency), constipation or diarrhea, excessive gas or bloating, stool that is tarry (black), or other than a normal brown color.
4. Inform patients who are 40 years and older that they should routinely test their stool for occult blood every two years for screening of cancer of the colon, or more often if advised by the physician (if family history indicates). All patients older than 50 years should test annually for occult blood and have a colonoscopy.
5. Advise patients to include high-fiber foods in their diets, avoid fat (especially saturated fats) and cholesterol, and eat red meats sparingly.
6. Urge patients to eat from a variety of foods (from the food pyramid) and to eat four to six small meals rather than one or two large meals daily to promote better utilization of nutrients and more energy.
7. Suggest to patients that it is better to select snacks and beverages wisely such as fruits, vegetables, and juices over coffee/tea/soda and high-calorie sweets or chips.

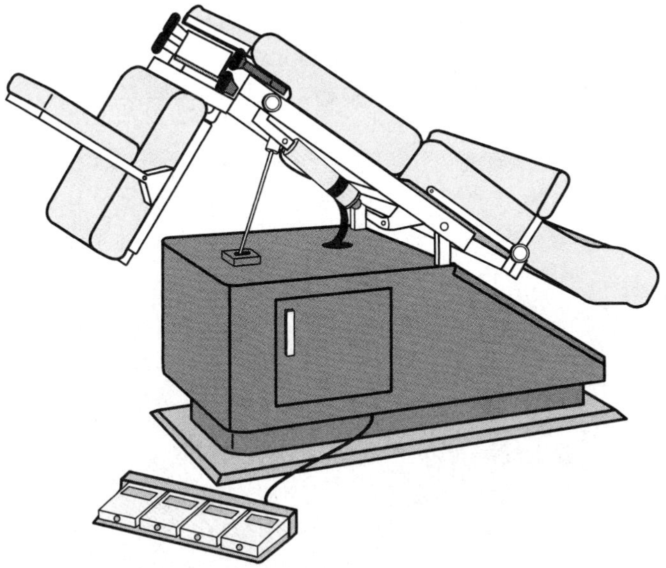

Figure 18-14 Proctologic table.

find this acceptable and it is more comfortable for the patient. You should ask about the physician's preference for patient position because there are many variations.

The physician may wish to view the intestinal mucosa after a normal bowel movement. More often, the patient is instructed to eat a light diet containing plenty of clear liquids and avoiding dairy products for 24 hours before the examination, and to have a plain cleansing enema the morning of, or two hours before, the examination. Still other physicians may wish patients to use laxatives the day before and an enema the night before and also the morning of the examination.

When making a diagnosis of hemorrhoids, fissures, and ulcerations, the physician usually begins investigative procedures by examining the anus and the interior of the rectum with a proctoscope. During the sigmoidoscopy, the physician may want to take a biopsy of questionable tissue from the sigmoid colon to aid in confirming the diagnosis. It is a good rule to have all possible necessary items available. When the patient has been prepared and the physician is ready to begin the examination, the medical assistant hands the necessary instruments and supplies to the physician as needed. Remember to advise patients to report any problems, such as bleeding, discharge, swelling, or any other unusual discomfort after the procedure. A biopsy laboratory request form must be completed and accompany the tissue to the laboratory. Containers for biopsy specimens have a formaldehyde solution to preserve the tissue until the analysis is done.

Whereas the proctosigmoidoscope examines the rectum and sigmoid colon with either a flexible or rigid scope, a procedure known as a **colonoscopy** (viewing the colon with a lighted scope) can be scheduled in the outpatient department of the hospital or endoscopy center or performed in the office or clinic. A flexible fiberoptic colonoscope is used, and the entire length of the large intestine (colon) can be examined for lesions such as tumors, polyps, fissures, and so on. Biopsies that consist of small tissue pieces can be removed with a snare-type instrument inserted through the colonoscope. The tissue is microscopically examined by a pathologist to determine whether a malignancy is present in the colon. The patient may receive a muscle relaxant/tranquilizer to facilitate the examination. (See "Endoscopic Procedures" later in this chapter.)

Patient Education

After sigmoidoscopy, patients should drink plenty of clear fluids to help relieve the usual abdominal discomfort and flatulence. Patients may also find relief in lying in a prone position with a pillow across their midabdominal area to aid in the passage of gas.

Fecal Occult Blood Test

Patients may be instructed to obtain three stool specimens at home to allow examination of a fecal sample for occult (hidden) blood. Occult blood slides, applicators, and envelopes will be given to the patient to take home (Figure 18-15). The patient will need to obtain two small stool samples from each of three separate bowel movements. Three separate samples are used to allow detection of blood from GI lesions that exhibit intermittent bleeding. The medical assistant's role is to instruct the patient about how to properly collect the stool specimens on the test slides, and then how to care and store the slides until they are returned to the office (see Procedure 18-4).

Critical Thinking

Phyllis Lomeli, a new patient of Dr. Reynolds, has been experiencing gastrointestinal problems. Dr. Reynolds has ordered fecal occult blood tests for the patient. What diet instructions does the medical assistant give to the patient? What directions and supplies does the medical assistant give to the patient? When the guaiac slides are returned, how does the medical assistant develop and interpret them?

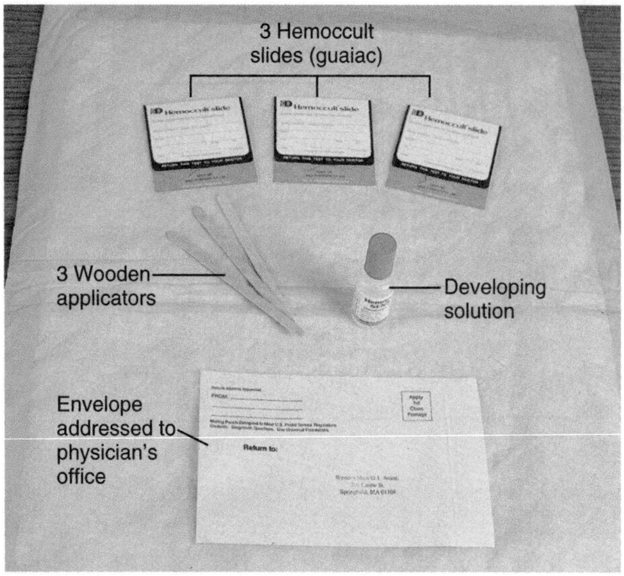

Figure 18-15 Supplies needed for the hemoccult test for fecal occult blood. The patient will take all supplies home except the developing solution.

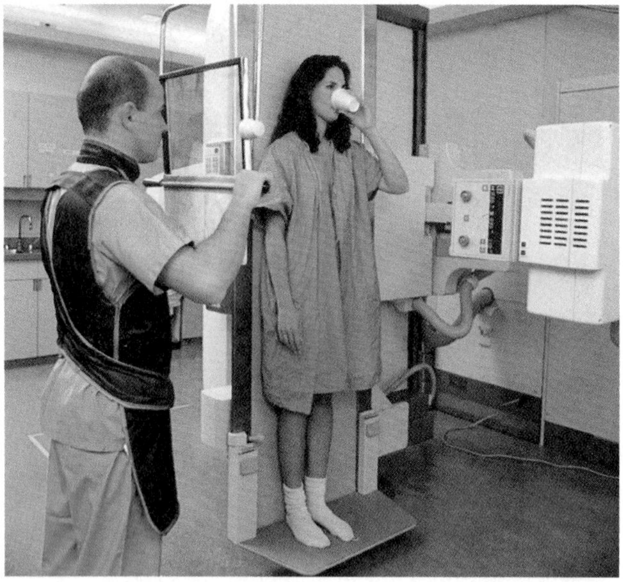

Figure 18-16 In a barium swallow test, barium sulfate is swallowed and radiographs are taken of the esophagus, stomach, and small intestine. This is also known as an upper gastrointestinal series.

Patient Education

Follow specific package instructions

The following steps should be followed two days before the fecal occult blood test and continued until three slides have been prepared:

1. Avoid red meats, processed meats, and liver. These release hemoglobin that can produce a false-positive result.
2. Avoid turnips, broccoli, cauliflower, and melons. These foods may contain a substance, peroxibase, that will cause a false-positive result.
3. Avoid aspirin, iron supplements, and large doses of vitamin C for seven days before the test. These substances may cause gastric bleeding that can mask bleeding from a lesion.
4. Consume a high-fiber diet. Fiber provides roughage to promote bowel movement and encourage bleeding from any lesion that may be present.
5. Do not begin test during menses, for three days after menses, or if bleeding from hemorrhoids.
6. Drink plenty of fluids to help avoid constipation.
7. Store slides at room temperature and protect from heat, sun, and fluorescent lights.

For patients who have daily bowel movements, this will not be a problem. For patients who have difficulty with daily elimination, it may take several days to collect the samples. Patients should not use laxatives unless directed by the physician.

Positive tests for occult blood require further testing, because occult blood testing is a screening tool only. Sigmoidoscopy and colonoscopy help to identify the source of bleeding. If a lesion is found either in the rectum or colon, a biopsy can be performed and sent to the laboratory for examination of cells for malignancy (see Procedure 18-4).

Radiographic Studies of the Digestive System. There are several diagnostic radiographic studies that can be performed to study digestive structures and functions for disease. They include the upper GI series (barium swallow) (Figure 18-16), lower GI series (barium enema), and the cholecystogram. Table 18-6 presents the purpose, patient preparation, and procedures for each of these studies.

TABLE 18-6 PATIENT PREPARATION AND PROCEDURE FOR RADIOGRAPHIC STUDIES OF THE DIGESTIVE SYSTEM

Test	Purpose	Patient Prep	Procedure	Time
Barium swallow (upper gastrointestinal [GI] series)	To study the esophagus, stomach, duodenum, and small intestine for disease (ulcers, tumors, hiatal hernia, esophageal varices)	Day before radiograph: 1. Light evening meal 2. NPO after midnight Day of test: 1. NPO Postprocedural: 1. Increase fluid intake 2. Take laxative as prescribed	1. The patient is asked to drink a flavored barium mixture while standing in front of the fluoroscope. 2. The radiologist observes the passage down the digestive tract 3. The patient is turned to various positions to allow good visualization of the intestine 4. Radiographs are taken	One hour
Barium enema (lower GI series)	To study the colon for disease (polyps, tumors, lesions)	Clear liquid one day prior (allowed: non-carbonated beverages, clear gelatin, clear broth, coffee and tea with sugar) No milk or milk products 8 oz water every hour until bedtime Prep kit: to include bottle of magnesium citrate, Dulcolax tab(s) Day before radiograph: 1. Late afternoon drink bottle of magnesium citrate 2. Early evening take Dulcolax tab(s) as prescribed 3. Light evening meal. NPO except water, after dinner Morning of procedure: 1. NPO 2. Cleaning enema Postprocedural instructions: 1. Increase fluid intake and dietary fiber 2. Report to physician if no bowel movement within 24 hours of test	1. The colon is filled with a barium sulfate mixture 2. The patient is turned in various positions to allow the barium to fill the colon. Air is injected to move the barium along the colon 3. When the colon is full, radiographs are taken	One to two hours
Cholecystogram	To study the gallbladder for disease (stones, duct obstruction), inflammation	1. Evening before test fat-free dinner 2. Patient takes dye tablets with 8 oz water 3. Cathartic or cleansing enemas may be prescribed 4. NPO after dinner and tablets	1. A series of radiographs is taken 2. A fatty meal may be given to stimulate the gallbladder to empty 3. Other radiographs can then be taken to check gallbladder function	One hour

SENSORY SYSTEM

The special senses of vision, hearing, **equilibrium** (balance), smell, touch, and taste permit the body to detect information about the environment. The eyes, ears, nose, taste buds, and skin are all sense organs that contain specialized receptor organs. See Table 18-7 for diseases and disorders and diagnostic tests and procedures for eyes and ears.

The Eye

The eye is the primary organ for sight and is one of the few organs of the body externally exposed. Its accessory structures—the eyelids, eyelashes, lacrimal ducts, and extrinsic muscles—provide protection for the eye. The anterior portion of the eyeball protrudes outward and the remainder is protected by the orbit.

The intraocular structures consist of some parts of the eye visible externally and parts visible only through an ophthalmoscope. The intraocular structures include the following:

- Sclera: white area covering the outside of the eye except over the pupil and iris
- Cornea: clear tissue covering the pupil and iris
- Iris: round disk of smooth and radial muscles giving the eye its color.

TABLE 18-7 SENSORY SYSTEM DISORDERS

	Laboratory Diagnostic Tests					
Disease/ Disorder	**Blood**	**Other**	**Radiography**	**Surgery**	**Medical Tests or Procedures**	**Treatment**
Amblyopia					• Ophthalmologic examination	• Cover the normal eye to force weaker eye to function
Cataract					• Ophthalmologic examination • Slit lamp	• **Phaco-emulsification** • Surgical extraction
Chalazion				• Excision		
Color blindness					• Ishihara color plates	
Conjunctivitis		• Culture and sensitivity of eye discharge		• Stained smears of conjunctival scrapings		• Antibiotic drops or by mouth • Ointment
Corneal abrasion					• Fluorescein stain	• Antibiotic ointment, dressing over affected eye
Diabetic retinopathy				• Laser	• Fluorescein • Angiogram	• Laser
Epistaxis	• Complete blood count			• Nasal	• Blood pressure cauterization	• Electrocautery
External otitis	• Complete blood count	• Culture and sensitivity of exudate			• Otologic examination	• Drug therapy • Laser (if severe)
Glaucoma					• Vision field testing • Ophthalmologic examination including intraocular pressure	• Dialysis • Kidney transplant
Impacted cerumen					• Otologic examination	• Removal with curette • Irrigation
Macular degeneration					• Ophthalmologic examination • **Amsler grid**	• Laser • Some untreatable
Ménière's disease					• Audiometry, magnetic resonance imaging	• Medication, surgery only if severe
Motion sickness						• Medication
Myopia					• Ophthalmologic examination	• Radial keratotomy
Nystagmus					• **Opticokinetic drum test** • Neurologic examination	• Directed at cause (inner ear or center nervous system
Hyperopia					• Astigmatoscopy	• Corrective lenses
Presbyopia					• Snellen chart	• Corrective lenses
Astigmatism					• Jaeger chart	• Corrective lenses
Nasal polyps				• Biopsy of polyp (lesion)	• Nasal examination	• Electrosurgery
Otitis media	• Complete blood count	• Culture and sensitivity of exudate		• Myringotomy • Tympanostomy	• Tympanography	• Antibiotics • Myringotomy

(continues)

TABLE 18-7 SENSORY SYSTEM DISORDERS (continued)

	Laboratory Diagnostic Tests					
Disease/ Disorder	**Blood**	**Other**	**Radiography**	**Surgery**	**Medical Tests or Procedures**	**Treatment**
Otosclerosis					• Audiometry • Rinne test	• Stapedectomy
Retinal detachment				• Laser or surgery to reattach	• Ophthalmologic examination	• Laser
Sinusitis	• Complete blood count	• Culture and sensitivity of exudate	• Sinus X-rays			• Antibiotics for bacterial infection
Strabismus					• Ophthalmologic examination • Neurologic examination	• Cover the normal eye to force weaker eye to function
Stye (Hordeolum)		• Culture and sensitivity if exudate present		• Incision and drainage		• Antibiotic ointment

- Pupil: round opening in the iris that changes size as the iris reacts to light and dark
- Anterior chamber: space between cornea and iris/pupil filled with clear fluid called aqueous humor
- Posterior chamber: space between the iris and lens that is filled with aqueous humor
- Lens: clear fibers enclosed in a membrane that refract and focus light to the retina
- Posterior cavity: the space in the posterior part of the eyeball filled with thick, gelatinous material called vitreous humor
- Posterior sclera: white opaque layer covering the posterior part of the eyeball
- Choroid layer: the layer between the sclera and retina containing blood vessels
- Retina: the inside layer of the posterior part of the eye that receives the light rays (visual stimuli)

The mechanism of vision occurs after impulses leave the retina and travel through the optic nerves to the brain. At the optic chiasm, the nerve fibers cross and continue to the thalamus. These fibers synapse with other neurons that send the impulses to the right and left visual area of the occipital lobe of the brain. Because the tracts cross at the optic chasm, the stimuli coming from the right visual fields are translated in the visual area of the left occipital area, and the stimuli coming from the left visual fields are translated in the visual area of the right occipital lobe. See Table 18-8 for common eye disorders. See Figures 18-17 and 18-18 for anatomy of the eye.

TABLE 18-8 DESCRIPTION OF EYE DISORDERS

Refraction and Other Disorders:

- *Astigmatism.* Irregular lens curvature or cornea shape causing improper focusing of objects.
- *Cataract.* Lens loses its transparent nature caused by changes in its proteins. Usually brought on by aging.
- *Color blindness.* Inability to distinguish among colors. Caused by an absence of a cone photopigment, a genetic disorder.
- *Conjunctivitis.* Caused by a bacterial infection or irritant resulting in irritated and reddened conjunctiva. If caused by bacteria, conjunctivitis is highly contagious. See Figure 18-20.
- *Corneal abrasion.* Caused by an injury to the cornea by a foreign body resulting in pain, tearing, redness, and possible infection.
- *Diabetic retinopathy.* Diabetes mellitus causes damage to the retina because the disease causes vascular changes. This is the leading cause of blindness in the United States.
- *Glaucoma.* Condition caused by increased intraocular pressure due to a buildup of aqueous humor. This results in mild visual disturbances with little or no pain but can lead to blindness if untreated.
- *Nearsightedness (Myopia).* Caused by an elongated eyeball and the image is focused in the front of the retina resulting in the inability to focus on objects at a distance.
- *Farsightedness (Hyperopia).* Caused when the eyeball is shortened and the image is focused behind the retina causing distance vision to be fuzzy.
- *Presbyopia.* Attributed to the aging process when the lens loses its elasticity and the ability to accommodate. Vision is hampered when items are close.
- *Retinal detachment.* Complete or partial separation of the retina from the choroid layer of the eye, leading to blindness. See Figure 18-19.
- *Stye (hordeolum).* Inflamed sebaceous gland of the eyelid caused by bacterial infection. Erythema and tenderness at site are common symptoms. See Figure 18-21.

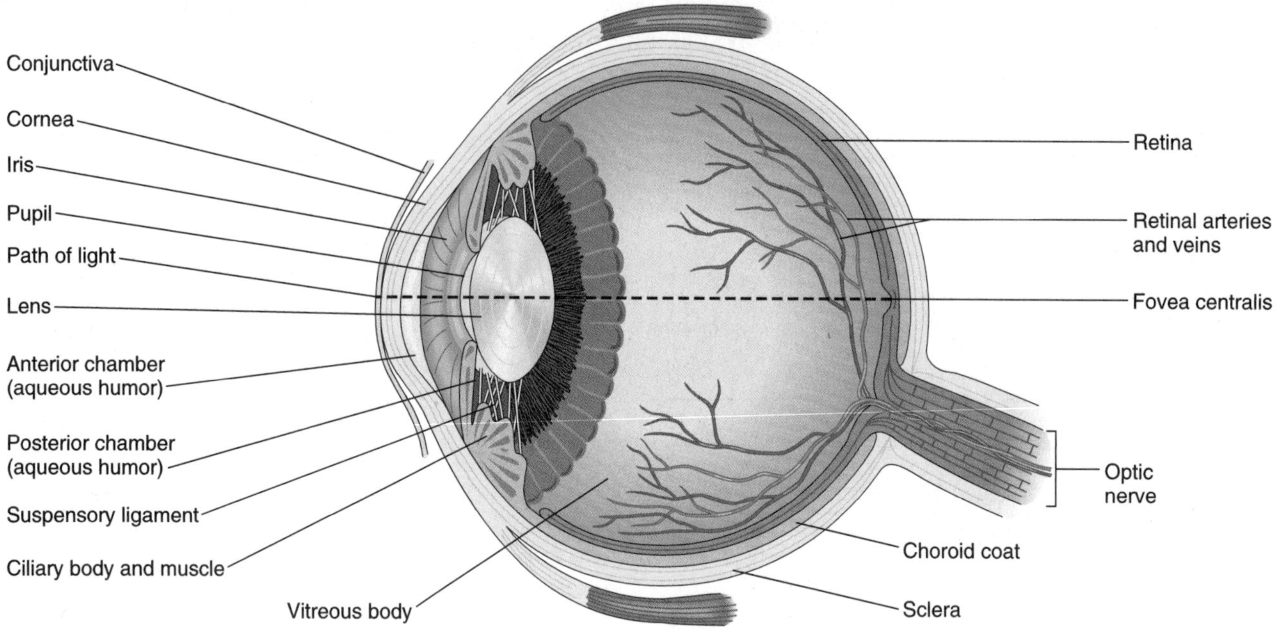

Figure 18-17 The eyeball—cross section view.

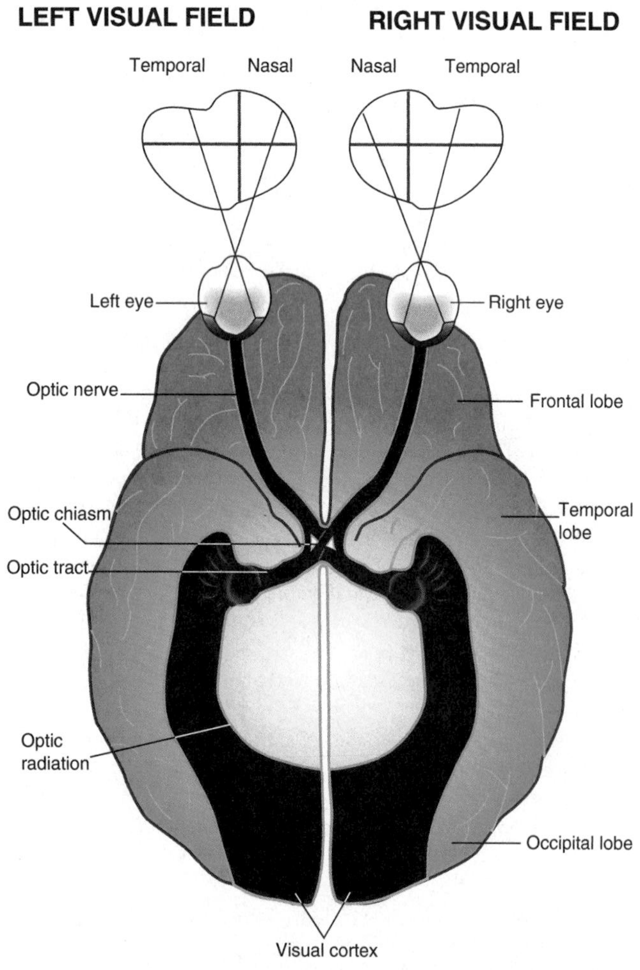

Figure 18-18 The visual pathways of the eye.

Signs and symptoms that are common to eye diseases and disorders are pain or burning in or around the eye, decreased visual acuity, and any visual changes such as seeing sudden flashes of light, which may indicate retinal detachment (Figure 18-19).

Measuring Visual Acuity. A procedure commonly performed by the medical assistant is the measuring of a patient's visual acuity. This is only a screening process used when errors in refraction are suspected. The procedure must be performed in a well-lighted, quiet area. While performing the procedure, the medical assistant must observe the patient for any action that may indicate difficulty with vision. These actions would include squinting, wiping of the eyes, or leaning toward the chart. In near-vision acuity, these actions would include holding the card nearer or farther than the stated position. The commonly used chart for distance visual acuity is the Snellen chart for the adult. Near-vision is commonly checked by using the Jaeger card.

The Jaeger chart used for checking clear vision is a small card that is held by the patient between 14 and 16 inches from the eye. The medical assistant measures the distance for accuracy. This is the distance from which a person with normal vision is able to read printed material such as a newspaper. The Jaeger test consists of a series of reading material, the letters of which gradually become smaller. Record the last line number that the patient can easily read. The patient is checked with and without corrective lenses and each eye is checked separately.

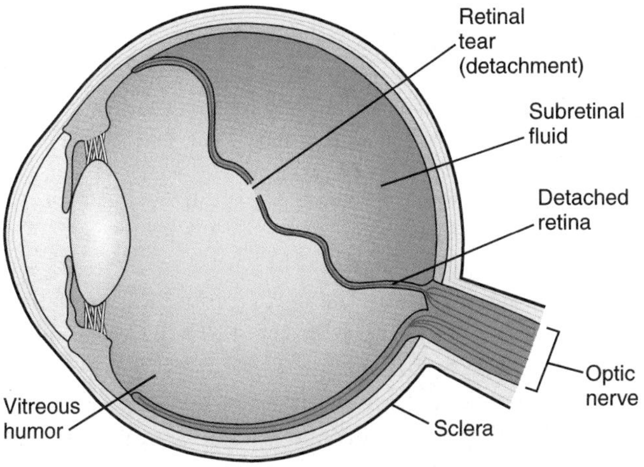

Figure 18-19 Detachment of retina.

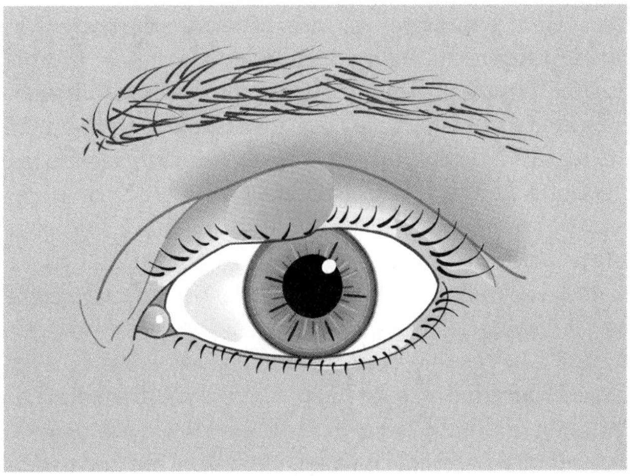

Figure 18-21 Stye (hordeolum).

Errors in refraction is the term used to designate visual acuity abnormalities. The common visual abnormalities include myopia (nearsightedness), the ability to see only near objects clearly; hyperopia (farsightedness), the ability to see only distant objects clearly; and astigmatism, uneven curvature of the cornea resulting in a scattering of light rays producing blurry vision. Presbyopia (associated with the aging process) is an increase in farsightedness and a loss of lens elasticity that is necessary to accommodate for near vision. See Figure 18-22.

The Snellen chart consists of the alphabet letters in various combinations starting at the top with a large E, and descending sized letters by line toward the bottom. Each line is labeled with the visual acuity measurement. The Snellen chart for children has pictures. Non–English-speaking patients may use a directional chart.

Recording Visual Acuity. Visual acuity, both near and far, is recorded in a fraction format. The numerator indicates the 20-foot distance between the patient and the chart. The

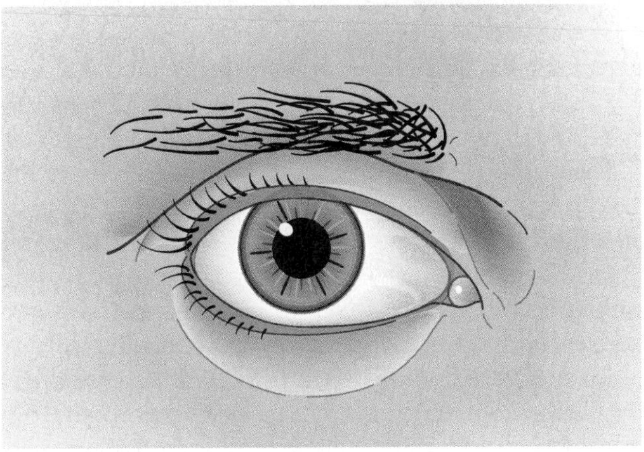

Figure 18-20 Conjunctivitis.

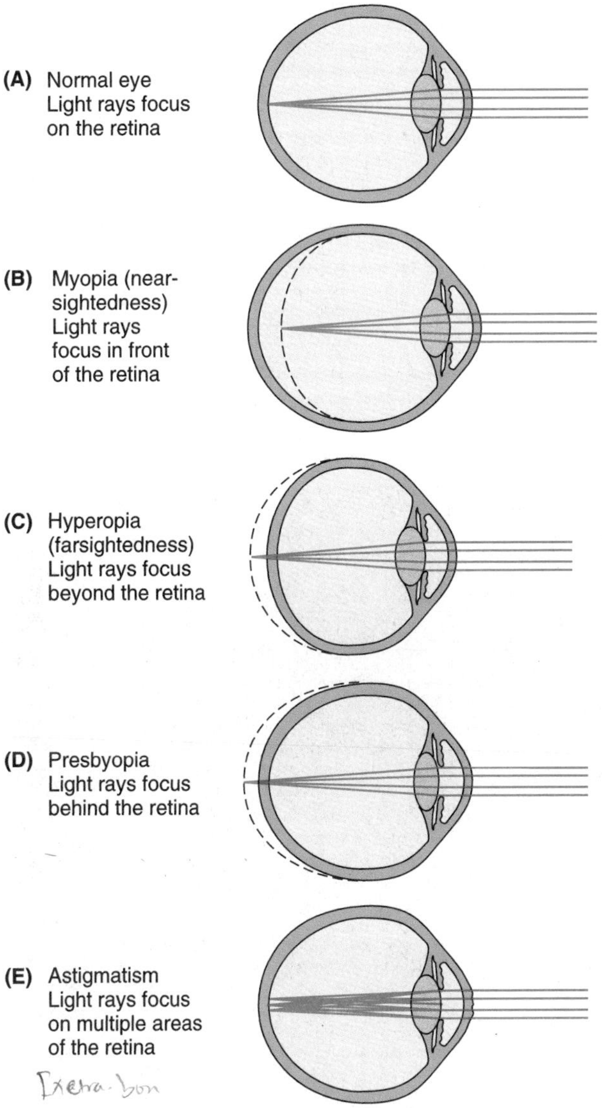

Figure 18-22 (A) Normal eye vision. (B) Myopia. (C) Hyperopia. (D) Presbyopia. (E) Astigmatism.

denominator indicates the visual acuity of the patient in relationship to the normal seeing eye. Normal vision is 20/20. This means that at 20 feet the eye is seeing what the normal eye would see at 20 feet. Should the vision be 20/30, this indicates that the eye is seeing at 20 feet what the normal eye would see at 30 feet away. A visual acuity of 20/15 indicates that the eye is seeing at 20 feet what the person with normal visual acuity would be able to see at 15 feet. Vision is recorded on the patient chart as right eye, left eye, and both eyes.

Example: Right 20/20 Left 20/20 Both 20/20

Patients should be screened with and without their corrective lenses and results recorded as such in patients' records.

Color Vision. Checking color vision is not part of a routine examination. This procedure is usually performed on people who must distinguish color as part of their occupation (e.g., truck drivers, pilots, and salespeople). A commonly used color vision test is the Ishihara color graph. The Ishihara is a book containing pages composed of varying sized and colored circles. Inside the circles are numbers or lines that can be traced. The patient is seated for the procedure with the book held 14 to 16 inches away and is instructed to identify the numbers as the page is turned or is instructed to trace the line from the indicated starting point to the end. Inability to see the number or follow the line may indicate color blindness. Should this occur, the medical assistant must inform the physician as to what number(s) could not be seen. The patient is referred to an ophthalmologist.

The medical assistant will be responsible for assisting the physician in ophthalmologic examinations and performing the tests for visual acuity. Diagnostic procedures for the special senses involve the use of specialized instruments. The use of the **ophthalmoscope** (lighted instrument used to view inside patient's eye) (Figure 18-23) assists in identifying disease-related problems. The interior of the eye can be examined.

See Procedures 18-5, 18-6, 18-7, 18-8, 18-9, and 18-10 for specialty procedures for the eye.

Critical Thinking

List the steps the medical assistant must follow when performing the visual acuity test on a 9-year-old child and a 3-year-old toddler.

The Ear

The structures of hearing and equilibrium are divided into the external ear, the middle ear, and the inner ear. The external ear includes the pinna **(auricle)** and the external auditory canal. The pinna is mostly cartilaginous tissue with a small amount of adipose tissue in the earlobe. The external auditory canal is about 1 inch in length and

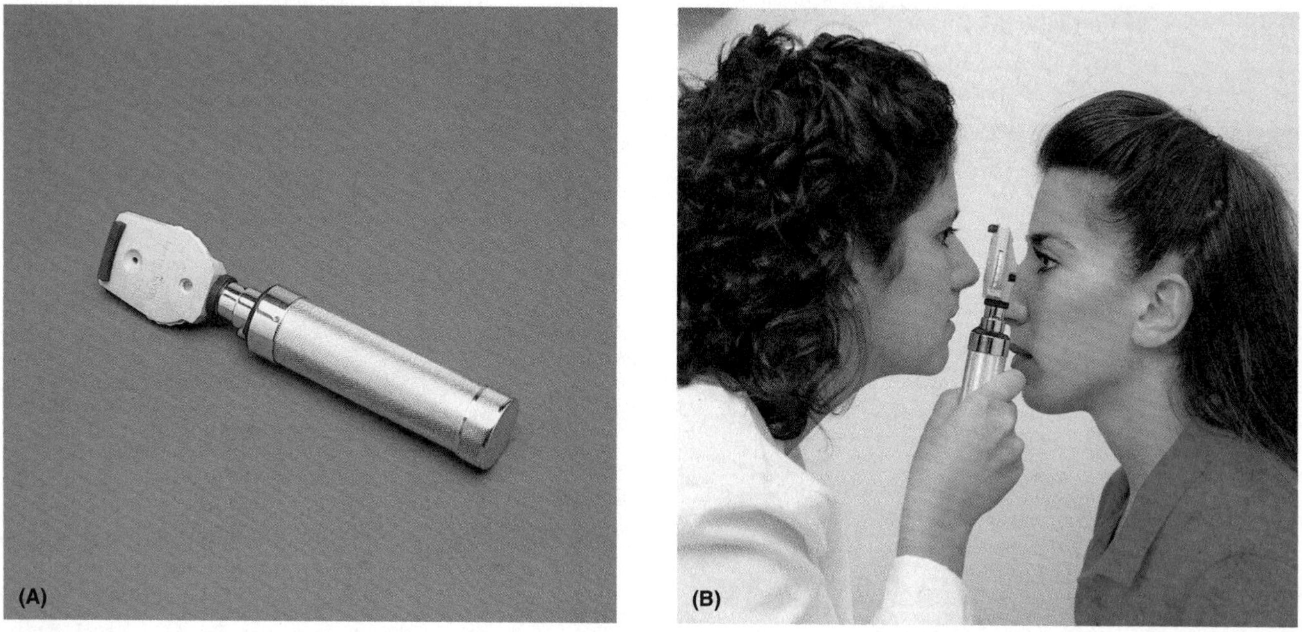

Figure 18-23 (A) The ophthalmoscope is used to identify eye disorders. (B) Here, the physician uses the ophthalmoscope to view the interior of the patient's eye.

contains hair and wax (cerumen)-producing glands. The external ear and middle ear are separated by the tympanic membrane (eardrum).

The middle ear, also called the tympanic cavity, is a small space containing three bones, the malleus (hammer), incus (anvil), and stapes (stirrup). Next to the stapes is the oval window that leads to the inner ear. The eustachian tube connects the middle ear to the throat.

The inner ear is the most sophisticated part of the ear. It is responsible for both hearing and equilibrium (balance). The inner ear consists of a fluid-filled sterile space housing the vestibule, the semicircular canals, the round window, and the cochlea. The structures in the vestibule are responsible for maintaining equilibrium during movement of the head. The semicircular canals assist the body to adjust to changes in direction. The movement of fluid in this area can cause symptoms of dizziness. The cochlea is the organ of hearing.

The outer ear (auricle/pinna) picks up sound waves that are sent through the external auditory canal to the tympanic membrane. The membrane vibrates in reaction to the sound striking it. These vibrations pass through the three tiny middle ear bones through the oval window and into the fluid in the cochlea. Receptor cells respond and transfer the sounds into electrical impulses that travel to the brain via the acoustic nerve. The receiving area of the brain for auditory impulses is in the temporal lobe. See Figure 18-24.

Diseases or conditions of the ear, if left untreated, can cause damage to nerves and tissues and can result in some degree of hearing impairment, from mild to deafness. Table 18-9 describes common diseases of the ear.

TABLE 18-9 EAR DISORDERS

- *External otitis (swimmer's ear).* Inflammation of ear canal. Symptoms are itchiness and crusting of ear canal.
- *Otitis media.* Acute infection of the middle ear usually caused by bacteria. Symptoms are pain, fever, discharge, and decreased hearing acuity.
- *Otosclerosis.* Conduction deafness caused by hardening of the stapes.
- *Ménière's disease.* Characterized by deafness, vertigo, nausea, and tinnitus. Probable cause is edema of the labyrinth.
- *Impacted cerumen.* Caused by accumulation of hardened cerumen that has built up against the tympanic membrane. Impaired hearing and tinnitus can result.

Measuring Auditory Ability. The simple methods of measuring hearing (gross hearing) are usually performed by the physician. The patient may be instructed to place a finger in one ear while the physician whispers one or two words in the other. The patient is then asked to repeat the words. A ticking watch may be placed by the patient's ear to ascertain hearing. A vibrating tuning fork may be placed on the mastoid process behind the ear and then on top of the head. The patient is asked if the sound vibrations could be heard or felt. This procedure will identify nerve or conduction deafness (Figure 18-25). Conduction deafness occurs when the sound

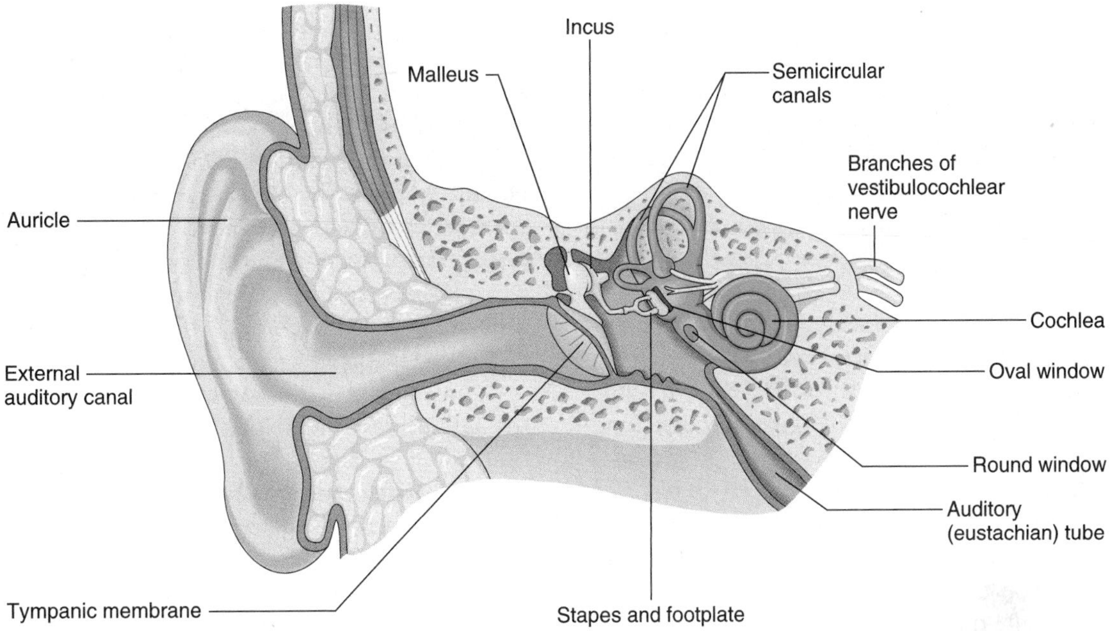

Figure 18-24 The ear.

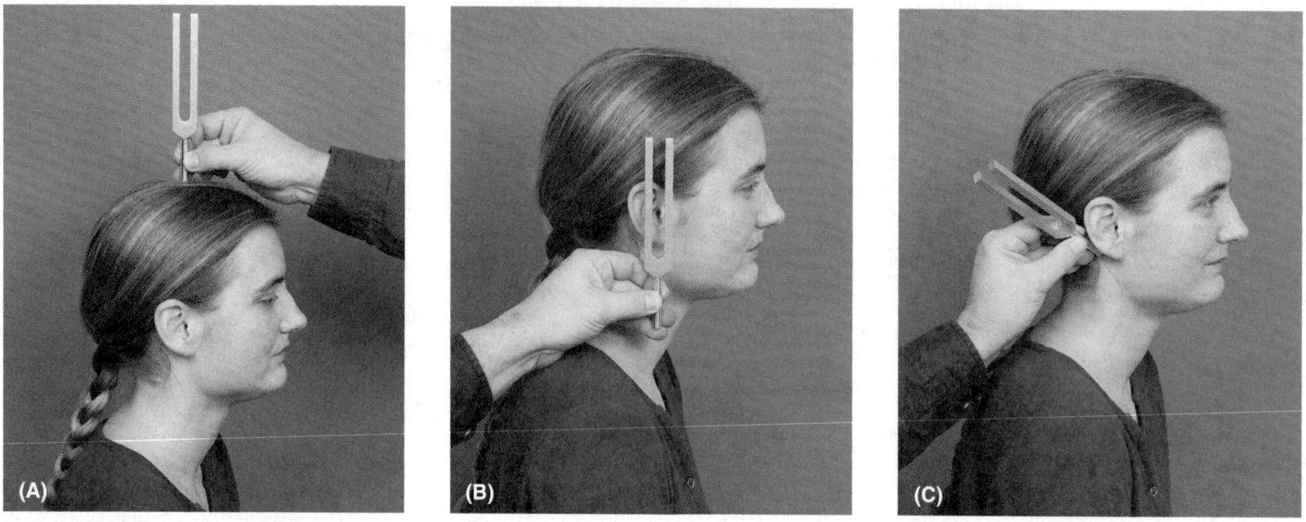

Figure 18-25 (A) The physician holds the tuning fork against the crown of the patient's head to determine which ear can hear the sound. (B) To check air conduction of sound, the physician holds the tuning fork 1 inch from the patient's auditory meatus. (C) The physician places the tuning fork on the bony prominence (mastoid bone) behind the patient's ear to check bone conduction of sound.

wave is not transmitted to the middle ear. This type of deafness may be a result of the presence of impacted ear wax (cerumen) in the ear canal or a scarred tympanic membrane.

Cerumen, or ear wax, is a substance secreted by glands at the outer third of the ear canal. In some individuals it can accumulate and block the canal and become impacted (pressed firmly against the tympanic membrane). The sound waves cannot pass through the hardened cerumen to the middle ear, and hearing loss (conduction hearing loss) results.

To remove impacted cerumen, the physician may use a curette. The patient may have had ear drops prescribed before the physical removal of the impacted cerumen. The drops are instilled in an effort to soften the cerumen to facilitate its removal. An ear irrigation may be performed by flushing the ear canal with warm water or a solution ordered by the physician. Commercial solutions are also available for patients to use at home (see Procedure 18-12).

A scarred tympanic membrane can occur from a ruptured or perforated tympanic membrane. This can occur from untreated acute otitis media or traumatic rupture. With acute otitis media, the tympanic membrane is red and bulges with serous or purulent fluid behind it. The pressure of the fluid on the tympanic membrane may be so great that the membrane ruptures and drainage can be seen in the ear canal. The perforation or rupture will probably heal, but a small scar on the membrane will remain. Repeated ruptures from acute otitis media will cause repeated scarring and diminished hearing function (conduction hearing loss). A culture and sensitivity of the drainage (purulent or serous) will indicate to which antibiotic the microorganism is sensitive.

A myringotomy is a surgical incision into the tympanic membrane to remove accumulated fluid caused by infection. Because the procedure is surgical in nature, the tympanic membrane can be incised to allow the fluid to drain. When done this way, scarring is minimized because the incision is done with a scalpel in a controlled location and will heal with less scarring. Tubes may be placed in the opening (tympanostomy) made by the myringotomy to equalize pressure and prevent fluid from accumulating. See Chapter 15.

Nerve deafness is a result of injury along the course of the nerves leading from the inner ear to the auditory centers of the brain.

A more complex procedure to measure hearing may be performed by the medical assistant, but often by an audiologist, using an audiometer. A quiet room with no distractions is required for the procedure to be accurate. The patient is seated facing away from the medical assistant and the audiometer, then ear phones are placed over the ears. The patient is instructed to raise a hand when a sound is heard. The audiometer has two dials, one for the various wavelengths and the other for wave intensity. Starting at the lowest pitch, the intensity is increased until the patient responds to the sound. The next pitch is then tested in the same manner. This process continues until the highest pitched sound is tested. The results are obtained by noting the number of intensity at which the sound was heard. When performing the procedure, the medical assistant must not develop a pattern that can be detected by the patient. The ears should be tested in an

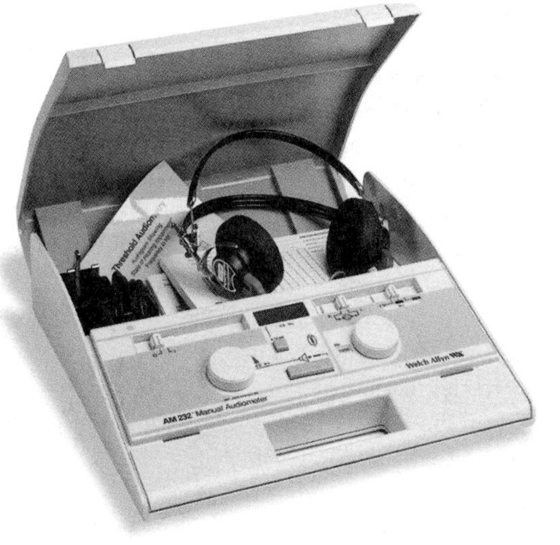

Figure 18-26 Manual audiometer.

alternating fashion to ensure accuracy. See Procedure 18-11 and Figure 18-26.

The medical assistant employed in an industrial medical facility may be required to monitor hearing of some employees. If this is the case, care must be taken to have the hearing test performed before the employee goes to work for the day. Hearing loss may result from the day's activities in some noisy facilities even when ear plugs are worn.

Tympanometry is a procedure used to ascertain the ability of the middle ear to transmit sound waves and is

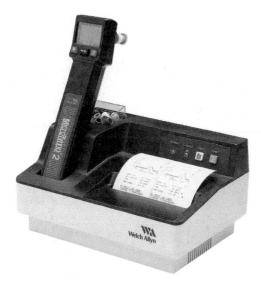

Figure 18-27 A portable tympanometric instrument shown with charger. A printout of the tympanogram can be seen. Testing is done in one second and is useful for diagnosing otitis media and other middle ear conditions such as patency of tympanostomy tubes and otosclerosis.

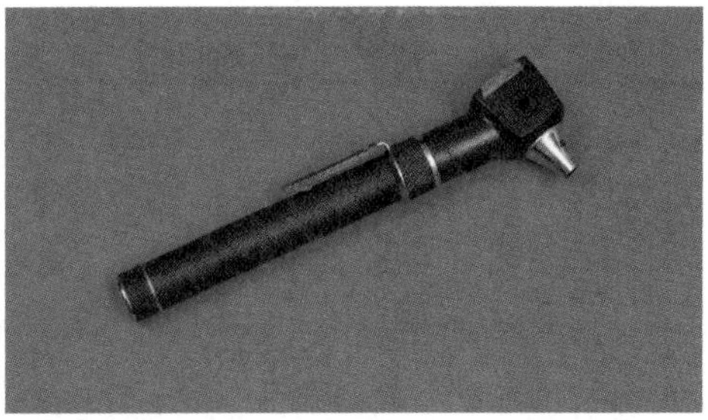

Figure 18-28 The otoscope is used to examine the patient's tympanic membrane.

commonly performed on children to diagnose middle ear infections. A probe is inserted into the ear canal to measure the air pressure of the ear canal in relation to the air pressure found in the middle ear. Tympanogram is the recording produced by this procedure. The waves and peaks are measured providing an indication of possible middle ear abnormalities (Figure 18-27).

The medical assistant or the physician may perform the audiometry test. Diagnostic procedures for the ear involve the use of specialized instruments, including the **otoscope** (lighted instrument to examine the tympanic membrane), which assists in identifying disease-related ear problems (Figure 18-28).

Procedures 18-11, 18-12, and 18-13 describe steps in audiometry and ear irrigation and instillation.

The Nose

The physician inspects the exterior surface of the patient's nose for skin lesions such as **rosacea,** squamous or basal cell carcinoma, and other dermatologic problems. The physician examines and palpates to determine if the nose is patent and for the patients ability to breathe in and out through the nose (through each nostril). The mucus membrane is checked for polyps, superficial blood vessels, or a foreign body. The septum is noted for deviation. Epistaxis is a common problem and it can be treated with electrocautery and/or nasal packing. Procedures 18-14, 18-15, and 18-16 are specialized procedures and examinations for the nose.

RESPIRATORY SYSTEM

The respiratory process is all important to the life process. **External respiration** allows for the exchange of carbon dioxide and oxygen across the cell walls into the airspaces of the lungs. **Internal respiration** is the exchange of these gases at the cellular levels of the organs.

The respiratory process begins with air entering the nose or mouth, where it passes through the pharynx, down into the trachea, into the **bronchi,** and then enters the lungs. Gas exchange takes place when the blood filters through the **alveoli** (smallest air sacs in the lungs) (Figure 18-29). See Table 18-10 for respiratory diseases and disorders and Table 18-11 for a description of respiratory disorders.

Signs and Symptoms of Respiratory Conditions and Disorders

If a patient's chief complaint indicates a respiratory condition or disorder, medical attention is essential. Some signs and symptoms include:

- Dyspnea
- Chest pain
- Fatigue
- **Hemoptysis**
- Chills and fever
- Hoarseness
- Wheezing
- Cough, productive or nonproductive

Irrigations of the nose, collection of sputum specimens, and assisting with pulmonary tests are the roles of the medical assistant.

Diagnostic Tests

A fundamental test, auscultation of the chest, is used to check for abnormalities in breathing rate and quality. Chest x-rays are useful in helping to diagnose tuberculosis (Figure 18-30), lung lesions, pneumonia, and other respiratory conditions. Cultures of sputum can help diagnose infections in the respiratory tract. Bronchoscopy is used to take a sample of lung tissues (biopsy) for help in the determination of lung cancer and for culture of lung abcesses, washing, and irrigation.

Arterial blood gases measure the amount of oxygen and carbon dioxide in the arterial blood. Higher amounts of carbon dioxide and lower amounts than normal of oxygen indicate poor lung functions.

See Procedures 18-17, 18-18, 18-19, 18-20 and 18-21 for specialized respiratory examinations and procedures.

Spirometry

The measurements of air flow, volume, and capacity are known as pulmonary function tests (PFTs). The patient's height, age, and sex are used in the PFT. Many times the physician will have the PFT performed before the administration of a **bronchodilator** and again after the bronchodilator. This is useful in evaluating the

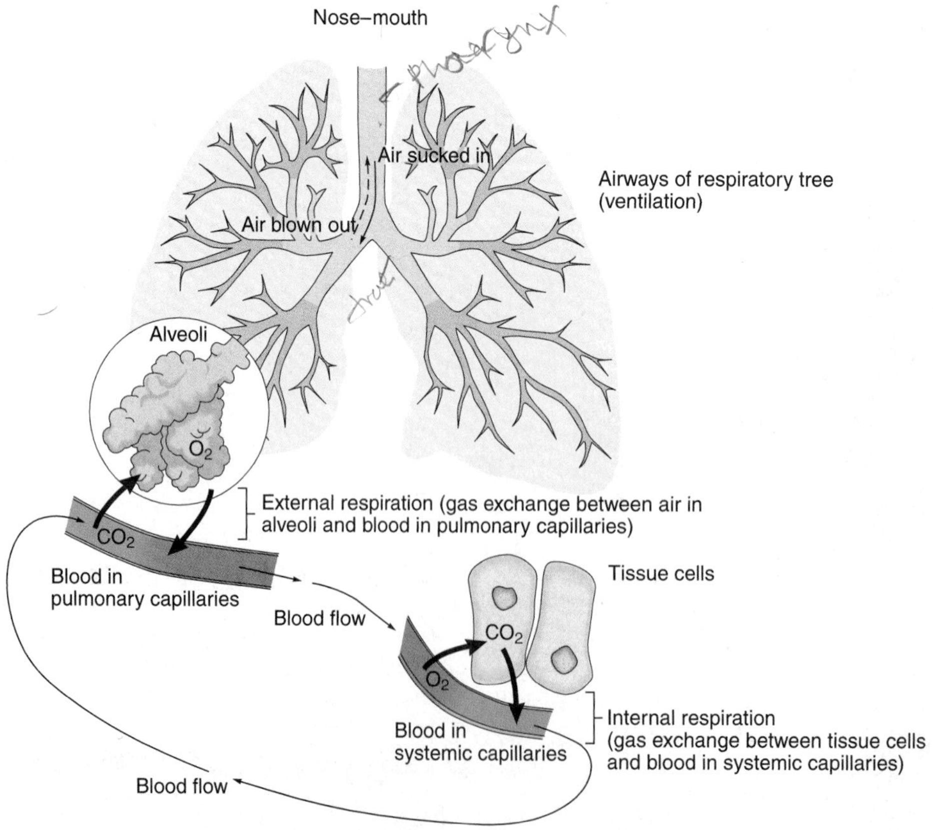

Figure 18-29 Gas exchange in the lungs and tissues.

TABLE 18-10 RESPIRATORY SYSTEM DISORDERS

	Laboratory Diagnostic Tests					
Disease/ Disorder	**Blood**	**Other**	**Radiography**	**Surgery**	**Medical Tests or Procedures**	**Treatment**
Acute or adult respiratory distress syndrome (ARDS)	• Complete blood count • Blood chemistry • Prothrombin time • Partial thromboplastin time • Arterial blood gases	• Electrocardiogram • Urinalysis	• Chest radiograph	• Tracheotomy		• Antibiotics • Ventilator • Oxygen
Asthma	• Complete blood count • Arterial blood gases	• Sputum analysis	• Chest radiograph		• Pulmonary function tests • Skin testing for allergies	• Medication (bronchodilators) • Metered-dose inhaler • Treatment of hypersensitivity
Bronchitis	• Complete blood count	• Sputum culture and analysis	• Chest radiograph		• Bronchoscopy	• Antibiotics if secondary bacterial infection occurs
Emphysema	• Complete blood count • Arterial blood gases		• Chest radiograph		• Pulmonary function tests • Pulse oximetry	• Bronchodilators
Epistaxis	• Complete blood count			• Nasal cauterization	• Blood pressure	• Packing of nose, cautery
Influenza	• Complete blood count		• Chest radiograph			• Symptomatic • Antibiotics if secondary bacterial infection occurs
Laryngitis		• Throat culture			• Laryngoscopy	• Throat lozenges Analgesics
Lung cancer	• Complete blood count	• Sputum cytology	• Chest radiograph	• Biopsy of lung tissue	• Bronchoscopy	• Surgery • Chemotherapy • Radiation
Nasal polyps				• Biopsy of lesions	• Nasal examination	• Surgical excision
Pharyngitis	• Complete blood count	• Throat culture				• Lozenges • Gargling
Pleurisy	• Complete blood count		• Chest radiograph			• Taping of chest • Antibiotics if bacterial • Analgesics
Pneumonia	• Complete blood count	• Blood culture • Sputum smear	• Chest radiograph			• Antibiotics if bacterial • Symptomatic treatment if viral
Severe acute respiratory syndrome (SARS)	• Complete blood count • Blood chemistry • Serum antibodies for SARS	• Throat or nasopharyngeal swab • Viral culture	• Chest radiograph			
Sinusitis	• Complete blood count	• Culture and sensitivity	• Sinus radiographs		• Nasal examination	• Decongestants • Antibiotics
Tonsillitis	• Complete blood count • Streptococcal antibody test	• Throat culture		• Tonsillectomy		• Antibiotics
Tuberculosis	• Complete blood count	• Sputum culture • Acid fast smear of sputum	• Chest radiograph	• Biopsy of lung tissue	• Tuberculin skin test: Mantoux tine	• Multiple antituberculosis medications

TABLE 18-11 DESCRIPTION OF RESPIRATORY DISORDERS

- *Acute or adult respiratory distress syndrome (ARDS).* A life-threatening condition that occurs when there is severe fluid buildup and hemorrhage in the lungs. ARDS is breathing failure that can occur in critically ill patients with underlying illnesses. There is a high mortality rate. Patients may need to be placed on isolation precautions (see Chapter 10).
- *Asthma.* Inflammation and spasm of the smooth muscle of the bronchi brought on by an allergen or emotional upsets. Characterized by dyspnea and wheezing.
- *Bronchitis.* Inflammation of the bronchi, caused by viral or bacterial infection with a dry, painful cough, progressing to a productive cough of greenish yellow sputum. Symptoms include cough, slight fever, chills, malaise, and soreness under the sternum.
- *Emphysema.* Enlargement of the alveoli due to lost elasticity, usually brought on by a long-time irritant, such as cigarette smoking. Results in dyspnea, chronic cough, weight loss, and the appearance of a "barrel chest."
- *Epistaxis.* A nosebleed. May be caused by trauma, chronic sinus irritation, drug abuse (esp. "snorting" drugs), hypertension, blood disorders, and high altitude.
- *Influenza.* A viral infection of various strains of the upper respiratory tract (URI). Sudden onset of chills, fever, cough, sore throat, gastrointestinal disorders are common. Can range from mild to life-threatening.
- *Laryngitis.* Hoarseness, cough, aphonia caused by infections from nose or throat.
- *Lung cancer.* Cancer that may appear in trachea, air sacs, and other lung tubes.
- *Nasal polyp.* A tumor of the nose that can bleed easily. Should be removed surgically.
- *Pharyngitis.* Inflammation of the pharynx caused by a bacteria, virus, or an irritant. Difficulty in swallowing, pain, redness, and inflammation of the pharynx are some of the symptoms. Streptococcus is the most common bacterial infection; influenza virus and the common cold virus are the most common viruses involved. May be accompanied by fever, malaise, and headache.
- *Pleurisy.* Inflammation of the pleura caused by bacteria or viruses. Symptoms include pain, fever, cough, chills, and dyspnea.
- *Pneumonia.* Inflammation of the lungs caused by bacteria, fungi, viruses, and chemical irritants. Usually has sudden onset and is characterized by chills, fever, chest pain, cough, and purulent sputum. Symptoms include sore throat, fever, and lymphadenopathy.
- *Severe acute respiratory syndrome (SARS).* An acute viral respiratory illness that begins with fever, headache, body aches, general malaise, and diarrhea. There may be mild respiratory symptoms at the onset. Most patients will experience development of pneumonia. The virus is spread by close person-to-person contact (i.e., kissing, hugging, sharing eating or drinking utensils, talking to someone within 3 feet [respiratory droplets] and touching someone directly). The patient may be placed on isolation precautions (see Chapter 10).
- *Sinusitis.* Inflammation and infection of a sinus or sinuses. May be caused by allergies, bacteria, viruses, or polyps.
- *Tonsillitis.* Inflammation of the tonsils usually caused by streptococcus. Tonsils become red and enlarged causing severe pharyngitis and fever.
- *Tuberculosis.* Inflammatory infiltrations, formation of tubercles, abscesses, fibrosis, and calcification. Can lead to infection of other body systems.

effectiveness of the medication. See Procedure 18-19 and Figure 18-31.

A commonly used tool in the medical office or clinic, **spirometry** (test to measure lung capacity) assists the physician in the evaluation of signs and symptoms of pulmonary disease by measuring the air capacity (air flow and volume) of the lungs. Three components of lung functions are measured:

1. Forced virtual capacity (FVC), which represents the volume of air that can be exhaled from the lung after the lung is filled with air to meet its total capacity
2. Forced expiration volume at one second (FEV), which is the volume of gas forcibly exhaled from the lungs the first second of expiration
3. Mean expiration flow (FEF) rate, which is a measure on a volume–time curve

Most spirometers are computerized, and thus automatically calculate the lung functions.

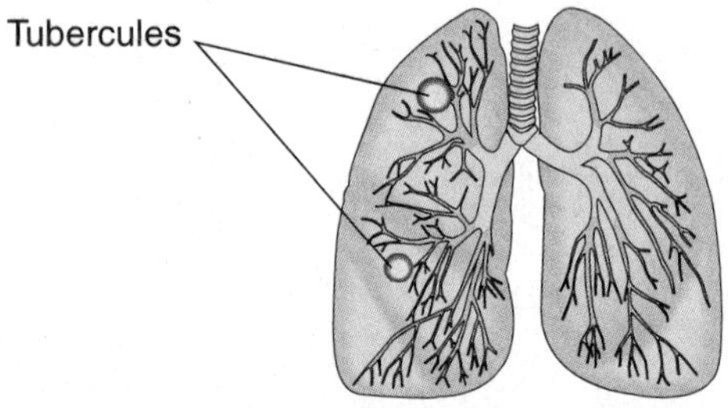

Figure 18-30 Tuberculosis.

Peak Expiratory Flow Rates

Peak expiratory flow rates (PEFRs), as part of pulmonary function studies, help determine the extent of a patient's asthma condition. The PEFR is the measurement of the fastest rate of the flow of air that is exhaled from the lungs. It is measured with a peak flow meter. The PEFR is lower in an individual experiencing an asthma attack caused by impaired expiration and trapped air in the lungs.

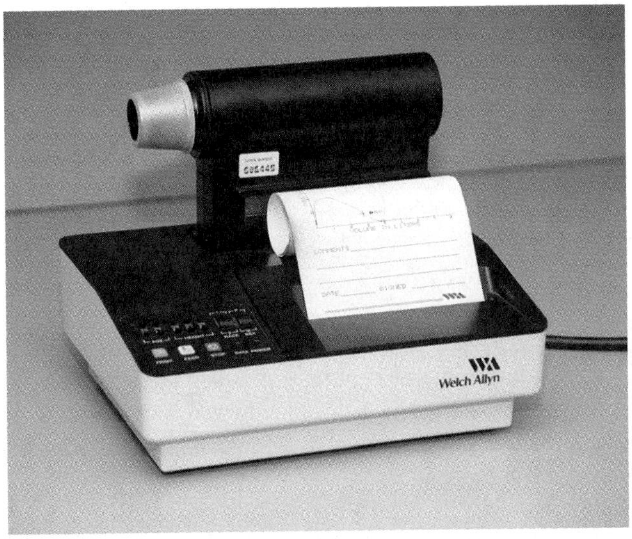

Figure 18-31 The spirometer is used to measure pulmonary function.

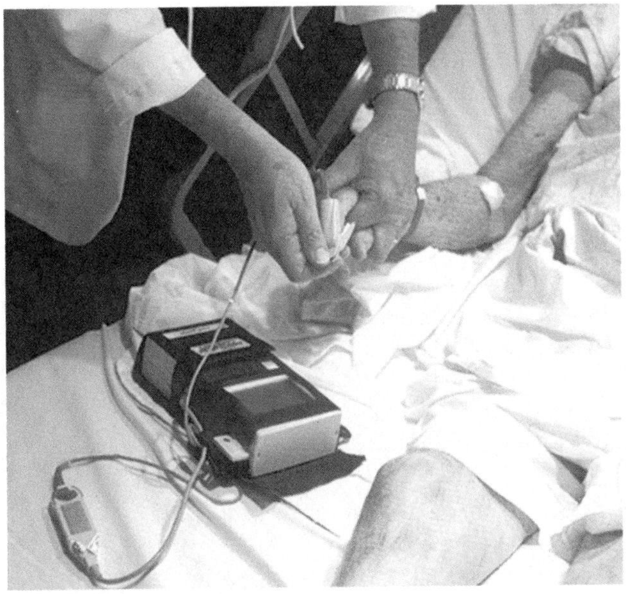

Figure 18-32 Apply the sensor to the selected site—in this case, the finger.

Pulse Oximetry

Pulse oximetry is another test that uses a small probe with an infrared light. The probe is placed on the earlobe, toe, finger, or bridge of the nose. It evaluates the amount of oxygen saturation in the blood. This is helpful because cyanosis is not manifested until the saturation of oxygen is less than 85%. Pulse oximetry is useful in the diagnosis and evaluation of impaired respiratory and cardiac functions. A reading less than 95% indicates hypoxemia. It is not unusual for a patient being tested for sleep apnea to experience a pulse oximetry of under 75%.

The appropriate body part is selected, and a clip (sensor) is placed on it (typically the finger). One side of the sensor is an infrared light, and a photo detector is on the other side. The infrared light passes through the tissues and blood vessels and the detection measures the amount of light absorbed by hemoglobulin. This is a noninvasive procedure done to measure the amount of hemoglobin and can be performed on any patient, but especially those with impaired heart and lung function. Postoperative patients are attached to an oxygen pulse oximeter in the recovery room. The patient is likely to have shallow, less effective respirations because of the anesthesia or narcotics. The patient must not be wearing nail polish. See Procedure 18-20 and Figure 18-32.

MUSCULOSKELETAL SYSTEM

The muscular and skeletal systems interact to coordinate the supporting framework and movements of the body. The musculoskeletal system includes bones, joints, muscles, and surrounding tissue. The skeletal system provides support, protection for vital organs, and allows for the attachment of ligaments, tendons, and muscles. The muscular system gives the body form and shape and is responsible for the coordination of movement.

Bones of the skeletal system store minerals for later use by the body. They are classified according to their shape. Characteristics of bones are their marking, which provides for the attachment of muscles, joining of another bone, and which allows for the passage of nerves and blood vessels. The skeletal system is divided into two parts: the **appendicular skeleton** (126 bones) and the **axial skeleton** (80 bones).

One of the top four reasons a patient visits a physician is for back pain. During the visit, the physician will evaluate the patient for contributory factors for the pain by assessing the patient for any deformities, asymmetry, and signs of restricted motion. The physician will do a functional assessment by observing the patient's **gait** (manner of walking) for indications of decreased mobility and postural changes associated with aging or injury. Flexion tests are done with a goniometer to detect the degree of resistance applied to a given force, thus defining restricted motion and the amount of discomfort associated with movement. Supine straight leg raising (SLR) tests are done to detect the amount of hamstring flexibility and can assess sciatic nerve damage.

There are more than 600 muscles in the body. Muscles are composed of bundles of muscle fibers, each with the ability to contract and relax. Any disease process that disrupts the balance between the muscular and skeletal systems severely hampers a person's ability to move effectively and painlessly. See Tables 18-12, 18-13, and 18-14.

TABLE 18-12 MUSCULOSKELETAL SYSTEM DISORDERS

Disease/ Disorder	Laboratory Diagnostic Tests: Blood	Laboratory Diagnostic Tests: Other	Radiography	Surgery	Medical Tests or Procedures	Treatment
Carpal tunnel syndrome	• Erythrocyte sedimentation rate • Uric acid • Complete blood count			• Surgical repair	• Electro-myography	• Cortisone injection • Physical therapy • Antiinflammatory drugs • Splinting • Surgery
Dislocation			• X-ray of affected joint	• Reduction		• Reduction with anesthesia if necessary • Surgical tightening of ligaments
Gout	• Uric acid • Complete blood count • Erythrocyte sedimentation rate	• Synovial fluid analysis • Urinalysis	• Skeletal x-rays			• Bed rest • Ice to affected joint(s) • Antiinflammatory agents • Analgesics • Corticosteroids • Antigout drugs
Herniated disk			• Myelogram • Computerized tomography (CT) • Magnetic resonance imaging (MRI)			• Muscle relaxants • Analgesics • Brace for affected disk • Epidural injection(s) of corticosteroids • Surgical incision and release
Osteoarthritis	• Complete blood count • Sedimentation rate		• Skeletal x-rays including vertebrae • CT scan • MRI			• Physical therapy • Antiinflammatory drugs • Analgesics • Muscle relaxants • Corticosteroid injection into affected joint • Surgery to replace knee, hip, or shoulder • Spinal fusion
Osteoporosis	• Serum calcium • Alkaline phosphatase • Estrogen level • Total protein • Creatinine	• Urine calcium • Urine creatinine	• Bone scan	• Bone biopsy		• Calcium supplements • Vitamin D supplements and sunshine • Drug therapy • Weight-bearing exercises
Rheumatoid arthritis	• Rheumatoid factor • Antinuclear antibody test • Lupus erythematosis test • Erythrocyte sedimentation rate • Complete blood count	• Synovial fluid analysis	• Skeletal x-rays	• To correct deformity		• Antiinflammatory drugs • Corticosteroids • Immunosuppression drugs • Splinting of affected joints • Exercises • Replacement of joint with artificial joint
Rickets	• Serum phosphorus • Vitamin D • Creatinine	• Urine calcium • Urine phosphorus • Urine creatinine	• Skeletal bone scan	• Bone biopsy		• Vitamin D and calcium supplements • Sunlight exposure
Spinal curvatures Scoliosis Lordosis Kyphosis			• X-rays of spine			• Exercise • Brace • Spinal fusion • Body cast

TABLE 18-13 MUSCULAR/CONNECTIVE TISSUE DISORDERS

Disease/ Disorder	Laboratory Diagnostic Tests: Blood	Laboratory Diagnostic Tests: Other	Radiography	Surgery	Medical Tests or Procedures	Treatment
Back Pain		• Urinalysis	• X-ray of vertebrae	• May be necessary	• Computerized tomography (CT) • Magnetic resonance imaging (MRI)	• Treatment depends on diagnosis • Analgesics • Antiinflammatory medications • Exercise • Epidural corticosteroids • Electronic stimulation device
Bursitis			• MRI • X-ray of affected joint for calcium deposits	• Excision of bursa wall		• Moist heat • Immobilization • Antiinflammatory medications • Local injection of corticosteroids
Fibromyalgia	• Rheumatoid arthritis antibody		• Skeletal x-rays		• Electromyography	• Antiinflammatory medications may be useful • Physical therapy • Medication for sleep disturbances (antidepressants) • Counseling • Exercise
Strain, sprain			• X-rays of affected body part to rule out fracture	• May be necessary		• Cold wet packs to area • Antiinflammatory medications • Elevate and rest affected part • Immobilization or movement of affected part (per physician's recommendation) • Physical therapy
Tendonitis			• Arthrogram			• Moist heat • Antiinflammatory medications • Local injection of corticosteroids • Physical therapy

NOTE: Physical therapy should be encouraged from the onset. Patient can prevent further damage. Provide patient education.

Diagnostic procedures involving the skeletal system involve the extensive use of various forms of radiographs and visual examination techniques. A bone biopsy may be ordered when additional diagnostic data are required. The muscular system employs the use of electrical stimulation to measure the neuromuscular activity and strength of muscles.

Therapeutic treatment of muscular system injuries caused by trauma is clinically handled by the use of hot and cold therapy and physical therapy including ultrasound therapy. These procedures are discussed in Chapter 21.

Fractures, Casting, and Cast Removal

Closed fractures of the wrist, forearm, fingers, lower legs, or upper arm are often treated in the ambulatory care setting. (See Table 18-15 for other types of fractures. Also refer to Chapter 9.)

Types of casting materials used are the plaster, synthetic or plastic cast, and the air cast. Plaster casts are formed by wetting bandage rolls impregnated with calcium sulfate and molding it to the injured body part. Synthetic casts are formed by using tapes with either a polyester,

TABLE 18-14 DESCRIPTION OF SKELETAL AND MUSCULAR DISORDERS

Bone

- *Carpal tunnel syndrome.* Causes pain and weakness of hand and fingers. May cause **paresthesia** of hand and fingers. Caused by compression of the median nerve against the carpal bones. Usually results from repetitive tasks (such as word processing or rolling hair).
- *Cleft palate.* Congenital disorder caused by nonunion of the maxillary bones. Surgical repair needed to close palate.
- *Fractures.* Break in a bone classified according to angle, usually caused by trauma or pathology.
- *Herniated disk.* A rupture of the cushioning mass between two intervertebral disks of the spine most often caused by injury. Causes back pain that may radiate into buttock(s) and down leg.
- *Osteoporosis.* Diminished bone mass caused by lack of calcium deposits in the bone, predisposing patients to fracture.
- *Paget's disease.* Chronic disease marked by a high rate of bone destruction and irregular bone repair. The new bone fractures easily. Cause unknown but may be hereditary.
- *Rickets.* Abnormal bone softening caused by inadequate utilization of vitamin D, inadequate intake or loss of calcium. One symptom is night fever (known as osteomalacia in adults).
- *Spinal curvatures.* Spinal defects with exaggerated curves caused by diseases of the spine, faulty posture, or congenital malformations.
  Scoliosis—right or left sideways curvature of the spine.
  Lordosis—inward curvature of the lower spine (swayback).
  Kyphosis—outward curvature of the upper spine (hunchback).

Joints

- *Dislocation.* A bone forcibly displaced from its joint usually caused by trauma.
- *Gout.* Form of arthritis caused by metabolic disturbances in purine metabolism resulting in uric acid crystal deposits in the joints. Causes periodic attacks of arthritis pain and joint inflammation.
- *Osteoarthritis.* Common, chronic inflammatory process of the joints, with overgrowth of bone and spur formation. Accompanies aging. Causes swollen joints and pain.
- *Rheumatoid arthritis.* More serious and crippling form caused by inflammation of the synovial tissues of several joints, may be caused by antigen–antibody reaction. Systemic symptoms include fatigue, temperature elevation, sensory disturbances, pain, and joint deformities.

Muscle Disorders

- *Back pain.* Localized discomfort usually in the lumbar area caused by stretching or straining of muscles.
- *Bursitis.* Inflammation of the cavity found in connective tissue of a joint that is lined with synovial fluid usually caused by trauma.
- *Fibromalagia.* Discomfort of muscles, tendons, ligaments, and soft tissues brought on by trauma, strain, and emotional stress.
- *Spasm.* Sudden involuntary muscle contraction.
- *Sprains.* Caused by trauma to a joint with torn ligament if severe.
- *Strain.* Trauma to a muscle from violent contraction.
- *Tendonitis.* Inflammation of tendons and attachments caused by trauma such as strain.

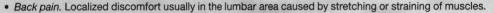

cotton combination, fiberglass, or plastic resin imbedded in the tape. Air casts are a type of inflatable immobilizer and are used for sprains and postcast support. The type of casting material used is dependent on physician preference and the body part to which a cast is being applied. Synthetic casts are lighter, stronger, and more water resistant.

- *Short arm cast (SAC)*. Extends from the fingers to just below the elbow. (Fracture or dislocation of wrist and forearm.)
- *Long arm cast (LAC)*. Extends from the fingers to the axilla, with a bend at the elbow. (Fracture of the upper arm.)
- *Long and short leg casts*. Extend from the thigh to the toes (LLC) or from below the knee to the toes (SLC) and usually include a walking heel.

The medical assistant's role in cast application and removal is to set up supplies and assist the physician. Patient teaching of cast care is also a primary function of the medical assistant. Procedures 18-21 and 18-22 outline steps in applying a plaster cast and assisting in cast removal. See Figures 18-33, 18-34, and 18-35.

NEUROLOGIC SYSTEM

The nervous system functions to coordinate the activities of body systems and allows for the body to adapt to its internal and external environment. Diagnosis and treatment of the brain, spinal cord, and **peripheral nerve** (nerves away from spinal cord) disorders are often difficult because of the interdependence of one part of the system on another.

The physician will screen the patient during a physical examination for neurologic signs and symptoms. The

TABLE 18-15 TYPES OF FRACTURES

Fractures can be simple, or closed, so called because the bone is broken with no penetration of the skin; or they can be compound, or open, so called because the broken bone has protruded through the skin and there is an open wound in addition to the fracture.

Two of the most common fractures are both simple fractures: Colles fracture and Potts fracture. Colles fracture is a fracture of the lower end of the radius. Potts fracture is a fracture of the lower part of the fibula and-the malleolus of the tibia.

Fractures are described by their characteristics:

Greenstick. The bone is bent on one side and fractured on the other.

Oblique. The bone is fractured and runs obliquely to the axis of the bone.

Transverse. The bone is fractured at a right angle to the axis of the bone.

Comminuted. The bone is splintered into fragments.

Impacted. The bone is fractured into fragments and the fragments have been driven into the interior of another bone.

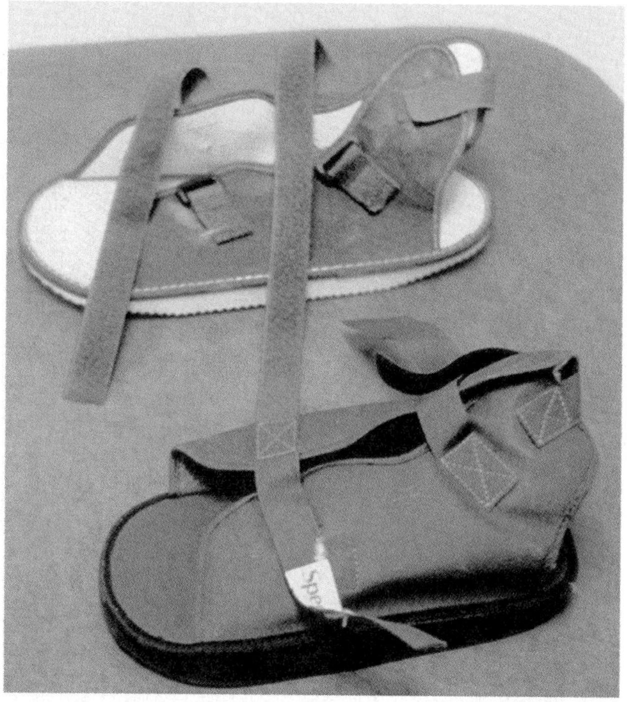

Figure 18-34 If the cast is on a lower extremity, and the patient will be ambulating, provide a cast boot for transfer.

medical assistant's role in a neurologic screening is to observe and evaluate the patient's mental status and to assist or perform other tests as directed by the physician. Most of the examination is performed in conjunction with the complete physical examination, but it can also be done when a patient is exhibiting specific signs and symptoms of a neurologic problem such as lack of sensation, seizures, confusion, paralysis, or **aphasia** (inability to speak).

The equipment and supplies used in a neurologic screening are those that test the patient's reflexes, touch, sense of smell, and degree of coordination to name a few (Figure 18-36). The physician pays particular attention to symmetric strength and notes unequal weakness on either side of the body. A patient's sex and body build will be considered when examining muscle mass and tone. Table 18-16 describes neurologic diagnostic procedures; Table 18-17 outlines neurologic disorders.

Procedures performed to confirm a diagnosis of a neurologic problem or disease are limited to the use of various radiograph and electrical impulse studies. The

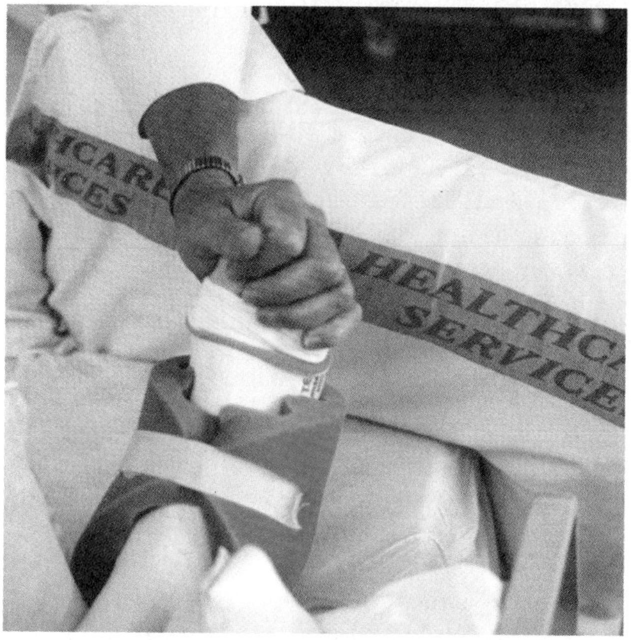

Figure 18-33 Ask the patient if she can feel you touching the extremities distal to the immobilized area.

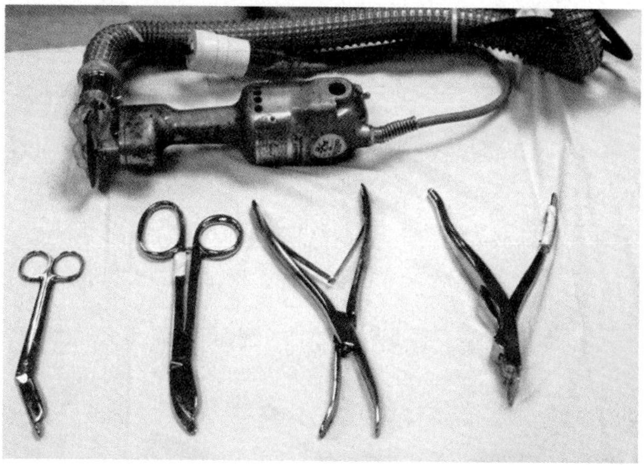

Figure 18-35 Cast cutter, cast splitter, and bandage scissors.

Patient Education

Cast Care Guidelines

The medical assistant should instruct the patient on managing and caring for a cast.

- Allow the casting material to dry by exposing it to the air and keeping it uncovered, even during the night. Applying pressure to the cast before drying can result in tissue damage under the pressure area.
- Elevate the casted extremity to aid in reducing swelling and pain. This allows for a better fitting cast, and thus less discomfort.
- Observe the fingers or toes for changes in color, temperature changes, and decreased sensation, pain, or tingling. This is called nerve and circulation assessment and could indicate the cast is too tight.
- Do not place objects into the cast to scratch irritated skin. A break in the skin will provide a breeding ground for bacteria. Do not use powder or creams.
- Do not get the cast wet. This could lead to a malformation of the cast, thus misalignment of the extremity and break down of the skin. Cover with waterproof covering when bathing. If the cast gets wet, dry it with a hair dryer.
- Cleaning a cast can be accomplished by using a damp cloth.
- When decorating a cast, use only water-soluble paints or marking pens. This allows the cast to breathe, thus avoiding tissue damage.
- Do not cut or trim the cast. Use a type of masking tape if there is a sharp edge, or use nail file to smooth rough edge.
- Notify the physician if any of the following occurs:
  1. A bad odor coming from the cast. This may indicate an infection.
  2. Numbness, tingling, severe pain, difficulty moving, severe swelling, or cold fingers or toes. The cast may be too tight.
  3. A burning sensation over a bony area. The cast may be too tight.
  4. Bleeding or pink to red discoloration on the cast. There may be bleeding from a wound under the cast.

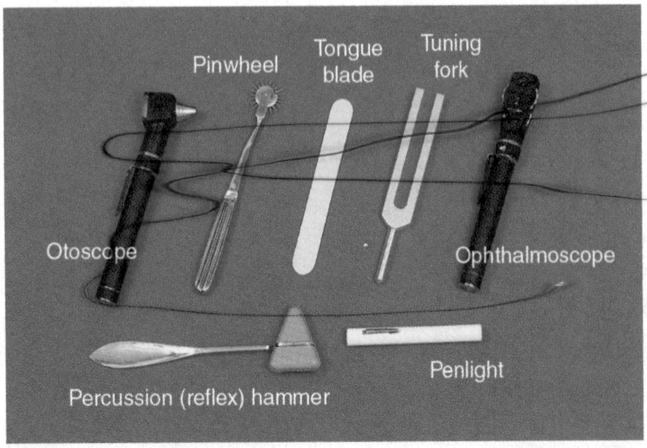

Figure 18-36 Supplies used in a neurologic examination.

medical assistant will assist the physician during certain procedures. Patient teaching by the medical assistant before a procedure and active reinforcement during a procedure will promote patient cooperation. Procedure 18-23 outlines steps involved in removing cerebrospinal fluid from the lumbar area.

Components of a Neurologic Screening

During the neurologic screening examination, various functions are observed. Procedure 18-24 outlines the steps involved in a neurologic screening examination:

- Mental status:
  - Level of consciousness (alert)
  - Memory (recall of past and present)

TABLE 18-16 NEUROLOGIC SYSTEM DISORDERS

Disease/ Disorder	Laboratory Diagnostic Tests: Blood	Laboratory Diagnostic Tests: Other	Radiography	Surgery	Medical Tests or Procedures	Treatment
Bell's palsy	• Complete blood count		• Magnetic resonance imaging (MRI) of brain			• Warm moist heat • Facial exercises • Analgesics • Eye patch if unable to close eye
Cerebral vascular accident (CVA) (stroke)			• Cerebral angiography • Computerized tomography (CT) • MRI	• To remove clots	• Electroencephalography • Lumbar puncture	• Anticoagulant therapy • Physical therapy • Speech therapy • Tissue-plasminogen activator (TPA)
Epilepsy			• CT • MRI		• Electroencephalography	• Antiepilepsy medication
Herpes zoster	• Varicella-zoster antibody				• Culture of cell scrapings from lesion	• Analgesics • Steroids • Antiviral medication (Acyclovir, Famvir)
Multiple sclerosis			• Brain scan • CT • MRI		• Lumbar puncture	• Steroids • Medications: experimental • Physical therapy • Muscle relaxants • Assistive devices
Rabies	• Complete blood count					• Wash wound immediately with soap and water • Antirabies injections • Medication for convulsions
Reye's syndrome	• Complete blood count • Serum ammonia	• Liver function studies		• Liver biopsy • Brain biopsy	• Lumbar puncture • Examination of cerebrospinal fluid	• Supportive • Physical therapy
Sciatica	• Blood serum		• Myelogram • CT • MRI	• Spinal fusion • Diskectomy (if caused by herniated disk)		• Physical therapy • Massage • Exercise • Analgesics • Antiinflammatory • Surgery
Tic douloureux				• Biopsy of trigeminal nerve		• Analgesics • Surgery to dissect the trigeminal nerve
West nile virus	• Complete blood count		• MRI		• Neurologic work-up	• No specific treatment

- Cognition (ability to calculate and remember current events)
- Mood (is it appropriate for the conversation)
- deational content (hallucinations)

- Cranial nerve function:
  - Cranial nerve I: aroma identification
  - Cranial nerve II: visual acuity, visual fields, optic disk
  - Cranial nerves III, IV, and VI: extraocular eye muscles
  - Cranial nerve V: sensations of the face, scalp, teeth
  - Cranial nerve VII: facial expressions, taste

- Cranial nerve VIII: ear—hearing and equilibrium
- Cranial nerves IX and X: gag reflex, saliva secretion, voice, slowing of heartbeat
- Cranial nerve XI: neck and shoulder muscle
- Cranial nerve XII: tongue

Patient Education

Review post–spinal tap instructions:

1. Remain in a prone position for two to three hours to allow tissues to close over the puncture site and minimize cerebrospinal fluid (CSF) leakage and to allow CSF to be replenished.
2. Increase fluid intake because this helps to replace fluid loss.
3. Report any severe headaches or alterations in neurologic status (paralysis, numbness, and tingling).

The physician continues with the neurologic examination by checking the patient for the following:

- Cerebral function:
  - Memory
  - Muscle coordination
  - Sensory interpretation
  - Posture and gait
- Motor function:
  - Muscle tone
  - Strength
  - Muscle mass
  - Twitching
- Sensory function:
  - Touch (pain, light touch, vibration, position sense)
- Deep tendon reflexes:

  Extremities:
  - Upper—biceps, triceps
  - Lower—quadriceps, achilles

  Additional tests:
  - Angiography provides visualization of the circulation of the blood throughout the brain.

TABLE 18-17 DESCRIPTION OF NEUROLOGIC DISORDERS

- *Bell's palsy.* Paralysis of seventh cranial nerve caused by an acute inflammation. Usually characterized by unilateral facial paralysis and pain, but it can be bilateral.
- *Cerebral vascular accident (CVA).* Loss of blood supply to the brain (anoxia). May be caused by a ruptured or clogged blood vessel or clot in the brain and hypertension. Symptoms include sudden loss of consciousness and paralysis. Also referred to as a stroke.
- *Epilepsy.* Episodes of seizures caused by changes in electrical brain potentials that result in disturbed brain impulses or function.
- *Headache.* Diffuse pain in different parts of the head. May be acute or chronic with varying degree of pain and may be caused by a variety of reasons.
- *Herpes zoster.* An acute infectious viral disease caused by varicella zoster virus. Painful vesicular eruptions. Known as "shingles."
- *Meningitis.* Inflammation of the membranes of the spinal cord or brain. Symptoms include a stiff neck, headache, anorexia, and irregular fever. Caused by either a bacterium or a virus.
- *Multiple sclerosis.* Chronic progressive disease characterized by **demyelination** (destruction of nerve covering) of nerve fibers. The cause is unknown. First symptoms are visual disturbances and muscle weakness.
- *Parkinson's disease.* A slowly progressive disease, usually occurring in later life, caused by a degeneration of brain cells due to lack of dopamine in the brain. Muscle rigidity and akinesia are common symptoms.
- *Rabies.* Caused by a virus and transmitted to humans by scratches or bites from animals infected with the virus. The disease infects the brain and spinal cord and causes acute encephalitis. It is often fatal.
- *Reye's syndrome.* A neurologic illness usually seen in young children after a viral infection such as influenza, varicella, Epstein–Barr. There may be a connection between the viral infection and aspirin. Cause is unknown, but characteristic symptoms include vomiting, rash, lethargy and neurologic involvement, seizures, and coma.
- *Sciatica.* Severe pain in the leg along the course of the sciatic nerve felt at the back of the thigh and running down the inside of the leg. Caused by compression of the nerve by a ruptured intervertebral disk or osteoarthritis. Characterized by sharp, shooting pain running down back of thigh. Leg movement aggravates the pain.
- *Tic douloureux.* Degeneration of or pressure on the trigeminal nerve (fifth cranial) causing severe stabs of pain that radiate from the angle of the jaw along one of the branches. Pain may be felt in the eye, lip, nose, tongue. Pain may come and go for hours.
- *West Nile virus.* A potentially serious illness that affects the central nervous system. Symptoms may include headache, stupor, disorientation, tremors, convulsions, and coma. Spread by infected mosquitoes when bitten by them.

- Computerized tomography (CT) helps to diagnose hemorrhage and tumors. See Chapter 20.
- Electroencephalography (EEG) records the electrical activity of the brain and helps to diagnose seizures and tumors.
- Magnetic resonance imaging (MRI) helps to diagnose tumors and hemorrhage. See Chapter 20.

CIRCULATORY SYSTEM

The circulatory system is composed of the heart and a complex network of blood vessels. Their function is to pump and transport the blood to all parts of the body, thus supplying oxygen and removing waste products from body tissues. Table 18-18 reviews circulatory system disorders and diagnostic procedures; Table 18-19 provides a description of disorders of the circulatory system.

The variety of diagnostic procedures used to determine the patient's diagnosis are necessary because of the complexity of the cardiovascular system. The medical assistant assists with and performs some of the procedures used for clinical diagnosis. Electrocardiogram (ECG) procedure is explained in Chapter 25.

BLOOD AND LYMPH SYSTEM

The blood and lymph are excellent indicators of many underlying diseases. As blood circulates through body tissues and organs, it deposits nutrients and removes wastes. Failure to accomplish this leaves the body in a disease state. Blood cells include erythrocytes, leukocytes, and platelets, and each has its own function. Studying the results of laboratory findings assists the physician in making a diagnosis.

Lymph is important because of its filtering properties. The body's immune system relies heavily on the fact that the lymph passes through the lymph glands and bacteria and other substances are filtered out. Table 18-20 describes diseases and disorders diagnostic procedures for blood and lymphatic system; Table 18-21 describes certain blood and lymph system disorders.

Common laboratory and diagnostic procedures requested by the physician include some of the following:

- *Complete blood count* (CBC). A routine test that includes a hemoglobin, hematocrit, and red and white blood cell count.

TABLE 18-18 CIRCULATORY SYSTEM DISORDERS

	Laboratory Diagnostic Tests					
Disease/ Disorder	**Blood**	**Other**	**Radiography**	**Surgery**	**Medical Tests or Procedures**	**Treatment**
Angina pectoris			• Ultrasonography • Angiography • Cardiac catheterization	• Coronary artery bypass • Angioplasty	• Electrocardiography • Stress test	• Nitrogycerin • Coronary artery bypass surger • Angioplasty with stent • Lifestyle changes
Congestive heart failure			• Chest x-ray	• Removal of part of myocardium	• Electrocardiography • Venous pressure	• Medication • Heart transplant • Lifestyle changes
Coronary artery disease	• Electrolytes • Chemistry, low-density lipoprotein, high-density lipoprotein, cholesterol • triglycerides		• Angiography • Thallium stress test • Cardiac catheterization		• Electrocardiography	• Medication • Coronary artery bypass surgery • Lifestyle changes
Essential hypertension	• Electrolytes	• Urinalysis • Kidney function	• Chest x-ray		• Electrocardiography • Blood pressure	• Medication • Lifestyle changes
Mitral valve stenosis			• Ultrasonography • Echocardiography • Cardiac catheterization	• Valvotomy	• Electrocardiography	• Valve replacement

(continues)

TABLE 18-18 CIRCULATORY SYSTEM DISORDERS (continued)

Disease/ Disorder	Laboratory Diagnostic Tests: Blood	Laboratory Diagnostic Tests: Other	Radiography	Surgery	Medical Tests or Procedures	Treatment
Myocardial infarction	• Cardiac enzymes • Complete blood count		• Thallium stress test • Cardiac catheterization • Ultrasonography		• Electrocardiography	• Oxygen • Medication • Lifestyle changes
Pericarditis	• Complete blood count • Erythrocyte sedimentation rate • Cardiac enzymes • Bacterial antibodies	• Urinalysis • Blood culture	• Chest x-ray		• Electrocardiography	• Medication • Antibiotics • Pericardio-centesis
Rheumatic fever	• Complete blood count • Streptococcal antibodies • Erythrocyte sedimen-tation rate (ESR) • Cardiac enzymes • Kidney function • Liver function	• Throat culture	• Echocardiography		• Electrocardiography	• Antibiotic therapy
Thrombo-phlebitis	• Bleeding and clotting time • Complete blood count	• Urinalysis	• Doppler ultrasonography • Angiography • Radioactive fibrinogen	• Thrombectomy		• Elevation of affected limb • Medication (anticoagulant) • Support hose
Varicose veins			• Venography • Doppler ultrasonography	• Ligation and stripping		• Elastic stockings • Sclerotherapy • Ligation and stripping

TABLE 18-19 DESCRIPTION OF CIRCULATORY SYSTEM DISORDERS

- *Angina pectoris.* Chest pain caused by lack of oxygen to the myocardium. Usual cause is coronary arteriosclerosis.
- *Congestive heart failure.* A syndrome characterized by the heart's inability to pump blood adequately to the body tissues. Characterized by congestion in the lungs, or edema of lower extremities, dyspnea on exertion, cough, and related edema.
- *Coronary artery disease.* Arteriosclerosis of the coronary arteries leading to impaired blood flow to the myocardium. Complete occlusion leads to myocardial infarction. May also be caused by thrombus in a coronary artery. Angina pectoris is the name of the chest pain that occurs due to lack of oxygen to the myocardium.
- *Essential hypertension.* Consistently increased blood pressure of unknown cause.
- *Mitral valve stenosis.* Narrowing of mitral valve obstructing flow from atrium to ventricle. Usual cause is a rheumatic heart disease as a result of a streptococcal infection (throat or scarlet fever). Thrombi can form.
- *Myocardial infarction.* Death of myocardial tissue caused by anoxia to the myocardium. Symptoms include dyspnea, chest pain, nausea, vomiting, and diaphoresis.
- *Pericarditis.* Inflammation of the pericardium. Caused by tuberculosis, pyogenic organisms, uremia, and myocardial infarction. Characterized by fever, dry cough, dyspnea, and palpitations.
- *Rheumatic fever.* A systemic disease affecting the heart, joints, and central nervous system after a Group A beta-hemolytic streptococcal infection. May occur without symptoms. Symptoms include fever, migratory joint pain, pericarditis, and heart murmur.
- *Thrombophlebitis.* An inflammation of a vein with thrombus formation, may be caused by trauma. Symptoms include pain and swelling in affected vein.
- *Varicose veins.* Enlarged, twisted, and engorged veins, commonly occurring in the saphenous veins but may occur in any vein in the body. Caused by conditions that hamper venous return, such as pregnancy, standing for long periods of time, and obesity. Symptoms include pain in feet and ankles, swelling, and leg ulcers.

TABLE 18-20 BLOOD AND LYMPH SYSTEM DISORDERS

Disease/ Disorder	Laboratory Diagnostic Tests: Blood	Laboratory Diagnostic Tests: Other	Radiography	Surgery	Medical Tests or Procedures	Treatment
Anemias	• Serum iron • Complete blood count • Red blood cell count • Serum B_{12}	• Gastric analysis	• Ferrokinetic studies • Radioactive B_{12}		• Bone marrow	• Depends on cause • Increase dietary intake of iron or folic acid • Vitamin B_{12} injections
Hodgkin's disease	• Complete blood count • Liver function		• Chest radiograph • Lymphangiography	• Lymph node biopsy	• Bone marrow	• Radiation • Chemotherapy
Infectious mono-nucleosis	• Complete blood count • Monoscreen • Heterophile antibody • Epstein–Barr virus • Liver function					• Analgesics • Rest
Leukemia	• Complete blood count • Liver function • Platelet count • Bleeding time			• Bone marrow transplant	• Bone marrow	• Chemotherapy • Bone marrow transplant
Lymphedema			• Lymphangiography			• Antibiotics • Surgery • Lymphedema therapy

- *Differential.* Distinguishes among the various types of white blood cells.
- *Erythrocyte sedimentation rate* (sedimentation rate or erythrocyte sedimentation rate [ESR]). Done to time the speed of red blood cells settling to the bottom of a test tube.
- *Platelet count.* The number of platelets in a blood specimen.
- *Liver function studies.* Measure coagulation factors, prothrombin, and fibrinogen necessary for blood coagulation.
- *Schilling test.* Radioactive vitamins B_{12} and intrinsic factor measured in 24-hour urine specimen.

Procedures to collect blood specimens and venipuncture are explained in Chapter 28; hematology is discussed in Chapter 29.

TABLE 18-21 DESCRIPTION OF BLOOD/LYMPH SYSTEM DISORDERS

- *Anemias.* All anemias are manifested by a reduction in circulating red blood cells and the amount of hemoglobin, which is the volume of packed red blood cells per 100 ml blood. Symptoms include pallor of the skin, nailbeds, and mucous membranes; weakness; vertigo; headache; drowsiness; and general malaise.

  Iron deficiency. Lack of reserve iron in the body and in red blood cells that lack hemoglobin resulting from inadequate dietary intake of iron, iron **malabsorption** (poor absorption of nutrients), blood loss, or pregnancy.

  Pernicious anemia. Lack of intrinsic factor in the stomach secretions (hydrochloric acid). Vitamin B_{12} cannot be absorbed. Red cells cannot develop properly.

  Sickle cell anemia. A hereditary chronic anemia characterized by abnormal red blood cells causing lysis of the cells and the formation of clumps in the blood vessels, impairing circulation. Not curable.
- *Hodgkin's disease.* An idiopathic malignancy of the lymphatic system causing enlargement of lymphatic tissue, spleen, and liver. Symptoms include fever and night sweats. Often curable.
- *Leukemia.* Overproduction of abnormal and immature white blood cells. Cause is unknown. Symptoms include anemia, fatigue, fever, and joint pain.
- *Lymphedema.* Abnormal accumulation of lymph in the extremities caused by obstruction of the lymphatics. Symptoms include edema in arms or legs.

INTEGUMENTARY SYSTEM

The integumentary system consists of the skin and its associated structures, such as hair, nails, nerve endings, and the sebaceous (oil) and sudoriferous (sweat) glands. This system provides protection for the body against invasion of microorganisms and trauma and helps regulate body temperature. Nerve endings sense pressure, touch, and pain. Structurally, the skin consists of two layers (Figure 18-37), which function differently from one another to perform specific activities.

- Epidermis is the outer layer of the skin that is composed of squamous epithelium and produces keratin and the pigment melanin.
- Dermis is the inner layer of the skin made up of connective tissue and contains blood vessels, nerve endings, and glands. Provides strength and elasticity.
- Subcutaneous connective tissue (hypodermis) is the layer on which the skin and muscles lie and consists of elastic and fibrous connective tissue and adipose tissue. Guards against heat loss and provides insulation.

Skin disorders frequently produce a **lesion** (injury or wound) unique to a specific skin disease, thus allowing for the diagnosis to be based on the appearance of the lesion, the patient's history, allergies, emotional well-being, and inherited diseases. If the lesion appears suspicious, the physician may perform a **biopsy** for tissue analysis. This procedure aids in the diagnosis and treatment of specific skin disorders. Table 18-22 describes integumentary system diseases and diagnostic procedures; Table 18-23 describes skin disorders of the integumentary system.

Diagnostic procedures involving the skin range from the simple to the complex. Simple observations such as skin color, texture, size and shape of a lesion, and patient history can lead to a quick diagnosis. Confirmatory procedures such as clinical studies of urine and blood, culture of a purulent lesion, radiographs, and biopsies of the affected tissues can further delineate the disease.

The clinical procedures most commonly performed by the medical assistant concerning the skin are obtaining wound cultures, the application of a sterile dressing to the wound site, and allergy skin testing.

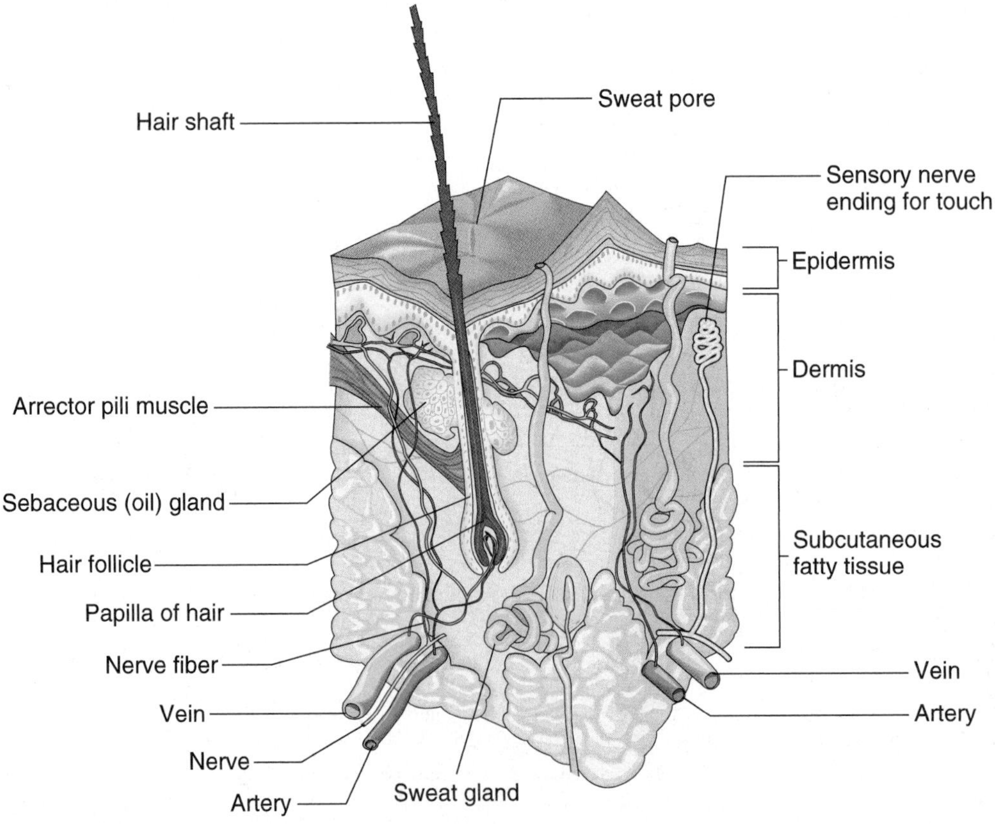

Figure 18-37 Cross-section of skin.

Allergy Skin Testing

Medical assistants often perform allergy skin testing. When performing allergy skin tests, the likelihood of severe allergic reaction is a distinct possibility. Emergency treatment must be available immediately and consists of the following: (1) notify physician immediately; (2) have patient lie down; (3) have epinephrine, benadryl, and corticosteroid injections ready to be administered; and (4) check patient's vital signs.

There can be a broad range of inflammatory responses to allergens. Some responses include urticaria (hives), swelling at the injection site, pruritis (itchiness), and redness. A response or reaction can be immediate, life-threatening, and systemic in nature. The allergen reaches the circulatory system triggering a massive release of substances (histamine) that can produce severe airway obstruction, vasodilation, hypotension, laryngeal edema, and shock. See Chapter 9.

Scratch Test. The back and arms are used for the scratch test type of allergy testing. The skin surface is numbered in rows approximately two inches apart so that they can be identified. A small scratch is made on the surface of the skin and the **allergen** (a substance that causes allergy) is placed on the scratch. As many as 50 allergens can be used at one time. A reaction to the allergen usually occurs within a half-hour. If the patient is allergic to a substance, a **wheal** or hive will develop at the scratch site. The site is compared with a scratch test with no allergens introduced into it, but rather an allergy-free fluid. The physician will read the results, which are graded on a scale from 2 to 4. A number 2 reaction indicates a wheal larger than the control scratch reaction (which is minimal). A number 3 is given to a larger reaction, and a 4 is given to a reaction in which there are extensions of the wheal beyond the usual circumscribed area of the injection. The allergen extract should be wiped away from the scratch area that is exhibiting a number 4 reaction.

TABLE 18-22 INTEGUMENTARY SYSTEM DISORDERS

	Laboratory Diagnostic Tests					
Disease/ Disorder	**Blood**	**Other**	**Radiography**	**Surgery**	**Medical Tests or Procedures**	**Treatment**
Abscess (furuncle, carbuncle)	• Complete blood count • Blood glucose	• Culture and sensitivity of wound exudate		• Incision and drainage		• Antibiotics • Incision and drainage
Acne		• Culture of skin lesions				• Antibiotics • Steroids • Retin-A
Corn, callus, wart (verucca), mole (nevus)				• Excisional biopsy • Electrocautery		• Surgical excision
Dermatitis	• Serum IgE			• Biopsy of lesion		• Depends on cause
Dermato-phytosis		• Culture			• Wood's rays (ultraviolet rays)	• Antifungal medication
Impetigo	• Complete blood count	• Gram stain of discharge from lesion				• Antibiotics
Melanoma			• Chest x-ray	• Biopsy of lesion		• Surgical excision • Chemotherapy
Psoriasis				• Skin biopsy		• Medication • Light therapy
Scleroderma	• Sedimentation rate • Rheumatoid arthritis factor • Antinuclear antibodies	• Urinalysis • Kidney function tests	• Gastrointestinal x-ray • Chest x-ray	• Tissue biopsy		• Medication
Skin cancer				• Biopsy of lesion		• Surgical excision • Laser therapy • Radiation therapy

TABLE 18-23 DESCRIPTION OF SKIN DISORDERS

- *Abscess.* **Furuncle** "Boil." Acute circumscribed infection of the subcutaneous tissues and surrounding tissues caused by staphylococci. **Carbuncle.** A circumscribed inflammation and infection of the skin and deeper tissues accompanied by fever, leukocytosis, and sometimes prostration. Caused by staphylococcus and common in patients with diabetes.
- *Acne.* Chronic inflammatory disease caused by blocked sebaceous glands, characterized by **comedones** (blackheads), papules, and pustules.
- *Corn and Callus.* Thickening and hyperplasia of the **stratum corneum** (outermost skin layer) caused by pressure or friction to the affected area.
- *Dermatitis.* Caused by a specific irritant characterized by **erythema** or redness as in inflammation.
- *Dermatophytosis.* A highly contagious infectious fungus infection of the skin. Common on hands and feet. When feet are infected, it is known as athlete's foot or tinea pedis.
- *Herpes Zoster.* An acute infectious disease caused by varicella-zoster virus. Characterized by inflammation of the ganglia of the spinal or cranial nerves. Painful, vesicular eruptions occur along the course of the nerves.
- *Impetigo.* Contagious small pustules caused by a staphylococci or streptococci or a combination of both and spread by direct contact.
- *Melanoma.* A malignant pigmented mole. Virulent and invasive. Can be caused by ultraviolet light exposure.
- *Nevus.* A mole. Usually congenital.
- *Psoriasis.* Chronic, genetically determined dermatitis, characterized by flat, reddened areas with silvery scales.
- *Scleroderma.* Progressive thickening of the skin involving collagen tissue. Systemic involvement occurs. Cause is unknown.
- *Skin cancer.* Malignant lesions on the skin surface caused by exposure to ultraviolet rays.
- *Verruca.* A wart. Caused by a virus.

Patch Test. The suspected allergen is placed on the skin and is covered with a square of cellophane and held in place by tape. As many as 25 tests can be done at one time and results are read in 24 to 96 hours.

Patient Education

Teach patients that the following may be warnings of skin cancer (melanoma, basal cell, and squamous cell carcinoma):

1. change in size, shape, or color of mole or wart
2. scaliness
3. oozing or bleeding
4. pain

Teach patients to avoid exposure to the sun and to use a high number sunscreen even during winter months and overcast days. Early detection is necessary for successful treatment. Treatment is by surgical excision or electrosurgery (see Chapter 19, Assisting with Office/Ambulatory Surgery).

Intradermal Test. A small dose (0.1 cc) of an allergen is injected intradermally. Ten to 15 tests can be done simultaneously on each arm, and the patient can experience a severe reaction more quickly. This test is always done on the patient's forearm.

Radioallergosorbent Test (RAST). The RAST laboratory test is obtained by venipuncture and uses radioisotopes to measure minute, specific antibodies present in the circulating blood. Scratch, patch, and intradermal testing provide immediate information about allergies and is less expensive.

After any type of allergy skin test, the patient is told to remain in the office for 20 to 30 minutes to watch for an allergic reaction. If a reaction occurs, emergency medications and supplies must be readily available.

Medical Assistant Responsibilities. Common procedures with which the medical assistant can assist the physician are the cutaneous punch biopsy and wart and mole removal. The prime responsibilities of the medical assistant are to follow the principles of surgical **aseptic** technique, infection control, and standard precautions; provide the physician with the required supplies as needed; safely handle and transport the biopsy specimen; and document in the patient record that the biopsy was sent to the laboratory.

Endoscopic Procedures. An endoscope is an instrument or device that is used to observe the inside of a hollow organ or cavity (to view within). Procedures can be done on many internal organs without surgical intervention by using an endoscope. These are known as fiberoptic endoscopic procedures or endoscopy, and they can be performed through a natural body opening or a small incision. A light source (fiberoptics) at the end of the endoscope permits the physician to observe within the body cavity for disorders such as polyps, tumors, cysts, stenoses, calculi, and malignancies. Biopses and cultures can be taken during the procedure. Small lesions, such as polyps, can be totally removed during endoscopy. Photos can be taken for documentation also.

The medical assistant must be certain that the patient has signed a consent form before the procedure and that the patient has followed the preparatory instructions. Table 18-24 lists endoscopic procedures, their importance in diagnosis, and patient preparation.

TABLE 18-24 ENDOSCOPIC PROCEDURES

Endoscopic Procedure	Importance in Diagnosis	Patient Preparation
Proctosigmoidoscope (views sigmoid colon and rectum)	Detects polyps, rectal abscesses, tumors, fissures, and fistulas.	Bowel preparation: 3-day special diet Laxative and enemas NPO after midnight the night prior
Colonoscopy (views entire colon)	Detects polyps, tumors, bleeding, malignancies. Can take biopsies, remove polyps, take photos, take cultures.	Clear liquids for 2 days before NPO after 10:00 PM Night before bowel preparation: laxatives and enemas
Bronchoscopy (examines bronchial tree)	Detects lesions, obstructions, malignancies. Can take cultures.	NPO for 12 hours before examination
Colposcopy (examines the cervix and vagina after an abnormal Pap test)	Biopsy lesions for abnormal cells.	No dietary restrictions
Cystoscopy (examines the urethra and bladder)	Identify lesions in the bladder, urethra, enlarged prostate gland. Biopsy photos.	No dietary restrictions
Arthroscopy (examination and repair of joints)	Detects torn ligaments, examine for synovial problems. Surgery can be performed to repair joint.	NPO after 10:00 PM
Laparoscopy (examines the peritoneal cavity, abdomen, and pelvis)	Detects endometriosis, cysts, fibroids, ectopic pregnancies. Surgery can be performed such as oophorectomy, biopsy, tubal ligation, and so on.	NPO after 10:00 PM
Esophagogastroduodenoscopy (EGD) (examines esophagus, stomach, and duodenum)	Detects abnormalities in the esophagus, stomach, and duodenum such as hiatal hernia, stenoses, tumors, ulcers, erosion. Biopsies, brushings, photos.	NPO after 10:00 PM
Endoscopic retrograde cholangiopancreatography (examines the liver, gallbladder, bile ducts, and pancreas)	Helps diagnose problems in the liver, gall bladder, bile ducts, and pancreas such as cholelithiasis, stenoses, and malignancies of these organs and structures.	NPO after 10:00 PM
Gastroscopy	Examines stomach for ulcers, lesions, and malignancies.	NPO after 10:00 PM
Gastroduodenoscopy	Examines stomach and duodenum for lesions such as tumors, polyps, structures, and ulcers.	NPO after 10:00 PM

Procedure 18-1 Performing a Urine Drug Screening

STANDARD PRECAUTIONS:

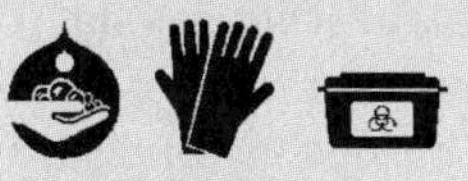

PURPOSE:

To accurately obtain a urine specimen from a patient for traces of drugs.

EQUIPMENT/SUPPLIES:

Urine Drug Kit (provide at least two choices)
Gloves
Biohazard waste container

PROCEDURE STEPS:

1. Ask patient to show a photo identification (ID) and have patient sign a consent form, keeping copies for the patient file. RATIONALE: Only the person scheduled to take the test will be able to do so.
2. Wash hands and explain procedure to the patient.
3. Supply at least two collection kits from which the patient can choose one. RATIONALE: By patient choosing a kit, it eliminates patient claiming wrong urine sample was tested.
4. Have patient remove unnecessary outer garments, empty pockets, and wash and dry hands. RATIONALE: Patient cannot substitute another specimen.
5. Instruct patient to collect at least 40 ml urine in the collection container.
6. Put on gloves. Record temperature of specimen, volume, and any contamination. RATIONALE: If fresh, specimen should be at least 98.6°F.
7. Label specimen and have patient initial specimen lid.
8. Seal specimen kit bag and have patient initial. RATIONALE: Kit bags are tamper-proof.
9. Secure sample in a locked container until pickup.
10. Collector and donor will need to sign off on the test collection procedure to document all procedure steps were followed.
11. Remove gloves and dispose of in biohazard waste container.
12. Wash hands.
13. Document procedure in patient's chart.

DOCUMENTATION

7/29/20XX 8:30 AM Urine collected for drug screening. Temperature of specimen 98.4°F. Patient initialed specimen lid. Specimen taken to laboratory and given to technician. B. Abbott, RMA

Procedure 18-2 Performing a Urinary Catheterization on a Female Patient

STANDARD PRECAUTIONS:

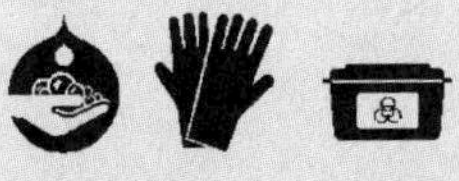

PURPOSE:

To obtain a sterile urine specimen for analysis or to relieve urinary retention.

EQUIPMENT/SUPPLIES:

Catheter kit (commercially available) containing:
- Sterile gloves
- Betadine® solution or swabs
- Lubricant
- Sterile cotton balls
- Sterile urine container with label
- Sterile 2 × 2 gauze sponges
- Forceps
- Sterile absorbent plastic pad

Additional items needed:
- Sterile catheter (size and type as ordered by physician)
- Biohazard waste container
- Laboratory requisition form
- Waxed paper bag

PROCEDURE STEPS:

1. Identify the patient and explain the procedure.
2. Wash hands and assemble supplies.
3. Place unopened catheter kit on Mayo stand near the patient.
4. Provide adequate lighting.
5. Have patient disrobe below the waist; provide a drape.
6. Position patient into a dorsal recumbent position on an examination table. RATIONALE: This allows for access to the urinary meatus.
7. Drape patient with sheet exposing only external genitalia.
8. Open outer wrapping of sterile kit. This becomes a sterile field.
9. Place sterile absorbent plastic pad under patient's buttocks. Touching only the corners, empty contents of tray onto sterile field. Add sterile catheter to field.
10. Ask patient to keep knees apart. RATIONALE: This position provides good visualization of the urinary meatus.
11. Apply sterile gloves.
12. Pour Betadine over three cotton balls in appropriate compartment of the kit or open Betadine swabs.
13. Open urine specimen container.
14. Apply sterile lubricant to a gauze sponge and place tip of catheter in lubricant.
15. Instruct patient to breathe slowly and deeply during procedure. RATIONALE: This helps the patient relax the abdominal and pelvic muscles and facilitates easier insertion of the catheter.
16. Spread labia with nondominant hand. Dominant hand remains sterile. With dominant hand and sterile forceps, wipe genitalia with each of the three antiseptic soaked cotton balls, with a front to back motion. First, wipe the right labia using front to back motion. Discard cotton ball into waxed paper bag that is placed away from sterile area. Second, wipe the left labia repeating procedure and last, wipe down the center discarding cotton ball after each wipe. Discard forceps. Continue to hold labia apart until catheter is inserted. RATIONALE: Holding labia open will keep urinary meatus from becoming contaminated from labia while inserting catheter.
17. Place sterile catheter tray between the patient's leg, touching only the sterile surfaces of tray.
18. Using sterile gloved hand, pick up catheter and hold it about 3 to 4 inches from lubricated end. The other end of the catheter should go into the sterile catheter tray.
19. Gently insert lubricated tip of catheter into urinary meatus approximately 6 inches or until urine begins to flow. Move nondominant hand to hold catheter in place.
20. Interrupt urine flow by clamping or pinching off. RATIONALE: Stop flow of urine while specimen container is positioned.
21. Position end of catheter into urine specimen container.

(continues)

Procedure 18-2 (continued)

22. Collect specimen by releasing clamp and collecting approximately 60 ml urine.
23. Allow remaining urine to flow into basin until flow ceases. Pinch catheter closed.
24. Remove catheter gently and slowly.
25. Dry area with remaining cotton balls.
26. Tighten lid on the urine specimen container.
27. Remove procedure items.
28. Position patient for comfort.
29. Assist patient in sitting up or relaxing in a horizontal recumbent position. Offer tissues and sink for hand cleansing.
30. Help patient to sit on edge of table. Check patient's color and pulse.
31. Discard disposable items per Occupational Safety and Health Administration (OSHA) guidelines.
32. If collecting specimen for analysis, label specimen container and attach to completed laboratory requisition form.
33. Assist patient from examination table.
34. Clean room and table. Remove gloves and discard in biohazard waste container.
35. Wash hands.
36. Document procedure in patient's chart including the amount of urine collected. Document that specimen was sent to outside laboratory (if appropriate).

DOCUMENTATION

9/07/20XX 10:15 AM Catheterized with straight catheter to relieve urinary retention. 700 ml clear urine obtained. W. Slawson, CMA

Procedure 18-3 Performing a Urinary Catheterization on a Male Patient

STANDARD PRECAUTIONS:

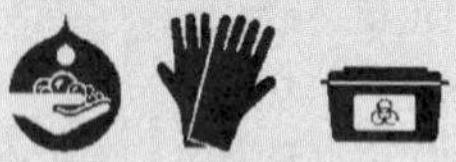

PURPOSE:

To obtain a sterile urine specimen for analysis or to relieve urinary retention.

EQUIPMENT/SUPPLIES:

Catheter kit (commercially available) containing:
- Sterile gloves
- Fenestrated drape
- Betadine solution, or Betadine swabs
- Lubricant
- Sterile cotton balls
- Sterile urine container with label
- Sterile 2 × 2 gauze sponges
- Forceps
- Sterile absorbent plastic pad

Additional items needed:
- Sterile catheter (size and type as ordered by physician)
- Biohazard waste container
- Laboratory requisition form
- Waxed paper bag

PROCEDURE STEPS:

1. Identify the patient and explain the procedure.
2. Instruct patient to breathe slowly and deeply during procedure. RATIONALE: This helps the patient relax the abdominal and pelvic muscles and facilitates easier insertion of the catheter.
3. Wash hands and assemble supplies.
4. Place unopened catheter kit on Mayo stand near the patient.

(continues)

Procedure 18-3 (continued)

5. Provide adequate lighting.
6. Have patient disrobe below the waist; provide a drape.
7. Position patient into a dorsal recumbent position on an examination table. RATIONALE: This allows for access to the urinary meatus.
8. Drape patient with sheet exposing only external genitalia.
9. Open outer wrapping of sterile kit. This becomes a sterile field.
10. Place sterile underpad under patient's penis touching only corners. Empty contents of tray onto sterile field. Add sterile catheter to field (Figure 18-38A). RATIONALE: Provides sterile field.
11. Wash hands. Put on sterile gloves.
12. Open fenestrated drape and, being careful not to contaminate drape or gloves, position drape opening over penis. Figure 18-38B.
13. Apply sterile lubricant to a sterile gauze sponge and place tip of catheter in lubricant.
14. With nondominant hand, hold the penis below the glans. In uncircumcised males, the glans must be pulled pack to expose the meatus. This is done entirely with the nondominant hand. RATIONALE: The dominant hand remains sterile so as not to contaminate remaining sterile equipment.
15. With the dominant hand, take the sterile forceps and a cotton ball that has been dipped in Betadine®, clean around the meatus in a circular motion from center toward outside. Use all three cotton balls or Betadine® swabs (Figure 18-39). RATIONALE: Assures that as many microorganisms as possible will be removed from the meatus and surrounding areas before insertion of sterile catheter.
16. With the dominant hand, take catheter out of lubricant; while holding the penis upright and straight with the nondominant hand, insert

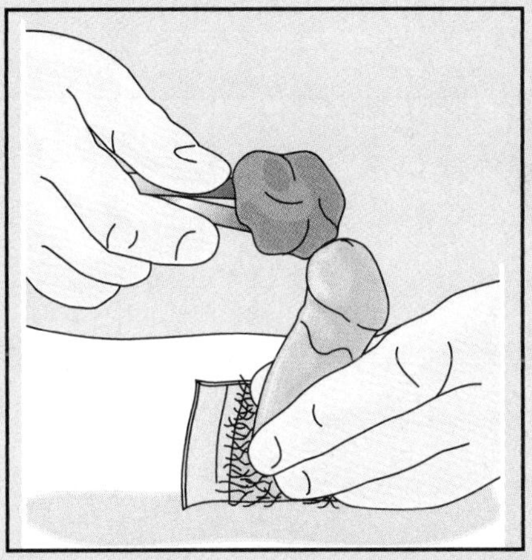

Figure 18-39 With the dominant hand, take the sterile forceps and a cotton ball dipped in Betadine® and clean around the meatus in a circular motion from center toward outside. Use all three cotton balls and Betadine®.

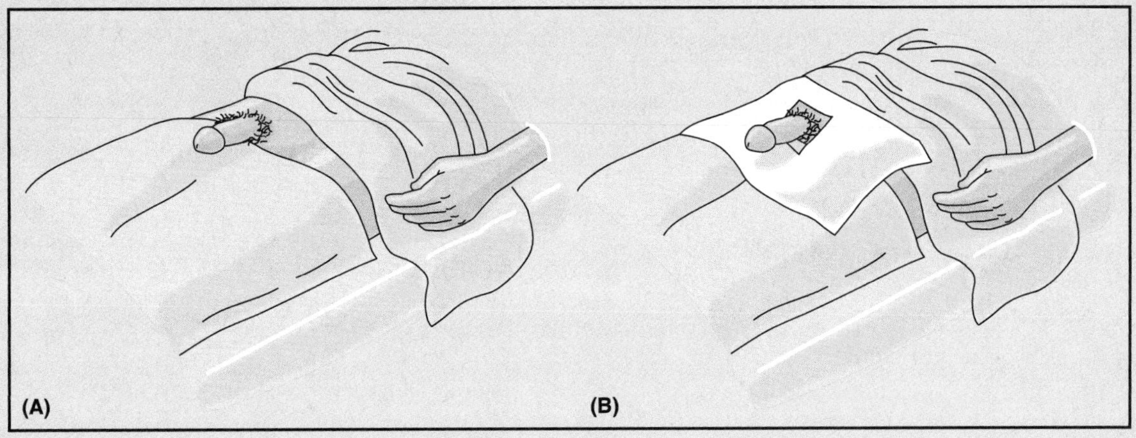

Figure 18-38 (A) Place sterile underpad under patient's penis. (B) Open fenestrated drape. Being careful not to contaminate drape or gloves, position drape opening over penis.

(continues)

Procedure 18-3 (continued)

the catheter approximately 6 inches until the urine flows into the sterile kit. See Figure 18-40A. RATIONALE: Holding the penis upright and straight facilitates insertion of the catheter. CAUTION: Do not force catheter. If problems arise attempting insertion, do not continue with procedure. Notify physician.

17. Obtain a specimen if ordered. See Figure 18-40B.
18. After urine flow ceases, remove catheter gently and slowly.
19. Dry penis with remaining cotton ball(s).
20. Position patient for comfort.
21. Discard disposable items per OSHA guidelines.
22. If collecting specimen for analysis, label specimen container and attach to completed laboratory requisition form.
23. Assist patient from examination table.
24. Clean room and table. Remove gloves and discard in biohazard waste container.
25. Wash hands.
26. Document procedure in patient's chart including the amount of urine collected. Document that specimen was sent to outside laboratory (if appropriate).

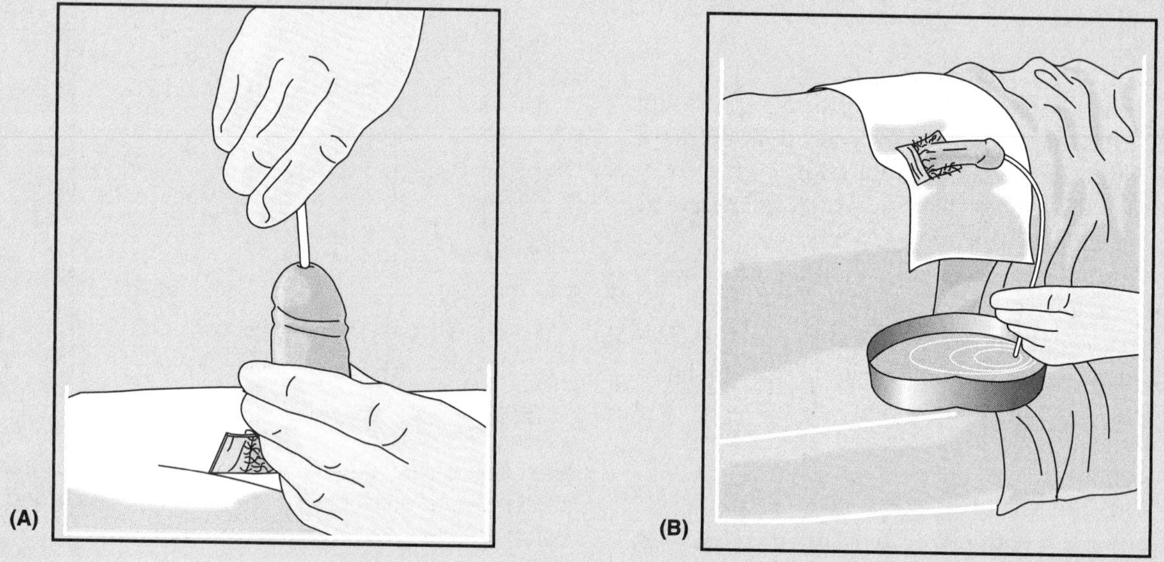

Figure 18-40 (A) With the dominant hand, take catheter out of lubricant; while holding the penis upright and straight with the nondominant hand, insert the catheter approximately 6 inches until the urine flows into the sterile kit. (B) Obtain a specimen if ordered.

DOCUMENTATION

9/07/20XX 10:15 AM Catheterized with straight catheter to relieve urinary retention. 700 ml clear urine obtained. W. Slawson, CMA

Procedure 18-4 Fecal Occult Blood Test

STANDARD PRECAUTIONS:

PURPOSE:

To test feces for occult blood.

EQUIPMENT/SUPPLIES:

Three occult slide test kits containing three slides, applicators, and envelope

PROCEDURE STEPS:

1. Check expiration dates on occult slides. RATIONALE: Outdated slides can give an inaccurate reading.
2. Identify the patient.
3. Fill out all information on the front flap of all three slides (Figure 18-41).
4. Explain the stool collection process; the patient will need to:
   a. Keep slides at room temperature away from sunlight. RATIONALE: Sunlight destroys effectiveness of guaiac paper and could result in an inaccurate result.
   b. Place date on front flap, then open it.
   c. Use one end of the wooden applicator to apply a thin smear of the stool sample from the toilet to Box "A." NOTE: *Do not collect during menstrual cycle or if hemorrhoids are present.*
   d. Repeat the procedure using the other end of the applicator, taking a specimen from a different section of the same stool and applying a thin smear to Box "B." RATIONALE: Occult blood may be distributed differently throughout the bowel movement.
   e. Dispose of the applicator in a waste container.
   f. Close the cover after air drying overnight.
   g. Repeat the process with the next two bowel movements, on subsequent days.
5. Provide the patient with an envelope to return the slides to the physician's office. Review with patient instructions on diet and medication (Figure 18-42). Caution patient not to mail slides to the office. RATIONALE: Slides are considered biohazardous material.
6. Record that the test kit and instructions were given to patient.

Developing the fecal occult slide

When the patient returns the fecal occult samples to the office, the medical assistant will be

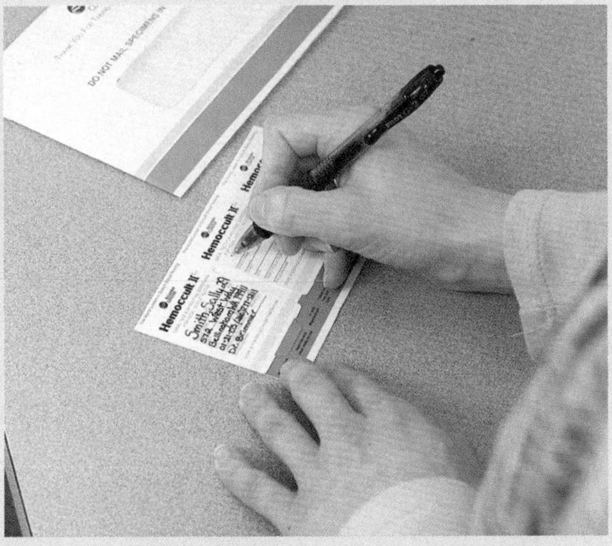

Figure 18-41 The medical assistant writes the patient's name, the date, and the specimen number on each occult slide.

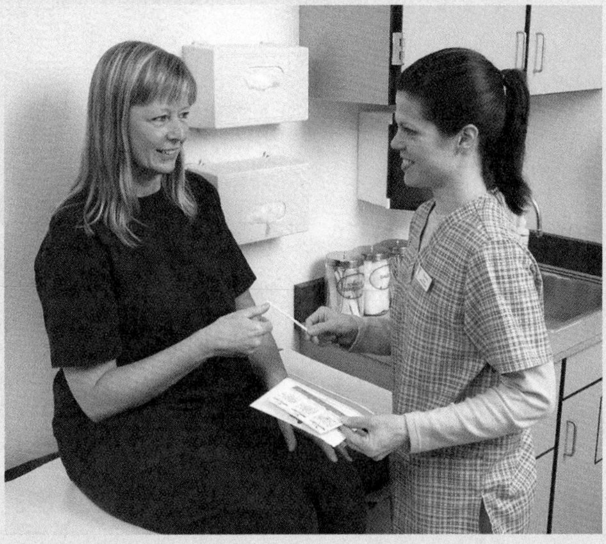

Figure 18-42 The medical assistant explains the process to the patient.

(continues)

Procedure 18-4 (continued)

responsible for developing the slides. Although most slides may be stored for up to 14 days before developing, the medical assistant should develop them as soon as possible because the patient may have already stored them for several days. Test results are important to ensure prompt treatment should a problem be discovered.

EQUIPMENT/SUPPLIES:

Prepared fecal slides from patient
Good lighting
Occult blood developer
Reference card that accompanies kit
Gloves
Biohazard waste container

PROCEDURE STEPS:

1. Check the expiration date on the developer.
2. Apply gloves and lay a surface protector (paper towels).
3. Open the window flap on the back of the slide.
4. Apply two drops of the developer to each Box "A" and "B," directly over each smear (Figure 18-43). RATIONALE: Paper contains the chemical guaiac, which will help identify occult blood.
5. Interpret the results within 30 to 60 seconds or as manufacturer directs. Record the results.
6. A positive reaction will have a blue halo appear around the perimeter of the specimen. Any blue color is positive.
7. Perform the quality-control procedure by processing the positive and negative monitor strip on each slide to confirm the test system is functional. RATIONALE: Failure of the positive strip to turn blue or negative strip to remain neutral indicates faulty supplies. Recheck expiration dates on slide and developer. Repeat test if necessary.
8. Dispose of all supplies according to OSHA guidelines.
9. Remove gloves and dispose in biohazard waste container.
10. Wash hands.
11. Document results in patient's chart.

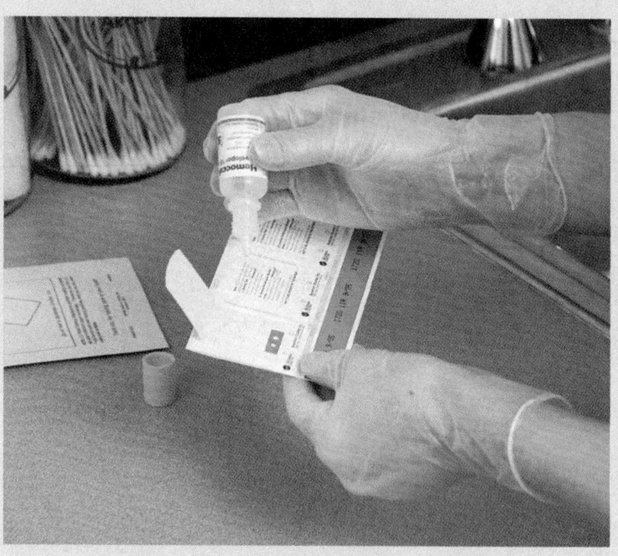

Figure 18-43 The medical assistant places developing solution on the slides.

DOCUMENTATION

1/14/20XX 2:00 PM Given 3 occult slides, 3 wooden applicators and an envelope with instructions. Instructed patient in dietary restrictions, the collection of the stool specimens and to keep the slides at room temperature away from sunlight. Patient instructed to bring specimens to office. J. Guerro, CMA

5/12/20XX 3:00 PM Three hemoccult slides returned. Results: all three slides negative. Reported to Dr. Woo. Dr. Woo wants patient notified of results and to remind patient to make an appointment with her gastroenterologist for a colonoscopy. Spoke to patient. Understands slides were negative for hidden blood in the stool. She will make an appointment for a colonoscopy. W. Slawson, CMA

Procedure 18-5 Performing Visual Acuity Testing Using a Snellen Chart

STANDARD PRECAUTIONS:

PURPOSE:

To perform a visual screening test to determine a patient's distance visual acuity.

EQUIPMENT/SUPPLIES:

Snellen eye chart placed at eye level (appropriate for age and reading ability of patient)
Pointer
Occluder
Alcohol wipes

PROCEDURE STEPS:

1. Wash hands and assemble equipment.
2. Prepare a well-lighted room, free from distractions and with a distance mark 20 feet from the eye chart. Be certain there is no glare on the chart.
3. Explain the procedure to the patient. Patients should be tested with their glasses or contact lenses, unless otherwise indicated by the physician.
4. Instruct the patient to stand behind the mark and cover the right eye with the **occluder** (Figure 18-44). Instruct the patient to keep the left eye open under the occluder and not to apply pressure to the eyeball. RATIONALE: Closing of the eye not being tested may cause the person to squint when reading the chart.
5. Stand next to the chart and point to row 3 instructing the patient to read each letter with the left eye, verbally identifying each letter read (Figure 18-45). If unable to read line 3, go to line 2 or 1. RATIONALE: Pointing to each row helps the patient to focus on one row of letters at a time. Beginning at row 3 saves time.

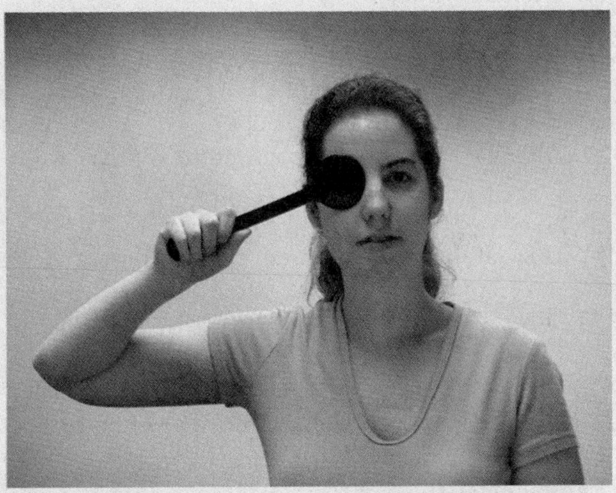

Figure 18-44 The patient covers the right eye with the occluder, keeping the eye open under the occluder.

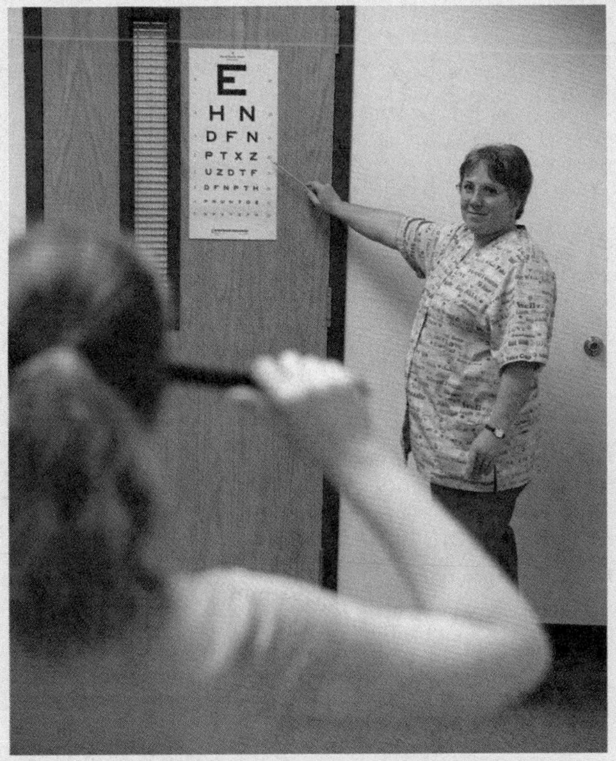

Figure 18-45 The patient uses the left eye to read the letters on the chart. The patient is instructed to start with row 3. Here she is reading row 4.

(continues)

Procedure 18-5 (continued)

6. Record the results at the smallest line the patient can read with two or fewer errors. Vision is recorded as right eye, left eye, both eyes.

   Examples: Right eye 20/25; Left eye 20/20; Both eyes 20/20

   RATIONALE: Visual acuity is recorded as a fraction. The number above the line on the chart is the distance the patient is standing from the chart. The number below the line on the chart is the distance from which a person with normal vision can read that row of letters.
7. Record the patient's reaction during the test. RATIONALE: Leaning forward, squinting or straining, or eye tears may indicate eye problems.
8. When finished with the examination of the left eye, use the same procedure to test the right eye.
9. Disinfect occluder. Wash hands. Record the results.

DOCUMENTATION

4/14/20XX 1:15 PM Visual acuity checked using Snellen chart. Results: right 20/30; left 20/20; both 20/20. B. Abbott, RMA

Procedure 18-6 Measuring Near Visual Acuity

STANDARD PRECAUTIONS:

PURPOSE:
To measure the near vision of the patient.

EQUIPMENT/SUPPLIES:
Appropriate near visual acuity chart
3 × 5 cards or occluder

PROCEDURE STEPS:

1. Wash hands.
2. Identify patient.
3. Explain procedure to patient; provide occluder. RATIONALE: To obtain patient cooperation.
4. Position patient in a comfortable position.
5. Position the near visual acuity card 14 inches from the patient by measuring with a tape measure. RATIONALE: To obtain accurate results.
6. Have patient lightly (no pressure) cover the left eye with the occluder. RATIONALE: Pressure will cause blurring of the other eye.
7. Have patient read the paragraphs printed on the card.
8. Once patient has reached a line where more than two mistakes are made, note the visual acuity for that eye (allow the patient to repeat the line to verify acuity).
9. Repeat the process to measure the left eye.
10. Repeat the process to measure both eyes.
11. Record the result in the patient chart. Results-are charted 14/14 for normal near visual acuity.
12. Discard the 3 × 5 card or disinfect the occluder. RATIONALE: To prevent microorganism cross-contamination.
13. Wash hands.
14. Record results.

DOCUMENTATION

7/22/20XX 4:00 PM Near visual acuity checked. Results: 14/14. J. Guerro, CMA

Procedure 18-7 Performing Color Vision Test Using the Ishihara Plates

STANDARD PRECAUTIONS:

PURPOSE:

To assess a patient's ability to distinguish between the colors red and green.

Patient education:

1. Explain that the purpose of the test is to determine if the patient has a color vision deficiency.
2. Show patient plate number 12 as an example of the test process.

EQUIPMENT/SUPPLIES:

Ishihara plates (1–12) (Figure 18-46)

PROCEDURE STEPS:

1. Wash hands and assemble the equipment in a room lighted by daylight. RATIONALE: Direct sunlight or electric light may produce errors in the results because of an alteration in the appearance of shades of color.
2. Hold each plate 75 cm or 30 inches from the patient and tilted so that the plane of the plate is at a right angle to the line of the patient's vision.
3. Record the number given by the patient on each plate.
4. Assess the patient's readings and record. RATIONALE: If 10 or more plates are read correctly, the color vision is regarded as normal.
   Source for error: Test plates should be kept covered when not in use. Undue exposure to sunlight causes a fading of the color plates, thus leading to inaccurate test interpretation.

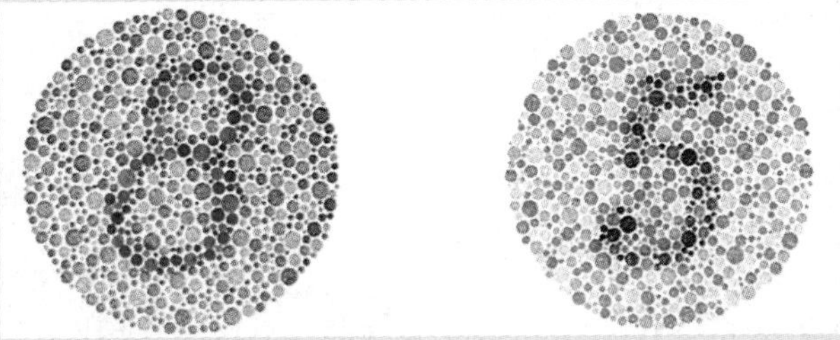

Figure 18-46 Ishihara plates are used to assess the patient's ability to distinguish between the colors red and green.

DOCUMENTATION

3/12/20XX 11:00 AM Color vision test performed using Ishihara plates. Twelve plates read correctly. L. Carlson, RMA

Procedure 18-8 Performing Eye Instillation

STANDARD PRECAUTIONS:

PURPOSE:

To treat eye infections, soothe irritation, anesthetize, and dilate pupils. Ophthalmic medication is supplied in liquid or ointment form. Use separate medication for each eye, if both are affected.

EQUIPMENT/SUPPLIES:

Sterile eye dropper for single use
Sterile ophthalmic medication as ordered by the physician, either drops or ointment
Sterile cotton balls
Sterile gloves
Tissues

PROCEDURE STEPS:

1. Wash hands.
2. Assemble supplies using sterile technique.
3. Check medication carefully as ordered by the physician, including expiration date. Read label three times.
4. Identify patient.
5. Explain procedure to the patient and inform the patient that instillation may temporarily blur vision.
6. Position the patient in a sitting or lying position.
7. Instruct the patient to stare at a fixed spot during instillation of the drops.
8. Prepare medication using either drops or ointment.
9. Have the patient look up to the ceiling and expose the lower conjunctival sac of the affected eye by using fingers over a tissue to pull down (Figure 18-47).
10. Place the number of drops ordered in the center of the lower conjunctival sac or a thin line of ointment in the lower surface of the eyelid being careful not to touch the eyelid, eyeball, or eyelashes with the tip of the medication applicator. Carefully replace cover on bottle. Discard dropper.
11. Have the patient close the eye and roll the eyeball. RATIONALE: Movement distributes the medication evenly.
12. Blot excess medication from eyelids with cotton ball from inner to outer canthus.
13. Dispose of supplies.
14. Wash hands.
15. Record procedure in patient's chart.

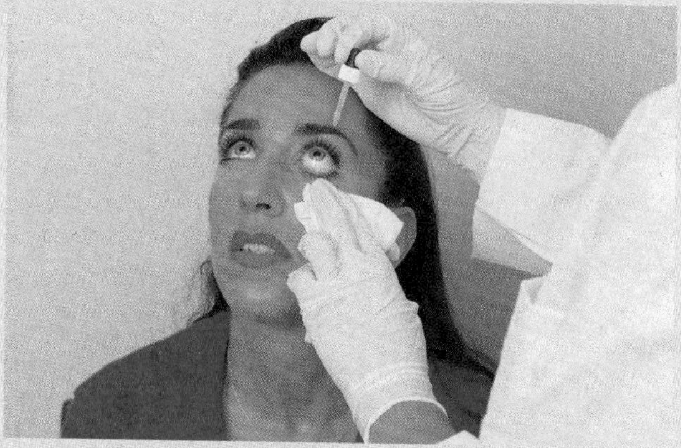

Figure 18-47 When instilling medication into the patient's eye, the patient should look up to the ceiling and the medical assistant should pull down on the lower lid. Contact with the eyeball should be avoided.

DOCUMENTATION

9/12/20XX 11:30 AM Ophthalmic drops (two) instilled in right eye. Eye red and swollen. No exudate noted. J. Bloom, RMA

Procedure 18-9 Performing Eye Patch Dressing Application

STANDARD PRECAUTIONS:

PURPOSE:
To apply a sterile eye patch.

EQUIPMENT/SUPPLIES:
Tape
Sterile eye patch
Sterile gloves

PROCEDURE STEPS:
1. Wash hands and assemble supplies.
2. Identify patient.
3. Explain the procedure. Ascertain if patient has a ride home. RATIONALE: Monovision is misleading, and the patient cannot see well enough to drive himself or herself.
4. Position the patient in a sitting or supine position.
5. Instruct the patient to close both eyes during the application of the patch. Prepare sterile area by opening the sterile package and using the inside of the package as a sterile field. Apply sterile gloves.
6. Place the patch over the affected eye using sterile gloves.
7. Secure the patch with three to four strips of transparent tape diagonally from mid-forehead to below the ear.
8. Remove gloves.
9. Wash hands.
10. Document the procedure and provide verbal and written care instructions to the patient.

DOCUMENTATION

8/1/20XX 2:30 PM Sterile eye patch applied to right eye. Eye appeared red. No exudate seen. Patient instructed not to drive with eye patch on. Wife to drive patient home. J. Bloom, RMA

Procedure 18-10 Performing Eye Irrigation

STANDARD PRECAUTIONS:

PURPOSE:
To irrigate the patient's affected eye.
a. To cleanse debris
b. To cleanse discharge
c. To remove chemicals
d. To apply antiseptic
e. To apply warmth for comfort

EQUIPMENT/SUPPLIES:
Sterile irrigation solution as ordered by the physician
Sterile bulb syringe (rubber)
Kidney-shaped basin to catch irrigation solution
Sterile cotton balls
Sterile gloves
Biohazard waste container
Towel
Pillow

(continues)

Procedure 18-10 (continued)

PROCEDURE STEPS:

1. Wash hands and assemble supplies. NOTE: If both eyes need to be irrigated, use separate equipment for each eye. RATIONALE: Avoid cross contamination.
2. Identify patient.
3. Explain the procedure to the patient.
4. Position the patient in a supine position.
5. Check expiration date on solution bottle.
6. Check label three times. Warm solution to body temperature (98.6°F).
7. Tilt head toward affected eye. Place towel on patient shoulder. RATIONALE: Avoid cross contamination of unaffected eye by allowing the solution to flow from the affected eye into the kidney basin.
8. Place the basin beside the affected eye. RATIONALE: Allows for the solution to drain into a catch receptacle.
9. Put on sterile gloves.
10. Moisten two to three cotton balls with irrigation solution and clean the eyelids and eyelashes of the affected eye from inner to outer canthus. Discard after each wipe.
11. Expose the lower conjunctiva by separating the eyelid with your index finger and thumb.
12. Have the patient stare at a fixed spot.
13. Irrigate the affected eye with sterile solution by resting the sterile bulb syringe on the bridge of the patient's nose, being careful not to touch the eye or conjunctival sac with the syringe tip. Allow the stream to flow from the inside canthus to the outer corner of the eye (Figure 18-48). RATIONALE: This avoids a flow of solution into the unaffected eye causing cross contamination.
14. After irrigation, dry the eyelid and eyelashes with sterile cotton balls. The physician will add a staining solution to check for corneal abrasion.
15. Discard supplies in biohazard container if discharge or exudate is present.
16. Remove gloves.
17. Wash hands and document procedure.

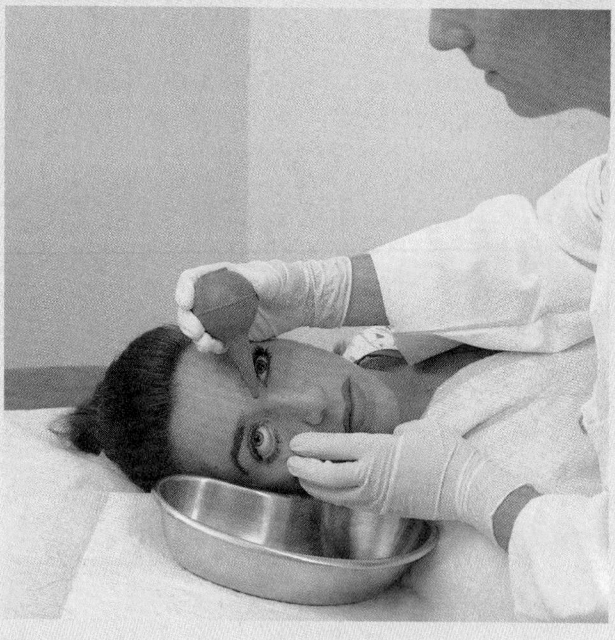

Figure 18-48 The medical assistant irrigates the patient's eye. Note that the solution will go from inner to outer canthus. The patient is turned toward the affected eye.

DOCUMENTATION

11/26/20XX 10:00 AM Right eye irrigated with 100 ml sterile normal saline (100°F). Eye appears slightly red. No exudate noted. Fluorescein stain (stain strip used for diagnosis and detecting foreign bodies or lesions on the cornea) instilled into right eye by Dr. Woo. Patient seemed to tolerate procedure well. Says she has "no discomfort." K. Bloom, RMA

Procedure 18-11 Assisting with Audiometry

STANDARD PRECAUTIONS:

PURPOSE:

To assist in testing patient for hearing loss.

Patient education:

1. Explain the use and purpose of the audiometer and that the test measures frequency of sound waves and ability of patient to hear various frequencies of sound waves (one frequency at a time).
2. When the patient hears a new frequency, he or she is to signal the tester.

EQUIPMENT/SUPPLIES:

Audiometer with head phones
Quiet room

PROCEDURE STEPS:

1. Wash hands and assemble equipment and supplies.
2. Prepare room. Test must be held in a room without outside noises. RATIONALE: Outside interference may cause inaccurate test results, especially in the lower frequencies, which are more difficult to hear.
3. Identify and explain procedure to patient.
4. Position patient in a comfortable sitting position.
5. Have patient put on head phones. The procedure is done on each ear separately.
6. If the medical assistant has been thoroughly trained to do the procedure, the physician will authorize the medical assistant to perform the audiometry. The audiometer is started at low frequency. The patient indicates when the sound is heard and the medical assistant plots it on the graph (the audiogram) (Figure 18-49).
7. The frequencies gradually increase until completed.
8. The other ear is checked in the same manner.
9. The results are given to the physician for interpretation.
10. Equipment is cleaned following manufacturer's instructions.
11. Wash hands.
12. Document procedure on patient's chart.

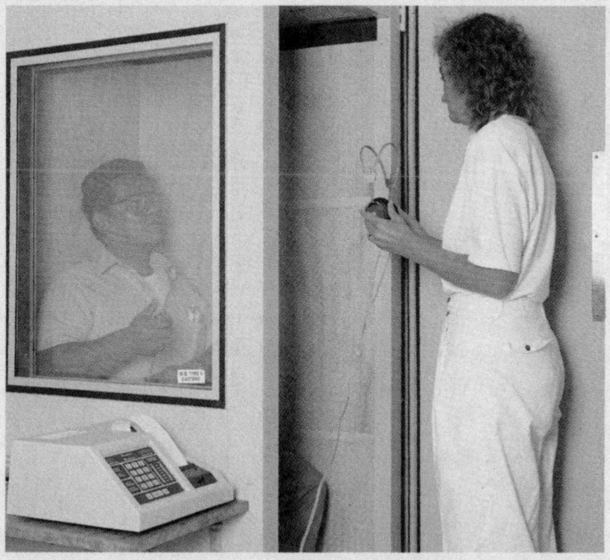

Figure 18-49 The patient presses the handheld control button each time he hears a sound. The medical assistant plots sounds heard on the audiogram.

DOCUMENTATION

4/12/20XX 2:00 PM Audiometry performed. Results given to Dr. Woo. B. Abbott, RMA

Procedure 18-12 Performing Ear Irrigation

STANDARD PRECAUTIONS:

PURPOSE:

To remove impacted cerumen, discharge, or foreign materials from the ear canal as directed by the physician.

EQUIPMENT/SUPPLIES:

Irrigation solution as ordered by the physician warmed to (98.6–103°F)
Ear irrigation syringe or bulb
Ear basin or emesis (catch) basin
Basin for warmed solution
Towel
Cotton balls
Otoscope

PROCEDURE STEPS:

1. Wash hands and assemble equipment.
2. Identify patient.
3. Explain the procedure and inform the patient that during the procedure a minimal amount of discomfort and dizziness may be experienced caused by solution coming into contact with the tympanic membrane. Be sure physician has examined the ear before irrigation. RATIONALE: Avoids perforation of tympanic membrane.
4. Place the patient in a sitting position and use an otoscope to visualize the affected ear. Have patient tilt head toward affected ear.
5. Cleanse the outer ear with a wet cotton ball moistened with irrigation solution.
6. Gently pull the auricle upward and back to straighten the ear canal.
7. Tilt the patient's head slightly forward and to the affected side (Figure 18-50). RATIONALE: This position allows the solution to flow into the basin by gravity.
8. Place towel on the patient's shoulder of the affected side.
9. Place the ear basin under the affected ear and have the patient hold the basin in place.
10. Check label of solution three times for correctness and also check the expiration date of the solution.
11. Pour the solution into a basin and fill the syringe with the warmed irrigation solution as prescribed by the physician. Use about 30 to 50 cc solution at a time to warm the instrument. (Repeat Step 5.)
12. Straighten the external auditory canal by pulling back and upward on the auricle for adults.
13. Expel air from syringe and gently insert the syringe tip into the affected ear, being careful not to insert too deeply. Do not occlude external auditory canal. Direct the flow of the solution upward toward roof of canal. RATIONALE: This will avoid injury to the tympanic membrane and prevent occlusion of external auditory canal, allowing solution to drain out.
14. Repeat the irrigation allowing the solution to drain from the ear, noting the return. Allow for free flow of return each time. Check with the patient about any discomfort or pain. Do not continue if pain is present.

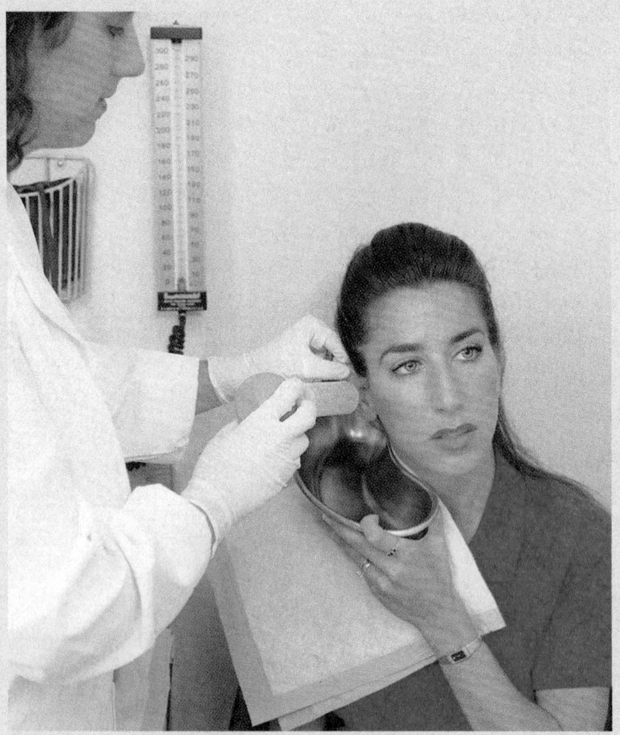

Figure 18-50 When irrigating the patient's ear, the affected ear is tipped to facilitate the flow of solution. The tip of the syringe does not occlude the opening to the external auditory canal.

(continues)

Procedure 18-12 (continued)

15. Dry the outer ear and visualize the inner ear with the otoscope to verify the procedure has removed or dislodged the foreign body.
16. Notify the physician the procedure has been completed.
17. When the procedure is completed, remove the ear basin and towel.
18. Have patient lie on affected side on examination table for ear to continue draining.
19. Provide dry cotton balls to the patient to catch any further drainage if directed by the physician.
20. Dispose of supplies.
21. Wash hands.
22. Document the procedure noting return and amount. Provide postcare instructions:
    a. Report any pain or dizziness to the physician.
    b. Do not insert any foreign object (i.e., cotton applicator) into the ear canal.

DOCUMENTATION

6/4/20XX 3:30 PM Left ear irrigated with normal saline (100°F). Three pieces (size of pencil eraser) of cerumen in solution returns. No complaints of pain or dizziness. Inner ear and tympanic membrane appear clear. Dr. King notified of results. W. Slawson, CMA

Procedure 18-13 Performing Ear Instillation

STANDARD PRECAUTIONS:

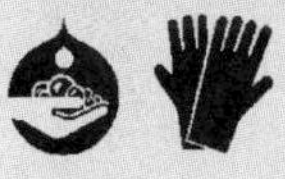

PURPOSE:

To soften impacted cerumen, fight infection with antibiotics, or relieve pain.

EQUIPMENT/SUPPLIES:

Otic medication as prescribed by the physician
Sterile ear dropper
Cotton balls
Gloves

PROCEDURE STEPS:

1. Wash hands and assemble supplies.
2. Identify patient.
3. Explain procedure to the patient.
4. Position patient to either lie on unaffected side or in sitting position with head tilted toward unaffected ear. RATIONALE: Facilitates flow of medication.
5. Check otic medication three times against the physician's order and check expiration date of the medication. RATIONALE: Only otic medication can be used in the ear. Checking the medication three times minimizes medication error.

(continues)

Procedure 18-13 (continued)

6. Draw up the prescribed amount of medication.
7. Gently pull the top of the ear upward and back (adult) or pull earlobe downward and backward (child) (Figure 18-51).
8. Instill prescribed dose of medication (number of drops) by squeezing rubber bulb on dropper into the affected ear.
9. Have the patient maintain the position for about five minutes to retain medication.
10. When instructed by the physician, insert moistened cotton ball into external ear canal for 15 minutes. RATIONALE: Moistened cotton ball will not absorb medication and will help retain medication in ear.
11. Dispose of supplies.
12. Wash hands.
13. Document procedure.

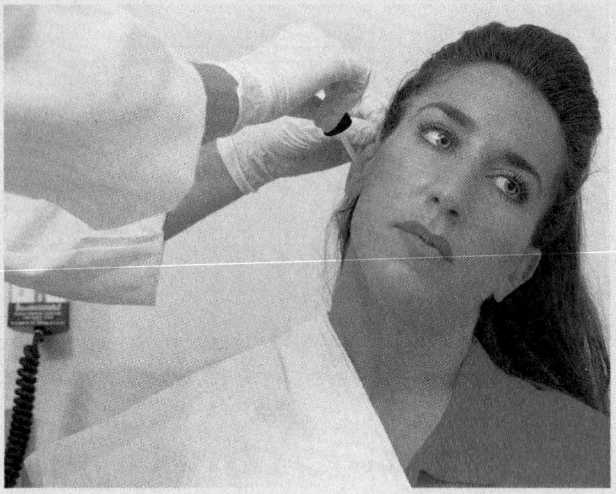

Figure 18-51 When instilling drops into patient's ear, have the patient tilt head so the affected ear is uppermost.

DOCUMENTATION

12/10/20XX 4:00 PM Otic solution (four drops) instilled into patient's right ear. Moistened cotton ball inserted in ear. No exudate noted. W. Slawson, CMA.

Procedure 18-14 Assisting with Nasal Examination

STANDARD PRECAUTIONS:

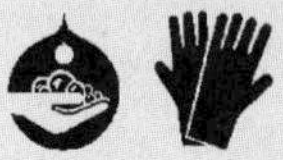

PURPOSE:

To assist the physician with the nasal examination when looking for polyps, engorged superficial blood vessels, and to assist in the possible removal of a foreign body.

Patient education:

When a foreign object is involved, instruct the patient not to blow the nose or to attempt to remove the object because this could cause tissue damage or push the object deeper into the nasal passage.

EQUIPMENT/SUPPLIES:

Nasal speculum
Light source
Gloves
Bayonet forceps
Kidney basin

PROCEDURE STEPS:

1. Wash hands and assemble supplies.
2. Identify patient.
3. Explain the procedure to the patient.
4. Place the patient in a sitting position.
5. Reassure the patient.

(continues)

Procedure 18-14 (continued)

6. Hand the physician equipment and supplies as needed.
7. Clean equipment and dispose of supplies per OSHA guidelines.
8. Wash hands.
9. Document procedure noting foreign object if applicable.

DOCUMENTATION

2/4/20XX 4:30 PM Nasal examination done by Dr. Woo. Small polyp noted in left nostril. Arrangements made with Bayside Surgery for polyp removal on 2/10. B. Abbott, RMA

Procedure 18-15 Cautery Treatment of Epistaxis

STANDARD PRECAUTIONS:

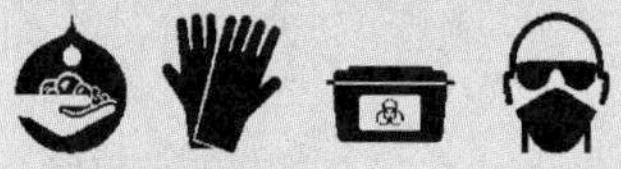

PURPOSE:

Patient education:

Depending on the location and severity of the nosebleed, the physician will decide to either pack the nasal canal or chemically cauterize the vessel. Generally, chemical cautery is attempted first; if that fails, nasal packing using endoscopy is performed. If cauterization is performed, patients should be instructed to not blow their nose or otherwise irritate/disturb the scab that will form. Cautery will sting, and the patient should be appropriately prepared.

EQUIPMENT/SUPPLIES:

Vienna nasal speculum
Light source (hands free)
Gloves
Bayonet forceps
Epinephrine
Silver nitrate sticks
Cotton balls
Cotton med cup
Local anesthetic (such as zylocaine with epinephrine or cocaine 4%)
Antibiotic/antiseptic ointment (such as triamcinolone)

PROCEDURE STEPS:

1. Wash hands, assemble equipment/supplies, and apply gloves.
2. Identify the patient and explain the procedure.
3. Give the patient a catch basin and tissue; have the patient lie down.
4. Assist the physician to visualize the area of treatment.
5. Assist the physician by handling him or her the supplies and instruments as directed.
6. Assist the physician with applying the anesthetic (a syringe and needle may be used to remove xylocaine from the vial and inject it into the med cup). The cotton-tipped applicators are then soaked in the anesthetic and applied to the nasal membranes.
7. Assist the physician and the patient during cautery.
8. Instruct the patient on postprocedure care.
9. Clean the equipment and dispose of contaminated supplies according to Standard Precautions and OSHA guidelines.
10. Wash hands.
11. Document the procedure.

DOCUMENTATION

8/6/20XX 2:45 PM Patient treated for epistaxis with silver nitrate cautery. Instructions given to avoid blowing nose or otherwise irritate/disturb the scab and to call/return immediately if nose begins to bleed again. J. Guerro, CMA

Patient Education

Nasal Irrigation

Advise the patient that commercial nasal irrigation kits are available at the pharmacy or department store, or the patient can make her own solution of salt and warm water (1/2 teaspoon to a pint). Use a bulb-type syringe for irrigation. Instruct patient not to blow nose for five minutes after the irrigation. This could force the solution into the sinuses or ears and possibly cause an infection in either or both.

Procedure 18-16 Performing Nasal Instillation

STANDARD PRECAUTIONS:

PURPOSE:

To provide medication to the nasal membranes as ordered by the physician.

Patient education:

1. Instruct the patient to keep the head tilted back during the procedure to allow the medication to cover the nasal tissues.
2. Do not blow nose immediately after treatment. Medication would be forced out of nose.

EQUIPMENT/SUPPLIES:

Medication as ordered by physician
Medicine dropper (sterile)
Tissues

PROCEDURE STEPS:

1. Wash hands and assemble equipment.
2. Identify patient.
3. Explain procedure to the patient.
4. Position the patient with the head lower than the shoulders.
5. Draw medication into dropper after checking medication three times and checking expiration date.
6. Place the dropper over the center of the outside of the affected nostril. Care should be taken not to touch the inside of the nostril. RATIONALE: Touching the inside of the nostril will lead to contamination of the dropper.
7. Repeat the procedure for the other nostril if required. Dispose of dropper; recap medication container using sterile technique.
8. Instruct the patient to remain in position for five minutes.
9. Provide cotton balls or gauze sponges to the patient when the patient returns to a sitting position. RATIONALE: Medication may still drain from the nostrils.
10. Dispose of the supplies per OSHA guidelines.
11. Wash hands.
12. Document the procedure.

DOCUMENTATION

4/13/20XX 6:00 PM Neosynephrine nasal drops (three drops) instilled into each nostril.
W. Slawson, CMA

Procedure 18-17 Administer Oxygen by Nasal Cannula for Minor Respiratory Distress

STANDARD PRECAUTIONS:

PURPOSE:

To provide a low dose of concentrated oxygen to a patient during periods of respiratory distress (e.g., chronic obstructive pulmonary disease).

Patient education:

1. Demonstrate the position of the nasal prongs of the cannula into the nose. They face upward and the tab rests above the upper lip.
2. Describe how to clear the oxygen cylinder valve by turning it counterclockwise.
3. Oxygen supports combustion and a fire can start with oxygen in use. Friction, static electricity, a spark, or a lighted cigarette or cigar can cause ignition.

EQUIPMENT/SUPPLIES:

Portable oxygen tank with stand
Disposable nasal cannula with connecting tube
Flowmeter
Pressure regulator

PROCEDURE STEPS:

1. Wash hands and explain procedure to the patient.
2. Identify patient.
3. Open the cylinder one full turn, counterclockwise.
4. Check the pressure gauge. RATIONALE: This will determine the amount of pressure in the cylinder.
5. Attach the nasal cannula to the tubing, and then to the flowmeter.
6. Adjust the flow rate according to the physician's order (oxygen is a medication).
7. Check for oxygen flow through the cannula.
8. Place the tips of cannula into the nares no more than 1 inch (Figure 18-52).
9. Adjust the tubing around the patient's ears (Figure 18-53) and secure it under the chin.

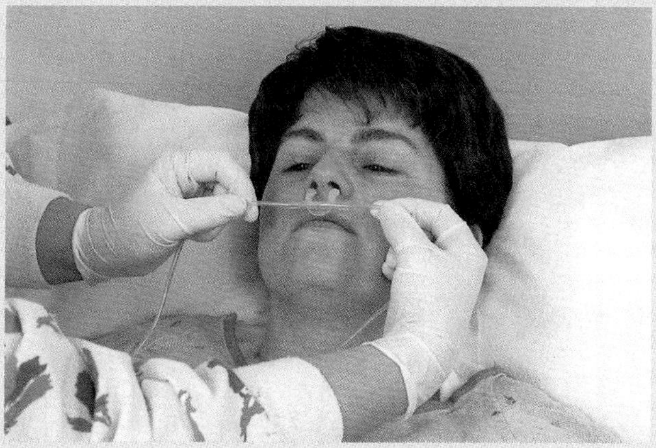

Figure 18-52 Insert cannula prong into nostrils.

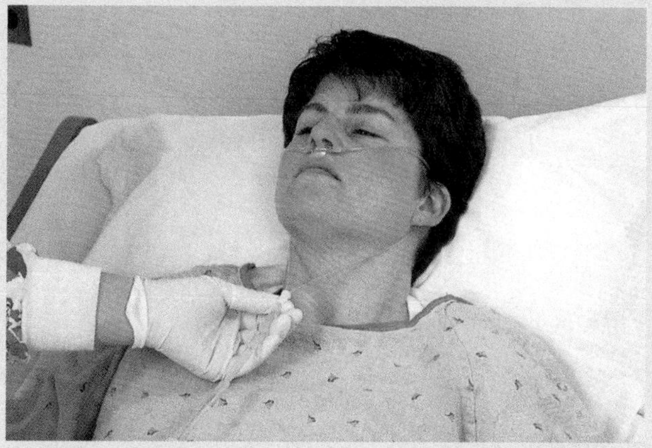

Figure 18-53 Adjust tubing.

(continues)

Procedure 18-17 (continued)

10. Answer patient's questions.
11. Wash hands.
12. Document the procedure.
    Note: Oxygen is usually humidified to prevent drying of respiratory mucosa (Figure 18-54).

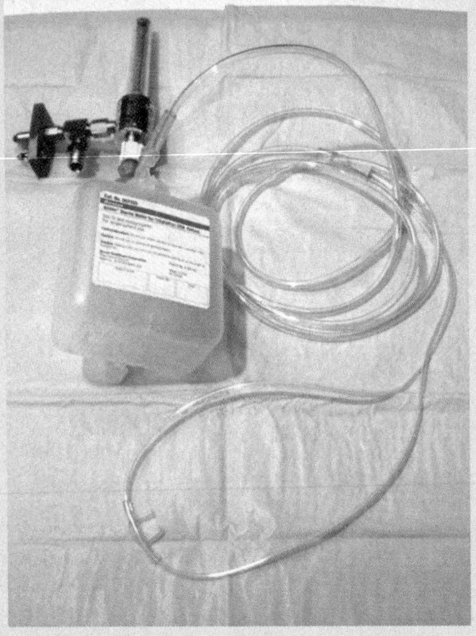

Figure 18-54 Nasal cannula and oxygen tubing attached to a humidifier.

DOCUMENTATION

4/19/20XX 2:45 PM Oxygen 3 L/minute by nasal cannula. Color slightly improved. Less cyanosis. J. Guerro, CMA

Procedure 18-18 Instructing Patient in Use of Metered Dose Nebulizer

STANDARD PRECAUTIONS:

PURPOSE:

To instruct a patient in the correct use of a handheld **nebulizer,** a device that delivers a fine mist of medication with or without the use of oxygen to the respiratory tract including the lungs.

Patient education:

1. Remind the patient to inhale slowly.
2. Close the mouth and lips around the mouthpiece.

(continues)

Procedure 18-18 (continued)

3. Clean the inhaler by rinsing the mouthpiece in warm water.
4. Adhere to prescribed dose.

EQUIPMENT/SUPPLIES:

Handheld nebulizer containing medication ordered by the physician

PROCEDURE STEPS:

1. Wash hands and assemble equipment.
2. Identify patient.
3. Check medication order three times (Figures 18-55 and 18-56).
4. Demonstrate the use of the equipment to the patient, and then have the patient repeat the demonstration.
5. Instruct the patient to sit upright and exhale fully.
6. Holding the nebulizer, close the mouth, lips, and teeth around the mouthpiece.
7. Tilting the head back, instruct the patient to take a deep breath and at the same time push the bottle against the mouthpiece.
8. Instruct the patient to continue to inhale until the lungs are full.
9. Remove the mouthpiece and slowly exhale.
10. Repeat Steps 4 through 7 if the physician has ordered more than one dose.
11. Check patient for adverse reactions.
12. Wash hands.
13. Document patient was given instructions and has demonstrated to you the use of the nebulizer.

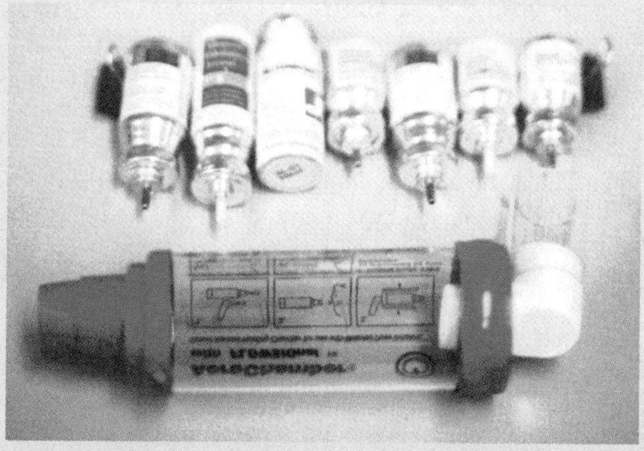

Figure 18-55 Metered-dose nebulizer and medications.

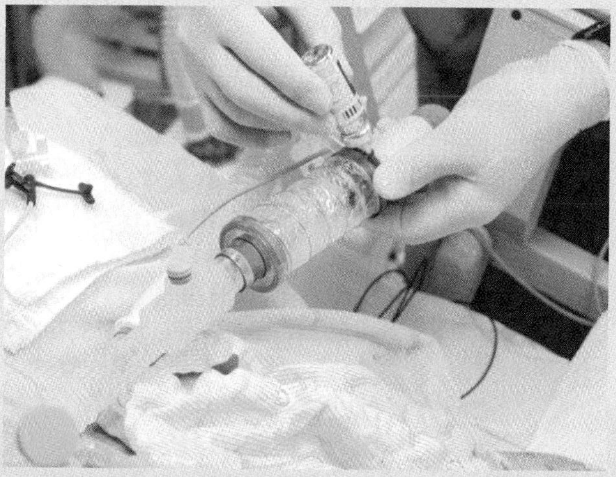

Figure 18-56 Preparation of a metered-dose nebulizer and medication.

DOCUMENTATION

4/19/20XX 2:45 PM Instructed in use of handheld metered dose nebulizer. Patient performed procedure well. No adverse reactions noted. W. Slawson, CMA

Procedure 18-19 Spirometry Testing

STANDARD PRECAUTIONS:

PURPOSE:
To prepare a patient for a spirometry to obtain optimum test results.
Patient education:
1. Reinforce the importance of good posture during the process.
2. When blowing into the mouthpiece, the lips must seal tightly around it.
3. Explain the parameters needed for successful completion of the test.
   Parameters:
   - Patient must inhale deeply and quickly and exhale quickly and forcibly until no air can be expelled.
   - Patient must refrain from the use of bronchodilators for 24 hours before test.
   - Explain to the patient that maximum effort is required for accurate test results.

EQUIPMENT/SUPPLIES:
Spirometer
Disposable mouthpiece

PROCEDURE STEPS:
1. Wash hands and assemble equipment.
2. Identify the patient.
3. Explain the procedure and equipment to the patient. Allow the patient to breathe into the machine to become acquainted with the equipment. See Figure 18-32.
4. Place the patient in a comfortable position (sitting/standing). Loosen tie or collar.
5. Instruct the patient not to bend at the waist when blowing into the mouthpiece.
6. Reinforce the inhalation process (deep breaths to fill the lungs to maximum capacity).
7. Instruct the patient to continue to blow into the mouthpiece until instructed to stop.
8. Be supportive and encouraging throughout the test.
9. Wash hands.
10. Attend to patient's needs.
11. Place the test results on the patient's chart after being reviewed by the physician.

DOCUMENTATION
12/22/20XX 4:00 PM Spirometry performed. Results given to Dr. Woo. J. Guerro, RMA

Procedure 18-20 Pulse Oximetry

STANDARD PRECAUTIONS:

PURPOSE:
To measure arterial oxyhemoglobin saturation (S_aO_2) within seconds by using an external sensor.

EQUIPMENT/SUPPLIES:
Pulse oximeter
Sensor
Soap and water or alcohol wipe
Nail polish remover, if needed

(continues)

Procedure 18-20 (continued)

PROCEDURE STEPS:

1. Wash hands and assemble equipment.
2. Identify the patient.
3. Explain the procedure.
4. Select a site for the sensor (finger commonly used).
5. If patient has poor circulation, use another site (bridge of nose, earlobe, or forehead).
6. Clean site with alcohol wipe. Remove nail polish if necessary. Wash with soap and water.
7. Apply sensor (finger is placed within a clip) (see Figure 18-32).
8. Connect sensor to oximeter with a sensor cable.
9. Turn on oximeter. A tone and a pulse fluctuation can be heard. Adjust volume.
10. Alarms can be set to alert medical assistant to levels either too high or too low.
11. Check pulse manually and compare with oximeter. They should be the same.
12. Note results per manufacturer's instructions.
13. Notify supervisor of abnormal results (less than 95%).
14. Document procedure noting type of sensor used and the site of application and the results.
15. Plug in oximeter for recharging when not in use so the battery does not get low. NOTE: When measuring, cover the sensor with a towel to eliminate sensor's exposure to light. It could interfere with the sensor and give incorrect results.

DOCUMENTATION

3/16/20XX 4:00 PM Pulse oximetry 98%. G. Underwood, CMA

Procedure 18-21 Assisting with Plaster Cast Application

STANDARD PRECAUTIONS:

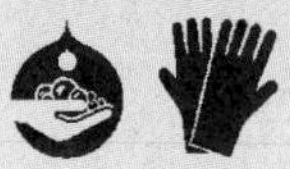

PURPOSE:

To assist physician in cast application.

EQUIPMENT/SUPPLIES:

Cast material:
Plaster bandage roll or synthetic tape
Container of warm water, which is lined with plastic or cloth to catch loose plaster
Water
Stockinette (3-inch width for arms, 4-inch width for leg casts)
Webril (sheet wadding) padding rolls
Bandage scissors
Rubber gloves
Sponge rubber for padding

PROCEDURE STEPS:

1. Identify the patient and provide the patient with an explanation of the procedure.
2. Answer any questions about the injury or cast application.
3. Wash hands and assemble the equipment and supplies.
4. Position the patient in a sitting position or as required by the physician. Proper alignment must be maintained.

(continues)

Procedure 18-21 (continued)

5. Put on gloves and drape patient around the procedure.
6. Clean and dry the area to be casted, as directed by the physician. Chart any areas of bruising, redness, or open areas. RATIONALE: Appropriate documentation of skin condition is needed to assist in evaluation of the extremity at a later time.
7. Pad bony prominence with sponge rubber. RATIONALE: To protect from pressure.
8. Provide the correct width of stockinette for the area on which cast is being applied. RATIONALE: A stockinette that is too large will form creases, thus allowing for injury to tissues.
9. Provide physician with correct width of webril rolls. RATIONALE: Webril (soft cotton bandage) provides protection to the patient's skin preventing pressure sores. Folds in the padding could lead to irritation of the skin.
10. Place the bandage in the container of warm water for five seconds. Remove from water and gently squeeze to remove excess water. Do not wring.
11. Assist with the application of the cast material as requested by the physician.
12. Reassure patient as needed.
13. After cast application, clean any plaster off patient, review cast care instructions, and provide written instructions for cast care and isometric exercises (if prescribed by the physician). Reinforce any precautions given by the physician. RATIONALE: Reviewing possible complications with the patient enhances the immediate reporting of circulatory impairment and infection.
14. Discard water down the sink drain being cautious to keep plaster from going down the drain. (Allow plaster to settle to bottom of basin first.) Discard plaster into trash receptacle.
15. Clean work area.
16. Remove gloves and wash hands.
17. Schedule patient for next appointment to have cast checked.
18. Document the procedure.

DOCUMENTATION

12/14/20XX 2:00 PM Plaster cast applied to left arm by Dr. King. Fingers warm to touch. Patient says there is no tingling or numbness in her fingers. Instructed about cast care, exercises, and reporting of circulatory impairment and infection. Sling applied. S. Walsh, RMA

Procedure 18-22 Assisting with Cast Removal

STANDARD PRECAUTIONS:

PURPOSE:
To assist the physician with the removal of a cast.

EQUIPMENT/SUPPLIES:
Cast cutter
Cast spreader
Bandage scissors
Bag for disposing of cast materials
Drape

PROCEDURE STEPS:
1. Wash hands.
2. Drape patient and area.
3. Explain the cast removal process to the patient. The cutter vibrates and does not spin. Some pressure and warmth may be experienced. RATIONALE: Explaining the procedure reduces apprehension and fears about being cut with the blade.
4. Reassure the patient that skin color and muscle tone will improve with therapy.
5. Hand the physician the equipment as requested.
6. After the procedure, provide written instructions for postcare.
7. Clean equipment.
8. Wash hands.
9. Document cast removal and appearance of body part from which cast was removed.

DOCUMENTATION

6/12/20XX 2:45 PM Cast removed from left arm by Dr. King. Arm seems slightly atrophied. Skin color good, circulation seems good. Patient given skin care instructions. Appointment for physical therapy scheduled for 6/14/XX at 3:00 PM. W. Slawson, CMA

Procedure 18-23 Assisting the Physician during a Lumbar Puncture or Cerebrospinal Fluid Aspiration

STANDARD PRECAUTIONS:

PURPOSE:
To assemble supplies and position the patient for removal of cerebrospinal fluid from the lumbar area, which will be sent to the laboratory for analysis.

EQUIPMENT/SUPPLIES:
Drape
Xylocaine 1–2%
Syringe and needle for anesthetic
Sterile gloves
Disposable sterile lumbar puncture tray (to include):
- Skin antiseptic with applicator—povidone–iodine
- Adhesive bandage
- Spinal puncture needle

(continues)

Procedure 18-23 (continued)

Three or four test tubes with corks or tops
Drape
Manometer
Laboratory requisition
Examination light
Gauze sponges

PROCEDURE STEPS:

1. Reinforce physician's explanation of the procedure and answer questions.
2. Verify the patient has signed a consent form.
3. Patient should be instructed to empty the bladder and bowel.
4. Wash hands and set up sterile field for the physician.
5. Cleanse the puncture site with antiseptic soap and water. Rinse.
6. Position the patient in a lateral recumbent position with the back at the edge of the examination table and a small pillow under the head (fetal position). RATIONALE: Patient's alignment of the spine is best achieved in a horizontal position.
7. Drape patient for warmth and privacy.
8. Have the patient draw the knees up to the abdomen and grasp onto knees (Figure 18-57A) and flex chin on chest. RATIONALE: Position allows for easier needle insertion into the subarachnoid space of the spinal cord because this position widens the spaces between the lumbar vertebrae. Procedure is performed at the fourth intervertebral space of the lumbar region (Figure 18-57B).
9. The physician will swab the puncture site with antiseptic such as Betadine®.
10. The physician drapes area with fenestrated drape.
11. Assist physician to aspirate anesthetic.
12. Help the patient maintain this position until the needle has been inserted into spinal canal. RATIONALE: Movement by the patient could produce trauma to the spinal cord area.
13. Remind patient to breathe evenly, not to hold his breath or talk, because this may interfere with the pressure reading.
14. At the physician's direction, have the patient straighten his legs. RATIONALE: Muscle tension can give false pressure reading. The physician reads manometer.
15. Physician collects spinal fluid.
16. After the procedure has been completed, the physician will apply an adhesive bandage to the puncture site. The patient is placed in a prone position for two to three hours, or as directed by the physician. RATIONALE: This helps prevent cerebrospinal fluid from leaking through the puncture site.
17. Apply gloves. Cap specimens tightly.
18. Label samples with date, patient's name, and number CSF (#1, #2, #3).
19. Send the labeled specimen to the laboratory with the appropriate laboratory requisition. Store in incubator.
20. Clean area using standard precautions.
21. Remove gloves.
22. Wash hands.
23. Document procedure in patient's chart.

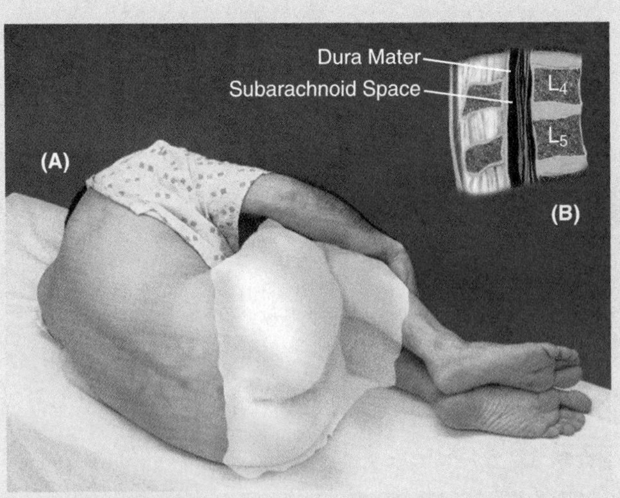

Figure 18-57 (A) Have the patient draw up the knees to the abdomen and grasp onto knees. Chin should flex on chest. (B) The site for the lumbar puncture.

DOCUMENTATION

6/12/20XX 3:10 PM Lumbar puncture performed by Dr. King. Three samples of cerebral spinal fluid obtained. Labeled #1, #2, #3. Taken to laboratory. Patient appeared to tolerate procedure. BP 142/82, P88. Patient instructed to remain flat for three hours and to drink increased amounts of fluids. J. Guerro, CMA

Procedure 18-24 Assisting the Physician with a Neurologic Screening Examination

STANDARD PRECAUTIONS:

PURPOSE:

To determine a patient's neurologic status.

EQUIPMENT/SUPPLIES:

Percussion hammer
Safety pin or sensory wheel
Material for odor identification
Cotton ball
Tuning fork
Flashlight
Tongue blade
Ophthalmoscope

PROCEDURE STEPS:

1. Wash hands.
2. The mental status examination can be done by the medical assistant when taking the patient's medical history by observing the following: When taking patient's history, pay special attention to level of awareness, memory, cognition, and mood. When the patient answers questions during the history taking, note if behavior is appropriate for the circumstances.
3. The physician will check reflexes using the percussion hammer.
4. The physician checks the patient's sensory abilities; responses to skin sensations using a safety pin or sensory wheel and cotton ball; and patient's ability to recognize the form of solid objects by touch (key, coin, paper clip). The physician also checks cranial nerves, performs finger to nose test, and checks patient's ability to touch heel to shin and ability to run the heel down opposite shin.
5. Assist the patient as needed during and after the examination.
6. Document procedure in patient's chart.

DOCUMENTATION

8/22/20XX 3:20 PM Assisted Dr. Woo with neurologic screening examination. Made appointment for patient to see Dr. Sullivan, neurologist, on 9/4/XX at 3:00 PM. J. Backus, RMA

Case Study 18-1

Corey Bayer is a 15-year-old patient at City Health Care. He sustained an injury to his right wrist today during soccer practice. Dr. Rice has examined him and ordered a radiograph of the right forearm. The results show that Corey has sustained a Colles' fracture of the right wrist. Dr. Rice asks you to prepare the equipment to apply a cast.

CASE STUDY REVIEW

1. Describe cast application. What are the medical assistant's responsibilities?
2. After Corey's cast application, describe the cast care instructions that will be given to Corey and his mother.

Case Study 18-2

Dr. Rice has scheduled Anita Blanchette for a spirometry test and wants you to telephone her the day before the test to prepare her so optimal results are obtained.

CASE STUDY REVIEW

1. What information can you give to Anita before her spirometry to obtain the best test results?

SUMMARY

Medical assistants are a vital link in the team of health care providers. A thorough knowledge and understanding of the various body system examinations and clinical procedures routinely performed as part of patient care will enhance the quality of care given.

Some of the specialty procedures will be performed on a routine basis in the ambulatory care setting; others will only be performed occasionally and perhaps only in the larger settings that offer specialized and primary care. Sometimes, to feel comfortable assisting with the less common procedures, medical assistants may need to broaden their base of knowledge by conducting independent research. Medical assistants who are willing to constantly expand their clinical understanding will not only fine-tune their professional skills, but will derive greater satisfaction from their job performance.

STUDY FOR SUCCESS

To reinforce your knowledge and skills of information presented in this chapter:

- ❑ Review the Key Terms
- ❑ Practice the Procedures
- ❑ Consider the Case Studies and discuss your conclusions
- ❑ Answer the Review Questions
  - ❑ Multiple Choice
  - ❑ Critical Thinking
- ❑ Navigate the Internet by completing the Web Activities
- ❑ Practice the StudyWARE activities on your student CD
- ❑ Apply your knowledge in the Student Workbook activities
- ❑ Complete the Web Tutor sections
- ❑ View and discuss the DVD situations

REVIEW QUESTIONS

Multiple Choice

1. What are the elevated skin lesions affecting the epidermis caused by the papillomaviruses called?
   a. scleroderma
   b. moles
   c. calluses
   d. warts
2. What is the disorder that is characterized by discomfort of the muscles, tendons, ligaments, and soft tissues brought on by trauma, strain, and emotional stress?
   a. carpal tunnel syndrome
   b. bursitis
   c. gout
   d. fibromyalgia
3. What type of fracture has its bone fragments driven into each other?
   a. greenstick
   b. impacted
   c. oblique
   d. comminuted
4. What disease is caused by a degeneration of brain cells caused by lack of dopamine, bringing about muscle rigidity and akinesia?
   a. multiple sclerosis
   b. Bell's palsy
   c. Parkinson's disease
   d. tic douloureux

5. An acute circumscribed infection of the subcutaneous tissues caused by staphylococcus is a:
   a. comedone
   b. carbuncle
   c. furuncle
   d. psoriasis

Critical Thinking

1. What would be the advantage of catheterizing a patient for urinalysis and culture and sensitivity?
2. What is the use and purpose of the audiometer? How is the test administered?
3. Explain the rationale when doing an eye irrigation that the flow of the irrigating solution is from the inside canthus to the outer canthus of the eye.
4. Differentiate among bronchitis, emphysema, and asthma.
5. What is the medical assistant's role when assisting in spirometry?
6. What are the cast care guidelines that the medical assistant gives to the patient?
7. When a mental status examination is given, what five areas are being reviewed?
8. Explain the medical assistant's role when assisting with a lumbar puncture.

WEB ACTIVITIES

Use the Internet to search for information from a medical site to find answers to the following:

1. Using a search engine of your choice, go to Web MD and gather information about the following conditions:
   kidney stones
   polycystic kidneys
   Describe the etiology of and treatment of each.
2. Search for possible treatments for sleep apnea.
   http://www.breathingdisorders.com
   http://www.sleepapnea.org
3. What are some long-term harmful effects of cigarette smoking?
   Check this website for information:
   http://www.tobaccofreekids.org
4. The National Digestive Diseases Clearinghouse is a useful source for learning about acute and chronic pancreatitis.
   What are the signs and symptoms of acute pancreatitis? How is a diagnosis made by the physician? What is the most common cause of chronic pancreatitis?
5. Adolescent cases of bacterial meningitis have increased since the 1990s.
   Is a particular group of adolescents at greater risk than other groups? How can meningitis be prevented?

THE DVD HOOK-UP

DVD Series
Skills Based Series

Program Number
6

Chapter/Scene Reference
- *Vision and Hearing Tests*

This chapter discusses the proper techniques for assisting with specialty examinations.

The selected scenes from today's DVD program illustrated various procedures that are used to test the patient's vision and hearing.

When measuring distant vision, the program featured two separate charts that can be used to measure distant vision in children.

1. What were the names of the charts?
2. Which chart should be used for younger children? Which chart should be used for older children?
3. The procedure for measuring visual acuity in this chapter talks about using an occluder to cover the eye when testing vision. The scene for measuring visual acuity in the DVD program illustrates a patient using a small paper cup to cover the eye. Are there any advantages to using a cup versus an occluder?

DVD Journal Summary

Write a paragraph that summarizes what you learned from watching today's DVD selected scene. Imagine that you are testing the eyes of a pilot. To pass the flight physical, the pilot has to have perfect eyesight. You notice that the pilot is really straining to see the eye chart. His acuity test showed less than perfect vision. He tells you his eyes are just strained from flying all day and asks you to alter the results. What would you do in this situation?

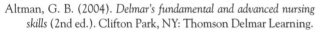

REFERENCES/BIBLIOGRAPHY

Altman, G. B. (2004). *Delmar's fundamental and advanced nursing skills* (2nd ed.). Clifton Park, NY: Thomson Delmar Learning.

Delaune, S. C., & Ladner, P. K. (2002). *Fundamentals of nursing standards and practice* (2nd ed.). Clifton Park, NY: Thomson Delmar Learning.

Neighbors, M., & Tannehill-Jones, R. (2000). *Human diseases*. Clifton Park, NY: Thomson Delmar Learning.

Roe, S. (2003). *Delmar's clinical nursing skills and concepts*. Clifton Park, NY: Thomson Delmar Learning.

Taber's cyclopedic medical dictionary. (2003). (22nd ed.). Philadelphia: FA Davis.

Tamparo, C., & Lewis, M. (2000). *Diseases of the human body* (3rd ed.). Philadelphia: FA Davis.

UNIT 6

Advanced Techniques and Procedures

CHAPTER 19

Assisting with Office/Ambulatory Surgery

OUTLINE

OBJECTIVES

The student should strive to meet the following performance objectives and demonstrate an understanding of the facts and principles presented in this chapter through written and oral communication.

1. Define the key terms as presented in the glossary.
2. Define surgical asepsis and differentiate between surgical asepsis and medical asepsis.

(continues)

KEY TERMS

Allergy
Anesthesia
Antibacterial
Approximate
Avascularization
Bandage
Betadine®
Caustic
Cautery
Contamination
Dressing
Epinephrine
Exudate
Fenestrated
Friable
Hibeclens®
Hydrogen Peroxide
Infection
Inflammation
Informed Consent
Isopropyl Alcohol
Ligature
Liquid Nitrogen
Mayo Stand/Instrument Tray
Ratchets
Silver Nitrate
Sitz Bath
Sodium Hydroxide
Sterile Field
Strictures
Suppurant
Surgery Cards
Surgical Asepsis
Suture
Swaged
Unsterile Field
Volatile

FEATURED COMPETENCIES

CAAHEP—ENTRY-LEVEL COMPETENCIES

Clinical Competencies

Fundamental Procedures

- Perform handwashing
- Wrap items for autoclaving
- Perform sterilization techniques
- Dispose of biohazardous materials
- Practice Standard Precautions

Specimen Collection

- Obtain specimens for microbiological testing

Patient Care

- Obtain vital signs
- Prepare and maintain examination and treatment areas
- Prepare patient for and assist with procedures, treatments, and office surgeries

General Competencies

Legal Concepts

- Identify and respond to issues of confidentiality
- Perform within legal and ethical boundaries
- Document appropriately

Patient Instruction

- Instruct individuals according to their needs
- Provide instruction for health maintenance and disease prevention

ABHES—ENTRY-LEVEL COMPETENCIES

Professionalism

- Maintain confidentiality at all times

(continues)

OBJECTIVES (continued)

3. List eight basic rules to follow to protect sterile areas.
4. Explain the sizing standards of suture material and the criteria used to select the most appropriate type and size.
5. Given a variety of surgical instruments, be able to identify each and describe its intended use.
6. Demonstrate the ability to select the most appropriate type of dressings for a given situation.
7. State advantages and disadvantages of Betadine®, Hibeclens®, isopropyl alcohol, and hydrogen peroxide when each is used as a skin antiseptic.
8. Define anesthesia, and explain the advantages and disadvantages of epinephrine as an additive to injectable anesthetics.
9. List five preoperative issues to be addressed in patient preparation and education.
10. List five postoperative concerns to be addressed with the patient and the caregiver.
11. Demonstrate applying sterile gloves.
12. Demonstrate setting up a surgical tray, including laying the field, applying supplies and instruments, pouring a sterile solution, using transfer forceps, and covering the sterile tray.
13. Explain what is meant by alternative surgical methods.

SCENARIO

It might be instructive to compare two different ambulatory care settings. At the multi-physician Inner City Health Care, minor surgery is performed on a routine basis. Certain days are dedicated to certain procedures. Because of the high volume of patients and different physician preferences, Inner City maintains two special rooms for minor surgery and has a large selection of instruments. At the smaller two-physician practice of Lewis and King, however, minor surgical procedures are less frequent and are conducted in the patient examination rooms.

FEATURED COMPETENCIES (continued)

- Be cognizant of ethical boundaries
- Be courteous and diplomatic
- Conduct work within scope of education, training and ability

Communication

- Adapt what is said to recipient's level of comprehension
- Serve as a liaison between Physician and others
- Use appropriate medical terminology
- Recognize and respond to verbal and non-verbal communication
- Principles of verbal and nonverbal communication
- Adaptation for individualized needs

Clinical Duties

- Prepare patients for procedures
- Apply principles of aseptic techniques and infection control
- Take vital signs
- Recognize emergencies
- Prepare and maintain examination and treatment area
- Assist physician with examinations and treatments
- Use quality control
- Wrap items for autoclaving
- Perform sterilization techniques

(continues)

INTRODUCTION

Office/ambulatory surgery differs from hospital surgery not only in complexity, but in the supplies, equipment, instruments, and personnel needed. Some office/ambulatory surgery is performed by the physician alone; some surgeries require the assistance of the medical assistant. Most ambulatory care settings do not need a large variety of surgical instruments, but will often need more than one of the more frequently used instruments. As a personal preference, special instruments may be purchased and maintained for a specific physician to use during a particular surgical procedure. These particular instruments are generally not used by the other physicians.

The equipment and supplies used in office/ambulatory surgery are usually portable and easily maintained. It is the larger practices that perform many office/ambulatory surgeries that can afford the space and expense of maintaining a special room just for that purpose. Often patient examination rooms serve as small surgical suites with portable ***Mayo stands/ instrument trays,*** *supplies, and equipment brought into the room for the procedure.*

Whether assisting with office/ambulatory surgery is a routine or an infrequent event for the medical assistant, it is nonetheless important to be knowledgeable about the use and care of instruments and the room, as well as patient preparation for the surgery. Medical assistants should also understand the preferences of each physician on staff to make the surgical procedure comfortable and effective for both patient and physician.

SURGICAL ASEPSIS

Regardless of the number and complexity of surgical procedures performed in the office or ambulatory care center, **surgical asepsis** must be strictly maintained. Surgical asepsis uses practices known as sterile techniques. The primary purpose of surgical asepsis is to prevent microorganisms from entering the patient's body during an invasive procedure. Some examples of invasive procedures include creating an opening in the skin such as a surgical incision, closing a wound such as a laceration, giving an injection, or inserting a sterile catheter into a sterile body cavity such as the urinary bladder.

Because microorganisms are on virtually every surface such as skin, instruments, surgical instrument trays, clothing, and even in the air, it is necessary to destroy as many as possible before any surgical procedure. Surgical asepsis or sterile technique prevents microorganism entry into the body during an invasive procedure and, therefore, helps to protect the patient from infection. Once the items and areas are sterilized, every precaution must be taken to prevent **contamination** of the sterile items or areas either from a nonsterile surface or from airborne contamination.

FEATURED COMPETENCIES (continued)

- Dispose of biohazardous materials
- Practice standard precautions

Legal Concepts

- Determine needs for documentation and reporting
- Document accurately
- Perform risk management procedures

Instruction

- Instruct patients with special needs
- Teach patients methods of health promotion and disease prevention

Spotlight on Certification

RMA Content Outline

- Asepsis
- Sterilization
- Instruments
- Clinical pharmacology
- Minor surgery

CMA Content Outline

- Principles of infection control
- Equipment preparation and operation
- Preparing/maintaining treatment areas
- Instruments, supplies and equipment

CMAS Content Outline

- Asepsis in the medical office
- Exam preparation
- Basic pharmacology

Living tissue surfaces such as skin cannot be sterilized but can be made as free of pathogens as possible before the use of a sterile covering. One example of this concept is the use of the surgical hand cleansing technique before applying sterile gloves (see Procedure 19-1). Another example of surgical asepsis is preparing the patient's skin with a surgical scrub solution before applying sterile drapes around the intended surgical site.

Refer to Chapter 10 for more complete information on the concepts of asepsis and aseptic techniques including hand cleansing for medical asepsis and methods of sterilization for surgical asepsis.

The differences between hand cleansing for medical asepsis as discussed in Chapter 10 (see Procedure 10-1) and hand cleansing for surgical asepsis are addressed in the following section.

Hand Cleansing for Medical and Surgical Asepsis

Hand cleansing for medical asepsis is defined as removing pathogenic microorganisms from the hands after contamination. Medical hand cleansing is used many times throughout the day to cleanse the skin after removing contaminated gloves, assisting with patient care, and touching unclean surfaces. Hand cleansing for surgical asepsis is defined as removal of as many microorganisms as possible before performing surgery or a sterile procedure. Hand cleansing for surgical asepsis consists of meticulously scrubbing hands, wrists, and forearms before applying sterile gloves. Both medical and surgical aseptic hand cleansing techniques are designed to prevent exposing patients, health care workers, and the public to potentially harmful microorganisms. A brushless/waterless surgical hand cleanser can be used after prewashing hands to remove debris from hands and nails. The brushless cleansing agent has an antimicrobial additive that contains alcohol. The agent must be completely dry before donning gown and gloves.

Proper protocol when assisting with surgery requires the use of surgical hand cleansing at the beginning of each workday, as well as before sterile techniques, with the complementary use of medical hand cleansing before leaving the office and when returning and between patients and procedures. Any opening in the medical assistant's skin should be covered with a sterile adhesive dressing, and gloves are worn during any direct patient contact. See Chapter 10 for information on Standard Precautions.

For a summary of how surgical hand cleansing differs from medical hand cleansing see Table 19-1.

STERILE PRINCIPLES

Sterile principles are a set of guidelines designed to designate what items and areas are considered sterile and what actions cause contamination. Some areas are logical and clear, some are subtle and less clear. It has already been

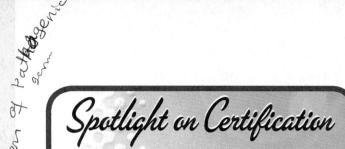

TABLE 19-1 DIFFERENCE BETWEEN MEDICAL AND SURGICAL HAND CLEANSING

Medical Hand Cleansing	Surgical Hand Cleansing
• Two-minute duration	• Two- to five-minute duration
• Wash hands and wrists	• Wash hands, wrists, and forearms to the elbows
• Hands should be held down during rinsing	• Hands should be held up during rinsing
• Scrub nails with brush; clean under nails with cuticle stick	• Scrub nails with brush and clean under each nail with cuticle stick
• Apply lotion*	• Do not apply lotion*
	• Glove for sterility

*The use of lotions is encouraged to help prevent chafing of the skin, especially with frequent hand cleansings. Nevertheless, studies have determined that lotions containing petroleum or mineral oil can break down latex and should be avoided if latex gloves are going to be worn within one hour after applying the lotion. If lotions are applied immediately before gloving, the use of water-based lotions is recommended. Of special interest to persons with latex sensitivities (see Chapter 10) is the fact that using lotions and creams containing petroleum products actually increases the amount of latex protein that is transferred from the gloves into the skin, thereby increasing the symptoms of latex sensitivity.

noted that some surfaces, such as skin, cannot be sterilized. In addition, large items such as instrument stands and their trays cannot fit into an autoclave for sterilization. To create sterile areas and surfaces where sterility is not possible, sterile barriers should be used; sterile gloves can be worn over the hands and sterile drapes can be applied to trays once both have been washed with disinfectant, rinsed, and dried.

Guidelines to protect sterile items and areas include:

- A sterile object may not touch a nonsterile object.
- Sterile objects must not be wet. Moisture will draw microorganisms into the sterile object.
- An acceptable border between a sterile area and a nonsterile area is 1 inch. The portion of a drape that hangs over the edge is considered nonsterile, no matter what its size. Sterile articles should be placed in the center of the **sterile field** and away from the edge as much as possible.
- Do not turn your back on a sterile field. If you cannot see the field, you cannot be aware of what touched it.
- Anything below the waist is considered contaminated. In support of this principle, all surgery trays should be positioned above the waist. All articles are to be held above the waist.
- All sterile objects (such as gloved hands) must be held in front and away from the body and above waist level.
- Do not cough, sneeze, or talk over a sterile field. Airborne particles may fall onto the sterile area and contaminate it.
- Do not reach over the sterile area. Contaminants may fall onto the area and clothing may touch, thereby contaminating the area. Spend as little time as possible reaching into the sterile area.
- Do not pass contaminated dressings or instruments over the sterile field.
- Arrange for the physician to place contaminated instruments into a separate container or area.
- Always be aware of actions to determine whether the sterile field has been contaminated. When in doubt, err on the side of safety.
- When opening sterile packages, the outer wrapper is contaminated. It should be opened without touching the inner contents, and the contents are then dropped onto the sterile field. Double wrapping can be used. (Refer to Chapter 10, Procedure 10-6.)
- Sterile solutions in bottles should be poured into sterile basins or cups on the sterile field without touching the rim of the bottle and without splashing solution onto the sterile field. If the sterile field is not polylined and becomes wet, it is considered contaminated, because when a field is wet it acts as a wick and draws microorganisms into the article. Using polylined drapes as sterile fields protects against contamination.

COMMON SURGICAL PROCEDURES PERFORMED IN PHYSICIANS' OFFICES AND CLINICS

All surgery has commonalities as well as specifics. The following specific surgery or surgical procedures includes lists of needed instruments, supplies, and equipment, as well as basic patient preparation and postoperative instructions for some of the more frequently performed surgeries. The following procedures are suggested protocol only, because physicians will have preferences and techniques unique to them and their practices.

This section includes a general procedure for assisting with surgery and is followed by specific office/ambulatory surgical procedures, including:

- Assisting with Office/Ambulatory Surgery (Procedure 19-5)
- Dressing Change (Procedure 19-6)
- Wound Irrigation (Procedure 19-7)
- Preparation of Patient's Skin before Surgery (Procedure 19-8)
- Suturing of Laceration or Incision Repair (Procedure 19-9)
- Sebaceous Cyst Excision (Procedure 19-10)
- Incision and Drainage of Localized Infections (Procedure 19-11)
- Aspiration of Joint Fluid (Procedure 19-12)
- Hemorrhoid Thrombectomy (Procedure 19-13)
- Suture/Staple Removal (Procedure 19-14)
- Application of Sterile Adhesive Skin Closure Strips (Steri-Strips) (Procedure 19-15)

ADDITIONAL SURGICAL METHODS

Additional surgical methods refer to those methods not requiring the use of a surgical knife or scalpel, but which use other methods of cutting or destroying, such as electric current, heat, freezing, chemicals, or laser beam. Which method is used is determined by the physician's preference.

Electrosurgery

Electrosurgery uses an electric current in a concentrated area to either cut or destroy tissue whenever pathologic examination is not required. The equipment for electrosurgery consists of a power source, usually a small boxed unit, and a detachable handheld applicator with removable tips. The tips are available in various sizes and are removable for cleaning and sterilizing.

Electrosurgery is useful in removing benign skin tags and warts. The main advantage of electrosurgery is that the bleeding is controlled through the cauterization of the blood vessels as the electric current is applied. The terms *electrocoagulation*, *electrofulguration*, *electrodessication*, *electroscission*, *electrosection*, and *eletrocautery* all refer to various uses of electric current to either coagulate blood vessels, destroy tissue either with a spark or by drying, or cut tissue. Disposable battery-operated units designed for one-time use are available.

Cautery. The word **cautery** comes from the term *caustic* and means the application of a **caustic** chemical or destructive heat. Electrosurgery, cautery, and electrocautery are often used interchangeably. The burning of tissue, either chemically or electrically, is known as cauterization. Sometimes during surgical procedures unnecessary bleeding can be controlled by use of electrosurgical equipment (Figure 19-1). Tissues that do not need to be pathologically examined, such as benign skin tags, can be destroyed using cauterization. Some common chemicals used to destroy tissue and stop bleeding are **silver nitrate, liquid nitrogen,** and **sodium hydroxide.**

Chemical Tissue Destruction. Silver nitrate is available in a solid form, impregnated on the end of a wooden applicator stick. Silver nitrate is especially useful inside the nose to cauterize **friable,** easily broken, blood vessels in the treatment of epistaxis (nosebleed).

Liquid chemical caustic agents such as sodium hydroxide are used to permanently destroy the growth plates of toenails whenever total and permanent removal of the toenail is necessary.

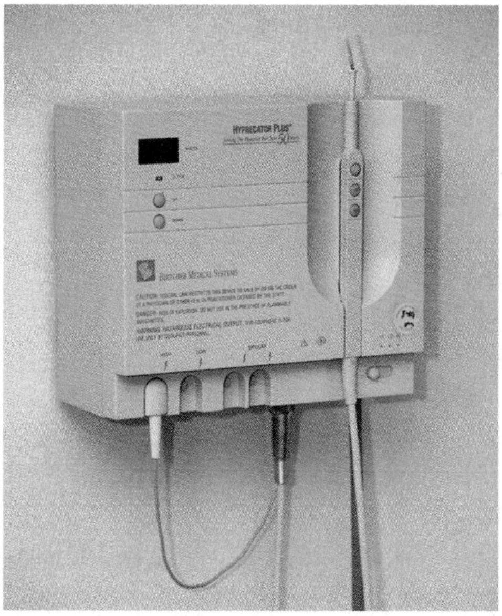

Figure 19-1 Electrosurgical equipment is used to destroy tissue, such as warts, or to coagulate blood vessels to decrease bleeding during surgery.

Electrical Tissue Destruction. Electrical burning of tissue is performed with the use of an electrical instrument. A wand on the end of a handheld apparatus is electrically heated and applied to tissues. The adjustable current is controlled by a foot pedal. Disposable battery-operated cautery units designed for one-time use are also available.

Cryosurgery

Cryosurgery refers to the destruction of tissue by freezing. Some types of tissues react differently to heat than cold in the rate of healing and level of scarring. The cryogenic substance most often used to destructively freeze tissue is liquid nitrogen. Liquid nitrogen, often incorrectly referred to as dry ice, is extremely **volatile** (easily evaporated) and must be kept in a covered insulated canister. Liquid nitrogen is obtained when nitrogen gas is compressed under cold temperatures into a liquid. It is most often used to destructively "freeze" warts. Liquid nitrogen may be applied to cervical erosions to facilitate the healing growth of normal tissue, to remove lesions on the anus, for cataract extraction, for retinal detachment, for prostate gland destruction, and for removal of superficial lesions in the nose and throat. Some units are for a single purpose use. There is less trauma, more control of bleeding, and less pain with cryosurgery.

Many patients experience pain with liquid nitrogen because it is actually colder than other chemical cryosurgery options. Liquid nitrogen is usually kept in a large canister in a central location in the office and carefully transferred to a small thermos for transport into the treatment room. The medical assistant must take care to keep the canister and thermos covered because of the volatile properties (evaporation rate) of the liquid nitrogen.

The cryogenic properties of solid liquid nitrogen make it useful for freezing warts and nevi. Nitrous oxide is another chemical used in cryosurgery. Nitrous oxide requires a gas cylinder, a regulator, a pressure gauge, and a cryogun with assorted tips. The nitrous oxide is applied in a more direct and controlled pattern because of the precision of the probes, and the nitrous oxide does not evaporate as readily as the liquid nitrogen. The tank, probes, and other supplies can be quite expensive, though. The nitrous oxide is not as cold as liquid nitrogen; therefore, although it is not as uncomfortable for the patient, it is not as destructive and therefore not appropriate for use with cancerous lesions, which must be completely destroyed. Because nitrous oxide is a carcinogen and Occupational Safety and Health Administration (OSHA) requires that all nitrous oxide systems have outside venting, this is not practical for most ambulatory clinics.

Bear in mind that all volatile gases are dangerous to inhale, and appropriate ventilation should be used. Refer to the Material Safety Data Sheet (MSDS) information (available in printed form or on the manufacturer's Web sites) for specific cautions.

Laser Surgery

Laser is an acronym for Light Amplification by Stimulated Emission of Radiation. The laser instrument converts light into an intense beam. By focusing the laser beam onto the target, the application can be extremely precise without damaging surrounding tissue. Over the past two decades, laser surgery has become less expensive, more readily available, and consequently much more widespread as a treatment of choice for surgery in dermatology, ophthalmology, nervons surgery, vascular surgery, plastic surgery, and others. Most specialty surgery is now using laser in various ways. With the advent of many physicians using laser technology in the ambulatory care setting, the medical assistant must be familiar with the dangers involved with laser surgery, and safety precautions must be implemented. Attending a laser education and safety workshop is recommended for all personnel intending to work with lasers.

The following precautions are designed to heighten awareness and serve as a safety guide:

- When the laser beam is focused on the target tissue, the cells explode and vaporize. Care should be taken not to inhale the vapors.
- Whenever high levels of electricity are used, care should be taken to avoid burns and to assure that the equipment is always in good working order.
- Safety glasses should be worn by the physician, medical assistant, and, if possible, the patient.
- If the patient has the skin prepared with flammable products such as alcohol-based antiseptics, the skin must be dry with no pooling of liquid. Read product label for alcohol and other flammable substances.
- Sterile water should be readily available to extinguish any fire if the laser beam accidently ignites cloth or paper in the area.

SUTURE MATERIALS AND SUPPLIES

Suture/Ligature

The word **suture** can be used as a verb to describe the motion of sewing or as a noun to describe the material used to sew. Suturing, or sewing, a wound is a common procedure in physicians' offices. The purpose is to **approximate,** or bring together the edges of a wound.

Suturing hastens healing and lessens scarring. Whether the wound is an accidental laceration or a surgical incision, the suturing process is basically the same. When suture material is used for tying off the ends of tubular structures during surgery, it is termed **ligature.** The terms *suture* and *ligature* both refer to suture material, but they are named according to their uses.

Most suture material used in office/ambulatory surgical procedures comes already fused, or **swaged,** to a needle and packaged in various lengths (Figure 19-2). These are also called atraumatic. Eighteen inches is a preferred length because it is short enough to be manageable yet long enough to complete most suturing procedures. Combinations of sizes and types of suture materials and sizes and shapes of needles are endless, but most physicians will use a select few. Selection of the many different suture materials and needles is based on the needs of the tissue and tissue healing. Suture ranges in size on a scale from the smallest gauge below 0 (aught) to the largest gauge above 0. The scale from 6–0 to 4 includes all sizes from the smallest to the largest:

6–0, 5–0, 4–0, 3–0, 2–0, 0, 1, 2, 3, 4

Sometimes 2–0 is labeled 00, 3–0 labeled 000, 4–0 labeled 0000, and so on. Ambulatory care settings use sizes 6–0 to 3–0.

If the tissue being sutured is delicate, as on the face or neck, the smaller suture material is used such as 6–0 or higher; the finer the stitch, the less scarring. Some sutures are made from materials that dissolve when they come in contact with the tissue enzymes. These are referred to as absorbable sutures. The original absorbable suture was called surgical gut or "cat gut." It was made from sheep intestinal tissue. Left "natural" or uncoated, it is called plain gut suture and will dissolve or be absorbed in about one to two weeks. If more time is needed to heal, surgical gut may be coated with chromion salts. It is then called chromion gut and allows for a longer period of healing to take place before dissolving. Absorbable gut suture is used

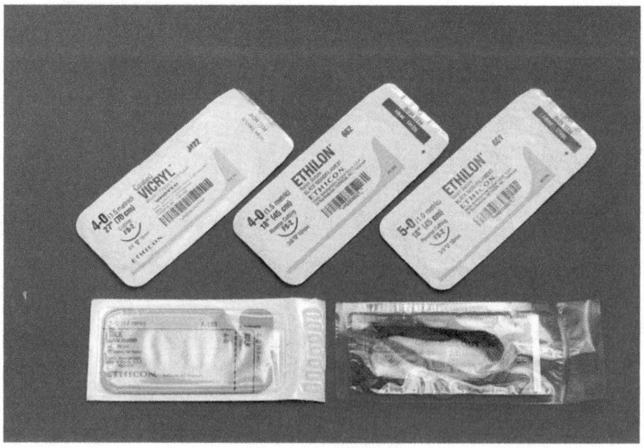

Figure 19-2 A display of a variety of prepackaged suture materials with needles of various sizes and shapes.

TABLE 19-2 SUTURING OPTIONS: MATERIALS, CHARACTERISTICS, AND APPLICATIONS

Suture	Types	Color of Material	Raw Material	Tensile Strength Retention *in Vivo*	Absorption Rate
Surgical gut suture	Plain	Yellowish tan Blue dyed	Collagen derived from healthy beef and sheep	Individual patient characteristics can affect rate of tensile strength loss.	Absorbed by proteolytic enzymatic digestive process.
Surgical gut suture	Chromic	Brown Blue dyed	Collagen derived from healthy beef and sheep	Individual patient characteristics can affect rate of tensile strength loss.	Absorbed by proteolytic enzymatic digestive process.
Coated VICRYL® (polyglactin 910) suture	Braided Monofilament	Violet Undyed (Natural)	Copolymer of lactide and glycolide coated with polyglactin 370 and calcium stearate	Approximately 65% remains at two weeks. Approximately 40% remains at three weeks.	Essentially complete between 56 and 70 days. Absorbed by slow hydrolysis.

Note: This chart is to be read across facing pages.

for underlying tissues where removal is not reasonable and areas where suture removal is inconvenient. Individual body chemistries will influence the exact absorption rate of both plain and treated gut suture. Surgical gut is rarely used anymore but has been replaced by man-made absorbable suture (such as Vicryl® and PDS® II). Suture is also made of nonabsorbable materials such as stainless steel, silk, cotton, nylon, and Dacron. Some are natural (cotton, silk) and some are synthetic/manmade (Dacron®, Ethilon®, Prolene®). Each type of suture material comes in a variety of options such as different colors for ease of visualization, braiding for additional elasticity and strength, and coatings for lubrications and to lessen irritability to tissues (see Table 19-2).

Suture Needles

The needles swaged (atraumatic) to the suture material are also varied (see Figure 19-2). In office/ambulatory surgery, the needles are usually curved. They are categorized according to size, shape, radius of curve, and type of point. Needles may be termed *cutting needles*, *round taper point needles*, or *blunt point needles*.

Staples

Many surgical incisions can be approximated using staples (made of stainless steel or titanium) and a stapler made for this purpose (Figure 19-3). The length, width, and number of staples depends on the tissue. They can be safely used, reduce blood loss, and reduce the length of time of the surgery. Wound healing is quicker, and there is less trauma. Staplers are made for specific types of tissues (e.g., blood vessels, skin, gastrointestinal tract, and so forth). It is more difficult to correct incorrectly placed staples than manually placed sutures.

Staple Removal

Staple removal (see Procedure 19-14) is done wearing sterile gloves and using sterile instruments. The staples are removed using a sterile prepackaged staple remover (Figure 19-4). The staple remover is carefully positioned under the staple and when the handle is squeezed, the staple flattens out and it can be carefully lifted out. Cleanse with an antiseptic solution such as Betadine® and pat dry. Be certain all staples have been removed by verifying the number that were inserted with the number you have removed.

INSTRUMENTS

Structural Features

Rarely does the phrase "form determines function" have as much meaning as when discussing surgical instruments. One can almost always correctly imagine function simply

Tissue Reaction	Contraindications	Frequent Uses	How Supplied	Color Code of Packets
Moderate	Being absorbable, should not be used where extended approximation of tissues under stress is required. Should not be used in patients with known sensitivities or allergies to collagen or chromium.	General soft tissue approximation or ligation, including use in ophthalmic procedures. Not for use in cardiovascular and neurologic tissues.	7–0 thru 3 with and without needles, and on LIGAPAK® dispensing reels 0 thru 1 with CONTROL RELEASE® needles	Yellow
Moderate	Being absorbable, should not be used where extended approximation of tissues under stress is required. Should not be used in patients with known sensitivities or allergies to collagen or chromium.	General soft tissue approximation or ligation, including use in ophthalmic procedures. Not for use in cardiovascular and neurologic tissues.	7–0 thru 3 with and without needles, and on LIGAPAK dispensing reels 0 thru 1 with CONTROL RELEASE needles	Beige
Minimal	Being absorbable, should not be used where extended time of approximation of tissue is required.	General soft tissue approximation or ligation, including use in ophthalmic procedures. Not for use in cardiovascular and neurologic tissues.	8–0 thru 3 with and without needles, and on LIGAPAK dispensing reels 4–0 thru 2 with CONTROL RELEASE needles 8–0 with attached beads for ophthalmic use	Violet

Note: This chart is to be read across facing pages.

(continues)

TABLE 19-2 SUTURING OPTIONS: MATERIALS, CHARACTERISTICS, AND APPLICATIONS (continued)

Suture	Types	Color of Material	Raw Material	Tensile Strength Retention *in Vivo*	Absorption Rate
MONOCRYL® (poliglecaprone 25) suture	Monofilament	Undyed (Natural)	Copolymer of glycolide and epsilon-caprolactone	Approximately 50–60% remains at one week. Approximately 20–30% remains at two weeks. Lost within three weeks.	Complete at 91–119 days. Absorbed by hydrolysis.
PDS® II (polydioxanone) suture	Monofilament	Violet Blue Clear	Polyester polymer	Approximately 70% remains at two weeks. Approximately 50% remains at four weeks. Approximately 25% remains at six weeks.	Minimal until about 90th day. Essentially complete within 210 days. Absorbed by slow hydrolysis.
PERMA-HAND® silk suture	Braided	Black White	Organic protein called fibroin	Progressive degradation of fiber may result in gradual loss of tensile strength.	Gradual encapsulation by fibrous connective tissue.
Surgical stainless steel suture	Monofilament Multifilament	Silver metallic	316L stainless steel	Indefinite.	Nonabsorbable.
ETHILON® nylon suture	Monofilament	Black Undyed (Clear)	Long-chain aliphatic polymers nylon 6 or nylon 6,6	Progressive hydrolysis may result in gradual loss of tensile strength.	Gradual encapsulation by fibrous connective tissue.
NUROLON® nylon suture	Braided	Black Green Undyed (Clear)	Long-chain aliphatic polymers nylon 6 or nylon 6,6	Progressive hydrolysis may result in gradual loss of tensile strength.	Gradual encapsulation by fibrous connective tissue.
MERSILENE® polyester fiber suture	Braided	Green White	Polyester polyethylene terephthalate	No significant change known to occur *in vivo*.	Gradual encapsulation by fibrous connective tissue.
ETHIBOND® extra polyester fiber suture	Braided	Green White	Polyester polyethylene terephthalate coated with polybutilate	No significant change known to occur *in vivo*.	Gradual encapsulation by fibrous connective tissue.
PROLENE® polypropylene suture	Monofilament	Clear Blue	Isotactic crystalline stereoisomer of polypropylene	Not subject to degradation or weakening by action of tissue enzymes.	Nonabsorbable.

Note: This chart is to be read across facing pages.

by close examination of the instrument's design. Handles designed to be squeezed between the thumb and finger are called "thumb" handles. "Ring" handles are designed for the insertion of the thumb and finger into rings. **Ratchets** are locking mechanisms located between the rings of the handles and are used for locking the instrument closed. Ratchets are designed to close in varying degrees of tightness. Serrations are the crevices etched into the surfaces of the jaws of hemostats, some forceps, and needle holders. The serrations provide a more secure grip during use with slippery tissues without actually puncturing the tissue. For the purposes of puncturing tissue, forceps with teeth are an option. Teeth may be numerous or few but are always sharp and should approximate tightly when the instru-

Tissue Reaction	Contraindications	Frequent Uses	How Supplied	Color Code of Packets
Slight	Being absorbable, should not be used where extended approximation of tissues under stress is required, such as in fascia.	General soft tissue approximation or ligation. Not for use in cardiovascular or neurologic tissues, microsurgery, or ophthalmic procedures.	6–0 thru 2 with and without needles 3–0 thru 1 with CONROL RELEASE needles	Coral
Slight	Being absorbable, should not be used where prolonged approximation of tissues under stress is required. Should not be used for placement of vascular prostheses and artificial heart valves.	All types of soft tissue approximation, including pediatric cardiovascular and ophthalmic procedures.	9–0 thru 2 with needles 4–0 thru 1 with CONTROL RELEASE needles 9–0 thru 7–0 with needles 7–0 thru 1 with needles	Silver
Acute inflammatory reaction	Should not be used in patients with known sensitivities or allergies to silk.	General soft tissue approximation or ligation, including cardiovascular, ophthalmic, and neurologic procedures.	9–0 thru 5 with and without needles, and on LIGAPAK dispensing reels 4–0 thru 1 with CONTROL RELEASE needles	Light blue
Minimal acute inflammatory reaction	Should not be used in patients with known sensitivities or allergies to 316L stainless steel, or constituent metals such as chromium and nickel.	Abdominal wound closure, hernia repair, sternal closure and orthopedic procedures including cerclage and tendon repair.	10–0 thru 7 with and without needles	Yellow-ochre
Minimal acute inflammatory reaction	Should not be used where permanent retention of tensile strength is required.	General soft tissue approximation or ligation, including use in cardiovascular, ophthalmic, and neurologic procedures.	11–0 thru 2 with and without needles	Mint green
Minimal acute inflammatory reaction	Should not be used where permanent retention of tensile strength is required.	General soft tissue approximation or ligation, including use in cardiovascular, ophthalmic, and neurologic procedures.	6–0 thru 1 with and without needles 4–0 thru 1 with CONTROL RELEASE needles	Mint green
Minimal acute inflammatory reaction	None known.	General soft tissue approximation or ligation, including use in cardiovascular, ophthalmic, and neurologic procedures.	6–0 thru 5 with and without needles 10–0 and 11–0 for ophthalmic (green monofilament) 0 with CONTROL RELEASE needles	Turquoise
Minimal acute inflammatory reaction	None known.	General soft tissue approximation or ligation, including use in cardiovascular, ophthalmic, and neurologic procedures.	7–0 thru 5 with and without needles 4–0 thru 1 with CONTROL RELEASE needles	Orange
Minimal acute inflammatory reaction	None known.	General soft tissue approximation or ligation, including use in cardiovascular, ophthalmic, and neurologic procedures.	6–0 thru 2 (clear) with and without needles 10–0 thru 8–0 and 6–0 thru 2 (blue) with and without needles 0 thru 2 with CONTROL RELEASE needles	Deep blue

Note: This chart is to be read across facing pages.

ment is closed. To help delicate tips match up properly, some thumb instruments may have a guide pin built into the handle. Box-lock is the name given to a special type of hinge found on most ring-handled instruments, especially grasping instruments such as hemostats, forceps, and needle holders. Because the box-lock provides strength and aids in the prevention of warping, most instruments with ratchets also need the box-lock hinge. Other features include prongs, hooks, and loops (Figure 19-5).

Categories and Uses

Several companies publish and distribute large pictoral catalogs of well over 30,000 medical-surgical instruments.

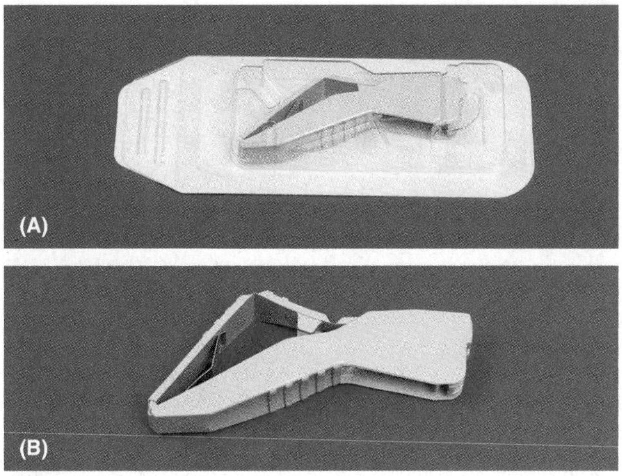

Figure 19-3 Disposable prepackaged skin stapler (A) in package; (B) out of package.

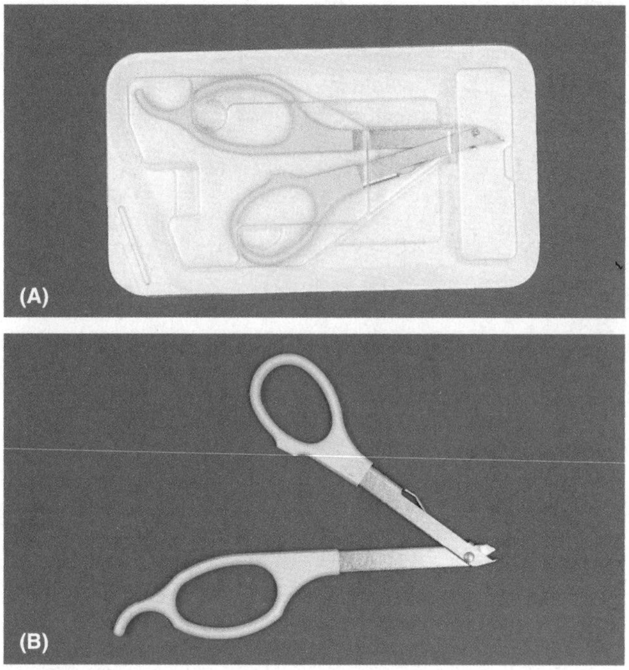

Figure 19-4 Disposable staple remover (A) in package; (B) out of package.

Categories of Instruments

Cutting	Scissors and scalpels
Grasping/Clamping	Hemostats, forceps, clamps, and needle holders
Dilating/Probing	Specula, scopes, probes, retractors, and dilators

A glance through these references shows the many choices available. For ease of discussion, learning, and cataloging, most surgical instruments are placed according to their uses into three basic categories.

Instruments designed for specific purposes within medical specialties often do not readily fit into any one group and are called specialty instruments. This group includes long-handled gynecologic instruments, as well as other instruments designed to meet specific needs within specialty practices.

Scissors and Scalpels. Most of the cutting instruments are scissors. Scissors have ring handles, two blades, and vary in size, shape, and function. Because scissors have two blades, the word *scissors* is always plural. Bandage scissors have one rounded tip to allow insertion under a bandage without causing injury to the patient. The two most common styles are the Lister bandage scissors and the finer finger bandage scissors (Figure 19-6).

Operating scissors are used to cut tissues and generally have very sharp blades. The blades may be curved or straight, and the tips may be sharp, blunt, or a combination of each. They are described as sharp/sharp (s/s), blunt/blunt (b/b), or sharp/blunt (s/b) (Figure 19-7A). A special type of scissors, the Mayo dissecting scissors, may be straight or curved, with curved more often used, but are never described as sharp or blunt because the tips are specifically designed to be neither but have a beveled edge with slightly rounded points (Figure 19-7B). Useful, delicately bladed scissors are iris scissors, originally named for usefulness in eye surgery but now widely used in many procedures. Iris scissors may be either curved or straight (Figure 19-8A). Suture scissors, also called stitch or stitch removal scissors, have a distinctively notched blade to facilitate the insertion of one tip under a suture (Figure 19-8B).

The scalpel is the knife used to cut the skin. The scalpel is actually a blade secured to a handle that, when combined, becomes a surgical knife or scalpel. Disposable one-piece units are also available. The most common blade sizes are #10, #11, and #15, with #11 often referred to as a "stab blade" because of its sharp point (Figure 19-9A). Handles vary in size, but the most popular are the sturdy #3 and #3L (long) and the more delicate #7 (Figure 19-9B).

Hemostats, Forceps, Clamps, and Needle Holders. Grasping and clamping instruments are the largest of the instrument categories. These instruments are used for many different tasks. Included in this category are the towel clamps or clips, needle holders, and forceps. Many forceps also have locking mechanisms called ratchets. Forceps may have ring handles or use a squeeze concept like a

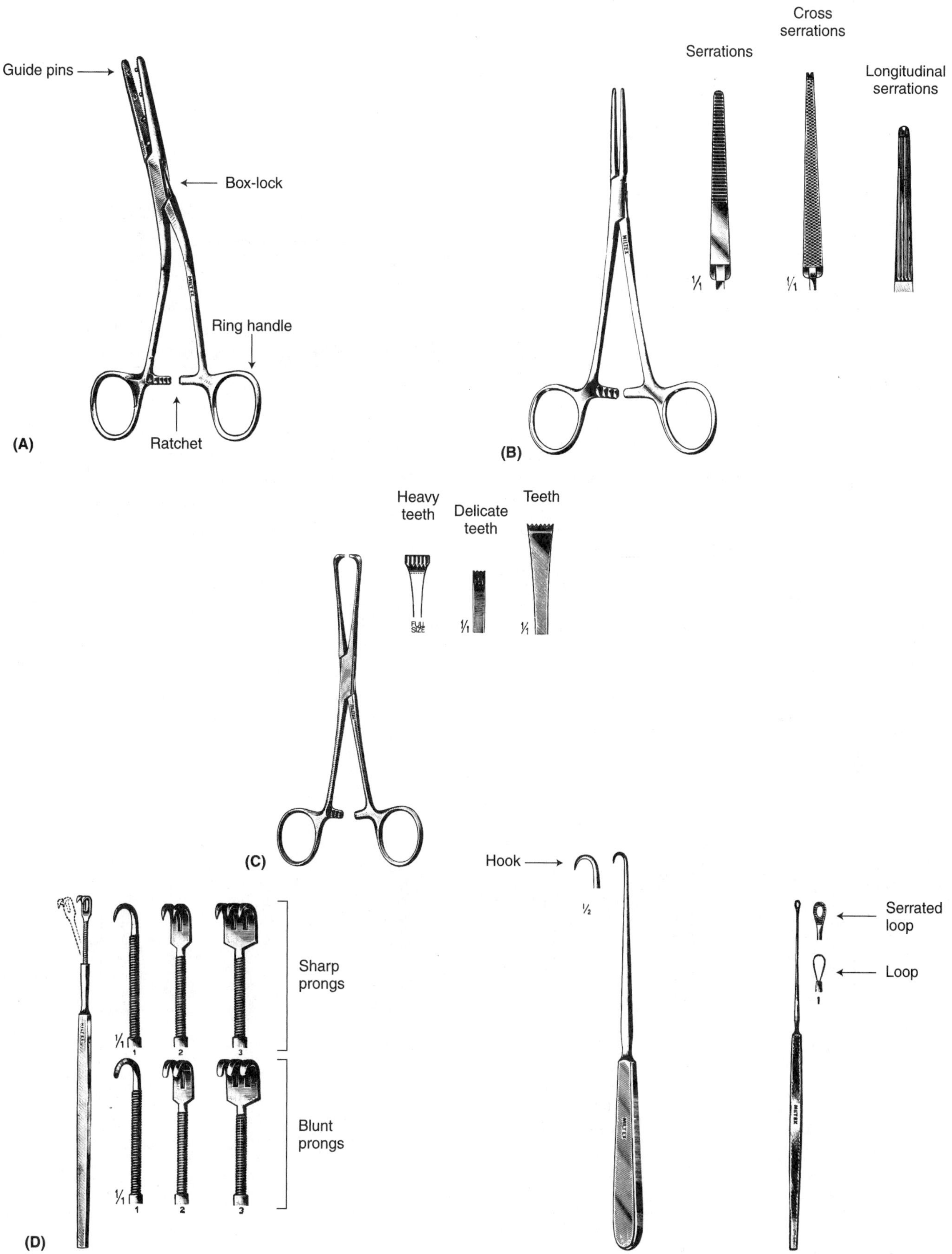

Figure 19-5 Structural features of instruments include (A) ratchets, box-locks, pins, and ring handle; (B) serrations; (C) teeth; (D) prongs, hooks, and loops. (Courtesy of Miltex, Inc.)

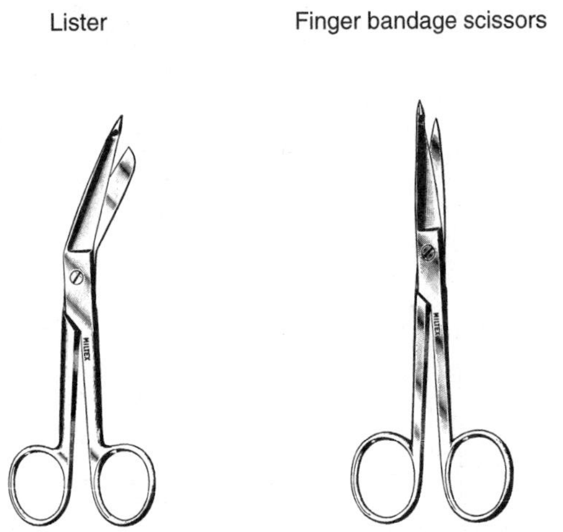

Figure 19-6 Bandage scissors: Lister bandage scissors, small; Knowles finger bandage scissors, straight. (Courtesy of Miltex, Inc.)

tweezer. Forceps number in the hundreds, but most offices need only a select few. Like the word *scissors*, the word *forceps* is always plural. Hemostatic forceps, or hemostats, are used to grasp and clamp blood vessels. Their name means literally to "stop blood." Because blood vessels are slippery, hemostatic forceps have serrations for grasping and ratchets for locking tightly. Mosquito hemostatic forceps have fine tips, with serrations along the entire length of the tips. The Kelly hemostats have serrations only along partial length of the tips. The Kelly hemostatic forceps are sturdier, and some hemostatic forceps have teeth. All types may be straight or curved (Figure 19-10).

Allis tissue forceps are of a similar design to hemostatic forceps but have unique angular jaws with teeth. Another type of grasping instrument are thumb forceps, sometimes referred to as "pick-ups." Thumb forceps do not have ring handles or ratchets but are more like the common tweezers. Thumb forceps with teeth are called tissue forceps because of their ability to grasp tissue. Dressing forceps (plain) do not have teeth and are useful for dressing wounds and applying sterile skin closure strips. Dressing forceps are also used to insert sterile gauze packing strips into wounds to facilitate drainage. The Adson, a special type of thumb forceps, is easily differentiated by the shape. Adsons may have teeth or be plain and have a finer tip.

The Lucae bayonet-type forceps, used in nose and ear procedures, have a thumb handle and are curved to allow the simultaneous use of other instruments and scopes and to facilitate viewing. In contrast, the Hartman ear forceps, duckbill ear alligator-type forceps, and the Hartman nasal dressing forceps have ring handles but also are bent for ease in ear and nose procedures. See Figure 19-11 for examples of each.

Splinter forceps do not have teeth and are used for pulling splinters. Many splinter forceps such as the plain splinter forceps and the Walter are of the thumb-handled style, but the physician's splinter forceps have ring handles and the Virtus have a spring-type handle (Figure 19-12).

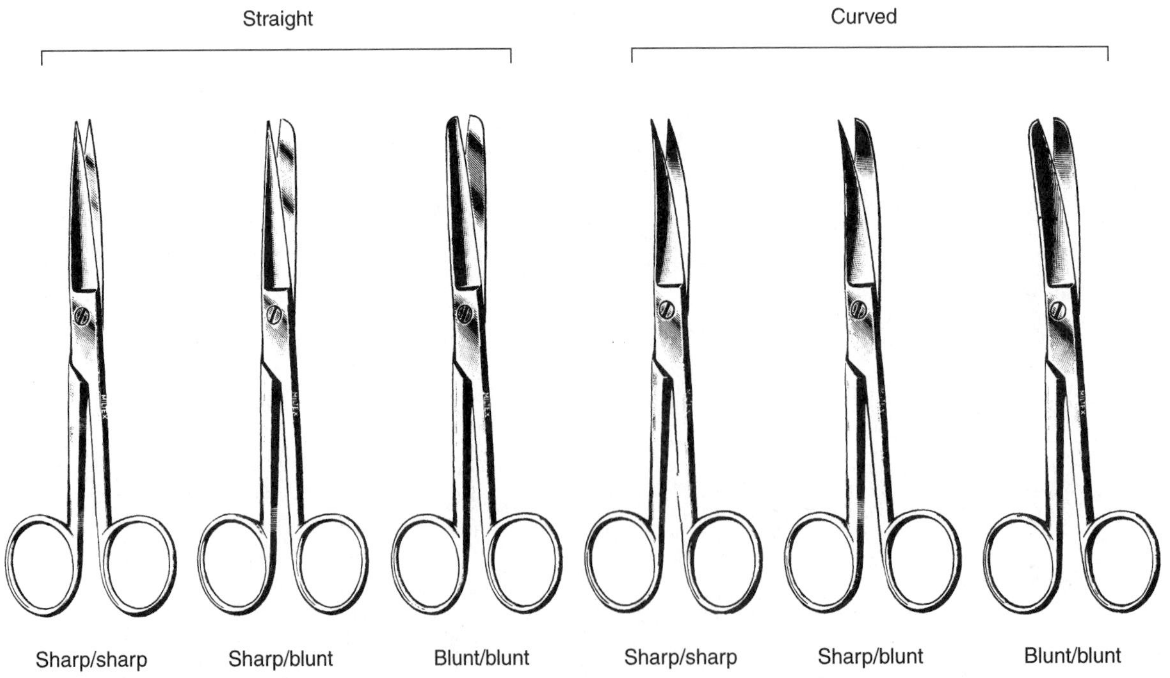

Figure 19-7A Standard operating scissors. (Courtesy of Miltex, Inc.)

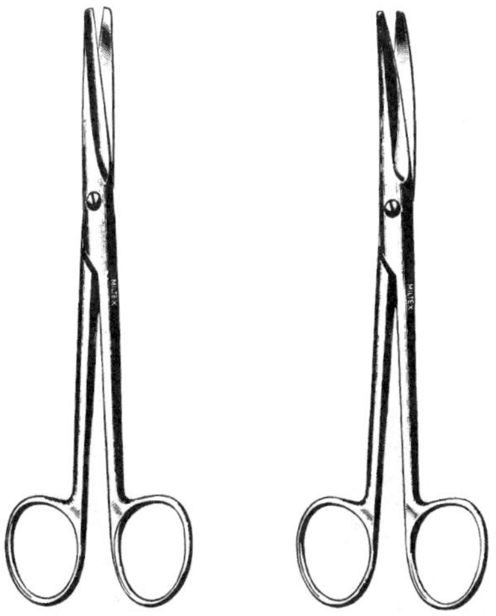

Figure 19-7B Mayo dissecting scissors. (Courtesy of Miltex, Inc.)

Sponge forceps such as the Foerster may have rings on the tips and, as the name implies, are used to hold surgical gauze sponges. The sponge forceps may have long handles making them useful for gynecological procedures and are then called uterine sponge forceps. Many medical offices will use the uterine sponge forceps as transfer forceps (Figure 19-13). See "Basic Surgery Setup" section later in this chapter.

Towel clamps are used to attach surgical field drapes to each other and in some situations, such as when bisecting the vas deferens in a vasectomy, to clamp onto dissected tissue. In the case of a vasectomy, the Backhaus towel clamp is used to hold the dissected section of the vas deferens (Figure 19-15).

Needle holders are ratcheted instruments similar to hemostats but with a wider and more stout jaw. Often called needle drivers, they are designed to hold the needle firmly without crushing it while suturing. Most needle holders have a vertical ditch in the center of the jaw to disperse tension and help prevent slipping of the needle. Needle holders such as the Crile-Wood may have a special groove in which to place the needle during suturing. Some needle holders come in various sizes and some are equipped with a cutting edge that eliminates the need for a separate scissors to cut the suture material (Figure 19-14).

Specula, Scopes, Probes, Retractors, and Dilators. The category of dilators and probes includes specula that are designed for enlarging and exploring body orifices (Figure 19-16). The vaginal speculum is available in various lengths and widths and may be made of metal or disposable plastic. The most common instrument for enlarging the nostril is the Vienna nasal speculum. This instrument is used with the Lucae bayonet forceps to perform procedures within the nose.

Scopes are defined as lighted instruments used for viewing. The otoscope, used to visualize the ear canal and eardrum, has a small light aimed into an ear speculum. Ear specula may be disposable or reuseable. If reused, they are sanitized, chemically disinfected, rinsed, and dried between uses. Proctoscopes, anoscopes, (Figure 19-17) and rigid sigmoidoscopes are used for viewing the rectum, anus, and the sigmoid portion on the large intestine and have guides called obturators to ease insertion. The light source for the proctoscopes and anoscopes is usually a separate lamp. Although the light sources cannot be sterilized, they can be meticulously disinfected. The speculum portion that is inserted into the rectum may

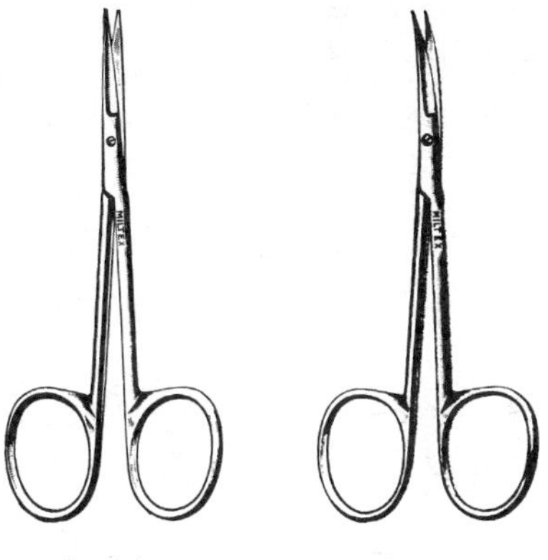

Figure 19-8A Iris scissors. (Courtesy of Miltex, Inc.)

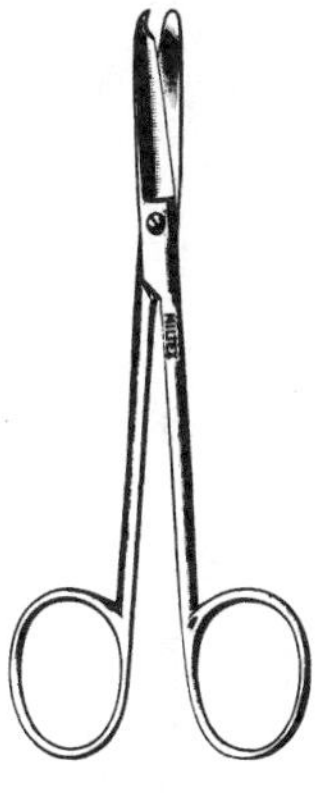

Figure 19-8B Suture or stitch removal scissors. (Courtesy of Miltex, Inc.)

be disposable plastic or made of metal. Both the metal speculum and its obturator may be sanitized and sterilized in the autoclave.

There is another group of scopes that are long, flexible, and are much more complex, and use fiber-optic light sources. Fiber-optic scopes are considered to be medical equipment rather than surgical instruments. Although considered to be medical equipment, these flexible scopes are inserted into body cavities and must be sanitized and sterilized between uses.

Probes are slender instruments used to probe into a hidden area, body cavity, or wound. Sounds are long, slender probing instruments used to determine the size and shape of the area being probed or to detect the presence of an unseen foreign body. Sounds may be calibrated in centimeters or inches (Figure 19-18).

Retractors used in office/ambulatory surgery are often called skin hooks and are used to hook onto and retract the edges of a wound to facilitate better viewing. Skin hooks are fine-tipped and delicate. As with all of the finer surgical instruments, special care should be taken to avoid damaging the delicate tips (Figure 19-19).

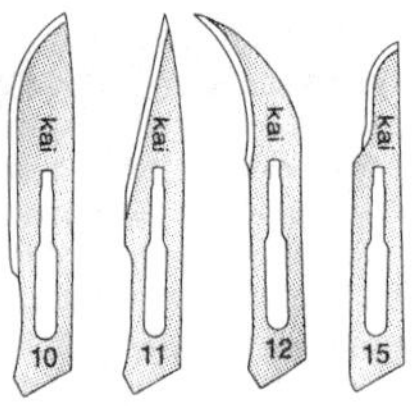

Figure 19-9A Surgical blades: #10, #11, #12, #15. (Courtesy of Miltex, Inc.)

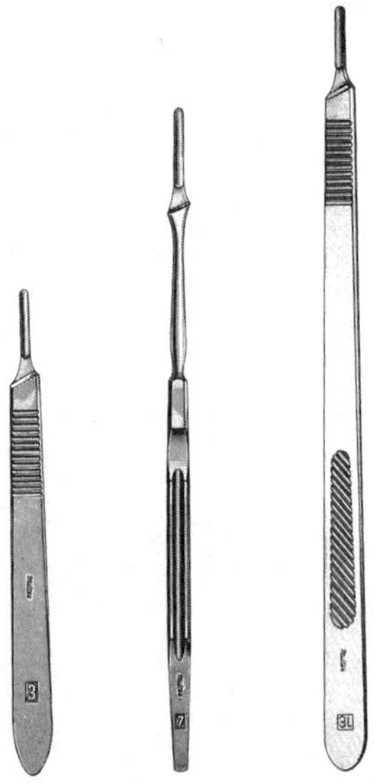

Figure 19-9B Scalpel handles: #3, #7, #3L. (Courtesy of Miltex, Inc.)

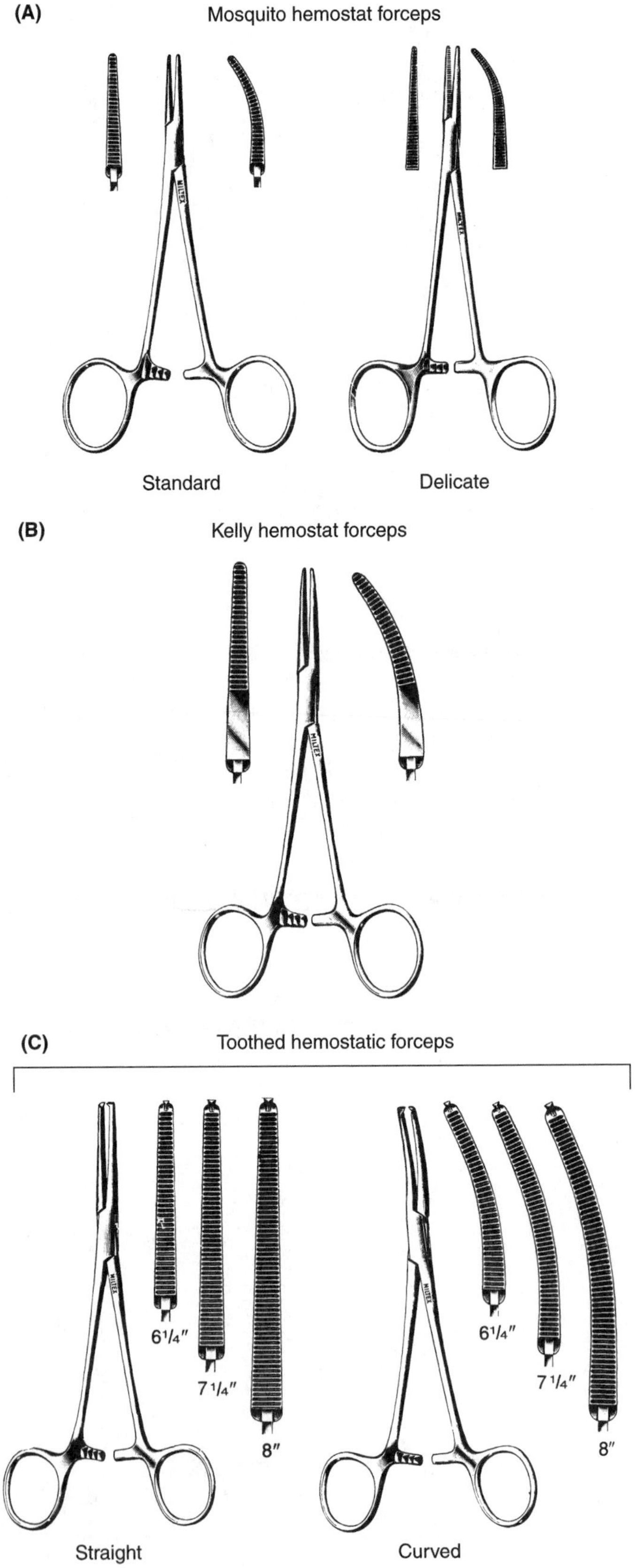

Figure 19-10 Hemostatic forceps include (A) mosquito hemostat forceps; (B) Kelly hemostat forceps; and (C) toothed hemostatic forceps. (Courtesy of Miltex, Inc.)

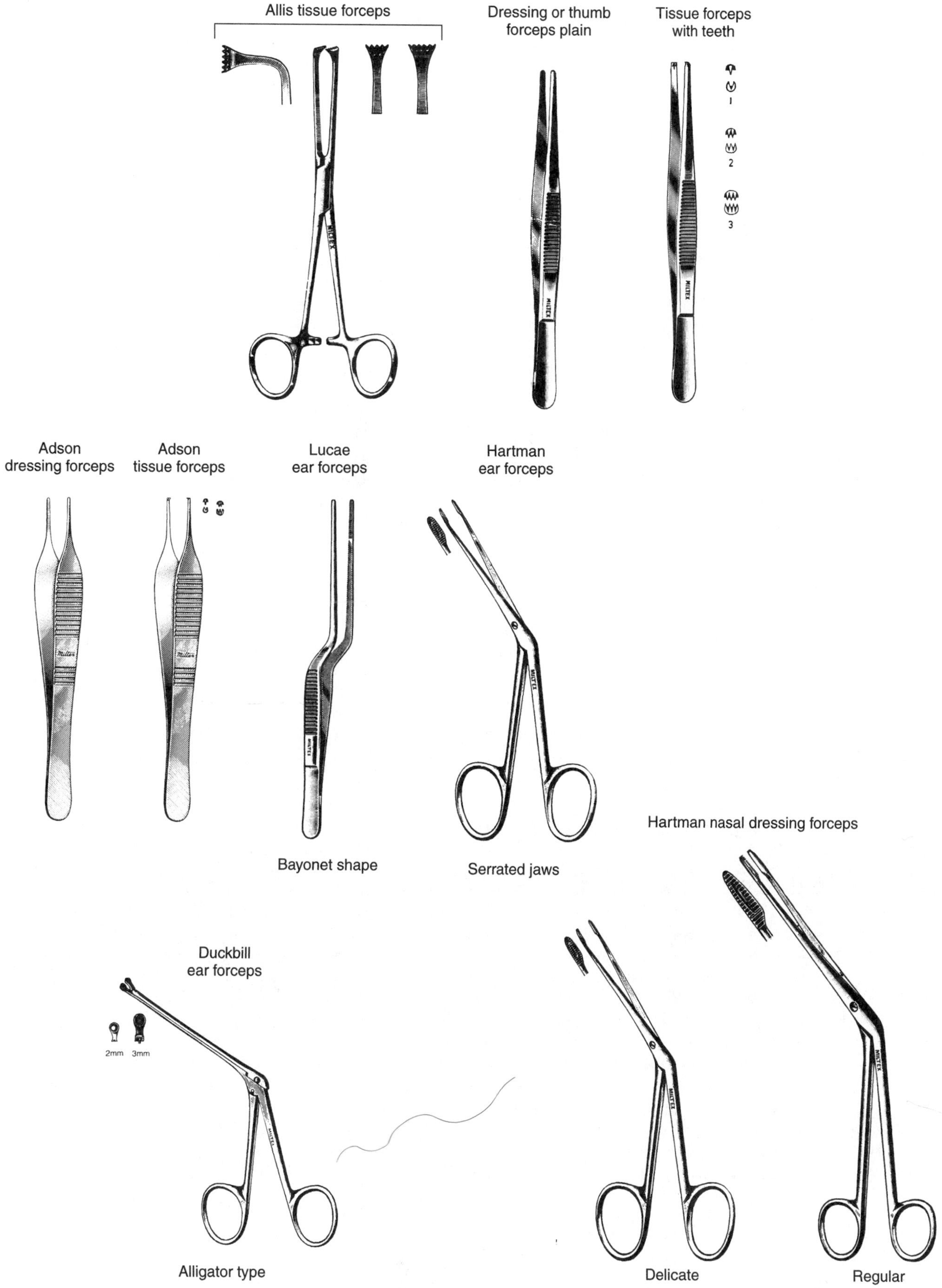

Figure 19-11 Tissue and dressing forceps. (Courtesy of Miltex, Inc.)

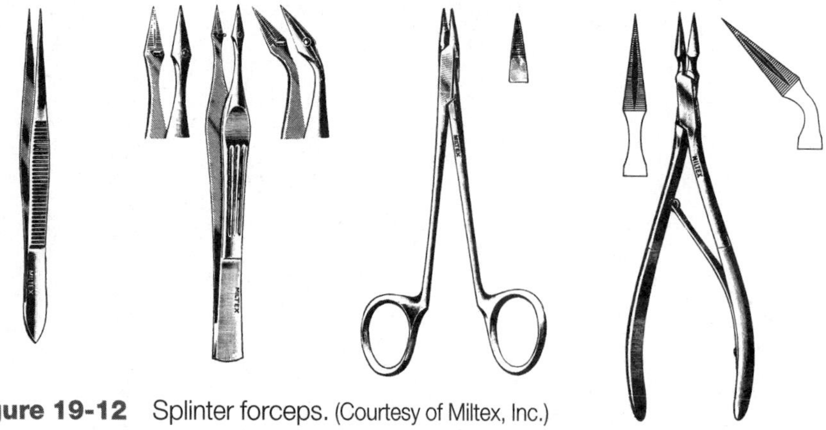

Figure 19-12 Splinter forceps. (Courtesy of Miltex, Inc.)

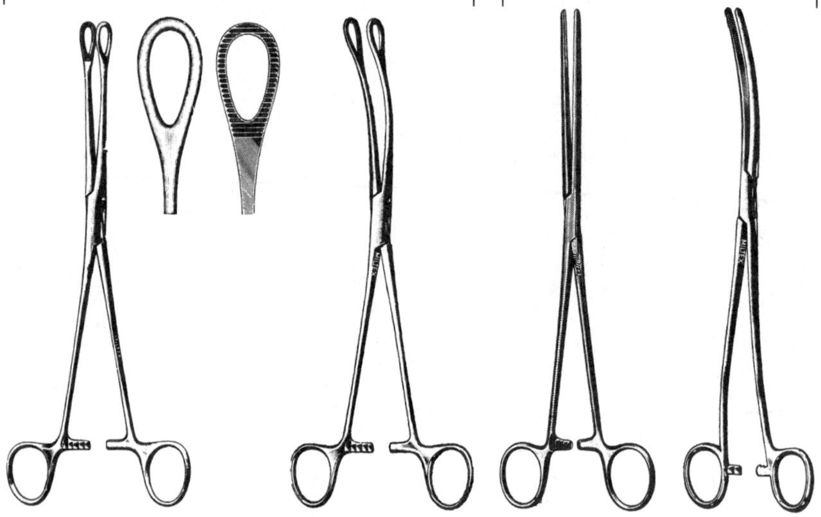

Figure 19-13 Sponge forceps. (Courtesy of Miltex, Inc.)

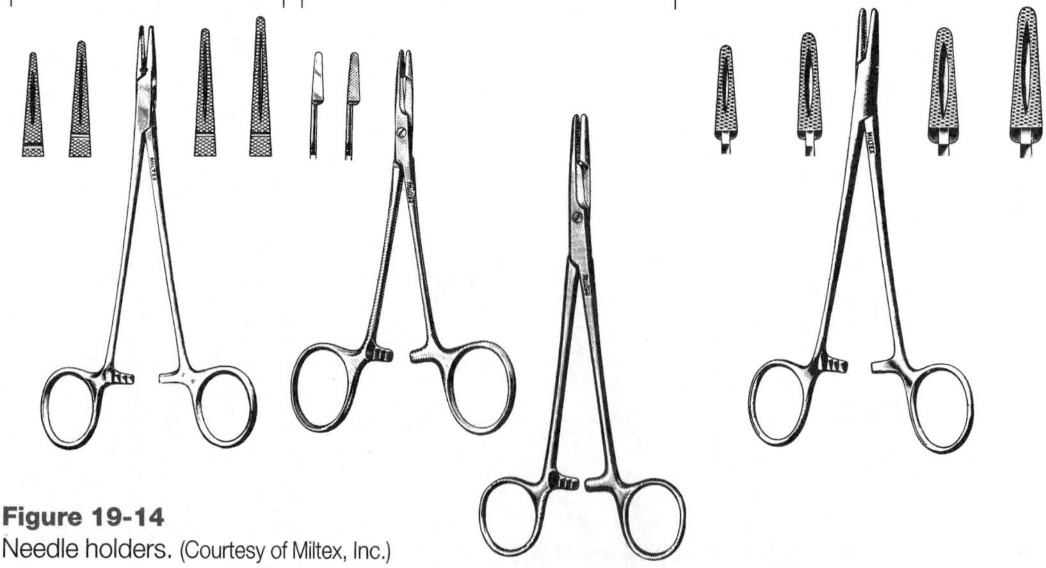

Figure 19-14
Needle holders. (Courtesy of Miltex, Inc.)

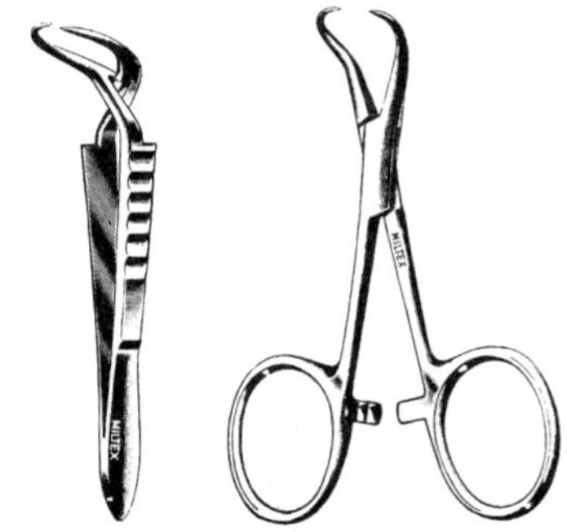

Figure 19-15 Towel clamps. (Courtesy of Miltex, Inc.)

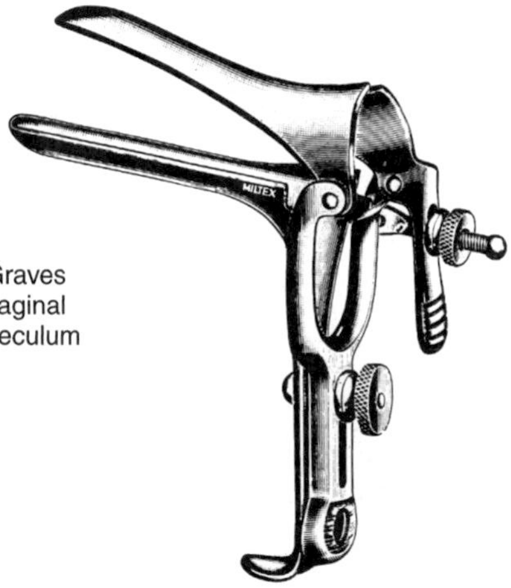

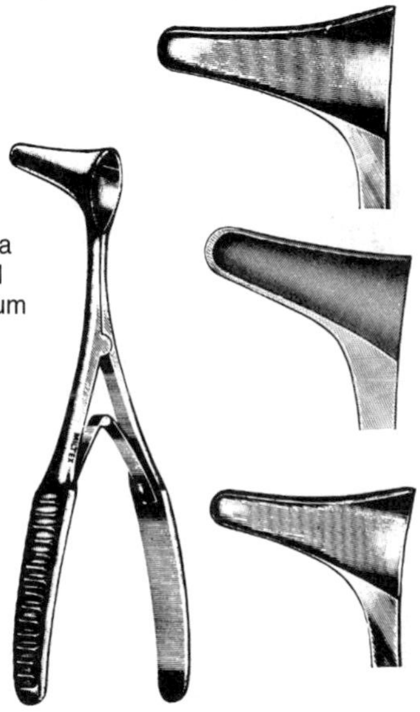

Figure 19-16 Specula and scopes are used to explore body openings by widening for better viewing. (Courtesy of Miltex, Inc.)

Dilators are double-ended metal rods with smooth, rounded tips, ranging in calibrated sizes from small to large. Dilators are inserted into narrowed or constricted ducts and tubes for the purpose of gradually dilating or enlarging the opening. Hegar uterine dilators are used to dilate the cervix to gain access to the inside of the uterus. Esophageal dilators are used to relieve **strictures,** or narrowing, of the esophagus. Urethral dilators are used to relieve strictures of the urethra (Figure 19-20).

Care of Instruments

Medical/surgical instruments require special care to prevent excessive wear and tear and unnecessary damage. Careful and frequent inspections will determine when instruments need to be replaced or repaired. Some basic rules and rationales include:

- Immediately after use, soiled instruments should be soaked. This prevents blood and other body fluids from drying onto the working surfaces of the instruments.
- Soak solutions should be about room temperature and contain a neutral pH detergent with a protein/blood solvent. The proteins in the body fluids will not coagulate on the instruments in cool water and the neutral pH detergent will help prevent spotting and corrosion of the metals. Solvents will help break up the blood and proteins in the body fluids.
- Soak basins should be plastic to prevent damaging points and edges. If a metal soak basin is used, placing a towel on the bottom as padding will help prevent damage to the instruments.
- Heavy-duty rubber gloves should be worn when cleaning instruments to lessen the likelihood of being stuck or cut with the sharp points and edges.
- Delicate instruments should be separated from heavier instruments to prevent the delicate instruments from being bent or otherwise damaged.
- Sharp instruments should be carefully separated from the other instruments and washed with extreme caution. The danger of being cut or punctured is greater when cleaning sharp instruments than at most other times, and the sharp instruments are usually the most contaminated.

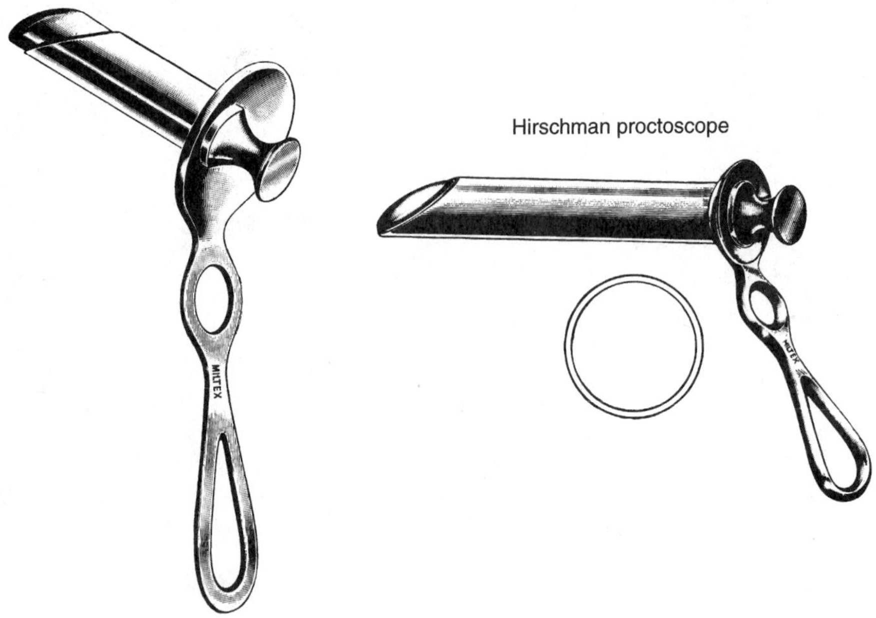

Figure 19-17 Scopes and specula are used to expose body orifices by opening for better viewing. (Courtesy of Miltex, Inc.)

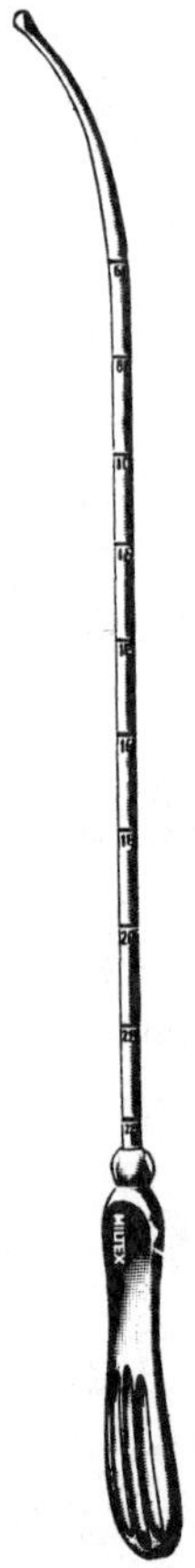

Figure 19-18 Uterine sound. (Courtesy of Miltex, Inc.)

- A soft bristle brush should be used to scrub hinges, ratchets, and serrations. The brush should be firm enough to clean crevices thoroughly yet soft enough to prevent scratching instruments. Instruments with multiple parts must be taken completely apart.
- Immediately after sanitization, instruments should be thoroughly rinsed and dried to prevent spotting and water damage.
- Carefully inspect all surfaces, edges, and points. Check for nicks, dulling, and warping. Test blades for sharpness. Be sure the instrument is not bent or pitted. Handles should also be checked for nicks that may snag and tear surgical gloves, thus disrupting the protective barrier and causing contamination.
- Damaged or malfunctioning instruments should be repaired or replaced.

Ultrasonic Cleaning. Surgical instruments can be cleaned (sanitized) by using an ultrasonic cleaner. Instruments are placed into an ultrasonic container with special cleaning solution. Sound waves vibrate to loosen debris and contaminants. Place instruments with ratchets or hinges into the cleaner in an open position. The articles, when finished, are rinsed well, dried, and wrapped for sterilization. The process of sanitizing contaminated instruments by ultrasound is safe for all instruments including delicate instruments. Follow manufacturer's directions for use and care of the ultrasonic cleaner.

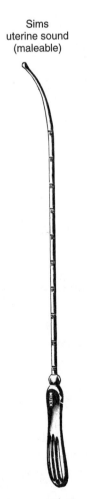

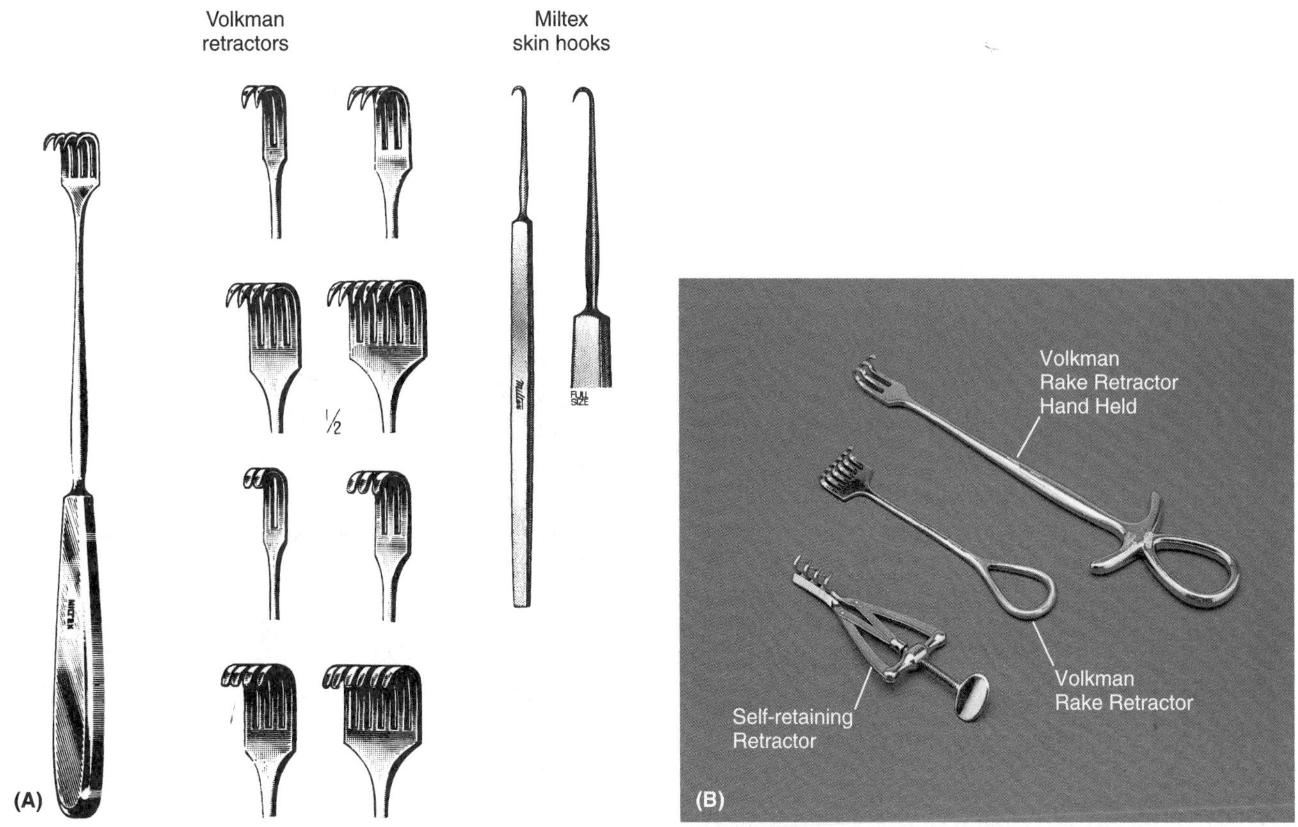

Figure 19-19 Various types of retractors (sharp and blunt). (Courtesy of Miltex, Inc.)

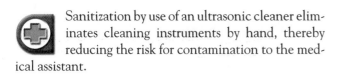

Sanitization by use of an ultrasonic cleaner eliminates cleaning instruments by hand, thereby reducing the risk for contamination to the medical assistant.

- Instruments should be processed in the cleaner for the full recommended cycle time, usually 5 to 10 minutes.
- Place instruments in open position into the ultrasonic cleaner. Make sure that sharps blades and points do not touch other instruments.
- All instruments have to be fully submerged.
- Do not place dissimilar metals (stainless, copper, chrome plated) in the same cleaning cycle.
- Change solution frequently—at least as often as the manufacturer recommends.
- Rinse instruments thoroughly with water after ultrasonic cleaning to remove ultrasonic cleaning solution.

Chemical "Cold" Sterilization. This type of sterilization is sometimes referred to as "cold" sterilization, which indicates that heat-sensitive items such as fiber-optic

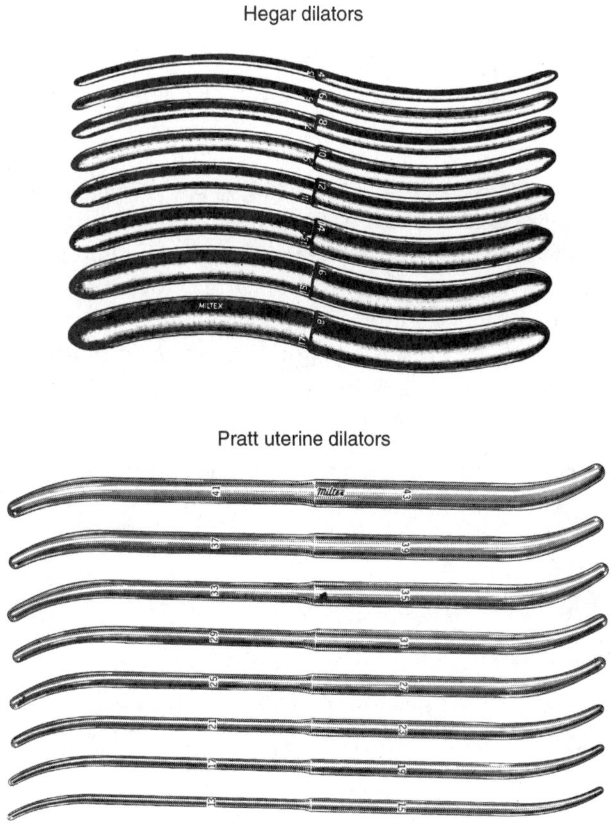

Figure 19-20 Two types of dilators (arranged smallest to largest). (Courtesy of Miltex, Inc.)

endoscopes and delicate cutting instruments can be immersed in a chemical solution. The chemicals used are reliable and capable of destroying bacteria and their spores and, used in strict accordance with the manufacturer's instructions regarding length of immersion time, sterility can be assured.

See Procedure 10-5 for cold sterilization and disinfection and sanitization procedures.

SUPPLIES AND EQUIPMENT

The supplies necessary for office/ambulatory surgery are often disposable and should be replenished as needed. Most medical/surgical supply companies have catalogs and Web sites available for ordering and many companies have sales representatives who make regular stops or are available by telephone or E-mail to assist in the ordering process. Sales representatives are familiar with the products their company markets and are extremely useful as a resource. Samples of new products are often available for trial, and optional choices are always offered. Medical/surgical supply companies frequently offer special prices for larger quantity purchases. If a medical/surgical supply item is being used frequently and storage space is available, buying in larger quantities might be more cost-effective. If a product currently being used is not meeting expectations, requesting optional trial products is usually the first step toward finding a better product. Following are some of the more commonly used supplies associated with office/ambulatory surgery.

Sponges and Wicks

Surgical sponges are prepackaged squares of folded gauze used in surgery. Within the physician's office, sponges are most often referred to by their size. A gauze square measuring 4 inches by 4 inches is called a 4 × 4 (Figure 19-21). The other most common sizes are 3 × 3 and 2 × 2. The gauge sponges are either packaged in individual peel-apart packages of two or may be purchased in non-

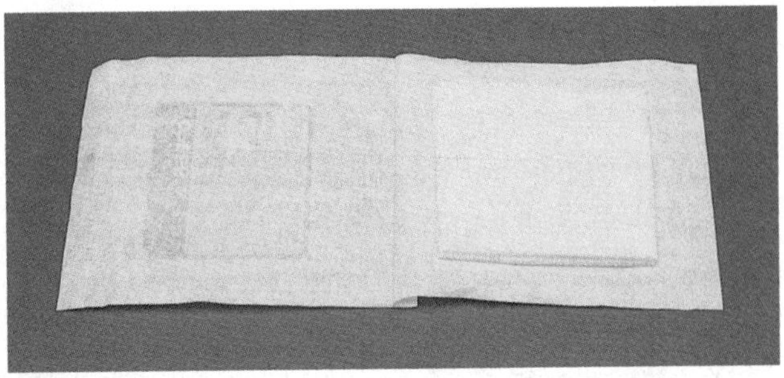

Figure 19-21 Peel-apart sterile open package of 4 × 4 gauze. These are also referred to as 4 × 4s or, in surgery, as surgical sponges.

sterile bulk packages of one hundred. The individual packages are convenient, sterile, and useful for most purposes but cost more per sponge than the nonsterile bulk packages. For larger surgical needs, the medical assistant may wrap several bulk sponges together and autoclave them for later use. Most sponges are simply folded gauze, but some have cotton or rayon pads embedded in them to increase absorption ability and to create a softer texture. The medical assistant and the physician using the sponge will probably have a preference among the different types and uses. Gauze sponges are used in wound cleansing, in skin preparation, as absorbable sponges during surgery, as dressings and coverings, and for padding. The ambulatory care setting may prefer to have different sizes and types in stock to meet different needs.

Sterile surgical wicks or wound packing strips are used when an infected wound needs to remain open for drainage. The wicking material is made of narrow strips of gauze packaged in long lengths in opaque glass bottles. The most recognizable trade name is Iodoform®. The Iodoform® is sterile and packaged in multiple-use bottles. Extreme care should be taken to prevent contamination during removal of individual lengths. The bottle is opened using sterile technique, sterile dressing forceps are inserted into the bottle, the strip is cut to the desired length using sterile scissors, and the lid is applied without compromising the sterility of the remaining wicking material in the bottle.

Solutions/Creams/Ointments

Many different soaps and solutions are available and effective as skin cleansers, preoperative scrubs, paints, soaks, and antiseptics. **Betadine®** (povidone-iodine) is a well-known antiseptic and is available as a surgical soap called a "scrub" and as a nonsoap solution for preoperative skin preparation/paint. Betadine® comes in multiple-use bottles, in single use, and in individually packaged swabs. **Hibeclens®** is another effective antiseptic that does not have the staining tendencies of iodine. Medical/surgical supply companies will have names and samples of other products. Consideration should be made to cost, effectiveness, ease of use, shelf life, and personal preferences. **Isopropyl alcohol,** a 70% alcohol solution, is of limited medical/surgical use, although because of its rapid volatility rate and its ability to dissolve oils, it is still preferred for skin preparation before injections and venipuncture. Isopropyl alcohol is available in bottles for use with cotton/rayon balls or in convenient individually packaged pledgets. Isopropyl alcohol can be irritating and is not effective as a preoperative skin preparation. **Hydrogen peroxide** is a noncaustic mildly effective skin antiseptic. It bubbles on contact with mucous membranes and other moist skin surfaces, dissolving blood and proteins, and has a mechanical cleansing action. Hydrogen peroxide is ineffective as a skin prep before surgery but is useful for cleaning after surgery. Many physicians do not recommend using hydrogen peroxide on surgical wounds because of its abrasive "scrubbing action," which can cause increased scarring and irritations. Do not use or recommend the use of hydrogen peroxide without consulting your physician delegator.

Antibacterial creams and ointments are sometimes applied topically on wounds to aid healing. Antibacterial creams are usually white, water-based, and nongreasy. Antibacterial ointments are usually clear and oil based. If a wound requires thorough cleaning between dressing changes, an antibacterial cream is preferred because of the ease of removal.

Some examples of sterile solutions are sterile saline, sterile distilled water, and Betadine® solution.

Silvadene® is brand name of a sterile cream used on burns and other abrasion wounds. It is an excellent antibacterial cream, but must be applied 1/8- to 1/4-inch-thick to help ensure that the dressing does not absorb all the cream, thus drying out the wound. Sterile tongue blades are handy to apply the Silvadene® cream to large area burns. Silvadene should be thoroughly removed and reapplied fresh with each dressing change. Silvadene is available by prescription only and comes in small tubes for individual use, as well as larger jars for multiple use. Silvadene is fairly expensive and when using a multiple use jar, as with any multiple-use container, extreme caution must be taken to avoid contamination of the product.

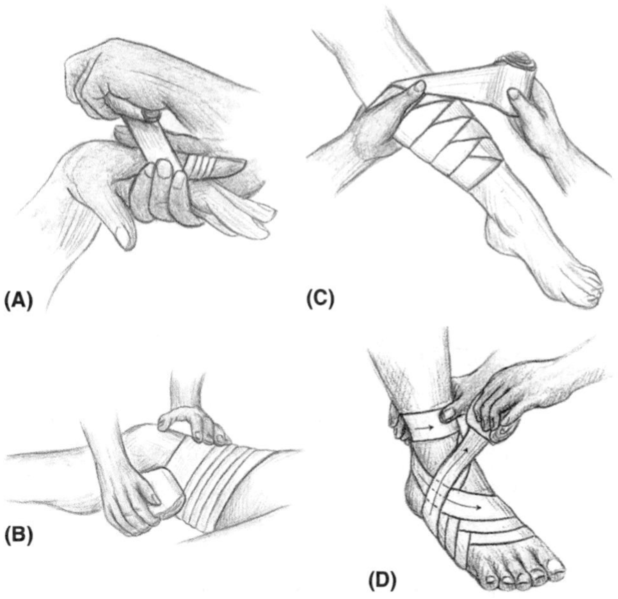

Figure 19-22 Bandage-wrapping techniques illustrating the circular, spiral, and figure-eight turns. (A) Circular turns are wrapped around a body part several times to anchor a bandage or to supply support. (B) Spiral turns begin with one or two circular turns, then proceed up the body part, with each turn covering two-thirds the width of the previous turn. (C) Reverse spiral turns begin with a circular turn. Then the bandage is reversed or twisted once each turn to accommodate a limb that gets larger as the bandaging progresses. (D) Figure-eight turns crisscross in the shape of a figure eight and are used on a joint that requires movement.

Dressings and Bandages

Dressings are defined as the sterile material applied directly onto the surface of a wound or surgical site. **Bandages** are defined as the supportive material applied over the top of dressings and are not sterile. A dressing, being sterile, should be handled with care to avoid contamination of the wound. Often a nonstick pad or topical medication will be applied to the wound to prevent the dressing from adhering to the wound.

Dressings are usually made of gauze and need to completely cover the wound. Dressings must be adequately absorbent for any wound drainage.

Bandages are used to keep dressings in place, to provide padding and protection, and to immobilize. Bandaging may consist of rolled gauze wrapped around the wound area with an additional sturdier wrap applied overall. An elastic bandage may provide additional support, and a triangular bandage, sling, brace, or splint provides even more. A unique type of bandage is the tubular gauze bandage. Tubular gauze bandages are used to cover appendages such as fingers, arms, toes, and legs and come in various sizes according to the size of the body part being covered. Refer to Chapter 9 for further information about wounds and bandages. See Figure 19-22 for examples and illustrations of various bandage-wrapping techniques.

Anesthetics

The word **anesthesia** means the loss of feeling or sensation. An anesthetic is any mechanism that causes this loss of feeling. The application of extreme cold can be an anesthetic because it causes numbness to nerve endings and thus the loss of feeling. Anesthetics may be inhaled, topically applied or sprayed, or injected either directly into a vein (intravenously), the spinal column (intrathecally), or locally (subcutaneously) into the tissues at the site of the surgical procedure.

Injectable Anesthetics. Most anesthetics used in office/ambulatory surgery are administered locally through injection into the subcutaneous tissues. The nerves exposed to the anesthetic become temporarily unable to conduct sensations and feelings to the brain, thereby causing a lack of pain sensation in the area during the surgery. All synthetic local anesthetics have names that end in *-caine*. Some of the most common are Xylocaine (lidocaine), Novacaine (procaine), Marcaine, and Carbocaine. Local anesthetics are available in single-dose vials or ampules of 10 ml, but most medical offices prefer the cost-effectiveness of multiple-dose vials containing 30 to 50 ml. Local anesthetics are also available in varying strengths such as 0.5%, 1%, and 2%.

Injectable anesthetics may contain an additive called **epinephrine.** It has a red label. Epinephrine causes vasoconstriction and is used when reduced blood flow to the area is desired. The medical assistant is often delegated the responsibility of filling the syringe with the prescribed amount and strength of the ordered anesthesia or may assist the physician in drawing up the medication. Be sure to identify the drug and dose for the physician.

Anytime the medical assistant draws up a medication for the physician or pours a solution into a prep basin on the sterile tray, the original vial or bottle that the medication or solution comes from should be brought into the procedure room with the surgical/procedure tray and other supplies. The physician should check the vial and container before using the medication or solution to be sure it is exactly what he or she ordered. A good practice is to set the vial or container on the counter within plain view for the physician to see. Often the physician will verbally confirm what medication is in the syringe or what solution is in the prep basin before using them.

Anesthetics with epinephrine should not be used on fingers, toes, noses, or earlobes because of the vasoconstriction action they have. Patients with circulatory complications may have even more restrictions/cautions on the use of epinephrine. This is one of the reasons it is important to bring the vial into the procedure room with the patient.

Drawing Techniques. If the physician plans to inject the anesthesia before applying sterile gloves, either the medical assistant or the physician may draw up the medication. The filled syringe is then placed on the side, rather than directly on the sterile field. This allows the physician to anesthetize the patient before beginning the sterile procedure. After the anesthesia has taken effect, the physician will perform a surgical hand cleansing, apply sterile gloves, and begin the surgery.

When the physician applies sterile gloves before injecting the anesthesia, the sterile syringe may be placed directly on the sterile field either empty or filled. One person wearing sterile gloves may handle the syringe and draw up the medication while another person not wearing sterile gloves holds the vial. This method requires either that the syringe and needle be applied directly to the sterile tray or handed directly to a "sterile" person. The medical assistant may draw up the anesthesia under sterile process when he or she sets up the sterile tray. As stated previously, if the tray contains a filled syringe, the vial from which it was drawn should accompany the tray into the procedure room and be set on the counter for the physician to verify. Refer to Chapter 24 for the specific techniques for drawing up medications.

Topical Spray Anesthetics. Not all anesthesia is injectable. Topical (applied to the surface) anesthetics are available in liquid and spray. The most common topical anesthetic used in the medical office is ethyl chloride spray. Ethyl chloride freezes the skin to allow for simple piercing or lancing. The anesthetic action usually only lasts for a few seconds; therefore, the procedure must be performed quickly. One example for the use of ethyl chloride spray is to briefly numb an area before an injection. A lesion that is infected is extremely painful to inject with a local anesthetic; however, by using ethyl chloride spray before the injection, the patient is able to remain still. Ethyl chloride spray may also be used before installing intravenous lines.

See Table 19-3 for a summary of supplies and equipment.

PATIENT CARE AND PREPARATION

Patient Preparation and Education

If the patient is having a planned surgical procedure performed, there is time for patient preparation. Patients may need to modify their diet, adjust medication, acquire special supplies, adjust their personal home and work situations, obtain prior approval from their insurance, and prepare for the postoperative period. If the patient is having an unplanned procedure performed, such as a laceration repaired, there is less time for preparation. In either case, the medical assistant will need to follow an established protocol about wound care, patient education, patient health consideration, and consent. In the case of an accidental wound, the medical assistant needs to determine the cause of the wound and the date of the last tetanus injection. See Chapters 10 and 23 for specific information about tetanus and immunization schedules. The medical assistant must also check to determine whether the patient has allergies or sensitivities of any kind, particularly to medication and medically related substances.

Diet modifications include abstaining from eating and drinking for several hours before the surgical procedure, as well as restricting the types and amounts of certain foods or liquids consumed before and directly after

TABLE 19-3 SUPPLIES AND EQUIPMENT COMMONLY USED IN MINOR SURGERY

Item	Use/Description
Sponges	Used in wound cleansing, skin preparation, as absorbable sponges during surgery, as dressings and coverings, and for padding. Also called 4 × 4s. Typically made of folded gauze, though some have cotton or rayon pads embedded in them to increase absorption.
Wicks	Used when an infected wound needs to remain open for drainage. Wicking material is made of narrow strips of gauze packaged in long lengths in opaque glass bottles, which should be opened using sterile technique.
Solutions	Used as skin cleansers, preoperative scrubs, paints, soaks, and antiseptics. Most common are Betadine®, an antiseptic often used in soap form as a scrub; Hibeclens®, an effective antiseptic without iodine's staining properties; isopropyl alcohol, a 70% alcohol solution favored for skin preparation before injections and venipuncture but not effective as a preoperative skin preparation; hydrogen peroxide, a mildly effective abrasive skin antiseptic.
Creams and ointments	Antibacterial. May be used topically on wounds to promote healing. Creams are water-based; ointments are oil-based.
Dressings	Sterile material applied directly onto surface of a wound or surgical site. Usually made of gauze. Must be adequately absorbent and completely cover the wound.
Bandages	Nonsterile supportive materials applied over dressings to keep the dressing in place. May be rolled gauze, elastic bandage, or tubular gauze bandage.
Anesthetics	A mechanism used to cause the loss of feeling. May be inhaled, topically applied, sprayed, or injected directly into a vein, the spinal column, or locally into the tissues at the site of the surgical procedure.

the procedure. When patients are aware of special dietary needs after surgery, they can shop early and be prepared. An example of a medication treatment includes prescribing an antibiotic to be taken as a precaution against acquiring an infection after surgery or adjusting anticoagulant medications to prevent excessive bleeding during surgery. Each clinic, physician, procedure, and patient will have individual requirements and preferences. The patient might be required to obtain special supplies for the convalescent period. For instance, immediately after a vasectomy a scrotal support is usually recommended. Crutches or special foot coverings might be necessary after foot or leg surgery. Specific wound dressing and bandages might need to be purchased before the surgery in anticipation of the postoperative need. Having another person accompany the patient to the clinic for the surgery is required for the safe return home. Knowing the planned period for recovery allows the patient to make the necessary arrangements for work, child care, and other personal situations.

Informed Consent

Before a surgical procedure, the patient's written consent must be obtained. In many medical and all surgical procedures, a written, **informed consent** form must be signed. An informed consent is a document that may be created specifically for a particular procedure or that may be an established document available for duplication. An informed consent document informs the patient of the medical or surgical procedure to be performed; describes to the patient, in lay terms, the actual procedure; cites alternative treatments; and lists the possible undesirable outcome and risks involved in the procedure. See Chapter 7 for additional information on informed consent.

The cost of the procedure is also important information. Some insurances and Medicare require the patient sign an Advanced Beneficiary Notice (ABN) if their out-of-pocket expenses are going to be above a certain amount. It is always a good idea to discuss financial arrangements with all patients before an elective procedure or surgery. Some offices will have the bookkeeper or office manager come into the examination room to sit down with the patient and go over the forms and financial arrangements. Any questions the patient has about the surgery should be answered completely by the physician and an assessment should be made that the patient understands the answers. Even in the best of circumstances, results cannot be guaranteed. Most of the difficult situations between physicians' practices and patients come from misunderstandings about unexpected outcomes. If patients are informed completely, even unplanned results are better tolerated.

Medical Assisting Considerations

The general health and condition of the patient before surgery is important when planning the recovery. A frail, weak man living alone may need home health care after even a simple surgical procedure. Some people may not be able to follow standard preoperative or postoperative instructions. The recovery may depend on the availability of supplies beyond what the patient can financially afford. If difficult circumstances can be identified before the surgery, arrangements can be made with home health care services, community assistance services, or friends and family.

Cardio Pulmanary weakn-
ess happen if the patient
receîved a general
anesthetie if she/he is
elderly. the Cause arise
hyptension or hypoxia
lack of O_2

istory
asked
s and
anes-
onary
lderly,
lation
poxia.
blood
about

Postoperative instructions should be written and clearly understood by the patient. If the patient has a caregiver at home, the postoperative instructions should be clearly understood by the caregiver as well. The telephone number of the clinic and an after-hours number should be written on the postoperative instructions and brought to the attention of the patient and caregiver. It is good practice to plan to call patients within the first postoperative day to check on their condition.

Wounds, Wound Care, and the Healing Process

There are many different types of wounds based on the type of injury incurred. Wounds may be classified as open or closed, accidental or intentional (surgical).

Lacerations, incisions, avulsions, and punctures are all examples of open wounds (Figure 19-23).

Ecchymosis, contusion, and hematoma are all examples of closed wounds. They are caused by a blunt trauma that damages underlying tissues but leaves the skin intact (Figure 19-24).

Wounds are classified as superficial if the injury does not extend deeper than the subcutaneous tissues.

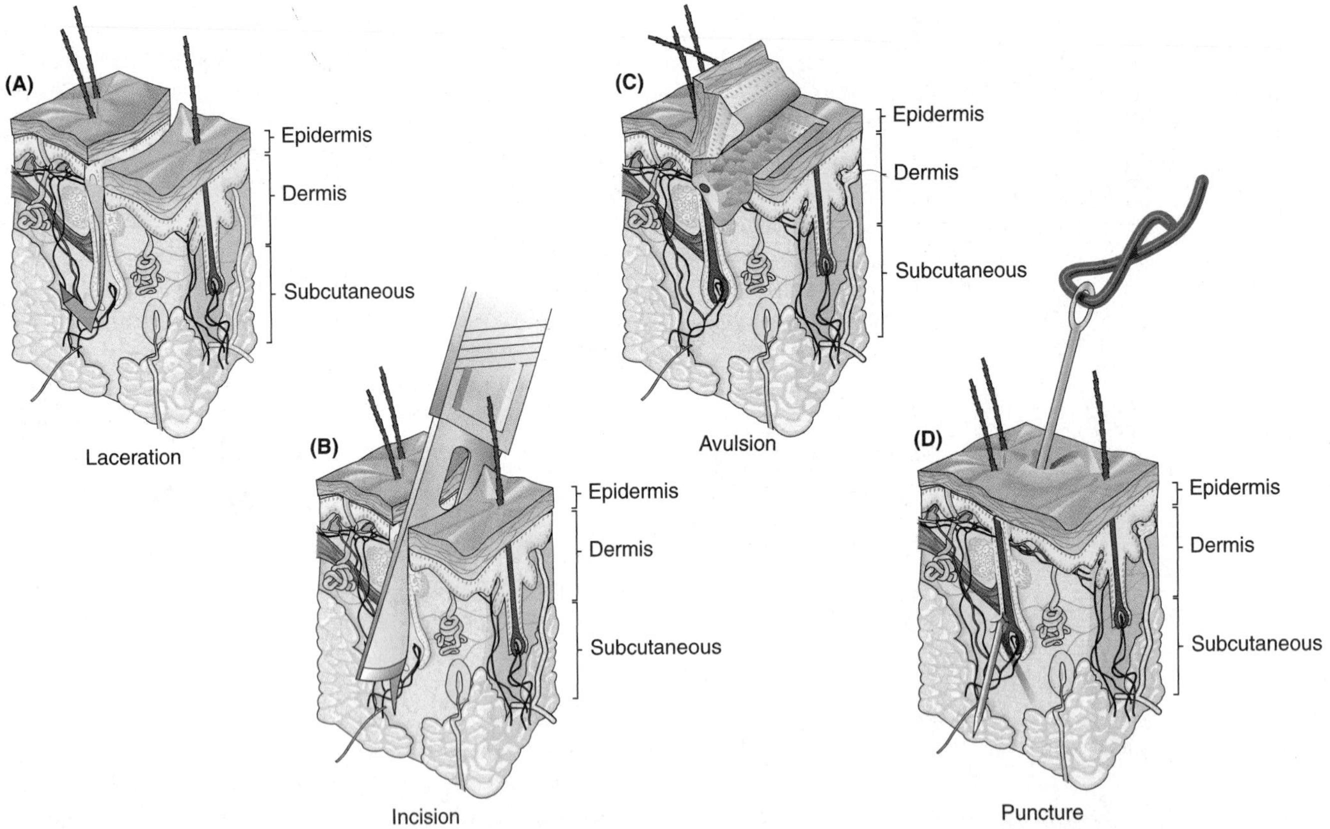

Figure 19-23 Open wounds. (A) Lacerations are accidental tearing of the body tissue usually made by sharp objects. The torn flesh may be smooth or jagged and is often difficult to clean and suture properly. There may be extensive bleeding. Paper cuts are examples of lacerations. (B) Incisions are intentional cuts typically made with a scalpel for surgical procedures. (C) Avulsions are accidental tearing away of a part or structures of the skin. (D) Punctures are holes or wounds made by a pointed object and can be either accidental or intentional. Puncture wounds have little bleeding because the point of entry is small. These wounds are typically not much larger than the instrument entering the skin. A puncture wound may also be the result of stepping on a nail.

~~The~~ Inflammation is the body's natural reaction to trauma.
- inflamed tissue will become infected if the trauma is cause Pathogen
- the best treatment for infect is Prevention & advis patient keep ~~clean~~ the wound clean

...ns, ...nows ...er. The ...und are an impo... ...ord and for proper insurance reimbursement. A typical description of a patient wound that is an intermediate laceration might be, "patient sustained a deep 3.5-cm laceration to the anterior surface of the right knee caused by a fall onto a rock." A puncture wound might be described as, "patient presents with a 2-cm deep puncture wound on the plantar surface of the left foot obtained from stepping on a rusty nail." Both statements describe not only the size, depth, location, and type of wound, but also the causative factor.

Patient Education

The basic signs of inflammation are redness, heat, swelling, pain, and loss of function. Any one or more of these may be present in varying intensities during an inflammatory process. Most wounds will have a mild inflammation described as slightly red or pink, mild warmth, slightly tender to the touch, and mildly swollen. The symptoms are caused by increased blood supply to the traumatized area and the infiltration of white blood cells in reaction to the trauma. Patients should be taught to watch for an increase in the intensity of redness, pain, swelling, and heat or any drainage, fever, or lymph gland swelling, which can indicate an infection from invading pathogens. The patient should be given instructions as to what actions to take if these symptoms of infection are noticed. The instructions should include a name and telephone numbers to call during the day or night. The medical assistant should reassure the patient not to hesitate to contact the center or physician if infection is suspected.

Inflammation is the body's natural reaction to trauma. Inflammation is also a normal process of wound healing. Occasionally, inflamed tissue will become infected if the trauma is caused by a pathogen. Although a certain degree of inflammation is expected, prevention of infection is a primary goal (see Chapter 10).

See Chapter 9 for further description of wounds and emergency care of wounds.

The best treatment for infection is prevention. Instructing the patient about proper wound care is extremely important. Encourage the patient to keep the wound clean and dry. In certain circumstances, the physician may prescribe a warm soak solution or the application of a topical antibacterial medication. If the wound becomes infected and a **suppurant** is present, the physician may order a wound irrigation (see Procedure 19-7). Wound irrigation removes the accumulation of purulent exudate that impairs and delays healing. After the irrigation, a dry sterile dressing is applied (see Procedure 19-6). Protecting the wound from further trauma and contamination will also aid in the healing process. Opinions will differ on whether a wound is best left open to air or covered with a dressing. Most health care providers will agree that covering a wound is preferred whenever contamination is likely. See Procedure 19-6.

BASIC SURGERY SETUP

Preparing for surgery includes assembling supplies and equipment, setting up the surgery tray, getting the patient and room ready, and preparing to assist during surgery. The specific instruments, supplies, and equipment needed for each surgery should be listed on individual **surgery cards.** These cards may be 3 × 5 or 5 × 7 cards stored in a card file or full sheets of procedures compiled in a manual or notebook. Procedures can be found on the computer. Each physician will have individual sets for each surgical procedure performed. Information on the surgery card or computer should include physician glove size, standing preoperative and postoperative instructions, and any additional information specific to the physician's needs or to the surgical procedure. The card file, whether manual or computerized, should be updated whenever changes are made and may be a responsibility of the medical assistant.

TABLE 19-4 GUIDELINES FOR STERILE TRAY SETUPS

- Set up the sterile surgery tray just before the surgery to allow less chance of accidental contamination.
- Immediately after the tray is set up, cover it with a sterile drape.
- Once the tray is prepared and covered, move it directly into the surgery area rather than leaving it in a common area.
- Inform the patient and others in the surgery room that the tray is sterile and should not be touched. Patients are often curious about instruments and may attempt to look under the cover if not cautioned against it.
- If the medical assistant is interrupted while preparing the tray and it becomes necessary to leave the tray unattended, cover the tray and move it out of traffic paths to prevent it from being bumped.

Basic Rules and Concepts for Setup of Surgical Trays

In addition to basic sterile principles, the guidelines in Table 19-4 will help ensure the sterile field remains sterile.

SURGERY PROCESS

For ease in understanding the individual tasks involved in office surgery, Table 19-5 provides generic steps for setting up the surgical tray, preparing the room, preparing the patient, assisting with the surgery, and the terminal care process of the room and equipment. Table 19-5 is intended as a quick checklist only and does not include all the specific details necessary for each surgery. Refer to the individual surgical procedures that follow for more details.

PREPARATION FOR SURGERY

The following procedures are used in preparation for minor surgery:

- Applying Sterile Gloves (Procedure 19-1)
- Setting Up and Covering a Sterile Field (Procedure 19-2)
- Opening Sterile Packages of Instruments and Supplies and Applying Them to a Sterile Field (Procedure 19-3)

TABLE 19-5 PREPARATIONS FOR OFFICE/AMBULATORY SURGERY

Tray Setup

1. Wash hands.
2. Reference surgery card, manual, or computer.
3. Gather equipment and supplies.
4. Sanitize and disinfect Mayo instrument tray.
5. Set up sterile field.
6. Place sterile instruments and supplies on the sterile field.
7. Apply sterile gloves.
8. Arrange instruments and supplies in an organized and logical manner.
9. Medication may be drawn up with assistance (optional).
10. Recheck tray for accuracy and completeness.
11. Remove gloves.
12. Cover and transport tray.
13. Add sterile solution (skin antiseptic) to tray if required.

Room Preparation

In preparing a room for a surgical procedure, all equipment should be clean and in good working order. Be certain to have spare parts such as light bulbs and filters readily available. Turn on equipment before the procedure to make sure all is working properly.

1. Check room equipment (light, stool, equipment, examination table, waste receptacle).
2. Check room supplies (tissue, extra gloves, and so on).
3. Arrange accessory supplies on the side counter in a logical order (pathology specimen bottle containing preservative, laboratory requisition, sterile glove package, dressings/bandages, postoperative medications, and instructions).

Patient Preparation

1. Wash hands.
2. Greet patient and ensure identity.
3. Escort the patient to the procedure room and offer restroom facilities.
4. Discuss the patient's compliance to preoperative instructions.
5. Explain the procedure again and address any questions.
6. Review postoperative instructions.
7. Check for signed informed consent form and financial forms.
8. Have the patient remove appropriate clothing and position the patient on the examination table. Offer a drape, gown, pillow, and blanket for comfort.
9. Prepare the skin for the surgical procedure (see Procedure 19-8).

(continues)

TABLE 19-5 PREPARATIONS FOR OFFICE/AMBULATORY SURGERY (continued)

Assisting with the Surgery

1. Remove the sterile cover from the surgical tray while the physician applies sterile gloves.
2. Assist the physician with stool and lamp adjustment as needed.
3. If the medical assistant did not perform the skin preparation, assist the physician as needed during skin preparation and draping. The equipment and supplies for skin preparation are separate from the surgery tray and equipment (see Procedure 19-8).
4. Adjust the instrument tray and equipment around the physician.
5. Assist with drawing up local anesthetic or other medication as needed.
6. Apply clean gloves for protection or sterile gloves to assist.
7. Surgery begins.
8. The medical assistant either assists with sterile procedure or supports the patient as needed.
9. After surgery, assist with or perform dressing of wound.
10. Clean patient if necessary.
11. Dispose of biohazardous waste materials.
12. Remove contaminated gloves; wash hands.
13. Assist the patient after surgery.

Assisting the Patient after Surgery

1. Check patient vital signs.
2. Remain with patient to ensure patient safety. Allow patient to rest if necessary.
3. Assist patient off examination table and assist with clothing as necessary.
4. Review written postoperative instructions with patient and caregiver. Dressing should be kept clean and dry. Patient should report any signs of infection.
5. Clarify any medication orders with patient and caregiver.
6. If not previously arranged, schedule follow-up appointment.
7. Document postoperative instructions in patient record.

Terminal Care of the Room and Equipment

1. Apply barrier gloves, gown, and goggles (if appropriate).
2. Dispose of drapes, table cover, pillowcase, and so on. Use biohazardous waste receptacle whenever appropriate.
3. Transfer contaminated surgical tray to cleanup area.
4. Using forceps, isolate sharps from surgical tray and dispose of them into designated sharps container.
5. Place instruments into a soak solution.
6. Sanitize Mayo instrument tray and all surfaces (examination table, stool, counter, lamp, machinery, and equipment).
7. Dispose of contaminated barrier gloves and apply protective gloves.
8. Disinfect all surfaces (examination table, stool, counter, lamp, machinery, and equipment).
9. Allow to air dry.
10. Sanitize, dry, wrap, and sterilize instruments.
11. It is the medical assistant's responsibility to make certain there are enough of each instrument and surgical sets.

Note: During most surgical procedures, if tissue is excised, it is placed in a biopsy specimen jar containing formalin (a preservative) and sent to the pathology laboratory with an appropriately completed requisition (Figure 19-25).

- Pouring a Sterile Solution into a Cup on a Sterile Field (Procedure 19-4)
- Preparation of Patient Skin before Surgery (Procedure 19-8)

Setting up surgical trays for specific surgeries is addressed in a later section of this chapter.

Critical Thinking

You are setting up a sterile surgical tray and have already applied your sterile gloves before you realize you forgot to place the suture package on the tray. You have several options. What are they and what are the advantages and disadvantages of each?

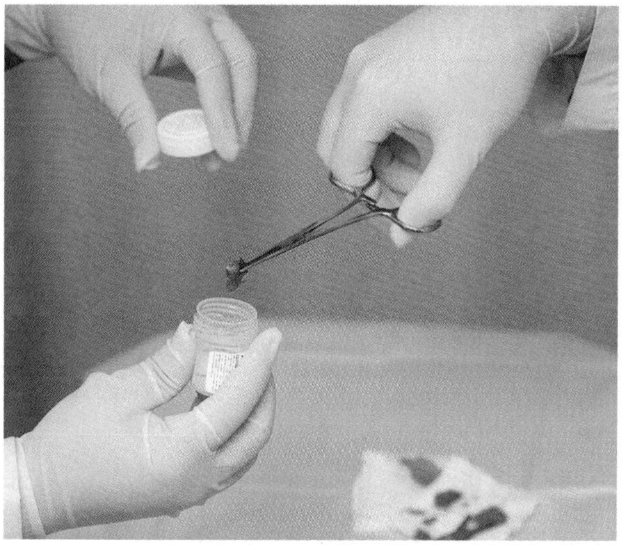

Figure 19-25 The doctor places biopsy tissue into specimen jar. The specimen will be sent to the pathology laboratory for examination.

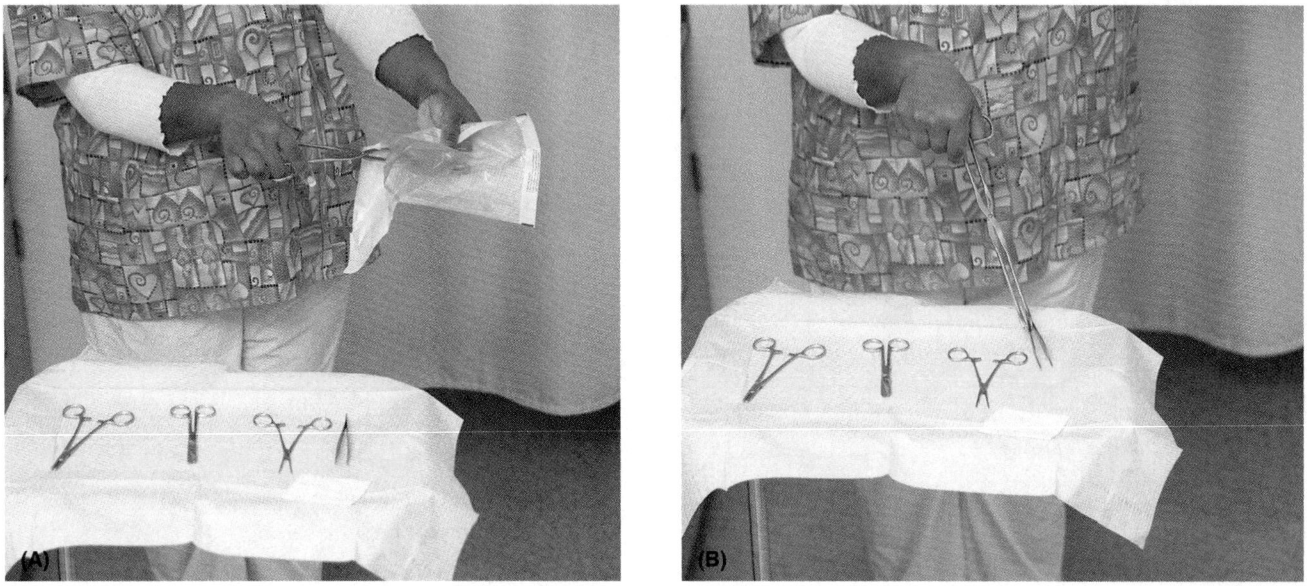

Figure 19-26 (A) If sterile gloves have been removed, use dry sterile transfer forceps to apply or rearrange sterile items on the Mayo stand. (B) Instruments and supplies may be moved around using dry sterile transfer forceps if necessary. (Note: Tray is below the waist for reader viewing.)

Using Dry Sterile Transfer Forceps

Occasionally after a sterile tray has been set up and sterile gloves removed, an additional item needs to be applied to or removed from the tray. The use of dry sterile transfer forceps allows sterile items to be applied or sterile items on the tray to be rearranged without the application of another pair of sterile gloves (Figure 19-26). The practice of using wet sterile transfer forceps is no longer recommended. Instead, when the use of sterile transfer forceps is needed, dry sterile transfer forceps are unwrapped, used only once, and then reprocessed for sterilization and subsequent use.

Procedure 19-1 Applying Sterile Gloves

STANDARD PRECAUTIONS:

PURPOSE:

Because hands cannot be sterilized, everyone performing sterile procedures must wear sterile gloves. This procedure provides direction on how to apply sterile gloves without compromising sterility.

EQUIPMENT/SUPPLIES:

Packaged pair of sterile gloves of appropriate size
Flat, clean, dry surface

PROCEDURE STEPS:

1. Remove rings and watch. Wash hands using surgical asepsis. RATIONALE: Rings and watches can snag and tear gloves, and therefore interfere with barrier protection.
2. Inspect glove package for tears or stains (Figure 19-27A). RATIONALE: Tears and stains indicate that the gloves are no longer considered sterile and must be disposed of or used for a nonsterile purpose.
3. Place the glove package on a clean, dry, flat surface above waist level. RATIONALE: Using a contaminated surface could compromise the sterility of the sterile package.
4. Peel open the package taking care not to touch the sterile inner surface of the package. Do not allow the gloves to slide beyond the sterile inner border (Figure 19-27B). RATIONALE: Care must be taken to maintain the sterility of the gloves.

(continues)

Procedure 19-1 (continued)

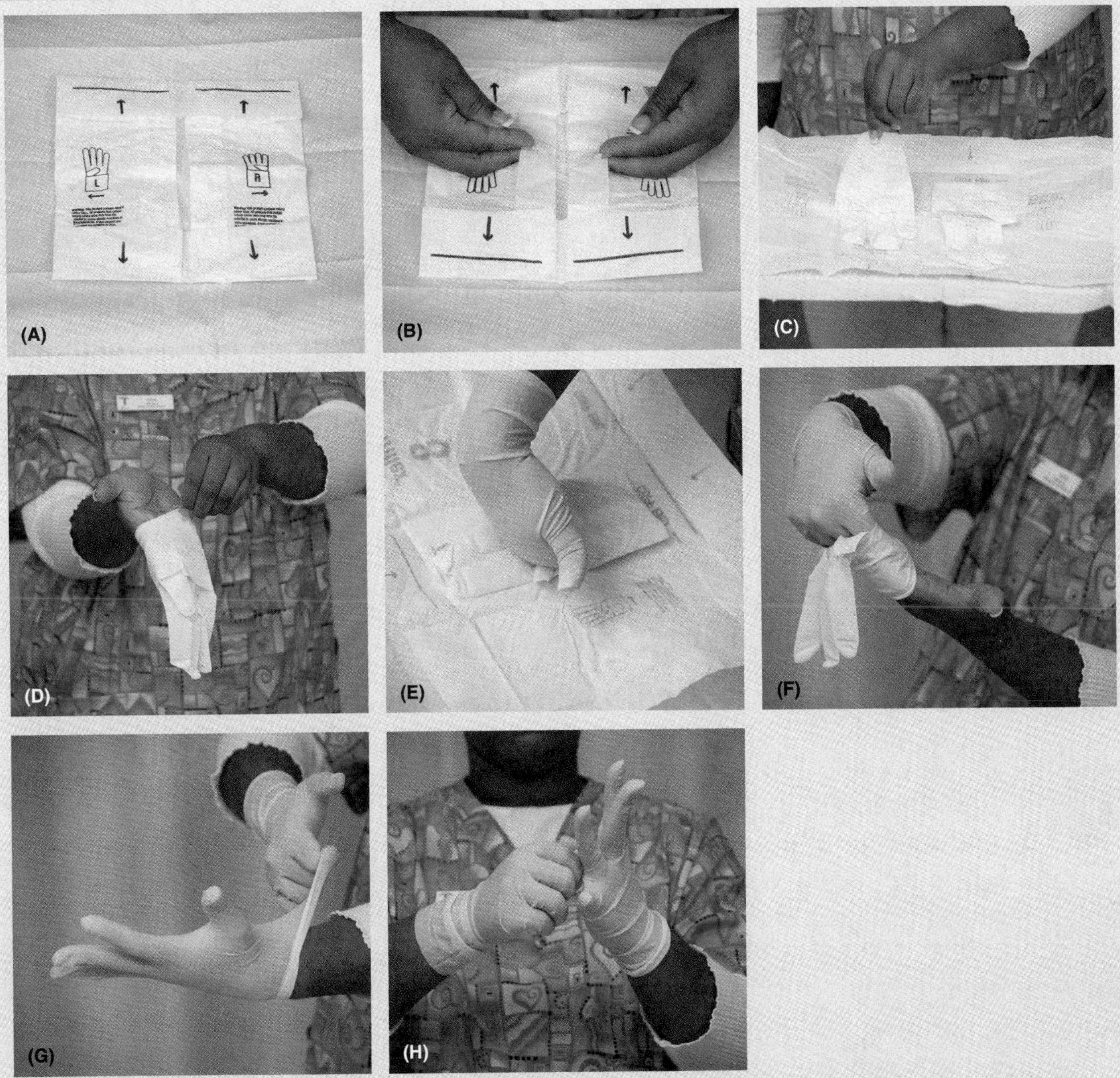

Figure 19-27 (A) Sterile gloves often are packaged with right and left clearly marked. (B) Using only the fingertips, reach in from each side and grasp the edges of the paper. Pull out and lay paper flat without touching any area except the very edges. (C) With the nondominant hand, grasp the *inner* cuffed edge of the opposite glove. Pick the glove up and step away from the sterile area, keeping your hands above your waist and away from your body. (D) With palm up on the dominant hand, slide the hand into the glove. (E) Step back to the sterile area. With the gloved hand, pick up the glove for the remaining hand by slipping four fingers under the outside of the cuff. (F) With palm up, slip the second hand into the glove. Keep the gloved thumb in a "hitchhiking" position. (G) Keeping hands above the waist and away from the body, pull on the second glove. (H) Adjust gloves if desired, staying away from the wrist area. Keep gloved hands above the waist and away from the body.

(continues)

Procedure 19-1 (continued)

5. The gloves should be opened with the cuffs toward you, the palms up, and the thumbs pointing outward. If the gloves are not positioned properly, turn the package around, being careful not to reach over the sterile area or touch the inner surface or the gloves. RATIONALE: Sterile gloves are packaged in this position for ease in application.
6. With the index finger and thumb of the nondominant hand, grasp the *inner* cuffed edge of the opposite glove. The glove should be picked straight up off the package surface without dragging or dangling the fingers over any nonsterile area (Figure 19-27C). RATIONALE: Picking up the glove by grasping the inner cuff prevents the outer glove from becoming contaminated. Strict adherence must be made to the sterile principles listed in the beginning of this chapter.
7. With the palm up on the dominant hand, carefully slide the hand into the glove. Do not allow the outside of the glove to come in contact with anything and stand away from sterile package. Always hold the hands above the waist and away from the body with palms up (Figure 19-27D). RATIONALE: Keeping the palm up allows the glove to remain sterile in the palm area if it rolls slightly on the back of the hand.
8. With the gloved hand, pick up the glove for the remaining hand by slipping four fingers under the *outside* of the cuff. Lift the second glove up, keeping it held above the waist and away from the body. Do not allow the glove to drag across the package or touch nonsterile surfaces (Figure 19-27E). RATIONALE: The outside of the second glove is sterile and may only be touched by another sterile surface.
9. With the palm up, slip the second hand into the glove. Do not allow the outside of the gloves to touch nonsterile skin and be especially mindful of the thumb (Figure 19-27F).
10. Adjust the gloves on the hands as needed, but avoid touching the wrist area. Keep gloved hands above the waist and away from the body. Do not touch nonsterile surfaces with the gloved hands (Figure 19-27G, H).

Procedure 19-2 Setting Up and Covering a Sterile Field

STANDARD PRECAUTIONS:

PURPOSE:

Disposable sterile field drapes or sterile towels are used to isolate a sterile area or field, as well as to cover the sterile field for use in surgery and sterile procedures. They are available in convenient peel-apart packages, fanfolded for ease of use, and often are two-tone in color to aid in differentiating one side from the other. Cloth drapes may be packaged separately and sterilized fanfolded.

NOTE: A variety of materials, both disposable and nondisposable, can be used to set up and cover a sterile field. All material has certain criteria to be safe for use and all have advantages and disadvantages. For example, woven textile fabrics are moisture retardant and are effective barriers to microbial penetration. Polylined paper disposable drapes are excellent barriers against microorganisms and moisture. Many times medical office preference is determined by financial consideration.

EQUIPMENT/SUPPLIES:

Disposable sterile polylined field drapes (two) or reuseable sterile towels (two) (muslin or linen with water-repellent finish)

Mayo instrument tray/stand positioned above the waist with stem to the right

Sterile transfer forceps (if needed)

(continues)

Procedure 19-2 (continued)

PROCEDURE STEPS:

1. Wash hands.
2. Sanitize and disinfect a Mayo instrument tray. Adjust tray to above waist level and have the stem to the right.
3. Select an appropriate disposable sterile field drape and place the drape package on a clean, dry, flat surface.
4. Open the package exposing the fanfolded drape. Assure that the cut corners of the drape are toward you; turn the package if necessary (Figure 19-28A). RATIONALE: Sterile field drapes are fanfolded and positioned within the package to facilitate ease of use.
5. With thumb and forefinger of one hand, carefully grasp the top cut corner without touching the rest

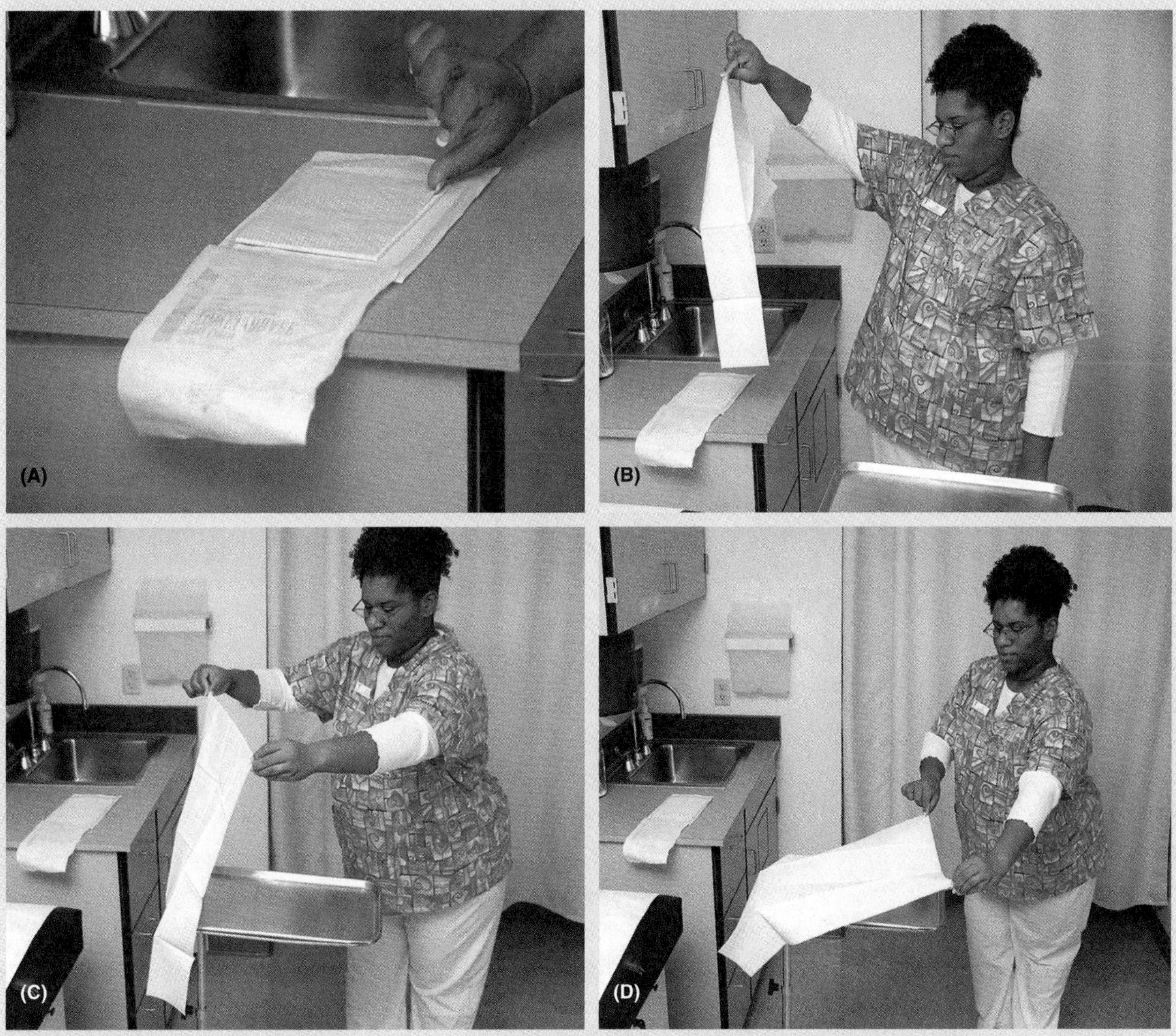

Figure 19-28 (A) Open the sterile drape package onto a flat, dry surface 90 degrees perpendicular to the Mayo tray. Grasp the corner of the sterile drape. (B) Pull the drape straight up, allowing it to unfold. Do not shake it out. (C) Carefully grasp another corner of the drape and apply the drape to the Mayo tray by pulling it toward you. Do not reach over the field; do not allow the "top" surface to touch anything. (D) Continue laying the drape as a sterile field.

(continues)

Procedure 19-2 (continued)

of the drape or towel and pick the drape or towel up high enough to assure that as it unfolds it does not drag across a nonsterile area (Figure 19-28B). RATIONALE: The drape or towel will naturally unfold as it is lifted, so care must be taken to assure that it is lifted quickly and allowed to unfold without touching a nonsterile surface.

6. Holding the drape or towel above waist level and away from the body, grasp the opposing corner so that both corners along the long edge of the drape are being held.
7. Keeping the drape or towel above waist level and away from the body, reach over the Mayo tray with the drape or towel. Take care that the lower edge of the drape or towel does not drag across the tray (Figure 19-28C). RATIONALE: Sterile principles state that sterile items should be kept above the waist and not touch other objects.
8. Gently pull the drape or towel toward you as it is laid onto the tray (Figure 19-28D). If adjustment is needed to center the drape or towel, do not touch the center of the drape or towel, or reach over the sterile field. Walk around or reach underneath the tray to move it or make adjustments. RATIONALE: The corners/edges that hang over the tray are no longer considered sterile.
9. After setting the instruments and supplies on the tray, it must be covered.
10. To cover the sterile field with a second sterile drape or towel, follow Steps 4 through 7; then instead of pulling the drape or towel toward you (as described in Step 8), which would necessitate reaching over the sterile field, apply the covering drape or towel by holding it up in front of the field. Adjust the lower edge so it is even with the lower edge of the field drape or towel (see Figure 19-29K). With a forward motion, carefully lay the cover over the sterile field (see Figure 19-29L). RATIONALE: Reaching over the sterile field would contaminate the tray.

Procedure 19-3 Opening Sterile Packages of Instruments and Supplies and Applying Them to a Sterile Field

STANDARD PRECAUTIONS:

NOTE: Sterile instruments and supplies are packaged in a manner that allows them to be opened and accessed without compromising sterility. Refer to other sections of this chapter for the specific steps of wrapping techniques, sterile gloving, and setting up sterile fields. The "wrapping twice" method of double wrapping was used in preparing the surgical packs for this procedure. Prepackaged items such as gauze squares should be in peel-apart packs.

PURPOSE:

To open sterile packages of surgical instruments and supplies and place them onto a sterile field using sterile technique.

EQUIPMENT/SUPPLIES:

Mayo instrument tray draped with sterile field
Sterile gloves
Wrapped-twice sterile surgical instruments
Prepackaged sterile surgical supplies

PROCEDURE STEPS:

1. Assemble supplies.
2. Wash hands and set up sterile field (see Procedure 19-2).

(continues)

Procedure 19-3 (continued)

3. Position package of surgical instruments on palm of nondominant hand with outer envelope flap on top. RATIONALE: This will facilitate opening the pack while protecting its sterile contents.
4. Grasping the taped end of the top flap, open the first flap away from you. Do not touch the inside of the flap (Figure 19-29A).
5. Grasping just the folded back tips of the side flaps, pull the right-sided flap to the right. Then pull the left-sided flap to the left, taking care not to reach over the package (Figure 19-29B and C). RATIONALE: Pulling the tips of the flaps toward each side allows the inner portion of the package to be exposed without contamination.
6. Pull the last flap toward you by grasping the folded-back tip taking care not to touch the inner contents of the package. RATIONALE: Pulling the last tip toward you allows you to avoid reaching over the inner contents of the package.
7. Gather all of the loose edges together to obtain a snug covering over your nondominant hand. Close your covered hand over the inner package and carefully apply the inner package to the sterile field (Figure 19-29D and E). RATIONALE: Gathering the loose edges prevents them from being dragged across the sterile field.
8. Open peel-apart packages using sterile technique by grasping both edges of the flaps and pulling them

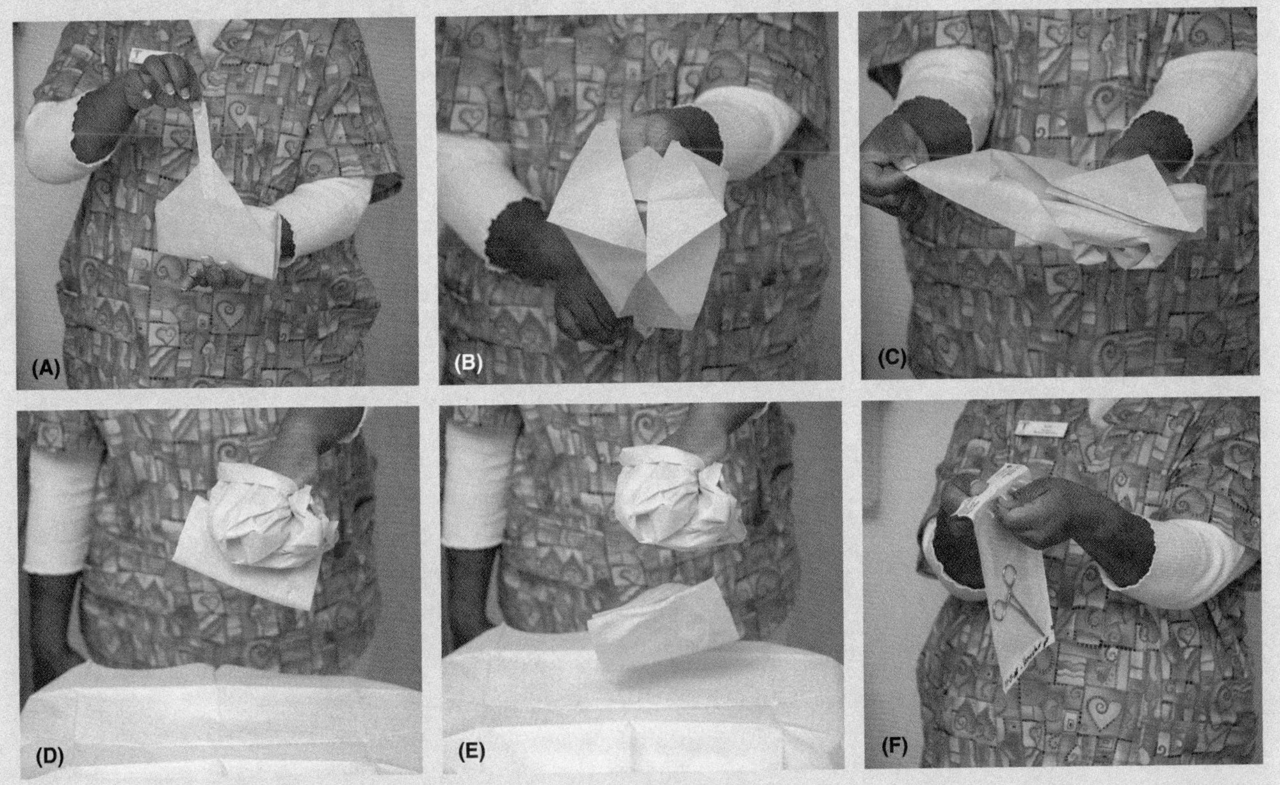

Figure 19-29 (A) To open a twice-wrapped pack, grasp the taped end of the top flap and open the first flap away from you. You should be standing back from the sterile field. (B) Allow the pack to unroll on your hand. Do not touch the inside of the flap. Notice the medical assistant's thumb is under the flap, where she can securely grasp the inner pack. (C) Grasp just the folded back tips of the side flaps. First pull the right-sided tip to the right, then, reaching around or under, pull the left-sided tip to the left. Do not reach over the package. (D) Gather the loose edges together to form a snug covering over your nondominant hand. Securely grasping the inner pack, step toward your sterile field and invert your hand. (E) Release the inner pack onto the center of the sterile field. Step back. (F) Open peel-apart packages using sterile technique, exposing sterile items gradually.

(continues)

Procedure 19-3 (continued)

apart in a rolling down motion, keeping both hands together (Figure 19-29F). The sterile item should be exposed gradually between the two peel-apart edges (Figure 19-29G). The sterile inner contents may then be offered to the sterile-gloved physician or applied to the sterile field using a flipping motion, or dropped as shown in Figure 19-29H, taking care not to contaminate either the package contents or the field.

9. Apply sterile gloves. Arrange instruments and supplies (Figure 19-29I) in an organized and logical manner according to the physician's preference (Figure 19-29J). RATIONALE: Instruments should be arranged in the order of use. All handles should be pointed toward the user. Instruments should be separated as much as possible within the space of the field so entanglement of instruments is not a problem.
10. Apply the sterile field cover (Figure 19-29K and L) (see Procedure 19-2). RATIONALE: A sterile cover will need to be applied if the surgical tray will not be used immediately, needs to be moved, or if the medical assistant leaves the tray unattended.

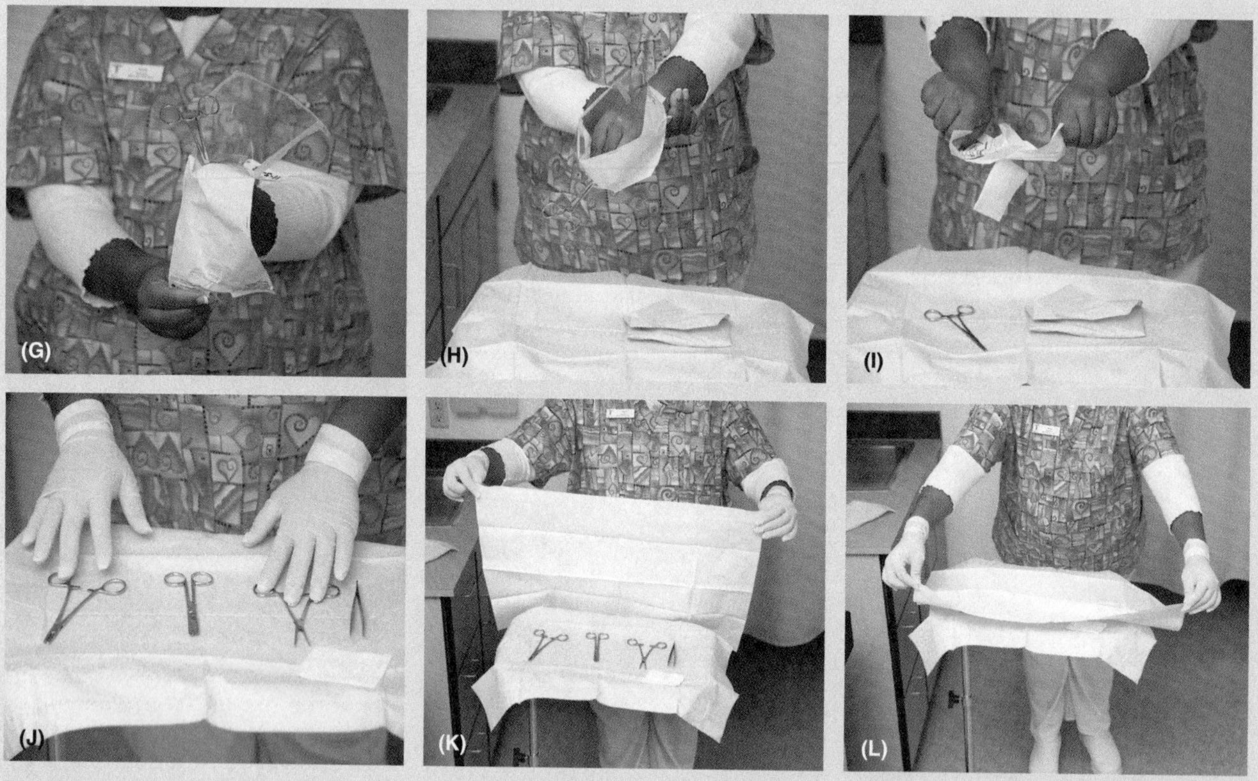

Figure 19-29 (continued) (G) Continue to peel back the sides of the package while securely holding onto the tip of the instrument. (H) Hold the sides of the package over your hand, step toward the Mayo tray and apply the instrument, handle first, onto the sterile field. (I) Apply other supplies as needed. (J) Arrange instruments and supplies according to physician's preference. (K) Apply the sterile drape cover to the surgical tray in a similar manner as the field was laid, except apply away from you. (L) Assure that the edges of the cover align with the edges of the field drape before applying the cover. Do not attempt to adjust the cover after it is laid.

Critical Thinking

You have removed a double-wrapped instrument pack from the autoclave and notice a small tear in the outermost wrap. The innermost wrap appears to be intact. What would your action be? Why?

Procedure 19-4 Pouring a Sterile Solution into a Cup on a Sterile Field

STANDARD PRECAUTIONS:

NOTE: Occasionally, sterile solutions will need to be poured into a sterile cup that has been placed onto the sterile tray. The solution is sterile, but the outside of the container is not; therefore, special precautions need to be taken to pour the solution into the cup without contaminating the sterile field. The solution is always poured after the tray has been moved into the surgical area to avoid spilling during transport.

PURPOSE:

To pour a sterile solution into a cup on a sterile tray in a sterile manner.

EQUIPMENT/SUPPLIES:

Covered sterile surgical tray with a sterile cup in upper right corner
Container of sterile solution (as ordered)

PROCEDURE STEPS:

1. Wash hands.
2. Transport the surgical tray into the surgical area before pouring the solution; or, the surgical tray can be set up for immediate use in the surgical area. RATIONALE: The solution may tip and spill during transport.
3. Read the label of the solution container three times and check the expiration date. RATIONALE: To eliminate the possibility of pouring the wrong solution or an outdated solution.
4. Remove the cap from the solution container taking care not to touch the inner surface of the cap. Place the cap upside down on a nonsterile surface to avoid touching the inner surface of the cap with a nonsterile surface. When the cap is held in the hand, hold it right side up. RATIONALE: Touching the inside of the cap with either your hand or a nonsterile surface will contaminate the inside of an otherwise sterile container.
5. Read the label again to assure accuracy. Place palm over the label to protect the label from stains. Pour a small amount of the solution into a bowl, cup, or sink that is outside the sterile field. RATIONALE: This action will cleanse the lip of the container.

NOTE: If the surgical tray is set up in a surgical area, the solution can be poured before covering the surgical tray with a sterile drape or towel.

6. Carefully pull back the upper right corner of the tray cover to expose the cup. Take care to only touch the corner tip of the cover and not reach over the exposed field. RATIONALE: Touching the underside of the cover or reaching over the exposed sterile field will contaminate the sterile surgical tray.
7. Approaching from the corner of the tray and using the cleansed side of the lip of the container, pour the needed amount of solution into the sterile cup (Figure 19-30). Precaution should be taken to avoid splashing, spilling, reaching over the field, or touching any of the sterile surfaces. RATIONALE: Splashing or spilling of the solution would cause the sterile field drape to become wet, which may cause contaminants to "wick" from the metal tray into the sterile field. Use of a polylined sterile field drape will create a barrier to avoid wicking.
8. Replace the corner of the drape cover using sterile technique or cover with a sterile drape or towel.
9. Replace the cap of the solution container using sterile technique.

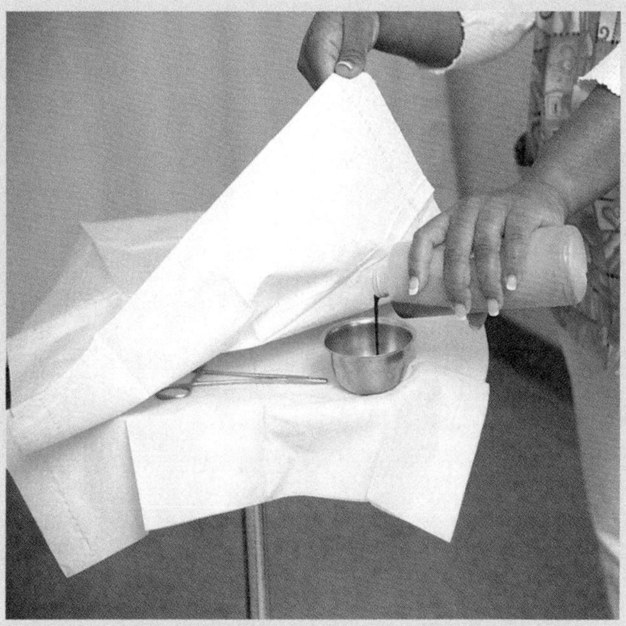

Figure 19-30 Approaching from the corner of the Mayo stand, pour the needed amount of solution into the sterile cup. Use the cleansed side of the container lip for pouring.

Procedure 19-5 Assisting with Office/Ambulatory Surgery

STANDARD PRECAUTIONS:

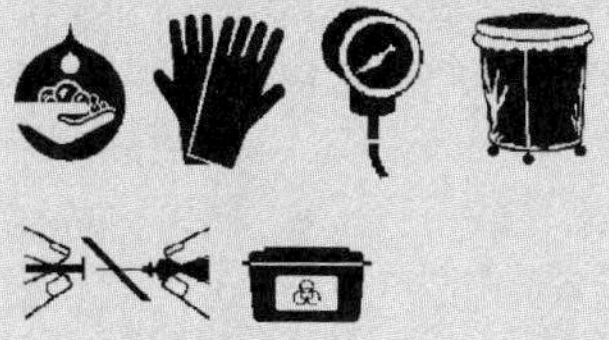

PURPOSE:

To maintain sterility during surgical procedures that require surgical excision.

EQUIPMENT/SUPPLIES:

Mayo stand:

- Needles and syringe for anesthesia
- Prep bowl/cup
- Betadine® solution
- Gauze sponges
- Scalpel and blade
- Operating scissors
- Fenestrated drape
- Hemostats (curved and straight)
- Thumb dressing forceps
- Thumb tissue forceps
- Needle holder
- Suture pack
- Transfer forceps

Side table (unsterile field):

- Sterile gloves (in package)
- Labeled biopsy containers with formalin
- Appropriate laboratory requisition
- Anesthesia vial
- Alcohol wipes
- Dressing, tape, bandages
- Biohazard container
- Betadine®

PROCEDURE STEPS:

1. Check room and equipment for readiness and cleanliness.
2. Wash hands.
3. Set up side table of nonsterile items. RATIONALE: Nonsterile items cannot be placed onto a sterile field because they will contaminate it.
4. Perform surgical asepsis hand cleansing.
5. Set up sterile field on a Mayo stand or on a clean, dry, flat surface (see Procedure 19-2).
6. Add sterile items (see Procedure 19-3).
7. Apply sterile gloves. Arrange instruments according to use. Remove gloves.
8. Cover the sterile field with a sterile towel if not being used immediately.
9. Identify patient, explain the procedure, and prepare the patient. Refer to patient preparation in Table 19-4.
10. Prepare patient's skin. Refer to Procedure 19-8.
11. Remove the sterile cover from the sterile setup as the physician applies sterile gloves. Lift the towel by grasping the tips of the corners farthest away from you and lifting toward you. Do not allow arms to pass over sterile field. RATIONALE: Avoids crossing over sterile field.
12. Assist the physician as necessary, being certain to follow the principles of surgical asepsis.
    - The physician will inject the local anesthetic, apply Betadine® or other antiseptic to the surgical site, apply sterile drapes, and begin the surgery.
    - The medical assistant will hold the vial of anesthesia while the physician withdraws the appropriate dose.
    - Adjust the instrument tray and equipment around the physician.
    - Assure a good light source.
    - Comfort and support patient emotionally.
    - Assist with the surgery as directed by the physician (sterile gloves must be worn).
    - Hand instruments to the physician and receive used intruments from the physician and place in a basin or container out of patient's sight.
    - If necessary, hold biopsy container to receive specimen being excised. Do not contaminate the inside of the container. Hold the cover facing down. Tightly place cover on the container. Assist with or apply sterile dressing to the operative site.
13. Assist patient as necessary. Refer to Assisting the Patient after Surgery in Table 19-4.
14. The specimen container must be tightly covered; labeled with the patient's name, date, type, and source of specimen; and sent to the laboratory accompanied by the appropriate laboratory requisition.

(continues)

Procedure 19-5 (continued)

15. Wearing appropriate personal protective equipment (PPE), clean surgical or examination room.
    - Dispose of used gauze sponges in biohazard container and knife blades and other disposable sharps in puncture-proof sharps container.
    - Rinse used surgical intruments; soak, sanitize, and sterilize for reuse. See Chapter 10.
    - Remove gloves and other PPE and dispose of per Occupational Safety and Health Administration (OSHA) guidelines.
16. Wash hands.
17. Document in the patient's record that the specimen was sent to the laboratory.

DOCUMENTATION

8/12/20XX 2:30 PM Skin tag from left axilla excised by Dr. King. Biopsy specimen in its entirety sent to laboratory. J. Guerro, CMA

Critical Thinking

Dr. Woo asks you to assist him in repairing the laceration on Jaime Carrera's hand. Though you are unsure, you think you may have noticed a tiny hole in the palm of your left glove. What is your next step?

Procedure 19-6 Dressing Change

STANDARD PRECAUTIONS:

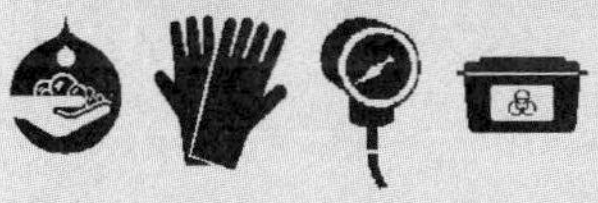

NOTE: After most surgical procedures have been completed, the wound is usually covered with a dry sterile dressing (DSD) that may need to be removed periodically so that the wound can be checked for healing or for suture removal. Another dry sterile dressing may then be applied. Burns require daily dressing changes.

PURPOSE:

To remove a wound dressing and apply a dry sterile dressing.

EQUIPMENT/SUPPLIES:

Sterile field:

Several sterile gauze sponges and other dressing material as needed or prepackaged sterile dressing kit

Sterile bowl with Betadine® solution or prepared sterile Betadine® swab sticks

(continues)

Procedure 19-6 (continued)

Sterile dressing forceps
Sponge forceps

Side area (unsterile field):

Nonsterile gloves
Sterile gloves
Container of sterile water
Cotton-tipped applicators
Sterile adhesive strips
Antibacterial ointment/cream as ordered
Tape
Sponge forceps
Bandage scissors
Waterproof waste bag
Biohazard waste container

PROCEDURE STEPS:

1. Wash hands.
2. Prepare sterile field. Add gauze sponges, bowl with solution, and forceps.
3. Position a waterproof bag away from sterile area.
4. Pour Betadine® solution into sterile bowl or use swab sticks.
5. Identify the patient and explain the procedure.
6. Reassure and comfort the patient as needed.
7. Loosen tape on dressing by pulling tape toward wound, or cut off bandage if necessary.
8. Put on nonsterile gloves or use forceps.
9. Carefully remove bandage; place in biohazard waste container. Do not pass over sterile field. RATIONALE: Passing dirty (used) dressing over sterile field contaminates it.
10. Remove dressing, taking care not to cause stress on the wound (Figure 19-31A).
    a. If stuck to the wound, pour small amounts of sterile water or hydrogen peroxide over dressing; allow to soak for a short time. Remove dressing when loose enough to remove without resistance. Note type and amount of drainage if present.
11. Place used dressing in waterproof bag without touching inside or outside of bag. RATIONALE: Dirty (used) dressing can contaminate bag.
12. Assess wound and note any drainage or signs of infection. Remove and discard gloves in waterproof bag.
13. Wash hands.
14. Apply sterile gloves.

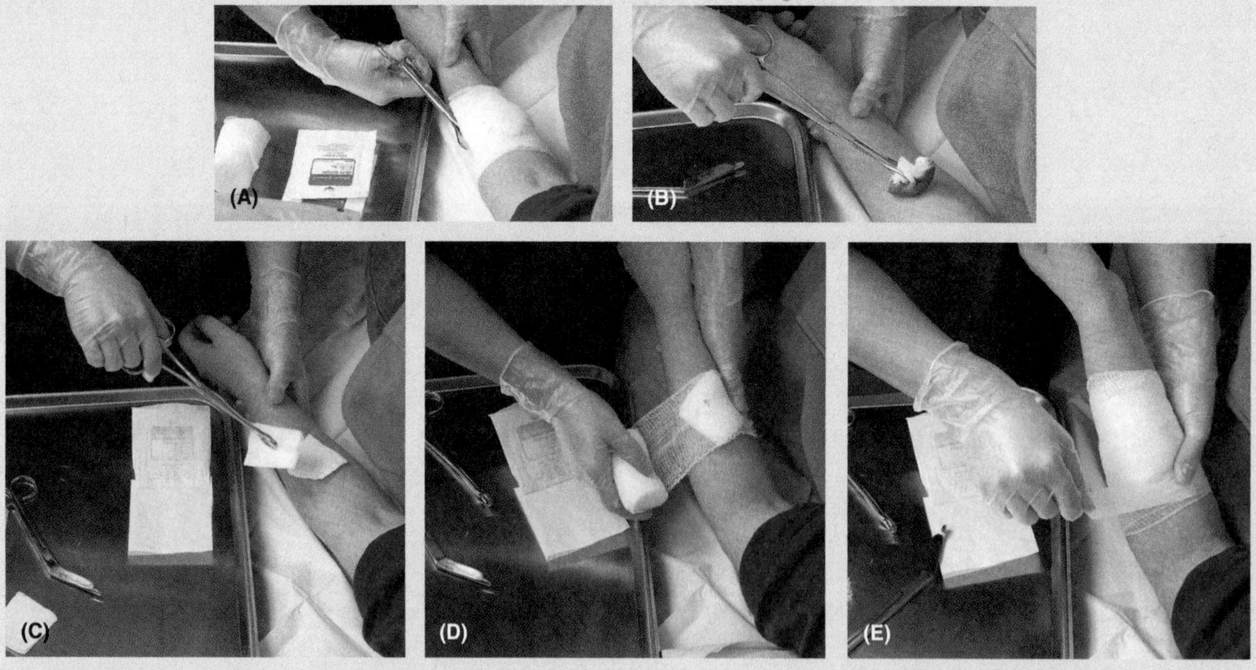

Figure 19-31 To change a dressing: (A) Gently remove dressing. Do not cause stress on wound. (B) Clean wound with Betadine® solution. (C) Using dressing forceps, a hemostat, or sterile gloves apply sterile gauze sponge(s) to wound. (D, E) Secure dressing with elastic bandage and adhesive tape or roller bandage.

(continues)

Procedure 19-6 (continued)

15. Clean the wound with antiseptic solution as ordered (Figure 19-31B).
16. Dispose of used gauze in waterproof bag.
17. Using sterile cotton-tipped applicators, apply cream/ointment as ordered. Using sterile forceps, apply sterile gauze sponge(s) to wound (Figure 19-31C).
18. Remove gloves, dispose of in waterproof bag.
19. Secure dressing with roller bandage and adhesive tape (Figure 19-31 D, E) or elastic bandage.
20. Dispose of waterproof bag in biohazard container.
21. Wash hands.
22. Document procedure and describe wound appearance (i.e., discharge, signs of infection, healing, and so on).

DOCUMENTATION

11/24/20XX 10:30 AM Dressing change to laceration left forearm. Small amount (dime-size) of serosanguinous discharge noted. No signs of redness or swelling in incisional area. DSD applied. Says she "feels fine and that my arm hurts very little." J. Guerro, CMA

Procedure 19-7 Wound Irrigation

STANDARD PRECAUTIONS:

PURPOSE:

To irrigate a wound to remove the accumulation of excessive exudate that impairs and delays healing.

EQUIPMENT/SUPPLIES:

On mayo tray:
Sterile gloves in package
Sterile irrigation kit (irrigating syringe, basin, and container for solution)
Sterile dressing material in package
Side area/unsterile field:
Waterproof pad
Sterile solution for irrigation (per physician's order)
Nonsterile gloves
Waterproof waste bag

PROCEDURE STEPS:

1. Check the physician's order. Select the correct solution and appropriate solution strength. (It should be at least body temperature.)
2. Identify your patient and explain the procedure.
3. Wash hands.
4. Place the waterproof pad under the body part that will be irrigated.
5. Have the patient position himself or herself in such a way that directs the flow of the solution into the wound and not into the basin.
6. Don nonsterile gloves, remove the dressing, and dispose into waterproof waxed bag.
7. Note the wound's appearance, color, amount of discharge, and odor to the discharge. RATIONALE: Allows ongoing assessment of the wound.
8. Remove and discard gloves into biohazard container.
9. Wash hands.
10. Maintaining sterile technique, open the sterile irrigation tray and the dressings. Use the inner kit wrapping as a sterile field.
11. Pour the irrigation solution into the sterile solution bowl or container. (Should be at least room temperature.) RATIONALE: Room temperature solution is more comfortable for the patient.
12. Don sterile gloves.

(continues)

Procedure 19-7 (continued)

13. Place the sterile basin against the edge of the wound. RATIONALE: The basin will collect the irrigation solution.
14. Fill the irrigating syringe (or bulb syringe) with the solution and carefully wash out the wound with the flow of solution.
15. Continue to fill the syringe and continue to wash out the wound until the solution becomes clear and there is no drainage noted.
16. Dry the wound edge with sterile gauze.
17. Reassess the wound.
18. Apply a dry sterile dressing.
19. Remove gloves. Dispose in biohazard container.
20. Wash hands.
21. Document.

DOCUMENTATION

8/6/20XX 2:30 PM Dressing removed from abdominal wound. Wound red and filled with serosanguinous exudate. Irrigated with 500 ml sterile normal saline (fluid returns were clear). Wound slightly red and clean-appearing after irrigation. Wound dried with sterile 4 × 4s. Dry sterile dressing applied. Patient states, "I feel much better now that my wound has been cleaned out. That only hurt a little." Patient says she does not want anything for pain. W. Slawson, CMA

Procedure 19-8 Preparation of Patient Skin before Surgery

STANDARD PRECAUTIONS:

NOTE: The skin contains many microorganisms and the patient's skin must be prepared before surgery to remove as many of the microorganisms as possible. Wound infection results when microorganisms enter the body. Because it is impossible to sterilize the skin, the operative site and an area surrounding it are scrubbed, shaved (hair harbors microorganisms), washed, and painted with an antiseptic such as Betadine® solution. A skin prep self-contained unit is a sponge applicator with a cylinder of antiseptic solution inside. One brand is known as DuraPrep. It contains iodophor and isoprophyl alcohol. The medical assistant can use the unit with nonsterile gloves. The unit is compressed, the seal to the inner cylinder is broken, and the sponge end becomes the applicator. The mixture is thick and should be allowed to dry and not be blotted. Because it contains alcohol, which can be a fire hazard, the site must be dry before draping. The chemical action decontaminates the patient's skin.

PURPOSE:

To remove as many microorganisms as possible from patient's skin before surgery.

EQUIPMENT/SUPPLIES:

Absorbent pads
Drape
Disposable prep kit (includes: antiseptic solution, several sponges, razor, and a container for water, or self-contained skin-prep unit)
Sterile water

(continues)

Procedure 19-8 (continued)

Sterile bowl
Sterile gloves for medical assistant and physician (two pairs)
If kit is unavailable, equipment needed is:
Sterile bowls (two)
Antiseptic solution
Sterile gauze sponges
Sterile razor
Basin for soiled sponges

PROCEDURE STEPS:

1. Wash hands.
2. Assemble equipment.
3. Identify patient.
4. Explain procedure, provide privacy, and drape patient if appropriate. Before the patient is prepped and draped for the procedure, ask the patient to state the location of the surgical site. Some facilities require that the appropriate site be marked with an indelible ink pen to be certain the correct site is identified.
5. Provide good light source.
6. Position patient for comfort and exposure of site.
7. Wash hands.
8. Protect area under preparation site with absorbent pads.
9. Put on sterile gloves or use sterile transfer forceps.
10. Open kit.
11. Apply antiseptic soap (Betadine®) with 4 × 4 sponges, beginning at operative site and moving outward in a circular motion from the center to away from center of prepared area. RATIONALE: Work from cleaner to least clean areas to prevent contamination.
12. Discard used sponges as necessary.
13. Using razor and holding skin taut, shave hair away from operative site, following hair growth pattern. RATIONALE: This prevents accidental nicks. Nicked skin can cause infection.
14. When hair has been removed, scrub again in a circular fashion as in Step 11 for about two to five minutes.
15. Rinse shaved area with sterile water and dry with a sterile 4 × 4 gauze sponge.
16. Remove and appropriately discard absorbent pad, 4 × 4 sponges, disposable prep kit, and gloves. RATIONALE: This removes used supplies and equipment from prepped skin area and avoids contamination.
17. Wash hands.
18. Using sterile transfer forceps, remove a sterile towel to place under operative site. RATIONALE: Placing a sterile towel under the operative area keeps site free from contamination.
19. Cover with a sterile towel. Instruct patient not to touch the area.
20. Pour antiseptic solution (Betadine®) into the sterile bowl. Physician will put on sterile gloves or will use sterile transfer forceps and using a sterile 4 × 4 gauze sponge will paint the operative site with the antiseptic solution. Let dry, drape patient with **fenestrated** drape, and commence with the surgical procedure.

Procedure 19-9 Suturing of Laceration or Incision Repair

STANDARD PRECAUTIONS:

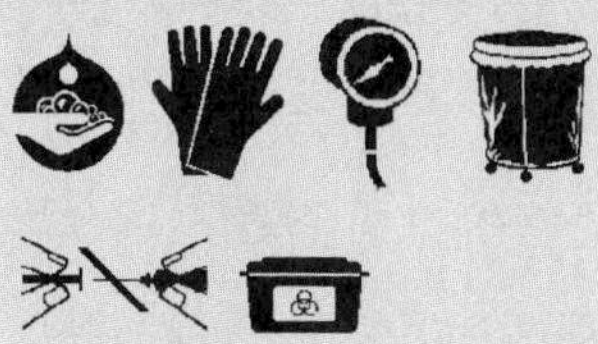

PURPOSE:

Suturing is recommended if a laceration or incision is gaping, bleeding uncontrollably, or is located on the face, neck, or a bend of a body part or extends deep into underlying tissue. Suturing facilitates healing by approximating the edges. Suturing decreases scarring, helps decrease the likelihood of infection, and promotes healing. The wound and the surrounding area must be meticulously cleaned of any dirt and debris. Many physicians have standard orders for wound cleaning before suture repair of either a laceration or incision-type wound such as a 10-minute soak in Hibeclens® solution.

EQUIPMENT/SUPPLIES:

Surgical tray:

Syringe and needle for anesthetic
Hemostats (curved)
Adson tissue forceps
Iris scissors (curved)
Suture material and needle
Needle holder
Gauze sponges

Side table (unsterile field):

Anesthetic as ordered by the physician
Dressings, bandages, and tape
Splint/brace/sling (optional)
Sterile gloves in package

PROCEDURE STEPS:

1. Wash hands.
2. Identify the patient and explain the procedure. Check for signed consent forms.
3. Reassure and comfort the patient as needed.
4. Assess cause of wound and its severity.
   - Determine any known allergies and last tetanus booster.
   - Identify any health concerns to avoid possible complications.
   - Soak wound in an antiseptic solution as ordered by physician.
   - Clean and dry wound.
   - Position patient comfortably, lying down.
5. Assist the physician as needed.
6. Support the patient as needed.

Give postoperative care:

7. Apply sterile gloves.
8. Clean area around the wound and dry wound with sterile 4 × 4s or sterile towels.
9. Dress/bandage/splint wound following physician's preference.
10. Remove gloves.
11. Wash hands.
12. Check patient's vital signs.
13. Explain wound care to the patient (and caregiver) and provide written instructions including symptoms of infection and after-hours phone number.
14. Assist the patient with any concerns or questions.
15. Arrange for follow-up appointment and medication as ordered.
16. Don personal protctive equipment.
17. Dispose of supplies per OSHA guidelines. Clean room, sanitize instruments, and sterilize for reuse.
18. Wash hands.
19. Document the procedure.

DOCUMENTATION

11/17/20XX 10:15 AM Patient sustained a 2 × 1.5-cm laceration on right knee. Wound soaked in Hibeclens® solution and water for 10 minutes, and then dried. Dr. King sutured the laceration after injecting xylocaine (1%) into laceration site. Ten nonabsorbable Ethicon sutures used to close wound. Dry sterile dressing applied to wound. Given a prescription for Perodan, 1 tab PO of 4-6h prn for pain, and Amoxicillin 500 mg PO of 6 h. Postoperative instructions reviewed and she appears to understand. Last tetanus 12 years ago. Tetanus injection given I.M. right deltoid (0.5 cc). W. Slawson, CMA

Procedure 19-10 Sebaceous Cyst Excision

STANDARD PRECAUTIONS:

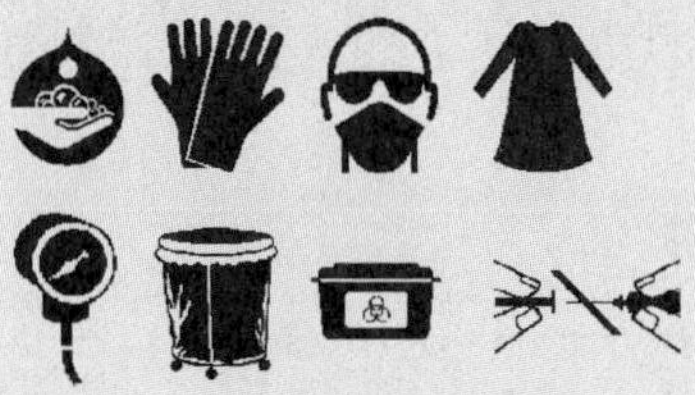

NOTE: A sebaceous cyst is a benign retention cyst, sometimes called a "wen." Sebaceous cysts are caused by an oil duct becoming "plugged," which causes the sebum (oil) to accumulate in the gland. Eventually the oil gland becomes distended. Sebaceous cysts that become inflamed or infected need to be removed. The patient may also elect to have a noninflamed sebaceous cyst removed if it is unsightly or located in a bothersome area. Incision and drainage of a sebaceous cyst is usually not the treatment of choice because they tend to recur if the entire cyst is not completely excised. Ideally, the entire cyst sac is removed intact, but occasionally the sac ruptures during removal and large amounts of malodorous biohazardous sebum can be expelled. In preparation for this occurrence, extra gauze sponges and gloves should be available.

PURPOSE:

To remove an inflamed or infected sebaceous cyst. To remove a sebaceous cyst that is not inflamed or infected but is located on an area of the body where the cyst is unsightly or where it may become irritated from rubbing.

EQUIPMENT/SUPPLIES:

Sterile field:

- Syringe/needle for anesthesia
- Iris scissors (curved)
- Mosquito hemostat (curved)
- Scalpel blade and handle
- Needle holder
- Suture material with needle
- Tissue forceps (two)
- Mayo scissors (curved)

Side area (unsterile field):

- Skin prep supplies
- Gauze sponges (many) (sterile, unopened)
- Fenestrated drape (a drape with an opening) in package
- Antiseptic solution as ordered
- Gloves (sterile and nonsterile)
- Personal protective equipment (PPE)
- Anesthesia as directed
- Dressing, bandages, tape
- Biohazard waste container
- Safety razor (optional)
- Alcohol pledgets
- Sterile culture tube (optional)

PROCEDURE STEPS:

1. Wash hands.
2. Identify the patient and explain the procedure.
3. Reassure and comfort the patient as needed.
4. Determine any known allergies and last tetanus booster.

(continues)

Procedure 19-10 (continued)

5. Check for signed consent form.
6. Identify any health concerns to avoid possible complications.
7. Position the patient comfortably, lying down.
8. Perform the skin preparation as directed. (See Procedure 19-8.)
9. Wear appropriate PPE including goggles if cyst is infected. RATIONALE: Purulent material may drain out of the wound.
10. Assist physician to inject the anesthesia by holding the vial while the physician withdraws the appropriate amount of anesthesia. Continue to assist while the physician excises the cyst and sutures the surgical incision.
11. Support patient during surgery.

Give postoperative care:

12. Apply sterile gloves.
13. Clean area around the wound.
14. Dress and bandage as directed.
15. Dispose of items per OSHA guidelines. Remove gloves.
16. Wash hands.
17. Check the patient's vital signs.
18. Explain wound care to the patient (and caregiver) and provide written instructions including symptoms of infection.
19. Assist the patient with any concerns or questions.
20. Arrange for follow-up appointment and medication as ordered.
21. Document the procedure and that the culture specimen was sent to laboratory if appropriate.

DOCUMENTATION

5/12/20XX 2:00 PM Infected sebaceous cyst (0.5 × 0.5 cm) excised by Dr. King. Moderate amount of purulent exudate noted as cyst ruptured during removal. Specimen of exudate obtained and sent to the laboratory for culture and sensitivity. Five nonabsorbable sutures used to close the incision. Wound cleansed with Betadine®; dry sterile dressing applied. Patient given verbal and written instructions on caring for the dressing and for watching for signs of infection. BP 118/74, P 88. Skin color good. Will call office for results of culture and sensitivity and to discuss the need for antibiotic therapy. Will return on 5/22/20XX or sooner if necessary. W. Slawson, CMA

Procedure 19-11 Incision and Drainage of Localized Infection

STANDARD PRECAUTIONS:

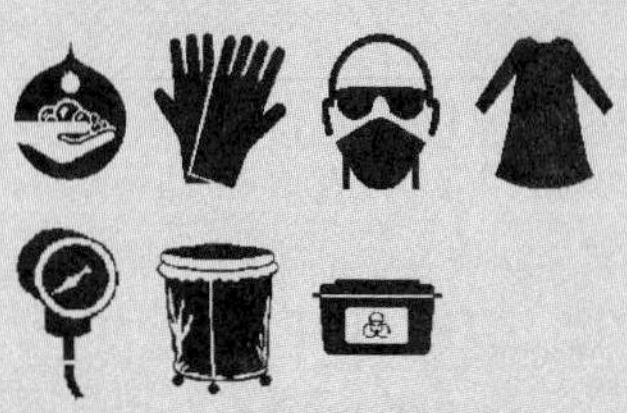

NOTE: An abscess is a localized accumulation of pus surrounded by inflamed tissue. The body attempts to isolate pus into a pocket or abscess as a means of protecting itself by walling off the pathogens and preventing them from spreading throughout the body. Incision and drainage is the procedure of cutting into an area (often an abscess) for the purposes of draining the fluid/material. A culture of the exudate can be done to iden-

(continues)

Procedure 19-11 (continued)

tify microorganisms. Rather than suturing or otherwise closing the wound, the physician may place a gauze wick or a latex penrose drain into the wound to facilitate continued drainage. The most commonly used type of wick is Iodoform. Iodoform is available in 5-yard lengths and widths of ¼, ½, and 1 inch. Iodoform is packaged sterile in glass bottles under the Johnson & Johnson brand name of Nu Gauze. Care must be taken when removing the desired length from the bottle to avoid contaminating the remaining gauze. To accomplish this, the medical assistant might hold the bottle and remove the lid to allow the physician to reach into the bottle with a sterile thumb dressing forceps and pull out the desired length. Sterile scissors are then used to cut the strip without contaminating the remaining wick. The Iodoform is packed into the wound with a short length exposed. After several hours or days of continued draining, the wick may be removed, and the wound allowed to heal. The patient may be prescribed an appropriate antibiotic.

The medical assistant should exercise caution by wearing appropriate PPE including goggles when assisting with this procedure because the exudate can be heavy and contains pathogenic microorganisms.

PURPOSE:

To incise and drain an abscess or other localized infection.

EQUIPMENT/SUPPLIES:

Surgical tray:
- Syringe/needle for anesthesia
- Scalpel blades and handles
- Thumb forceps
- Mosquito hemostat (optional)
- Gauze sponges (many) (sterile, unopened)
- Fenestrated drape
- Tissue forceps (two)
- Mayo scissors
- Iris scissors
- Antiseptic solution such as Betadine® in sterile cup

Side area (unsterile field):
- Skin prep supplies
- Gloves (sterile and nonsterile)
- Personal protective equipment (PPE)
- Anesthesia as directed
- Dressing, bandages, and tape
- Specimen container with preservative/requisition (optional)
- Biohazard waste container
- Extra gauze sponges
- Iodoform gauze wick or latex penrose drain
- Alcohol pledget
- Antiseptic solution
- Sterile culture tube

PROCEDURE STEPS:

1. Wash hands.
2. Identify the patient and explain the procedure.
3. Reassure and comfort the patient as needed.
4. Determine any known allergies and last tetanus booster.
5. Check for signed consent form.
6. Identify any health concerns to avoid possible complications.
7. Position the patient comfortably, lying down.
8. Put on PPE, including goggles.
9. Perform the skin preparation as directed. (See Procedure 19-8.)
10. Assist the physician as needed to inject the anesthesia by holding the vial while the appropriate amount is aspirated for injection. The physician will incise the abscess and either Iodoform gauze or a latex penrose drain will be inserted into the wound to encourage drainage. Specimen taken for culture and sensitivity.
11. Support the patient as needed.

Give postoperative care:

12. Apply sterile gloves.
13. Clean area around the wound with sterile 4 × 4s or sterile towels.
14. Dress and bandage as directed. Several thicknesses of dressing material will be needed to absorb **exudate,** or the accumulated fluid in a cavity.
15. Dispose of items per OSHA guidelines. Remove gloves.
16. Wash hands.
17. Check the patient's vital signs.
18. Explain wound care to the patient (and caregiver) and provide written instructions such as to apply warm moist compresses to wound. Explain to watch for symptoms of infection.
19. Assist the patient with any concerns or questions.
20. Arrange for follow-up appointment and medication as ordered.
21. Document the procedure.

DOCUMENTATION

6/20/20XX 10:00 AM Incision and drainage of an abscess (2 × 1 cm) on the left buttock. Large amount purulent exudate noted. Wound packed with 1/2-inch iodoform gauze and DSD applied with large amount of 4 × 4s and abdominal dressings. Culture tube with specimen of exudate sent to laboratory with a requisition for C&S so that the appropriate antibiotic can be prescribed. BP 138/92, P 100. Postoperative wound care explained to patient and given written instructions as well. BP 142/72, P 88. J. Guerro, CMA

Critical Thinking

While assisting during an incision and drainage of a localized infection on Abagail Johnson's left leg, you notice there is a large amount of exudate that discharges from the incisional site. What, if any, precautions should you take?

Procedure 19-12 Aspiration of Joint Fluid

STANDARD PRECAUTIONS:

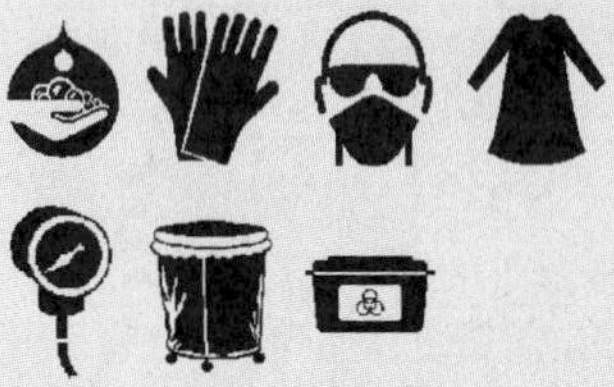

NOTE: The most common reason for aspirating fluid is to remove excess fluid from a joint, often the knee. A long sturdy needle is inserted into the joint capsule and fluid is removed. Often a long-acting anesthetic and cortisone are injected at the same time. The fluid can be diagnostically examined for blood, pus, and fatty substances and also cultured for infective pathogens. After surgery the patient may be placed on antiinflammatory medications to treat the inflammation and antibiotics if the culture is positive for pathogens.

PURPOSE:

To remove excess synovial fluid from a joint after injury.

EQUIPMENT/SUPPLIES:

Surgical tray:

- Syringe/needle for anesthesia
- Gauze sponges
- Sterile basin for aspirated fluid
- Fenestrated drape (optional)
- Syringe/needle for drainage
- Sturdy hemostat or needle driver

Side area (unsterile field):

- Skin prep supplies
- Gloves (sterile and nonsterile)
- Personal protective equipment (PPE)
- Anesthesia as directed
- Cortisone medication as directed
- Culture tube
- Pathology requisition
- Specimen container
- Biohazard waste container
- Extra gauze sponges (sterile, unopened)
- Alcohol pledgets
- Dressing, bandages, and tape
- Biohazard specimen transport bag

(continues)

Procedure 19-12 (continued)

PROCEDURE STEPS:

1. Wash hands.
2. Identify the patient and explain the procedure.
3. Reassure and comfort the patient as needed.
4. Determine any known allergies, last tetanus booster, and which joint will be aspirated.
5. Check for signed consent form.
6. Identify any health concerns to avoid possible complications.
7. Position the patient comfortably, lying down.
8. Put on PPE if needed.
9. Perform the skin preparation as directed (see Procedure 19-8).
10. Assist the physician by holding the vial as anesthesia is aspirated. The physician will inject anesthesia and then insert a long, sturdy needle into the synovial sac and aspirate fluid with a large syringe. The aspirated fluid will be put into a sterile bowl as the syringe fills with fluid. A hemostat is used to remove the syringe from the needle, leaving the needle in the joint. The syringe is reapplied to the needle, and the process continues until excess fluid is removed.
11. Support the patient as needed.

Give postoperative care:

12. Apply sterile gloves.
13. Clean area around the wound with sterile 4 × 4s or sterile towels.
14. Dress and bandage as directed.
15. Dispose of items per OSHA guidelines. Remove gloves.
16. Wash hands.
17. Check the patient's vital signs.
18. Explain wound care to the patient (and caregiver) and provide written instructions including symptoms of infection.
19. Assist the patient with any concerns or questions.
20. Arrange for follow-up appointment and medication as ordered.
21. Apply gloves and eye/mouth protection if sending specimen to laboratory. Place aspirated fluid into a sterile container and cover tightly.
22. Send labeled specimen container and requisition to the pathology laboratory after placing specimen in transport bag.
23. Document the procedure.

DOCUMENTATION

10/12/20XX 11:30 AM Left knee aspirated. 250 ml clear fluid withdrawn after injection of anesthetic. Sent to pathology department. Patient says she "feels better." Bandage applied to aspiration site. Postoperative verbal and written directions given. BP 118/64, P 72. Follow-up appointment made for discussion about results of analysis of fluid sent to laboratory. B. Abbott, RMA

Procedure 19-13 Hemorrhoid Thrombectomy

STANDARD PRECAUTIONS:

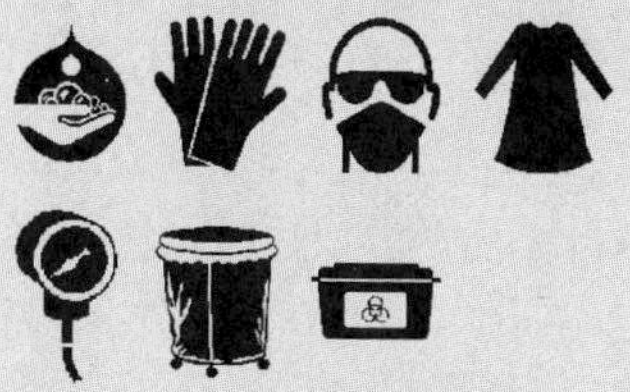

NOTE: Hemorrhoids are dilated or varicose veins in the rectum, either internal or external. Sometimes a blood clot can form in a protruding portion of the hemorrhoid and the vessel can become inflamed. The hemorrhoid is incised with a scalpel blade and the clot removed with a hemostat forceps. Suturing is not usually necessary. Soaking the area in a **sitz bath** can aid in healing. Hemorrhoidectomy can be performed in much the same manner as a hemorrhoid thrombectomy, and the supplies and equipment are similar. The anal sphincter is dilated, the hemorrhoid pedicle is tied, and then each hemorrhoid is removed with either laser, electrosurgery, or cryosurgery. Another alternative is to ligate the internal hemorrhoids after visualizing the area with an anoscope. Two rubber bands are placed around the pedicle of each hemorrhoid. They will slough off after a week to 10 days because of the loss of blood supply to them (**avascularized** hemorrhoid).

PURPOSE:

To incise inflamed hemorrhoids and remove thrombus. To remove hemorrhoids with laser, electrosurgery, cryosurgery, or banding.

EQUIPMENT/SUPPLIES:

Surgical tray:

- Syringe/needle for anesthesia
- Mosquito hemostat (curved)
- Sterile basin
- Gauze sponges
- Rubber bands
- Fenestrated drape

Side area (unsterile field):

- Skin prep supplies
- Gloves (sterile and nonsterile)
- Personal protective equipment (PPE)
- Anesthesia as directed
- Biohazard waste container
- Extra gauze sponges
- Soft absorbent pad, similar to sanitary napkin
- T-bandage (to hold pad in place)

PROCEDURE STEPS:

1. Wash hands.
2. Identify the patient and explain the procedure.
3. Reassure and comfort the patient as needed.
4. Determine any known allergies and last tetanus booster.
5. Check for signed consent form.
6. Identify any health concerns to avoid possible complications.
7. Position the patient comfortably, according to physician's preference; proctologic position for male and female patients is used.
8. Assist with adequate draping for patient comfort.
9. Apply PPE if necessary.
10. Perform the skin preparation as directed (see Procedure 19-8).
11. Assist the physician to aspirate the appropriate amount of local anesthesia. After administering the anesthesia, the physician will either band or excise the hemorrhoids with a scalpel. Suturing is usually not necessary.
12. Support the patient as needed.

Give postoperative care:

13. Assist the physician in placing the soft absorbent pad against the wound. It may be held in place with a T-shaped bandage.
14. Dispose of used items per OSHA guidelines. Remove gloves and wash hands.
15. Assist the patient as needed.
16. Check the patient's vital signs.
17. Explain wound care to the patient (and caregiver) per physician. Sitting in a tub of warm water is soothing and aids healing. Provide written instructions including signs of complications such as excessive bleeding or pain.
18. Assist the patient with any concerns or questions.
19. Arrange for follow-up appointment and medication as ordered.
20. Document the procedure.

DOCUMENTATION

3/17/20XX 1:00 PM A. Thrombus removed from hemorrhoid. Perineal pad applied and secured with a T-binder. Patient tolerated the procedure well. BP 110/70, P 88. Postoperative instructions, verbal and written, given to patient. Prescription for Percodan, 1 tab p.o. q 4-6 h prn given to patient. Return appointment made for 4/4/20XX. W. Slawson, CMA

B. Internal hemorrhoids removed with electrosurgical equipment. Very little bleeding noted. Perineal pad and T-binder applied. Patient tolerated procedure well. BP 110/68, P 72. Postoperative instructions given to patient (verbal and written). Prescription for Percodan 1 tab. p.o. q 4-6 h prm given to patient. Return appointment made for 4/4/20XX. W. Slawson, CMA

Procedure 19-14 Suture/Staple Removal

STANDARD PRECAUTIONS:

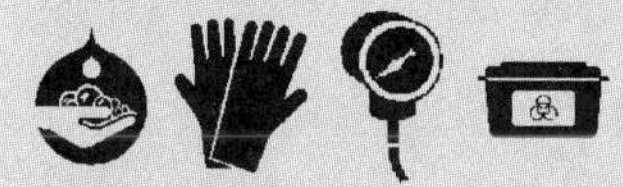

NOTE: Many minor surgical procedures require that suturing be done to approximate the skin edges to promote healing. Because these sutures or staples are nonabsorbable, they must be removed when the wound has healed. The patient will return to the office or clinic to have the sutures or staples removed. The medical assistant will remove the dressing and check the wound. The physician will also check the wound for degree of healing and determine that the sutures/staples can be removed.

PURPOSE:

To remove sutures from a healed surgical wound (as per physician).

EQUIPMENT/SUPPLIES:

(See Figure 19-32.)
Gauze sponges
Bandage scissors
Biohazard waste container
Tape
Forceps
Suture removal kit (suture scissors or staple remover, thumb forceps, and 4 × 4s)
Sterile latex gloves
Antibiotic cream if ordered

PROCEDURE STEPS:

1. Identify patient.
2. Wash hands.
3. Glove and remove bandage. Dispose in biohazard container.
4. Wash hands.
5. Open suture or staple removal kit.
6. Apply sterile gloves.
7. If removing sutures: Using thumb forceps, gently pick up one knot of a suture. Gently pull upward toward suture line. RATIONALE: Less pressure is exerted on suture line.

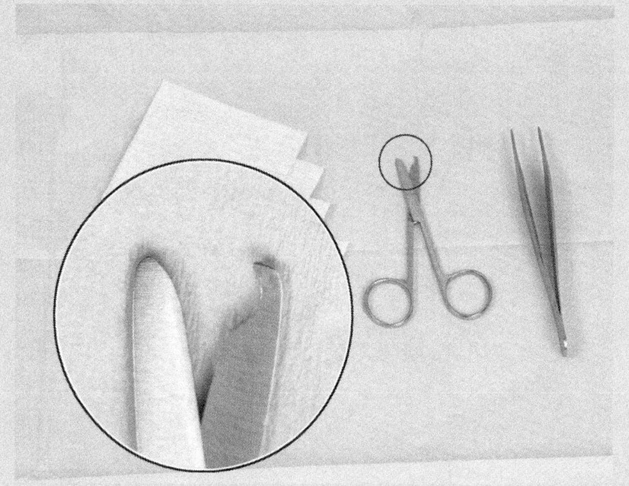

Figure 19-32 Equipment and supplies for suture removal.

(continues)

Procedure 19-14 (continued)

Using suture removal scissors, cut one side of the suture as close to skin as possible (Figure 19-33A and B). RATIONALE: Holding knot with forceps and cutting suture as close to skin as possible, the suture will be pulled out from under the skin, avoiding contamination of the wound.

8. If removing staples: Gently apply instrument to staple. Gently squeeze handle of staple remover until staple is pinched outward and upward. Pull up.
9. Remove all sutures/staples in the same manner, noting number of sutures/staples removed. Dispose of the sutures/staples on a sterile gauze sponge. Examine the wound to be certain all sutures have been removed.
10. Apply antibiotic cream to area as ordered.
11. Apply dry sterile dressing if ordered by the physician (see Procedure 19-6).
12. Remove gloves.
13. Dispose of used items per OSHA guidelines.
14. Wash hands.
15. Check patient's vital signs if indicated.
16. Explain wound care and provide written instructions to patient.
17. Arrange follow-up appointment if necessary.
18. Document the procedure.

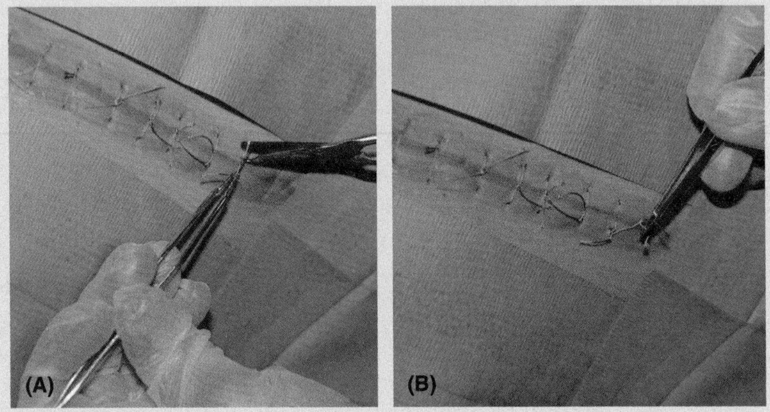

Figure 19-33 To remove sutures: (A) Grasp suture knot with thumb forceps. Place curved tip of suture removal scissors just next to skin under the suture. Clip. (B) Gently pull the suture knot up and toward the incision with thumb forceps to remove.

DOCUMENTATION

11/27/20XX 2:30 PM Ten sutures removed from right forearm. Wound appears clean, well healed. No discharge seen. Edges of wound well approximated. B. Abbott, RMA

OR

11/27/20XX 2:30 PM Six staples removed from right forearm. Wound appears clean, well healed. No discharge seen. Edges of wound well approximated. B. Abbott, RMA

Procedure 19-15 Application of Sterile Adhesive Skin Closure Strips

STANDARD PRECAUTIONS:

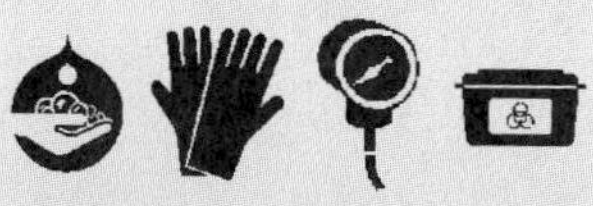

NOTE: On occasion, a superficial wound does not require sutures. However, the edges of the wound can be drawn together and sterile strips of adhesive are used to hold the edges of the wound together to facilitate healing.

PURPOSE:

To approximate the edges of a wound after the removal of sutures. Sometimes used in lieu of sutures or to give additional support along with sutures.

EQUIPMENT/SUPPLIES:

Sterile field:

Suture removal instruments (as indicated)
Sterile adhesive skin closure strips
Iris scissors (straight)
Adson dressing forceps
Tincture of benzoin (optional)
Sterile cotton-tipped applicators (for tincture of benzoin)

Side area (unsterile field):

Sterile gloves
Dressings, bandages, and tape

PROCEDURE STEPS:

1. Identify the patient and explain the procedure.
2. Position patient comfortably.
3. Wash hands and apply gloves.
4. Remove bandages and dressings. See Procedure 19-6.
5. Clean and dry wound. See Procedure 19-6.
6. Assess the need for skin closure strips and alert the physician as indicated.
7. Remove gloves.
8. Wash hands.
9. Open container of tincture of benzoin.
10. Apply sterile gloves.
11. Apply tincture of benzoin to edges of wound if directed. Use sterile cotton-tipped applicator, taking care not to let it come into contact with the actual wound. RATIONALE: Tincture of benzoin is applied to the periphery of the sutures to prepare it for application of the skin closure strips and to provide a better sticking surface and aid in easier removal with less skin irritation.
12. Open package of skin strips. Cut to size if needed. Remove strips from packaging one at a time using dressing forceps.
13. Apply one end of a skin closure strip to one side of the wound. Place the first strip over the center of the wound (Figure 19-34A).
14. Secure the end to the skin by carefully pressing.
15. Stretch the strip across the edge of the wound and secure on the other side in the same manner. This motion should bring the edges together without puckering the skin.
16. Apply the next two closure strips at halfway points between the first strip and each end of the wound (Figure 19-34B).
17. Continue in this manner until the edges are approximated. Keep wound edges in alignment.

Give postoperative care:

18. Dress and bandage if necessary.
19. Dispose of used items per OSHA guidelines.
20. Remove gloves and wash hands.
21. Check the patient's vital signs, if indicated.
22. Explain wound care to the patient (and caregiver) and provide written instructions including symptoms of infection.
23. Assist the patient with any concerns or questions.
24. Arrange for follow-up appointment and medication as ordered.
25. Document the procedure.

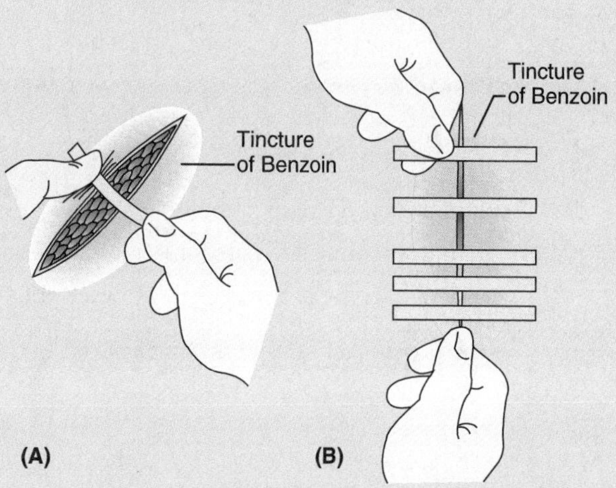

Figure 19-34 To apply skin closure strips: (A) Apply first strip in center of incision. (B) Apply closures to each side of center.

DOCUMENTATION

3/17/20XX 4:00 PM Nine skin closure strips applied to wound on shoulder after tincture of benzoin applied to skin around sutures. Suture line approximated well; no puckering of skin noted. Wound appears clean and to be healing. No redness or swelling. Patient says there is "very little discomfort." B. McQuestion, RMA

Case Study 19-1

Cele Little, an 84-year-old patient at Inner City Health Care, is having office surgery performed on Thursday morning. Her sister, Dottie Tate, also a patient and also in her 80s, will come with Cele. A friend from the local senior citizen center has offered to drive them to the center and home again. Dottie is more nervous about the procedure, the removal of a bothersome cyst, than Cele. After talking with the sisters about the procedure, clinical assistant Wanda Slawson, CMA, MLT, realizes this and wants to reassure Dottie but also wants her to be prepared to be caregiver to Cele.

CASE STUDY REVIEW

1. Where should Wanda begin in her communication with the two sisters?
2. What specific advice should Wanda give Cele and Dottie before the procedure?
3. What instructions should Wanda give the sisters to follow after the procedure?

Case Study 19-2

Letisha Brown has been scheduled to have a nevus excised from her upper back.

CASE STUDY REVIEW

1. Explain how you would prepare her for the surgery.
2. Explain how you would care for her after the surgery.
3. What will become of the excised nevus? Explain your actions.

SUMMARY

In assisting with surgery in the ambulatory care setting, the medical assistant needs to know sterile principles and understand the difference between medical and surgical asepsis. Knowledge of suture materials, instruments, and other supplies such as dressings and bandages is also critical. In preparing for surgical procedures, the medical assistant's communication skills will be needed, for patients can be apprehensive and will require both reassurance and education. In addition to understanding the basic process and preparations for assisting with minor surgery, the medical assistant should also be aware of the steps involved in some of the more common surgical procedures.

STUDY FOR SUCCESS

To reinforce your knowledge and skills of information presented in this chapter:

- ❑ Review the Key Terms
- ❑ Practice the Procedures
- ❑ Consider the Case Studies and discuss your conclusions
- ❑ Answer the Review Questions
  - ❑ Multiple Choice
  - ❑ Critical Thinking
- ❑ Navigate the Internet by completing the Web Activities
- ❑ Practice the StudyWARE activities on your student CD
- ❑ Apply your knowledge in the Student Workbook activities
- ❑ Complete the Web Tutor sections
- ❑ View and discuss the DVD situations

REVIEW QUESTIONS

Multiple Choice

1. Which of the following describes the primary purpose of surgical asepsis?
   a. to prevent microorganisms from collecting on the Mayo stand
   b. to prevent microorganisms from causing inflammation
   c. to prevent microorganisms from entering the body during an invasive procedure
   d. to prevent microorganisms from multiplying
2. A basic rule to follow to protect sterile items is:
   a. a sterile object may touch a nonsterile object under certain circumstances
   b. it is safe to turn your back on the sterile field if you leave plenty of room between you and the field
   c. provide the physician a separate container for contaminated instruments
   d. gloved hands are held at the same height as the hip bone
3. Which of the following is the smallest size suture material?
   a. 0
   b. 2–0
   c. 4–0
   d. 1
4. Which of the following is an example of absorbable suture material?
   a. vicryl
   b. nylon
   c. silk
   d. cotton
5. What is the purpose of adding epinephrine to the local anesthetic?
   a. to prevent an allergic reaction
   b. to reduce blood flow in the operative site through vasoconstriction
   c. to reduce patient discomfort during the procedure
   d. to maintain patient vital signs
6. Which of the following actions might the physician take if a sebaceous cyst were infected?
   a. remove the cyst
   b. do a biopsy of the cyst
   c. perform cryosurgery on the cyst
   d. incise and drain the cyst

Critical Thinking

1. What would be the rationale behind leaving a wound open rather than suturing it? On what basis would this decision be made?
2. While you are preparing a patient for surgery, he confides in you that he doesn't have anyone to drive him home, but he only lives three miles away and plans to drive himself. How do you respond?
3. You have thoroughly explained the postoperative instructions to the patient and caregiver. Are written instructions also necessary? Why or why not?
4. While pouring a sterile solution into a bowl on the sterile field, you accidentally splash a very tiny amount of the solution onto the field. What is your next step? Explain your actions.

WEB ACTIVITIES

Search the Internet to explore the most current ambulatory surgical procedures for hemorrhoids, cataracts, and cholelithiasis.

1. Using a search engine of your choice, go to a Web site about ambulatory care.
   a. Look for the criteria that the patient must meet after surgery to be discharged.
   b. What are some common complications that can occur in the ambulatory center after any surgical procedure?
   c. Name two other surgeries other than those listed in your book that can be performed in an ambulatory center. Discuss them.
   d. List three to four advantages and disadvantages of ambulatory surgery.

REFERENCES/BIBLIOGRAPHY

Association of Surgical Technologists, Inc. (2001). *Surgical technology for the surgical technologists.* Clifton Park, NY: Thomson Delmar Learning.

Phillips, N. (2004). *Barry and Kohn's operating room technique* (10th ed.). St. Louis, MO: Mosby.

Taber's cyclopedic medical dictionary (20th ed.). (2005). Philadelphia: FA Davis.

THE DVD HOOK-UP

DVD Series	Program Number
Skills Based Series	**14**

Chapter/Scene Reference
- *Entire program*

This chapter discussed the proper technique for assisting with minor surgical procedures.

Today's DVD program illustrated how to assist with a sebaceous cyst removal. Eileen called the patient the day before the procedure to make certain that the patient was going to be there the day of the surgery. Eileen gave the patient some important information that he needed to know before having the surgery. The day of the surgery, Eileen escorted the patient back to the physician's office so that the physician could explain the procedure. Once the physician was finished explaining the procedure, Eileen took over and gave the patient his prescriptions and home-care instructions. Eileen had many duties during the procedure and had additional duties immediately after the procedure.

1. Why is it so important to contact the patient the day before the surgery?
2. What type of phone instructions did Eileen give the patient before the surgery date?
3. What type of instructions did Eileen give the patient the day of the surgery, before having the procedure? Why did Eileen give the patient instructions before the procedure?

DVD Journal Summary

Write a paragraph that summarizes what you learned from watching today's DVD program. What did you think about the testimony of the other medical assistant named Eileen regarding her first experience assisting the physician with a surgery? Would you have quit after the physician raised his voice and scolded you in front of the patient? What do you need to do now, while you are still in school, to ascertain that you do not break sterility when you get into the industry?

CHAPTER 20

Diagnostic Imaging

OUTLINE

OBJECTIVES

The student should strive to meet the following performance objectives and demonstrate an understanding of the facts and principles presented in this chapter through written and oral communication.

1. Define key terms as presented in the glossary.
2. Describe safety precautions for personnel and patients as they relate to ionizing radiation treatments.
3. Explain how fluoroscopy is used and explain its benefits.
4. Describe the various positions used during X-ray procedures.
5. Describe four X-ray procedures that require patient preparation.
6. Discuss the uses of ultrasonography, positron emission tomography, computerized tomography, magnetic resonance, and flat plates.
7. Discuss how radiographs are stored.
8. Explain the differences among radiology, radiation therapy, and nuclear medicine.
9. Recall four possible side effects of radiation.

KEY TERMS

Cathode
Claustrophobia
Dosimeter
Echocardiogram
Esophageal Varices
Fluoroscope
Ionizing Radiation
Isotope
Noninvasive
Oscilloscope
Palliative
Radioactive
Radiograph
Radiolucent
Radionuclides
Radiopaque
Radiopharmaceuticals
Stomatitis
Transducer

FEATURED COMPETENCIES

CAAHEP—ENTRY-LEVEL COMPETENCIES

Patient Care

- Prepare patient for and assist with procedures, treatments, and minor office surgeries
- Screen and follow-up test results

Legal Concepts

- Identify and respond to issues of confidentiality
- Perform within ethical and legal boundaries
- Document appropriately
- Demonstrate knowledge of federal and state health care legislation and regulations

Patient Instruction

- Instruct individuals according to their needs

ABHES—ENTRY-LEVEL COMPETENCIES

Professionalism

- Conduct work within scope of education, training and ability

Communication

- Adapt what is said to recipient's level of comprehension
- Adaptation for individualized needs

Clinical Duties

- Prepare patients for procedures
- Apply principles of aseptic techniques and infection control
- Prepare and maintain examination and treatment area

(continues)

SCENARIO

In the radiology department of Inner City Hospital, there are several patients waiting to have their procedures performed. Wanda Slawson, CMA, brings Don Waite to the department for an excretory urography formally known as intravenous pyelogram. She is careful to make certain that Mr. Waite has been properly prepared for the procedure. She does not want the procedure to have to be repeated because of the inconvenience and anxiety it may cause Mr. Waite, nor does she want there to be additional expense and time spent repeating the procedure.

FEATURED COMPETENCIES (continued)

- Use quality control
- Perform selected tests that assist with diagnosis and treatment
- Screen and follow up patient test results

Legal Concepts

- Document accurately
- Maintain licenses and accreditation
- Monitor legislation related to current healthcare issues and practices

Instruction

- Instruct patients with special needs

INTRODUCTION

*Radiology is a branch of medicine concerned with **radioactive** substances, including **radiographs,** radioactive **isotopes,** and **ionizating radiation.** There are three specialties into which radiology can be classified: diagnostic radiology, radiation therapy, and nuclear medicine. All the specialties are extremely valuable tools that can be used to diagnose and treat diseases.*

*X-rays were named when a German physicist, Wilhelm Roentgen, discovered them in 1895. He received the first Nobel Prize in physics for his discovery. Roentgen noticed while working with a **cathode** ray tube that the rays of energy emitted could pass through skin, paper, wood, and other solid materials. Because he didn't know what the rays were, he called them X-rays.*

Radiologic procedures are not often performed in an office setting; rather, they are taken in the radiology department of a hospital, clinic, or a freestanding facility outside of the hospital or clinic.

Some radiographs, such as those looking for a fractured bone, require no preparation, whereas others, such as an excretory urography or a computerized axial tomography (CAT) scan, require special preparation.

Spotlight on Certification

RMA Content Outline
- Patient education
- Physical examinations

CMA Content Outline
- Safety precautions
- Examinations
- Medical imaging

CMAS Content Outline
- Exam preparation

RADIATION SAFETY

X–rays, though invisible to the human eye, are extremely powerful and can be a benefit or can be dangerous and harmful. Exposure to radiation can destroy tissue and permanently damage the eyes, bone marrow, and the skin. They are also harmful to the developing embryo and fetus, causing severe anomalies and death.

Benefits from X-rays are the information obtained from them that can be used to diagnose and manage a patient's disease. The diagnostic benefits outweigh the risks that may result from X-ray exposure. Radiographers are educated to be certain that patients receive as low a dose of radiation as possible to obtain a useful radiograph, and that they and patients are protected from exposure to radiation that is not necessary. Radiation is rarely used during pregnancy because of the danger it poses to the fetus and embryo. The first trimester is the most critical because severe congenital anomalies can be the result of the fetus's or embryo's exposure to radiation. Women are routinely asked if there is a possibility of their being pregnant. X-rays of fertile women should be taken only when necessary and with a minimal exposure to the fetus or embryo. If a radiologic examination is necessary, a radiologic physicist would calculate the dosage of radiation to estimate how little radiation to which the fetus or embryo should be exposed. In the past, there was a guideline stating that X-rays of fertile women should not be done until 10 days after the onset on their last menstrual period. The thinking was that it was unlikely that women could be pregnant during these 10 days. This guideline is now considered to be outdated because the ovum for the next menstrual cycle is its most susceptible during this 10-day period.

In some states, medical assistants and other health care professionals who are not licensed to take radiographs are not allowed by law to take or assist with radiologic procedures. Licensure in those states (about 35 states) is

Critical Thinking

What are the effects of radiation on a fetus or an embryo?

Critical Thinking

What do some state laws require of personnel who take X-rays?

mandated because of the possibility of severe injury to an unlicensed individual and to patients. In some states, a limited license is required. The medical assistant must take additional training and is limited to "skeletal films" (arms, legs, and so forth). Education and training in radiologic techniques is of utmost importance for the safety of the patient and health care worker. Medical assistants must have a basic understanding of radiology and radiology safety to instruct patients in the correct preparation for procedures and to keep patients and themselves safe. They must protect themselves from radiation exposure by not participating in procedures for which they have not been adequately educated and trained.

Personnel in the X-ray department and others who are exposed to X-rays must wear a **dosimeter,** a small badge-like device worn above the waist. The dosimeter contains a strip of film that measures the amount of X-ray to which a person is exposed. The dosimeter film is read on a regular basis, and radiation exposure is reported to a supervisor. Exposure can come from the X-ray beam itself or from scattered rays that are produced when going through the patient's body.

Patients must wear lead aprons over the reproductive organs, and technicians must shield themselves with lead aprons and gloves if they are assisting, but shields are not necessary when standing behind the lead wall working the control panel. In addition, walls in rooms where X-rays are taken are lead-lined to absorb scattering rays.

X-RAY MACHINE

There are three main parts to an X-ray machine: the table, the X-ray tube, and the control panel. The tube is where the X-rays are produced, and then come out as a beam of X-ray. Lead surrounds the tube except for the area where the beams of X-ray are sent out. The table on which the patient lies is movable in several directions, even upright or angled. The control panel is positioned behind a lead wall especially designed for shielding the radiographer from X-rays when an X-ray is being taken (Figure 20-1).

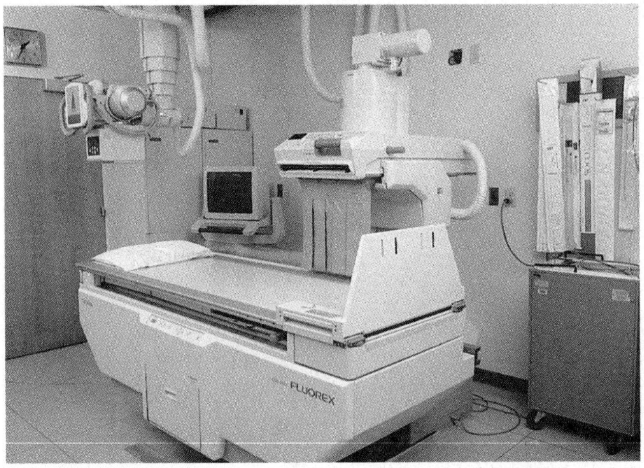

Figure 20-1 Radiographic room prepared for procedure.

Photographic film is placed beneath or behind the patient's body and a radiograph, X-ray film, is produced by sending X-rays from the tube of the machine through the body and onto the film. After the film is processed, an image is created (see Figure 20-4A and B). Bone is denser than skin and other soft tissues, and therefore can absorb more X-rays. The image of the hand bones on the X-ray film is white due to absorption of the X-rays.

CONTRAST MEDIA

Various body structures are of different densities. Bone is denser than skin and, therefore, can absorb more X-rays, leaving fewer to be picked up by the X-ray film. Thus, an X-ray film of bone will appear white. A lung is less dense, and the X-rays can penetrate lung tissue. The lung appears black on the radiograph. If X-rays do not penetrate a structure easily, it is termed **radiopaque;** if they penetrate readily, it is termed **radiolucent.** Contrast media are radiopaque and help to obtain a radiographic image of an internal organ or structure that ordinarily would be difficult to see because the contrast media cause the organs or structures of the body to absorb more radiation (see Figure 20-2).

Some commonly used contrast media are barium sulfate, iodine compounds, air, and carbon dioxide. Barium is a chalky compound, and when mixed with water, can be swallowed by the patient or administered as an enema by a radiologic technician. It is not absorbed by the body. It is used for upper and lower gastrointestinal (GI) series of X-rays (see Figure 20-3). The patient is told to drink extra fluids to flush out barium after the procedure. Iodine salts are radiopaque and are used for kidney, gallbladder, and thyroid examinations. Some individuals are allergic to the iodine salts used as contrast media. Patients are asked whether they have any allergies, particularly allergies to foods that contain iodine, such as fish.

Air and carbon dioxide are used to visualize the spinal cord and joints but have been replaced by use of the magnetic resonance imaging (MRI) machine.

PATIENT PREPARATION

By law, without special education and training about X-rays, the medical assistant's role in X-ray procedures in most states will be limited to patient preparation information and explanations about what the patient can anticipate. A thorough knowledge of the procedure that the physician has ordered is essential, and the medical assistant must be certain that patients understand the preparation they are about to undertake. Verbal explanations should be followed up with written instructions. Many patients, fearful of what the ordered X-ray will show, are anxious and frightened and can easily forget verbal instructions. Proper preparation is essential for the best results on the radiographs. Repeating a procedure because of inadequate preparation results in increased patient anxiety, time, expense, and inconvenience (Table 20-1).

POSITIONING THE PATIENT

The correct patient position is important for obtaining the best quality radiograph and the type of examination that is necessary will determine patient position. Some basic views are:

- Anteroposterior view (AP)—the anterior surface of the body faces the X-ray tube and X-rays are directed from the front toward the back of the body.
- Posteroanterior view (PA)—the posterior surface of the body faces the X-ray tube and X-rays are directed from back to front (see Figure 20-4A, B).
- Lateral view—X-rays pass through the body from one side to the opposite side.
- Right lateral view (RL)—X-rays are directed through the body from the left to the right side. The right side of the body is next to the film.
- Left lateral view (LL)—X-rays are directed through the body from the right to the left side. The left side of the body is next to the film.
- Oblique view—the body is positioned at an angle.
- Supine view—the body is lying face up, on the back.
- Prone view—the body is lying face down, on the abdomen.

FLUOROSCOPY

Fluoroscopy is the process of using a **fluoroscope** to view internal organs and structures of the body so that they may be seen in motion immediately by the radiologist. The patient is usually given a contrast medium and placed between the X-ray tube and the fluoroscope. Fluoroscopy is used for procedures such as cardiac catheterization and for viewing the function of the stomach and intestinal structures to detect any abnormalities. A television screen and camera are usually available so the radiographer can watch and take photos of the body system(s) in operation (see Figure 20-5).

DIAGNOSTIC IMAGING

Positron Emission Tomography (PET)

PET is a radiographic procedure using a computer and a radioactive substance. The radioactive substance is injected into the patient's body and gives off charged particles. They combine with particles in the patient's body to produce color images that tell the amount of metabolic activity there is in an organ or structure.

PET imaging is primarily a diagnostic medical imaging modality. It makes use of specialized, intravenously injected **radiopharmaceuticals** that emit positrons, which can be detected out of the body due to high-energy releases. Specialized detectors arranged around the patient sense the energy and map the location from which it originated inside the body. These radiopharmaceuticals can be chemically designed to localize in the heart, brain, or certain types of tumors throughout the body. A clinical image is formed by the accumulation of positron emissions in a target organ. The patient's emission pattern forms a clinical image. This image is compared with the normal distribution by the nuclear medicine physician.

Generally, low to moderate doses are used to diagnose disease in patients. Certain nuclear medicine treatment studies use specialized radiopharmaceuticals that will isolate in the area to be treated. These agents emit their energy locally, irradiate tissue, and usually do not leave the body, unlike diagnostic radiopharmaceuticals. The properties and intent of diagnostic radiopharmaceuticals are different from therapeutic radiopharmaceuticals (see Figure 20-6A–C).

TABLE 20-1 SOME EXAMPLES OF X-RAY PROCEDURES, THEIR PURPOSE, PATIENT PREPARATION, AND THE PROCEDURE

Test	Purpose	Patient Preparation	Procedure
Angiography	To visualize the inside of blood vessel walls. Helps to diagnose heart attacks, stroke, and aneurysm (Figure 20-2).	NPO six to eight hours before examination.	1. Contrast medium (iodine) injected into an artery or vein. 2. Catheter threaded to the appropriate site. 3. Digital angiography can be done and stored on computer disk.
Barium swallow (upper gastrointestinal [GI] series)	To study the esophagus, stomach, duodenum, and small intestine for disease (ulcers, tumors, hiatal hernia, **esophageal varices**) (Figure 20-3).	Day prior: Light evening meal. NPO after midnight. Day of test: NPO. Postprocedural: Increase fluid intake. Take laxative as prescribed.	1. The patient is asked to drink a flavored barium mixture while standing in front of the fluoroscope. 2. The radiologist observes the passage down the digestive tract. 3. The patient is turned to various positions to allow good visualization of the intestines. 4. Radiographs are taken.
Barium enema (lower GI series)	To study the colon for disease (polyps, tumors, lesions).	Prep kit (usually supplied by physician's office) to include bottle of magnesium citrate and Dulcolax tablet(s). Day prior: 1. Clear liquid allowed: carbonated beverages, clear gelatin, clear broth, coffee and tea with sugar. No milk or milk products. 2. 8 oz. of water every hour until bedtime. 3. Late afternoon, drink bottle of magnesium citrate. 4. Early evening, take Dulcolax tablet(s) as prescribed. 5. Light evening meal. NPO except water after dinner. Morning procedure: NPO, cleansing enema Postprocedural: 1. Increase fluid intake and dietary fiber. 2. Report to physician if no bowel movement within 24 hours of test.	1. The colon is filled with a barium sulfate mixture. 2. The patient is turned in various positions to allow the barium to fill the colon. Air is injected to move the barium along the colon. 3. When the colon is full, radiographs are taken.
Cholangiography	To view the bile ducts for possible calculi or lesions.	May have cleansing enema one hour before examination. Meal preceding examination is withheld.	Contrast medium injected and radiograph of bile ducts is taken.
Cholecystography	To study the gallbladder for disease (stones, duct obstruction), inflammation.	1. Evening before test, fat-free dinner. 2. Patient takes dye tablets with 8 oz. of water. 3. Cathartic or cleansing enemas may be prescribed. 4. NPO after dinner and tablets.	1. A series of radiographs is taken. 2. A fatty meal may be given to stimulate the gallbladder to empty. 3. Other radiographs can then be taken to check gallbladder function.
Cystography	To view the urinary bladder for lesions, calculi.	Day prior: Light evening meal. Laxative in evening. NPO after midnight.	Contrast medium injected and radiograph of the urinary bladder is taken.
Hysterosalpingography	To view the uterus and fallopian tubes for blockage and lesions. To check for pelvic masses.	Laxative evening before. Cleansing enema day of exam. Meal prior to examination is withheld.	Contrast medium injected and radiographs taken of uterus and fallopian tubes. Carbon dioxide may also be used.
Excretory urography	Visualization of kidneys, ureters, and bladder to detect kidney stones, lesions, strictures of urinary tract.	Eat a light evening meal and nothing after midnight. A laxative and enema are used to clean out the intestines to prevent a blocked view of the ureters behind the intestines.	A contrast medium of iodine salts is given intravenously after it has been determined that the patient is not allergic to iodine (see Chapter 18).
Mammography	To detect abnormalities in the breast, especially breast cancer.	Do not wear lotion, deodorant, or powders. Remove clothing from waist up. No contrast medium required.	Breast is positioned on the mammograph and compressed to flatten it. Two radiographs are taken of each breast, from the side and from above.
Retrograde pyelography	To view the kidneys and urinary tract for abnormalities.	Drink four to five glasses of water before examination unless sedated, then NPO.	Contrast medium injected and radiographs taken of the kidneys and urinary bladder.

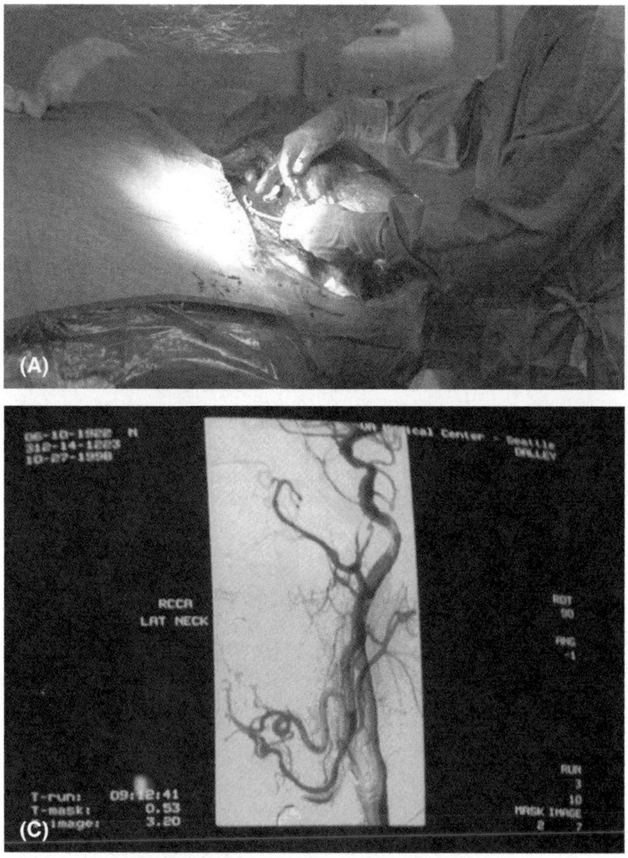

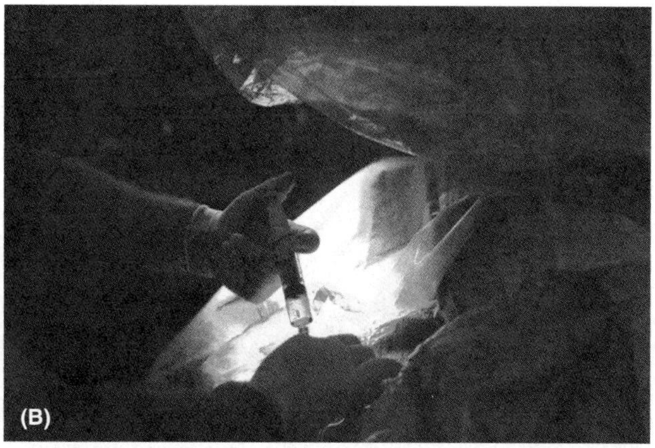

Figure 20-2 Angiography. (A) An intra-arterial catheter is inserted. (B) Radiopaque contrast material is injected. (C) The arteries are visualized.

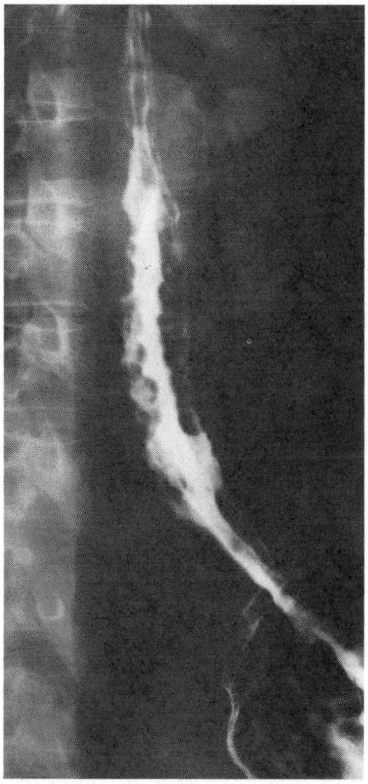

Figure 20-3A Barium swallow showing esophageal varices.

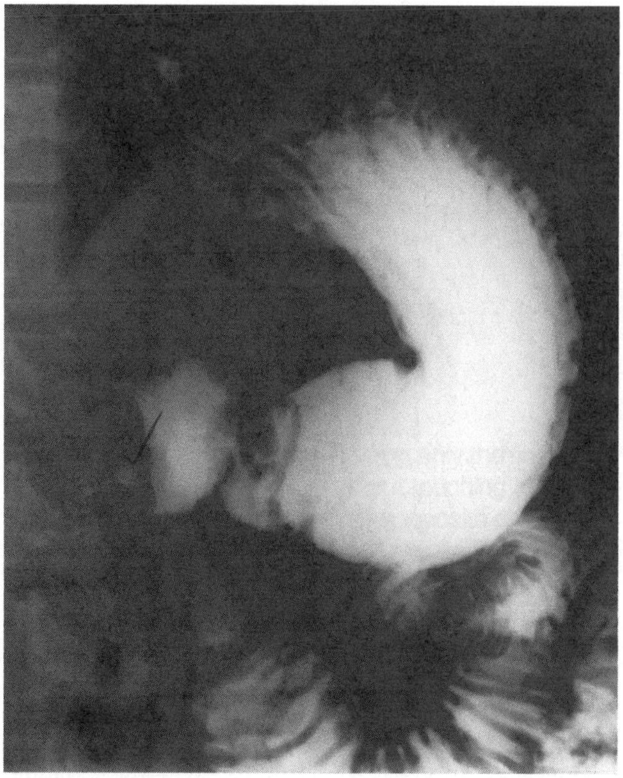

Figure 20-3B Barium swallow showing duodenal ulcer.

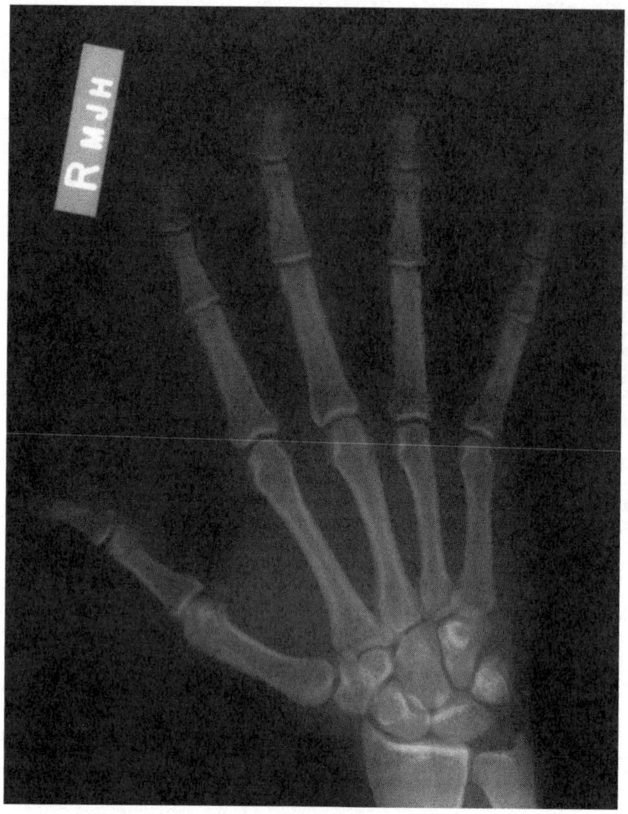

Figure 20-4A Posteroanterior view of a hand. Note that there appear to be dark spaces between the bones. This is because the bones (denser) pick up the X-rays (absorb them) and are white. The soft tissue (less dense) does not absorb the X-rays and is dark.

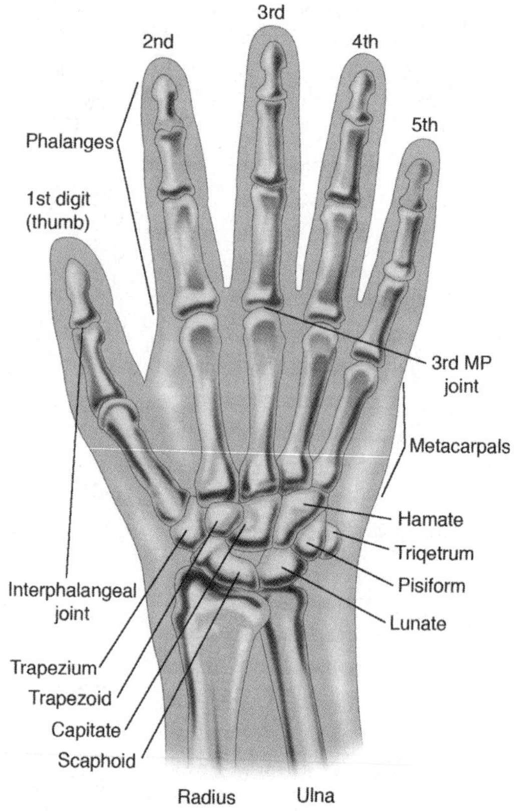

Figure 20-4B PA hand.

Computerized Tomography (CT)

A computerized tomograph uses a small amount of radiation. The beams penetrate body tissues to produce a series of cross-sectional images of the body part being examined. It allows images of structures that cannot be seen with regular X-rays. It is a noninvasive test that usually requires no preparation and uses the computer with a minimal amount of radiation. It rotates 360 degrees around the patient to obtain cross-sectional images that can be viewed on a monitor and on film. It is ideal for early detection of tissue tumors such as childhood cancers and abdominal tumors, and it helps in directing radiation therapy for tumor masses. On occasion, a contrast medium is injected for a better view of internal structures. If contrast medium is used, the patient must be NPO (have nothing by mouth) for four hours before being placed onto a motorized table that moves the body part to be examined into a scanner that surrounds that part of the patient. In 15 to 20 minutes, an entire body can be scanned (Figures 20-7A–D).

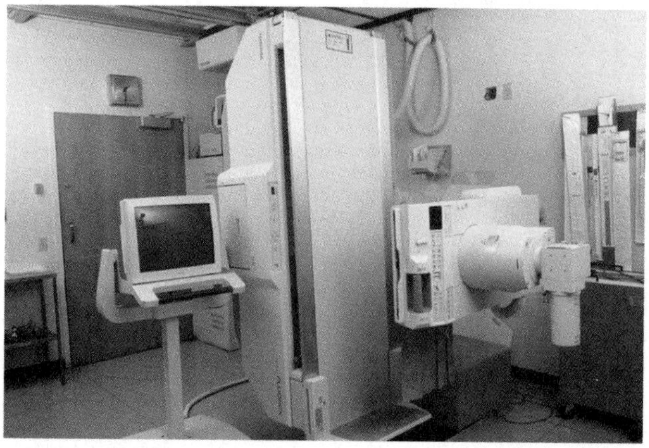

Figure 20-5 Fluoroscopic room ready for upper gastrointestinal study.

Magnetic Resonance Imaging (MRI)

Images produced by MRI are of exceptionally high quality. No ionizing radiation is used, and it is a noninvasive, safe, and painless procedure. All body areas can be viewed by the MRI, but it is especially helpful for soft tissues. It is good for the spine, pelvis, and joints and is superior for visualizing the brain. The examiner can see through

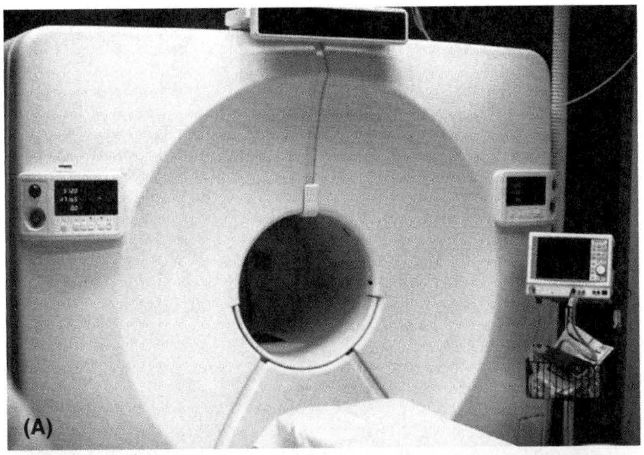

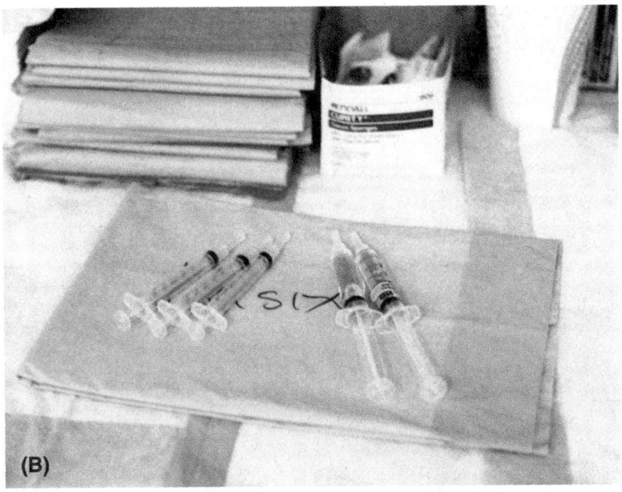

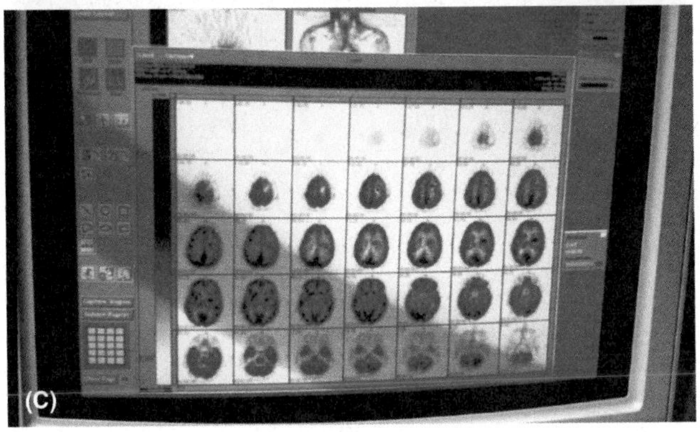

Figure 20-6 (A) Position emission tomography (PET) scanner. (B) Medications ready for injection. (C) PET scan output images.

fluid-filled tissue with exceptional detail using an MRI machine. The computer forms the visual image.

The patient lies on a table inside a cylinder-shaped machine in which there is an electromagnet. The machine is sealed with the patient inside. Some patients who suffer from **claustrophobia** (fear of closed in places) may need medication to help relieve symptoms of anxiety. Open MRI machines are available and are particularly useful for those patients who are too apprehensive to be sealed in the traditional MRI machine.

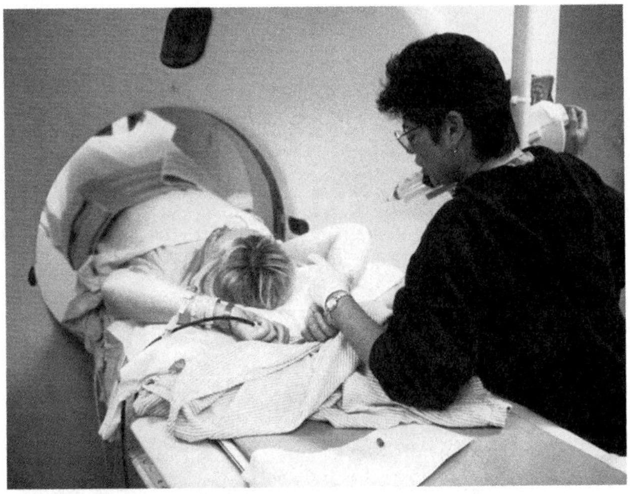

Figure 20-7A Computed tomography (CT) scanning. Instruct patient to lie still.

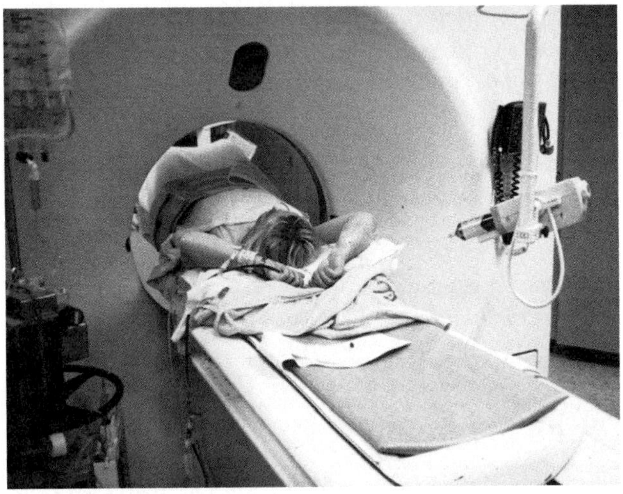

Figure 20-7B Instruct patient to breathe deeply and relax during procedure. Reassure patient that whirring and clicking sounds are normal.

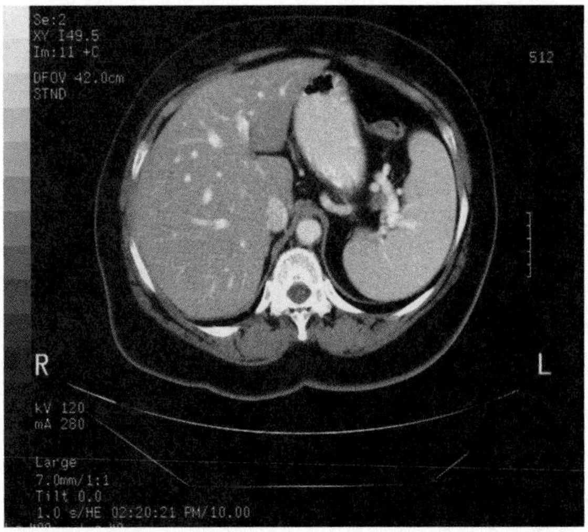

Figure 20-7C The positive contrast seen in the text and the-highlighted hepatic vessels, inferior vena cava, aorta, and splenic artery denotes the administration of intravenous contrast media in this CT scan.

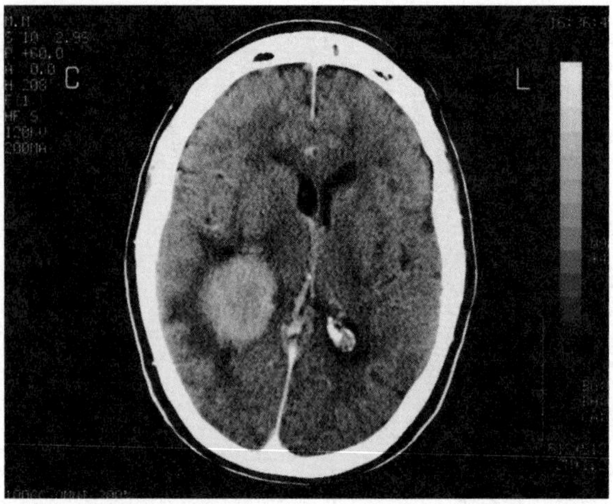

Figure 20-7D Axial CT scan demonstrates a meningioma surrounded by edema.

Some drawbacks to the MRI are that it cannot be used for patients who have pacemakers or other metal clips left in place on internal structures or organs as part of a surgical procedure. An MRI is not as useful as conventional radiographs or a CT scan for diagnosing fractured bones.

Patients are told to remove all objects that have metal: watches, belts, hairpins, rings, other metal jewelry, and credit cards because of the strong magnet in the MRI machine. Loose, comfortable clothing without zippers or snaps should be worn. The procedure takes about 45 minutes to an hour, during which time the patient must remain still. The technician, although not in the room with the patient, has a camera and microphone with which to communicate with the patient. An intermittent tapping sound can be heard throughout the procedure and earphones are available if the patient wants them (see Figure 20-9).

Flat Plates

Flat plates are also known as "plain" films because they require no special technique or the use of contrast medium. This type of X-ray is used on various parts of the body and is helpful in diagnosing problems in the skull, abdomen, chest, sinuses, and bone.

Ultrasonography

Ultrasonography, CT, and MRI allow for greater imaging detail than conventional radiographs. Ultrasonography, or ultrasound, has been available longer than the others. High-frequency sound waves (inaudible to the human ear) are used to image internal soft tissues. It can be used to help diagnose problems in the abdominal organs, the liver, and gallbladder. It cannot be used for skeletal structures or the lungs. An **echocardiogram,** an ultrasound of the heart, can view it and determine the size, shape, and position of the heart and the motion made by the valves opening and closing. Ultrasound has advantages over other methods of viewing internal organs and structures in that it uses no X-rays and allows for continuous viewing while organs and structures are in motion.

During ultrasound, a **transducer** is used with a coupling agent and sound waves are emitted from the

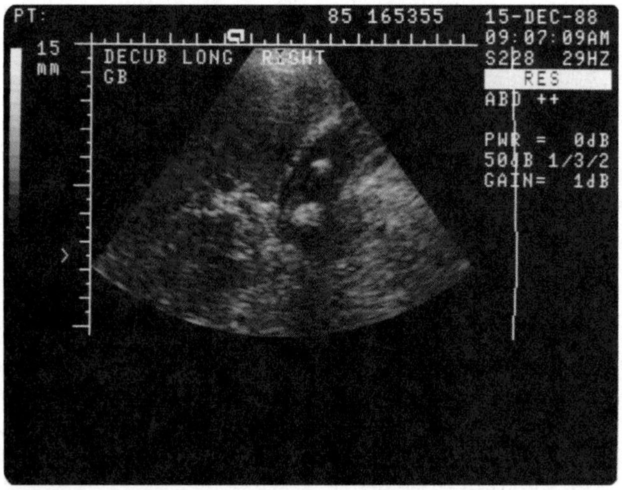

Figure 20-8 Sonogram of gallbladder with gallstones.

Patient Education

MRI

1. Determine if the patient has followed the preparation instructions if there were any.
2. Explain the procedure and what the patient can expect.
3. Have patient remove all metal objects (jewelry, watch, and so on). The magnet in the MRI machine is strong and metal can disrupt images.
4. Have patient urinate before the procedure because it takes about 45 minutes and patient cannot move during that time.
5. Explain to patient that machine makes humming and tapping noises.
6. Tell patient that the intravenous contrast medium may be slightly uncomfortable when injected into vein.
7. Remind patient to lie still and not to move.
8. Tell patient that there is a microphone for communication between the patient and technician.

head of the transducer. The transducer is placed firmly on the patient's body over the organ to be examined. The sound waves pass through the skin and bounce off the body's tissues and are reflected back to the transducer. These echoes are displayed on an **oscilloscope,** showing a visual pattern or picture. The image or record produced is known as a sonogram or echogram. A permanent film for the patient's record and videotape can also be made.

Ultrasonography, because it is **noninvasive** (procedure does not puncture skin or enter the body), is widely accepted for obstetrical use. Gestational age can be determined, congenital anomalies detected, multiple fetuses noted, ectopic pregnancy diagnosed, and fetal size and position determined (see Chapter 14).

Ultrasound takes 15 to 45 minutes, and the preparation depends on the body part being examined. An obstetrical ultrasound may require the patient to have a full bladder to push aside the intestines. An ultrasound of the gallbladder and liver require the patient to have had nothing to eat or drink for 8 to 12 hours before the examination. The patient must remain still unless requested to change positions (Figure 20-8). Therapeutic ultrasonography is discussed in Chapter 21.

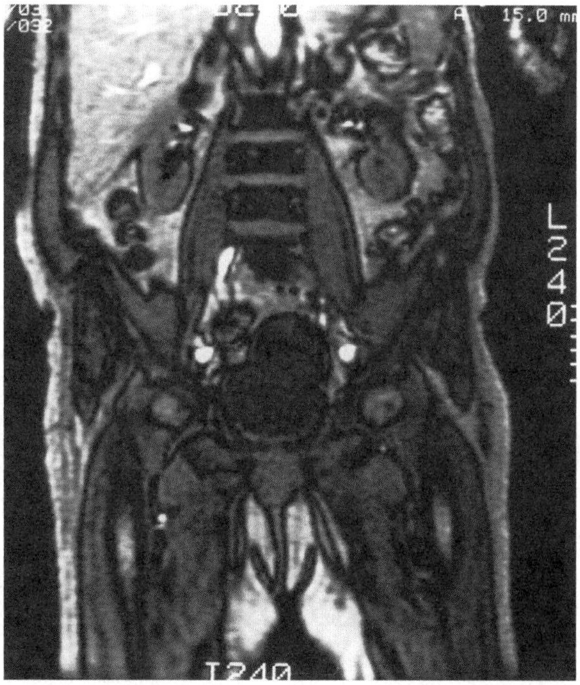

Figure 20-9 Coronal image of abdomen acquired during a breath hold in this magnetic resonance image.

Mammography

More than any other X-ray, the mammogram must be of the highest resolution and contrast. High resolution and contrast call for an increase in exposure to radiation, but mammography currently is safer than ever because of strong regulations (the only fully regulated radiography examination by the federal government) and improved technology. The machine currently used for mammography must meet stringent requirements. They are used with special screens, film, and cassettes. Currently, the equipment can produce high-resolution and extremely high-contrast images with exposures that are lower than ever. Digitalization helps improve images. Although some newer mammography equipment is digitalized, according to some experts, it produces images that are only slightly better than those produced by nondigitalized equipment. Researchers continue to seek ways to reduce the exposure of X-rays to the patient even further. See Chapter 14 for more information on mammography, particularly Figures 14-6 and 14-7.

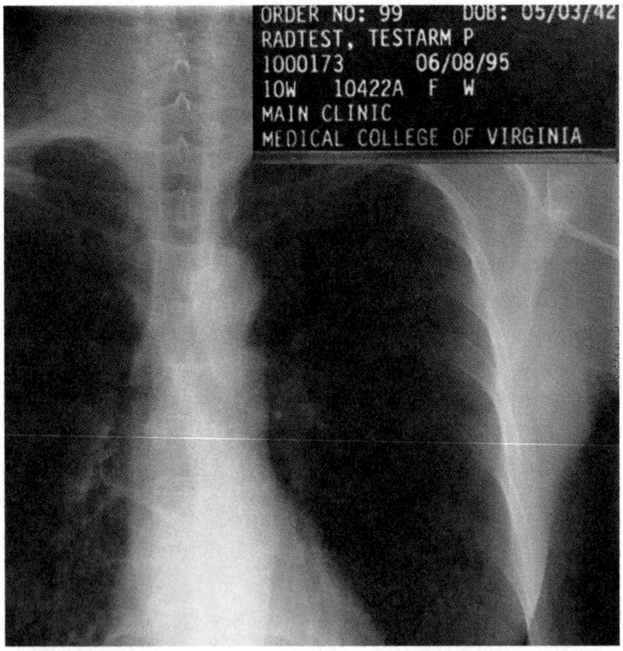

Figure 20-10A Radiograph showing patient identification information.

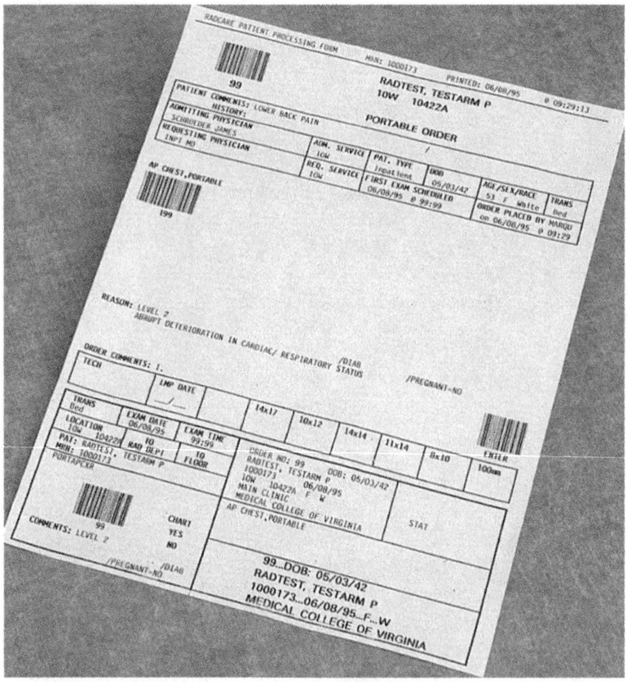

Figure 20-10B Sample requisition form.

Filing Films and Reports

Because radiographs are part of the patient's permanent record, they must be safeguarded from the environment. Such conditions as heat, moisture, and light can damage them. Processed films are stored in special envelopes with the patient's name, date, and identification number marked on the outside. They are stored in a cool, dry place. The films are the property of the hospital or other facility where the films were taken and usually remain where they were taken. Storage on-site makes them accessible for future use for comparison purposes and eliminates the possibility of their being lost if they were allowed to be taken away from the facility where they were processed. Written reports of the findings are prepared by the radiologist and sent to the patient's physician(s) (Figure 20-10).

RADIATION THERAPY

Radiation therapy is generally used to treat tumors that cannot be surgically removed or are inaccessible for surgical removal, and for treatment of a malignant tumor that was surgically excised but a portion of the tumor remains. When used to treat inaccessible or inoperable tumors, the treatment is considered **palliative** treatment. The treatments shrink the tumor, thereby lessening the symptoms. The treatments can be either external, with direct radiation aimed through the surface of the skin to an area within the body, or internal, using various applications of radioactivity such as seeds or beads that are planted inside the body and left there for a certain amount of time. The aim with radiation therapy is to interfere with cell growth and to disrupt the DNA. The object is to destroy as many of the malignant cells as possible without harming healthy cells surrounding the tumor. The side effects can be nausea, vomiting, hair loss, anorexia, bone marrow suppression, and **stomatitis.**

Critical Thinking

Describe how radiation therapy helps to destroy malignant neoplasms.

NUCLEAR MEDICINE

Nuclear medicine is the branch of medicine involved with the use of radioactive (emits rays or particles from nucleus) substances for diagnosis, therapy, and research. Specific training is necessary for this speciality.

Radioactive substances are administered to the patient either by mouth or by injection. The radioactive compounds, known as **radionuclides,** travel to an organ or area in the body that attracts them and creates an image of that area.

If the radionuclide is in an area that is abnormal, such as a tumor, it is referred to as "hot." If it does not concentrate in the abnormality, but surrounds it instead, this is known as a "cold" area. Both hot and cold areas are suggestive of abnormalities.

Case Study 20-1

Gloria McDermott is scheduled to have a GI series of X-rays next week because of persistent reports of stomach pain that is unrelieved by the prescription medication Dr. King has prescribed for her.

CASE STUDY REVIEW

1. How will you explain to her the purpose of the test?
2. What will you tell her about how to prepare for the examination?

Case Study 20-2

Raymond Brunnelle has had a series of X-rays, a GI series, a cholecystogram, and an MRI of his abdomen. He has scheduled an appointment with a gastroenterologist and asks you to get all of the films for him.

CASE STUDY REVIEW

1. What is your response to his request?
2. Explain why they should be kept on-site.

SUMMARY

Radiology and diagnostic imaging are helpful in the diagnosis and treatment of diseases and conditions because procedures can be done to visualize internal structures and their functions. Radiation is not without its risks to personnel and patients, but by following specific safety precautions, the health and safety of all involved can be safeguarded.

The three specialty areas are radiology, radiation therapy, and nuclear medicine.

STUDY FOR SUCCESS

To reinforce your knowledge and skills of information presented in this chapter:

- ❑ Review the Key Terms
- ❑ Consider the Case Studies and discuss your conclusions
- ❑ Answer the Review Questions
  - ❑ Multiple Choice
  - ❑ Critical Thinking
- ❑ Navigate the Internet by completing the Web Activities
- ❑ Practice the StudyWARE activities on your student CD
- ❑ Apply your knowledge in the Student Workbook activities
- ❑ Complete the Web Tutor sections

REVIEW QUESTIONS

Multiple Choice

1. Which of the following radiologic procedures does *not* require a contrast medium?
   a. hysterosalpingogram
   b. mammogram
   c. cholecystogram
   d. angiogram
2. A cholecystogram requires which type of contrast medium?
   a. air
   b. tablets
   c. carbon dioxide
   d. radionuclides
3. A cholangiogram will examine:
   a. upper GI tract
   b. lower GI tract
   c. bile ducts
   d. kidneys and ureters
4. In which of the following positions does the posterior aspect of the body face the X-ray tube and the anterior face the film?
   a. oblique
   b. anteroposterior
   c. posteroanterior
   d. prone
   e. supine
5. The radiologic procedure of choice for brain imaging is:
   a. computerized tomography
   b. positron emission tomography
   c. magnetic resonance imaging
   d. ultrasonogram
   e. thermography

Critical Thinking

1. Describe the purpose of a lead apron and lead-lined walls in the radiology department.
2. For what is thermography used?
3. How are X-rays used to diagnose?
4. How are X-rays used to treat patient diseases or conditions?
5. What is contrast media? How is it used and why?
6. To whom do X-ray films belong once they are taken and processed?
7. What special precautions should be taken when a patient is having an excretory urography, especially the initial time?

WEB ACTIVITIES

1. Visit the American Society of Radiologic Technicians at http://www.asrt.org and view "Obesity May Affect Mammography." What is available at this site?
2. Use Google to find a Web site for "The history of MRI." Describe how long it took for the first MRI to produce one image.
3. Using a search engine of your choice, locate information about how CAT scans work. What is the fundamental concept of how a CAT scan operates?
4. Using a search engine of your choice, find information about how nuclear medicine works. Name three types of techniques that use nuclear medicine. How is an image obtained?
5. Locate a Web site about medical radiation safety. Find a guide about radiation protection for the patient. What are the benefits and risks of a mammogram? Excretory urogram (IVP)?

REFERENCES/BIBLIOGRAPHY

Carlton, R. R., & Adler, A. M. (2001). *Principles of radiographic imaging: An art and a science* (3rd ed.). Clifton Park NY: Thomson Delmar Learning.

Cornuelle, A., & Gronefeld, D. (1998). *Radiographic anatomy positioning: An integrated approach.* Stanford, CT: Appleton and Lange.

Cowling, C. (1998). *Radiographic positioning procedures, Volume II: Advanced imaging procedures.* Clifton Park NY: Thomson Delmar Learning.

Early, P. J., & Sodee, D. B. (1995). *Principles and practice of nuclear medicine* (2nd ed.). St. Louis: Mosby-Year Book.

Greathouse, J. (1998). *Radiographic positioning procedures, Volume I: Basic positioning and procedures.* Clifton Park NY: Thomson Delmar Learning.

Metler, F. A., Jr., & Guiberteau, M. J. (1997). *Essentials of nuclear medicine imaging* (4th ed.). Philadelphia: WB Saunders.

Taber's cylopedic medical dictionary. (22nd ed.). (2003). Philadelphia: FA Davis.

CHAPTER 21

Rehabilitation and Therapeutic Modalities

OUTLINE

OBJECTIVES

The student should strive to meet the following performance objectives and demonstrate an understanding of the facts and principles presented in this chapter through written and oral communication.

1. Define the key terms as presented in the glossary.
2. Define rehabilitation medicine and explain its importance in patient care.
3. Discuss the importance of correct posture and body mechanics, and demonstrate how to safely transfer patients and lift or move heavy objects using proper body mechanics.
4. Describe safety precautions and techniques used when helping a patient to ambulate and demonstrate how to assist the patient to safely stand and walk.
5. Demonstrate how to safely care for the falling patient.
6. Describe assistive devices and the importance of each in helping patients to ambulate.

(continues)

KEY TERMS

Abduction
Activities of Daily Living (ADL)
Adduction
Ambulation
Assistive Device
Atrophy
Body Mechanics
Circumduction
Contracture
Cryotherapy
Dorsiflexion
Eversion
Extension
Flexion
Gait
Gait Belt
Goniometer
Goniometry
Hemiplegia
Hyperextension
Inversion
Modalities
Muscle Testing
Plantar Flexion
Pronation
Range of Motion (ROM)
Rehabilitation Medicine
Rotation
Supination
Thermotherapy
Ultrasound
Vasoconstriction
Vasodilation

FEATURED COMPETENCIES

CAAHEP—ENTRY-LEVEL COMPETENCIES

Patient Care

- Prepare patient for and assist with procedures, treatments, and minor office surgeries

Patient Instruction

- Instruct individuals according to their needs

ABHES—ENTRY-LEVEL COMPETENCIES

Communication

- Be impartial and show empathy when dealing with patients
- Adapt what is said to recipient's level of comprehension
- Adaptation for individualized needs

OBJECTIVES (continued)

7. Demonstrate how to measure patients for a walker, crutches, and a cane and help them ambulate safely with each device.
8. Describe the ambulation gaits used with crutches.
9. Discuss the safety precautions and techniques used when pushing a wheelchair.
10. Explain the importance of joint range of motion and the method used to measure joint movement.
11. Explain the importance of therapeutic exercise and the types of therapeutic exercises used in patient rehabilitation.
12. Describe electromyography and its purpose.
13. Explain the purpose of the electrostimulation of muscle.
14. Explain the body's physiologic reactions to heat and cold therapeutic modalities.
15. Be able to identify and describe the various types of hot and cold modalities, and describe how ultrasound works.

SCENARIO

In a large urgent care center such as Inner City Health Care, a team of therapists is responsible for providing patients with a high level of rehabilitative care. However, the clinical medical assistants at Inner City also are involved on a daily basis in the care of patients who have experienced injuries such as fractures or severe back pain. Clinical medical assistant Wanda Slawson, CMA, MLT, and clinical medical assistant Bruce Goldman, CMA, are often responsible for transferring patients and getting them safely from the reception area to the examination room and from wheelchair to examination table. Although acutely aware of the needs and safety of the patient, Wanda and Bruce also make sure they protect themselves by using proper body mechanics, by observing good posture, by using their arm and leg muscles and not their back muscles, and by always bending from the hips and knees, not the waist. Wanda's and Bruce's observation of these important principles protects their health and ensures the safety of their patients.

INTRODUCTION

Physical disability affects millions of people in the United States, regardless of age, race, or socioeconomic status. Every year thousands of people survive strokes, head or spinal cord injury, or other debilitating illness or injury that leaves them unable to perform complete independent function. Some of these individuals recover completely. Others recover to their fullest ability, living the rest of their lives with some type of disability. Still other patients experience chronic conditions such as arthritis or severe back pain that incapacitates them to the extent they cannot work or completely care for themselves.

***Rehabilitation medicine** is a field of medical disciplines that uses physical and mechanical agents to aid in the diagnosis, treatment, and prevention of diseases or bodily injuries. Its goal is to aid in the restoration of those functions that have been affected by the patient's condition. For those who have experienced permanent loss of ability, it seeks to find practical substitutions for that loss, whereas assisting patients to make the most of their remaining abilities.*

Most rehabilitation services are prescribed by the physician in charge of a patient's care and, depending on the patient's condition, can include a recommendation to one or several rehabilitation specialists. Most likely, that specialist will be a physical therapist, occupational therapist, speech therapist, or sports medicine specialist, although the field of rehabilitation medicine is certainly not limited to these four areas of specialty.

Professional rehabilitation therapists, in whichever field they practice, are specifically trained and licensed in their field of expertise to assess, plan, and execute the patient's treatment in an overall effort to restore that patient to the highest level of physical and social independence possible. The medical assis-

Spotlight on Certification

RMA Content Outline
- Patient education
- Therapeutic modalities

CMA Content Outline
- Patient instruction
- Patient education
- Principles of operations

CMAS Content Outline
- Communication

TABLE 21-1 SOME OF THE SPECIALIZED FIELDS OF REHABILITATION MEDICINE

Physical Therapy/ Physiotherapy	The treatment of disorders with physical and mechanical agents and methods to restore normal function after injury or illness.
Occupational Therapy	The use of activities to help restore independent functioning after an injury or illness.
Speech Therapy	The diagnosis and treatment of speech disorders.
Sports Medicine	A branch of medicine that specializes in the treatment and prevention of injuries caused by athletic participation.

tant, as a member of an interdisciplinary health team, can use medical assisting skills to enable patients to regain normal or near-normal function after an illness or injury. See Chapter 7 for Legal Considerations and for information on the American with Disabilities Act (ADA).

THE ROLE OF THE MEDICAL ASSISTANT IN REHABILITATION

As a medical assistant, you may find yourself working in one of the rehabilitation fields. Such opportunities might include an ambulatory care setting with a specialty in physical therapy or sports medicine, an orthopedic surgeon's practice, the occupational or speech therapy department of a large suburban hospital, or other outpatient clinic or medical office. For the more chronically ill, nursing homes and rehabilitation hospitals also focus on restoring patients to as much independence as possible.

Even if you do not work in the field of rehabilitation and therapeutic modalities, you may be referring patients for treatments and perhaps even performing insurance coding or rehabilitative and therapeutic modalities. Either way, a good working knowledge of the field is important for a well-rounded understanding of today's medical treatments.

Whatever the rehabilitation setting, you will most likely find that you are a member of an interdisciplinary team of health care professionals who bring a broad knowledge base to patient care (Table 21-1). However, the physician is responsible for prescribing any type of rehabilitative medicine.

It is important to remember that patients seeking rehabilitation treatment may have undergone a tremendous loss of physical ability, leaving them vulnerable to feelings of helplessness. They may be able to perform only limited **activities of daily living (ADL)** or normal daily self-care such as brushing their teeth, getting dressed, and eating. Perhaps they cannot even do the simple tasks we take for granted everyday, leaving them completely dependent on another person for help.

Understanding and encouragement are vital to the recovery process of these patients. While working with disabled persons, remember that certain tasks may be challenging to them. More than likely they are acutely aware of their impairment and feel frustrated at their loss of function and discouraged about the future. Some patients may also suffer some speech impairment, making communication difficult or impossible. Respect for their dignity will build their self-esteem and have a positive effect on their treatment.

PRINCIPLES OF BODY MECHANICS

Much of the medical assistant's work with disabled persons will require great physical effort, particularly if patients are incapable of lifting or moving themselves. Moving patients or heavy, awkward objects can be hazardous for the patient, as well as the caregiver if not performed correctly.

Body mechanics is the practice of using certain key muscle groups together with good body alignment and proper body positioning to reduce the risk for injury to both patient and caregiver. Always be conscious of using proper body mechanics, not just on the job, but in everything that requires moving, lifting, pushing, or pulling heavy or awkward objects.

Posture

Practicing good body mechanics starts with good posture. Good posture protects the entire body, particularly the back, whether standing, sitting, or lying down.

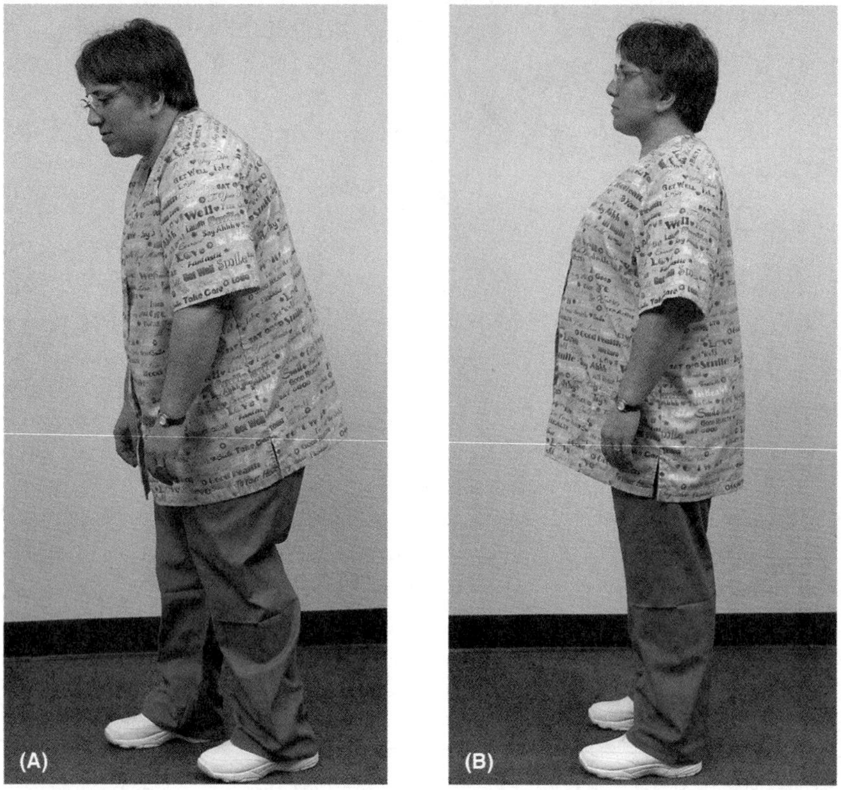

Figure 21-1 (A) A medical assistant demonstrating poor posture. (B) Good posture not only looks more professional but can prevent back injuries.

Glance at yourself sideways in a full-length mirror. When standing, does your posture most resemble that in Figure 21-1A or 21-1B? When the body's muscle groups and body parts are in proper alignment, as shown in Figure 21-1B, the body is said to be in balance. Good balance is important for your body to function at its best. It enables you to lift, push, and pull easily and safely.

Frequently check your posture by reminding yourself to keep your chin and chest up, shoulders back, pelvis tilted slightly inward, feet straight and shoulder-width apart, and weight evenly distributed to both legs with a slight bend in your knees.

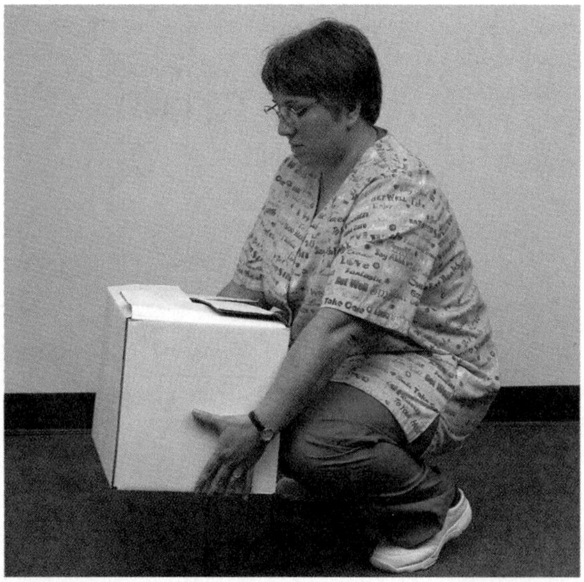

Figure 21-2 Provide a good base of support by keeping the back straight and feet apart.

Using the Body Safely and Effectively

The spine is a flexible rod, designed to bend in many directions and hold the back steady. However, the muscles of the back are small and not meant for lifting heavy loads. They can be easily damaged if called on to work beyond their natural ability. The muscles in the arms and legs, however, are large and were designed for heavy work. Rely on these muscles when lifting and carrying heavy objects, bending over or bending down, or moving patients.

It is important to keep several basic rules in mind whenever performing any task:

- Keep the back as straight as possible and feet shoulder-width apart to provide a good base of support (Figure 21-2).

- Always bend from the hips and knees, which enables the largest muscles of the legs to do the hard work, but *never* bend from the waist (Figure 21-3).
- Pivot the entire body instead of twisting it.
- Use the body's weight to push or pull any heavy object.
- Obtain help if unable to move a patient or object that is too heavy.
- Hold heavy objects close to the body (Figure 21-4).
- Make sure the path is clear and the area to receive the object is ready before lifting or moving it.
- Get into the habit of wearing a body support if a job includes much lifting (Figure 21-5).

Lifting Techniques

When lifting patients or moving or lifting heavy objects, certain techniques should be used to prevent back injury:

- Get as close as possible to the object or person being lifted, because this allows the center of gravity to be maintained over the base of support.
- Keep the feet apart, one slightly in front of the other, and knees slightly bent.
- Use the large muscles of the legs and arms to lift, not back muscles.
- Keep the back straight to transfer the workload to larger arm and leg muscles.

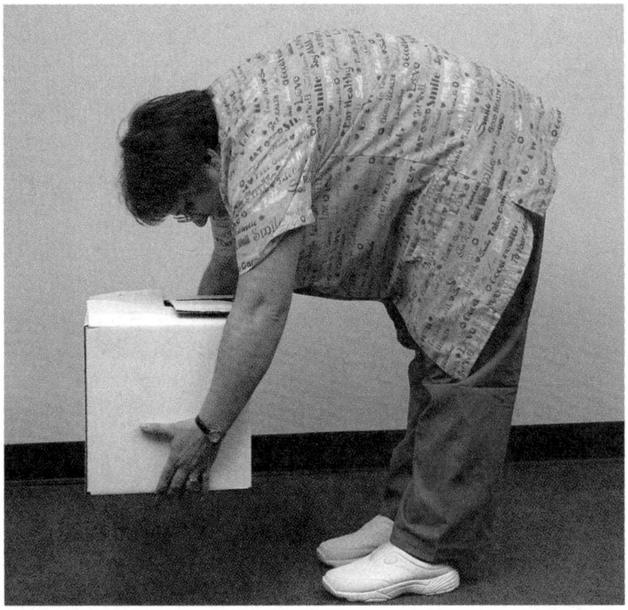

Figure 21-3 Never bend from the waist.

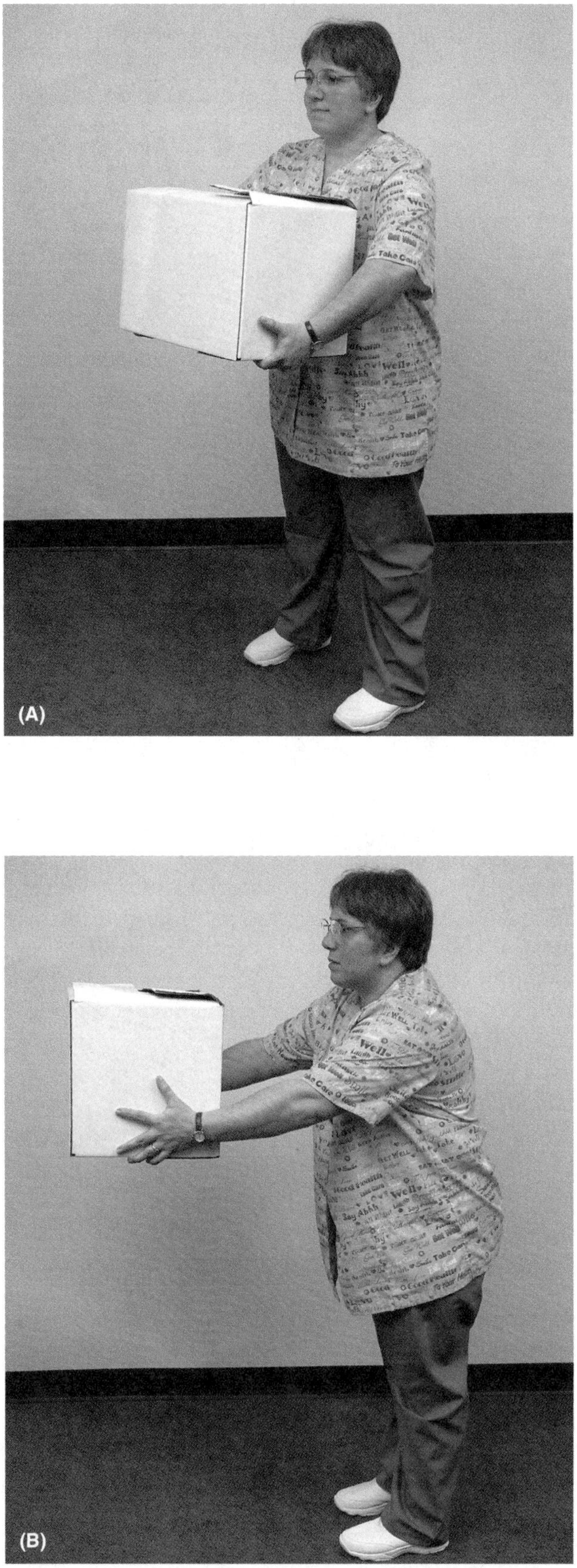

Figure 21-4 (A) When carrying heavy objects, hold them close to the body. (B) Never carry heavy objects out in front.

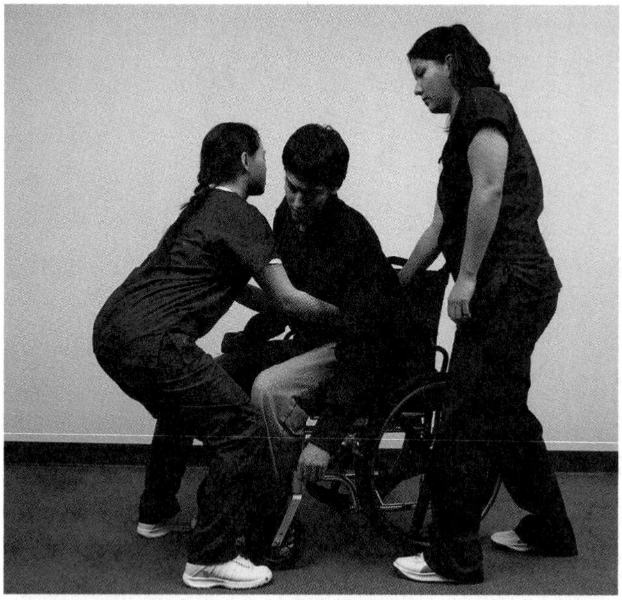

Figure 21-5 When a patient or object is too heavy, get help if necessary. Consider wearing a body support to protect the back if a job requires frequent lifting.

- Bend from the hips and knees, squat down, and push up with leg muscles.

TRANSFERRING PATIENTS

It may be necessary to transfer patients if they cannot walk or lift themselves. Such patients may have a wide variety of disabilities, from severe back pain to **hemiplegia,** or paralysis of one side of the body resulting from a stroke, accident, or other condition. The frail older adults also require particular care when being transferred, because they are more prone to bruising and broken bones.

As a safety precaution, it is important to remember good body mechanics when transferring patients. The act of lifting and moving someone can throw off one's center of gravity, and therefore the base of support. Provide a wider base of support by moving the feet further apart and bending slightly, using strong arm and leg muscles to lift.

Before beginning any transfer, observe certain precautions:

- Make sure the equipment is stable and firm. Lock the brakes of the wheelchair and make sure the examination table or other surface will not move during the transfer.
- Check that there are no obstructions to trip over when making the transfer.
- Take small shuffling steps, and avoid crossing the feet.
- It is best if the transfer surfaces being used are close to the same height. If possible, lower the examination table or bed to the height of the wheelchair.
- Position the equipment according to the patient's physical limitations or disability. If the patient is stronger on one side, make sure that is the side on which the transfer will take place. It not only makes the transfer easier, it gives the patient more confidence.
- Always use a **gait belt,** a safety belt worn around the patient's waist, when transferring a patient. Lift the patient by grasping the belt from underneath and lifting up. Never lift a patient by the arms, or under the armpits, because this could cause injury to you and the patient.
- Take advantage of any assistance the patient can provide in lifting and moving.
- Never have patients put their arms around your neck or on your shoulders, because it could cause you to be injured.
- Make sure both you and the patient are wearing footwear that will not slip or hinder the transfer process in any way. If a prosthesis or brace is involved, make sure it is secure and will not present a problem.
- Thoroughly explain to the patient what you intend to do, and make sure the patient understands what to expect during the transfer. Instructions need to be simple and repeated when necessary.
- Practice good body mechanics. Get close enough to the patient so you can lift with your legs. Always bend at the hips instead of the waist.
- Ascertain beforehand whether assistance will be needed with the transfer.
- Finally, take sufficient time when completing each step. Many patients will want to help themselves. Respect their courage, but remember that safety is of the utmost importance.

See Procedure 21-1 for proper steps in transferring patients from a wheelchair to an examination table. Procedure 21-2 outlines steps for transfer from examination table to wheelchair.

ASSISTING PATIENTS TO AMBULATE

Despite great strides that have been made in recent years to provide access for disabled persons, **ambulation,** or walking, is a functional activity that still provides the ultimate level of independence and freedom. For many patients, being able to ambulate again gives them tremendous satisfaction, because the act of walking more than anything else signifies their return to wellness. Some patients take months to walk again by undergoing exercises and treatment designed to strengthen specific muscles. They may still need help while in our office.

Before assisting with any type of ambulation, there are several safety issues to remember:

- Make sure the patient is ready to walk. If a patient has trouble sitting well, or cannot balance once standing up, walking should not be attempted.
- The patient should be wearing good shoes that are flat, supportive, and have a rubber sole.
- Check to be certain there are plenty of handholds or railings within easy reach should the patient become unstable during walking.
- A gait belt provides a firm hold on the patient should the patient require assistance with stability at any time. For the patient just starting to walk, this device should be used and held by the caregiver throughout the session.
- Monitor the patient when standing and throughout the ambulation session for signs of fatigue and vertigo.
- Ambulate only as long as the patient has strength. Never push the patient beyond endurance.
- Never hurry a patient.
- Be ready should a patient start to fall. Generally, patients will fall toward their weaker side, but sometimes their legs lose stability and they go straight down.

Procedures 21-3 and 21-4 detail the steps involved in assisting patients to stand and walk and in caring for a falling patient.

ASSISTIVE DEVICES

For some patients, the extent of their physical disability may determine that ambulation is only possible with the help of an **assistive device,** or walking aid such as a walker, crutches, or cane. For others, their physical disability is such that mobility is not possible at all without the use of a wheelchair.

Some assistive devices provide stability and support, whereas others require more coordination. Depending on the patient's condition, one assistive device may be used until the patient has gained enough strength and coordination to move on to another type of assistive device, with the ultimate goal of walking unaided. The device a patient needs depends both on the disability and the patient's recuperation curve and is prescribed after careful evaluation by the attending physician or other health professional (Table 21-2).

Whatever device a patient will be using, medical assistants may be called on to measure the patient for the correct size and provide instruction in its proper use and care. Once the patient has become proficient on level surfaces, provide instruction on sitting, standing, turning around, and negotiating stairs, curbs, ramps, doors, and other obstacles. In addition, patients should be taught how to protect themselves should they fall and how to get back up.

Walkers

Walkers are best used for patients who require maximum assistance with balance and coordination, because they provide stability and support when the patient is standing or walking. They provide patients with the ability to ambulate independently with confidence. To use one, patients must be strong enough to be able to hold themselves upright while leaning on the walker.

Various styles of walkers are available. The two most widely used walkers are those that have rubber tips on the legs (stationary walkers), and those with wheels on the bottom of the legs (rolling walkers). Walkers that have wheels can be easily pushed ahead by the patient while walking and are best for patients who primarily need a walker for balance.

Most walkers are made of aluminum and are lightweight; most can be easily folded for storage or transport. The major disadvantage is that they must be used on level ground and cannot be used on stairs. Walkers are also difficult to use when attempting to go through doorways and in small areas around the house.

Fitting a Walker. Most walkers can be adjusted for a proper fit. The height of the handgrip should be adjusted to the individual patient just below the patient's waist, or at the top of the femur so the elbow can be bent at a 30-degree angle when the patient is standing with hands on the handgrip (Figure 21-6).

Procedure 21-5 provides steps for assisting a patient to ambulate with a walker.

Crutches

Crutches provide the ambulating patient with a great deal more mobility and flexibility. They provide good stability and support, whereas allowing for a broad range of gait patterns and ambulating speeds.

TABLE 21-2 TYPES OF ASSISTIVE DEVICES

Assistive Device	Features	Patient Requirements
Walkers		
Standard	• Adjustable • Rubber tips	• Requires upper body strength • Provides maximum stability and support • Excellent for older adults
Rolling	• Legs have wheels • Otherwise same as regular walker	• Good for patients who need walker only for balance and not support
Crutches		
Axillary	• Wooden or steel • Worn under axillae	• Requires good upper body strength and balance • Not recommended for older adults • Best for younger persons with lower extremity or hip fractures that will heal in a short time • Provides greatest range of ambulation
Forearm (Lofstrand or Canadian)	• Shorter than axillary crutches • Has metal cuff worn around forearm	• Less stable than axillary crutches • Best for long-term crutch use • Reduces stress on axillary vessels and nerves • Requires upper body strength and more stability and coordination • Provides most maneuverability of all crutches
Platform	• Platform affixed to a crutch • Patient bears weight on forearm	• Best for patients with severe arthritis or poor use of hands • Does not require as much upper body strength • Requires good balance
Canes		
Standard	• Single leg • Curved handle • Rubber tip	• Good for patients with only one good arm, lateral instability, or balance conditions
Quad (four-point)	• Single cane resting on a platform with four legs • Rubber tips on legs	• Better for patients with more severe conditions • Does not require as much coordination, but still requires balance and upper body strength in one arm
Walkcane or Hemiwalker	• Has four legs that come all the way up to a handlebar • Rubber tips on all legs	• Provides most stability of all canes • Best for hemiplegic patients who require extra support on one side

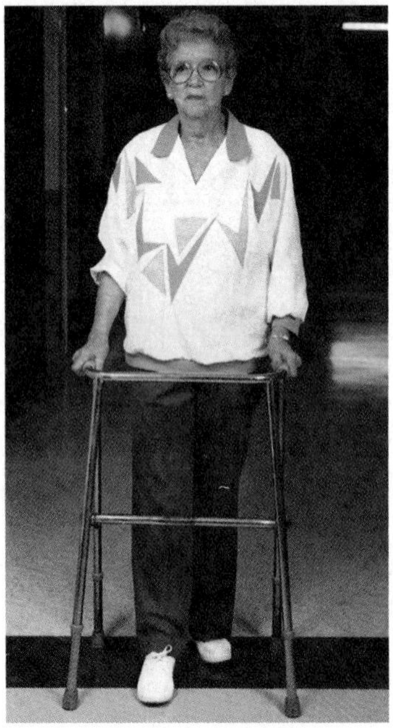

Figure 21-6 Proper fit for a walker. Note the patient's elbows are flexed at a 30-degree angle.

Three basic types of crutches are prescribed, depending on the patient's physical limitations and abilities: axillary crutches, forearm crutches (also called Lofstrand or Canadian crutches), and platform crutches (Figure 21-7).

Axillary crutches are made of wood or aluminum and are used primarily for individuals who need crutches temporarily while a lower extremity heals. Axillary crutches are ideal for stronger patients and pediatric patients who have minor injuries, but they are not recommended for frail older adults because upper body strength and balance are both required to use them (Figure 21-8). These crutches are easily transported and can be used to maneuver on stairs or in tight places.

Forearm crutches, or Lofstrand or Canadian crutches as they are also known, are shorter and provide less stability than axillary crutches. Forearm crutches are fixed with a metal or hard plastic cuff that fits around the patient's forearm. The weight is borne almost exclusively on the hand grip, requiring a great deal of upper body strength and coordination to use. This type of crutch is generally

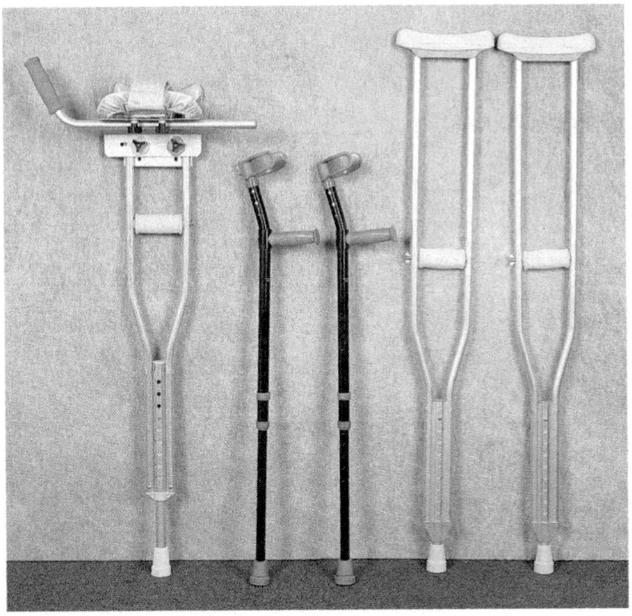

Figure 21-7 Types of crutches, from left to right: platform, forearm or Lofstrand, and axillary.

recommended for patients who will need crutches permanently or for a long period because they do not put any pressure on the axillary vessels and nerves (Figure 21-9).

The *platform crutch* is a third type of crutch that is recommended for patients who cannot grip the handles of other types of crutches or bear weight through their wrists or hands. The crutch has a platform attached to the top that includes a hand grip. It is high enough for the patient to use with the elbow bent at a right angle. The patient bears his or her weight completely on the forearm, which requires stability, strength, and coordination. The platform crutch is an ideal substitute for a cane when a patient only requires minimal weight transfer but cannot bear weight on or grip with the hands (Figure 21-10).

Measuring a Patient for Axillary Crutches. To determine the right height of the crutches, the patient should stand tall. Be sure the patient is wearing good walking shoes. Adjust the height of the crutch so it is about two to three fingers, or 2 inches below the patient's axillae, or armpits (Figure 21-11). Adjust

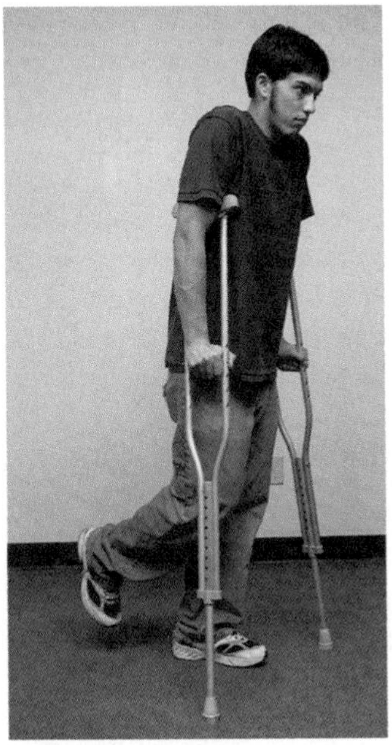

Figure 21-8 Patient using axillary crutches.

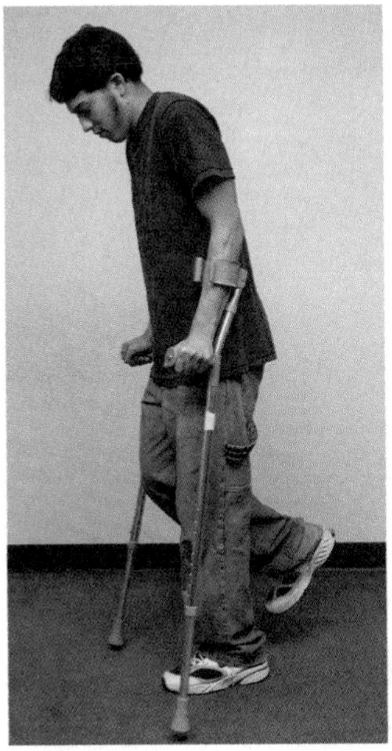

Figure 21-9 Patient using Lofstrand or forearm crutches.

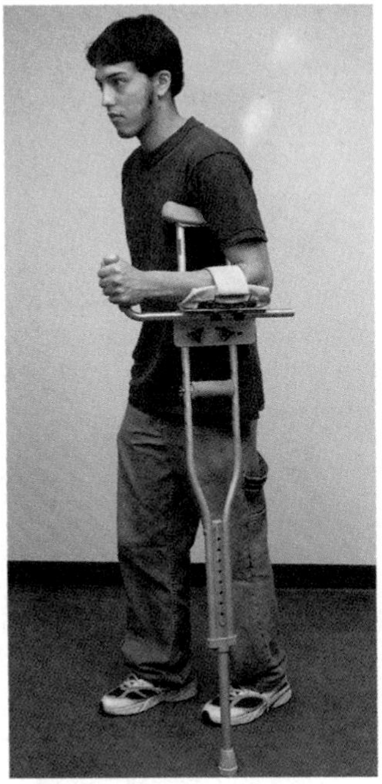

Figure 21-10 Patient using a platform crutch. This crutch is an ideal substitute for a cane if the patient cannot bear weight in his upper arm or on his hand.

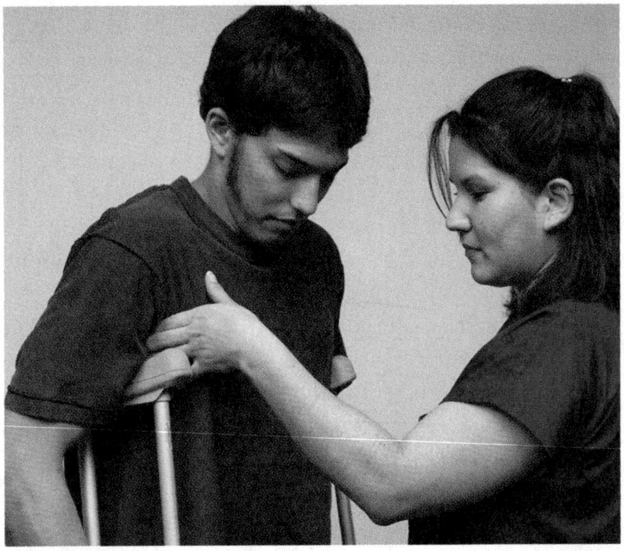

Figure 21-11 Measuring for axillary crutches. Note the height is about two to three fingers below the patient's armpit.

the hand grips so the patient's elbows are bent at about a 20- to 30-degree angle. Position the crutch tips about 2 inches lateral and 6 inches anterior to the foot. When the patient is standing correctly, the crutch tips and patient's feet should form a triangle (Figure 21-12).

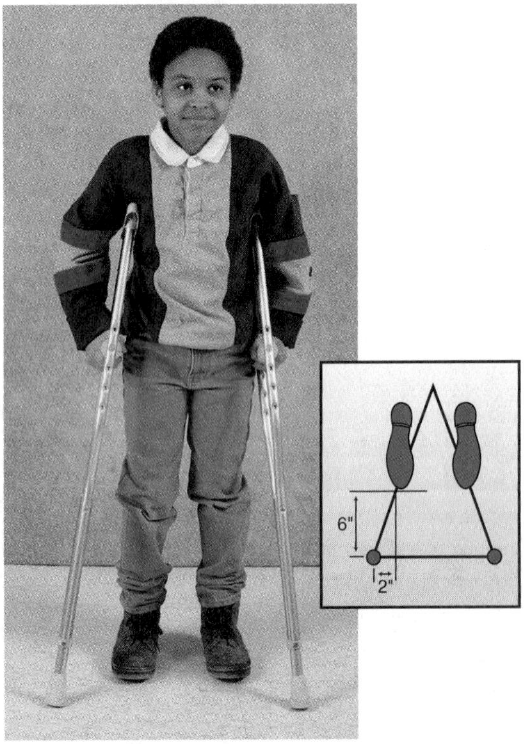

Figure 21-12 The distal end of the crutch should be 2 inches lateral and 6 inches anterior to the foot to form a triangle.

Procedure 21-6 indicates steps for teaching patients to ambulate with axillary crutches.

Crutch-Walking Gaits. The type of **gait,** or walk, a patient uses depends on the patient's injury and condition and is determined by the physician or licensed therapist. In crutch-walking gaits, each time the patient's foot or crutch touches the ground it is called a *point.* There are five gaits that are commonly used in crutch ambulation. The number of points in the gait relates to the number of feet and crutch tips that are on the ground at the same time.

Common crutch-walking gaits include two-point, three-point, four-point, swing-to, and swing-through gaits.

Two-Point Gait. There are two types of two-point gaits:

1. The first type is a nonweight-bearing gait. Patients place the crutch tips about 18 inches in front of them. They push off, taking the weight off their body and transferring it to their hands, then bring their strong leg forward past the crutches.
2. The second gait, called the two-point alternating gait, is used when the patient can bear weight on both legs. The opposite foot and crutch are advanced forward at the same time (Figure 21-13). This gait is a more advanced gait and is used after the four-point gait has been mastered.

Three-Point Gait. This gait is used when the patient can only bear partial weight on one leg, or just touch that foot to the floor. Both the crutches and the weak leg are advanced at the same time. The body weight is then transferred forward to the crutches, and the stronger leg is advanced and placed slightly in front of the crutches (Figure 21-14).

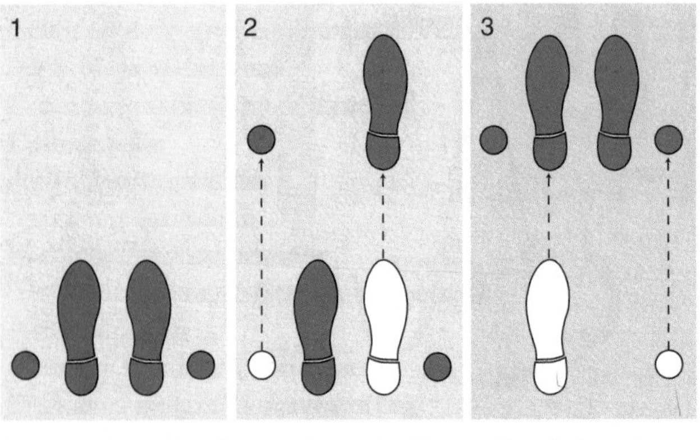

Figure 21-13 Two-point gait. The patient is bearing weight on both legs.

Patient Education

When instructing patients in the use of axillary crutches, impress on them the importance of putting all their weight on their hands, not on the armpits. Many patients using crutches for the first time mistakenly put the pressure on their armpits, which can damage the axillary nerve. Also reinforce the need for wearing flat, nonskid shoes when using crutches.

Throw rugs and other obstacles in the home or work area are a danger to patients on crutches. Remind them to have such hazards removed. Teach patients to check crutches daily for the following:

- Check that the wing nuts that adjust the crutches are tight.
- Check the crutch tips for wear and tear.
- Check the foam pads of the hand grips and armpit rests for tears.

Four-Point Alternating Gait. This is a slower gait that is used for patients who can bear weight on both legs and move each leg separately. The patient moves one crutch forward, then the opposite foot. The patient then moves the other crutch forward, then the opposite foot (Figure 21-15).

Swing-To Gait. Patients start with the crutches at their side. They move both crutches forward, transfer their weight forward, and swing both feet together up to the crutches.

Swing-Through Gait. Start with the crutches at the side. Move both crutches forward. Transfer the weight and swing both feet through the crutches, stopping slightly in front of the crutches.

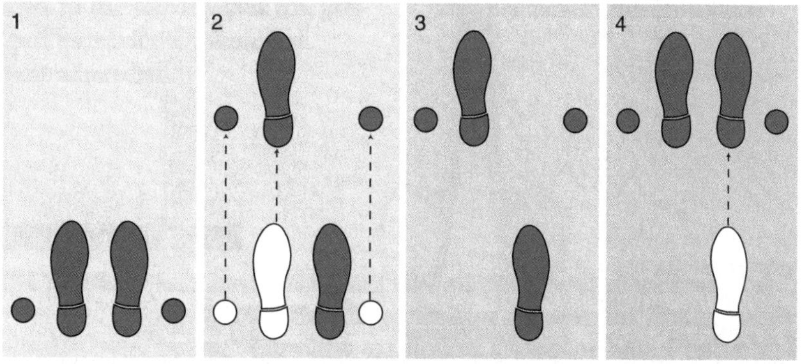

Figure 21-14 Three-point gait. The left leg is the weaker leg and bears no weight.

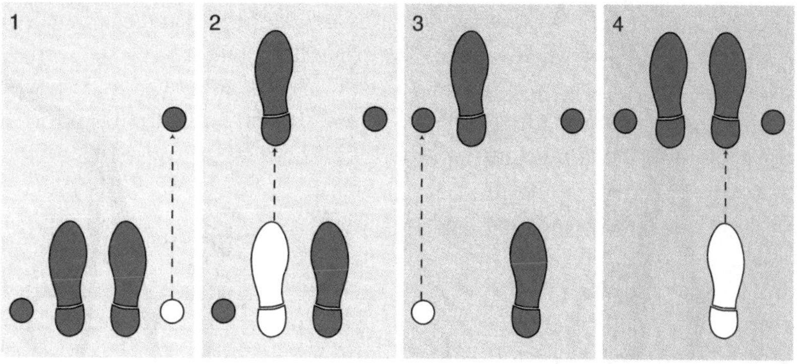

Figure 21-15 Four-point gait. The patient is bearing weight on both legs.

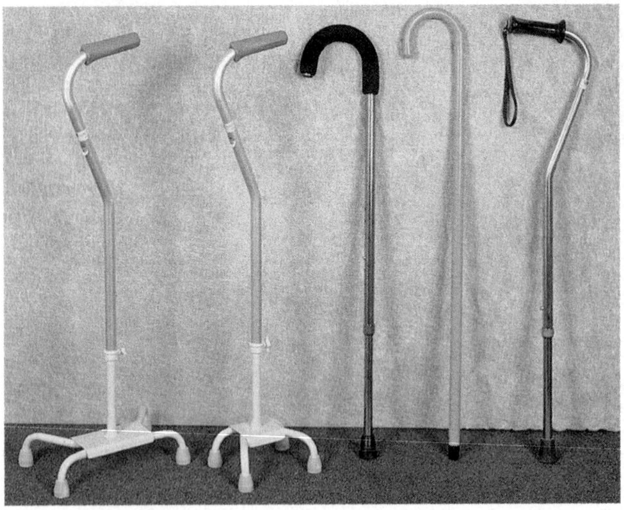

Figure 21-16 Types of standard canes: (A) quad canes; (B) single-tip canes.

Sitting. The patient backs into a straight chair with armrests until the seat of the chair touches the back of the legs. Crutches are held in the hand on the strong side and opposite the weak leg. With the other hand the patient can grasp the armrest of the chair and lower slowly into the chair.

Standing. The patient holds both crutches in the hand on the strong side, moves forward in the chair, grasps the armrest with the hand on the weaker side, then pushes up to a standing position.

Canes

A cane is used when the patient has one weak side and will need this assistive device for a longer period than crutches. It is also useful for patients who have a general but minor weakness on one side or those who have poor balance.

Canes come in three basic types, are made of either aluminum or wood, and have rubber tips. Some are adjustable and some are not (Figure 21-16). The first type of cane is called a *standard* (Figure 21-17), or single-tipped cane. It has a curved handle for gripping, and the newer canes have a hand grip attached. The standard cane is used for patients with less severe walking conditions and needs a small amount of support.

The second type of cane is a four-legged, or *quad* cane. It is a single cane that rests on a four-legged platform, provides stability and a wide base of support, and is for patients with more severe walking difficulties.

The third type of cane is a *walkcane*. It has four legs and a handlebar for gripping and provides the best support of all canes. This type of cane is also referred to as a Hemiwalker because it is ideal for hemiplegic patients who need the extra stability of this wide base. When the cane is the correct height, the elbow is flexed at a 20- to 30-degree angle.

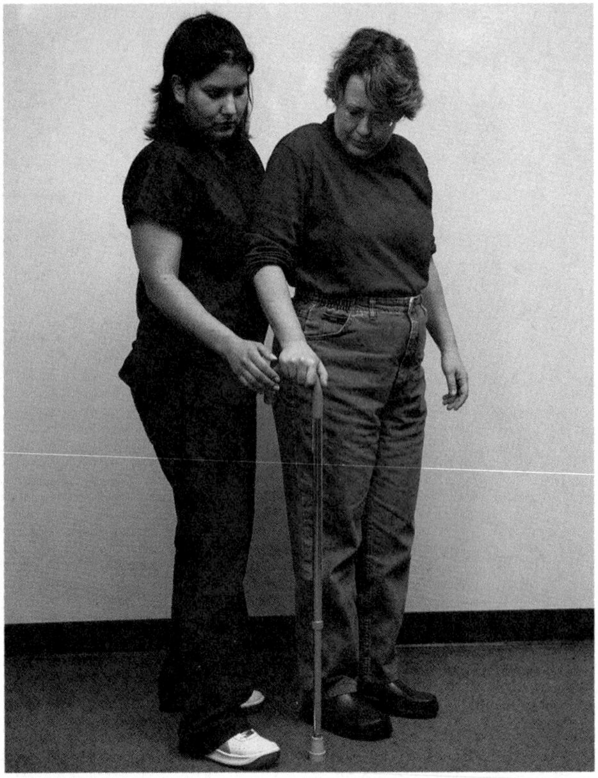

Figure 21-17 A standard cane being used by a hemiplegic patient.

Procedure 21-7 outlines the steps for teaching a patient how to walk safely with a cane.

Wheelchairs

Wheelchairs are mobile chairs that enable patients with severe ambulation conditions, or no ability to ambulate at all, to otherwise get around. Some must be moved manually, either by the patient or by someone else. Others are motorized and can be controlled completely by the patient (Figure 21-18).

Many advancements in wheelchair design over the years have enabled patients with chronic conditions to no longer be restricted to a home or hospital environment. Today, all public buildings and many private ones have handicapped access ramps as an alternative to stairs, remote-controlled doors, elevators that can accommodate a wheelchair, and other amenities that enable wheelchair patients to get around almost as well as if they were ambulating.

There are many types of wheelchairs and modifications that can be tailored to suit a patient's particular

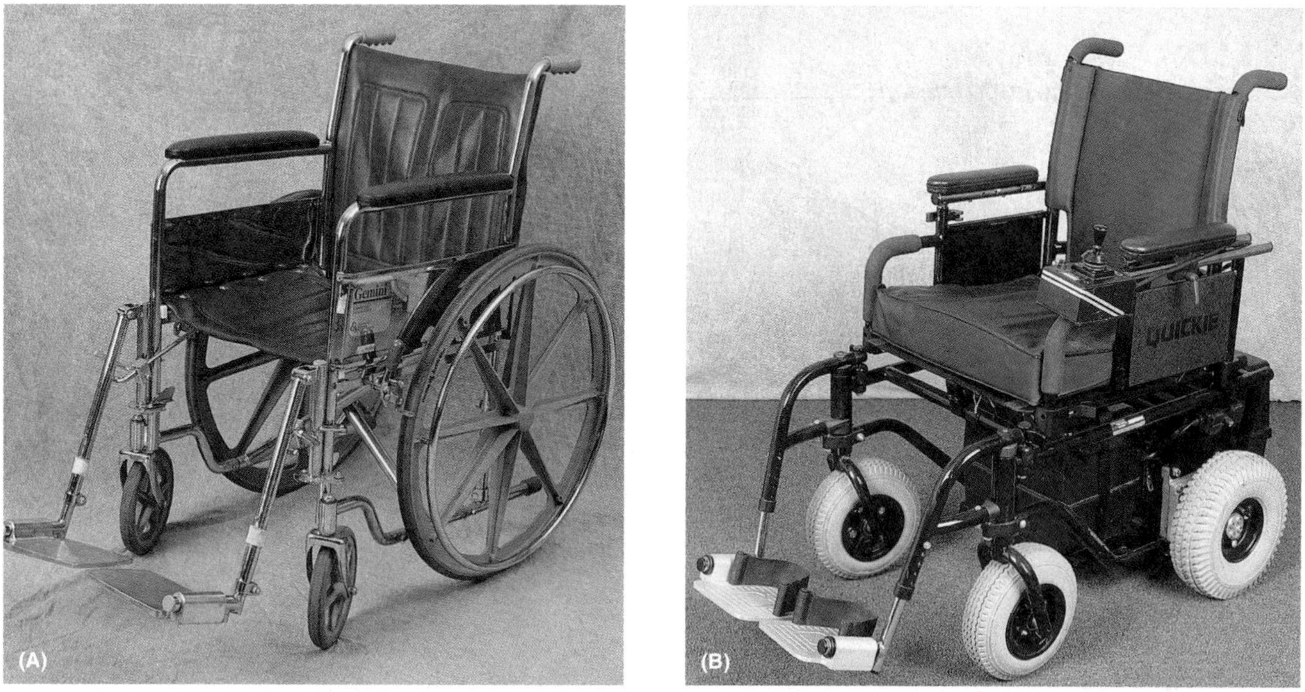

Figure 21-18 (A) A manual wheelchair. (B) A motorized wheelchair.

disability and lifestyle. There are even wheelchairs that enable patients to take part in sports activities. Many car manufacturers can modify a van to accommodate a wheelchair, and some are equipped to allow wheelchair patients to drive.

Patients who will be using a wheelchair for a long time are taught how to maintain it. Depending on their abilities, they check it regularly to make sure all the parts are working correctly, and, if they are able, to make any necessary repairs. Patients are taught to use the wheelchair safely and maneuver into and out of difficult spaces.

If a patient is being pushed by someone else, that individual must learn basic safety rules for transporting a patient:

- Make sure that the brakes are locked when transferring a patient into and out of a wheelchair, and if a patient must be left alone in the wheelchair for any length of time, lock the brakes.
- Make sure the patient's feet are placed on the footrests when the wheelchair is in use.
- Be certain the patient feels safe (Figure 21-19).
- Always back into and out of elevators.
- Stay to the right in corridors.
- Back down slanted ramps.

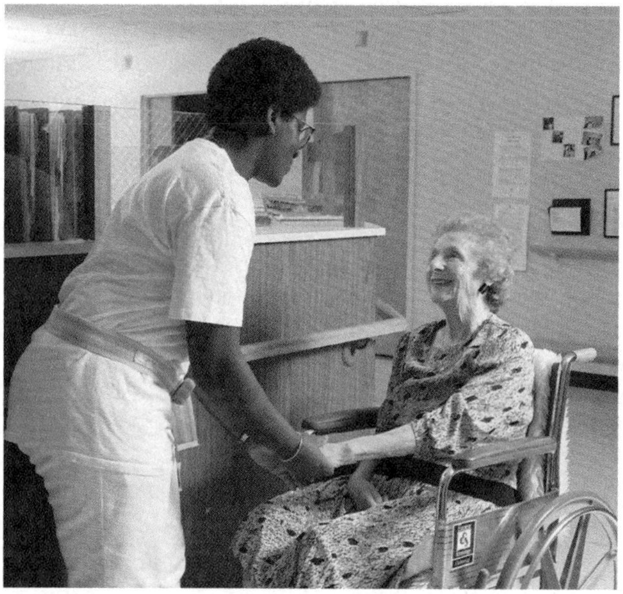

Figure 21-19 Be certain the patient feels safe.

THERAPEUTIC EXERCISES

Range of Motion

The musculoskeletal system is a complex joining of bones, joints, ligaments, and tendons. Not only does it give structure to the body and protect the body's vital organs, it allows for movement so we can carry out a multitude of activities.

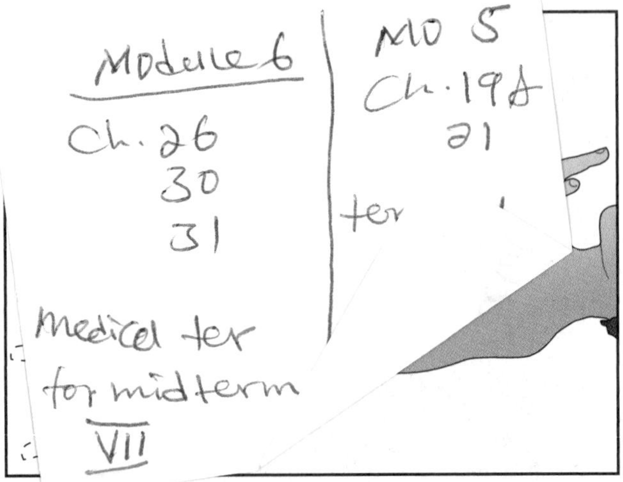

Figure 21-20 Joint mobility is measured against standard ranges of motion and is always expressed in degrees.

TABLE 21-3 TERMINOLOGY OF JOINT MOVEMENT	
Abduction	Motion away from the midline of the body
Adduction	Motion toward the midline of the body
Circumduction	Circular motion of a body part
Dorsiflexion	Moving the foot upward at the ankle joint
Eversion	Moving a body part outward
Extension	Straightening of a body part
Flexion	Bending of a body part
Hyperextension	A position of maximum extension, or extending a body part beyond its normal limits
Inversion	Moving a body part inward
Plantar Flexion	Moving the foot downward at the ankle
Pronation	Moving the arm so the palm is down
Rotation	Turning a body part around its axis
Supination	Moving the arm so the palm is up

The bones of almost all the joints of the body are designed to move as well, each joint having its own **range of motion (ROM).** ROM refers to the amount of movement that is present in a joint.

Normal ROM varies between people and depends on several factors, such as age, sex, and whether the motion being performed is passive (assisted motion) or active (voluntary motion). There is a standard ROM for all movable joints, and it is this standard that is used when evaluating the joint movement of a particular patient.

The measurement of joint motion is called **goniometry.** Joint movement is measured with an instrument called a **goniometer** and is always expressed in degrees. For example, the average person lying flat with arms to the sides can move the elbows from a 20-degree hyperextension (extending the arm beyond its normal limits) to 0-degree extension, through to 150 degrees of flexion, or bending (Figure 21-20).

ROM evaluation is one of several tools used when developing a therapeutic program for a patient.

As a medical assistant, you need to be familiar with ROM exercises. ROM exercises are designed to maintain joint mobility and are either performed passively (someone else does the movement) or actively (the patient does the movement).

Joint movement has a special vocabulary. It is helpful to learn the terms and their definitions, as shown in Table 21-3.

Before performing ROM exercises on a patient, the therapist will need to observe some general precautions:

- Always move the patient's limbs gently, within pain tolerance and the flexibility of the limb.
- Use slow, careful movements that allow the muscles time to adjust to the movement.
- Always support the limb above and below the joint.
- It is best to perform passive ROM with the patient in the supine position.
- ROM should never cause pain. If the patient reports pain at any time, the ROM exercises should be discontinued until a physician or other health care professional can determine the source of pain.
- Repeat each movement several times or as prescribed by the physician.

Muscle Testing

The other tool used for evaluating the movement abilities of a patient is muscle testing. Whereas goniometry focuses on joint movement, **muscle testing** evaluates the motion, strength, and task potential of a given muscle. *ROM* testing for muscles determines how flexible and resilient a muscle may be. *Strength testing* shows how hard a muscle can work. *Task potential* of a muscle means how well a muscle can aid in accomplishing a given activity. As a medical assistant, you may assist with testing the patient for joint mobility, posture, and strength of muscles.

Types of Therapeutic Exercise

Without constant exercise, the musculoskeletal system would deteriorate. Joints would become stiff and **contractures,** or deformities, could develop. Muscles would **atrophy,** or shrink and lose strength. Bones would lose vital minerals such as calcium and phosphorus. And the body's overall circulation would decrease, which would, in turn, create a separate set of unhealthy conditions.

Like drugs, exercise has a powerful and systemic effect on the body. It involves the function of joints, bones, muscles, nerves, tendons, ligaments, as well as the circulatory and respiratory systems. Therapeutic exercises are prescribed after careful evaluation by a trained specialist and are tailored to each patient depending on that patient's individual condition and rehabilitation goals. It is the role of the medical assistant to understand the goals and objectives of the therapeutic exercise program to better support and encourage patients to complete their program.

Whereas an athlete uses exercise to build strength and endurance to attain a certain level of performance, therapeutic exercises are prescribed for a variety of therapeutic and preventive effects. They are used most commonly for therapeutic reasons to correct or prevent deformities, regain body movement after an accident or disease, restore joint motion after immobility, improve neuromuscular coordination, and improve or develop ADLs.

Exercise is also used for another important reason: It can prevent many common problems brought on by inactivity, such as those problems associated with respiration and circulation.

A variety of exercise programs are used for therapeutic or preventive purposes:

1. *Active exercises*, which are self-directed and performed by the patient without assistance
2. *Passive exercises*, which are performed by another person with no voluntary participation from the patient
3. *Assisted exercises*, which help the patient voluntarily move weakened muscles with the use of an assistive device, such as a therapy pool
4. *Active resistance exercises*, which provide voluntary movement against various types of manual or mechanical pressure to increase muscle strength

Electromyography

Electrical activity of a muscle can be recorded on a graph or film to help to determine how well muscles contract. An electromyograph is the instrument used to test the electrical activity of a muscle. An electrode (using a small gauge needle) is inserted through skin into the muscle, and measurements can be made as to muscle strength.

Electrostimulation of Muscle

An electric current of low voltage can help to stimulate muscles to exercise by innervating the sensory and motor nerves for that muscle. It is helpful for a patient who has nerve damage to the muscle and cannot voluntarily move the muscle. The purpose is to prevent atrophy of the muscle and help to restore muscle function.

The low current of electricity passing through the patient's muscle acts similarly to the patient's own nerves causing the muscle to contract and relax. The stimulation is helpful to retrain a patient after experiencing an injury to a muscle or muscle group.

THERAPEUTIC MODALITIES

Sometimes, therapeutic exercise is not the best or only way to restore injured or painful joints and tissues. A patient's condition may respond equally well to certain physical agents, called **modalities,** which take advantage of the properties of heat, cold, electricity, light, and water to improve circulation, minimize pain, and correct or alleviate muscular and joint malfunction.

Many modalities have been around for centuries, and some can easily be performed by the patient or caregiver at home. Modalities can be used locally to treat a small area at a time or systemically to alter a patient's temperature or soothe many groups of painful muscles or joints. The patient's condition and rehabilitation program both influence the modality or combination of modalities used.

A physician's order is required for any therapeutic modality.

Heat and Cold

Heat, or **thermotherapy,** acts on the body by causing **vasodilation** (dilation of the blood vessels). The effect of heat increases circulation to an area and acts to speed up the repair process. Heat can be used to:

- Relax muscle spasms
- Relieve pain in a strained muscle or sprained joint
- Relieve localized congestion and swelling
- Increase drainage from an infected area
- Increase tissue metabolism and repair

However, because heat dilates the blood vessels and increases circulation, it also acts to speed up the inflammatory process, which can lead to more serious problems, such as increased bleeding and swelling. Heat should not be used longer than its prescribed length of time.

Cold applications, or **cryotherapy,** are used to constrict blood vessels and slow or stop the flow of blood to an area. This process, also called **vasoconstriction,** slows down the inflammatory process, which can reduce or prevent swelling of inflamed tissues, reduce bleeding, numb the pain sensation by acting as a topical anesthetic, and reduce drainage to an area.

By understanding how heat and cold affects the body, it is easier to observe whether they are having the desired therapeutic effect. Heat and cold modalities can be extremely effective, which is why they are so widely used for treating certain physical conditions. However, the effects of heat and cold modalities depend on several conditions: the type of modality used, the length of time it is applied, the patient's condition, and the area or areas being treated.

Precautions for Heat and Cold Applications. When applying either heat or cold modalities, you need to take certain precautions to avoid injury. If misused, any therapeutic modality can actually cause more damage to the site it is trying to heal. Before starting any treatment, keep the following precautions in mind:

- Infants and patients who cannot report a burning sensation should be watched carefully. Infants and older adults are particularly susceptible to burns.
- Heat and cold sensitivity varies with the patient; check patients frequently and never leave them alone.
- Never have a patient lie on a heating pad, because severe burning can result. Place a rubber cover over the heating pad if using with moist dressings.
- Always wrap appliances with cloth before applying them to the skin.
- Only soak or immerse patients in water between 104°F and 113°F (40–45°C). Temperatures of 116°F (47°C) or greater can cause burning.
- Never use heat within the first 48 hours of an acute inflammatory process and never apply heat to newly burned skin.
- Watch carefully persons with impaired circulation; cardiovascular, renal, sensorineural, or respiratory conditions; or osteoporosis.
- Lack of sensation to a therapy may mean impaired circulation to an area and the patient may be unable to report a burning sensation.
- As heat concentrates in metal materials, have patients remove all jewelry and other metal objects and administer the treatment on nonmetal tables and chairs.

Moist and Dry Heat Modalities

Moist Heat Therapies. Moist heat refers to heat modalities that feel moist against the skin. Moist heat penetrates better than dry heat and aids in improving circulation, relaxation, and mobility.

Hot Soaks. Hot soaks are generally used for soaking the extremities and can be administered easily at home by the patient or caregiver. The patient's body part is gradually immersed in plain or medicated water no hotter than 110°F (44°C) for a short time, usually no more than about 15 minutes. The patient should be positioned to be comfortable. Observe the patient's skin for excessive redness and, if noticed, remove the limb at once. Always dry the skin carefully by patting, not rubbing, it.

Total body immersion in hot water can be administered in a whirlpool bath or special Hubbard tank. This treatment is often prescribed to promote relaxation, circulation, and movement of limbs in preparation for exercise. The mechanical action of agitating water moving over the body in a whirlpool is called hydromassage and can both relax muscles and stimulate circulation. The Hubbard tank is a bit larger and provides room for limited body exercise without the effects of gravity.

Hot Compresses and Packs. A hot compress is usually applied to a small area, and is prepared by soaking and wringing out either a square of gauze or other absorbent material (such as a clean washcloth) and applying it for a limited time to the affected area (Figure 21-21). Hot compresses can be administered easily at home. A hot pack is used for a larger area and generally involves the use of a professional hot pack administered in the clinical setting. This type of hot pack is soaked in hot water, removed with tongs and drained, and placed over larger areas such as the back or shoulders.

Paraffin Wax Bath. This type of treatment is most often used for chronic joint disease, such as rheumatoid arthritis. The bath mixture of seven parts paraffin to one part mineral oil is heated to melting (about 127°F) and the body part is dipped in the mixture several times until a thick coat of wax builds up. The body part is then wrapped

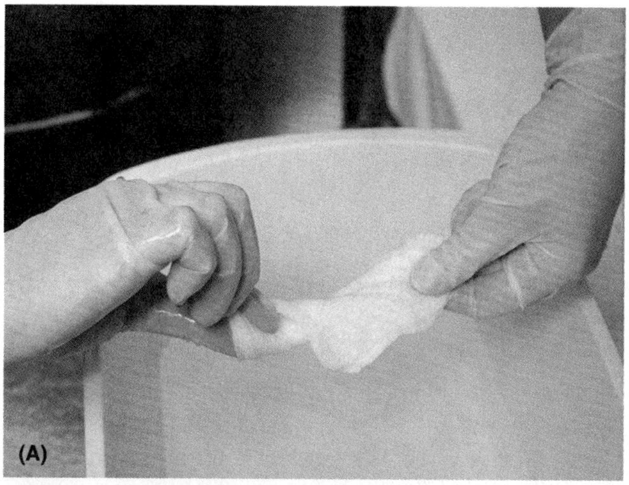

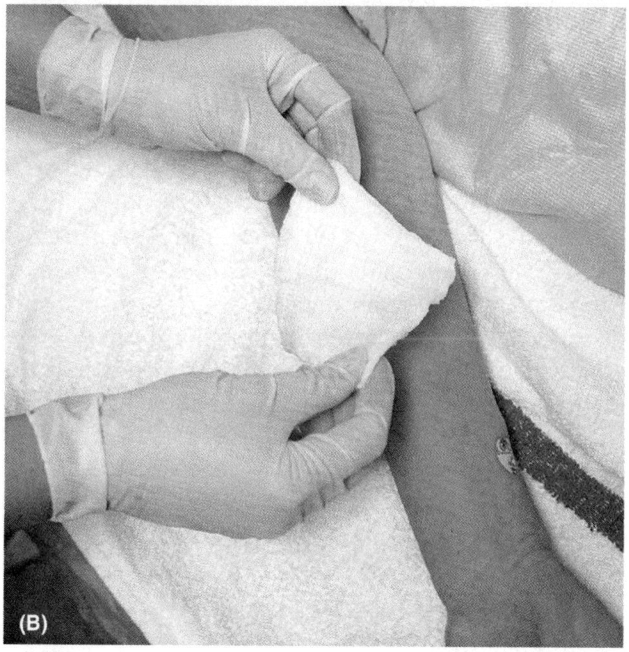

Figure 21-21 (A) Dip hot compresses frequently into a basin of hot water to keep them warm. (B) Apply compresses directly to the skin. Note: Limb will be wrapped in a towel that will then be covered with a blue plastic wrap. This helps keep the compress hot.

in foil, cloth, or plastic wrap to help insulate the heat, then left on for 30 minutes or less. Once peeled off, the circulatory effects of this treatment can last up to several hours. It is an excellent modality for warming up joints before ROM or other exercises. This modality, ordered by a physician, will be carried out in the physical therapy department by a professional therapist.

Dry Heat Therapies. Dry heat applications feel dry against the skin and do not penetrate like moist heat. They are used more to improve circulation for the purposes of relieving swelling and healing wounds, as well as to relax muscles and reduce muscle spasms. Most dry heat modalities can also be performed easily by the patient or caregiver at home.

Heating Pads and Packs. Heating pads and commercially prepared packs are used for smaller areas and should always be covered with a cloth before applying against the skin. Never let a patient lie directly on a heating pad, because burns can result. Set the switch on the heating pad to a low or medium setting and observe the proper time of exposure.

An Aquamatic K-Pad® is a commercial pad that is safer to use than a heating pad or commercially prepared packs because you can maintain a constant temperature and regulate that temperature more carefully. It is a pad with tubes that are filled with distilled water and heated by a control unit. The pad must be covered and left on the patient for no more than about 30 minutes.

Moist and Dry Cold Modalities

Moist Cold Therapies. Moist cold therapies refer to cold modalities that feel moist against the skin. Moist cold, as with moist heat, penetrates better than dry cold and is used to prevent swelling or edema, relieve pain or tenderness, and reduce body temperature. Most cold therapies can be performed easily at home by the patient or caregiver.

Cold Compresses and Packs. Cold compresses are used for smaller areas, and cold packs are used for larger areas. For a cold compress, immerse the cold cloth, gauze, or other clean material in a basin filled with ice and cold water. Wring out the cloth and apply it to the affected area. Keep the cloth cold by immersing it several times throughout the treatment. Cold or ice packs are administered in the same manner.

Dry Cold Therapies. Dry cold treatments are used for all the same reasons as a moist cold treatment but are better for bleeding and acute injuries. Dry cold is also an excellent therapy for sprains, strains, burns, or bruises.

The temperature used depends on the area being treated and the method used, as well as the patient's tolerance for cold temperatures. In general, the colder the temperature, the shorter the duration of exposure.

Ice Packs. Dry cold treatments include ice packs and commercially prepared chemical ice packs. Always cover the pack with cloth before applying it to the skin (Figure 21-22). Generally, ice packs can be kept on the body longer than heat packs, about 30 minutes. See also Chapter 9. A commercial ice pack can be used for smaller areas

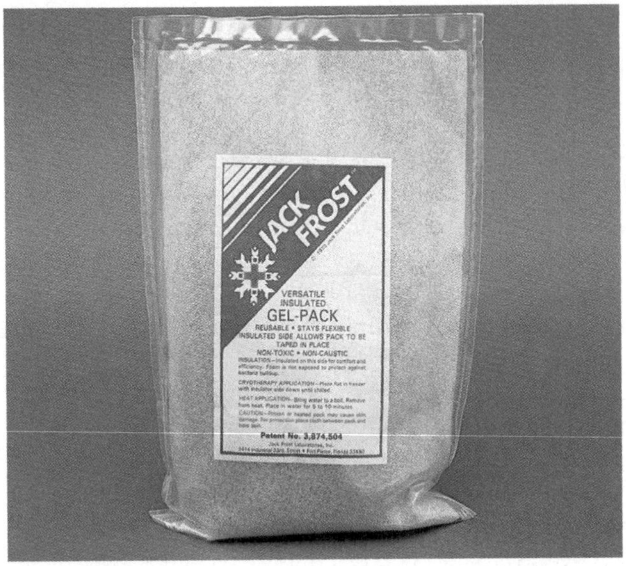

Figure 21-22 A chemical ice pack. These should be covered with a cloth before applying to the skin.

Critical Thinking

How do heat and cold affect the body's physiology and for what conditions should each be used?

and can usually be chilled in the freezer. Because they do not freeze and become solid, these ice packs are pliable, making them ideal for contouring to the body part being treated.

Deep-Tissue Modalities

Ultrasound. **Ultrasound** is a high-frequency acoustic vibration that is part of the electromagnetic spectrum, and its frequencies are beyond the perception of the human ear. This type of treatment uses high-frequency sound waves that are converted to heat in the deeper tissues.

Ultrasound is an effective form of treatment for chronic pain or acute injuries such as sprains or strains.

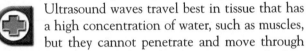

Patient Education

Neither heat nor cold applications should be left on the skin for prolonged periods, because both can have counterproductive effects if not monitored carefully. When applying heat or cold, periodically check the skin for signs of paleness or redness. If the patient experiences any tingling reaction, discontinue the application. Report the observations, and document.

It relaxes muscle spasms, increases the elasticity of tissue such as tendons and ligaments, and stimulates circulation, which, in turn, speeds up the healing process.

Ultrasound waves travel best in tissue that has a high concentration of water, such as muscles, but they cannot penetrate and move through tissue such as bone that has a low water content. In fact, ultrasound treatment must be used carefully near bones, particularly those near the surface, because their waves are capable of concentrating in one area and causing damage.

Because ultrasound waves cannot be conducted through air, a special gel is applied to the skin surface that acts as a conduit. The sound waves are generated through an applicator that is rubbed over the gel. This applicator must be kept moving to prevent any internal damage caused by too high a concentration of sound waves. The duration of treatment lasts anywhere from 5 to 15 minutes, depending on the condition being treated and the recommendation of the physician or other health care provider. It is important to note that, because of its potential dangers, ultrasound treatment should only be administered if the medical assistant or other caregiver is specially trained in its safe and effective use.

Procedure 21-1 Transferring Patient from Wheelchair to Examination Table

STANDARD PRECAUTIONS:

PURPOSE:

To move a patient safely from a wheelchair to the examination table.

EQUIPMENT/SUPPLIES:

Stool with rubber tips and a handle for gripping
Gait belt

PROCEDURE STEPS:

1. Wash hands.
2. Identify the patient and introduce yourself. Explain to the patient what you are going to do.
3. Place the wheelchair next to the examination table and lock the brakes. **CAUTION:** The side nearest the examination table should be the patient's stronger side to allow the patient to balance on that leg during the transfer.
4. Place the gait belt snugly around the patient's waist and tuck the excess end under the belt (Figure 21-23A).
5. Move the footrests up and out of the way. Have the patient place feet on the floor. Newer wheelchairs have removable footrests. Taking them off enables you to put the wheelchair closer to the examination table. There is also less chance of being bumped or bruised by the wheelchair.
6. Position the stool in front of the examination table as close to the wheelchair as possible (Figure 21-23B).
7. Have the patient move to the edge of the wheelchair.
8. Stand directly in front of the patient with your feet slightly apart. Bending at the hips and knees, grasp the gait belt and have the patient place his or her hands on the armrests of the wheelchair so he or she can push up when you give the signal (Figure 21-23C). If the patient does not have

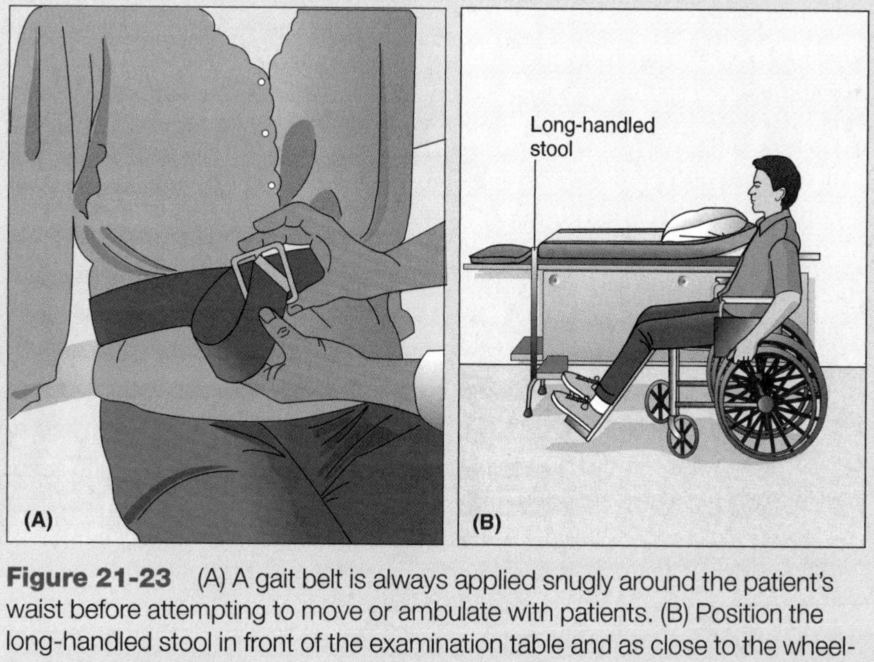

Figure 21-23 (A) A gait belt is always applied snugly around the patient's waist before attempting to move or ambulate with patients. (B) Position the long-handled stool in front of the examination table and as close to the wheelchair as possible.

(continues)

(continues)

Procedure 21-1 (continued)

the upper body strength to push off, simply let his or her arms rest in front of him or her.

9. Give a signal and lift the gait belt upward, pushing with your knees. If the patient has the strength in his or her legs, he or she should push with his or her legs in addition to pushing up with his or her arms.
10. Still grasping the gait belt, have the patient step onto the stool with the foot closest to the examination table, and pivot so his or her back is to the examination table (Figure 21-23D). Make sure the buttocks are lifted slightly higher than the bed. Support the patient's weaker, outer leg with your leg furthest from the examination table.
11. Have the patient grasp the stool handle and place his or her other hand on the examination table.
12. Gently ease the patient to a sitting position on the examination table.
13. Position the patient on the examination table as necessary.
14. Move the wheelchair and stool out of the way.

Modification: Two-Person Transfer

1. Place the gait belt snugly around the patient's waist and tuck the excess end under the belt.
2. Have one person stand in front of the patient and the other to the side, next to the examination table.
3. Both persons should grasp the gait belt from underneath. Have the patient place his or her hands on the armrests of the wheelchair.
4. On one person's signal, both persons pull the patient straight up. The patient should also push up with his or her hands, but if he or she does not have the upper body strength to push off, simply let his or her arms rest in front of him or her (Figure 21-24).
5. The person nearest the examination table moves the wheelchair out of the way, whereas the other pivots the patient and has the patient place his or her stronger leg on the stool. If the patient has the upper body strength, he or she should also grasp the handle of the stool.
6. On one person's signal, both persons lift the patient onto the examination table.
7. Position the patient on the examination table as necessary.

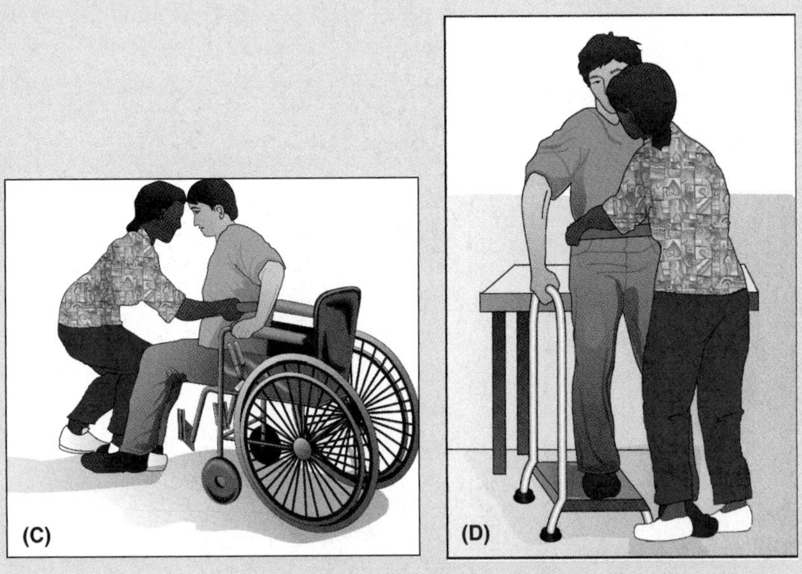

Figure 21-23 (C) Before lifting, observe proper body mechanics to avoid injuring yourself or the patient. (D) Check that the patient's foot is firmly placed on the stool before completing the transfer.

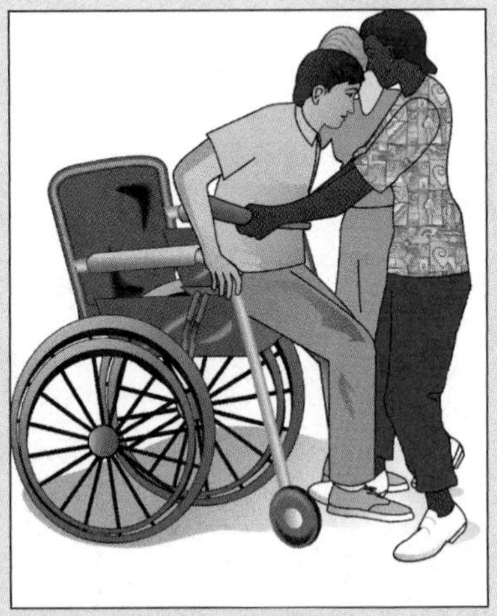

Figure 21-24 A two-person transfer when the patient does not have the upper body strength to help move himself or herself.

Procedure 21-2 Transferring Patient from Examination Table to Wheelchair

STANDARD PRECAUTIONS:

PURPOSE:
To move a patient safely from the examination table to a wheelchair.

EQUIPMENT/SUPPLIES:
Stool with rubber tips and a handle for gripping
Gait belt

PROCEDURE STEPS:
1. Wash hands.
2. Identify the patient and introduce yourself. Explain to the patient what you are going to do.
3. Position the wheelchair next to the examination table and lock the brakes. NOTE: Place the wheelchair so it is closest to the patient's stronger side so the patient can transfer his or her weight onto the stronger foot as he or she gets down.
4. Position the stool next to the wheelchair.
5. Assist the patient to rise to a sitting position. Place the gait belt snugly around the patient's waist and tuck the excess end under the belt.
6. Place your arm under the patient's arm and around his or her shoulders, and your other arm under his or her knees. Pivot the patient so his or her legs are dangling over the side of the examination table.
7. Keeping a hand on the patient, move so you are directly in front of him or her.
8. Grasp the patient by placing your hands under the gait belt. Plant your feet shoulder's width apart and bend your knees so you will have a strong base of support.
9. On your signal, pull the patient slightly toward you so his or her feet come down onto the stool. The patient should push off the examination table and grasp the stool handle for support.
10. Still grasping the gait belt, have the patient step onto the floor with his or her strong leg, and pivot at the same time so his or her back is to the wheelchair.
11. Have the patient grasp the armrests of the wheelchair.
12. Bending from your knees and hips, gently lower the patient into the wheelchair and make sure he or she is comfortably seated.
13. Lower the footrests and place his or her feet on them.

Procedure 21-3 Assisting the Patient to Stand and Walk

STANDARD PRECAUTIONS:

PURPOSE:
To help a patient ambulate safely.

EQUIPMENT/SUPPLIES:
Gait belt

PROCEDURE STEPS:
1. Wash hands.
2. Identify the patient and introduce yourself. Explain to the patient what you are going to do.
3. Lock the brakes on the wheelchair, if the patient is using one. Place the patient's feet on the floor and move the foot plates out of the way.
4. Instruct the patient to slide forward in the chair.

(continues)

Procedure 21-3 (continued)

5. Place the gait belt around the patient's waist and tuck the excess end under the belt.
6. Standing directly in front of the patient, grasp the gait belt from underneath and assist him or her to stand on your signal. At the same time, have the patient push up on the armrests of the wheelchair.
7. Steady the patient momentarily and watch for balance, strength, and skin color. If necessary, take his or her pulse.
8. If the patient appears steady and has balance, strength, and good skin color, proceed by standing slightly behind and to the side of the patient's weaker side.
9. Grasp the gait belt with one hand and place the other hand on the patient's bent arm for support. Note the gait belt is grasped with your fingers under the belt, palm up and elbow bent (Figure 21-25).
10. Start with the same foot as the patient and keep in step with him or her.
11. Document the procedure including date, time, duration of ambulation, response of patient, and instructions given.

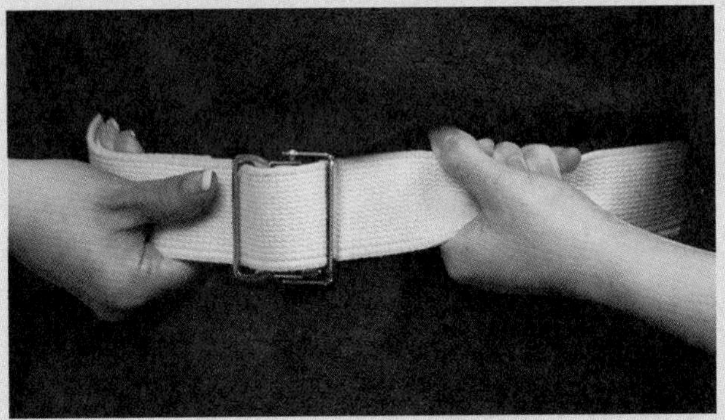

Figure 21-25 Firmly grasp the gait belt from underneath, with the palm up and elbow bent.

Modification: Two-Person Assist with Ambulation

1. Perform the preceding Steps 1 through 5.
2. Have a person stand on either side of the patient. Grasp the gait belt from underneath with one hand, and place the other hand on the patient's back for support.
3. During ambulation, there should be a person on either side of the patient and slightly behind (Figure 21-26). Both persons should be grasping the gait belt throughout the ambulation session.
4. Document the procedure including date, time, duration of ambulation, response of patient, and instructions given.

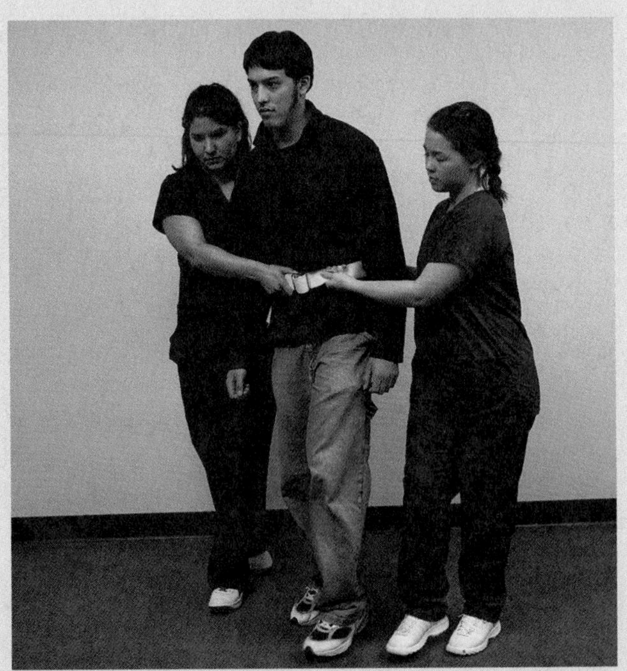

Figure 21-26 When two persons are assisting with ambulation, have them stand on either side of the patient.

DOCUMENTATION

7/14/20XX 2:30 PM Patient states she has been doing "fairly well" in physical therapy. She says she walks short distances, about 10 feet. Assisted with ambulation. Seems steady on her feet. Says she feels "very good." W. Slawson, CMA

DOCUMENTATION

7/14/20XX 2:30 PM Patient has been to physical therapy a total of 15 times. Dr. Woo wants patient to ambulate to see her progress. Assisted patient to ambulate with another person assisting. Did very well. Walked about 100 feet. Color remained good. P 100. B. Beckus, RMA

Procedure 21-4 Care of the Falling Patient

PURPOSE:
To help the patient fall safely to avoid injury.

EQUIPMENT/SUPPLIES:
Gait belt (should already be on patient)

PROCEDURE STEPS:

1. Keep a firm hand on the gait belt. **CAUTION:** Never grab clothing, because it can shift and become unstable.
2. If the patient falls backward, widen your stance to become a more stable base of support for him or her to fall against (Figure 21-27). Gently guide the patient to the floor, call for assistance, and take his or her pulse.
3. If the patient falls to either side, steady him or her back onto his or her feet. To do this, you will need to move your foot in the direction he or she is falling. Inquire whether the patient would like to terminate the ambulation session and check for signs of fatigue. If necessary, call for assistance. Check blood pressure and pulse.
4. Should the patient fall forward, support him or her around the waist. Step forward with your outer leg and gently lower him or her to the floor, making sure to protect him or her from injury (Figure 21-28). Call for assistance and take blood pressure and pulse.
5. Have the patient examined by a doctor before moving him or her again.
6. Document the fall in an incident report.

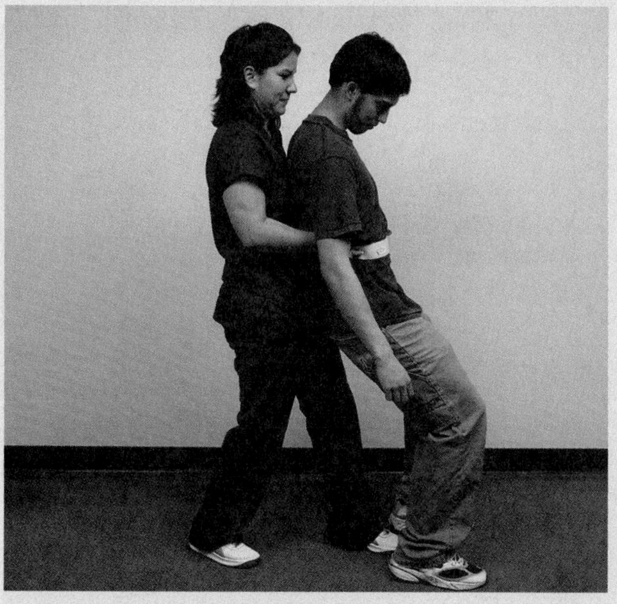

Figure 21-27 Support a falling patient with a wide base of support.

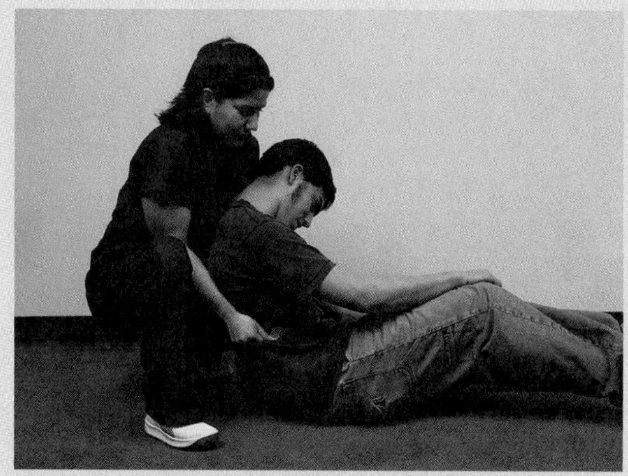

Figure 21-28 Ease the falling patient to the floor and try to protect the head.

DOCUMENTATION

1/21/20XX 11:30 AM Patient walking to exam room with assistance. Suddenly began to fall forward with knees buckling. Says she feels "faint." Eased to the floor gently. Did not strike any body parts during fall. BP 110/60, P 108 (lying on floor). BP and pulse rechecked when patient placed in wheelchair. BP 120/78, P 92. Dr. King notified. B. Abbott, RMA

Procedure 21-5 Assisting a Patient to Ambulate with a Walker

STANDARD PRECAUTIONS:

PURPOSE:

To allow a patient to ambulate independently and safely with a walker.

EQUIPMENT/SUPPLIES:

Walker
Gait belt

PROCEDURE STEPS:

1. Wash hands.
2. Identify the patient and introduce yourself. Explain to the patient what you are going to do.
3. Apply the gait belt snugly around the patient's waist and tuck the excess end under the belt.
4. Check the walker to be sure the rubber suction tips are secure on all the legs. Check the handrests for rough or damaged edges that could cut or pinch the patient. The adjustments should be tightened so they will not slip.
5. Be sure the patient is wearing good walking shoes with a rubber sole.
6. Check the height of the walker. The handrests should be level with the tip of the patient's femur, and the elbows should be flexed at a 30-degree angle.
7. Position the patient inside the walker, and instruct the patient to hold onto the handles while keeping the walker in front of him or her.
8. Position yourself behind and slightly to the side of the patient.
9. Have the patient lift the walker and place all four legs of the walker in front of him or her so the back legs are even with the patient's toes.
10. Instruct the patient to lean forward and transfer his or her weight so that he or she steps into the walker, first with his or her stronger leg, then the weaker leg. Make sure he or she brings his or her stronger leg past the weaker leg.
11. Monitor the patient carefully. Be alert for signs of fatigue and be ready to catch the patient if he or she should fall.
12. If the walker has rollers, the patient simply rolls the walker ahead a comfortable distance, then walks into it. The patient can also walk normally with a rolling walker by simply rolling it in front and leaning into the gait, using the walker for support.
13. Document the date, time, duration of ambulation, response of patient, and instructions given.

DOCUMENTATION

2/12/20XX 1:35 PM Patient assisted with ambulation using a walker for the first time after surgery. Did well. Walked to reception desk and back. No change in color. P 100. J. Guerro, CMA

Procedure 21-6 Teaching the Patient to Ambulate with Crutches

STANDARD PRECAUTIONS:

PURPOSE:
To teach the patient how to ambulate safely using crutches.

EQUIPMENT/SUPPLIES:
Crutches
Gait belt

PROCEDURE STEPS:

1. Wash hands.
2. Identify the patient and introduce yourself. Explain to the patient what you are going to do.
3. Assemble the crutches and be sure they are in good working order. Make sure there are rubber suction tips on the bottom ends, and that they are not worn or torn. Check the bar and handrest to be sure they are covered with padding, and that the padding is not cracked or worn. Be sure the wing nuts are tight.
4. Check the measurement of the crutches. Pediatric crutches must be used for pediatric patients.
5. Apply the gait belt and assist the patient to stand and place the crutches under the armpits.
6. Instruct the patient to carry his or her weight completely on his or her hands and not on his or her armpits.
7. Have the patient put all his or her weight on his or her good leg, and bend the weak leg slightly so it will not drag on the floor as he or she walks.
8. Assist the patient with the required gait.
9. Wash hands.
10. Document the date, time, duration of ambulation, and instructions given.

DOCUMENTATION

3/24/20XX 4:45 PM Crutches adjusted to patient's height. Three-point gait used. Tolerated well. J. Guerro, CMA

Procedure 21-7 Assisting a Patient to Ambulate with a Cane

STANDARD PRECAUTIONS:

PURPOSE:
To teach patients how to walk safely with a cane.

EQUIPMENT/SUPPLIES:
Appropriate cane for patient
Gait belt

PROCEDURE STEPS:

1. Wash hands.
2. Ascertain what type of cane the physician or therapist indicates your patient is to be using and assemble the equipment.
3. Identify the patient and introduce yourself. Explain to the patient what you are going to do.
4. Check the cane to be sure the bottom has a rubber suction tip. If a quad or walkcane is to be used, make sure all the legs have rubber suction tips.

(continues)

Procedure 21-7 (continued)

5. Apply the gait belt snugly around the patient's waist if needed and tuck the excess end under the belt. Assist the patient to a standing position.
6. Place the cane relatively close to the body to the side of the foot of the strong leg. Adjust the cane so the handle is at the level of the patient's hip joint (Figure 21-29).
7. During weightbearing, the patient's elbow should be flexed 20- to 30-degrees.
8. The cane and the involved leg are advanced simultaneously.
9. Have the patient move the weak leg forward while transferring the weight to the cane.
10. Have the patient move the strong leg forward past the cane.
11. Follow along behind and to the side of the patient's weak side.
12. Wash your hands.
13. Document the date, time, duration of ambulation, response of patient, and instructions given.

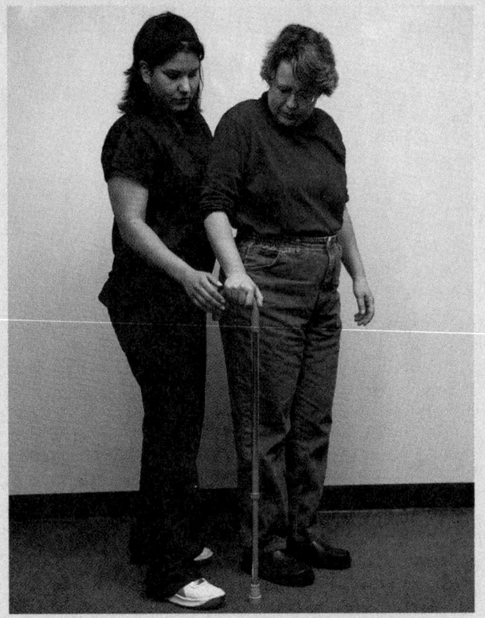

Figure 21-29 In placing the cane, be sure the handle comes to the top of the patient's hip and elbow is flexed 20 to 30 degrees.

DOCUMENTATION

4/17/20XX 10:30 AM Standard cane adjusted to patient's hip joint. Ambulated about 100 yards and seemed to tolerate it well. W. Slawson, CMA

Case Study 21-1

It is a mild summer afternoon in the city of Carlton, the home of Inner City Health Care. The softball season is in full swing, and Inner City has treated its share of players and spectators who have had minor injuries. On this particular Tuesday, Bill Schwarz, a regular patient, comes in late in the day in obvious pain. Bruce Goldman, the clinical medical assistant on duty, quickly gets the patient into a wheelchair. From the patient's description of the situation and the pain, Bruce suspects a sprained ankle. Dr. Woo is on call and available to examine the patient immediately and asks Bruce to transfer Bill from the wheelchair to the examination table.

CASE STUDY REVIEW

1. What are some of the general principles the medical assistant should observe during any transfer?
2. Summarize the steps involved in transferring the patient from the wheelchair to the examination table.
3. Summarize the steps involved in transferring the patient from the examination table to the wheelchair.

Case Study 21-2

After diagnosing Mr. Schwarz with a sprained left ankle, Dr. Woo has prescribed an Ace bandage to the ankle, crutches, and an ice pack to be applied to the ankle. He has also given Mr. Schwarz a prescription for pain relievers and has recommended that Mr. Schwarz stay off his feet as much as possible. He is to keep the leg elevated with an ice pack on it.

CASE STUDY REVIEW

1. Explain what you would tell Mr. Schwarz about applying the ice pack to his ankle at home.

SUMMARY

Rehabilitation medicine is a field of medical disciplines that specializes in both preventing disease or injury and restoring physical function. It uses a combination of physical and mechanical agents to aid in the diagnosis, treatment, and prevention of diseases or bodily injury, including exercise and a variety of treatment modalities.

Much of what a medical assistant might do on the job in this field involves some form of lifting or moving of heavy objects. It is important to remember to use good body mechanics to prevent back or other injury. When transferring patients, good body mechanics ensures the safety of both caregiver and patient. If necessary, get someone to help with the transfer.

Helping the patient to ambulate safely after a period of sedentary recuperation is an important part of a rehabilitation program. If they are not able to ambulate on their own, patients can be fitted for a variety of assistive walking devices, including walkers, crutches, and canes. Crutch walking, by far the most common use of an assistive device, can be done using one of several walking patterns, or gaits, depending on the patient's condition, strength, and stability. Whatever assistive device is used, it is important that the patient be measured correctly for that device and taught how to periodically check it for safety.

In addition to ambulation, there are a number of other types of therapeutic exercises. Depending on the patient's condition, an exercise program can be prescribed after evaluating the patient's joint ROM and muscle strength. Joints and muscles must be exercised regularly to avoid muscle atrophy or joint contractures, as well as improve circulation and maintain or improve overall health. ROM and other exercises can be performed either by the caregiver, the patient, or a combination of the two.

In addition to exercise, a variety of therapeutic modalities might also be used as part of the patient's rehabilitation program. The various properties of heat, cold, light, electricity, and water act on the body to improve circulation, minimize pain, or correct or alleviate joint and muscle malfunction. Heat dilates the blood vessels, thereby increasing circulation to an area

(continues)

SUMMARY (continued)

and speeding up the repair process. Cold constricts the blood vessels, slowing circulation and therefore the inflammatory process. Ultrasound and other electrical diathermies use an electrical current to create heat in the deeper tissues of the body. It is important to understand how each modality affects the physiologic functioning of the body and observe certain safety precautions to avoid injuring the patient.

STUDY FOR SUCCESS

To reinforce your knowledge and skills of information presented in this chapter:

- ❑ Review the Key Terms
- ❑ Practice the Procedures
- ❑ Consider the Case Studies and discuss your conclusions
- ❑ Answer the Review Questions
  - ❑ Multiple Choice
  - ❑ Critical Thinking
- ❑ Navigate the Internet by completing the Web Activities
- ❑ Practice the StudyWARE activities on your student CD
- ❑ Apply your knowledge in the Student Workbook activities
- ❑ Complete the Web Tutor sections
- ❑ View and discuss the DVD situations

REVIEW QUESTIONS

Multiple Choice

1. Brushing teeth, getting dressed, and eating are referred to as:
   a. rehabilitation medicine
   b. activities of daily living
   c. body mechanics
   d. occupational therapy
2. Hemiplegia is defined as:
   a. inability of the patient to ambulate properly
   b. severe back pain
   c. paralysis of one side of the body
   d. confinement to a wheelchair
3. Ambulatory assistive devices include:
   a. gait belts
   b. walkers, canes, and crutches
   c. wheelchairs
   d. stools with handholds
4. Motion away from the midline of the body is called:
   a. adduction
   b. pronation
   c. extension
   d. abduction
5. Supination involves:
   a. placing the patient in the supine position
   b. moving the arm so the palm is up
   c. bending a body part
   d. straightening a body part

Critical Thinking

1. Define rehabilitation and explain its importance in patient care.
2. If a patient should fall to the side, what action would you take to ensure safety?
3. Describe the procedure for measuring for axillary crutches.
4. What kind of patient would need a forearm crutch?
5. In crutch-walking gaits, what is a *point*?
6. Describe the five different types of crutch gaits.
7. List the six safety rules for transporting a patient in a wheelchair.
8. What is joint range of motion, how is it measured, and how is the measurement expressed?
9. Describe how ultrasound works and identify the patient conditions for which it is an effective treatment.

WEB ACTIVITIES

Access information online about the Americans with Disabilities Act of 1990.

1. To what group of people does the act apply?
2. What does the act provide for these individuals?
3. Does the act have any influence over access to physicians' offices and clinics? Explain.

REFERENCES/BIBLIOGRAPHY

Hegner, B., & Caldwell, E. (2004). *Nursing assistant: A nursing process approach* (9th ed.). Clifton Park, NY: Thomson Delmar Learning.

Norkin, C. C., & White, D. J. (1995). *Measurement of joint motion: A guide to goniometry* (2nd ed.). Philadelphia: FA Davis.

O'Sullivan, S. B., & Schmitz, T. (2000). *Physical rehabilitation: Assessment and treatment* (4th ed.). Philadelphia: FA Davis.

Taber's cyclopedic medical dictionary. (22nd ed.). (2003). Philadelphia: FA Davis.

Weiss, R. C. (1999). *The physical therapy aide: A work text*. Clifton Park, NY: Thomson Delmar Learning.

THE DVD HOOK-UP

DVD Series	Program Number
Skills Based Series	**7**

Chapter/Scene Reference
- *Entire program*

This chapter discusses the medical assistant's role in assisting with various types of modalities and rehabilitation therapy.

In the first scene of this program, Carla, the medical assistant, helped Jerry through the door. She noticed that Jerry was having a difficult time maneuvering the crutches and the door at the same time, so she took that opportunity to conduct some patient education.

1. Do you think that Carla should have waited until the patient was in the examination room to instruct the patient? Why or why not?
2. In general, what is the public's attitude about rehabilitative therapy?
3. Why does the patient start with the weak leg first, when using a cane or walker?

DVD Journal Summary

Write a paragraph that summarizes what you learned from watching today's DVD program. Many times when a patient has an injury to an extremity, it prohibits him or her from being able to shower properly. What will you do if another coworker starts talking to you about the way a patient looks or smells?

CHAPTER 22

Nutrition in Health and Disease

OUTLINE

OBJECTIVES

The student should strive to meet the following performance objectives and demonstrate an understanding of the facts and principles presented in this chapter through written and oral communication.

1. Define the key terms as presented in the glossary.
2. Describe the relation of nutrition to the functioning of the digestive system.
3. Identify the seven basic nutrient types.
4. Explain the relation and balance among the three energy nutrients.
5. Distinguish between water-soluble and fat-soluble vitamins.
6. Discuss herbal supplements.
7. Explain the reason for nutrition labels on food packaging.
8. Read and interpret nutrition facts and ingredients on three food packages.
9. Discuss various therapeutic diets, and explain how each can help to control a particular disease state or accommodate a change in the life cycle.

KEY TERMS

Amino Acid
Antioxidant
Ascorbic Acid
Basal Metabolic Rate (BMR)
Beriberi
Calorie
Carotene
Catalyst
Cellulose
Cheilosis
Cholecalciferol
Cobalamin
Coenzyme
Digestion
Diuretic
Electrolytes
Extracellular
Fat-Soluble
Folic Acid
Glycogen
Homeostasis
Major Mineral
Metabolism
Niacin
Nutrient
Nutrition
Oxidation
Pellagra
Preservative
Processed Food
Pyridoxine
Riboflavin
Saturated Fat
Scurvy
Thiamin
Tocopherol
Trace Mineral
Water-Soluble
Xerophthalmia

FEATURED COMPETENCIES

CAAHEP—ENTRY-LEVEL COMPETENCIES

Patient Instruction

- Provide instruction for health maintenance and disease prevention

ABHES—ENTRY-LEVEL COMPETENCIES

Instruction

- Teach patients methods of health promotion and disease prevention

SCENARIO

This morning at Inner City Health Care, clinical medical assistant Wanda Slawson, CMA, was conferring with Dr. Rice on three of the center's patients whose diets needed modification. With the help of Dr. Rice, Wanda was putting together dietary plans for patients Edith Leonard, who is in her early 70s and is losing weight because she is not eating well enough or often enough; Corey Boyer, who is in the prime of adolescence and capable of eating large quantities of food with little nutritional value; and Annette Samuels, who recently discovered she was pregnant. All these patients have different nutritional requirements, and Wanda wants to encourage all to review and modify their diets.

INTRODUCTION

The human body is in a constant state of fluctuation. The outside environment is constantly changing, and the body requires ***homeostasis,*** *or a continual internal environment, which, in turn, gives us a requirement for nutrients. The nutrients we take into our bodies replenish the materials we have used. In this way, homeostasis is maintained, and our bodies have a relatively balanced internal environment.* ***Nutrition*** *is the study of the taking of nutrients into the body and how the body uses them.*

The normal healthy individual will consume and use close to what the body needs to stay healthy. However, some individuals either do not consume enough nutrients or consume too much of a particular type of nutrient. These are poor diets that can cause particular disease states, and the diet must be modified to return the patient to good health. In addition, specific disease states, such as diabetes mellitus, warrant a change from a normal diet to control the progress of the disease. The human body also goes through many changes in a lifetime and with these changes come new nutritional needs.

This chapter explores the balance of nutrients required for good health and examines therapeutic modifications to the diet that should take place at various life stages or in the presence of disease. The astute medical assistant will recognize the role of nutrition in maintaining health and will use a knowledge of nutritional principles to encourage patients to adopt a healthy lifestyle.

Spotlight on Certification

RMA Content Outline
- Disorders of the body
- Patient education

CMA Content Outline
- Developmental stages of the life cycle
- Patient instruction
- Basic principles (Nutrition)
- Special needs (Nutrition)

CMAS Content Outline
- Communication

NUTRITION AND DIGESTION

Nutrition includes ingestion, digestion, absorption, and metabolism of food. It is known that good nutrition has resulted in longer life spans and healthier individuals through the control of preventable diseases. The food eaten by an individual is used to build and repair cells and tissues of the body. Therefore, it is important to have knowledge and information about nutrition and to make appropriate food choices for optimum health. The

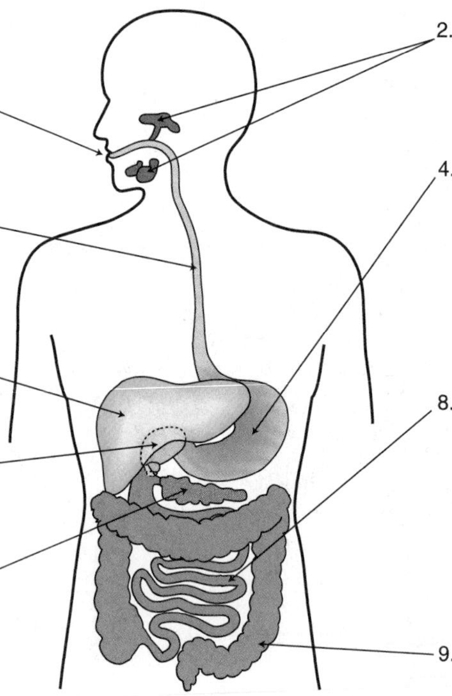
1. Mouth: Teeth and tongue begin mechanical digestion by breaking apart food.
2. Salivary Glands: Begin chemical digestion as salivary amylase begins to change starch to maltose.
3. Esophagus: Peristalsis and gravity move food along.
4. Stomach: Hydrochloric acid prepares the gastric area for enzyme action. Pepsin breaks down protein into smaller proteins. In children, rennin breaks down milk proteins. Lipase acts on emulsified fats.
5. Liver: Produces bile.
6. Gallbladder: Stores bile and releases it into small intestine to emulsify fats.
7. Pancreas: Enzymes are released into the small intestine. Amylase breaks down starch. Lipase breaks down fats. Pancreatic proteases break down proteins.
8. Small Intestine: Produces enzymes, prepares foods for absorption, lactase converts lactose, maltase converts maltose, sucrase converts sucrose to simple sugars. Peptidases further reduce proteins to amino acids.
9. Large Intestine: Absorbs water and some other nutrients, and collects food residue for excretion.

Figure 22-1 The digestive system.

well-nourished individual is less susceptible to infection and disease.

Patient education is important especially when the normal diet must be modified to treat the patient's illness. The medical assistant can answer patient questions only through a knowledge of good nutrition and what constitutes the therapeutic diets prescribed by the physician.

Digestion involves the physical and chemical changes that the body makes to food to make it absorbable. Absorption is the transfer of the nutrients from the gastrointestinal tract into the bloodstream. Without absorption, the body would not receive the nutrients. Figure 22-1 shows the digestive system and its basic functions.

TYPES OF NUTRIENTS

Nutrients serve many purposes in the body. Some nutrients can provide energy for the body to perform activities such as the pumping of the heart, the division of cells, or the contraction of muscles. Nutrients also provide building blocks so that proteins or phospholipids can be made within the body, or they can act as catalysts to help processes such as the clotting mechanism proceed at a faster rate. Essentially, ingested substances that help the body stay in its homeostatic state can be called **nutrients.**

Nutrients can be divided into two groups: those that provide energy and those that do not. Table 22-1 shows examples of each of these two groups. Those that provide energy are composed of three types: carbohydrates, fats (lipids), and proteins. Each of these three substances is used in ways other than making energy, but it is important to remember that these are the only substances from which the body can derive energy. Nutrients that do not provide energy are also important and perform other vital functions as described previously. These nutrients include vitamins, minerals, water, and fiber.

TABLE 22-1 TYPES OF NUTRIENTS

Energy Nutrients	Other Nutrients
Carbohydrates	Vitamins
Lipids (Fats)	Minerals
Proteins	Water
	Fiber

Nutrients are divided into two groups: those that provide energy and those that do not. Both groups are essential to good health.

Energy Nutrients

The three energy nutrients—carbohydrates, fats, and proteins—have one thing in common: all can be converted into energy.

Carbohydrates. Carbohydrates are made up of carbon, hydrogen, and oxygen. Although many compounds are made up of these three elements, it is the ratio of these elements that is important. Carbohydrates are made up of units called sugars. The scientific term for sugar is *saccharide*, and carbohydrates can exist as monosaccharides, disaccharides, or polysaccharides.

A monosaccharide is composed of a single unit of sugar whereas disaccharides have two units of sugar. Together, monosaccharides and disaccharides are known as simple sugars. Examples of monosaccharides are glucose, fructose, and galactose. Glucose is the sugar that the body uses most efficiently, thus most ingested sugar is broken down in the intestines and converted to glucose in the liver. Fructose is found largely in fruits, whereas galactose is a product of lactose digestion. Examples of disaccharides are lactose, maltose, and sucrose. Lactose is found primarily in milk or milk products. Maltose is a product of starch breakdown. Sucrose is one of the sweetest sugars and is what we commonly refer to as table sugar. It occurs naturally in many fruits and vegetables, as well as sugar cane and the sugar beet, which are commercial sources of refined sugar.

Polysaccharides are also known as complex carbohydrates. They are made up of many units of sugar connected together. The most common polysaccharides are starches, glycogen, and fiber. Starches are the most important dietary complex carbohydrate. **Glycogen** is only ingested in small quantities, but is an important carbohydrate form for storage of glucose in the body. Fiber is a special polysaccharide because it cannot be digested.

Because the simple sugars are composed of only one or two units of sugar, their digestion takes little time, and absorption occurs soon after ingestion. The body initially experiences a large increase in sugar concentration in the blood, which is brought down to within a normal range by the release of insulin. The complex carbohydrates require more time to digest, and as a result there is a slow absorption of the single-carbohydrate units as the larger starch molecule is broken down. This is demonstrated in Figure 22-2. In this case, there would be a moderate increase in the sugar levels in the blood, and this would continue for a longer period. A continuous level of sugar in the bloodstream is necessary for a constant energy supply.

Fats. Fats, also called lipids, are also composed of carbon, hydrogen, and oxygen, but in a ratio different from

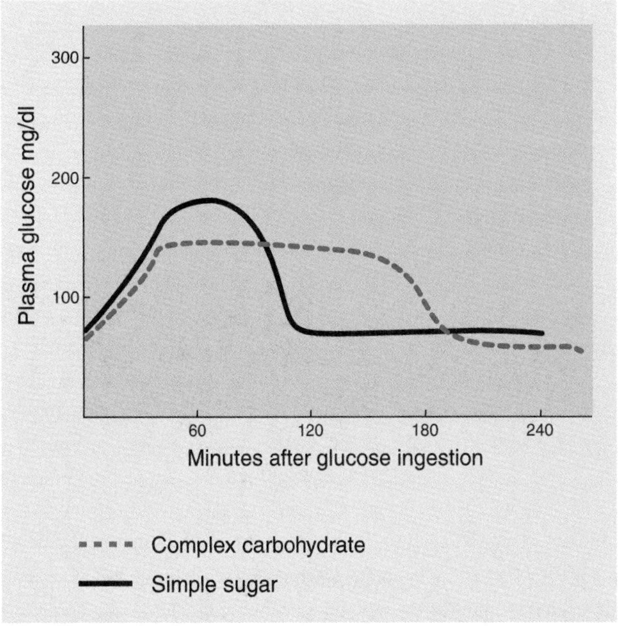

Figure 22-2 This graph shows how complex carbohydrates (red broken line) and simple sugar (black line) are used by the body (in minutes) after glucose ingestion. Simple sugar peaks to approximately 120–160 mg/dl in 60 minutes and returns to a normal level within 120 minutes. Complex carbohydrates (red broken line) never increase to more than approximately 130–140 mg/dl during a 60-minute period; that level is maintained for the next 120 minutes, and then returns to normal.

Digestion

carbohydrates. They exist as triglycerides in the body. A triglyceride has three fatty acids attached to a glycerol molecule (Figure 22-3). The fatty acid component of a triglyceride has several important characteristics. The first is whether it is essential to the diet. The only true essential fatty acid in the human diet is linoleic acid, and all other fatty acids the body requires can be derived from this. Another important characteristic of fatty acids is saturation. When a fatty acid is saturated, every carbon molecule on the fatty acid holds as many hydrogens as possible. If it does not hold all the hydrogens possible, it is called unsaturated. The more unsaturated the fatty acid, the more liquid the fat. For example, lard has saturated fatty acids and a thick consistency compared with corn oil, which has relatively unsaturated fatty acids and a thin consistency. If an unsaturated fat is hydrogenated, combined with hydrogen, it becomes more saturated. **Saturated fats** are more common in foods from animal sources than from plant sources. Generally, saturated fatty acids tend to increase the level of fats and cholesterol in the blood.

Trans unsaturated fatty acids (trans fats) are unhealthy fats because they increase low-density lipoproteins

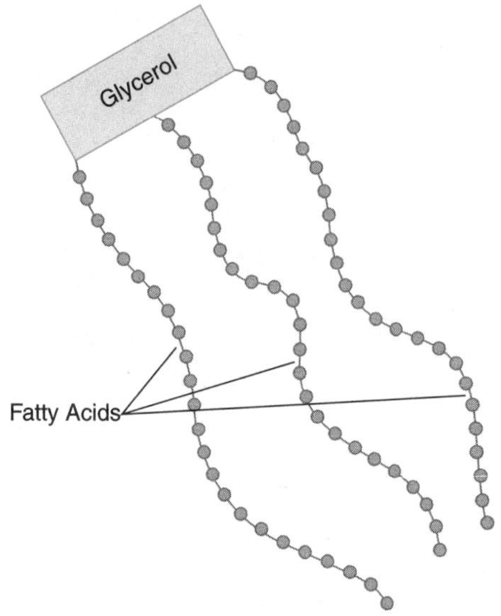

Figure 22-3 A triglyceride has three fatty acids attached to a glycerol molecule.

(LDL), bad cholesterol, and decrease high-density lipoproteins (HDL), good cholesterol.

Trans fats are produced by a process known as hydrogenation. Vegetable oil (liquid) is heated and hydrogen is added to it. This makes the product solid at room temperature. It gives certain foods a longer shelf life (stays fresh longer) and a better taste. The process, however, turns healthy fat (vegetable oil) into unhealthy fat, trans fats.

Trans fats are found in meat and dairy products, as well as stick margarine, solid shortening, and many commercially prepared foods. Foods that are considered convenience foods such as snacks, potato chips, cookies, crackers, and cakes are high in trans fats. Margarine, fast foods, cereal, doughnuts, and french fries are also examples. Experts recommend that the daily amount of trans fats be as close to zero as possible. The FDA requires that all food packaging labels show the amount of trans fats per serving in the product by January, 2006. Some companies have already begun to display trans fat amounts on their labels. Table 22-2 shows some common foods and their grams of total fat and trans fat per serving.

Patient Education

Trans Unsaturated Fatty Acids

- Use of a margarine that is soft at room temperature is lower in trans fat. Some margarines are available that are entirely trans fat free.
- Olive oil is a wise choice for salads and for dipping bread, and butter is a better option than margarine, especially if the trans fats are not listed on the label.
- Olive oil and canola oil are best for sautéing and frying.
- Make foods from scratch to avoid trans fats. Foods such as breads, dips, salad dressings, cereals, and soups can be made without hydrogenated fats.

If a food label lists hydrogenated oil or shortening as one of its main ingredients (usually one of the first listed ingredients), it has a large amount of trans fats in it. Avoid the product altogether, or eat only small amounts.

Proteins. Although protein is also composed of carbon, hydrogen, and oxygen, it contains one more important element: nitrogen. The basic structural unit of protein is the **amino acid.** There are 22 amino acids in proteins. Eight of these are needed in the diet for the body to function normally. One more, histidine, is essential only during childhood. The rest of the amino acids can be synthesized from the eight, provided that they are present in adequate quantities. A complete protein is so named because it has all eight of the essential amino acids. An incomplete protein does not contain all of these. The best sources for complete proteins are meats and animal products such as milk and eggs. Most plants provide only incomplete proteins and must be combined with complementary incomplete proteins to obtain all eight amino acids (Figure 22-4).

Although protein is described as an energy nutrient, its main function is not to provide energy but to provide amino acids to be used as building components of body proteins, which can be used as enzymes, hormones, and as the basic structural unit in all body tissues and cells. The body uses carbohydrates and fats as its primary energy sources; however, when these are in short supply, the body diverts its use of protein for structural purposes to use it as an energy source. This has detrimental effects on the body.

Deficiencies in protein usually occur together with deficiencies in total Calories. Failure to thrive is a lack of protein in infants and young children.

TABLE 22-2 GRAMS OF FAT PER SERVING OF SOME COMMON FOODS

Product	Serving Size	Total Fat	Saturated Fat	Trans Fat
Butter	1 tbsp	10.8	7.2	0.3
Cake (pound)	1 slice	16.4	3.4	4.3
Cookies (filled with cream)	3	6.1	1.2	1.9
Doughnut	1	18.2	4.7	5.0
French fries (fast-food)	Medium	26.9	6.7	7.8
Granola bar	1 bar	7.1	4.4	0.4
Margarine (stick)	1 tbsp	11.0	2.1	2.8
Margarine (tub container)	1 tbsp	6.7	1.2	0.6
Mayonnaise	1 tbsp	10.8	1.6	0.0
Milk (whole)	1 cup	6.6	4.3	0.2
Potato chips	Small bag	11.2	1.9	3.2
Ramen noodle soup	42 g	7.2	3.2	0.9
Shortening (solid)	1 tbsp	13.0	3.4	4.2
Wheat crackers	50 g	10.0	2.0	4.0

Source: Food and Drug Administration Center for Food Safety and Applied Nutrition; U.S. Department of Agriculture National Nutritional Database.

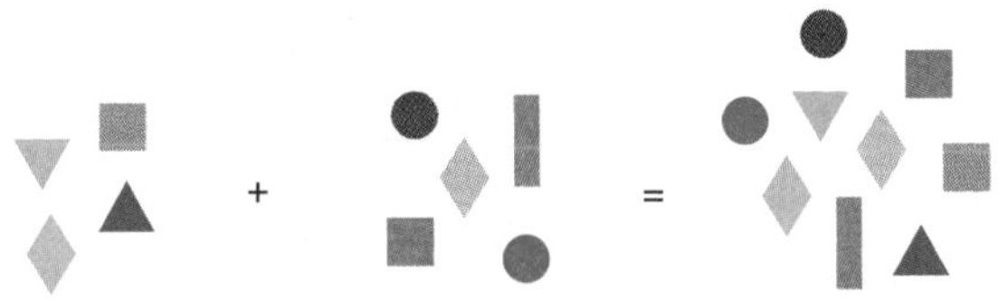

Figure 22-4 Some foods, such as grains and dairy products, may not have all the essential amino acids when considered separately. Combined, however, these form a complete protein and therefore are considered complementary.

Energy Balance. Although all of the energy nutrients are capable of supplying energy to the body, they do so in different ways and in varying amounts. The amount of energy that a substance is able to supply can be measured in large **Calories.** Nutrition is discussed in terms of the large Calorie, which is always capitalized to distinguish it from the small calorie. The large Calorie (abbreviation: C or Cal) is also expressed as a kilocalorie (abbreviation: kcal). One thousand small calories equal one large Calorie or one kilocalorie.

Carbohydrates and proteins both give four Calories for each respective gram. So, if 10 g pure carbohydrate were ingested, it would yield 40 Calories.

$$\underset{\text{carbohydrate}}{10\text{ g}} \times \frac{4\text{ Calories}}{\text{gram of carbohydrate}} = 40\text{ Calories}$$

Similarly, if 10 g protein were used for energy, it would yield 40 Calories.

$$\underset{\text{protein}}{10\text{ g}} \times \frac{4\text{ Calories}}{\text{gram of protein}} = 40\text{ Calories}$$

Fats, in comparison, yield nine Calories for every gram of fat. Fats, therefore, are a more energy-rich food source than carbohydrates or proteins because they give more Calories for every gram used. If 10 g fat were used, it would yield 90 Calories.

$$\underset{\text{fat}}{10\text{ g}} \times \frac{9\text{ Calories}}{\text{gram of fat}} = 90\text{ Calories}$$

The total of all changes, chemical and physical, that take place in the body is called **metabolism.** The metabolic rate concerns itself with the changes in the body with respect to energy. It is the balance between the energy that is brought into the body and the energy used by the body. Energy is used during every action of the body, including voluntary activities such as walking or riding a bicycle and involuntary activities such as breathing and cellular repair.

The level of energy required for activities that occur when the body is at rest is called basal metabolism. The **basal metabolic rate (BMR)** will vary according to several factors. For example, the BMR will be higher in individuals with leaner body mass because it takes more energy to fuel the muscles than it does to store fat. BMR will also be higher for individuals in a period of high growth rate such as children and pregnant women.

Ideally, an individual will take in as many Calories as the body will use each day. When a person takes in more Calories than will be used, the body will store the excess energy in the form of fat. When a person uses more energy than is brought into the body, the body breaks down these stores. When the stores of fat are depleted, the body will start to break down its protein structures.

For an optimal energy balance in the body, the largest percentage of Calories in the diet should come from carbohydrates. Ideally, the percentage should be 50 to 60% of total calories consumed. The percentage of Calories attributable to fat should not be greater than 30%, with a percentage closer to 20% being preferred. Proteins should make up 10 to 20% of Calories in the diet.

Take note that these values are the percentage of the total Calories derived from each energy nutrient—not the percentage of grams. This distinction is important because of the difference in Calories derived from each energy nutrient. Figure 22-5 gives an example of these calculations.

Label for Mystery Food:	*Amount Per Serving*
Calories	149
Total Fat	9g
Total Carbohydrate	14g
Total Protein	3g

The first calculation to make is one that converts grams to Calories.

$$9 \text{ grams of fat} \times \frac{9 \text{ Calories}}{\text{gram}} = 81 \text{ Calories due to fat}$$

$$14 \text{ grams of carbohydrate} \times \frac{4 \text{ Calories}}{\text{gram}} = 56 \text{ Calories due to carbohydrate}$$

$$3 \text{ grams of protein} \times \frac{4 \text{ Calories}}{\text{gram}} = 12 \text{ Calories due to protein}$$

The next calculation is to find the percentage of total Calories due to each of the energy nutrients.

$$\frac{81 \text{ Calories due to fat}}{149 \text{ total Calories}} = 54\%$$

$$\frac{56 \text{ Calories due to carbohydrate}}{149 \text{ total Calories}} = 38\%$$

$$\frac{12 \text{ Calories due to protein}}{149 \text{ total Calories}} = 8\%$$

Figure 22-5 Calculations of percentages of total calories due to fat, carbohydrate, or protein.

In many cultures outside of the United States, rice, bread, and noodles are the basis of the diet. In the United States, we have available great amounts of food from the dairy and meat groups. Unfortunately, dairy products and meats, although containing many good nutrients, also contain a great deal of fat. Studies have shown that many Americans are obese (as defined as weight being at least 20% greater than what their ideal weight should be). The U.S. diet is too high in fat, has too many calories, has too much salt and cholesterol; and has insufficient amounts of complex carbohydrates and fiber. As a result, many illnesses and diseases occur, such as heart disease, high blood pressure, diabetes, and cancer.

Because obesity in the United States has become such a serious problem, there has been much interest in modifying the U.S. Department of Agriculture's pyramid for ideal weight. Health experts believe that the emphasis on 6 to 11 servings from the bread, cereal, rice, and pasta groups (carbohydrates) is a contributing factor to obesity. Ongoing studies and research has led to redesign of the pyramid with less emphasis on the carbohydrate group and more emphasis placed on the fruits, vegetables, whole grains, legumes, and nuts (see Figure 22-6).

The new food pyramid has specific information about portions and calories. It can help individuals get individualized nutrition and exercise advice.

Each color on the pyramid represents a food group.

- *Orange* represents grains. The recommendation is to eat 5–8 ounces of grain per day, 3 of which should be from whole grain breads, pasta, rice, cereal, or crackers.
- *Green* represents vegetables. For a low calorie per day intake, 2 1/2 cups of vegetables should come from all 5 vegetable groups several times a week.
- *Red* represents fruits. Two cups daily is the recommended intake.
- *Yellow* represents oils. Most oil should come from nuts, fish, vegetable oil, while limiting butter, lard, stick margarine, and shortening.
- *Blue* represents milk. Three cups per day of fat-free or low fat milk or milk products.
- *Purple* represents beans and meat. Choose lean meat and poultry and use fish, beans, nuts, seeds, and peas.
- The *action figure* represents physical activity.

The new government Web site allows individuals to input their age, gender, and activity level. By doing so, they get a recommendation about their personal daily calorie intake and physical activity level.

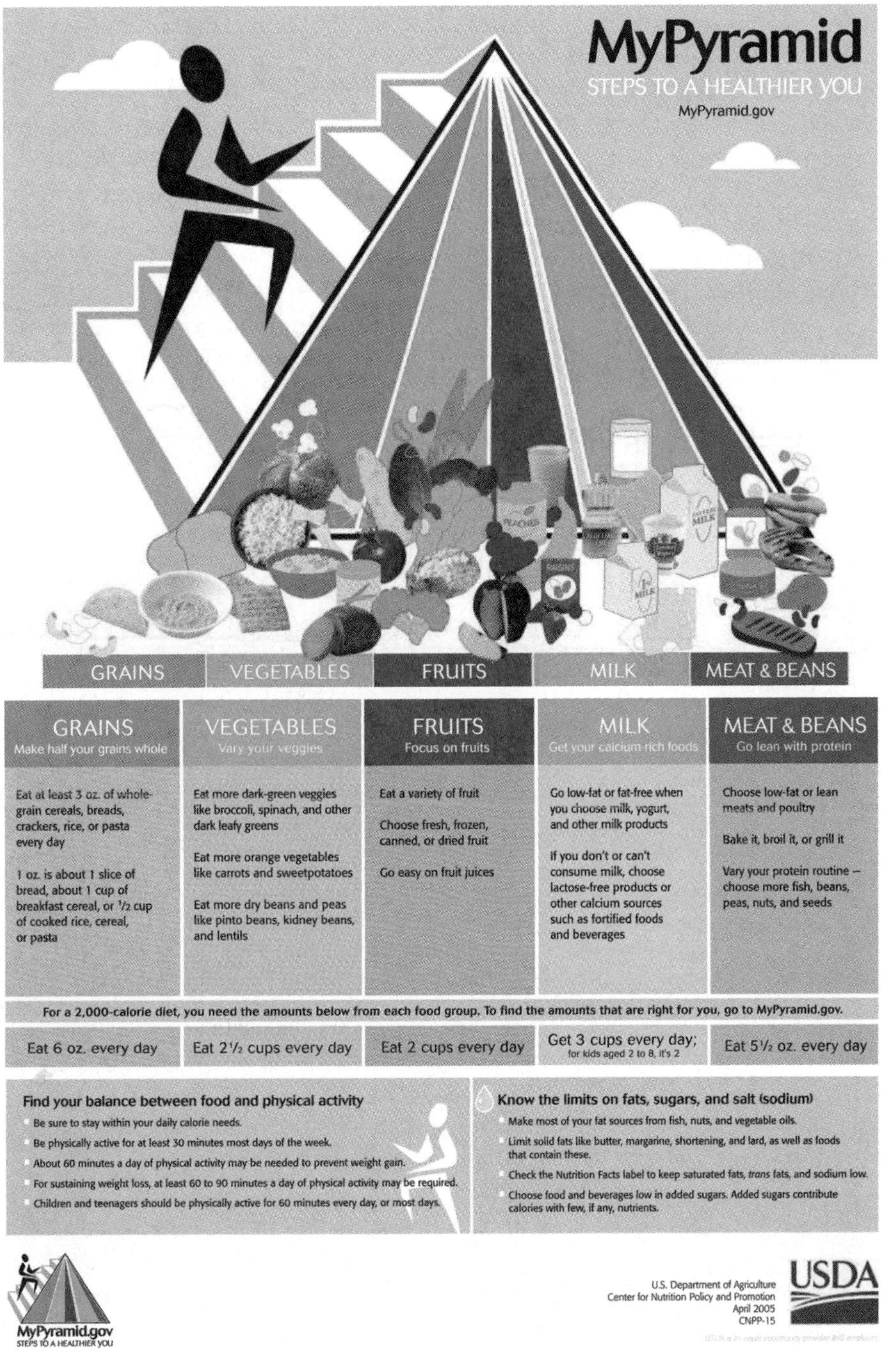

Figure 22-6 The U.S. Department of Agriculture's guide to a balanced diet takes the shape of a pyramid. The foundation of a good diet is made up of a balance between food and physical activity. (Courtesy of U.S. Department of Agriculture.)

Other Nutrients

There are many other nutrients essential to maintaining good health. Although they do not provide the body with energy, they perform a variety of necessary functions. They include vitamins, antioxidants, herbal supplements, minerals, water, and fiber.

Vitamins. Vitamins are a class of nutrient in which each specific vitamin has a function entirely its own. They are complex molecules and are required by the body in minute quantities. Vitamins were first named as letters of the alphabet. These names have been supplemented with chemical names and both should be learned. Vitamins generally have one of two functions: to facilitate cellular metabolism by acting as a coenzyme with a catalyst, and to act as a component of tissue structure. A **catalyst** allows a chemical reaction to proceed at a much quicker rate and without as much energy input, and the **coenzyme** is the nonprotein part that acts with it. Neither a catalyst nor its coenzyme is used in the reaction, thus each can be used again and again. Vitamins that work with catalysts are only needed in minute quantities.

Vitamins are divided into two classes based on solubility. The vitamins that are not soluble in water are said to be fat soluble. This is important because the **fat-soluble** vitamins are not carried into the bloodstream easily and are stored in fatty tissue, especially the liver. The **water-soluble** vitamins are not so easily stored, and blood levels must be maintained by constant dietary intake. Toxicity can occur with high doses of either type of vitamin but is more likely to occur with the fat-soluble vitamins because they are stored in the body. The vitamins are listed in Table 22-3.

There are four fat-soluble vitamins, which include vitamins A, D, E, and K. The first one, vitamin A, has two forms. The form that is used by the body is retinol, which

TABLE 22-3 VITAMIN SOURCES AND FUNCTIONS

Name	Food Sources	Functions	Deficiency/Toxicity
Fat-Soluble Vitamins			
Vitamin A (carotene or retinol)	Animal Liver Whole milk Butter Cream Cod liver oil Plants Dark green leafy vegetables Deep yellow or orange fruit Fortified margarine	Antioxidant Dim light vision Maintenance of mucous membranes Growth and development of bones	Deficiency Night blindness **Xerophthalmia** Respiratory infections Bone growth ceases Toxicity Cessation of menstruation Joint pain Stunted growth Enlargement of liver
Vitamin D (cholecalciferol)	Animal Eggs Liver Fortified milk Plants None	Bone growth	Deficiency Rickets Osteomalacia Osteoporosis Poorly developed teeth Muscle spasms Toxicity Kidney stones Calcification of soft tissues
Vitamin E (alphatocopherol, betatocopherol, deltatocopherol, gammatocopherol)	Animal None Plant Wheat germ Margarines Salad dressing Nuts	Antioxidant	Deficiency Neurologic defects Destruction of red blood cells (RBCs) Toxicity Hypertension
Vitamin K (phytonadione)	Animal Egg yolk Liver Milk Plant Green leafy vegetables Cabbage	Blood clotting	Deficiency Prolonged blood clotting Toxicity Hemolytic anemia Jaundice
Water-Soluble Vitamins			
Thiamin (vitamin B_1)	Animal Liver Eggs Fish Pork Beef Plants Whole and enriched grains Legumes	Coenzyme in oxidation of glucose	Deficiency Beriberi Gastrointestinal tract, nervous and cardiovascular system problems Toxicity None

(continues)

TABLE 22-3 (continued)

Name	Food Sources	Functions	Deficiency/Toxicity
Riboflavin (vitamin B_2)	Animal Poultry Milk Fish Plants Green vegetables Cereals Enriched bread	Aids release of energy from food	Deficiency **Cheilosis** Glossitis Photophobia Toxicity None
Pyridoxine (vitamin B_6)	Animal Pork Milk Eggs Plants Whole grain cereals Legumes	Synthesis of nonessential amino acids Conversion of tryptophan to niacin Antibody production	Deficiency Irritability Depression Dermatitis Toxicity Liver disease Rare
Vitamin B_{12} (cobalamin)	Animal Seafood Meat Eggs Milk Plants None	Synthesis of RBCs Maintenance of myelin sheaths	Deficiency Degeneration of myelin sheaths Pernicious anemia Toxicity None
Niacin (vitamin B_3, nicotinic acid)	Animal Milk Eggs Fish Poultry	Transfers hydrogen atoms for synthesis of adenosine triphosphate	Deficiency **Pellagra** Toxicity Vasodilation of blood vessels
Folacin	Animal None Plants Spinach Asparagus Broccoli Kidney beans	DNA synthesis Synthesis of RBCs Protein metabolism	Deficiency Depression Glossitis Macrocytic anemia Neural tube defects Toxicity None
Biotin	Animal Milk Liver Plants Legumes Mushrooms	Coenzyme in carbohydrate and amino acid metabolism Niacin synthesis from tryptophan	Deficiency None Toxicity None
Pantothenic acid (vitamin B_5)	Animal Eggs Liver Salmon Plants Mushrooms Cauliflower Peanuts Yeast	Metabolism of carbohydrates, lipids, and proteins Synthesis of acetylcholine	Deficiency None Toxicity None
Vitamin C (ascorbic acid)	Fruits All citrus Plants Broccoli Tomatoes Brussel sprouts Potatoes	Prevention of scurvy Formation of collagen Healing of wounds Release of stress hormones Absorption of iron	Deficiency Scurvy Muscle cramps Ulcerated gums Toxicity Increase uric acid level Hemolytic anemia Kidney stones

Vitamins are divided into two classes based on water solubility: fat-soluble and water-soluble vitamins.

is found in animal foods. The form found in plants is carotene. **Carotene** is converted into retinol in the body. Vitamin A is part of the pigment rhodopsin found in the eye and is responsible in part for vision, especially night vision. Vitamin A also gives strength to epithelial tissue and is required for healthy skin and mucous membranes. It is also an antioxidant. Sources of vitamin A include animal fats, butter, and cheese.

Vitamin D, also called **cholecalciferol,** is the fat-soluble vitamin involved in the metabolism of calcium in the body. It not only helps with absorption of this important mineral, but also with formation and maintenance of bone tissue. Vitamin D can be made in the body with exposure to sunlight. Rickets, osteomalacia, and osteoporosis are diseases caused by a deficiency in vitamin D. When deficiencies occur, especially during childhood, malformation of the skeleton is seen. Sources of vitamin D include milk, cod liver oil, and egg yolk.

Another fat-soluble vitamin is vitamin E, or **tocopherol.** It too is an **antioxidant,** reducing the likelihood of **oxidation** of substances. This ability to reduce oxidation has recently led to suggestions that vitamin E may slow the aging process, but its true effectiveness is yet to be demonstrated. Vitamin E is found in lettuce and other green leafy vegetables, wheat germ, and rice.

Vitamin K is a fat-soluble vitamin required for the production of prothrombin. Prothrombin is one agent responsible for the clotting of blood. Deficiencies can result in prolonged blood clotting time and hemorrhage. Vitamin K is synthesized by intestinal bacteria, and bile is required for its absorption. About half of the body's requirement for vitamin K is fulfilled in this way. Sources of vitamin K include fats, fishmeal, oats, alfalfa, wheat, and rye.

Antioxidants. Antioxidants are an important topic in nutrition. Some think they are as important as the discussion about fats. Antioxidants are powerful and beneficial to us. The four primary antioxidants are betacarotene (vitamin A), vitamin C, vitamin E, and Selenium.

When our bodies use oxygen to burn (oxidize) food for energy, the process results in the formation of free radicals. Most times our bodies take care of the free radicals by producing enzymes to fight them.

If free radicals are excessive, health can be seriously impaired. Evidence has shown that excess free radicals cannot be fought successfully and the body cannot get rid of them.

The radicals attack the cells' DNA and blood vessel cells are attacked contributing to cardiovascular disease, strokes, arthritis, and cataracts are examples of some diseases that may be degenerative in nature and seen in older adults.

Free radicals are not only a by-product of oxidation, they form with exposure to environmental influences such as water and air pollution, cigarette smoke, and certain foods, like fried foods.

Antioxidants fight free radicals through those enzymes in our bodies, those we ingest in food, and those we take as supplements. Vitamins A (as betacarotene), C, E, and Selenium provide powerful benefits because they fight against oxidation that produces free radicals.

Vitamin C, or **ascorbic acid,** is a water-soluble vitamin. Vitamin C is a constituent of connective tissue and acts to hold cells together. A deficiency of vitamin C causes **scurvy,** in which the walls of the capillaries become so weakened that they burst. Vitamin C also helps with wound healing and with the absorption of iron. Sources include most fresh fruits (especially citrus fruits) and vegetables (especially tomatoes).

The last group of water-soluble vitamins is the B-complex vitamin. It is important to remember that each vitamin in the B-complex is a separate vitamin with distinct functions. Vitamin B_1, or **thiamin,** helps in the conversion of glucose to energy. The disease **beriberi** is caused by thiamin deficiency and is characterized by neuritis edema, and cardiovascular changes. Sources include whole grain cereals, peas, beans, vegetables, and brewer's yeast. Vitamin B_2, or **riboflavin,** is also involved in energy production and is important in the production of proteins and necessary for normal growth. Sources include eggs, liver, milk, brewer's yeast, and green vegetables. A third B-complex vitamin, **niacin,** works with both thiamin and riboflavin in the production of energy. Lack of niacin results in gastrointestinal and central nervous system disturbances. All three of these vitamins are important throughout the body.

Vitamin B_6, or **pyridoxine,** has an important role in protein metabolism, especially the synthesis of proteins. It is also important in the metabolism of fats and carbohydrates. Vitamin B_6 is found in rice, beans, and yeast. Another B-complex vitamin, **folic acid,** is involved in the formation of DNA and the formation of red blood cells. Folic acid is found in liver, yeast, and green leafy vegetables. Vitamin B_{12}, or **cobalamin,** is another vitamin important to the functioning of red blood cells. This vitamin is responsible for the synthesis of the heme portion of hemoglobin, and deficiencies in vitamin B_{12} result in the disease pernicious anemia. Because vitamin B_{12} is only found in animal foods such as liver, kidney, and dairy products, pernicious anemia may be a problem for some vegetarians. Pernicious anemia may also occur when there is decreased production of a factor required for vitamin B_{12} absorption. Other B-complex vitamins, pantothenic acid, vitamin B_5, and biotin, are generally responsible for energy metabolism.

Multivitamin supplements may help reduce the risk for certain diseases, especially in individuals who do not eat nutritionally sound diets. The B-vitamin folate eaten in food helps reduce the risk for development of cancer of the colon and is about as effective in reducing the risk for development of cancer of the colon in persons taking a supplement with folate in it. Some studies show a reduced risk for coronary artery disease in patients who take a multivitamin coupled with antioxidants. Researchers believe that B vitamins and antioxidants help keep plaque from forming in arteries.

Most patients who are healthy and eat a nutritious diet do not need a supplement in the form of a multivitamin. A balanced diet is the best overall source of nutrients. Some people may need a supplement because they are at risk for disease such as cancer and heart disease. Examples of people at high risk are patients who have a chronic illness such as AIDS or cancer; who have gastrointestinal problems that impair digestion or absorption; who are dieting; who are vegans or vegetarians; pregnant and breast-feeding women; and patients older than 50 years (many older than 50 years have difficulty absorbing B vitamins from food, and their level of vitamin D may be low because of lack of sunshine and eating poorly).

Patients should check with their physician before beginning to take multivitamin supplements.

Herbal Supplements. Herbs are medicinal plants and are also known as botanicals or phytomedicines. Many have been used as far back as Roman times and used as traditional herbal medicine.

Many patients use herbs for the treatment of illnesses and diseases and to maintain health. It is part of a movement toward alternative or complementary therapy. The herbal supplements can be found in health food stores, pharmacies, supermarkets, large outlet stores, through the mail, and on the Internet.

Herbs are made from dried plants and plant juices. Herbal teas are made by placing the herb into boiling water. Natural hormones can be found in soy products.

Some supplements are helpful; other supplements are harmful and are banned in several countries but may be available in the United States. The Food and Drug Administration (FDA) is exempt from having authority over dietary supplements, although under the Dietary Supplement Health and Education Act of 1994, the FDA must prove a product is unsafe before it can order its removal from store shelves. An example of an unsafe herbal supplement that the FDA proved to be harmful and removed from the shelves is ephedra. It was used as an anorectic and a bronchodilator, but it acts as a stimulant and can increase blood pressure and pulse to dangerous levels. Recently a federal judge struck down the FDA's year long ban on ephedra and supplements containing ephedra. A Utah supplement company challenged the ban that prompted the judge's ruling. The company said it is too soon to say whether it will put the product back on the shelves.

Be sure to ask patients about all substances or remedies they may be using, including herbs, vitamins, teas, or others. Most patients do not consider supplements to be medicines and may not think to mention them when asked what medications they are taking. Herbs can interact unfavorably with certain prescription and over-the-counter medications.

Minerals. Minerals differ from vitamins in two distinct ways. Whereas vitamins are complex molecules, minerals are singular elements. Another way that minerals differ from vitamins is that although vitamins are only required in minute quantities, some minerals are required in larger amounts. The foundation of the classification of minerals falls into two groups: major and trace minerals. No matter how small the quantity required of either a mineral or vitamin, all are vital to a healthy body. Some minerals are considered **electrolytes,** in that they become ionized and carry a positive or negative charge. The levels of these minerals in the bloodstream must be carefully balanced for the body to function in a healthy state.

There are seven **major minerals** (Table 22-4). They are calcium, phosphorus, sodium, potassium, magnesium, chlorine, and sulfur.

Calcium (Ca) is the mineral present in the largest quantity in the body because of its involvement in the structure of bone and teeth. It is also important in blood clotting, muscle contraction, and nerve conduction. Its levels in the blood must be kept at narrow limits to ensure that the nervous and muscular tissues can function. This is especially important for the beating heart tissue. When there is a deficiency of calcium in the diet, calcium is taken from the bones to keep the blood calcium levels constant. The resulting deficient peak bone mass may put a person at risk for osteoporosis. This condition develops when there is not enough calcium in the bones and the bones become porous and easily broken.

Women older than 60 years are at greater risk for osteoporosis than men. There are no symptoms of the disease, and the first indication for the patient is when he or she sustains a fracture caused by weakened bones.

Most adults in the United States older than 60 years do not take in enough calcium in their diets and risk development of osteoporosis. Dairy products contain high amounts of calcium, as do sardines, figs, oranges, almonds, greens, and beans.

Supplemental estrogen for menopausal women was once a common preventative for bone loss in older

TABLE 22-4 THE SEVEN MAJOR MINERALS AND THEIR FOOD SOURCES

Name	Food Sources	Functions	Deficiency/Toxicity
Calcium (Ca)	Milk exchanges Milk, cheese Meat exchanges Sardines Salmon Vegetable exchanges Green vegetables	Development of bones and teeth Permeability of cell membranes Transmission of nerve impulses Blood clotting Normal heart action	Deficiency Osteoporosis Osteomalacia Rickets Poor bone and teeth formation
Phosphorus (P)	Milk exchanges Milk, cheese Meat exchanges Lean meat	Development of bones and teeth Transfer of energy Component of phospholipids Buffer system	Deficiency (Same as calcium) Anorexia Weakness
Potassium (K)	Fruit exchanges Oranges, bananas Dried fruits Legumes	Contraction of muscles Maintaining water balance Transmission of nerve impulses Carbohydrate and protein metabolism	Deficiency Hypokalemia Toxicity Hyperkalemia
Sodium (Na)	Table salt Meat exchanges Beef, eggs Milk exchanges Milk, cheese	Maintaining fluid balance in blood Transmission of nerve impulses	Toxicity Increase in blood pressure
Chloride (Cl)	Table salt Meat exchanges Eggs	Gastric acidity Regulation of osmotic pressure Activation of salivary amylase	Deficiency Imbalance in gastric acidity Imbalance in blood pH
Magnesium (Mg)	Vegetable exchanges Green vegetables Bread exchanges Whole grains	Synthesis of adenosine triphosphate Transmission of nerve impulses Activator of metabolic enzymes Relaxation of skeletal muscles	Unknown, perhaps mental and emotional disorders
Sulfur (S)	Meat exchanges Eggs, poultry, fish	Maintaining protein structure Formation of high-energy compounds	Unknown

women. Since 2002, estrogen has not been given as often as a preventive measure because a large study by the Women's Health Initiative showed an increased risk for heart disease, stroke, cancer, and breast cancer in postmenopausal women who took estrogen.

Phosphorus (P) is another mineral important in bone formation. Phosphorus also is involved in numerous activities associated with energy metabolism, as well as maintaining a proper pH balance in the blood.

Sodium (Na) and potassium (K) are two minerals that act as electrolytes. Together they work to maintain proper water balance. They also help in maintenance of proper pH balance and are involved in nerve and muscular conduction and excitability. In addition, potassium is involved in protein synthesis and release of insulin from the pancreas.

Magnesium (Mg) is another mineral that is involved with energy metabolism. It also functions in nerve and muscle excitability and is stored in bone.

Chloride (Cl) is important in pH balance and is the major **extracellular** (outside the cell) anion. It is also a major component of gastric secretions in the form of hydrochloric acid.

The last major mineral is sulfur (S). It is a component of one of the amino acids, and therefore is found in protein. It is also involved in energy metabolism.

The **trace minerals** are required in smaller quantities but are as important as the major minerals. Some of the more important trace minerals include iron, copper, chromium, molybdenum, selenium, manganese, iodine, zinc, cobalt, and fluorine.

Iron is vital to life because of its role in the heme molecule, which carries oxygen to every cell in the body. Iron-deficiency anemia results when the diet is low in iron and is characterized by small, pale red blood cells. Iron is also part of the molecule myoglobin, found in muscle cells, and is involved in a number of metabolic reactions.

Copper, chromium, molybdenum, selenium, and manganese are trace minerals important as factors in a number of metabolic reactions. Selenium acts as an antioxidant and has been receiving much of the recent publicity that vitamin E has. Iodine is also involved in metabolism but is unique in that the only place that iodine is found is in the thyroid hormones. Without it, the thyroid gland would be unable to regulate the overall metabolism of the body.

Zinc is an important constituent of many parts of the body but most notable is its involvement with the immune system and growth of tissues. Deficiencies lead to decreased ability to heal and reduced immune resistance. Cobalt is part of vitamin B_{12} and is therefore important for the functioning of red blood cells. Fluorine is involved in calcified tissues. Its involvement in strengthening teeth has led to the fluoridation of most public water supplies. Its role in the prevention of osteoporosis has been suggested but is still under investigation.

Water. Water is the most important nutrient. The human body can go far longer without food than it can without water. Water has a multitude of functions in the body. It is the major solvent of the body and is the medium in which most biochemical reactions of the body take place. As a solvent, water also is essential for the removal of toxic waste from the body. In addition, it is an important component of many structures, the body being composed of 50% to 60% water. Being the major component of blood, water serves as a transporter. Another function of water is its lubricating role, especially in joints and in the digestive system. In addition, water helps control temperature within the body by eliminating excess heat through the evaporation of water secreted in the form of perspiration.

Because the body cannot efficiently store water, water that is lost daily must continually be replenished. Water is lost through perspiration, fecal material, urine, and respiration. Water can be replenished in part from foods that are ingested, but additional water should also be consumed. It is suggested that eight glasses of water be taken in per day. Although other beverages are important sources of water, it should be considered that caffeine and alcohol are **diuretics** and will cause the body to lose water through increased urinary output. Beverages containing these substances should not be counted in the eight glasses of water.

Fiber. Although most fiber is carbohydrate in composition, it is included in its own section because of its special characteristics. Fiber comes only from plant sources. An adequate supply of fruits, vegetables, and grains is necessary to ensure enough fiber in the diet. Fiber cannot be digested and therefore is not absorbed into the body. Although fiber is not digested, it is important for the proper functioning of the gastrointestinal tract because it adds bulk to the fecal material as it is passed through the intestines; therefore, it gives the muscles of the tract something against which to work. Lack of fiber in the diet has been implicated in such gastrointestinal disorders as diverticulitis and colorectal cancer.

There are several types of fiber. Most are carbohydrates and include **cellulose,** gums, mucilages, algal polysaccharides, pectins, and hemicellulose. Another important fiber, lignin, is not a carbohydrate. It is suggested that the diet contain 15 to 20 g fiber per day. The U.S. diet tends to be far below this suggestion, in part because of the consumption of processed foods. During processing, fiber is often removed. This is true with polished, or white rice where the husk has been removed. Fiber levels should be increased gradually to prevent gastrointestinal distress, which can include diarrhea or flatulence.

READING FOOD LABELS

When assisting patients to change or modify their diets, the medical assistant must be knowledgeable not only about types of nutrients, but about how these nutrients are expressed in the foods we eat. The nutritional analysis presented on a package's food label is a helpful guide to understanding levels of fat, cholesterol, sodium, carbohydrate, protein, and vitamins contained in a particular food.

Many of the foods we eat are **processed foods,** which are cooked or packaged with parts removed or ingredients added. We rely on the labels on the cans, bottles, and boxes to tell us what nutrients are inside. The government wants to make it easier for people to understand the labels.

The government also wants to prevent food companies from fooling people into thinking something has good nutrition when it really does not. Food companies often put words on their labels to make people believe a product is healthy. Words like "healthy" and "light" or "lite" are not adequately descriptive. To discover what is in the package and if it is healthy, it is important to read the nutrition label (Figure 22-7).

Items on the Nutrition Label

Serving Size. The nutrition information given is for one serving of the food. In this case, one serving is one-half cup of the food. The package contains four servings.

Calories. The label lists the number of calories per serving, as well as the number of calories from fat per serving. This number should be less than 30% of the total calories. For example, if the total calories is 100, the calories from fat should be 30 or less.

The Percentage (%) Daily Value. The percentage (%) daily value is the amount of a nutrient obtained by eating one serving of the product. The amount is given in a percentage based on a diet of 2,000 calories a day. For example, if the packaged food has 3 g fat, the total fat from eating one serving is 5% of the total fat that should be ingested in an entire day.

Sodium Cause a lot of disease & many other problems.

Nutrition Facts
Serving Size: 1/2 Cup
Servings Per Container: 4

Amount Per Serving	
Calories 100	Calories from Fat 30
	% Daily Value*
Total Fat 3g	**5%**
Saturated Fat 0g	**0%**
Cholesterol 0mg	**0%**
Sodium 340mg	**14%**
Total Carbohydrate 15g	**5%**
Dietary Fiber 1g	**4%**
Sugars 0g	
Protein 2g	

Vitamin A 0% • Vitamin C 0%
Calcium 0% • Iron 2%

*Percent Daily Values are based on a 2,000 calorie diet. Your daily values may be higher or lower depending on your calorie needs:

	Calories	2,000	2,500
Total Fat	Less than	65g	80g
Sat Fat	Less than	20g	25g
Cholesterol	Less than	300mg	300mg
Sodium	Less than	2,400mg	2,400mg
Total Carbohydrate		300g	375g
Dietary Fiber		25g	30g

Calories per gram:
Fat 9 • Carbohydrate 4 • Protein 4

Ingredients: Flour, Water, Yeast, Vegetable Oil, Salt, Artificial Flavor and Color.

Figure 22-7 Labels on food packages give facts about the ingredients and nutrition of the food in the package.

Fat and Cholesterol. Because it is important to eat a low-fat diet, the nutrition labels list both the total amount of fat and the amount of saturated fat per serving. Saturated fat comes from an animal source and contains more cholesterol than unsaturated fats, which come from vegetable sources. The cholesterol content is also listed. Trans fats must be listed by 2006.

Sodium. The amount of sodium per serving is listed. This category is especially important for patients on a sodium-restricted diet.

Carbohydrates. The total amount of carbohydrates per serving is listed together with the amount of carbohydrates that come from simple sugar. These two types of carbohydrates are separated for individuals who are trying to eat more complex carbohydrates and less simple sugar.

Other Information. The amount of fiber, protein, and only some vitamins and minerals are listed.

Patient Education

Encourage patients to read and evaluate food labels. Typically, they should look for:

- No fat or the lowest amount of fat, saturated fat, and trans fat. Calories from fat should not be more than 30% of total calories.
- No cholesterol or low cholesterol. Total cholesterol should be less than 300 milligrams (mg) per day.
- Low sodium content. Total sodium should be less than 2,400 mg per day.
- High fiber. Fiber intake should be as high as possible.
- Vitamins and minerals. Some vitamins and minerals occur naturally and sometimes they are added to food during processing.

Ingredients. The ingredients contained in a packaged food are listed on the label. The item that is in the largest quantity is listed first. For example, if a product lists flour first and water second, there is more flour than water in the product. **Preservatives,** or chemicals added to food to keep it fresh longer, and artificial flavors and colors are often added to processed foods.

Comparing Labels

Look at some labels from snack foods that people eat when they want something crunchy and salty. Figure 22-8 shows labels from potato chips, pretzels, and snack crackers. When comparing products, compare equal amounts.

Critical Thinking

Following is information from a label for peanut butter. Calculate the percentage of calories due to fat, protein, and carbohydrate.

Serving size	2 tbs.
Calories	204
Protein	9 g
Carbohydrates	6 g
Fat	16 g

Potato Chips
Nutrition Facts
Serving Size: 1oz. (28g/About 19 Chips)
Servings Per Container: 6

Amount Per Serving	
Calories 150	Calories from Fat 90
	% Daily Value*
Total Fat 10g	**15%**
Saturated Fat 2.5g	**13%**
Cholesterol 0mg	**0%**
Sodium 340mg	**14%**
Total Carbohydrate 15g	**5%**
Dietary Fiber 1g	**4%**
Sugars 1g	
Protein 2g	
Vitamin A 0% • Vitamin C 10%	
Calcium 0% • Iron 2%	

*Percent Daily Values are based on a 2,000 calorie diet. Your daily values may be higher or lower depending on your calorie needs:

		Calories 2,000	2,500
Total Fat	Less than	65g	80g
Sat Fat	Less than	20g	25g
Cholesterol	Less than	300mg	300mg
Sodium	Less than	2,400mg	2,400mg
Total Carbohydrate		300g	375g
Dietary Fiber		25g	30g

Calories per gram:
Fat 9 • Carbohydrate 4 • Protein 4

Ingredients: Potatoes, Vegetable Oil (Contains one or more of the following: Canola, Corn, Cottonseed, or Partially Hydrogenated Canola, Soybean or Sunflower Oil), Salt.

(A)

Pretzels
Nutrition Facts
Serving Size: 7 Pretzels (30g)
Servings Per Container: 9.4

Amount Per Serving	
Calories 120	Calories from Fat 10
	% Daily Value*
Total Fat 1g	**2%**
Saturated Fat 0g	**0%**
Cholesterol 0g	**0%**
Sodium 360mg	**15%**
Total Carbohydrate 24g	**8%**
Dietary Fiber 1g	**4%**
Sugars 1g	
Protein 3g	
Vitamin A 0% • Vitamin C 0%	
Calcium 0% • Iron 2%	

*Percent Daily Values are based on a 2,000 calorie diet. Your daily values may be higher or lower depending on your calorie needs:

		Calories 2,000	2,500
Total Fat	Less than	65g	80g
Sat Fat	Less than	20g	25g
Cholesterol	Less than	300mg	300mg
Sodium	Less than	2,400mg	2,400mg
Total Carbohydrate		300g	375g
Dietary Fiber		25g	30g

Calories per gram:
Fat 9 • Carbohydrate 4 • Protein 4

Ingredients: Unbleached Wheat Flour, Water, Corn Syrup, Partially Hydrogenated Vegetable Oil (Soybean), Yeast, Salt, Bicarbonates and Carbonates of Sodium.

(B)

Wheat Snack Crackers
Nutrition Facts
Serving Size: 25 Cracker (30g)
Servings Per Container: 7

Amount Per Serving	
Calories 150	Calories from Fat 70
	% Daily Value*
Total Fat 7g	**11%**
Saturated Fat 2g	**10%**
Cholesterol 0mg	**0%**
Sodium 310mg	**13%**
Total Carbohydrate 16g	**5%**
Dietary Fiber 1g	**4%**
Sugars 2g	
Protein 3g	
Vitamin A 0% • Vitamin C 0%	
Calcium 0% • Iron 4%	

*Percent Daily Values are based on a 2,000 calorie diet. Your daily values may be higher or lower depending on your calorie needs:

		Calories 2,000	2,500
Total Fat	Less than	65g	80g
Sat Fat	Less than	20g	25g
Cholesterol	Less than	300mg	300mg
Sodium	Less than	2,400mg	2,400mg
Total Carbohydrate		300g	375g
Dietary Fiber		25g	30g

Calories per gram:
Fat 9 • Carbohydrate 4 • Protein 4

Ingredients: Enriched Flour, Partially Hydrogenated Soybean and/or Cottonseed Oil, Dehydrated Potatoes, Steamed Crushed Wheat, Sugar, Salt, Natural and Artificial Flavors, Corn Syrup, Monosodium Glutamate, Dehydrated Cheddar Cheese, Dextrose, Nonfat Dry Milk, Artificial Color (Yellow 5, Yellow 6).

(C)

Figure 22-8 (A) An example of food label from potato chips. (B) An example of food label from pretzels. (C) An example of food label from snack crackers.

Critical Thinking

Evaluate your own diet. Write down every item you eat in a day and find the values of the nutrients contained in the foods. A medical dictionary is a good source for listing the nutrient value of selected foods. If you are eating prepared foods, read the package food label. Remember, you are trying to get an idea of your average daily diet, so do not change your diet for your analysis unless you plan to maintain it. What is the balance of your energy nutrients? Are you getting enough vitamins and minerals? Are you getting adequate fiber? What modifications could be made?

These products list the serving as 30 or 28 g. That is close enough to compare the labels.

In reviewing these labels, note the amount of fat and saturated fat in each item. It might be assumed that potato chips, which are fried, would be high in fat. It may be surprising that the snack crackers have high fat content. Pretzels are the clear winner for a low-fat snack.

Note that all three labels show "partially hydrogenated vegetable, canola, soybean, sunflower, or cottonseed oil." Although the labels show total fat, none of these labels shows the amount of trans fatty acids (TFA). The TFAs are included as part of the "total fat." The FDA has given food manufacturers until 2006 to list on the label the amount of TFAs in the food item. All three snack items contain TFAs. These snacks should be avoided or used sparingly.

In terms of sodium, calories, and sugar, pretzels have the most sodium, but all three are high in sodium.

All three are low in sugar. Their calories are nearly the same as are the amounts of fiber and protein. The pretzels have the most carbohydrates, and the crackers have the most artificial flavors, colors, and preservatives.

NUTRITION AT VARIOUS STAGES OF LIFE

As nutrients were discussed in the preceding sections, ranges of suggested normal requirements were offered. These ranges should be used as a guide, remembering that each individual is unique and there will be variations for requirements.

Pregnancy and Lactation

Pregnancy and lactation both cause marked changes in a woman's body and both require an increase in various nutrients. During pregnancy, not only does the growth of the fetus require additional nutrients, but the growth of the placenta, the increase in adipose tissue in the mother, the increased volume of blood, and the growth of breast tissue also require additional nutrients.

The increased demand for nutrients is not just a demand for Calories, but also for other specific nutrients to be increased, most notably protein. Protein requirements are nearly double during pregnancy. Because of the role vitamins play in metabolism and structure, they are needed in greater quantities than usual. In addition, calcium, phosphorus, and iron are needed in such high amounts that usually a vitamin supplement is prescribed. It is important that diet modifications are not simply an increase in Calories but include quality foods high in minerals, vitamins, and protein.

Pregnancy is an important time for both fetus and mother. It is normal and healthy for the mother to gain weight, and Calories should not be skimped at this time. During lactation, there is still a requirement for higher levels of nutrients; however, overall, it is not as high as during pregnancy. A baby is more likely to be healthy and develop normally if the mother has good nutritional habits during pregnancy and breast-feeding. A baby born to a mother who is malnourished may suffer from mental retardation and be of lower birth weight. Lower birth weight babies (less than 5.5 pounds) have a greater mortality rate than babies of normal weight.

> **Critical Thinking**
>
> Write a response to a teenage girl who refuses to gain weight during her pregnancy.

Breast-Feeding

There are several reasons why breast-feeding is encouraged. The nutrition the infant receives from breast milk is a perfect combination of water, lactose (sugar), fat, and protein. There are more than 100 ingredients in breast milk that are not found in formula milk. There are no allergic reactions to mother's milk. (On occasion, if the mother eats a particular food, the infant may react by being fussy.) Breast-fed babies receive antibodies to many diseases from their mothers. Mother and infant bond during breast-feeding.

The mother during the time that she breast-feeds her infant will continue to require nutritious foods taken from the food pyramid and will need to increase her intake of calories. If the mother consumes inadequate calories, the amount of milk produced will be decreased. When the mother terminates the period of breast-feeding (6 months is recommended for the greatest benefit to the infant), caloric intake should be reduced to avoid gaining weight.

Infancy

Infancy is a time of continuous growth, and many of the mother's nutritional requirements during pregnancy are still required by the baby after birth. In the first year of life, the baby will triple birth weight. The infant will need two to three times more Calories per kilogram (kg) of body weight than the normal adult. This is true for protein as well, and most of the vitamins and minerals are required at greater levels per kilogram. Most of these can be furnished with breast milk or formula; however, once iron stores have been used up, the infant will require an iron supplement, which is why pediatricians prescribe infant liquid iron supplement. Because of the high rate of growth, especially of the nervous system, infancy is an important time to be sure nutritional requirements are met.

Adolescence

During adolescence, individuals experience the greatest levels of growth. The period of growth varies from person to person, but generally begins sooner with girls. Except for times of pregnancy and lactation, the need for total nutrients is greatest at this stage of growth. At the end of the growth spurt, nutrient requirements decrease, and young adults must then also decrease the amount of food they consume.

Two particular nutrients that especially need to be altered during adolescence are iron and calcium. Iron requirements increase for the female individual as she begins menstruation. Calcium requirements increase for both male and female individuals as bone development is occurring at a rapid rate.

Older Adults

Aging is a natural process of the body. Although aging occurs in different stages and at different rates for each individual, some generalities can be made. As we age, our cellular metabolism tends to slow. Coupled with a general decline in physical activity, this results in a decreased requirement for Calories. At the same time, there may be an increase in nutrient requirement in special circumstances. There is always an increased requirement for nutrients, vitamins, and protein in particular during illness, especially the prolonged illness that may occur in older adults. With aging, there may be increased breakdown of cells; as a result, there is an increased requirement for nutrients that repair and build cells and tissues. There is also a need to ingest more nutrients because of decreased absorption within the digestive tract. Thus, although there is less need for Calories, there is more need for nutrient-rich foods.

This may become difficult for older adults for several reasons. One may be an individual's psychological state. Loneliness and depression affect many older adults, especially after the loss of a spouse. Older adults may not like the idea of eating alone. The economic status of the individual also may present problems, as after retirement income will generally decrease. Physiologically, taste tends to diminish with age and interest in food may decrease. In addition, problems with teeth and a decrease in salivary gland secretions may make eating painful. Many medications will cause a decrease in saliva production. Also, decreased motility in the gastrointestinal tract may lead to constipation, making eating uncomfortable. All these, as well as a general unwillingness to break old habits may make it difficult to change the diet to keep up with the body's aging process.

THERAPEUTIC DIETS

Thus far this chapter has examined the nutrient requirements of the body under normal conditions. There are times, however, when the body becomes diseased and nutrient requirements change. These changes may be because of disease states such as diabetes mellitus or conditions resulting from a poor diet such as obesity. Therapeutic diets are designed to overcome or control these conditions.

The diet can be modified in a number of ways. The number of overall Calories can be adjusted, or one type of nutrient may be restricted or encouraged. The consistency, texture, and spiciness of food may be varied. The frequency of eating may be increased or decreased. When counseling patients, remember that habits are hard to change. The medical assistant should be supportive and encouraging.

Weight Control

Overweight and underweight are both weight disorders. The problem in defining overweight or underweight stems from the fact that there is no ideal weight for an entire population. There is only an ideal weight for the individual. Ideal weight can depend on many factors including age, sex, lean muscle mass, bone structure, and physical activity. Obesity is generally considered more than 20% overweight. Height-weight tables now generally give ranges that vary more than 20 pounds. The ratio of fat tissue to lean muscle mass is a better indicator of whether individuals are at their ideal weight than a specific weight.

Individuals will gain weight if they consume more Calories than they need. Conversely, individuals will lose weight if they use more Calories than they ingest. In either case, the individual must bring the amount of Calories ingested into balance with the amount used. For the overweight individual, this means either decreasing Calorie consumption or increasing Calorie usage, or both. For the underweight individual, it usually entirely involves increasing Calorie consumption.

Weight loss has become a big business. However, individuals do not need to spend tremendous amounts of money to lose weight; patient education about low-Calorie, low-salt foods and a moderate exercise program are basic starting points for weight loss. Because losing more than one to two pounds a week can put an individual into nutritional deficiency, goals should not be set higher than this. Modifications made to the diet should then be maintained even after the weight is lost and should be continued throughout life. Losing weight takes much effort, and the patient needs constant encouragement and support from medical personnel and family.

Obesity has become a serious health problem. It is defined as severely overweight and having a body mass index (BMI) of 30 or above. BMI uses height and weight to calculate an individual's total amount of body fat.

Genetics may play a role in obesity. Several genes affect the rate at which the body burns calories. Playing a major role in obesity are family eating habits, other lifestyle habits, physical activity levels, and psychological factors such as stress and depression. Major causes are lack of physical exercise, oversized portions of high-fat foods, and the accessibility of fast foods. Many people eat more food than their bodies need.

Obesity causes increased risk for hypertension, heart and lung disease, hip and knee problems, certain cancers, and diabetes, and it shortens the life span.

Parents can be role models and teach their children to eat nutritious foods and not to consume more calories than their bodies need. Parents should provide nourishing foods, limit inactivity such as television and computer time, engage the entire family in regular exercise, eat at regular mealtimes at the table, and encourage the family to drink plenty (six to eight glasses) of water daily. By parents setting good examples when their children are young, the children will learn that healthy eating habits and regular exercise will improve the quality of life (fewer illnesses) and prolong the length of life.

The American Heart Association and the American Cancer Society are community resources available with information about reducing the risk for heart disease and cancer. Keeping weight under control and regular exercise helps prevent heart attacks, hypertension, and certain cancers.

Because there has been a great deal of media attention given to the problem of obesity and the diseases it can cause, many people are looking for a quick fix to lose weight. There are many claims that people can lose weight without exercising or eating healthy foods. Most claims about weight loss products are deceptive or false.

Individuals who want to lose weight must strive to eat a healthful diet over time. A healthful diet together with regular exercise can reduce their risk for hypertension, coronary artery disease, and certain cancers (colon and breast).

Diabetes Mellitus

Diabetes mellitus is a disease in which there is either reduced or no production of insulin, or in which there is reduced or no response to insulin. Approximately 5% of the population has diabetes mellitus in some form. Most patients with this disease are not dependent on insulin and can control their condition by monitoring diet and weight.

Normally, after a meal, the body secretes the hormone insulin, which makes its way to all cells of the body. Insulin signals the cells that the glucose is available and should be brought in so that it can be converted to energy. If the cells do not receive this signal, or do not respond to it, their ability to use glucose is markedly reduced. Because the body uses glucose as its main energy source, the ramifications of this affect almost every tissue of the body. In addition, the high levels of glucose that remain in the bloodstream put a tremendous strain on the kidney and other major body organs, causing problems such as myocardial infarction, vascular diseases, neuropathy, and infections.

The effects of diabetes mellitus can be controlled with a general goal of maintaining a regular level of glucose in the bloodstream, avoiding large fluctuations between high and low levels. There are several ways suggested to accomplish this. Total Calories need not be altered, unless the diabetic patient is overweight. However, the ratio of carbohydrate, fat, and protein must be closely monitored. Total carbohydrates should be increased, but simple sugars should be avoided. Because of the longer rate of digestion and absorption of complex carbohydrates, these will be released over a longer period and prevent a sudden high level of glucose in the bloodstream, and these are the type of carbohydrates diabetics need. Increasing fiber content also increases the time of absorption and decreases the likelihood of sudden increases in glucose levels in the bloodstream. Regular snacks may be added between meals to maintain levels of glucose. The trend is for patients to take charge of their own care. The role of educator for the medical assistant will be an important one to facilitate patient self-management.

Diabetes Type 2 and Obesity. Obesity has become epidemic in the last 10 years and is the most significant factor in the increase in diabetes. Children and young people who are obese are being diagnosed with diabetes type 2 at an extremely high rate. The longer individuals have diabetes, the greater their risk for development of the complications of the disease, heart disease, stroke, kidney disease, blindness, and infections. Diabetes is a major cause of death.

Prevention of diabetes type 2 is of utmost importance. Changes in lifestyle such as weight loss, regular exercise, and a nutritious diet can prevent diabetes type 2. If a patient has diabetes type 2, it can be controlled by diet and exercise and by medication. See Chapter 24 for more information about diabetes and insulin.

Cardiovascular Disease

Cardiovascular disease is currently the leading cause of death in the United States. The unfortunate aspect is that much of it is preventable. Cardiovascular disease encompasses a variety of problems. Two of these problems, hypertension and atherosclerosis, often work hand in hand to perpetuate one another until a myocardial infarction occurs. It is important to remember that the conditions leading up to a myocardial infarction do not occur overnight. They have been developing slowly over many years, often asymptomatically. These conditions can be reduced or prevented with lifestyle modifications such as a healthy diet, moderate exercise, cessation of smoking, and weight management. This section focuses on a healthy diet to prevent cardiovascular disease.

Hypertension, or increased blood pressure, is often of unknown cause. Sometimes it has a familial connection. When the blood pressure is only moderately increased, certain diet modifications can be used to reduce it. If it is severe, drug therapy may be used in conjunction with diet therapy. The largest diet factor in controlling increased blood pressure is restricting sodium, because it plays such an important role in maintenance of water levels in the body. An increased volume of blood and water will increase the pressure on the blood vessel walls. Eliminating sodium includes more than simply eliminating use of table salt. Foods that are particularly high in sodium include smoked meats, luncheon meats, olives, pickles, chips, crackers, catsup, and cheese. In some cases, eliminating foods with only moderate salt levels may be indicated. These may include certain meats, breads containing baking powder or baking soda, shellfish, and some vegetables.

Atherosclerosis is another condition that can lead to a myocardial infarction. Atherosclerosis is hardening of the arteries because of deposits of fatty substance. It should not be confused with arteriosclerosis, which is a hardening of the arteries because of loss of the elasticity of the arterial wall. Atherosclerosis leads to arteriosclerosis, which generally occurs because of a lack of exercise and increased blood cholesterol levels. The elasticity can be regained by increasing activity, although it should be started slowly and under a physician's guidance. Atherosclerosis and arteriosclerosis often occur together. Smoking and hypertension will increase the likelihood of development of both of these conditions.

The conditions of atherosclerosis and arteriosclerosis facilitate each other. The fatty deposits associated with atherosclerosis tend to occur at points of damage to the inner walls of the artery. One of the causes of this damage is high pressure at points where there may be narrowing because of deposits that are already there, or because of the constriction of blood vessels due to nicotine. Carbon monoxide brought into the bloodstream during smoking also causes damage to the arterial walls. The deposits and hardening increase the blood pressure, which, in turn, causes more damage and more deposits. It is a cycle that is difficult to stop. The best solution is prevention.

Fats and cholesterol in the diet have been strongly implicated in atherosclerosis. It is not only total fat that is important, but also types of fat ingested. The effect of high levels of fats and cholesterol in the diet will vary among individuals, and the factor in atherosclerosis is the levels of these substances in the bloodstream. Some individuals are able to ingest high amounts of fat and cholesterol without the body maintaining high levels of it in the blood. Unfortunately, this is not the case for everyone, and fat and cholesterol levels in the bloodstream must be closely monitored. Fat levels are measured by looking at triglycerides and lipoproteins. Lipoproteins are a complex made of fatty acids and proteins and are used to carry fat and cholesterol in the bloodstream. LDLs are used by the body to transport fats and cholesterol to the body tissues. These are the lipoproteins more likely to deposit cholesterol and fat into the arterial wall. HDLs carry fats and cholesterol to the liver to be broken down and used. These lipoproteins are more likely to remove fats and cholesterol from the deposits in the arterial walls. HDL levels can be increased by exercise.

The Nurses' Health Study, done by Harvard University, showed that there was an association between the intake of hydrogenated fats (trans fats) and heart disease. The women who consumed high levels of foods that contained hydrogenated fats experienced a much greater risk for having a heart attack than the women who consumed few hydrogenated fats. Harvard School of Public Health researchers have found that hydrogenated fats are responsible for the thousands of premature heart disease deaths in the United States every year. Trans fats have also been implicated in increasing the risk for type 2 diabetes.

If total serum cholesterol and LDL levels are found to be increased, the individual must modify the diet, and if severe enough, drug therapy may be indicated. The percentage of Calories from fat should be kept to less than 30% of total daily dietary intake, with less than a third of these coming from saturated fats. Cholesterol consumption should be less than 300 mg per day.

If a person experiences a myocardial infarction, it is important that the heart muscle be allowed to rest to facilitate proper healing. This includes bed rest, initially with a gradual progression to limited activity over about a two-week period. Then the patient is allowed to resume full activity. Rehabilitation consists of cessation of smoking; control of hypertension; weight reduction through a low-fat, low-calorie diet; and a program of exercise. All help to improve myocardial function.

Cancer

Some substances ingested or inhaled are thought to be carcinogenic. For example, nitrites that are found in foods such as smoked ham or bacon are thought to cause cancer of the stomach and esophagus. Smoking tobacco, although not a food, has been implicated in cancers of the mouth and esophagus. High fat in the diet has been shown to be associated with cancer of the breast, uterus, and colon.

High fiber in the diet may protect from colon cancer. Foods with vitamins A and C protect from cancer of the stomach, lung, and bladder. Fruits and vegetables, legumes, and foods with soy may protect from certain cancers.

Wise choices of foods from the food pyramid, avoiding foods with known carcinogens, keeping weight under control, and practicing a healthy lifestyle will improve the quality and length of life.

Cancer is a disease that comes in a variety of forms. It generally means that normal regulatory mechanisms within a cell have broken down. The result is that cells continue to grow in an unrestrained manner, diverting energy and nutrients from the patient's body to the cells' uncontrolled growth. There are many stages through which these cells may go, and they will go through them at varying rates. The ramifications of this new growth will vary depending on what types of cells are affected.

For these reasons, each cancer patient will have varying nutritional requirements. However, there are some generalities that can be made. First, there is definitely a need for increased Calories. Because the new growth has the ability to divert nutrients to itself, the result is the body receives fewer nutrients. It will then break down its own tissue. In addition, there is an increased need for nutrients to supply the immune system with energy and nutrients in its attempt to destroy the cancerous cells.

If the patient receives chemotherapy or radiation treatment, there is an even greater need for increased nutrients. These therapies are directed at killing cells that are rapidly dividing. This includes not only the cancerous cells, but also healthy cells such as those of the lining of the gastrointestinal tract and hair follicles. Increased nutrients are needed for repair and replacement of the lost cells, and protein levels in particular should be increased. Because of the disturbance of the gastrointestinal lining, digestion and absorption may also be decreased. It is important that the patient maintain as healthy a nutritional status as is possible, rather than having to make up for nutritional deficiencies.

The patient will likely experience loss of appetite, as well as nausea and vomiting. There are several ways to cope with this. First, food should be made as appealing as possible. Also, if the patient has difficulty swallowing, food can be liquefied in a food processor. Generally, food will be better tolerated if it is slightly chilled; extremes of temperature should be avoided. Several smaller meals may be easier to eat than three large meals.

DIET AND CULTURE

Medical assistants are likely to come into contact with patients from many different ethnic groups. Many of these patients will have diets based on traditional cultures, and some of the foods they eat, or the way they combine foods, may be unfamiliar to the medical assistant. Often, diets in other cultures are sensible ones, with foods chosen or combined to make up a complete protein. The medical assistant who has some knowledge of ethnic food choices can help reassure patients that the dietary changes they need to make are within the parameters of their own cultures. Table 22-5 presents some highlights of the food choices of different ethnic groups.

Vegetarian diets are also fairly common around the globe, including in the United States. With a good variety of grains, vegetables, fruits, and dairy products, a vegetarian diet can supply an individual with all the required nutrients. Pernicious anemia, a disease caused by

TABLE 22-5 SAMPLE FOOD CHOICES OF VARIOUS CULTURAL, RELIGIOUS, AND ETHNIC GROUPS

Culture/Region/Group	Diet and Food Choices
Native American	It is thought that approximately half of the edible plants commonly eaten in the United States today originated with the Native Americans. Examples are corn, potatoes, squash, cranberries, pumpkins, peppers, beans, wild rice, and cocoa beans. In addition, they used wild fruits, game, and fish. Foods were commonly prepared as soups and stews, and dried. The original Native American diets were probably more nutritionally adequate than their current diets, which frequently consist of too high a proportion of sweet and salty, snack-type, empty calorie foods. Native American diets today may be deficient in calcium, vitamins A and C, and riboflavin.

(continues)

TABLE 22-5 (continued)

Culture/Region/Group	Diet and Food Choices
U.S. Southern	Hot breads such as corn bread and baking powder biscuits are common in the U.S. South because the wheat grown in the area does not make good quality yeast breads. Grits and rice are also popular carbohydrate foods. Favorite vegetables include sweet potatoes, squash, green beans, and lima beans. Green beans cooked with pork are commonly served. Watermelon, oranges, and peaches are popular fruits. Fried fish is served often, as are barbecued and stewed meats and poultry. There is a great deal of carbohydrate and fat in these diets and limited amounts of protein in some cases. Iron, calcium, and vitamins A and C may sometimes be deficient.
Mexican	Mexican food is a combination of Spanish and Native American foods. Beans, rice, chili peppers, tomatoes, and corn meal are favorites. Meat is often cooked with the vegetable as in chili con carne. Corn meal is used in a variety of ways to make tortillas and tamales, which serve as bread. The combination of beans and corn makes a complete protein. Although tortillas filled with cheese (called enchiladas) provide some calcium, the use of milk should be encouraged. Additional green and yellow vegetables and vitamin C–rich foods would also improve these diets.
Puerto Rican	Rice is the basic carbohydrate food in Puerto Rican diets. Vegetables commonly used include beans, plantains, tomatoes, and peppers. Bananas, pineapple, mangoes, and papayas are popular fruits. Favorite meats are chicken, beef, and pork. Milk is not used as much as would be desirable from the nutritional point of view.
Italian	Pastas with various tomato or fish sauces and cheese are popular Italian foods. Fish and highly seasoned foods are common to Southern Italian cuisine, whereas meat and root vegetables are common to northern Italy. The eggs, cheese, tomatoes, green vegetables, and fruits common to Italian diets provide excellent sources of many nutrients, but additional milk and meat would improve the diet.
Northern and Western European	Northern and Western European diets are similar to those of the U.S. Midwest, but with a greater use of dark breads, potatoes and fish, and fewer green vegetable salads. Beef and pork are popular, as are various cooked vegetables, breads, cakes, and dairy products.
Central European	Citizens of Central Europe obtain the greatest portion of their calories from potatoes and grain, especially rye and buckwheat. Pork is a popular meat. Cabbage cooked in many ways is a popular vegetable, as are carrots, onions, and turnips. Eggs and dairy products are used abundantly.
Middle Eastern	Grains, wheat, and rice provide energy in these diets. Chickpeas in the form of hummus are popular. Lamb and yogurt are commonly used, as are cabbage, grape leaves, eggplant, tomatoes, dates, olives, and figs. Black, very sweet (Turkish) coffee is a popular beverage.
Chinese	The Chinese diet is varied. Rice is the primary energy food and is used in place of bread. Foods are generally cut into small pieces. Vegetables are lightly cooked, and the cooking water is saved for future use. Soybeans are used in many ways, and eggs and pork are commonly served. Soy sauce is extensively used, but it is salty and could present a problem with patients on low-salt diets. Tea is a common beverage, but milk is not. This diet may be low in fat.
Japanese	Japanese diets include rice, soybean paste and curd, vegetables, fruits, and fish. Food is frequently served tempura style, which means fried. Soy sauce (shoyu) and tea are commonly used. Current Japanese diets have been greatly influenced by Western culture.
Southeast Asian	Many Indians are vegetarians who use eggs and dairy products. Rice, peas, and beans are frequently served. Spices, especially curry, are popular. Indian meals are not typically served in courses as Western meals are. They generally consist of one course with many dishes.
Thailandese, Vietnamese, Laos, and Cambodian	Rice, curries, vegetables, and fruit are popular in Thailand, Vietnam, Laos, and Cambodia. Meat, chicken, and fish are used in small amounts. The wok (a deep, round fry pan) is used for sautéing many foods. A salty sauce made from fermented fish is commonly used.
Jewish	Interpretations of the Jewish dietary laws vary. Those who adhere to the Orthodox view consider tradition important and always observe the dietary laws. Foods prepared according to these laws are called kosher. Conservative Jews are inclined to observe the rules only at home. Reform Jews consider their dietary laws to be essentially ceremonial and thus minimize their significance. Essentially the laws require the following: • Slaughtering must be done by a qualified person, in a prescribed manner. The meat or poultry must be drained of blood, first by severing the jugular vein and carotid artery, then by soaking in brine before cooking. • Meat or meat products may not be prepared with milk or milk products. • The dishes used in the preparation and serving of meat dishes must be kept separate from those used for dairy foods. • A specified time, six hours, must elapse between consumption of meat and milk.

(continues)

TABLE 22-5 (continued)

Culture/Region/Group	Diet and Food Choices
Jewish (continued)	• The mouth must be rinsed after eating fish and before eating meat. • There are prescribed fast days—Passover Week, Yom Kippur, and Feast of Purim. • No cooking is done on the Sabbath—from sundown Friday to sundown Saturday. These laws forbid the eating of: • The flesh of animals without cloven (split) hooves or that do not chew their cud • Hind quarters of any animal • Shellfish or fish without scales or fins • Fowl that are birds of prey • Creeping things and insects • Leavened (contains ingredients that cause it to rise) bread during the Passover Generally, the food served is rich. Fresh smoked and salted fish and chicken are popular, as are noodles, egg, and flour dishes. These diets can be deficient in fresh vegetables and milk.
Roman Catholic	Although the dietary restrictions of the Roman Catholic religion have been liberalized, meat is not allowed its adherents on Ash Wednesday and Fridays during Lent.
Eastern Orthodox	Followers of this religion include Christians from the Middle East, Russia, and Greece. Although interpretations of the dietary laws vary, meat, poultry, fish, and dairy products are restricted on Wednesdays and Fridays and during Lent and Advent.
Seventh Day Adventist	Generally, Seventh Day Adventists are ovolacto-vegetarians, which means they use milk products and eggs, but no meat, fish, or poultry. They may also use nuts, legumes, and meat analogues (substitutes) made from soybeans. They consider coffee, tea, and alcohol to be harmful.
Mormon (Latter Day Saints)	The only dietary restriction observed by Mormons is the prohibition of coffee, tea, and alcoholic beverages.
Islamic	Adherents of Islam are called Muslims. Their dietary laws prohibit the use of pork and alcohol, and other meats must be slaughtered according to specific laws. During the month of Ramadan, Muslims do not eat or drink during daylight hours.
Hindu	To the Hindus, all life is sacred, and small animals contain the souls of ancestors. Consequently, Hindus are usually vegetarians. They do not use eggs because they represent life.
Vegetarians	There are several vegetarian diets. The common factor among them is that they do not include red meat. Some include eggs, some fish, some milk, and some even poultry. When carefully planned, these diets can be nutritious. They can contribute to a reduction of obesity, high blood pressure, heart disease, some cancers, and possibly diabetes. They must be carefully planned so they include all needed nutrients. Lacto-ovo vegetarians use dairy products and eggs but no meat, poultry, or fish. Lacto-vegetarians use dairy products but no meat, poultry, or eggs.
Vegans	Vegans avoid all animal foods. They use soybeans, chickpeas, and meat analogues made from soybeans. It is important that their meals be carefully planned to include appropriate combinations of the nonessential amino acids to provide the needed amino acids. For example, beans served with corn or rice, or peanuts eaten with wheat, are better in such combinations than any of them would be if eaten alone. Vegans can show deficiencies of calcium; zinc; vitamins A, D, and B_{12}; and, of course, proteins.
Zen macrobiotic diets	The macrobiotic diet is a system of 10 diet plans developed from Zen Buddhism. Adherents progress from the lower number diet to the higher, gradually giving up foods in the following order: desserts, salads, fruits, animal foods, soups, and ultimately vegetables, until only cereals—usually brown rice—are consumed. Beverages are kept to a minimum, and only organic foods are used. Foods are grouped as Yang (male) or Yin (female). A ratio of 5 : 1 Yang to Yin is considered important. Most macrobiotic diets are nutritionally inadequate. As the adherents give up foods according to plans, their diets become increasingly inadequate. These diets can be especially dangerous because avid adherents promise medical cures from the diets that cannot be attained, and thus medical treatment may be delayed when needed.

lack of cobalamin (vitamin B_{12}), is sometimes associated with vegetarian diets that do not contain enough animal product (see the section on vitamins in this chapter). One type of vegetarian, vegan, does not eat any product associated with animals, including milk or eggs. This type of diet is particularly susceptible to nutritional deficiencies.

In speaking with patients about diet and dietary changes, it is important to remember that patients choose their diets for a variety of reasons, including cultural, religious, or ethical beliefs. The medical assistant should respect the patient's reasons for following a certain diet while encouraging any modifications.

Case Study 22-1

Anita Ferguson is a new patient at Inner City Health Care. She is a sixteen-year-old girl who is four months pregnant and came to the urgent care center only a couple of weeks ago. After Wanda Slawson, CMA, took Anita's medical history, and after Anita was examined by the physician, Wanda set aside time to answer any questions Anita might have about her pregnancy. Anita is obviously scared; she wants the baby, but does not want her life to change. According to the history, Anita has lost a few pounds in the last two weeks.

CASE STUDY REVIEW

1. What patient education can Wanda provide to alert Anita to the importance of diet and weight gain during pregnancy?
2. What foods should Wanda encourage Anita to eat?
3. If Anita resists Wanda's suggestions and has not gained any weight by the next visit, how should Wanda proceed?

Case Study 22-2

Dr. Lewis prescribed a diabetic diet for Mrs. Johnson.

CASE STUDY REVIEW

1. Describe what is included in a diabetic diet.
2. Describe the patient education you would use to help Mrs. Lewis understand the diet and to help her reach her goal of improved health.

SUMMARY

Seven types of nutrients are required by the body for maintenance of good health. Carbohydrates, fats, and proteins provide energy for the body. Vitamins, minerals, fiber, and water cannot provide energy but are responsible for many vital processes within the body.

Some individuals take herbal supplements. Making the physician aware of which supplements is an important responsibility of the medical assistant.

Nutritional needs change at various points in the life cycle. During pregnancy, lack of nutrients can be detrimental to the development of the fetus and the health of the expectant mother. The need for nutrients is great during infancy and childhood, with the greatest need for total nutrients occurring during adolescence. During adulthood, the requirement for Calories decreases. With the decrease in basal metabolism that occurs with aging, the requirement for Calories decreases even more.

At times of disease, the diet of the individual must be modified to help relieve stress put on the body by the disease, to give energy to fight the disease, and, in cases where the disease is diet related, to decrease the severity of the disease.

It is important to have adequate nutritional intake during every stage of life. The healthier one is, the better one feels. Nutritional status should be examined and adjustments made if necessary with the goal of helping patients maintain a healthy body.

STUDY FOR SUCCESS

To reinforce your knowledge and skills of information presented in this chapter:

- ❑ Review the Key Terms
- ❑ Consider the Case Studies and discuss your conclusions
- ❑ Answer the Review Questions
  - ❑ Multiple Choice
  - ❑ Critical Thinking
- ❑ Navigate the Internet by completing the Web Activities
- ❑ Practice the StudyWARE activities on your student CD
- ❑ Apply your knowledge in the Student Workbook activities
- ❑ Complete the Web Tutor sections

REVIEW QUESTIONS

Multiple Choice

1. The transfer of nutrients from the gastrointestinal tract into the bloodstream is:
   a. ingestion
   b. digestion
   c. absorption
   d. elimination
2. Fats are considered a(n):
   a. mineral
   b. vitamin
   c. energy nutrient
   d. fiber
3. The total of all chemical and physical changes that take place in the body is called:
   a. homeostatis
   b. metabolism
   c. a catalyst
   d. an antioxidant
4. What is the significance for the physician in determining the patient's use of herbal supplements?
   a. The FDA has authority over these dietary supplements, therefore they are safe.
   b. They are unsafe if bought in a supermarket.
   c. They may interact with over-the-counter and prescription medications.
   d. They are not considered medicines. It is not significant to inform the physician.

5. Another name for vitamin C is:
   a. tocopherol
   b. caratene
   c. biotin
   d. ascorbic acid

Critical Thinking

1. For each of the following vitamins and minerals, suggest some symptoms that might appear if there were a deficiency:
   vitamin A
   vitamin K
   vitamin C
   thiamin
   riboflavin
   cobalamin (vitamin B_{12})
   calcium
2. Consider the functions of the various regions of the digestive system, and look up in a medical dictionary each of the following procedures. Describe the problems that might exist with the following procedures if diet modifications do not take place:
   colostomy
   gastroileostomy
   gastrectomy
3. Explain why a breakfast high in complex carbohydrates is an important goal.
4. Figure 22-5 shows calculations of percentages of total calories due to fat, carbohydrate, or protein. Are the percentages healthy or unhealthy? What are the recommended percentages of total calories due to fat, carbohydrate, or protein?
5. What are some things to consider when assessing the diet of an older adult?
6. Find five things a person can do to decrease the risk for heart disease. Compile a list from the class. How many of the items are associated with diet? How many of the items involve you?
7. Describe how the diet can be used to control diabetes mellitus. When a person becomes dependent on insulin, should the diet continue to be used?

WEB ACTIVITIES

1. Search community agencies on the Web for information about the following diseases and the role nutrition plays in prevention of the disease:
   a. diabetes mellitus
   b. arteriosclerotic heart disease
   c. hypertension
2. Explore the FDA's site and find the amount of trans fats in one serving of:
   a. apple pie
   b. a jelly doughnut
   c. shredded wheat
   d. ice cream
3. Explore the National Center for Chronic Disease Prevention and Health Promotion and Physical Activity at Web site (http://www.cdc.gov/nccdphp/dnpa/index.htm) and discuss with your classmates four diseases that can be prevented through nutrition and exercise. Explain how and why.
4. Using a search engine, find a site for discussion about anorexia nervosa and bulimia. Describe these eating disorders. Is there any treatment for them?
5. Visit http://www.healthmonitor.com to calculate your body mass index (BMI) and decide if it is within a healthy range.
6. Use this government Web site to help you determine how your dietary habits rate according to the new food pyramid: http://mypyramid.gov/.

REFERENCES/BIBLIOGRAPHY

Farrell, M. L. & Nicoteri, J. L. (2001). *Nutrition quick look nursing.* Clifton Park, NY: Thomson Delmar Learning.

Nicholson, C. R. (editor). *Harvard women's health watch.* (2004).

Roth, R. A., & Townsend, C. E. (2003). *Nutrition and diet therapy.* (8th ed.). Clifton Park, NY: Thomson Delmar Learning.

Spratto, G. R., & Woods, A. L. (2004). *PDR nurses drug handbook.* Clifton Park, NY: Thomson Delmar Learning.

CHAPTER 23

Basic Pharmacology

OUTLINE

Medical Uses of Drugs
Drug Names
History and Sources of Drugs
- Plant Sources
- Animal Sources
- Mineral Sources
- Herbal Supplements
- Synthetic Drugs
- Genetically Engineered Pharmaceuticals

Drug Regulations and Legal Classifications of Drugs
- Controlled Substance Act of 1970
- Prescription Drugs
- Nonprescription Drugs
- Proper Disposal of Drugs
- Administer, Prescribe, Dispense

Drug References and Standards
- How to Use the PDR
- Other Reference Sources

Classification of Drugs
Principal Actions of Drugs
- Factors That Affect Drug Action
- Undesirable Actions of Drugs

Drug Routes
Forms of Drugs
- Liquid Preparations
- Solid and Semisolid Preparations
- Other Drug Delivery Systems

Storage and Handling of Medications
Emergency Drugs and Supplies
- Bioterrorism

Drug Abuse
- Effects of Drug Abuse

KEY TERMS

Abuse
Administer
Anaphylaxis
Contraindication
Dispense
Pharmacology
Prescribe
Pruritus
Urticaria

OBJECTIVES

The student should strive to meet the following performance objectives and demonstrate an understanding of the facts and principles presented in this chapter through written and oral communication.

1. Define the key terms as presented in the glossary.
2. Recall five medical uses for drugs.
3. Describe three types of drug names and give an example, for one drug, of all three names.
4. List five sources of drugs.
5. Describe the Federal Foods, Drug, and Cosmetic Act and the Controlled Substance Act of 1970.
6. Name the five controlled substances schedules and describe appropriate storage of the substances.

(continues)

FEATURED COMPETENCIES

CAAHEP—ENTRY-LEVEL COMPETENICES

Legal Concepts

- Establish and maintain the medical record
- Document appropriately
- Demonstrate knowledge of federal and state health care legislation and regulations

ABHES—ENTRY-LEVEL COMPETENICES

Professionalism

- Conduct work within scope of education, training and ability

Clinical Duties

- Use quality control
- Maintain medication records

Legal Concepts

- Determine needs for documentation and reporting
- Document accurately

OBJECTIVES (continued)

7. Define the law in terms of administering, prescribing, and dispensing drugs.
8. Describe the four most commonly used sections of the *Physician's Desk Reference* (PDR).
9. Describe the principal actions of drugs and three undesirable reactions.
10. Describe routes of drug administration and drug forms.
11. Describe handling and storing of drugs.
12. List emergency drugs and supplies.
13. Recall commonly abused drugs and describe their physical and emotional effects.
14. Critique the legal role and responsibilities of the medical assistant.

SCENARIO

Policy at Drs. Lewis and King dictates that a patient medication history is taken on the first appointment, routinely updated, and reviewed whenever medication is prescribed, dispensed, or administered. Both administrative and clinical medical assistants work together to ensure that this policy is carried out. When making a patient appointment, administrative medical assistants ask patients to bring with them any medications (keeping them in the labeled container) that they are currently using. When taking or updating a patient history, clinical medical assistants Audrey Jones and Joe Guerrero ask a number of questions of patients regarding medications, prescription, over-the-counter, and herbal supplements, and gently probe to assure that patients include all medications in the history and describe any allergy or hypersensitivity they may have to certain drugs.

INTRODUCTION

Pharmacology *is the study of drugs, the science that is concerned with the history, origin, sources, physical and chemical properties, uses, and effects of drugs on living organisms. Medical assistants in the ambulatory care setting need to understand basic pharmacology including the uses, sources, forms, and delivery routes of drugs; must know and be able to implement the intent of the law regarding controlled substances and other medications; and must have a knowledge of drug classifications and actions to be able to caution patients when taking prescription or nonprescription drugs. In addition, the medical assistant must be able to educate patients about a drug's intended purpose and the correct way to take the drug for maximum effectiveness.*

This chapter provides an overview of pharmacology; it is considered a review for medical assistants who have had a formal course in the subject. Information on dosage, calculation, and medication administration can be found in Chapter 24.

Spotlight on Certification

RMA Content Outline
- Clinical pharmacology

CMA Content Outline
- Legislation
- Pharmacology

CMAS Content Outline
- Basic Pharmacology

MEDICAL USES OF DRUGS

A drug is defined as a medicinal substance that may alter or modify the functions of a living organism. There are five medical uses for drugs:

- *Therapeutic*. Used in the treatment of a condition to relieve symptoms. An example is an antihistamine that may be used in the treatment of an allergy.
- *Diagnostic*. Used in conjunction with radiology and other diagnostic imaging procedures to allow the physician to pinpoint the location of a disease process. An example is dye tablets used in the X-ray study of the gallbladder.
- *Curative*. Used to kill or remove the causative agent of a disease. An example is an antibiotic.
- *Replacement*. Used to replace substances normally found in the body. Hormones and vitamins are examples of replacement drugs.
- *Preventive or Prophylactic*. Used to ward off or lessen the severity of a disease. Examples are immunizing agents such as vaccines.

DRUG NAMES

Most drugs have three types of names: chemical, generic, and trade or brand name.

- The *chemical name* describes the drug's molecular structure and identifies its chemical structure.
- The *generic name* is the drug's official name and is assigned to the drug by the U.S. Adopted Names Council. A generic drug can be manufactured by more than one pharmaceutical company. When this is the case, each company markets the drug under its own unique trade or brand name. Generic name begins with a lowercase letter.
- A *trade or brand name* is registered by the U.S. Patent and Trademark Office and is approved by the U.S. Food and Drug Administration (FDA). The ® symbol following a drug's trade or brand name indicates that the name is registered and protected for 17 years. No other manufacturer can make or sell the drug during that time. Once the patent expires, any manufacturer can sell the drug under its generic name or a new trade name. The original trade name cannot be reused. The brand name begins with a capital letter.

Example:

Chemical name: 1, 4, 3, 6-dian hydrosorbitol-2, 5 dinitrate
Generic name: isosorbide dinitrate
Trade/Brand name: Sorbitrate®

When physicians prescribe a drug, they may use either the generic or trade name. It is not uncommon for physicians to prescribe the generic form of a drug because it is usually less costly for the patient. To reduce costs, some insurance companies will pay only for generic brands. Sometimes, physicians specify drugs by their trade names. Some states allow patients to request that their pharmacist dispense the generic drug equivalent unless the physician has specified that the drug be dispensed by its trade name. Also, in some states, a pharmacist may select a generic form of a drug if not specifically directed otherwise by the physician. Generic and trade name drugs have the same chemical composition and must adhere to identical FDA standards; therefore, according to most state laws, they can be used interchangeably. The drug label reflects the drug products dispensed.

HISTORY AND SOURCES OF DRUGS

Drugs prepared from roots, herbs, bark, and other forms of plant life are among the earliest known pharmaceuticals. Their origin can be traced back to primitive cultures where they were first used to evoke magical powers and to drive out evil spirits. Having discovered that certain plants were pharmacologically useful, a search was begun for sources of drugs.

Today this search continues. In addition to plants, drugs are derived from animals, minerals, and are produced in laboratories using chemical, biochemical, and biotechnologic processes.

Plant Sources

The leaves, roots, stems, or fruit of certain plants may contain medicinal properties. For example, the dried leaf of the foxglove plant *(Digitalis purpurea)* is a source of digitalis, a cardiac glycoside used in the treatment of certain heart conditions.

Herbals fit into this plant source category. The disadvantage of many natural herbals on the market today is that some drugs derived from plants may not be standardized. In any given crop, there may be plants that are more or less potent than their neighboring plants. This lack of consistency is related to the amount of sunshine and water a particular plant receives, as well as the nutrients in the soil. Another disadvantage of natural plant drugs is the pesticides that may be present. These may be man-made pesticides applied to the plants or taken up by the plant through the environment (soil, water, and air); they may also be natural pesticides originating from the plant itself to defend itself from molds, insects, and other threats. These pesticides all pose biologic threats to our chemical and biologic functions. These foreign chemicals can be interpreted by our bodies as irritants, free radicals, antigens, and antagonists. Patients should be cautioned to purchase only reputable, standardized, natural herbal products for these reasons.

Animal Sources

A number of essential extracts are obtained from tissues such as the pancreas and adrenal glands of animals. An example of a drug obtained from animals is insulin, a hormone that can be extracted from the pancreas of cows and hogs, though it is also made synthetically and by genetic engineering. Insulin is used in the treatment of diabetes mellitus. Two common compounds extracted from the adrenal glands of animals are adrenalin and cortisone.

Mineral Sources

Some naturally occurring mineral substances are used in medicine in a highly purified form. One such mineral is sulfur, which has been used as a key ingredient in certain bacteriostatic drugs. It is now prepared synthetically and used in the treatment of urinary and intestinal tract infections.

Herbal Supplements

With the increased interest in alternative or complementary medicine, many patients and some practitioners use herbal products for treatment, prophylaxis, and maintenance of health and care of disease. *Phytomedicine* is the term used to describe the use of plants to promote optimum health.

Native cultures since ancient times had great respect for their medicine men and women because they knew about plants and herbs for medicinal purposes. Such diseases and conditions as cardiac arrhythmia, pain, blood thinning, digestive upsets, and increased urinary output (diuresis) have been treated with success with herbal medicine.

European physicians use herbal medicines routinely in their practices and have had classes on the topic throughout medical school.

In the United States, it was not until 1974 that the FDA passed an act known as the Dietary Supplement Health and Education Act (DSHEA). The act examines any dietary supplement such as herbal products and may remove it from the market if it presents a significant or unreasonable risk for illness or injury when used according to its labeling or under ordinary conditions of use.

The DSHEA gathers and thoroughly reviews evidence about the pharmacology of a product, uses peer-review scientific literature on safety and effectiveness, examines adverse event reports, and includes public comments for information about associated health risks.

Self-medication with herbal products is less in the United States than worldwide, but sales in the United States have been increasing yearly. There has been an abundance of interest by the public in herbal products because of the media attention given to them and their benefits.

Many physicians combine herbal products (together with nutrition) in their practice(s), and certain herbal treatments have become part of the practitioner's treatment regimen.

Some examples of herbs and their uses are as follows: cascara—laxative; feverfew—headaches; garlic—antibacterial; licorice—gastritis, cough, menopause; St. John's Wort—depression and anxiety; and Saw Palmetto—prostate health.

There are risks associated with self-medication with herbal products. Patients need to be informed that taking certain medications together with herbal products can produce dangerous interactions. It is important for you as the medical assistant to gather information about all medications, prescriptions, over-the-counter medications, and herbals. Pregnant patients should inform their physician about what they are taking and should be cautioned about possible harm to the fetus (see Chapter 14).

The dietary supplement ephedra, also known as Ma huang, had been prohibited from being sold since April 2004 because, according to DSHEA of 1994, ephedra

> **Patient Education**
>
> If you want to use herbal therapy, you should find a qualified herbalist and work with him or her and your practitioner. Herbal products are not regulated or standardized by an agency or organization (see earlier for information about DSHEA). Report at once symptoms that seem unusual. Herbal products should be used for the shortest amount of time needed to obtain results. Keeping track of herbs taken, for what purpose they are being taken, and the effect on symptom control is important and provides information about which products are helpful and those that are not. Journals, newsletters, and the Internet can provide information about herbal medicine. These publications can be explored for information and are a valuable resource. Relevent publications include *Herbalgram, Phytomedicine, Alternative Medicine Alert,* and *Alternative and Complementary Medicine*.

presented an unreasonable risk for illness and injury. The herbal supplement had been promoted for use in weight loss and control and for enhancing performance in sports activities. Evidence showed modest effectiveness for weight loss with no clear health benefit. It was confirmed that, in many instances, the substance increased blood pressure and caused tachycardia, chest pain, myocardial infarction (MI), cerebral vascular accidents (CVA), seizures, psychosis, and death.

A federal judge struck down the ban on the sale of ephedra and ephedra-containing products which the FDA had put into effect a year ago. It is uncertain whether ephedra will become available again.

Synthetic Drugs

Synthetic drugs are artificially prepared in pharmaceutical laboratories. By combining various chemicals, scientists can produce compounds that are identical to a natural drug or create entirely new substances. An advantage of synthetic drugs over natural is the ability to standardize doses. Thousands of drugs are now produced synthetically. Examples are Motrin® (ibuprofen), Feldene® (piroxician), and Prilosec® (omeprazole).

Genetically Engineered Pharmaceuticals

Scientists are now capable of creating new strains of bacteria using a technique known as gene splicing. Through this process, hybrid forms of life have been created that benefit human beings by providing an alternative source of drugs, such as Humulin® (insulin) for the diabetic patient and interferon for use in treatment of cancer. These drugs can be manufactured in large quantities; thus, they are less expensive than natural substances.

DRUG REGULATIONS AND LEGAL CLASSIFICATIONS OF DRUGS

Qualified medical practitioners who prescribe, dispense, or administer drugs must comply with federal and state laws. The laws govern the manufacture, sale, possession, administration, dispensing, and prescribing of drugs. All drugs available for legal use are controlled by the Federal Food, Drug, and Cosmetic Act. The law protects the public by ensuring the purity, strength, and composition of foods, drugs, and cosmetics. It also prohibits the movement in interstate commerce of altered and misbranded food, drugs, devices, and cosmetics. Enforcement of the act is the responsibility of the FDA, which is part of the Department of Health and Human Services (DHHS).

Controlled Substance Act of 1970

One category of drugs—those with potential for abuse or addiction—is regulated by the Controlled Substance Act of 1970. It controls the manufacture, importation, compounding, selling, dealing in, and giving away of drugs that have the potential for abuse and addiction. The drugs are known as controlled substances and include heroin and cocaine and their derivatives; other narcotics, stimulants, and depressants. The Drug Enforcement Agency (DEA) of the U.S. Justice Department monitors and enforces the act, which is also known as the Comprehensive Drug Abuse Prevention and Control Act. Under federal law, physicians who prescribe, administer, or dispense controlled substances must register with the DEA and renew their registration as required by state law.

Applications for registration are made directly to the DEA Registration Section, P.O. Box 28083, Central Station, Washington, DC 20038-8083. A licensed physician is issued a registration that must be renewed at regular intervals (Figure 23-1). The renewal form is sent approximately two months before the expiration date.

Controlled Substances Schedules. Controlled substances are classified according to five schedules:

- *Schedule I* specifies drugs that have a high potential for abuse and are not accepted for medical use within the United States. Examples are heroin and lysergic acid diethylamide (LSD).
- *Schedule II* drugs include those that also have a high abuse potential but have an accepted medical use within the United States. Examples are amphetamines and cocaine. Because of their high potential for abuse, a special DEA Form #222 must be used to order these drugs. The form is not necessary for Schedule III and IV drugs. A written prescription is required for Schedule II drugs and it cannot be renewed.
- *Schedule III* drugs have a low-to-moderate potential for physical dependence, yet have a high potential for psychological dependency. Some examples are barbiturates and various drug combinations containing codeine and paregoric. Prescriptions for Schedule III drugs can be either written or oral. They can be refilled, but only five times within six months.
- Misuse or abuse of *Schedule IV* drugs can lead to limited physical or psychological dependency. Examples of these drugs include chloral hydrate and diazepam. Prescriptions for Schedule IV drugs may include refills, but refills are limited to five times within six months.
- *Schedule V* drugs have the lowest abuse potential of controlled substances. Some examples from this schedule are Lomotil® and Donnagel®. Some drugs from Schedule V may include refills, but refills are limited to five times within six months.

On occasion, the DEA will reclassify drugs and move them from one schedule to another.

So they can be readily identified, controlled substances are labeled with a large C with a Roman numeral inside it to indicate from which schedule the drug has come, for example, CII represents a Schedule II drug.

The physician's DEA number must appear on each prescription for controlled substances.

A copy of the federal law and a complete list of controlled substances and their schedules are available from any DEA office or online.

Storage of Controlled Substances. Federal law requires that all controlled substances be kept separate from other drugs. They must be stored in a well-constructed metal box or compartment that has a double lock. Controlled substances must be protected from possible misuse and abuse, and persons who administer controlled substances must record them in a separate record book. The book must be maintained on a daily basis and kept for a minimum of two to three years, depending on state laws. Patient name, address, date of administration of the controlled substance, drug name, dose, and route and method of administration must be included in the record. Record keeping applies only to persons who administer or dispense controlled substances.

Controlled substances (Schedule II) stored and used on the premises must be counted at the end of each workday, verified by two individuals for accuracy of count, and recorded on an audit sheet. An inventory record of Schedule II drugs must be submitted to the DEA every two years.

Because the increase in office and clinic drug theft and substance abuse, as well as the stringent federal laws that apply to storing, dispensing, and administration of controlled substances, many offices and clinics do not keep controlled substances (Schedule II) on the premises.

Medical Assistant Role and Responsibilities. Medical assistants are required to know the legalities that surround controlled substances. Medical assistant responsibilities may include:

1. Monitor the physician's DEA registration renewal date.
2. Maintain legally designated records and inventories of all drugs (Figure 23-2), including samples.
3. Provide security for all drugs, in particular controlled substances (Schedule II).
4. Provide security for prescription pads.
5. Properly destroy expired drugs and document.
6. Know and understand federal and state laws that regulate drugs, including all controlled substances and samples.

Prescription Drugs

State laws require that licensed practitioners who prescribe drugs must write and sign an order for the dispensing of drugs. This process is known as writing a prescription. Some examples of drugs that require a prescription are all of the controlled substances, except for Schedule I, and other categories such as digoxin, a cardiac drug, and epinephrine, a vasoconstrictor.

Medical assistants need to advise patients after the physician prescribes a drug. Patients should also read

READ INSTRUCTIONS BEFORE COMPLETING

APPLICATION FOR REGISTRATION
Under Controlled Substances Act of 1970

OMB NO.
1117-0014

DEA Form 224
(Nov. 1999)

USE BLACK INK

Name: Applicant or Business

(Last,

First, MI)

No registration will be issued unless a completed application form has been received (21 CFR 1301.13).

Taxpayer Identifying Number and/or Social Security Number

Proposed Business Address *(When using a P.O. Box you must also provide a street address)*

The Debt Collection Improvement Act of 1996 (PL 104-134) requires that you furnish your Federal Taxpayer Identifying Number to DEA. This number is required for debt collection procedures should your fee become uncollectable. If you do not have a Federal Taxpayer Identifying Number, use your Social Security Number.

City State Zip Code

Applicant's Business Phone Number Applicant's Fax Number

REGISTRATION CLASSIFICATION:

1. BUSINESS ACTIVITY: (X only one)

☐ RETAIL PHARMACY ☐ HOSPITAL/CLINIC ☐ PRACTITIONER- (Specify professional degree, e.g. DDS, DO, DVM, MD, etc.) →

☐ TEACHING INSTITUTION (Instructional purposes only) ☐ MID-LEVEL PRACTITIONER (MLP)- (Specify professional degree, e.g. PA, NP, OD, NH, AMB, AS, etc.) →

2. INDICATE HERE IF YOU REQUIRE ORDER FORM BOOKS. ☐

3. DRUG SCHEDULES: (X all that apply)

☐ SCHEDULE II NARCOTIC ☐ SCHEDULE II NON NARCOTIC ☐ SCHEDULE III NARCOTIC ☐ SCHEDULE III NON NARCOTIC ☐ SCHEDULE IV ☐ SCHEDULE V

4. ALL APPLICANTS MUST ANSWER THE FOLLOWING:

(a) Are you currently authorized to prescribe, distribute, dispense, conduct research, or otherwise handle the controlled substances in the schedules for which you are applying under the laws of the state or jurisdiction in which you are operating or propose to operate?

☐ Yes - State License No. ☐ Pending ☐ N/A

☐ Yes - State Controlled Substance No. ☐ Pending ☐ N/A

(b) MLP only: Applicant is authorized to engage in the following controlled substance activites by the **state** in which applicant practices.

	Prescribe	Administer	Dispense	Procure*
SCHEDULE II NARCOTIC	☐	☐	☐	☐
SCHEDULE II NON NARCOTIC	☐	☐	☐	☐
SCHEDULE III NARCOTIC	☐	☐	☐	☐
SCHEDULE III NON NARCOTIC	☐	☐	☐	☐
SCHEDULE IV	☐	☐	☐	☐
SCHEDULE V	☐	☐	☐	☐

*Procure means to individually obtain controlled substances by purchase or receipt of samples from a manufacturer or distributor. It does not include receipt of controlled substances from, or pursuant to an order from a collaborating or supervising physician.

↓ATTACH CHECK HERE↓

Continue on Reverse

ATTENTION → **FEE IS $210. FOR 3 YRS**

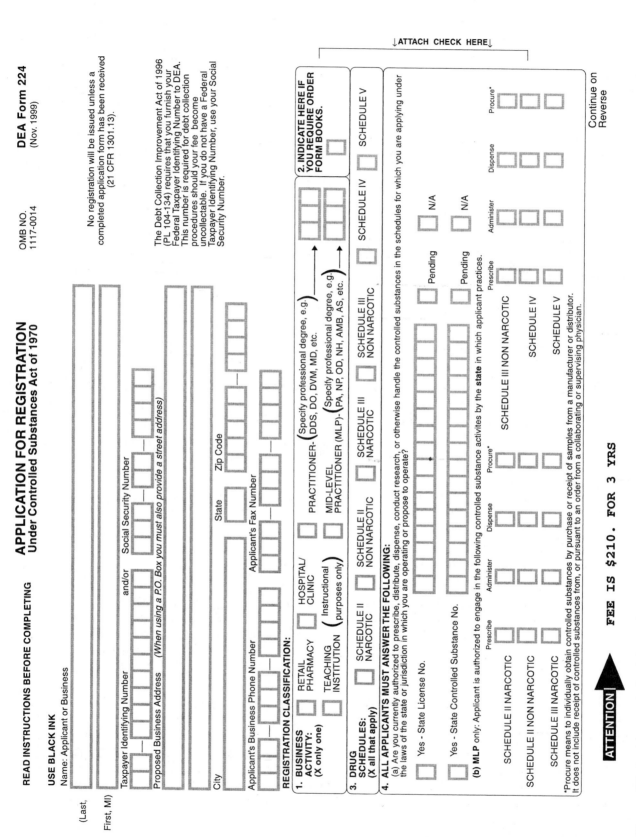

Figure 23-1 Licensed physicians who prescribe, administer, or dispense controlled substances must register with the Drug Enforcement Agency (DEA) of the U.S. Justice Department. The registration must be renewed at regular intervals. Shown here is Form 224 for a new application for registration with the DEA. Form 224(A) is for registration renewal.

4. CONTINUED

(c) Has the applicant ever been convicted of a crime in connection with controlled substances under state or federal law? ☐ YES ☐ NO

(d) Has the applicant ever surrendered or had a federal controlled substance registration revoked, suspended, restricted or denied? ☐ YES ☐ NO

(e) Has the applicant ever had a state professional license or controlled substance registration revoked, suspended, denied, restricted, or placed on probation? ☐ YES ☐ NO

(f) If the applicant is a corporation (other than a corporation whose stock is owned and traded by the public), association, partnership, or pharmacy, has any officer, partner, stockholder or proprietor been convicted of a crime in connection with controlled substances under state or federal law, or ever surrendered or had a federal controlled substance registration revoked, suspended, restricted or denied, or ever had a state professional license or controlled substance registration revoked, suspended, denied, restricted, or place on probation? ☐ YES ☐ NO

5. EXPLANATION FOR ANSWERING "YES" TO ITEM(S) 4(c), (d), (e), OR (f).
Applicants who have answered "yes" to item(s) 4(c), (d), (e), or (f) are required to submit a statement explaining such response(s). The space provided below should be used for this purpose. If additional space is needed, use a separate sheet and return with application.

6. PAYMENT METHOD (X only one)

FEES ARE NOT REFUNDABLE

☐ VISA ☐ MASTER CARD ☐ CHECK ☐ U.S. MONEY ORDER

Credit Card Number

Expiration Date

SIGNATURE OF CARD HOLDER

7. CERTIFICATION FOR FEE EXEMPTION

☐ MARK THIS BLOCK **IF APPLICANT NAMED HEREON IS A FEDERAL, STATE, OR LOCAL GOVERNMENT OPERATED HOSPITAL, INSTITUTION, OR OFFICIAL.**
The undersigned hereby certifies that the applicant named hereon is a federal, state, or local government operated hospital, institution, or official, and is exempt from payment of the application fee.

Signature of Certifying Official **(other than applicant)** **Date**

Print or Type Name of Certifying Official

Print or Type Title of Certifying Official

8. APPLICANT SIGNATURE (must be an original signature in ink)

Signature Date

I hereby certify that the foregoing information furnished on this application is true and correct.

Print or Type Name

Print or Type Title (e.g., President, Dean, Procurement Officer, etc...)

RETURN COMPLETED APPLICATION WITH FEE IN ATTACHED ENVELOPE

MAKE CHECK OR MONEY ORDER PAYABLE TO DRUG ENFORCEMENT ADMINISTRATION

UNITED STATES DEPARTMENT OF JUSTICE
DRUG ENFORCEMENT ADMINISTRATION
CENTRAL STATION
P.O. BOX 28083
WASHINGTON, D.C. 20038-8083

For information, call 1 (800) 882-9539

See "Privacy Act" Information on last page of application.

DEA Form **224** (Nov. 1999) **MAKE A COPY FOR YOUR RECORDS.**

Figure 23-1 (continued)

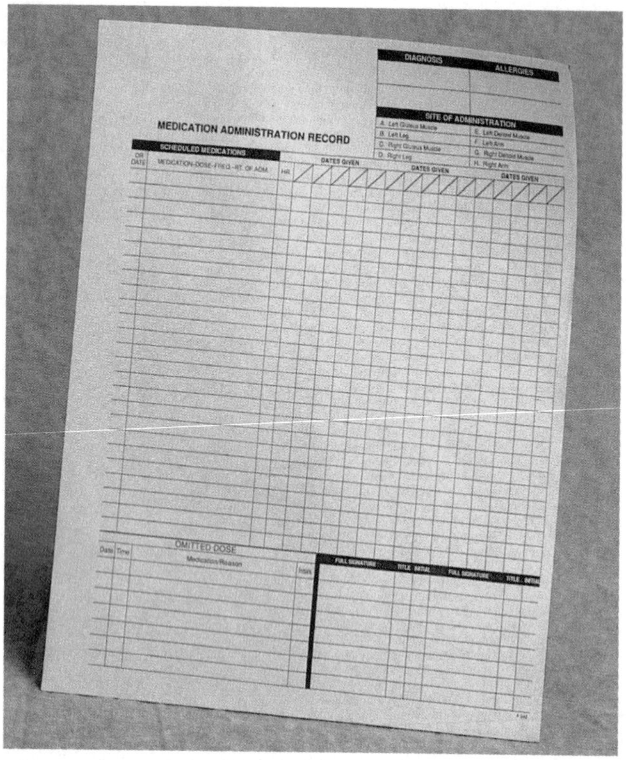

Figure 23-2 It is important to maintain patient medication records both for the safety of the patient and to protect the practice.

> ## Patient Education
>
> Guidelines for patients who take prescription medications include:
>
> 1. Take exactly as directed.
> 2. Inform the physician or the medical assistant of unusual or adverse reactions.
> 3. Continue to take the medication for the duration of the prescribed number of days, weeks, and so on.
> 4. If you want to discontinue the medication, inform your physician or the medical assistant.
> 5. Do not take other medications or herbs concurrently without checking with your physician or medical assistant.
> 6. Do not take someone else's prescribed medication.
> 7. Store all medications away from children.
> 8. Discard unused medication properly (flush liquids down the sink; flush pills and tablets flush down the toilet).
> 9. Heed warning labels on medication containers.

warning labels on medication containers (Figure 23-3). Prescription drugs are also called legend drugs.

Nonprescription Drugs

Drugs that are frequently referred to as over-the-counter (OTC) drugs fall into the category of nonprescription drugs. These drugs are readily accessible to the public. They do not require a prescription because the FDA considers them safe to use without a physician's advice. Examples of OTC drugs are aspirin, ibuprofen, and vitamins such as vitamin C and herbals. Although OTC drugs are considered safe, it is useful for the medical assistant to offer patients some guidelines (Figure 23-4).

Proper Disposal of Drugs

All drug labels contain an expiration date. When that date has been reached, the drug must be removed from the shelf and destroyed (Figure 23-5).

An expired drug cannot be dispensed nor administered because it could be harmful.

To destroy expired drugs, liquids and ointments can be rinsed down the drain and will be destroyed by the sewage system. Powdered drugs can be mixed with water and disposed of in the same manner. Pills and capsules can be flushed down the toilet. Vials and ampules of liquid drugs are opened and their contents poured down the drain.

If a medication is removed from its original container, it should not be used (for example, the patient refused the medication); do not replace it in the container. Dispose of it as outlined earlier.

Outdated and expired controlled substances (Schedule II) are handled differently. They must be returned to the pharmacy (as required by law). If a controlled substance (Schedule II) has been either dropped onto the floor (and is thus unfit to be given to a patient) or has spilled (if in liquid form), a witness should verify the action and proper documentation must take place.

The local DEA office and local police must be notified and the appropriate paperwork completed if there has been a loss or theft of a controlled substance (Schedule II).

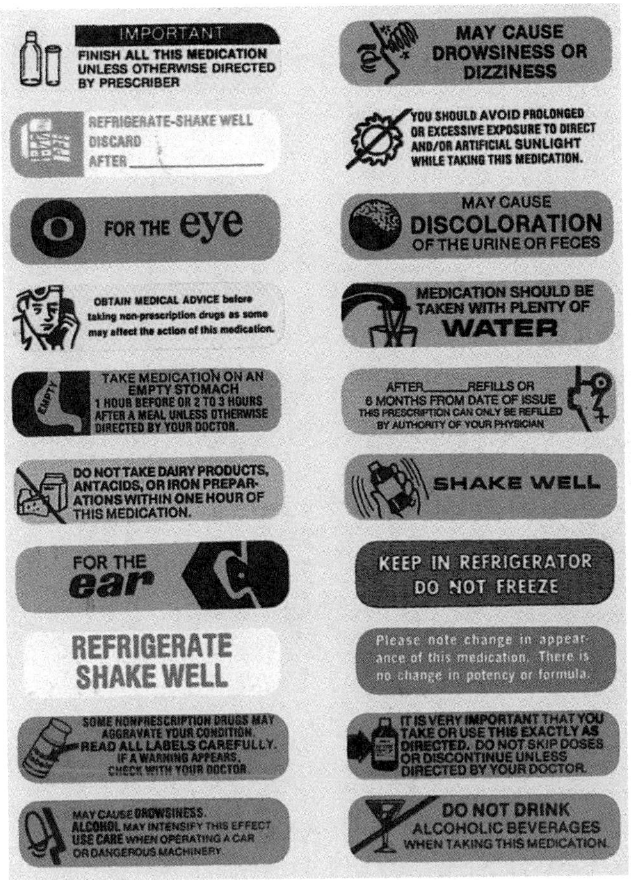

Figure 23-3 Warning labels are placed on prescription medication containers, and patients should be advised to read and adhere to the precautions or instructions.

Because patients are more aware and better informed about their health care needs, they are becoming more involved in making choices and decisions about their health care. When they choose to take over-the-counter (OTC) drugs, they need information and guidance. Over the past few years, some previous prescription drugs have been changed to OTC drugs. The safety of these drugs can only be assured if patients take them as directed.

Patients need to realize that OTC medications:

1. Can interact with other drugs (either prescribed, herbal, or other OTCs) and cause undesirable or adverse reactions or complications
2. May be used in lieu of seeking professional help and thereby interfere with the need for medical care
3. Can mask symptoms and exacerbate an existing condition
4. May have several active ingredients, which may be found to be undesirable
5. Have a safe minimum dose, which may not have the desired therapeutic effect

Figure 23-4 Guidelines for patients when taking nonprescription (over-the-counter) medications.

Patient Education

Many patients keep unused medications past their expiration date. This presents a potential health hazard, because some medications lose their potency after a period, whereas others become toxic. It is best to inform patients to discard any unused portion of medication by the stated date. Encourage patients to check their medicine cabinets at the same time every year so it becomes a routine practice.

Administer, Prescribe, Dispense

There are three ways to handle drugs in the physician's office or clinic: by prescribing, dispensing, or administering them. To **prescribe** a drug means that the licensed practitioner with prescriptive authority (physician, physician assistant, or nurse practitioner) gives a written order to be taken to the pharmacist to be filled. To **dispense** a drug means to give (hand over) the medication as ordered by the physician to the patient to be taken at another time. To **administer** a drug means to give it to the patient by mouth or injection or any other method of administration as ordered by the physician.

Although state laws vary, some states allow certain professionals including medical assistants to prepare and administer medications under the licensed practitioner's supervision. Usually, it is the physician and pharmacist who dispense medications. However, medical assistants can also dispense samples of drugs under the physician's direction. Although medical assistants act as the physician's agent when they prepare and administer medication, they are ethically and legally responsible for their own actions and can be subject to legal action should harm come to a patient. The law requires that individuals who prepare

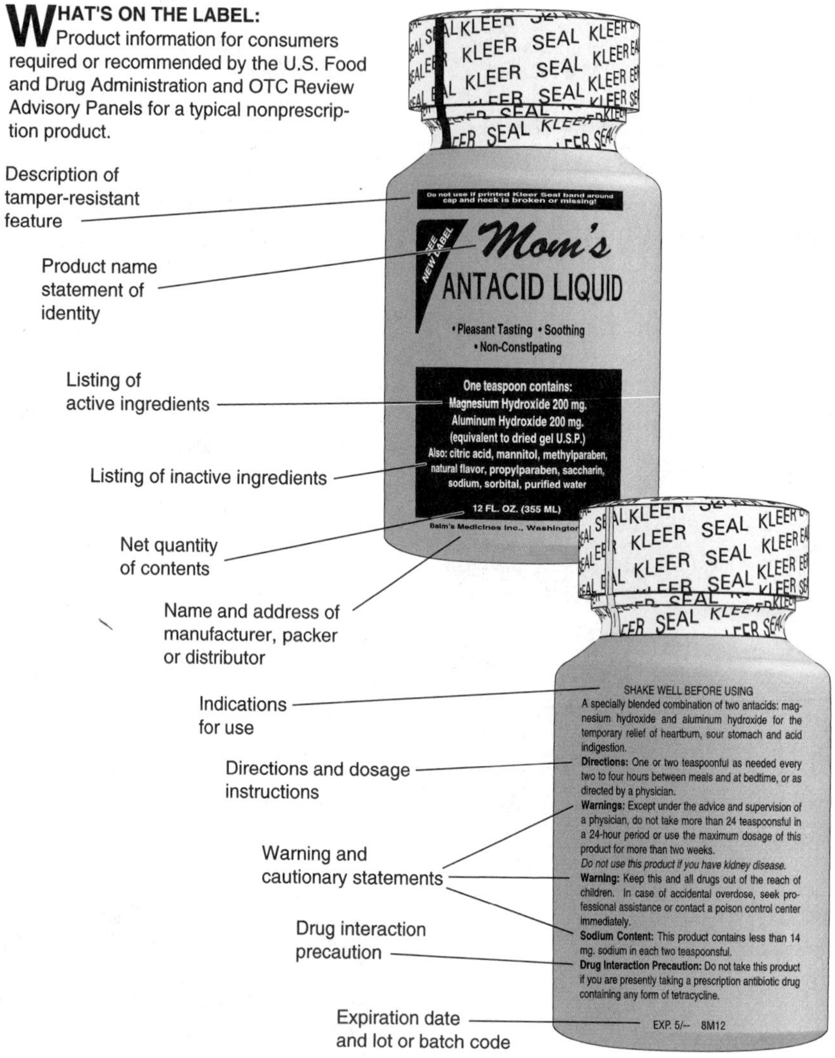

Figure 23-5 Medication labels contain valuable information essential to the safe and effective use of the drug. OTC, over-the-counter.

and administer medications know the medications and their side effects.

DRUG REFERENCES AND STANDARDS

The strength, purity, and quality of drugs differ depending on how they are manufactured. To control the differences, standards have been set. By law, the various drug products must meet standards that are set forth by the FDA. A special reference book, *United States Pharmacopeia/National Formulary,* lists the drugs for which standards have been established. The book is recognized by the U.S. government as the official list of drug standards, which are enforced by the FDA. Every five years the book is updated in an attempt to include all drug products in the United States. Naturals and herbals are not regulated.

Other useful books used as references include the *Compendium of Drug Therapy,* and *Desk Reference for Nonprescription Drugs,* and the *Physician's Desk Reference* (PDR), which is published annually by Medical Economics Company in cooperation with pharmaceutical companies. It is one of the most widely used reference books and is found in most offices and clinics. It is divided into seven sections of drug information, which are followed by other useful drug information such as a list of products, poison control 800 telephone numbers, conversion tables, and a guide to management of drug overdose (Figure 23-6).

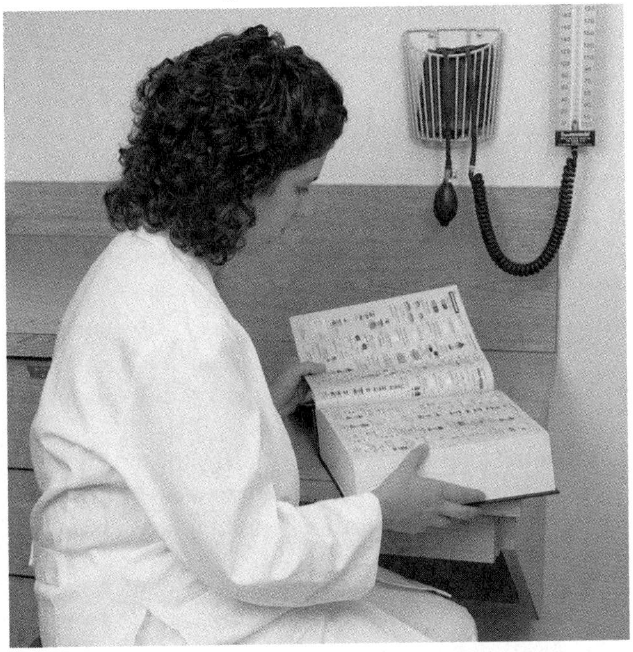

Figure 23-6 The *Physicians' Desk Reference* (PDR) is a valuable resource for the medical assistant who wishes to obtain information about a specific medication.

How to Use the PDR

The four most commonly used sections of the PDR list drugs according to:

- Brand name and generic name (pink section), section 2
- Classification or category (blue section), section 3
- Product information (white section), section 5
- Alphabetical arrangement by manufacturers (white section), section 1

The following guidelines will assist you as you learn to use the PDR.

1. If you know the brand name of the drug, turn to the pink section and locate the drug in the alphabetical listing. The manufacturer's name will be in parentheses, followed by a page number or two page numbers. The first number is the product identification page number. The second number is the product information section (white).

   Example: Look up Zithromax® capsules in a current PDR.

   Zithromax®
   [zi-th-rō-maks]
   (azithromycin capsules)
   (azithromycin tablets)
   (azithromycin oral syspension)
   for ORAL USE

   Note all the information provided about the drug.

   - *Description*. Gives the origin and chemical composition of the drug.
   - *Clinical Pharmacology*. Indicates the effect of the drug on the body and the process by which the drug exerts this effect.
   - *Indications*. States the various conditions, diseases, types of microorganisms, and so on, for which the drug is used.
   - *Contraindications*. States when the drug should not be given to a specified person.
   - *Warnings*. Gives the potential dangers of the drug.
   - *Precautions*. States the possible unfavorable effects that the drug may have on a patient.
   - *Adverse Reactions*. Lists the side effects of the drug.
   - *Dosage and Administration*. States the amount (usual daily dose for adults and children) and time sequence of administration.
   - *How Supplied*. Lists the various forms of the drug and their dosages.

2. If you know the classification of the drug, turn to the blue section and locate the category of the drug.

   Example: Antibiotics
   Macrolide
   Zithromax® capsules (Pfizer)

NOTE: All controlled substances listed in the PDR are indicated with the symbol C with the Roman numeral II, III, IV, or V printed inside the C to designate the schedule in which the substance is classified.

Example: Duramorph® C-II, morphine sulfate USP.

Other Reference Sources

On occasion, you may not find the drug that you are looking for listed in the PDR. When this happens:

- Refer to another drug reference book
- Ask a pharmacist about the drug
- Refer to the packet insert that comes in the drug package

The package insert that most manufacturers provide with their products is an important source of information about a particular drug. This is a brief description of the drug, including its clinical pharmacology, indications and usage, **contraindications** (any symptom or circumstance that indicates that the use of a particular drug is inappropriate when it would otherwise be advisable), warnings, precautions, drug interactions, adverse reactions, overdose, dosage, and administration. The package insert can be a valuable source of information about drugs that might not be listed elsewhere, or if a PDR is unavailable.

Information about some older medications, such as digoxin, can be found in the package insert because they may have been deleted from the current PDR.

CLASSIFICATION OF DRUGS

Drugs can be classified (arranged in groups) in a number of ways. Some examples are:

- Drugs used to treat or prevent disease (examples are hormones and vaccines) (See Figure 23-7)
- Drugs that have a principal action on the body (examples are analgesics and antiinflammatory drugs)
- Drugs that act on specific body systems or organs (examples are respiratory and cardiovascular drugs)
- Drug preparation (examples are suppository, liquid)

Table 23-1 shows a list of common drug classifications. See the Appendix for the 50 top prescribed brand name medications, or visit the following Web site: http://pharmacytimes.com/files/article.

PRINCIPAL ACTIONS OF DRUGS

In general, drugs may be grouped as follows: those that act directly on one or more tissues of the body; those that act on microorganisms; and those that replace body chemicals.

Certain drugs have selective action, such as stimulants, which increase cell activity, and depressants, which decrease cell activity.

Other drugs may have what is known as:

- *Local action*. The drug acts on the area to which it is administered.
- *Remote action*. A drug affects a part of the body that is distant from the site of administration.
- *Systemic action*. The drug is carried via the bloodstream throughout the body.
- *Synergistic action*. One drug increases or counteracts the action of another.

Factors That Affect Drug Action

The four principal factors that affect drug action are: absorption, distribution, biotransformation, and elimination. These factors depend on the individual patient, the form and chemical composition of the drug, and the method of administration.

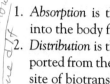

1. *Absorption* is the process whereby the drug passes into the body fluids and tissues.
2. *Distribution* is the process whereby the drug is transported from the blood to the intended site of action, site of biotransformation, site of storage, and site of elimination.
3. *Biotransformation* is the chemical alteration that a drug undergoes in the body.
4. *Elimination* is the process whereby the drug is excreted from the body. Elimination occurs via the gastrointestinal tract, respiratory tract, skin, mucous membranes, and mammary glands.

Undesirable Actions of Drugs

Most drugs have the potential for causing an action other than their intended action. For example:

1. *Side effect*. An undesirable action of the drug that may limit the usefulness of the drug.
2. *Drug interaction*. Occurs when one drug potentiates—increases—or diminishes the action of another drug. These actions may be desirable or undesirable. Drugs may also interact with various foods, alcohol, tobacco, and other substances.
3. *Adverse reaction*. An unfavorable or harmful unintended action of a drug, such as an allergic reaction.

A patient may experience an allergic reaction to a drug after administration. It is often mild and may exhibit itself in the form of a rash, **urticaria,** or **pruritus.** On occasion, a severe reaction or **anaphylaxis** can occur, which is hypersensitivity to a drug or other foreign protein. It is the least common allergic reaction but can become severe quickly and result in dyspnea and shock. Loss of consciousness and death can result. To help prevent an allergic reaction or minimize its risk, the medical assistant should attempt to ascertain before administration of every drug whether the patient has any known allergies. The medical assistant should be aware of signs and symptoms of allergic reaction and notify the physician immediately so that appropriate emergency treatment can be given. One or two injections of epinephrine usually reverses the life-threatening symptoms of anaphylaxis and is followed by administration of an antihistamine such as Benadryl®. In severe cases that do not respond to this treatment, oxygen and immediate transfer to the emergency department is necessary.

DRUG ROUTES

Drugs are manufactured in a variety of forms and for various purposes. The route of a drug refers to how it is administered to the patient, and thereby transported into the patient's body. Certain medications can be administered by more than one route, whereas others must be administered via a specific route.

The route of administration is determined by a number of factors. One factor is the action of the medication on the body, either local or systemic. Intravenous medication reaches the systemic circulation rapidly via the bloodstream and quickly becomes effective. Injections of medication and medications absorbed through mucous membranes such as suppositories and sublingual nitroglycerine are absorbed quickly. Oral medications take longer to act because they must be digested by the stomach and then be absorbed into the bloodstream.

Another factor in route selection is the physical and emotional state of the patient. The patient's consciousness level, emotional status, and physical restrictions are considered when selecting a route to administer medication.

A third factor to consider is the characteristics of the drug. An example is insulin. Insulin is destroyed by digestive enzymes; therefore, the route of administration must be by injection.

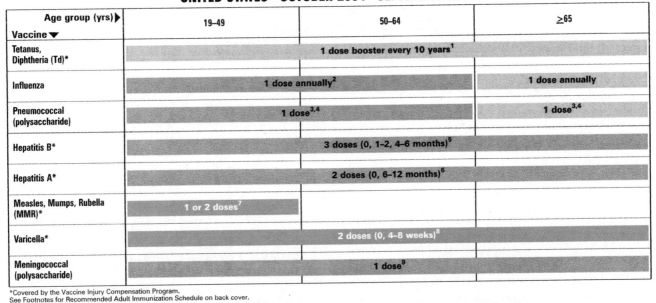

Recommended Adult Immunization Schedule by Vaccine and Age Group

UNITED STATES · OCTOBER 2004–SEPTEMBER 2005

Age group (yrs) ▶ / Vaccine ▼	19–49	50–64	≥65
Tetanus, Diphtheria (Td)*	1 dose booster every 10 years[1]		
Influenza	1 dose annually[2]		1 dose annually
Pneumococcal (polysaccharide)	1 dose[3,4]		1 dose[3,4]
Hepatitis B*	3 doses (0, 1–2, 4–6 months)[5]		
Hepatitis A*	2 doses (0, 6–12 months)[6]		
Measles, Mumps, Rubella (MMR)*	1 or 2 doses[7]		
Varicella*	2 doses (0, 4–8 weeks)[8]		
Meningococcal (polysaccharide)	1 dose[9]		

*Covered by the Vaccine Injury Compensation Program.
See Footnotes for Recommended Adult Immunization Schedule on back cover.

For all persons in this group — For persons lacking documentation of vaccination or evidence of disease — For persons at risk (i.e., with medical/exposure indications)

The Recommended Adult Immunization Schedule is Approved by the Advisory Committee on Immunization Practices (ACIP), the American College of Obstetricians and Gynecologists (ACOG), and the American Academy of Family Physicians (AAFP)

This schedule indicates the recommended age groups for routine administration of currently licensed vaccines for persons aged ≥19 years. Licensed combination vaccines may be used whenever any components of the combination are indicated and when the vaccine's other components are not contraindicated. Providers should consult manufacturers' package inserts for detailed recommendations.

Report all clinically significant postvaccination reactions to the Vaccine Adverse Event Reporting System (VAERS). Reporting forms and instructions on filing a VAERS report are available by telephone, 800-822-7967, or from the VAERS website at http://www.vaers.org.

Information on how to file a Vaccine Injury Compensation Program claim is available at http://www.hrsa.gov/osp/vicp or by telephone, 800-338-2382. To file a claim for vaccine injury, contact the U.S. Court of Federal Claims, 717 Madison Place, N.W., Washington, DC 20005, telephone 202-219-9657.

Additional information about the vaccines listed above and contraindications for immunization is available at http://www.cdc.gov/nip or from the National Immunization Hotline, 800-232-2522 (English) or 800-232-0233 (Spanish).

Figure 23-7 Vaccines are used to prevent disease as noted in Chapters 10 and 18. (Courtesy of Centers for Disease Control and Prevention. [2004]. Recommended adult immunization schedule—United States, October 2004–September 2005. *MMWR 53,* 1–4.)

(continues)

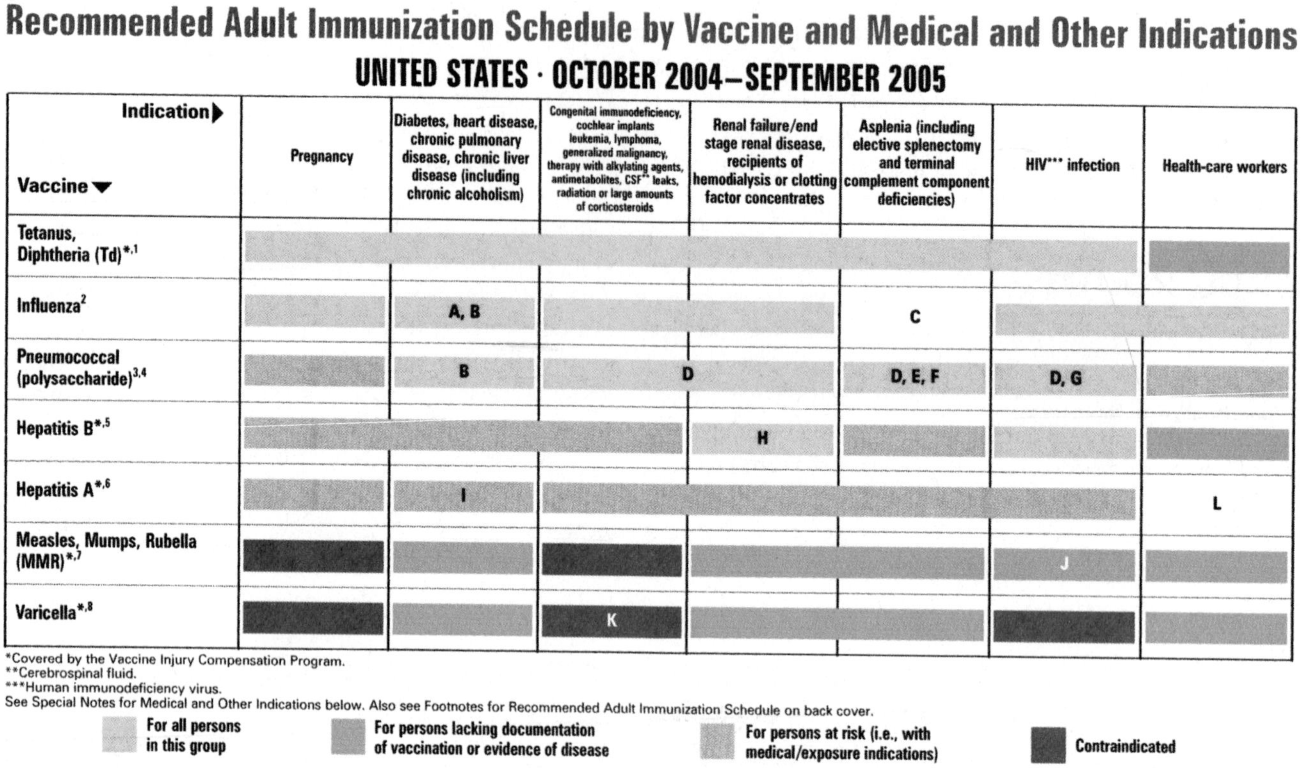

Recommended Adult Immunization Schedule by Vaccine and Medical and Other Indications
UNITED STATES · OCTOBER 2004–SEPTEMBER 2005
Indication
Vaccine
Pregnancy
Diabetes, heart disease, chronic pulmonary disease, chronic liver disease (including chronic alcoholism)
Congenital immunodeficiency, cochlear implants leukemia, lymphoma, generalized malignancy, therapy with alkylating agents, antimetabolites, CSF** leaks, radiation or large amounts of corticosteroids
Renal failure/end stage renal disease, recipients of hemodialysis or clotting factor concentrates
Asplenia (including elective splenectomy and terminal complement component deficiencies)
HIV*** infection
Health-care workers
Tetanus, Diphtheria (Td)*,1
Influenza2
A, B
C
Pneumococcal (polysaccharide)3,4
B
D
D, E, F
D, G
Hepatitis B*,5
H
Hepatitis A*,6
I
L
Measles, Mumps, Rubella (MMR)*,7
J
Varicella*,8
K
*Covered by the Vaccine Injury Compensation Program.
**Cerebrospinal fluid.
***Human immunodeficiency virus.
See Special Notes for Medical and Other Indications below. Also see Footnotes for Recommended Adult Immunization Schedule on back cover.
For all persons in this group
For persons lacking documentation of vaccination or evidence of disease
For persons at risk (i.e., with medical/exposure indications)
Contraindicated

Special Notes for Medical and Other Indications

A. Although chronic liver disease and alcoholism are not indications for influenza vaccination, administer 1 dose annually if the patient is aged ≥50 years, has other indications for influenza vaccine, or requests vaccination.

B. Asthma is an indication for influenza vaccination but not for pneumococcal vaccination.

C. No data exist specifically on the risk for severe or complicated influenza infections among persons with asplenia. However, influenza is a risk factor for secondary bacterial infections that can cause severe disease among persons with asplenia.

D. For persons aged <65 years, revaccinate once after ≥5 years have elapsed since initial vaccination.

E. Administer meningococcal vaccine and consider *Haemophilus influenzae* type b vaccine.

F. For persons undergoing elective splenectomy, vaccinate ≥2 weeks before surgery.

G. Vaccinate as soon after diagnosis as possible.

H. For hemodialysis patients, use special formulation of vaccine (40 μg/mL) or two 20 μg/mL doses administered at one body site. Vaccinate early in the course of renal disease. Assess antibody titers to hepatitis B surface antigen (anti-HB) levels annually. Administer additional doses if anti-HB levels decline to <10 mIU/mL.

I. For all persons with chronic liver disease.

J. Withhold MMR or other measles-containing vaccines from HIV-infected persons with evidence of severe immunosuppression (see *MMWR* 1998;47 [No. RR-8]:21–2 and *MMWR* 2002;51 [No. RR-2]:22–4).

K. Persons with impaired humoral immunity but intact cellular immunity may be vaccinated (see *MMWR* 1999;48[No. RR-6]).

L. No data to support a recommendation.

Figure 23-7 (continued)

The most frequently used routes of administering medication to the patient are oral and parenteral routes: oral medications are taken by mouth; parenteral generally by injection. Other routes of administration include:

- Direct application to the skin (lotions, creams, liniments, ointments, and transdermal [patch] systems)
- Sublingual (tablets, liquid, drops)
- Buccal (tablets)
- Rectal (suppositories, ointments)
- Vaginal (suppositories, creams, applications)
- Inhalation (sprays, aerosols)
- Instillation (liquid, drops)

FORMS OF DRUGS

Drugs are compounded in three basic types of preparations: liquids, solids, and semisolids. The ease with which a drug's ingredients can be dissolved largely determines the variety of forms manufactured. Some drug agents are soluble in water, others in alcohol, and others in a mixture of several solvents.

The method for administering a drug depends on its form, its properties, and the effects desired. When given orally, a drug may be in the form of a liquid, powder, tablet, capsule, or caplet. If it is to be injected, it must be in the form of a liquid. For topical use, the drug may be in the form of a liquid, powder, or semisolid. Oral and injectable medications are examples of preparations designed for internal use.

Footnotes

Recommended Adult Immunization Schedule · UNITED STATES · OCTOBER 2004–SEPTEMBER 2005

1. **Tetanus and diphtheria (Td).** Adults, including pregnant women with uncertain history of a complete primary vaccination series, should receive a primary series of Td. A primary series for adults is 3 doses; administer the first 2 doses at least 4 weeks apart and the 3rd dose 6–12 months after the second. Administer 1 dose if the person received the primary series and if the last vaccination was received ≥10 years previously. Consult recommendations for administering Td as prophylaxis in wound management (see *MMWR* 1991;40[No. RR-10]). The American College of Physicians Task Force on Adult Immunization supports a second option for Td use in adults: a single Td booster at age 50 years for persons who have completed the full pediatric series, including the teenage/young adult booster.

2. **Influenza vaccination.** The Advisory Committee on Immunization Practices (ACIP) recommends inactivated influenza vaccination for the following indications, when vaccine is available. *Medical indications:* chronic disorders of the cardiovascular or pulmonary systems, including asthma; chronic metabolic diseases, including diabetes mellitus, renal dysfunction, hemoglobinopathies, or immunosuppression (including immunosuppression caused by medications or by human immunodeficiency virus [HIV]); and pregnancy during the influenza season. *Occupational indications:* health-care workers and employees of long-term–care and assisted living facilities. *Other indications:* residents of nursing homes and other long-term–care facilities; persons likely to transmit influenza to persons at high risk (i.e., in-home caregivers to persons with medical indications, household/close contacts and out-of-home caregivers of children aged 0–23 months, household members and caregivers of elderly persons and adults with high-risk conditions); and anyone who wishes to be vaccinated. For healthy persons aged 5–49 years without high-risk conditions who are not contacts of severely immunocompromised persons in special care units, either the inactivated vaccine or the intranasally administered influenza vaccine (FluMist®) may be administered (see *MMWR* 2004;53[No. RR-6]).
Note: Because of the vaccine shortage for the 2004–05 influenza season, CDC has recommended that vaccination be restricted to the following priority groups, which are considered to be of equal importance: all children aged 6–23 months; adults aged ≥65 years; persons aged 2–64 years with underlying chronic medical conditions; all women who will be pregnant during the influenza season; residents of nursing homes and long-term–care facilities; children aged 6 months–18 years on chronic aspirin therapy; health-care workers involved in direct patient care; and out-of-home caregivers and household contacts of children aged <6 months. For the 2004–05 season, intranasally administered, live, attenuated influenza vaccine, if available, should be encouraged for healthy persons who are aged 5–49 years and are not pregnant, including health-care workers (except those who care for severely immunocompromised patients in special care units) and persons caring for children aged <6 months (see *MMWR* 2004;53:923–4).

3. **Pneumococcal polysaccharide vaccination.** *Medical indications:* chronic disorders of the pulmonary system (excluding asthma); cardiovascular diseases; diabetes mellitus; chronic liver diseases, including liver disease as a result of alcohol abuse (e.g., cirrhosis); chronic renal failure or nephrotic syndrome; functional or anatomic asplenia (e.g., sickle cell disease or splenectomy); immunosuppressive conditions (e.g., congenital immunodeficiency, HIV infection, leukemia, lymphoma, multiple myeloma, Hodgkins disease, generalized malignancy, or organ or bone marrow transplantation); chemotherapy with alkylating agents, antimetabolites, or long-term systemic corticosteroids; or cochlear implants. *Geographic/other indications:* Alaska Natives and certain American Indian populations. *Other indications:* residents of nursing homes and other long-term–care facilities (see *MMWR* 1997;46[No. RR-8] and *MMWR* 2003;52:739–40).

4. **Revaccination with pneumococcal polysaccharide vaccine.** One-time revaccination after 5 years for persons with chronic renal failure or nephrotic syndrome; functional or anatomic asplenia (e.g., sickle cell disease or splenectomy); immunosuppressive conditions (e.g., congenital immunodeficiency, HIV infection, leukemia, lymphoma, multiple myeloma, Hodgkins disease, generalized malignancy, or organ or bone marrow transplantation); or chemotherapy with alkylating agents, antimetabolites, or long-term systemic corticosteroids. For persons aged ≥65 years, one-time revaccination if they were vaccinated ≥5 years previously and were aged <65 years at the time of primary vaccination (see *MMWR* 1997;46[No. RR-8]).

5. **Hepatitis B vaccination.** *Medical indications:* hemodialysis patients or patients who receive clotting factor concentrates. *Occupational indications:* health-care workers and public-safety workers who have exposure to blood in the workplace; and persons in training in schools of medicine, dentistry, nursing, laboratory technology, and other allied health professions. *Behavioral indications:* injection-drug users; persons with more than one sex partner during the previous 6 months; persons with a recently acquired sexually transmitted disease (STD); all clients in STD clinics; and men who have sex with men. *Other indications:* household contacts and sex partners of persons with chronic hepatitis B virus (HBV) infection; clients and staff members of institutions for the developmentally disabled; inmates of correctional facilities; or international travelers who will be in countries with high or intermediate prevalence of chronic HBV infection for >6 months (http://www.cdc.gov/travel/diseases/hbv.htm) (see *MMWR* 1991;40[No. RR-13]).

6. **Hepatitis A vaccination.** *Medical indications:* persons with clotting factor disorders or chronic liver disease. *Behavioral indications:* men who have sex with men or users of illegal drugs. *Occupational indications:* persons working with hepatitis A virus (HAV)-infected primates or with HAV in a research laboratory setting. *Other indications:* persons traveling to or working in countries that have high or intermediate endemicity of hepatitis A. If the combined Hepatitis A and Hepatitis B vaccine is used, administer 3 doses at 0, 1, and 6 months (http://www.cdc.gov/travel/diseases/hav.htm) (see MMWR 1999;48[No. RR-12]).

7. **Measles, mumps, rubella (MMR) vaccination.** *Measles component:* adults born before 1957 can be considered immune to measles. Adults born during or after 1957 should receive ≥1 dose of MMR unless they have a medical contraindication, documentation of ≥1 dose, or other acceptable evidence of immunity. A second dose of MMR is recommended for adults who 1) were recently exposed to measles or in an outbreak setting, 2) were previously vaccinated with killed measles vaccine, 3) were vaccinated with an unknown vaccine during 1963–1967, 4) are students in postsecondary educational institutions, 5) work in health-care facilities, or 6) plan to travel internationally. *Mumps component:* 1 dose of MMR vaccine should be adequate for protection. *Rubella component:* Administer 1 dose of MMR vaccine to women whose rubella vaccination history is unreliable and counsel women to avoid becoming pregnant for 4 weeks after vaccination. For women of childbearing age, regardless of birth year, routinely determine rubella immunity and counsel women regarding congenital rubella syndrome. Do not vaccinate pregnant women or those planning to become pregnant during the next 4 weeks. For women who are pregnant and susceptible, vaccinate as early in the postpartum period as possible (see *MMWR* 1998;47[No. RR-8] and *MMWR* 2001;50:1117).

8. **Varicella vaccination.** Recommended for all persons lacking a reliable clinical history of varicella infection or serologic evidence of varicella zoster virus (VZV) infection who might be at high risk for exposure or transmission. This includes health-care workers and family contacts of immunocompromised persons; persons who live or work in environments where transmission is likely (e.g., teachers of young children, child care employees, and residents and staff members in institutional settings); persons who live or work in environments where VZV transmission can occur (e.g., college students, inmates, and staff members of correctional institutions, and military personnel); adolescents aged 11–18 years and adults living in households with children; women who are not pregnant but who might become pregnant; and international travelers who are not immune to infection.
Note: Approximately 95% of U.S.-born adults are immune to VZV. Do not vaccinate pregnant women or those planning to become pregnant during the next 4 weeks. For women who are pregnant and susceptible, vaccinate as early in the postpartum period as possible (see *MMWR* 1999;48[No. RR-6]).

9. **Meningococcal vaccine (quadrivalent polysaccharide for serogroups A, C, Y, and W 135).** *Medical indications:* adults with terminal complement component deficiencies or those with anatomic or functional asplenia. *Other indications:* travelers to countries in which meningococcal disease is hyperendemic or epidemic (e.g., the "meningitis belt" of sub-Saharan Africa and Mecca, Saudi Arabia). Revaccination after 3–5 years might be indicated for persons at high risk for infection (e.g., persons residing in areas where disease is epidemic). Counsel college freshmen, especially those who live in dormitories, regarding meningococcal disease and availability of the vaccine to enable them to make an educated decision about receiving the vaccination (see *MMWR* 2000;49[No. RR-7]). The American Academy of Family Physicians recommends that colleges should take the lead on providing education on meningococcal infection and availability of vaccination and offer it to students who are interested. Physicians need not initiate discussion of meningococcal quadrivalent polysaccharide vaccine as part of routine medical care.

Figure 23-7 (continued)

Liquid Preparations

Liquid preparations are those containing a drug that has been dissolved or suspended. Depending on the solvent used, the drug may be further classified as an aqueous (water) or alcohol preparation or as an aerosol or mist. When prescribed for internal use, liquid preparations other than emulsions are rapidly absorbed through the stomach or intestinal walls.

Solid and Semisolid Preparations

Tablets, capsules, caplets, troches or lozenges, suppositories, and ointments are examples of solid and semisolid preparations. These products offer great flexibility as a means of dispensing different dosages of drugs (Figure 23-8).

Other Drug Delivery Systems

Technologic advances have introduced new ways by which drugs can be introduced into the patient. In addition to the conventional preparations, the following miniature therapeutic systems offer special delivery of medication to targeted areas.

Transdermal System. The transdermal system of medication delivery consists of a small adhesive patch that may be applied to intact skin near the treatment site. For example, Transderm Scop®, used for preventing motion sickness, may be applied behind the ear; Nitro-Dur® (Figure 23-9), used for preventing angina pectoris, may be applied to the chest; Estraderm®, used to treat menopausal symptoms, may be applied to the trunk; and Nicoderm®,

TABLE 23-1 COMMON CLASSIFICATIONS OF DRUGS AND THEIR ACTIONS

Classification (with Phonetic Spelling)	Action	Examples of Drugs Commonly Used in Ambulatory Care Setting
Analgesic (an"al-je'sik)	An agent that relieves pain without causing loss of consciousness	acetaminophen (Tylenol) acetylsalicylic acid (aspirin) ibuprofen (Advil, Motrin)
Anesthetic (an"es-thet'ik)	An agent that produces numbness May be local or general depending on the type and how administered	lidocaine HCl (Xylocaine) } Both are local anesthetics procaine HCl (Novacaine) }
Antacid (ant-as'id)	An agent that neutralizes acid	Amphojel, Gelusil, Mylanta, Milk of Magnesia
Antianemic (an"ti-an-em'ic)	An agent that replaces iron	iron (imferon), ferrous sulfate
Antianxiety (an"ti-ang-zi'e-te)	An agent that relieves anxiety and muscle tension	benzodiazepines: diazepam (Valium) chlordiazepoxide HCl (Librium) alprazolam (Xanax)
Antiarrhythmic (an"te-a-rith'mik)	An agent that controls cardiac arrhythmias	lidocaine HCl (Xylocaine) propranolol HCl (Inderal)
Antibiotic (an"ti-bi-ot'ik)	An agent that is destructive to or inhibits growth of microorganisms	penicillins (Pentids, Duracillin, Polycillin, Pipracil, Augmentin)
Anticholinergic (an"ti-ko"lin-er'jik)	An agent that blocks parasympathetic nerve impulses	atropine, scopolamine, trihexyphenidyl HCl (Artane)
Anticholesterol (an"ti-ko"less'ter-ol)	An agent that reduces cholesterol	Zocor, Lipitor, Crestor
Anticoagulant (an"ti-ko-ag'u-lant)	An agent that prevents or delays blood clotting	heparin sodium, Dicumarol, warfarin sodium (Coumadin)
Anticonvulsant (an"ti-kon-vul'sant)	An agent that prevents or relieves convulsions	carbamazepine (Tegretol) phenytoin (Dilantin) ethosuximide (Zarontin)
Antidepressant (an"ti-dep-res'ant)	An agent that prevents or relieves the symptoms of depression	monoamine oxidase (MAO) inhibitors: isocarboxazid (Marplan), phenelzine sulfate (Nardil), tricyclic: amitriptyline HCl (Elavil), imipramine HCl (Tofranil), Sertraline HCl (Zoloft), paroxetine HCl (Paxil), trazodone (Desyrel), fluoxentine (Prozac)
Antidiarrheal (an"ti-di-a-re'al)	An agent that prevents or relieves diarrhea	Pepto-Bismol, Kaopectate, Diphenoxylate HCl (Lomotil)
Antidote (an-ti'dot)	An agent that counteracts poisons and their effects	naloxone (Narcan)
Antiemetic (an"ti-e-met'ik)	An agent that prevents or relieves nausea and vomiting	Tigan, Dramamine, Phenergan, Reglan, Marinol, Compazine
Antihistamine (an"ti-his'ta-min)	An agent that acts to counteract histamine	Dimetane, Benadryl, Seldane
Antihypertensive (an"ti-hi"per-ten'siv)	An agent that prevents or controls high blood pressure	methyldopa (Aldomet) clonidine HCl (Catapres) metoprolol tartrate (Lopressor)
Antiinflammatory (an"ti-in-flam'a-to-re)	An agent that counteracts inflammation	naproxen (Naprosyn) aspirin, ibuprofen (Advil, Motrin)
Antimanic (an"ti-man'ik)	An agent used for the treatment of the manic episode of manic-depressive disorder	lithium
Antineoplastic (an"ti-ne"o-plas'tik)	An agent that kills or destroys malignant cells	busuflan (Myleran) cyclophosphamide (Cytoxan)
Antipsychotic	An agent that helps in schizophrenia and chronic brain syndrome	haloperdol (Haldol) chlorpromazine (Thorazine)
Antipyretic (an"ti-pi-ret'ik)	An agent that reduces fever	aspirin, acetaminophen (Tylenol)
Antitussive (an"ti-tus'iv)	An agent that prevents or relieves cough	codeine, dextromethorphan (Pertussin, Romilar)

(continues)

TABLE 23-1 (continued)

Classification (with Phonetic Spelling)	Action	Examples of Drugs Commonly Used in Ambulatory Care Setting
Antiulcer (an"ti-ul'ser) (H_2 blockers)	An agent that relieves and heals ulcers by blocking hydrochloric acid	cimetidine (Tagamet) ranitidine (Zantac) omeprazole (Prilosec)
Bronchodilator (brong"ko-dil-a'tor)	An agent that dilates the bronchi	isoproterenol HCl (Isuprel) albuterol (Proventil)
Contraceptive (kon"tra-sep'tiv)	Any device, method, or agent that prevents conception	Envid-E 21, Ortho-Novum 10/11-21; 10/11-28 Triphasil-21, Ovral 28, Alesse, Levlen
Decongestant (de"con-gest'ant)	An agent that reduces nasal congestion or swelling	oxymetazoline (Afrin) phenylephrine HCl (Neo-Synephrine) pseudoephedrine HCl (Sudafed)
Diuretic (di"u-ret'ik)	An agent that increases the excretion of urine	chlorothiazide (Diuril) furosemide (Lasix) mannitol (Osmitrol)
Expectorant (ek-spek'to-rant)	An agent that facilitates removal of secretion from bronchopulmonary mucous membrane	guaifenesin (Robitussin)
Hemostatic (he"mo-stat'ik)	An agent that controls or stops bleeding	Humafac, Amicar, vitamin K
Hypnotic (hip-not'ik)	An agent that produces sleep or hypnosis	secobarbital (Seconal); chloral hydrate; ethchlorvynol (Placidyl)
Hypoglycemic (hi"po-gli-se'mik)	An agent that reduces blood glucose level	insulin; chlorpropamide (Diabinese); tolbutamide (Orinsase)
Laxative (lak'sa-tiv)	An agent that loosens and promotes normal bowel elimination	Metamucil powder, Dulcolax; Docusate sodium (Colace)
Muscle relaxant (mus'el re-lak'sant)	An agent that produces relaxation of skeletal muscle	Robaxin, Norflex, Paraflex, Skelaxin, Valium
Sedative (sed'a-tiv)	An agent that produces a calming effect without causing sleep	amobarbital (amytal) butabarbital sodium (Buticaps) phenobarbital
Tranquilizer (tran"kwi-liz'er)	An agent that reduces mental tension and anxiety	Diazapem (Valium) Alprazolam (Xanax); chlordiazepoxide (Librium)
Vasodilator (vas"o-di-la'tor)	An agent that produces relaxation of blood vessels; reduces blood pressure	isorbide dinitrate (Isordil); atenolol (Tenormin) nitroglycerin; diltiazem (Cardizem)
Vasopressor (vas"o-pres'or)	An agent that produces contraction of muscles of capillaries and arteries; increases blood pressure	metaraminol (Aramine) norepinephrine (Levophed)

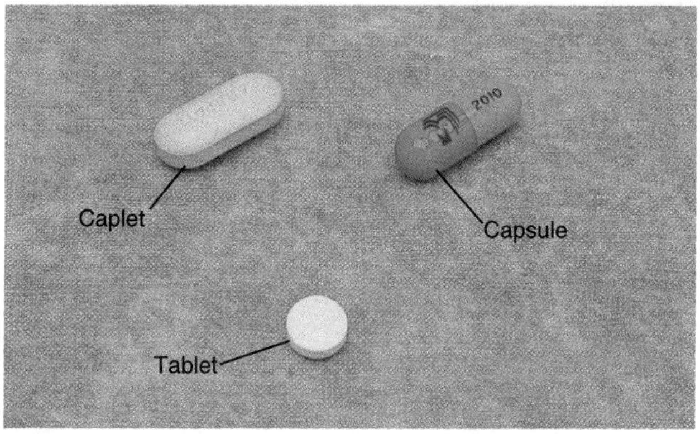

Figure 23-8 Drugs are manufactured in various forms, including solid preparations such as this caplet, capsule, and tablet.

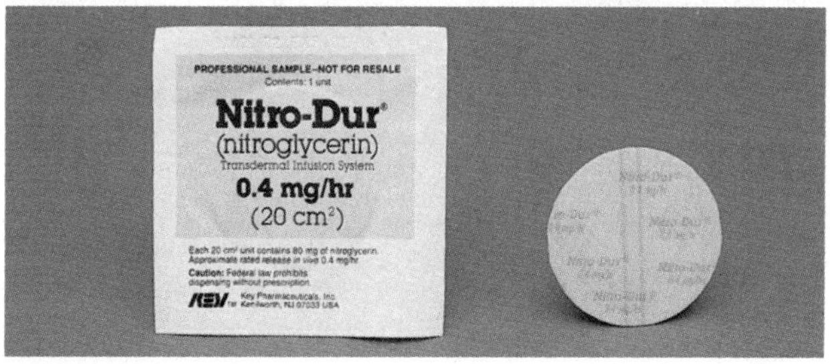

Figure 23-9 Nitro-Dur® is a transdermal system of delivering medication used for prevention and for long-term management of angina pectoris. It may be applied to the chest.

used to relieve the body's craving for nicotine, may be applied to any area above the waist. A transdermal system generally consists of four layers (Figure 23-10):

1. An impermeable backing that keeps the drug from leaking out of the system
2. A reservoir containing the drug
3. A membrane with tiny holes that controls the rate of drug release
4. An adhesive layer or gel that keeps the device in place

Inhalation Medications. Medication for respiratory diseases and conditions such as asthma, bronchiectasis (permanent dilation of one or more bronchi), bronchitis, and others may require treatment with inhalation medication from an aerosolized inhaler or a nebulizer. Some of the commonly prescribed medications are bronchodilators such as aminophylline, isuprel, epinephrine, and cortisone-type medications. Oxygen may be prescribed for hypoxia caused by respiratory diseases. Oxygen may be prescribed for cardiovascular collapse, congestive heart failure, and pneumonia among other examples. (See Chapter 18 for information about nebulizers and oxygen administration.)

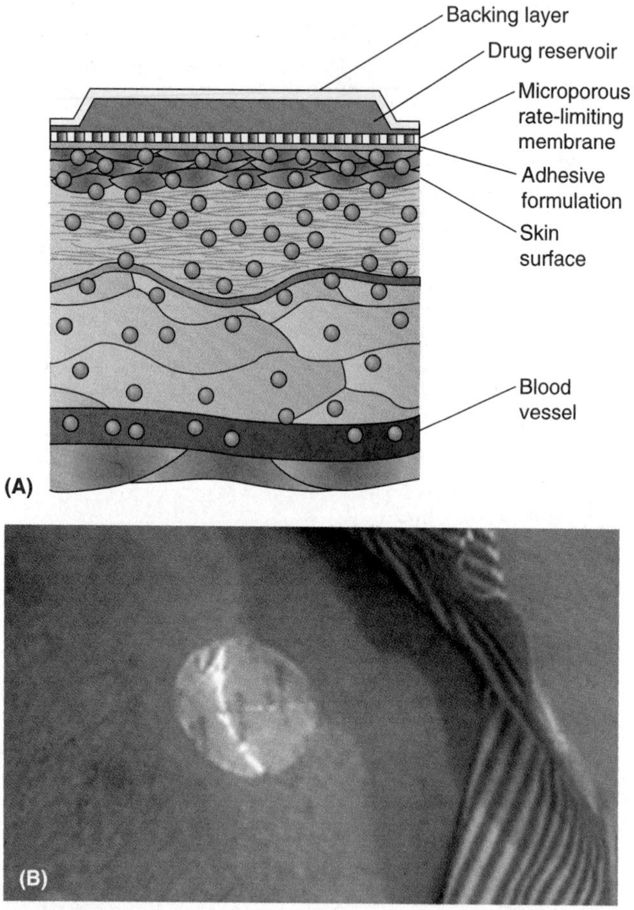

Figure 23-10 (A) The multilayer unit comprising TransdermNitro® delivers nitroglycerin into the bloodstream in a consistent, controlled manner for 24 hours. The thin unit contains a backing layer, a reservoir of nitroglycerin, a unique rate-limiting membrane, and an adhesive layer that has a priming dose of nitroglycerin. (B) The patch is applied to the skin. (Courtesy of Novartis.)

Eye-Curing Lens. Another innovative drug delivery system is one in which a drug, contained between two ultrathin plastic membranes, is placed inside the lower eyelid. It appears to cause little or no discomfort and provides a controlled release of the medication for an extended period. Pilocarpine, a miotic that causes contraction of the pupils, is being used in this method for the treatment of glaucoma.

Implantable Devices. Implantable devices are available in several shapes and sizes and are positioned just beneath the skin near blood vessels that lead directly to the area to be medicated. For example, an infusion pump that is about the size of a hockey puck can be implanted below the skin near the waist to provide continuous delivery of chemotherapy to patients with liver cancer or insulin to a diabetic. This device, which has a refillable drug reservoir, is connected by an outlet catheter to the patient's blood vessel. In addition to providing a continuous supply of medication, these devices have the advantage of delivering greater doses with fewer side effects than can be realized through the systemic route.

STORAGE AND HANDLING OF MEDICATIONS

Certain precautions should be followed if the ambulatory care setting keeps medications on the premises. The goal should be to store all medications in their original containers in a separate room in a locked cabinet. Many medications require storage in a certain manner, such as a dark area or in a dark container (to keep light away from them) or in the refrigerator. Some must be kept in glass containers only because plastic may react with the medication's chemical composition. The drug label indicates proper storage and handling for each medication.

Keep medications that are for internal use separated from those intended for external use.

Access to medications is simplified if they are organized in the storage area either according to their classification (diuretic, hormones) or according to the alphabet. Always check expiration dates.

EMERGENCY DRUGS AND SUPPLIES

The ambulatory care setting should maintain a tray, box, cabinet, or crash cart (see Chapter 9 for contents of crash cart) especially and solely for drugs and supplies needed in an emergency such as anaphylaxis or other form of shock. The drugs listed in Table 23-2 are a sample of some general drugs to keep readily available for emergencies.

Other supplies and equipment to keep together with the drugs on the emergency cart are:

- Intravenous materials such as IV fluids, needles, tubing, syringes, alcohol, swabs, constriction band, and tape
- Sphygmomanometer
- Stethoscope
- Oxygen and mask
- Airways
- Defibrillator
- Suction equipment (nasopharyngeal)
- Personal protective equipment

TABLE 23-2 EXAMPLES OF COMMON EMERGENCY DRUGS

Adrenalin (a-dren'a-lin) or **epinephrine** (ep-i-nef-rin)	A vasoconstrictor. Relieves anaphylactic shock.
Albuterol (al-bú-ter-ol)	A bronchodilator. Relaxes smooth muscle of the respiratory tract.
Benadryl (ben'a-dril)	An antihistamine that relieves allergic symptoms.
Compazine (com-pa'zeen)	An antiemetic. Relieves symptoms of nausea and vomiting.
Dextrose (deks'trose) 50%	Used for hypoglycemia to counteract hyperinsulinism.
Digoxin (di-jox'in)	Cardiac drug. Used for congestive heart failure, arryhthmias. Slows and strengthens heartbeat.
Diuril (di'ur-il)	Promotes excretion of urine.
Hydrocortisone (hi"dro-cort'i-zon)	An antiinflammatory. Used to suppress swelling and shock.
Insulin (in'sah-lin)	Diabetic coma.
Narcan (nar'can)	Antidote. Used in narcotic overdose.
Nitroglycerin (ni"tro-glis'er-in)	Vasodilator. Dilates coronary arteries. Used in treatment of angina pectoris.
Valium (val'e-um)	Antianxiety, muscle relaxant. Used to calm anxious patients and to relax muscles. Valium is a Schedule IV drug, and therefore must be kept in a locked cabinet.
Verapamil (ver-ap'a-mil)	For cardiac arrhythmia, stable and unstable angina.

Note: Ipecac syrup, no longer used to induce vomiting, has proven to be cardiotoxic, and several cases of aspiration have occurred.

Check the tray on a regular basis (weekly, monthly, depending on use) according to need. Check the oxygen tank and gauge. Replace items that have been used as soon as possible, and discard drugs and supplies that have reached their expiration dates. Document that the tray has been checked and updated. (See Chapter 9 for more information about emergencies and emergency drugs used in the office and other ambulatory areas.)

Bioterrorism

Bioterrorism is the name given to the use of biologic weapons (pathogenic microorganisms) to create fear in people. There are many biologic agents that can be used in an attempt to cause serious diseases. Most diseases can be treated with pharmaceutical agents such as antibiotics and antitoxoids.

The most dangerous disease threats are anthrax, botulism, pneumonic/bubonic plague, smallpox, and tularemia.

Anthrax, pneumonic/bubonic plague, and tularemia can all be treated with antibiotics. Botulism is treated with botulism antioxides supplied by public health authorities. Smallpox is treated by early vaccination (within four days). The Centers for Disease Control and Prevention has the vaccine.

Education plays a vital role in raising awareness and increasing the knowledge of health care professionals to aid them in being better prepared for threats to the public health. The World Health Organization, the Centers for Disease Control and Prevention, and state and local public health departments are excellent resources for more information about bioterrorism. (See Chapter 10 for more information on infectious diseases and Chapter 24 for information on antibiotics.)

DRUG ABUSE

There has been an enormous increase in the **abuse,** or misuse, of legal and illegal drugs. Any drug can be abused, whether it is penicillin, alcohol, or a controlled substance such as cocaine. Medical assistants, while caring for patients, may unexpectedly come in contact with patients who abuse or misuse drugs.

Medical assistants must be able to recognize the symptoms of drug abuse in a patient or coworker and report it to the physician. Health professionals, including physicians, are among the individuals who may have a problem with drug or alcohol abuse, and this must be reported to the proper professional association. Refer to Chapter 7 for more information on drug abuse.

There are many programs available for treatment of drug abuse. Detoxification and rehabilitation are examples of treatment programs.

Following are examples of drug types most commonly abused:

- Marijuana, LSD ("acid"), Mescaline
- Narcotics: cocaine, opioids, Oxycontin, Vicodin
- Amphetamines: Dexedrine®, Ritalin®
- Depressants: Valium®, alcohol
- Barbiturates ("barbs," "downers," "red devils"): Nembutal®, Seconal®
- Antitussives: Coricidin, Robitussin DM
- Solvents (inhaled): paint thinner, glue, gasoline

Effects of Drug Abuse

When an individual is directly under the influence of a particular substance, acute effects of drug abuse are evident. For example, the acute effects of amphetamines may include symptoms that affect the central nervous system, such as euphoria, excitement, anorexia, or insomnia. Dilated pupils, nervousness, talkativeness, agitation, tachycardia, fever, and chills are other symptoms of amphetamine abuse.

As an abused substance, cocaine is usually injected, sniffed, or snorted into the nose or smoked in a form called crack or freebase. It is absorbed through the mucous membrane. Effects begin within a few minutes, and then subside within an hour. Dilated pupils, increased blood pressure, tachycardia, and increased body temperature are symptoms of the acute effects of cocaine. Euphoria and excitement are probable reasons for its high abuse potential. Death comes from respiratory and circulatory failure.

Barbiturates are used medically as sedatives to relieve anxiety. Abuse effects include slurred speech, confusion, poor motor coordination, and impaired judgment. Coma and death result from high doses. Abrupt withdrawal can be fatal, and symptoms include apprehension, weakness, tremors, delirium, and convulsions.

LSD is a hallucinogenic agent with no medicinal benefit. It is an extremely potent drug causing altered perception and mood changes that range from euphoria to deep depression. Long-term use can cause chromosomal changes and prolonged adverse psychological effects such as suicide attempts.

Marijuana is usually used by smoking it in the form of a hand-rolled cigarette. Feelings of euphoria, relaxation, and drowsiness are the primary effects of the drug. Individuals lose inhibitions and may exhibit inappropriate behavior, poor coordination, and poor judgment. Hallucinations are possible. Tachycardia, increased appetite, and decreased pulmonary function are other symptoms that can occur and aggravate existing medical conditions such as heart disease or hypertension. Although marijuana has been shown to have some limited medicinal uses, in most states it remains classified as a Schedule I drug under the Federal Controlled Substance Act.

The same social pressures that influence young people to try alcohol are responsible for introducing people of all ages to the previously mentioned drugs and other chemical substances. Because it is easier to prevent drug abuse than it is to break an established habit, most efforts to combat drug abuse are directed at the young. However, people of all ages, including older people, may be or become abusers.

Case Study 23-1

Maria Jover reports vaginal discharge and discomfort. Dr. King confirms the diagnosis of a yeast infection by performing a smear and identifying the microorganism. Dr. King prescribes over-the-counter vaginal suppositories. After asking Maria if she has any questions, medical assistant Audrey Jones proceeds to help Maria understand the self-administration of this particular medication.

CASE STUDY REVIEW

1. The patient, Maria, asks Audrey Jones whether she can use some vaginal suppositories she bought last year. How should Audrey respond?
2. Maria tells Audrey that the last time she had a vaginal yeast infection she only used part of the recommended number of suppositories because the infection cleared up. How should Audrey respond?
3. Maria does not really like using suppositories. Should Audrey ask Dr. King to prescribe another form of medication for the yeast infection? What other forms might be available?

Case Study 23-2

Dr. Lewis keeps a small quantity of various controlled substances on the premises for use in an emergency situation.

CASE STUDY REVIEW

1. What are the legalities that surround controlled substances in so far as Joe Guerrero, the medical assistant, is concerned?
2. What are his responsibilities?

SUMMARY

Medical assistants must know state and federal laws that govern the distribution and administration of medications and understand their role and responsibilities in light of these laws. Knowledge of drug regulations, the legal classifications of drugs including controlled substances, and prescribing, administering, and dispensing of drugs is essential to ensure compliance with the law.

Available resources and reference books will provide valuable information about pharmaceutical products, their classifications, routes, forms, storage and handling, and side effects.

Emergency drugs and supplies should be available on a crash cart or a tray or cabinet for the sole use in an office emergency.

With the increase of drug abuse and misuse, it is important for medical assistants to recognize the signs of drug abuse in patients and coworkers and to report abuse to the physician or supervisor.

STUDY FOR SUCCESS

To reinforce your knowledge and skills of information presented in this chapter:

- ❑ Review the Key Terms
- ❑ Consider the Case Studies and discuss your conclusions
- ❑ Answer the Review Questions
  - ❑ Multiple Choice
  - ❑ Critical Thinking
- ❑ Navigate the Internet by completing the Web Activities
- ❑ Practice the StudyWARE activities on your student CD
- ❑ Apply your knowledge in the Student Workbook activities
- ❑ Complete the Web Tutor sections

REVIEW QUESTIONS

Multiple Choice

1. Which of the following drugs is commonly used in an emergency such as anaphylactic shock?
   a. lomotil
   b. interferon
   c. cytoxan
   d. epinephrine
2. Which of the following types of drugs do physicians prescribe most frequently?
   a. generic
   b. official
   c. chemical
   d. brand
3. An example of a drug that can be obtained from an animal is:
   a. digitalis
   b. insulin
   c. imferon
   d. sulfur
4. Which of the following is an example of a controlled substance?
   a. Nembutal
   b. Keflin
   c. Inderal
   d. Aldomet
5. After you have poured a medication and taken it to the patient, he refuses to take it. You should:
   a. give it to another patient who has the same medication prescribed
   b. return the refused medication to its original container
   c. save it for the next time the patient is due for another dose
   d. dispose of it down the sink and document

Critical Thinking

1. Drugs are derived from various sources. List five sources of drugs.

2. How does the Federal Food, Drug, and Cosmetic Act protect the public?
3. The _________ is recognized by the U.S. government as the official list of standardized drugs.
4. Describe the principal factors that affect drug action.
5. While preparing an injection of Demerol® (meperidine), you accidentally drop and break the ampule spilling its contents. Describe what actions you would take.
6. Name five emergency drugs that may be found on a crash cart or emergency tray. Describe the use and actions of each.
7. Under what circumstances can a medical assistant dispense stock medication?
8. Audrey Jones is considering taking a new position with a physician who is opening an office in another state. Audrey will be responsible for the clinical aspect of the practice. Where can Audrey find information about laws that apply to her in regard to administering medications? Where can she get information about the storage and handling on the premises of narcotics?
9. List several drug references and briefly describe the contents of the PDR.
10. After lunch, a newly hired medical assistant is helping you get Lenore McDonell back into her wheelchair after her physical examination. You strongly suspect that the medical assistant has been drinking alcohol, because she is uncoordinated in her movements and there is a strong odor of what seems to be alcohol on her breath. Describe your next action.

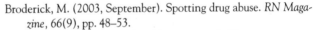

WEB ACTIVITIES

Explore on the Internet for information regarding the Drug Enforcement Agency.

1. Print a copy of Schedules I–V of the controlled substances.
2. Find to which schedule the following controlled substances belong: phencyclidine (PCP), amphetamines, cocaine, and heroin.
3. Using a search engine of your choice, gather information about over-the-counter (OTC) analgesics such as aspirin and nonsteroidal antiinflammatory drugs (NSAIDs).
   a. What risks can be associated with taking these drugs?
   b. Look for surveys that have been done by the National Consumers League on adults who used an OTC pain reliever in the past year.
   c. What percentage exceeded the recommended dose?
   d. What percentage had not spoken to a health care professional about possible risks associated with these products?

REFERENCES/BIBLIOGRAPHY

Broderick, M. (2003, September). Spotting drug abuse. *RN Magazine*, 66(9), pp. 48–53.

Centers for Disease Control and Prevention. *Public emergency preparedness and response*. Retrieved from http://www.bt.cdc.gov. Accessed December 2, 2004.

Spratto, G. R., & Woods, A. L. (2004). *Physician's desk reference—nurses drug handbook*. Clifton Park, NY: Thomson Delmar Learning.

Taber's cyclopedic medical dictionary (22nd ed.). (2003). Philadelphia: FA Davis.

U.S. Food and Drug Administration, Department of Health and Human Services. (2004, February 6). *FDA issues regulations prohibiting sale of dietary supplements containing ephedrine alkaloids and reiterates—it advises that consumers stop using these products*. Retrieved from http://www.cfisan.fda.gov/~lrd/fpephed6.html.

Wooten, J. M. (2003, April). Medicine cabinet staples are not without risks. *RN Magazine*, 66(4), p. 96.

World Health Organization. (n.d.). *Health aspects of biological and chemical weapons*. Retrieved from http://www.who.int. Accessed December 2, 2004.

CHAPTER 24

Calculation of Medication Dosage and Medication Administration

OUTLINE

Legal and Ethical Implications of Medication Administration
- Ethical Considerations
- The Medication Order
- The Prescription

Drug Dosage
- Age
- Weight
- Sex
- Other Factors

The Medication Label

Calculation of Drug Dosages
- Understanding Ratio
- Understanding Proportion
- Weights and Measures

Medications Measured in Units
- How to Calculate Unit Dosages
- Insulin
- Diabetes

Calculating Adult Dosages
- The Proportional Method
- The Formula Method

Calculating Children's Dosages
- Body Surface Area
- Kilogram of Body Weight

Administration of Medications
- The "Six Rights" of Proper Drug Administration
- Medication Error
- Patient Assessment

Administration of Oral Medications
- Equipment and Supplies for Oral Medications

Administration of Parenteral Medications
- Hazards Associated with Parenteral Medications
- Reasons for Parenteral Route Selection
- Parenteral Equipment and Supplies

IV Therapy

Site Selection and Injection Angle
- Marking the Correct Site for Intramuscular Injection

Basic Guidelines for Administration of Injections

Z-Track Method of Intramuscular Injection

Administration of Allergenic Extracts

Inhalation Methods of Medication Administration
- Implications for Patient Care
- Administration of Oxygen

KEY TERMS

Administering
Apnea
Body Surface Area (BSA)
Compounding
Dispensing
Hypoxemia
Meniscus
Nomogram
Parenteral
Phytomedicines
Precipitate
Retrolental Fibroplasia
Status Asthmaticus
Taut
Unit Dose

OBJECTIVES

The student should strive to meet the following performance objectives and demonstrate an understanding of the facts and principles presented in this chapter through written and oral communication.

1. Define the key terms as presented in the glossary.
2. Discuss the legal and ethical implications of medication administration.
3. Describe the medication order.
4. Describe the parts of a prescription.
5. Define drug dosage.
6. State what information is found on a medication label.
7. Understand ratio and proportion.
8. Use the metric, household, and apothecary systems of measurement and convert between metric and apothecary systems.
9. Understand units of medication dosage.
10. Correctly calculate dosages for adults and children.
11. List the guidelines to follow when preparing and administering medications.
12. Describe safe disposal of syringes, needles, and biohazard materials.
13. Understand intravenous therapy.
14. Describe site selection for administration of injections.
15. Understand allergenic extracts.
16. Describe inhalation medication and its administration.

FEATURED COMPETENCIES

CAAHEP—ENTRY-LEVEL COMPETENCIES

Fundamental Procedures

- Dispose of biohazardous materials
- Practice Standard Precautions

Patient Care

- Apply pharmacology principles to prepare and administer oral and parenteral (excluding IV) medications
- Maintain medication and immunization records

Legal Concepts

- Perform within legal and ethical boundaries
- Document appropriately
- Demonstrate knowledge of federal and state health care legislation and regulations

ABHES—ENTRY-LEVEL COMPETENCIES

Professionalism

- Conduct work within scope of education, training and ability

Clinical Duties

- Prepare and administer medications as directed by Physician
- Maintain medication records
- Dispose of biohazardous materials
- Practice standard precautions

Legal Concepts

- Determine needs for documentation and reporting
- Document accurately
- Monitor legislation related to current healthcare issues and practices

SCENARIO

At Drs. Lewis and King's practice, office policy dictates that a medicine card must be written out before the administration of any medication to a patient. Clinical medical assistant Joe Guerrero, CMA, is careful to check the physician's order, then prepare the medicine card before preparing and administering medication. He notes that the card contains the patient's name, the physician's order, and the date, time, and route the medication is to be administered. After giving the medication to the patient, Joe documents the fact in the patient file, and then, according to procedure, shreds the medicine card.

INTRODUCTION

Despite the fact that many ambulatory care centers use what is known as the unit dose type of medication preparation, there remains a responsibility for medical assistants to know and understand how to calculate dosages of medication and to safely administer them to patients.

This chapter addresses calculation of adult and pediatric dosages of medication using the metric and household systems. It also emphasizes the legal aspects of medication administration and discusses oral and parenteral medication administration.

LEGAL AND ETHICAL IMPLICATIONS OF MEDICATION ADMINISTRATION

Members of the health care profession who prepare and administer medications are ethically and legally responsible for their own actions. Under law, these individuals are required to be licensed, registered, or otherwise authorized by a physician.

Each state has enacted laws governing the practice of medicine, nursing, and pharmacy. These laws vary from state to state; therefore, it is essential that medical assistants become familiar with the laws of the state in which they are employed before administering any medication. In some states, the only health professional authorized to give injections, other than a physician, is a registered nurse, nurse practitioner, or physician's assistant. In other states, legislation gives physicians broad authority to delegate responsibility for administering medication to other health care workers such as medical assistants. Laws have been passed in some states specifying which qualified and properly educated and trained persons may perform certain medical acts.

Regardless of the differences in state authorization laws, the courts will not permit the careless action of health care workers to go unpunished, especially when such actions result in harm or death to the patient. Under the law, those administering medications are expected to be knowledgeable about the drugs that they administer and the effects the drug(s) may or will have on the patient. Many states have uniform disciplinary acts. Never administer a medication without thorough knowledge of the drug. It is the medical assistant's responsibility to know the information about a medication listed in Figure 24-1 before administering it to a patient.

1. Drug name (generic and brand)
2. Action
3. Uses
4. Contraindications
5. Warnings when indicated
6. Adverse reactions
7. Dosage and route
8. Implications for patient care
9. Patient teaching
10. Special considerations

Figure 24-1 Medical assistants should have a thorough knowledge of any medication they administer to a patient and should consult references such as the *Physician's Desk Reference* (PDR).

Spotlight on Certification

RMA Content Outline
- Clinical pharmacology

CMA Content Outline
- Disposal of biohazardous material
- Safety precautions
- Preparing and administering medications

CMAS Content Outline
- Basic Pharmacology

Ethical Considerations

Anyone who has access to medications may be tempted to use them for personal benefit. To do so is not only unethical, it is considered to be illegal. The conversion to personal use of medications intended for another is unethical and may cause harm to the patient. It is also unethical and illegal to take any medication that belongs to your employer, even aspirin or drug samples, without proper authorization.

The Medication Order

The medication order is given by the physician. It is for a specific patient and denotes the drug to be given, the dosage, the form of the drug, the time for or frequency

Parts of a Prescription

1. The physician's name, address, telephone number, and registration number.
2. The patient's name, address, and the date on which the prescription is written.
3. The *superscription* that includes the symbol Rx ("take thou").
4. The *inscription* that states the names and quantities of ingredients to be included in the medication.
5. The *subscription* that gives directions to the pharmacist for filling the prescription.
6. The *signature* (Sig) that gives the directions for the patient.
7. The physician's signature blanks. Where signed, indicates if a generic substitute is allowed or if the medication is to be dispensed as written.
8. REPETATUR 0 1 2 3 p.r.n. This is where the physician indicates whether or not the prescription can be refilled.
9. ☐ LABEL Direction to the pharmacist to label the medication appropriately.

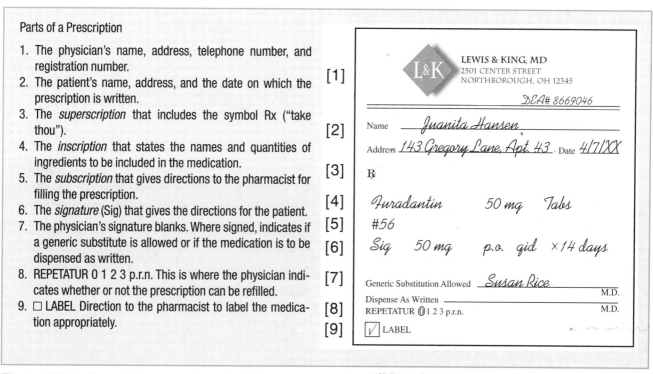

[1] [2] [3] [4] [5] [6] [7] [8] [9]

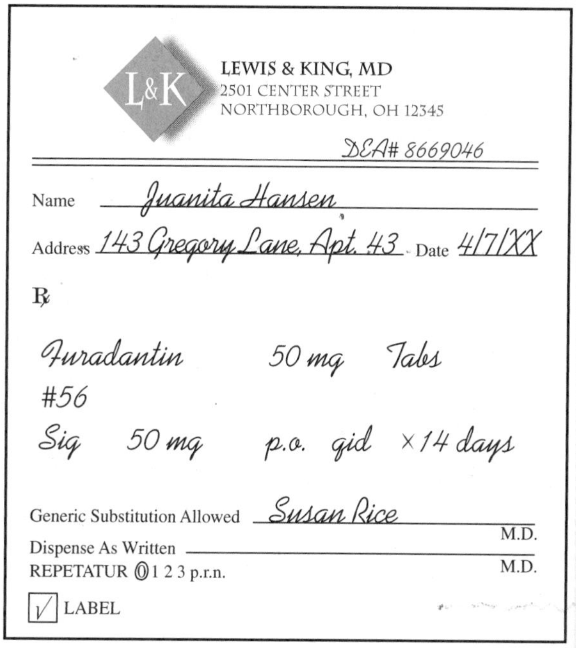
L&K
LEWIS & KING, MD
2501 CENTER STREET
NORTHBOROUGH, OH 12345
DEA# 8669046
Name Juanita Hansen
Address 143 Gregory Lane, Apt. 43 Date 4/7/XX
℞
Furadantin 50 mg Tabs
#56
Sig 50 mg p.o. qid ×14 days
Generic Substitution Allowed Susan Rice M.D.
Dispense As Written M.D.
REPETATUR 0 1 2 3 p.r.n.
☑ LABEL

Figure 24-2 Prescriptions are written legal documents that give directions for compounding, dispensing, and administering a medication. Prescriptions have nine distinct elements.

of administration, and the route by which the drug is to be given.

The Prescription

The prescription is a written legal document that gives directions for **compounding**, **dispensing**, and **administering** a medication to a patient. There are nine parts to a prescription (Figure 24-2).

The purpose of a prescription is to control the sale and use of drugs that can be safely and effectively used only under the supervision of a licensed physician. Federal law divides medicines into two main classes: prescription or legend medicines and over-the-counter (OTC) medicines. The prescription is written by the physician and signed with an ink pen. The pharmacist fills the prescription according to the physician's order. Once the prescription has been filled, the assigned prescription number and all other information may be entered into a computer. The hard copy of the prescription is filed and kept for a minimum of seven years. Schedule II controlled substances prescriptions (see Chapter 23 for a description of schedule II medications) are kept separate from other prescriptions and are stamped with a red C (C for controlled) and filed separately. Schedule III through V prescriptions are stamped with a red C and filed.

E-prescribing is the process of electronically accessing the patient's medical history, prescribing a medication, and selecting a pharmacy.

The Medicare Prescription Drug, Improvement and Modernization Act (MMA) of 2003 and the Health Insurance Portability and Accountability Act (HIPAA) of 1996 have recommended e-prescribing standards. Medications handled electronically have reduced the problems of medication errors. Patients enjoy the ease of e-prescriptions because they do not have to drop off the prescriptions and then return to pick it up. Some states already have e-prescriptions in patients' electronic medical records. However, the possibility of a breach in confidentiality exists whenever electronic medical records are used.

Prescriptions for Controlled Substances. Federal laws require that specific procedures be followed by the physician when prescribing controlled substances. See Table 24-1.

All prescriptions for controlled substances must be dated and signed on the date issued, bearing the full name and address of the patient and the name, address, and Drug Enforcement Administration (DEA) number

TABLE 24-1 REQUIREMENTS FOR PRESCRIPTIONS FOR CONTROLLED SUBSTANCES

	Verbal Order or Prescription	Written Prescription	Refills
Schedule I	NOT FOR MEDICINAL USE		
Schedule II	No	Yes	No
Schedule III	Yes	Yes	5× within 6 months
Schedule IV	Yes	Yes	5× within 6 months
Schedule V	Yes	Yes	Yes

(see Chapter 23) of the physician. The prescription must be written in ink or typewritten and signed by the physician's own hand.

Prescription Abbreviations and Symbols. It is important to be knowledgeable of the most common abbreviations used by the physician when an order for a prescription drug is given. The abbreviations are a clear and concise means of writing orders. This medical shorthand is an international language used by professional and nonprofessional people involved with patient care. All abbreviations in Table 24-2 should be memorized to enable medical assistants to prepare medications safely and accurately for administration.

The Joint Commission on Accreditation of Healthcare Organizations (JCAHO) requires that facilities comply with the JCAHO's minimum requirement for the banning of certain abbreviations, acronyms, symbols, and their *do not use* list. This ban, as part of JCAHO's 2004 patient safety goals, has been applied to protect patients from errors during documentation.

Abbreviations no longer allowed by JCAHO are as follows:

AD right ear
AS left ear
AU both ears
cc cubic centimeter
hs at bedtime
OD right eye
OS left eye
OU both eyes
sc subcutaneous
IU international unit
qd every day
qod every other day

DRUG DOSAGE

The dosage or dose is the amount of medicine that is prescribed for administration. It is determined by the physician or qualified practitioner who considers the following important factors: age, weight, sex, and other factors as well.

Age

The usual adult dose is generally suitable for the 20- to 60-year age group. Infants, young children, adolescents, and older adults require an individualized dosage regimen.

Weight

The average adult dosage is based on 150 pounds (about 68 kilograms). Individuals who weigh less or more than this should have the dosage based on **body surface area (BSA)** or kilogram of body weight.

Sex

Many medications are contraindicated during pregnancy and breast-feeding. It is important that these two factors be known before any dose of medication is prescribed.

Other Factors

There are other factors that determine the dosage of a medication including:

1. Physical and emotional condition of patient
2. Disease process, especially kidney disease because of impaired excretion
3. Presence of more than one disease process
4. Causative microorganism(s) and the severity of the infection
5. Patient's medical history, allergies, and idiosyncrasies
6. The safest method, route, time, and amount to effect the desired maximum result

THE MEDICATION LABEL

The medication label can be a source of valuable information to the medical assistant and the patient. Regardless of whether administering a prescription drug or taking a nonprescription product, an understanding of the information provided on the label is essential to the safe and effective use of any medicine. In addition to the name and address of the manufacturer, other important items of information on a medication label include:

- The trade or brand name for the medication
- The generic name (or listing of active and inactive ingredients)
- The National Drug Code (NDC) numbers that can be used to identify the manufacturer, the product, and the size of the container
- The dosage strength in a given amount of the medication
- The usual dosage and frequency of administration
- The route of administration
- Precautions and warnings
- The expiration date for the medication

Other information that may be on a medication label includes directions for storage and directions for mixing or reconstituting a powdered form of the drug.

CALCULATION OF DRUG DOSAGES

The preparation and administration of medications is one of the most important and critical tasks that medical assistants perform. Today, drugs are more potent and more likely to cause physiologic changes in the body; therefore, anyone who administers medications must do so with extreme care.

Incorrectly calculated or measured dosages are the leading cause of error in the administration of medications. A drug error is a violation of a patient's rights. It is important that medical assistants develop a working knowledge of mathematics to calculate or measure accurately a medication that is to be administered to a patient.

Each year medications kill about 14,000 hospital patients and injure another 750,000 according to the Institute of Medicine. About half of these deaths and injuries come from side effects; the other half are from errors. Because the majority of prescriptions are written in the physician's offices, the figures are likely to be proportionately higher. The Food and Drug Administration (FDA) has proposed a new rule that will become effective in 2006. All hospital prescriptions and all OTC medications, vaccines, and blood will require standardized and universal bar codes to help prevent medication errors. Reading the bar code with a scanner

TABLE 24-2 COMMON PRESCRIPTION ABBREVIATIONS AND SYMBOLS

Abbreviation or Symbol	Meaning
aa	of each
ac	before meals
ad lib	as desired
aq	water
bid	twice a day
$\bar{c}$	with
caps	capsules
dil	dilute
ʒ	dram
elix	elixir
Gm	gram
gr	grain
gt or gtt	drop (drops)
h	hour
IM	intramuscular
IV	intravenous
kg	kilogram
L	liter
liq	liquid
m or min	minim
mg	milligram
ml or ML	milliliter
mm	millimeter
NPO	nothing by mouth
non rep	do not repeat
$\bar{p}$	after
pc	after meals
per	by or with
po	by mouth
prn	as needed
pt	patient
q	every
qh	every hour
q (2, 3, 4) h	every (2, 3, 4) hours
qid	four times a day
qs	of sufficient quantity
Rx	take
$\bar{s}$	without
sol	solution
ss	one-half
stat	at once
tab	tablet
Tbs	tablespoon
tsp	teaspoon
tid	three times a day
tr	tincture
ung	ointment

Medication error categories:
1. Human errors = 42%
2. Labeling problems = 20%
3. Miscommunication = 19%
4. Drug name confusion = 13%
   and packaging/design = 6%

Source: http://www.fda.gov/cder/drug/MedErrors/mixed.pdf

can correlate the medication bar code with a patient identification bar code.

Understanding Ratio

Ratio is a method of expressing the relation of a number, quantity, substance, or degree between two similar components. For example, the relation of one to five is written 1:5. Note that numbers are side by side and separated by a colon.

In mathematics, a ratio may be expressed as a quotient, a fraction, or a decimal.

Ratio Expressed as a Quotient. A quotient is the number found when one number is divided by another number. The ratio one to five written as a quotient is 1 ÷ 5.

Ratio Expressed as a Fraction. A fraction is the process of dividing or breaking a whole number into parts. The ratio one to five written as a fraction is ⅕.

Ratio Expressed as a Decimal. A decimal is a linear array of numbers based on 10 or any multiple of 10. To express the ratio one to five as a decimal, divide the denominator (5) into the numerator (1).

$$\text{(denominator)}\quad 5\overline{)1.0}^{\;0.2}\quad \text{(numerator)}$$

The ratio may be expressed as:

A quotient	*A fraction*	*A decimal*
1 ÷ 5	⅕	0.2

Understanding Proportion

Proportion is a process of expressing the comparative relation between a part, share, or portion with regard to size, amount, or number. In mathematics, a proportion expresses the relation between two ratios. In setting up a proportion, the ratios are separated by : or an = sign. In this text, the equal sign (=) is used to separate ratios.

Example: 3 : 4 = 1 : 2
Read: Three is to four equals one is to two.

Patient Education

Patients should:
1. Question the physician, pharmacist, and staff administering the drug about the drug and its possible side effects.
2. Be sure the prescription has been written legibly. Many drugs sound alike (e.g., Ambien® for insomnia and Amen® for menstrual cycle control; Xanax® for anxiety and Xantac® for heartburn and ulcers; Fosamax® for osteoporosis and Flomax® for enlarged prostate).
3. Always check the label at the pharmacy to make sure it is clearly written.
4. Always check your medication at the pharmacy to be certain that the medication and directions are what you expect.
5. Have the physician or pharmacist explain the name and purpose of each new medication that is being prescribed. Be sure you understand.
6. Keep an updated list of all medications, prescriptions, OTC vitamins, minerals, and phytomedicines.
7. Take medications as directed, and do not discontinue use until the appropriate date as indicated by the physician.
8. Store medicines away from heat and humidity in their original containers.
9. Ask the physician or pharmacist what you should do if you miss a dose.

The four terms of a proportion are given special names. The *means* are the inner numbers or the second and third terms of the proportion.

Example: $3:4=1:2$ (4) (1)
means

The *extremes* are the outer numbers or the first and fourth terms of the proportion.

Example: $3:4=1:2$ (3) (2)
extremes

In a true proportion, the product of the means equals the product of the extremes.

Example: *means* (16) (1)

$8:16=1:2$

extremes (8) (2)

$16\times1=16$ (*means*)

$8\times2=16$ (*extremes*)

Solving for *x*. The proportion is a useful mathematical tool. When a part, share, or portion of the problem is unknown, then *x* represents the unknown factor. You can determine the unknown by solving for *x*. The unknown factor *x* may appear any place in the proportion.

Now solve for *x* in the problem: $3:4=x:12$.

1. Multiply the terms that contain the *x* and place the product to the left of the equal sign ($4x$).
2. Multiply the other terms and place the product to the right of the equal sign (36).
3. To find *x*, divide the product of *x* into the product of the other terms.

$$4x=36$$
$$x=\frac{36}{4} \text{ or } 36\div4$$
$$x=9$$

After finding the unknown factor, check your mathematical skills by determining if you have a true proportion. This technique is called proof or proving your answer. To prove your answer:

1. Place the answer you found for *x* back into the formula where *x* was.

$$3:4=9:12$$

2. Now multiply the means by the means, and the extremes by the extremes.
3. The results will equal each other.

Formula: $3:4=x:12$

Proof: $3:4=9:12$

$$4\times9=36$$
$$3\times12=36$$

Weights and Measures

There are two systems of measurement used in pharmacology to calculate dosages. These systems are metric and the household. The metric system is used throughout the world as the official language of communication in scientific and technical fields. It is based on the decimal system: the number 10 or multiples of 10.

Metric System Guidelines. The following guidelines are helpful when learning basic facts about the metric system:

1. Arabic numbers are used to designate whole numbers; e.g., 1, 250, 500, 1,000.
2. Decimal fractions are used for quantities less than one; e.g., 0.1, 0.01, 0.001, 0.0001.
3. To ensure accuracy, place a zero before the decimal point; e.g., 0.1, 0.001, 0.0001.
4. The Arabic number precedes the metric unit of measurement; e.g., 10 grams, 2 millimeters, 5 liters.
5. The abbreviation for gram should be capitalized (Gm) or written as (g) to distinguish it from grain (gr).
6. The abbreviation for liter is capitalized (L).
7. Prefixes are written in lowercase letters; e.g., milli, centi, deci, deka.
8. Capitalize the measurement and symbol when it is named after a person; e.g., Celsius (C).
9. Periods are no longer used with most abbreviations or symbols.
10. Abbreviations for units are the same for singular and plural. An *s* is not added to an abbreviation to indicate a plural.

The Seven Common Metric Prefixes. It is important to know common metric prefixes to have a solid foundation for determining metric equivalents. When a metric prefix is combined with a root of physical quantity, you arrive at multiples or submultiples of the metric system.

Example:

- **milli** (prefix): one-thousandth of a unit
  meter (root): a measure of length
  millimeter: one-thousandth of a meter

- **kilo** (prefix): one thousand units
  liter (root): a measure of volume
  kiloliter: one thousand liters
- **micro** (prefix): one-millionth of a unit
  gram (root): a measure of mass and/or weight
  microgram: one-millionth of a gram

Prefixes:

micro (mi'kro)	=	one millionth of a unit written as 0.000001
milli (mil'i)	=	one-thousandth of a unit written as 0.001
centi (sen'ti)	=	one-hundredth of a unit written as 0.01
deci (des'i)	=	one-tenth of a unit written as 0.1
deka (dek'a)	=	ten units written as 10
hecto (hek'to)	=	one hundred units written as 100
kilo (kil'o)	=	one thousand units written as 1000

Fundamental Units:
Following are the fundamental units of the metric system:

meter (m)	length
liter (L)	volume
gram (Gm, g)	mass and/or weight

The meter is the fundamental unit of length in the metric system and originally formed the foundation for the entire system. A meter is equal to 39.37 inches, which is slightly more than a yard, or 3.28 feet.

A millimeter is about the width of the head of a pin. It takes approximately 2½ centimeters to make an inch; a decimeter is approximately 4 inches.

Meter (m)	=	Length
1 millimeter (mm)	=	0.001 meter
1 centimeter (cm)	=	0.01 meter
1 decimeter (dm)	=	0.1 meter
1 meter (m)	=	1 meter
1 dekameter (dam)	=	10 meters
1 hectometer (hm)	=	100 meters
1 kilometer (km)	=	1,000 meters

The liter is the metric unit of volume. A liter is equal to 1.056 quarts, which is 0.26 gallon or 2.1 pints.

A milliliter is equivalent to one cubic centimeter (cc), because the amount of space occupied by a milliliter is equal to one cubic centimeter. The weight of one milliliter of water equals approximately one gram. It takes approximately 15 milliliters to make 1 tablespoon. It takes 15 or 16 minims to make one milliliter.

Liter (L)		Volume
1 milliliter (mL)	=	0.001 liter
1 centiliter (cL)	=	0.01 liter
1 deciliter (dL)	=	0.1 liter
1 liter (L)	=	1 liter
1 dekaliter (daL)	=	10 liters
1 hectoliter (hL)	=	100 liters
1 kiloliter (kL)	=	1,000 liters

The gram is the metric unit of mass and weight. It equals approximately the weight of 1 cubic centimeter or 1 milliliter of water. A gram is equal to approximately 15 grains or 0.035 ounce.

Gram (Gm, g)		Mass and Weight
1 microgram (μg)	=	0.000001 gram
1 milligram (mg)	=	0.001 gram
1 centigram (cg)	=	0.01 gram
1 decigram (dg)	=	0.1 gram
1 gram (Gm, g)	=	1 gram
1 dekagram (dag)	=	10 grams
1 hectogram (hg)	=	100 grams
1 kilogram (kg)	=	1,000 grams

The metric equivalents most frequently used in the medical field are:

Length	Volume
2½ centimeters (cm) = 1 inch	1,000 milliliters (mL) or 1,000 cubic centimeters (cc) = 1 liter (L)

Weight

1,000 micrograms (μg)	=	1 milligram (mg)
1000 milligrams (mg)	=	1 gram (Gm, g)
1000 grams (Gm, g)	=	1 kilogram (kg)
1 kilogram	=	2.2 pounds (lb)

Household Measurements. Household measurements are approximate measurements. They are more frequently used in the home than in the medical field, but the medical assistant should be familiar with the common household measurements listed in Table 24-3.

Because medications can be prescribed in either metric or household measurements, it is important to know equivalents between both to calculate the dose of prescribed medication. See Table 24-4.

Metric System Conversion. The process of changing into another form, state, substance, or product is known as conversion. In the metric system, changing from one unit to another involves multiplying or dividing by 10, 100, 1,000, and so forth. This can be done by the proportional method or by moving the decimal in the correct direction.

Proportional Method for Converting Metric Equivalents. There are six basic steps in the proportional method, plus

TABLE 24-3 COMMON HOUSEHOLD MEASURES

60 drops (gtt)	is equal to:	1 teaspoon (t or tsp)
1 dash	is equal to:	Less than ⅛ teaspoon
3 teaspoons (tsp)	is equal to:	1 tablespoon (T or tbsp)
2 tablespoons (tbsp)	is equal to:	1 ounce (oz)
4 ounces (oz)	is equal to:	1 juice glass
6 ounces (oz)	is equal to:	1 teacup
8 ounces (oz)	is equal to:	1 glass or cup
16 tablespoons or 8 ounces	is equal to:	1 measuring cup (c)
2 cups (c)	is equal to:	1 pint (pt)
2 pints (pt)	is equal to:	1 quart (qt)
4 quarts (qt)	is equal to:	1 gallon (gal)

Drop (gt) = approximate liquid measure depending on kind of liquid measured and the size of the opening from which it is dropped.

an additional step to prove the answer. The following example will serve as a model for future applications of the proportional method of converting metric equivalents.

Example:
Convert 1,500 milligrams to grams.

$$1{,}500\text{ mg} = \underline{\qquad}\text{ Gm, g}$$

Step 1. Because the unknown factor in the given formula is the number of grams contained in 1,500 milligrams, substitute the symbol *x* for grams in the equation.

Step 2. Setting up the proportion requires that you know metric equivalents. For example, in this problem you have to know that 1,000 milligrams (mg) = 1 gram (Gm, g).

Step 3. Since you know that 1,000 mg is equal to 1 Gm, you can create one-half of the equation. Write the equivalent and place it on the left of the equal sign.

$$1{,}000\text{ mg} : 1\text{ Gm} =$$

Step 4. Now that you have the left side of the equation, set up the right side by using the designated metric value 1,500 mg : *x* Gm. Always write the smallest equivalent as to the largest equivalent, for example, mg : Gm. By being consistent, it is less likely errors will occur.

$$1{,}000\text{ mg} : 1\text{ Gm} = 1{,}500\text{ mg} : x\text{ Gm}$$

Step 5. Note that you have an equal equation:

$$\text{mg} : \text{Gm} = \text{mg} : \text{Gm}$$

The first values on either side of the equal sign are milligrams, and the second values on either side are grams.

TABLE 24-4 APPROXIMATE EQUIVALENTS AMONG METRIC AND HOUSEHOLD SYSTEMS

Metric	Household
DRY	
60 mg	
1 Gm	¼ tsp
15 Gm	1 tbsp (3 tsp)
30 Gm	1 oz (2 tbsp)
—	1 lb (16 oz)
1 kg	2.2 lb
LIQUID	
	1 gt
1 mL (1 cubic centimeter)	15 gtt
5 mL	1 tsp
15 mL	1 tbsp (3 tsp)
30 mL	1 fl oz (2 tbs)
500 mL	(1 pt or 2 cups)
1,000 mL	4 cups (1 qt)
LENGTH	
2.5 cm	1 in
1 m	39.37 in

Step 6. Now solve for the unknown (*x*) by multiplication and division. Multiply the means by the means and the extremes by the extremes. **NOTE:** Once the proportion is correctly set up, simply use the numbers as you multiply and divide.

$$1{,}000 : 1 = 1{,}500 : x$$

$$1{,}000x = 1{,}500$$
$$x = 1{,}500 \div 1{,}000$$
$$x = 1.5$$

$$\begin{array}{r} 1.5 \\ 1{,}000\overline{)1{,}500.0} \\ \underline{1{,}000} \\ 500.0 \\ \underline{500} \end{array}$$

Step 7. To make sure the answer is correct, prove the work: Place the answer 1.5 Gm into the formula where *x* once was. Now multiply the means by the means and the extremes by the extremes.

$$1{,}000\text{ mg} : 1\text{ Gm} = 1{,}500\text{ mg} : 1.5\text{ Gm}$$
$$1{,}500 = 1{,}500$$

MEDICATIONS MEASURED IN UNITS

Medications such as insulin, heparin, some antibiotics, hormones, vitamins, and vaccines are measured in units. These medications are standardized in units based on their strengths. The strength varies from one medicine to another, depending on the source, condition, and method by which it is obtained.

How to Calculate Unit Dosages

When calculating medications that are ordered in units, use either the proportional method or the formula method.

The Proportional Method

Example:
The physician orders 4,000 USP units of heparin given deep subcutaneously. On hand is heparin 5,000 USP units per milliliter.

Step 1. Use the following proportion to calculate the dose:

Known unit on hand	:	Known dosage form	=	Dose ordered	:	Unknown amount to be given
5,000 U	:	1 mL	=	4,000 U	:	x mL
		5,000x	=	4,000		
		x	=	⅘ = ⅘ mL or 0.8 mL		

Use a tuberculin syringe to draw up 0.8 mL, or convert ⅘ mL to minims.

Step 2. Convert ⅘ mL to minims. NOTE: There are 15 or 16 minims per milliliter.
Multiply:

$$\frac{4}{5} \times \frac{15}{1} = \frac{4}{1} \times \frac{3}{1} = 12 \text{ minims}$$

Administer 12 minims (of 5,000 U/ML for correct dose of 4,000 units) to the patient.

The Formula Method

Example:
The physician orders 450,000 units of Bicillin 1M. On hand is Bicillin 600,000 units per milliliter.

Step 1. Use the following formula to calculate the dose:

$$\frac{\text{Dose ordered (desired)}}{\text{Dose on hand}} \times \text{Quantity (per mL)} = \text{Amount to give}$$

$$\frac{450{,}000 \text{ U}}{600{,}000 \text{ U}} \times 1 \text{ mL} = \frac{450{,}000\text{U}}{600{,}000\text{U}} \times 1 \text{ mL} = \tfrac{3}{4} \text{ mL}$$

Step 2. You may convert to minims. If you do, multiply ¾ by 16.

$$\frac{3}{4} \times \frac{16}{1} = 12 \text{ minims}$$

The patient will receive 12 minims of Bicillin 600,000 U for the ordered dose of 450,000 U.

Insulin

Insulin is a chemical substance (hormone) secreted by the beta cells of the islets of Langerhans in the pancreas. Insulin is necessary for the proper metabolism of blood glucose and maintenance of the correct blood sugar level. Inadequate secretion of insulin, as in the disease diabetes mellitus, results in hyperglycemia and subsequent excessive production of ketone bodies. Eventual coma can ensue.

Patients' needs are individualized according to the severity of their disease; treatment includes taking insulin, controlling diet, and exercise. The diet is well-balanced and consists of the correct number of calories distributed among carbohydrates, fats, and proteins. Patients are taught to monitor blood and urine glucose levels at home throughout the day, for the dosage of insulin taken depends on the amounts of glucose detected. Uncontrolled diabetes mellitus can result in serious complications such as circulatory problems, especially in the feet and legs, kidney disease, loss of vision, bedsores, infection, and gangrene. Special care of the feet is essential. The mouth and teeth require excellent oral hygiene.

Diabetes

The National Diabetes Data Group of the National Institutes of Health organized the various forms of diabetes into the following categories:

Type I	Insulin-dependent diabetes mellitus (IDDM)
Type II	Noninsulin-dependent diabetes mellitus (NIDDM)
Type III	Women who developed glucose intolerance in association with pregnancy
Type IV	Other types of diabetes associated with pancreatic disease, hormonal changes, adverse effects of drugs, or genetic or other anomalies

Individuals with Type I diabetes must take insulin injections on a regular basis to maintain life. The dosage

Patient Education

Encourage patients with diabetes to enroll in diabetic education classes, which are offered at most local hospitals. Patients also need to realize that treatment of diabetes is a lifelong commitment and that they must abide by everything that the hospital teaches.

of insulin is expressed in units and is individualized by the physician for each patient. The amount of insulin that a person must take is based on blood and urine glucose levels, diet, exercise, and the individual's needs (Tables 24-5 and 24-6).

It is *extremely important* that the *exact dosage of insulin be given to the patient*. Too little or too much insulin can cause serious problems ranging from a blood sugar level too low or too high, to coma, and even death. It may be the medical assistant's responsibility to administer insulin and to teach patients or their families how to administer insulin.

When administering insulin, the U-100 syringe (1 mL or LO-DOSE® ½ mL) is preferred. U-100 means there are 100 units of insulin per milliliter or cubic centimeter. Insulin dosage should always be expressed in units rather than in milliliters or cubic centimeters. For example, if the physician orders 30 units of U-100 NPH insulin, use a U-100 syringe and draw up 30 units of U-100 NPH insulin.

Precautions to Observe When Administering Insulin.

The following precautions must be observed when administering insulin:

- Be sure to use the proper insulin, the one ordered by the physician. Refer to Tables 24-5 and 24-6 for various insulin preparations.
- Do not substitute one insulin for another.
- Use the correct syringe, U-100.
- Dosage of insulin is always measured in units and is individualized for each patient.
- Check the label for the name and type of insulin, strength, and expiration date.
- Make sure the insulin has the proper appearance. Refer to Tables 24-5 and 24-6 for proper appearance of various insulins.
- When insulin is not in use, store it in a cool place and avoid freezing.
- When mixing insulins in one syringe, be certain they are compatible. NPH and Regular are compatible. Regular and lente are not compatible.
- Avoid shaking the insulin bottle. Roll gently in palms of hand to mix. This method prevents bubbles in the medication.
- Use a subcutaneous needle, but inject at a 90-degree angle.
- Insulin pens are available prefilled with 300 units of insulin.
- Use a site rotation system and select an appropriate site. Insulin injection sites must be rotated to prevent tissue damage. Record site used (Figure 24-3).

TABLE 24-5 INSULIN PREPARATIONS U-100

Rapid-Acting	Onset of Action	Appearance
Regular	30 minutes	Clear, colorless
Crystalline zinc	30–60 minutes	Clear, colorless
Semilente	90 minutes	Cloudy
Humulin R	15 minutes	Clear, colorless
Humalog	15 minutes	Clear, colorless
Velosulin	30 minutes	Clear, colorless
Novolin	30 minutes	Clear, colorless

TABLE 24-6 INTERMEDIATE-ACTING AND LONG-LASTING INSULIN: INSULIN PREPARATIONS U-100

	Onset of Action	Appearance
Intermediate-Acting		
NPH	½ hour	Cloudy
Lente	2½ hours	Cloudy
Novolin L	2½ hours	Cloudy
Novolin N	1½ hours	Cloudy
Humulin N	1 hour	Cloudy
Long-Acting		
Ultralente	4 hours	Cloudy
PZI (protamine zinc insulin)	4–8 hours	Cloudy
Insulin glargine	Constant concentration over 24 hours	Cloudy

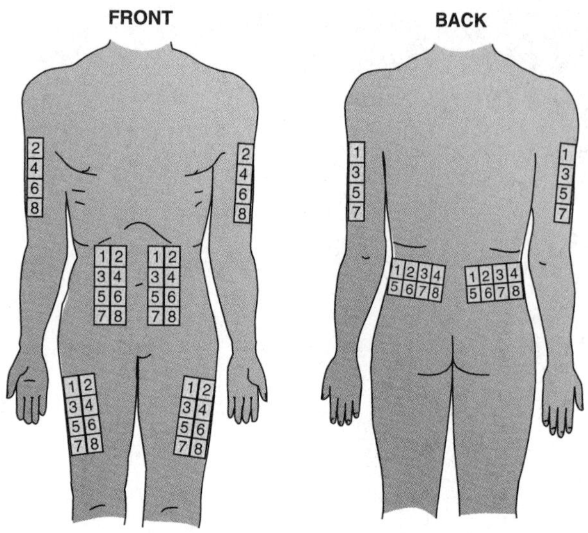

Figure 24-3 Sites and rotation for insulin administration.

- Do not massage after injection.
- Always follow the physician's order and office policy when mixing insulins.

CALCULATING ADULT DOSAGES

Two measures, weight and volume, are used to determine the amount of medication that is to be administered. The weight of a medication may be expressed as any of the following:

- milliequivalent (mEq)
- microgram (μg)
- milligram (mg)
- gram (Gm, g)
- unit

The volume of a medication may be expressed as a:

- milliliter (mL)
- minim (m)
- dram (dr)
- ounce (oz)
- by a variety of household measures, such as the teaspoon (tsp)

Many different methods can be used when calculating the dosage to be administered. Two of the most useful methods—the proportional method and the formula method—are described next.

The Proportional Method

Example:

The physician orders 0.2 Gm of Equanil tabs. The dose on hand is 400 mg tabs.

Step 1. Determine whether the medication ordered and the medication on hand are available in the same unit of measure.

Step 2. If the medication ordered and the medication on hand are not in the same unit of measure, convert so that both measures are expressed using the same unit of measure.

Conversion: To change 0.2 Gm to mg

$$1{,}000 \text{ mg} : 1 \text{ Gm} = x \text{ mg} : 0.2 \text{ Gm}$$

$$x = 200 \text{ mg}$$

or

$$\text{multiply } 0.2 \times 1{,}000 = 200$$

Step 3. Now use the following proportion to calculate the dosage. Remember that 0.2 Gm was converted to 200 mg.

Known unit on hand	:	*Known dosage form*	=	*Dose ordered*	:	*Unknown amount to be given*
400 mg	:	1 tab	=	200 mg	:	x tab

$$400 : 1 = 200 : x$$

$$400x = 200$$

$$x = \frac{200}{400} \text{ (Reduce fraction to lowest terms)}$$

$$x = \tfrac{1}{2} \text{ tab of 400 mg}$$

Step 4. Prove your answer. Place your answer in the original formula in the x position.

$$400 \text{ mg} : 1 \text{ tab} = 200 \text{ mg} : \tfrac{1}{2} \text{ tab}$$

$$200 = \tfrac{1}{2} \text{ of } 400$$

$$200 = 200$$

The Formula Method

Example:

The physician orders 0.2 Gm of Equanil tabs. The dose on hand is 400 mg tabs.

Step 1. Determine whether the medication ordered and the medication on hand are available in the same unit of measure.

Step 2. If the medication ordered and the medication on hand are not in the same unit of measure, convert so that both measures are expressed using the same unit of measure.

Conversion: To change 0.2 Gm to mg

$$1{,}000 \text{ mg} : 1 \text{ Gm} = x \text{ mg} : 0.2 \text{ Gm}$$
$$x = 200 \text{ mg}$$
or
$$\text{multiply } 0.2 \times 1{,}000 = 200$$

Step 3. Now use the following formula to calculate the dosage.

$$\frac{\text{Dose ordered (desired)}}{\text{Dose on hand}} \times \frac{\text{Quantity}}{1} = \frac{\text{Amount to give}}{\text{(form of drug)}}$$

$$\frac{D}{H} \times Q = \text{Amount to give}$$

The physician ordered 0.2 Gm of Equanil tabs (0.2 Gm converts to 200 mg). The dose on hand is 400 mg tabs.

$$\frac{200 \text{ mg}}{400 \text{ mg}} \times 1 \text{ tab} = \frac{200}{400} \text{ or } \tfrac{1}{2} \text{ tab}$$

Give ½ tab of 400 mg.

CALCULATING CHILDREN'S DOSAGES

Each child is an individual with differences in age, size, and weight. In the past, formulas such as Young's, Clark's, and Fried's rules were used to calculate pediatric dosages. These formulas determined what fraction of an adult dose was appropriate for a child. Because each child does not develop in the same way during a given time span, these formulas have been replaced by more exact methods of determining the correct dosage of medication for a child.

Today, there are two basic methods used to calculate children's dosages:

- According to kilogram of body weight
- According to BSA

The body weight method is generally the method of choice, because most medications are ordered in this way and it is easier to calculate. The BSA is an exact method, but one must use a formula and a **nomogram** (a device-graph that shows relation among numeric values) to determine a correct dosage.

Body Surface Area

The BSA is considered to be one of the most accurate methods of calculating medication dosages for infants and children up to 12 years of age. This method requires the use of a nomogram that estimates the BSA of the patient according to height and weight (Figure 24-4).

The body surface area is determined by drawing a straight line from the patient's height to the patient's weight. Intersection of the line with the surface area column is the estimated BSA. This figure is then placed in the following formula:

$$\frac{\text{BSA of child (m}^2\text{)}}{1.7 \text{ (m}^2\text{)}} \times \text{adult dose} = \text{child dose}$$

This formula is based on the average adult who weighs 140 pounds and has a body surface area of 1.7 square meters (1.7 m^2).

Example:

Marion Carrera is a 4-year-old child who is 40 inches tall and weighs 38 pounds (BSA 0.7). The physician has ordered Demerol for pain. The average adult dose of Demerol is 50 mg per mL. What dosage will be given to Marion according to the BSA method?

$$\frac{0.7 \text{ (m}^2\text{)}}{1.7 \text{ (m}^2\text{)}} \times \frac{50 \text{ mg}}{1} = \text{child's dose}$$

$$\frac{0.7 \text{ (m}^2\text{)}}{1.7 \text{ (m}^2\text{)}} \times \frac{50}{1} = \frac{35}{1.7} = 20.5 \text{ mg} = 20.5 \text{ or } 21 \text{ mg}$$

Now use the formula $\frac{\text{Desired}}{\text{Have}} \times$ Quantity to convert mg to ml.

$$\frac{21 \text{ mg}}{50 \text{ mg}} \times 1 = x \text{ mL}$$

$$\frac{21}{50} = 0.42 \text{ mL administered in a tuberculin syringe}$$

Kilogram of Body Weight

It may be the responsibility of the medical assistant to calculate the amount of dosage ordered by the physician according to the patient's body weight. Today, many medications are ordered in this manner; therefore, it is essential that you learn how to calculate dosage according to this method. The following example will guide you step by step through the mathematical process of calculating dosage according to kilogram of body weight.

There are 2.2 pounds in 1 kg.

Example:

The physician ordered an antiepileptic agent, Depakene (valproic acid) 15 mg/kg/day capsules for Clark Kipperley, who weighs 110 pounds. The medication is to be given in three divided doses.

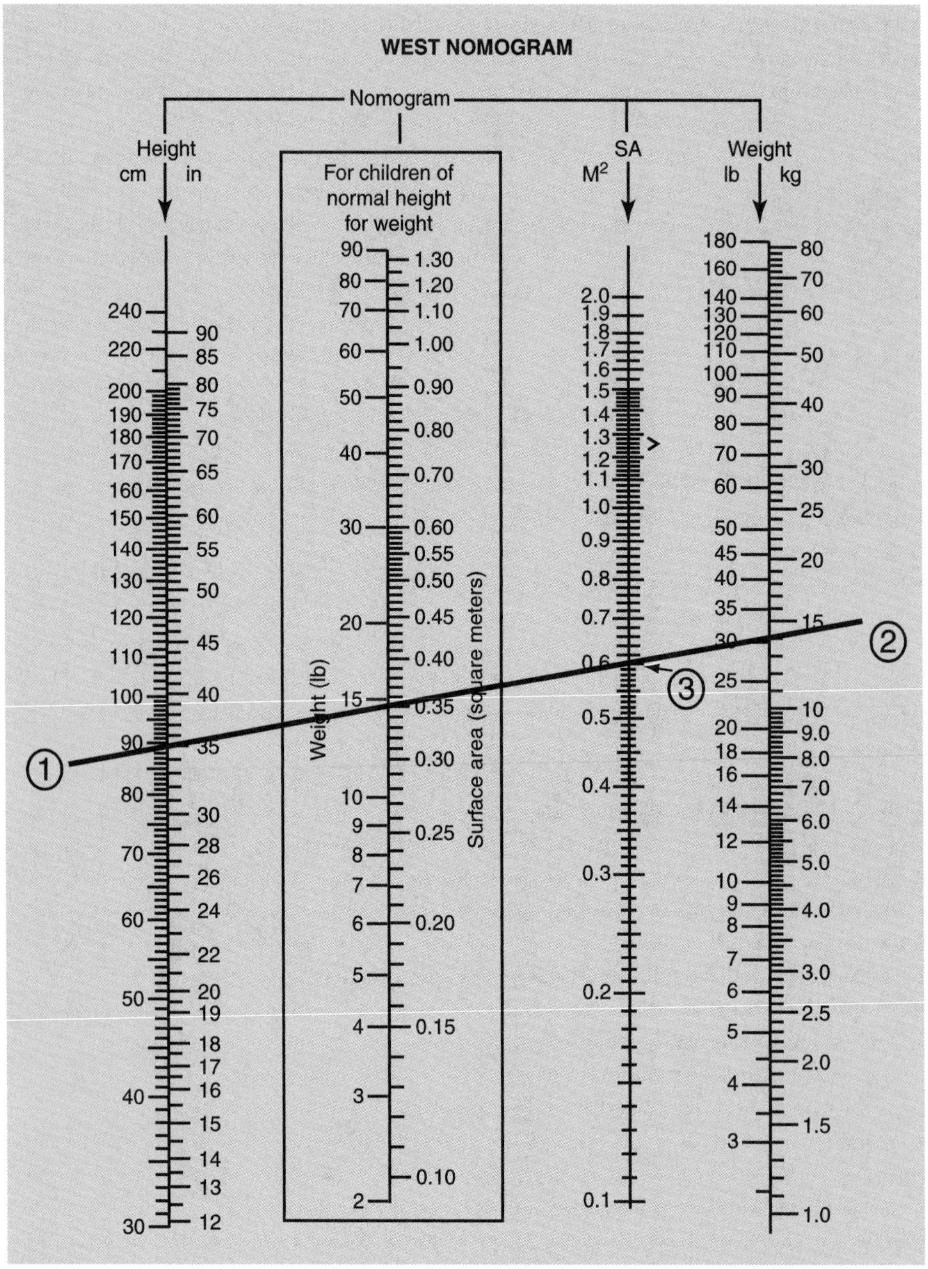

Figure 24-4 Body surface area (BSA) is determined by drawing a straight line from the patient's height (1) in the far left column to his or her weight (2) in the far right column. Intersection of the line with BSA column (3) is the estimated BSA (m^2). For infants and children of normal height and weight, BSA may be estimated from weight alone by referring to the enclosed area. (From Behrman, R. E., Kleigman, R. M., & Arvin, A. M. (1996). *Nelson textbook of pediatrics* (15th ed.). Philadelphia: WB Saunders, Reprinted with permission from Elsevier.)

Step 1. To express pounds in kilograms, divide the weight in pounds by 2.2. Convert the patient's weight to kilograms:

$$110 \div 2.2 = 50 \text{ kilograms}$$

Step 2. Now, calculate the prescribed dosage by placing 50 in the appropriate place:

15 mg/50/day

$$15 \times 50 = 750 \text{ mg/day}$$

Step 3. To determine the amount of each dose, divide 750 by 3 (divided doses).

$$750 \text{ mg} \div 3 = 250 \text{ mg}$$

Depakene is available in 250-mg capsules and 250-mg/5 mL syrup. The physician ordered the medication in capsules, so Clark will receive a 250-mg capsule every 8 hours for a total of 3 doses a day.

In the same example, use the proportional method to calculate kilogram of body weight.

Step 1. To convert 110 pounds to kilograms, set up the proportion as follows:

$$2.2 \text{ lb} : 1 \text{ kg} = 110 \text{ lb} : x \text{ kg}$$

Step 2. Now, solve for x.

$$2.2 : 1 = 110 : x$$
$$2.2x = 110$$
$$x = 50$$

Step 3. Now, calculate the prescribed dosage by placing 50 in the appropriate place: mg/50 kg/day

$$15 \times 50 = 750 \text{ mg/day}$$

Step 4. To determine the amount of each dose, divide 750 by 3 (divided doses).

$$750 \div 3 = 250 \text{ mg per dose}$$

ADMINISTRATION OF MEDICATIONS

Regardless of a medication's form or the route by which it is administered, certain basic guidelines must be followed. These guidelines are:

1. Practice medical asepsis. (See Chapter 10 for specific medical asepsis rules.) Wash your hands before and after administering a medication. Remember Occupational Safety and Health Administration (OSHA) guidelines and standard precautions. (See Chapter 10 for Standard Precautions.)
2. Work in a well-lighted area that is free from distractions.
3. Follow the "Six Rights" of proper drug administration (see following section).
4. Always check for allergies before administering any medication.
5. Give only drugs ordered by a licensed physician or practitioner who is authorized to prescribe medications.
6. Never give a medication if there is any question about the order.
7. Be completely familiar with the drug that you are administering before giving it to the patient. Look it up in the PDR.
8. Always check the expiration date on the medication label.
9. Never give a drug if its normal appearance has been altered in any way (color, structure, consistency, or odor); it may be outdated, contaminated, or stored incorrectly.
10. Make out a medication note (Figure 24-5) for medications, dose, route, and time exactly as ordered by the physician using the physician's order from the patient's record as a guide. Do not rely on memory.

A medication note is written out prior to administration of any medication to the patient in the ambulatory care setting. The information is taken directly from the physician's order sheet of the patient's record. An example follows.

Information needed:

Patient name: Abigail Johnson

Physician's order: Cardizem (diltiazem hydrochloride) 180 mg po stat. Winston Lewis, MD.

The medicine note is then used to be certain you have the correct patient, and to document the information on Mrs. Johnson's record. Following documentation, tear up the medication note and discard.

Room 3
Johnson, Abigail
Cardizem
180 mg
po
stat
10/24/XX – 10 A.M.

Figure 24-5 A medication note is used to prepare, administer, and record medications, dose, route, and time as ordered by the physician.

11. Give only those medications that you have actually prepared for administration. Trust only your own actions.
12. Do not allow someone else to give a medication that you have prepared. Depend on yourself to give the correct medication.
13. Once you have prepared a medication for administration, do not leave it unattended; it could be misplaced or spilled.
14. Be careful in transporting the medication to the patient. Do not spill or drop.
15. When administering oral medications, stay with the patient until you are certain that the medication has been taken, to be sure patient swallowed medication.
16. Shake (to mix) all liquid medications that contain a **precipitate** before pouring. A precipitate is a substance that separates from a solution if allowed to stand. This mixes the liquid for the proper medication.
17. When pouring a liquid medication, hold the measuring device at eye level or place it on a flat surface and squat down so you can observe it at eye level. Read the correct amount at the lowest level of the **meniscus**, which is the top surface of the column of liquid.
18. Do not contaminate the cap of a bottle while pouring a medication. Place the cap with the rim pointed upward to prevent contamination of that portion that comes into contact with the medication.
19. Keep all drugs not being administered in a safe storage place.
20. Carefully follow the procedural steps for the type of medication that you are giving or the type of procedure you are performing.
21. Always keep safety precautions in mind. The United States Department of Health and Human Services, Public Health Service, and Centers for Disease and Prevention Control recommend following standard precautions for prevention of hepatitis B and C viruses and human immunodeficiency virus and other bloodborne diseases (refer to Chapter 10 for specifics about Standard Precautions).

The "Six Rights" of Proper Drug Administration

The "Six Rights" have been developed as a checklist of activities to be followed by those who give medications. This easy-to-remember list should always be followed to ensure the proper administration of any drug:

1. *Right drug*. To be sure that the correct drug has been selected, compare the medication order with the label on the medication. A frequent check of the medication label is a good way to avoid a medication error. One should make a practice of reading the label on each of the following three occasions:

   First: When the medication is taken from the storage area.

   Second: Just before removing it from its container.

   Third: On returning the medication container to storage or before discarding the empty container.

2. *Right dose*. It is essential that the patient receive the right dose. If the dose ordered and the dose on hand are *not the same*, carefully determine the correct dose through mathematical calculation. When calculating dosage, it is advisable to have another qualified person verify the accuracy of your calculations before the medication is administered.
3. *Right route*. Check the medication order to be sure that you have the right route of administration (Figure 24-6A).
4. *Right time*. You are responsible for medicating the patient at the proper time. Check the medication order to ensure that a drug is administered according to the time interval prescribed. For a drug to be maintained at the proper blood level, care must be taken to administer it at the right time (see Figure 24-6B).
5. *Right patient*. Before administering any medication, always be sure that you have the right patient. A good safety practice is to correctly identify the patient on each occasion when you administer a medication. In a hospital, the patient's identification bracelet is always checked. In the ambulatory care facility, call the patient by name or ask the patient to state his or her name (see Figure 24-6C).
6. *Right documentation:* The recording process is the vital link between physician, patient, and medical assistant. It is an account of the essential data that are collected and preserved. The patient's chart is a legal document; therefore, all data should be recorded in ink or entered into the computer. The data should be accurate and clearly stated. It is important that certain data about drug administration be entered into the patient's chart (see Figure 24-6D):
   - Patient's name
   - Date and time of administration
   - Name of the medication and the amount (dosage) administered

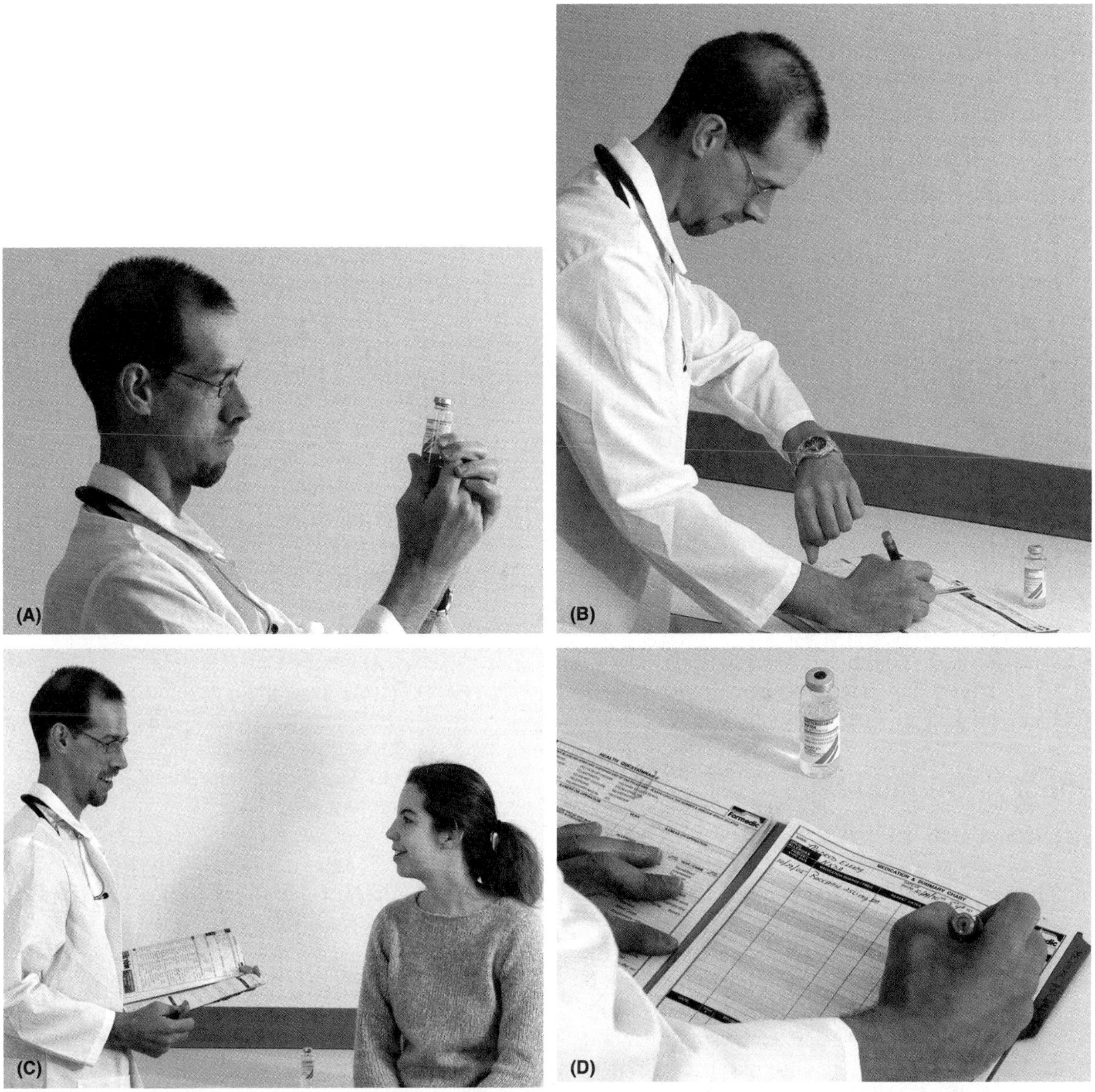

Figure 24-6 (A) Medical assistant checks the right drug, the right route, and the right dose of medication to administer. (B) Medical assistant checks for the right time to administer medication to the patient. (C) Medical assistant assesses patient before administering the medication. The medical assistant ascertains he has the right patient and asks the patient if she has any allergies. (D) Medical assistant documents administration of medication in patient's record.

- Route by which the medication was administered
- Any unusual reactions experienced by the patient
- Any complications in administering the drug (patient refusing to take the medication, difficulty in swallowing)
  - If the medication was *not* given, state why and dispose of the medication according to agency policy and federal and state laws
- Patient data, such as blood pressure, pulse, respirations, when appropriate
- Your name or initials and title

Medication Error

Medication errors should not happen when personnel follow the "Six Rights" of proper drug administration and the essential medication guidelines; however, honest

When a medication error occurs, follow standard procedure:

a. Recognize that an error has been made.
b. Stay calm. Assess the patient's condition and reactions to the medication.
c. Report the error immediately to the physician. Give the details of the mistake and the patient's reactions.
d. Follow the physician's order for correcting the error.
e. Document the error in the patient's record or the facility's record form:
   - Describe the type of error.
   - Describe the patient's reactions.
   - Describe the steps taken to correct the error.
   - State date, time, and your name.

mistakes will be made periodically. A medication error occurs when any of the following happen:

1. A drug is given to the wrong patient
2. The incorrect drug is given
3. The drug is given via an incorrect route
4. The drug is given at the incorrect time
5. The incorrect dose is administered
6. Incorrect data are entered on the patient's chart

Patient Assessment

Before administering any medication, carefully assess the patient's condition. An assessment should include, but is not limited to, the following conditions:

1. *Age*. Is the medication and route suitable for the patient at a particular stage in life? The stages of life include infancy, childhood, adolescence, adulthood, and old age. During infancy, early childhood, and old age, a smaller dose of medication may be required than would be appropriate for the other stages in life.
2. *Physical conditions*. Potential problems associated with the patient's physical condition must be considered. Female patients during pregnancy or while breastfeeding should not be given certain contraindicated medications.
3. *Body size*. The amount of medication given and size of the needle used are directly related to the size of the patient. Pediatric and geriatric patients usually have less subcutaneous and muscular tissue per BSA than the average adult (see Figure 24-4). Small, thin patients usually require less medication, and a shorter needle may be used to reach the appropriate tissue level. On the other hand, the large or obese patient may or may not require more medication than the average adult and a longer needle to reach the appropriate tissue level.
4. *Sex*. Consider differences that are related to the sex of the patient.
   - *Build*. Muscular patients generally have more muscular tissue. Obese patients have more adipose tissue. Always inspect and palpate muscle tissue with this in mind when determining the appropriate needle length to reach muscle tissue.
   - *Skin texture*. Some patients usually have tougher skin than others. A young person's skin might have more tone than that of an older adult. Slightly more force is required to penetrate skin that is tough or lacking in tone.
5. *Injection site*. Always inspect and palpate the skin before administering an injection. The following body areas should be avoided when choosing the site for an injection:
   - Any type of skin lesion
   - Burned areas
   - Inflamed areas
   - Previous injection sites
   - Any traumatized area
   - Scar tissue (vaccination, keloid)
   - Moles, warts, birthmarks, tumors, lumps, hard nodules
   - Nerves, large blood vessels, bones
   - Cyanotic areas
   - Edematous areas
   - Paralyzed areas
   - Arm on same side as mastectomy, or other lymphatic compromise

Correct injection sites are illustrated later in this chapter.

ADMINISTRATION OF ORAL MEDICATIONS

Oral medications are easily and economically administered with a high degree of safety. There are, however, several disadvantages associated with the oral route. For instance, the drug may:

- Have an objectionable odor/taste
- Cause discoloration of the teeth, mouth, and tongue
- Irritate the gastric mucosa
- Be altered by digestive enzymes
- Be poorly absorbed from the digestive system because of illness or nature of the medication

- Not be taken by the patient
- Have less predictable effects on the body when given orally than when given by the parenteral route (by injection)
- Not be able to be swallowed if in tablet, capsule, or caplet form

Equipment and Supplies for Oral Medications

Three measuring devices commonly used in the administration of oral medications are the medicine cup, the water cup, and the medicine dropper. The medicine cup (Figure 24-7) comes in various sizes and shapes, depending on its manufacturer and its intended use. Cups may be calibrated in fluid ounces, fluidrams, cubic centimeters, milliliters (mL), and tablespoons.

The water cup is a small plastic or paper cup that is disposable. The average water cup holds three ounces of liquid.

The medicine dropper (Figure 24-8) may be calibrated in milliliters, minims, or drops. Medicine droppers are often included with the bottle of medication. Uncalibrated droppers may be provided when the medicine is administered only in drops. The size of the drop varies with the size of the dropper opening, the angle at which it is held, the force exerted on the rubber bulb, and the viscosity of the medication.

It is important that the appropriate measuring device be selected for a medication and the prescribed dosage accurately measured. The selection of the measuring device depends on the physical structure of the medication (solid or liquid), the amount of medication prescribed, the size of the measuring device, and the calibrations on the container.

See Procedure 24-1 for administration of oral medications.

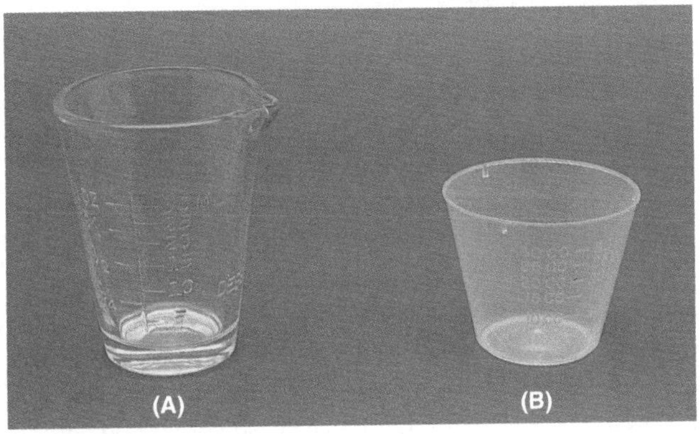

Figure 24-7 Medicine cups: (A) glass; (B) plastic.

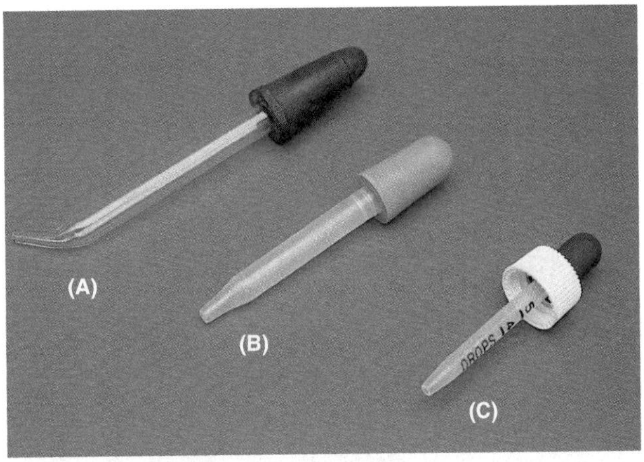

Figure 24-8 Various types of medicine droppers: (A) glass; (B) plastic; (C) plastic calibrated.

ADMINISTRATION OF PARENTERAL MEDICATIONS

The term **parenteral** is used to describe the injection of a substance into the body via a route other than the alimentary canal/digestive system. The most frequently used parenteral routes are:

- *Subcutaneous*. Just below the surface of the skin. A subcutaneous injection is usually given at a 45-degree angle.
- *Intramuscular*. Within the muscle. An intramuscular injection is given at a 90-degree angle, passing through the skin and subcutaneous tissue, and penetrating deep into muscle tissue.
- *Intradermal*. Within the dermal layer of the skin. An intradermal injection is given at an angle between 5 and 10 degrees.
- *Intravenous*. Within or into a vein.

Medications that have been prepared for use by injection are available in multiple-dose form (vials) and in unit dose form (ampules and cartridge-needle units). (See Figure 24-9.) **Unit dose** forms are premeasured amounts, packaged on a per-dose basis.

- *Ampule*. A small, sterile, prefilled glass container that usually holds a single dose of a hypodermic solution.
- *Cartridge-needle unit*. A disposable sterile cartridge containing a premeasured amount of medication. This unit is designed for use in a nondisposable cartridge-holder syringe such as the Tubex® or Carpuject®.

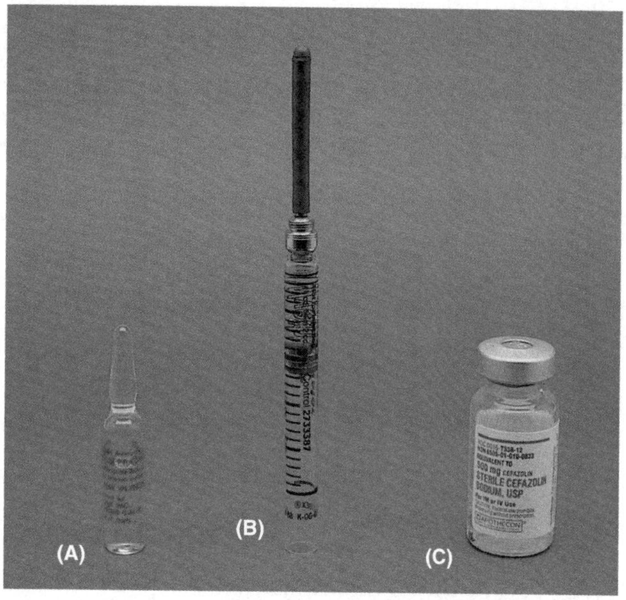

Figure 24-9 Medications given parenterally. (A) Ampule. (B) Sterile cartridge with premeasured medication. (C) Vial of powder for reconstitution.

- *Vial.* A small, sterile, prefilled glass bottle with rubber stopper containing a hypodermic solution.

Hazards Associated with Parenteral Medications

Injections of medications must be done with extreme care. Sterile technique must be used because the needle and medication are being introduced into the patient's body and microorganisms must not be transmitted. Appropriate site selection and proper technique assure effectiveness of the medication.

Additional dangers to be aware of when administering medications parenterally (by injection) include:

- Allergic reaction (if present) will be swift
- Injury to bone, nerve, or blood vessel
- Breaking of needle in tissue (rare)
- Injecting into a blood vessel instead of tissue. (This is avoided by checking for blood return, on aspiration.)

Reasons for Parenteral Route Selection

The parenteral route is selected because of:

- Rapid response time to medication
- Accuracy of dosage
- Need to concentrate medication in a specific body part or area (into a joint or local anesthetic)
- Inability to administer orally because the medication is destroyed by gastric juices, or the patient is incapable of taking medication orally

Because parenteral medications are intended for use by injection, they must be injected as liquids. Some medications are supplied in powder form and must be reconstituted to a liquid form for injection. See Procedure 24-8.

Because they must be in liquid form, the amount of parenteral medications is expressed in terms of volume (cubic centimeters, milliliters, minims, or ounces). The strength of the drug contained in the liquid is usually expressed in terms of its weight (milliequivalents, micrograms, milligrams, grams, grains, or units). Therefore, medications ordered for parenteral use are often ordered by both weight and volume.

Example:
Atropine sulfate injection (gr = weight; mL = volume)

$$0.4 \text{ mg } (\text{gr } \frac{1}{150}) \text{ per mL}$$

The parenteral route of drug administration offers an effective mode of delivering medication to a patient when a rapid and direct result is desired. The effect of a parenteral medication is faster than by the oral route; however, the accuracy of dosage calculation for both is important.

Parenteral Equipment and Supplies

Syringes. Syringes are classified as disposable, nondisposable, and as combinations of these two types. Most syringes used in ambulatory care are plastic. They also may be classified according to their intended use. In addition to the standard hypodermic syringes that are in general use, there are special-purpose syringes for irrigations or oral feedings, tuberculin syringes, and insulin syringes.

Disposable Syringes. Disposable syringes are those that are sterilized, prepackaged, nontoxic, nonpyrogenic, and ready for use. They are available as a syringe-needle unit and are generally enclosed in individual peel-apart packages of durable paper or clear plastic. They are available in sizes from 0.5 to 50 cubic centimeters. The 1-, 3-, and 5-cc syringes are the ones most often used when parenteral medications are administered.

A disposable syringe-needle unit consists of a syringe with an attached needle. The needle is covered by a hard plastic sheath to prevent it from accidentally penetrating the package or sticking the

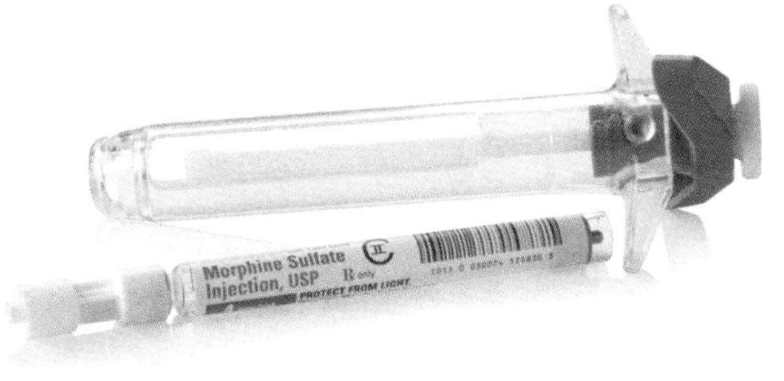

Figure 24-10 The Carpuject® is a type of cartridge-injection system with click-lock mechanism for safety. (Courtesy of Hospira, Inc.)

user. The unit may be sealed within a peel-apart package or encased in a rigid plastic container that has been heat sealed to ensure sterility. Labeling usually includes the manufacturer's name, type and size of the syringe, gauge and length of the needle, and a reorder number. Packages are usually color coded for ease of identification. Always read the label. Disposable syringes are generally preferred for the administration of parenteral medications because they ensure sterility and sharp needles. Also, disposable syringes eliminate the need for resterilizaton, which is costly, time-consuming, and possibly unsafe if not done properly.

Nondisposable Syringes. Nondisposable syringes are usually made of specially strengthened glass resistant to thermal shock. These units, consisting of round glass barrels with individually fitted plungers, are manufactured to exacting specifications.

Nondisposable glass syringes are available in sizes from 1 to 50 cubic centimeters. They may be used by physicians to perform special procedures such as paracentesis, thoracentesis, thoracotomy, and tracheotomy.

Combination Disposable/Nondisposable Cartridge-Injection Syringes. A cartridge-injection system, such as the plastic Carpuject® (Figure 24-10) or the metal Tubex® consists of a disposable cartridge-needle unit and a nondisposable cartridge-holder syringe. The cartridge-needle unit is factory sealed and sterile and contains a precisely measured unit dose of medicine. The cartridge-holder syringe may be made of durable chrome-plated brass or of plastic. These reusable syringes are designed for quick and safe loading and unloading of cartridge-needle units, which are manufactured in various sizes and dosage capacities and contain a wide range of medications (Figure 24-11A–E).

The combination of disposable/nondisposable syringe system is easy to use and convenient. When using this system, be careful to read the label and compare the medication order with the label. For example, the physician may order Demerol® 25 mg and the cartridge is 50 mg/cc. Give ½ cc and properly discard the other ½ cc according to office policy. Another person must witness the disposal of the Demerol®, which is a controlled substance.

Parts of a Syringe. The component parts of a syringe consist of a barrel, plunger, flange, tip (Figure 24-12), and a safety shield on a safety syringe (Figure 24-13B).

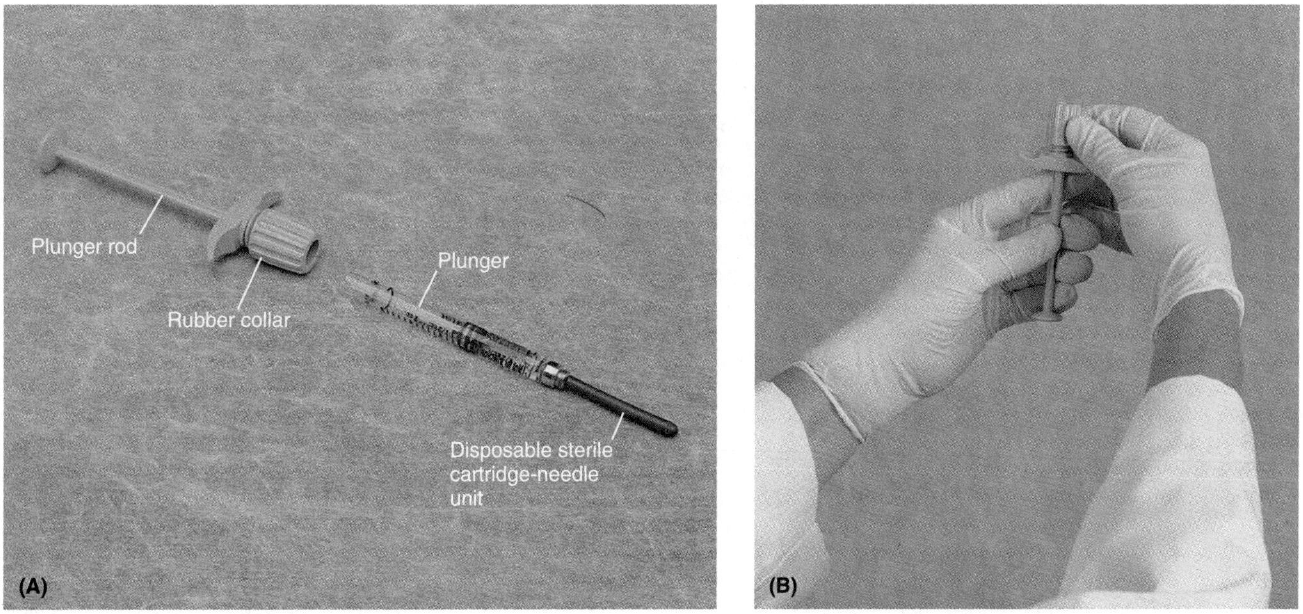

Figure 24-11 (A) Reusable cartridge holder with disposable sterile cartridge needle unit. (B) Turn ribbed collar to open position.

(continues)

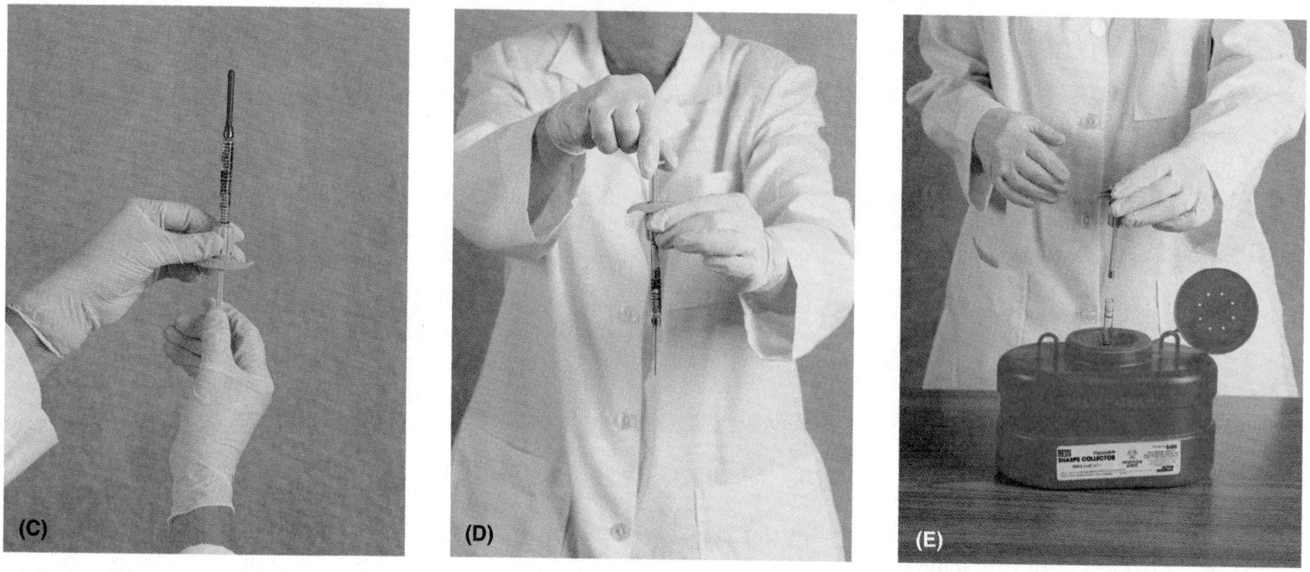

Figure 24-11 *(continued)* (C) Insert the sterile cartridge-needle unit into the open end of the injector. The ribbed collar is firmly tightened. The plunger of the injector and the plunger of the cartridge-needle unit are tightened and ready for use. (D) The medical assistant prepares to dispose of the cartridge-needle unit. The needle is not recapped. The plunger rod is disengaged by unscrewing. The ribbed collar is loosened. (E) The medical assistant holds the cartridge-needle unit over a sharps container and the unit drops into the container.

- The *barrel* is the part that holds the medication and has graduated markings (calibrations) on its surface for use in measuring medications.
- The *plunger* is a movable cylinder designed for insertion within the barrel; it provides the mechanism by which a medication (or other substance) is drawn into or pushed out of the barrel.
- The *flange* is at the end of the barrel where the plunger is inserted. It forms a rim around the end of the barrel where the plunger is inserted and has appendages against which one places the index and middle fingers when drawing up solution for injection. The flange also prevents the syringe from rolling when laid on a flat surface.

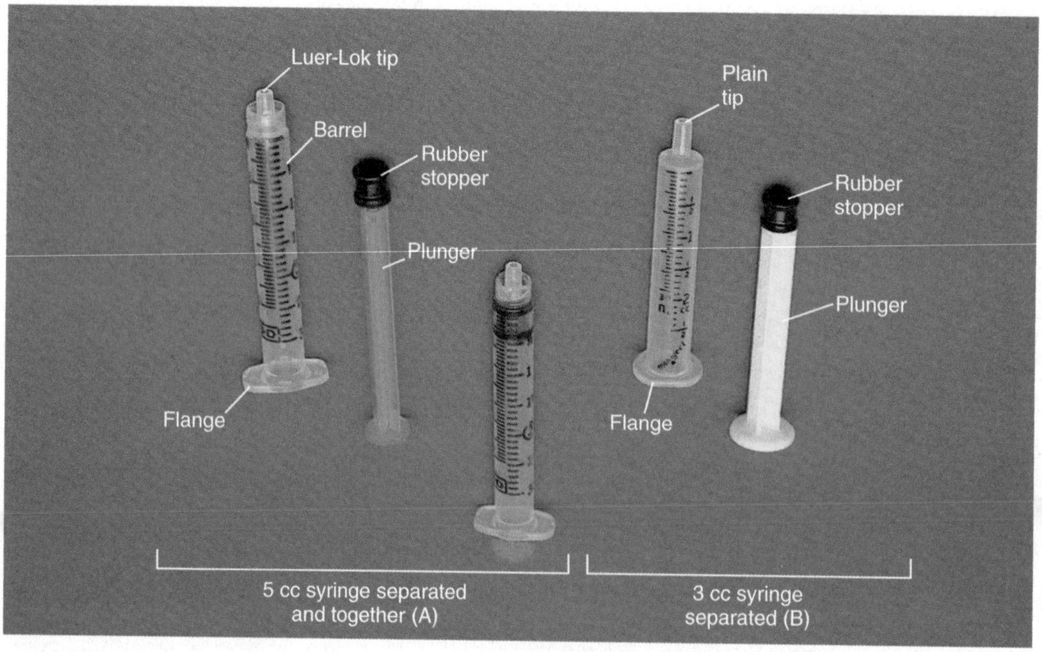

Figure 24-12 Parts of a syringe (A) A 5-mL syringe separated and unseparated with Luer-Lok® tip. (B) A 3-mL syringe separated with plain tip.

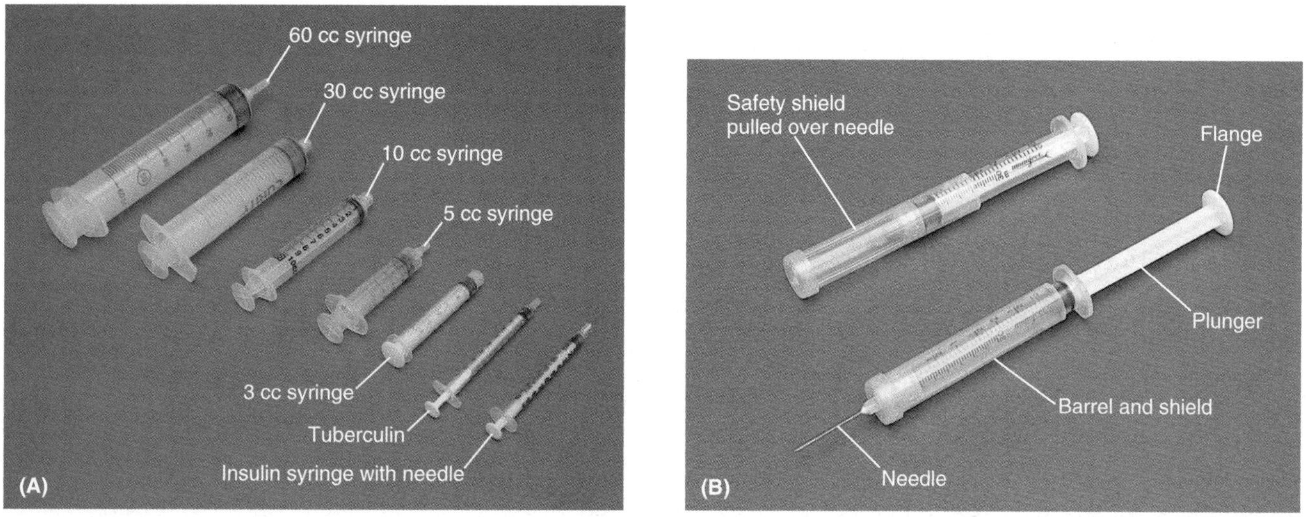

Figure 24-13 (A) Various sizes of disposable syringes. Note tuberculin and insulin syringes. (B) A type of safety syringe and needle.

- The *tip* is at the end of the barrel where the needle is attached.
- The safety shield is pulled over the needle while withdrawing it (Figure 24-13B). Safety needles have a mechanism to either sheath the needle, retract it, or blunt it.

The parts of a syringe that must remain sterile during the preparation and administration of a parenteral medication are the inside of the barrel, the section of the plunger that fits inside the barrel, and the syringe tip to which the needle is to be attached.

Types of Syringes and Uses. Syringes are named according to their sizes and uses. Table 24-7 lists the types, sizes, calibrations, and uses of syringes used in the administration of parenteral medications. Figure 24-13A shows various sizes of disposable syringes, and Figure 24-13B shows a type of safety needle and syringe.

One should always choose a needle with sufficient length to reach the desired tissue level (see Table 24-8). A large person may require a longer needle to reach the correct body tissue than would be required for a smaller person. The delivery of medication to the proper tissue level is important. A concentrated or irritating medication that is intended for deep intramuscular injection could be delivered instead into the subcutaneous tissue of an obese patient if one selects a needle that is too short. Such an inappropriate injection may cause a sterile abscess and necrosis. This unnecessary complication can be avoided by considering the size of the patient when choosing the length of the needle.

Needles. Both disposable and nondisposable needles are available for use with syringes. Of these, the most

TABLE 24-7 THE MOST FREQUENTLY USED SYRINGES FOR PARENTERAL MEDICATIONS

Type of Syringes	Size and Calibration	Typical Uses
Hypodermic	3 cubic centimeters Calibrated 0.1 15/16 minims/cubic centimeter	Intramuscular and subcutaneous injections
Hypodermic	5 cubic centimeters Calibrated 0.2	Venipuncture and intramuscular injections
Hypodermic	Larger sizes (10, 30, and 60 cubic centimeters)	Medical/surgical treatments, aspirations, irrigations, venipunctures, gavage (tube-to-stomach) feedings
Tuberculin	1 cubic centimeter Calibrated 0.1 and 0.01 16 minims/mL	To inject minute amounts for intradermal injections, allergy testing, allergy injections
Insulin	U-100 (0.5 cubic centimeters) U-100 (1 cubic centimeter)	Lo-Dose® administration of insulin Insulin administration

TABLE 24-8 SYRINGE-NEEDLE COMBINATIONS FOR VARIOUS PARENTERAL ROUTES

Subcutaneous Injection	Intramuscular Injection	Intradermal Injection
3-cc syringe/25G, 5/8 inch needle	3-cc syringe/23G, 1 inch needle	1-cc syringe/25G, 5/8 inch needle
3-cc syringe/26G, 3/8 inch needle	3-cc syringe/22G, 1 1/2 inch needle	1-cc syringe/26G, 3/8 inch needle
3-cc syringe/27G, 1/2 inch needle	3-cc syringe/21G, 1 1/2 to 2 inch needle	1-cc syringe/27G, 1/2 inch needle
U-100 (1 cc)/26G, 1/2 inch needle for insulin		

frequently used are disposable needles, which are individually packaged in sterile paper or plastic containers. Disposable needles and syringe-needle units are available with a color-coded sheath. The sheath protects the needle and identifies its gauge and length. Common needle gauges (G) range from 16 to 32, and their lengths vary from 3/8 to 2 inches. The needle's gauge is determined by the diameter of the lumen or opening at its beveled tip. The larger the gauge, the smaller the diameter of its lumen. For example, a 32-gauge needle is much smaller than a 16-gauge needle.

Nondisposable needles are made of high-quality stainless steel. They are equipped with a mounting hub that has a cylindrical opening designed to slip over the lock onto the tip of a syringe, such as a Luer-Lok®. See Figure 24-14 for various sizes and types of needles.

Parts of a Needle. Figure 24-15 shows the parts of a needle used to administer parenteral medications.

- The *point* is the sharpened end of the needle. The point is formed when the end of the shaft is ground away to form a flat, slanted surface called the *bevel*.
- The *lumen*, the hollow core of the needle, forms an oval-shaped opening when exposed at the beveled point.
- The hollow steel tube through which the medication passes is the *shaft*.
- The other end of the shaft attaches to the *hub*, which is part of the needle unit that is designed to mount onto the syringe.
- The point at which the shaft attaches to the hub is called the *hilt*.

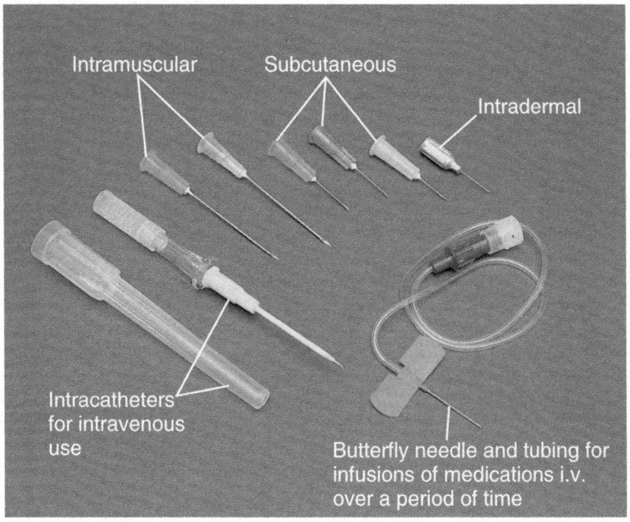

Figure 24-14 Various sizes and types of needles. Different colored hubs denote needle gauges.

The Safe Disposal of Needles and Syringes. The careless disposal of used needles and syringes may present a health risk to any person coming into contact with the used equipment. An accidental stick by a contaminated needle could transmit diseases such as hepatitis B, hepatitis C, syphilis, Rocky Mountain spotted fever, tuberculosis, malaria, varicella zoster, and human immunodeficiency virus (HIV). Used needles and syringes should be discarded in a rigid, puncture-proof container (Figure 24-16). Do not recap the needle after giving the injection. Do engage safety feature. Most needlesticks occur while recapping. Refer to Chapter 10 for OSHA regulations.

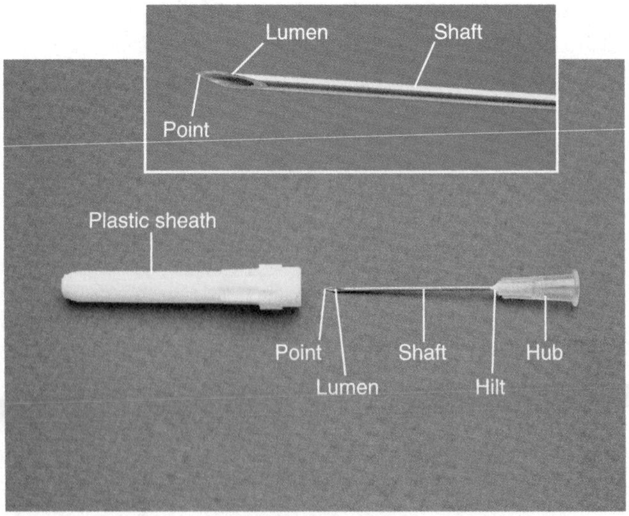

Figure 24-15 Parts of a needle and needle sheath. Inset shows point, lumen, and shaft.

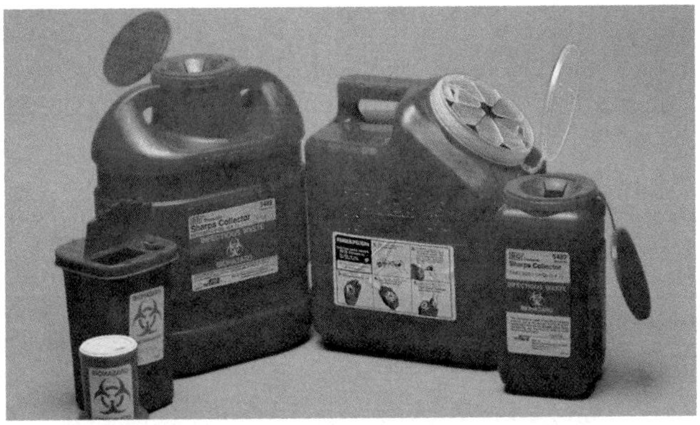

Figure 24-16 Place used needles, point down, in puncture-proof sharps containers.

Most sharps-related injuries (needlesticks) occur in the hospital with inpatients. However, any health care worker who administers parenteral medications is at risk for an injury. Other types of sharps-related injuries besides disposable needles include suture needles, butterfly needles, scalpel blades, phlebotomy needles, and IV catheter stylets.

A number of pathogens can enter the body during a sharps-related injury, but of greatest concern are hepatitis B and C viruses and HIV. (See Chapter 10 for details about these and other bloodborne pathogens).

The National Alliance for the Primary Prevention of Sharps Injuries (NAPPSI) consists of medical device makers, health organizations, and health care providers whose goal is the prevention of sharps-related injuries. Besides safety needles (see information on retractable needles in Chapter 10), laser scalpels, and needleless drug delivery systems such as patches and inhaled medications, a needleless injection system is available (fluid under pressure). There are glues and adhesives available to approximate surgical incisions. These alternative methods are helpful in reducing sharps-related injuries; however, phlebotomy and IV therapy still require a needle. Legal regulations (CDC and OSHA) require use of the safest needle available.

Proper use and disposal of sharps is the utmost importance to health care workers and others. Avoid needles if there are other methods available, and do not recap needles. Engage the safety mechanism and dispose of needles and syringes immediately after use.

Sharps Collectors. Sharps collector systems eliminate the need to reshield the needle, thereby reducing the risk for an accidental needlestick.

Needles are placed into the container as a whole unit after safety mechanisms are engaged. Sharps containers need to be within reach at any time injections are given.

IV THERAPY

The latest Commission on Accreditation of Allied Health Education Programs (CAAHEP) Standards and Guidelines for Medical Assisting Education Programs, are effective as of January 1, 2005. Included in the curriculum Content Requirements are principles of IV therapy.

IV therapy is usually performed by a physician or a registered nurse who will insert a needle or catheter into an appropriate vein and attach tubing to the catheter. The tubing is inserted into a glass or plastic container of fluid. The tubing is known as a basic administration set. A sterile dressing covers the skin surrounding the IV site.

The fluid is infused into the patient drop by drop. The administration set package states the drop factor. The rate of the IV flow is extremely important. It is crucial that the number of drops per minute be accurate. There is a mathematical formula to calculate the rate. Volume restriction can be critical with all patients and especially with neonatal patients. Excessive volume (too many drops per minute) can result in overhydration of the patient with possible cardiac and pulmonary consequences.

Factors essential for IV infusion are that the prescribed amount of fluid be infused, that the prescribed time for the infusion to be correct, and that the drop factor be calculated using a mathematical formula.

Electronic devices for infusions are mechanisms powered by battery, electricity, or a combination of both. These devices are safe and precise and can be programmed to infuse at a specific rate and signal when the infusion is complete. The device has alarms that alert the health care provider if there is a problem with air in the system or pressure in the line.

IV therapy or infusion is ordered by the physician for a variety of reasons and patient conditions. It allows medication to be given for a rapid response, replaces fluids and electrolytes that the patient may have lost through burns or vomiting and diarrhea, helps to increase blood pressure when the patient is in shock from blood or fluid loss, and is used for nutritional supplement and for blood or blood product administration. The advantages of IV infusion therapy are to have access to a vein whenever needed and to have a systemic effect in a short period. Veins are accessible for emergencies. The route is useful for unconscious patients and provides a rapid route to counteract poisonous substances or inappropriate medication response. Many times patients' veins collapse because of to their condition (dehydration, blood loss) and it may be difficult to locate a vein that can be accessed. Once the vein is found, the physician may order that the vein be kept open (keep vein open [KVO] or TKO [to keep open]) for immediate accessibility.

It is important to realize that IV infusion is an invasive procedure much like the phlebotomy procedure. The veins for IV infusion are similar to those used for venipuncture in the hands and arms.

Although IV therapy is not a procedure medical assistants usually perform, they must be knowledgeable about the procedure, understand the purpose for IV infusions, recognize the precautions concerning this invasive procedure, and realize that state laws vary regarding IV infusion and which professionals can be responsible for the procedure. All persons providing health care to patients are legally responsible for their own actions. See Chapter 28 for information regarding phlebotomy.

SITE SELECTION AND INJECTION ANGLE

The selection of a proper site for a subcutaneous, intramuscular, or intradermal injection and the correct angle of insertion for each will assure that the medication is delivered to the correct tissue type (see Figure 24-17).

A subcutaneous injection is given at an angle of 45 degrees just below the surface of the skin wherever there is subcutaneous tissue. The shaded areas in Figure 24-18A are usually used for subcutaneous injections because they are located away from bones, joints, nerves, and large blood vessels.

An intramuscular injection is given at a 90-degree angle, passing through the skin and subcutaneous tissue and penetrating deep into muscle tissue. Body areas normally used for intramuscular injections are the dorsogluteal area, ventrogluteal area, deltoid muscle, and vastus lateralis.

After locating an appropriate vein, an IV injection is given at a 25-degree angle penetrating the skin and introducing the needle into the vein. The antecubital, median cephalic, median basilic, and median cubital veins are common sites appropriate for IV injections. See Chapter 28 for more information about vein selection.

Intradermal injections are given at an angle between 10 and 15 degrees into the dermal layer of the skin. The body areas used for intradermal injections are the inner forearm and the middle of the back (see Figure 24-18B). The reasons for the use of these two sites are that the skin is thin and there is little hair.

Marking the Correct Site for Intramuscular Injection

To give a safe injection, it is necessary to become familiar with the anatomic structures associated with the injection site. With knowledge of where such structures are located, it is easier to mark injection sites that avoid bones, nerves, and large blood vessels.

Dorsogluteal Site. The dorsogluteal site is the traditional location for giving most (adult) deep intramuscular injections (Figure 24-19). Commonly referred to as the "upper outer quadrant of the buttocks," this descrip-

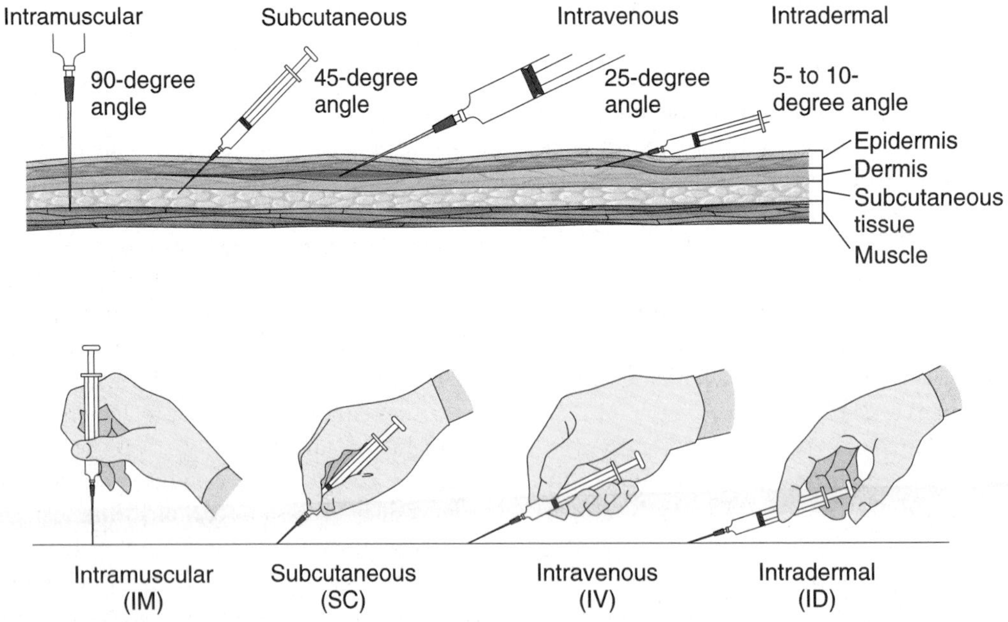

Figure 24-17 Angles of injection for intramuscular, subcutaneous, intravenous, and intradermal injections.

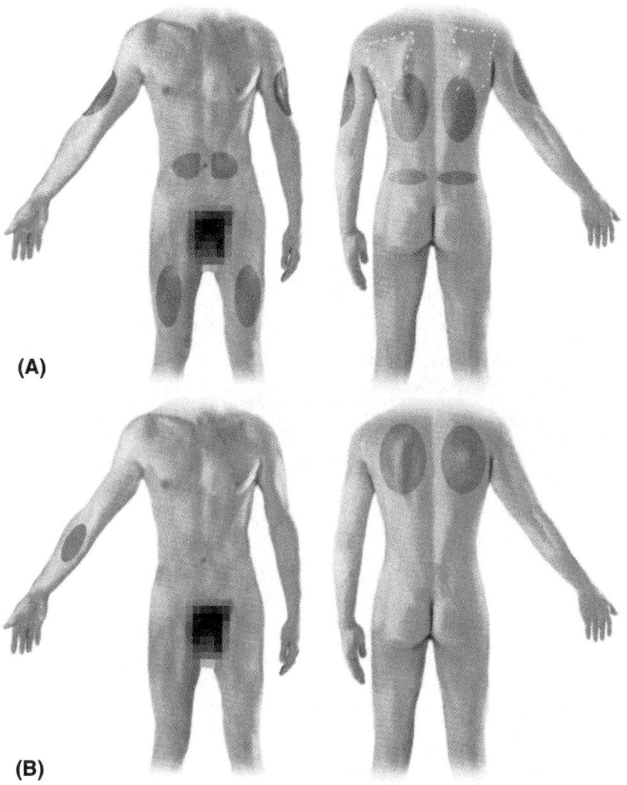

Figure 24-18 Injection sites: (A) subcutaneous. (B) intradermal.

tion can be easily misinterpreted and result in an injection into the inappropriate area. To locate the correct site for a dorsogluteal injection, locate the superior posterior iliac spine and place a small *x* on this spot. Then locate the greater trochanter of the femur and mark this spot. Draw (or imagine) a diagonal line between the two locations. The area above and outside this line and about 3 inches below the iliac crest is the correct location of the dorsogluteal site.

Extreme caution should be used when giving intramuscular injections in the dorsogluteal area. Improper site selection can result in damage to the sciatic nerve or injection into the superior gluteal artery or vein. This site is contraindicated for infants and is used only as a site of last resort in children because of less muscle development. This muscle mass may be degenerated in older adults, the nonwalking, or the emaciated patient (see Figures 24-19 and 24-23A).

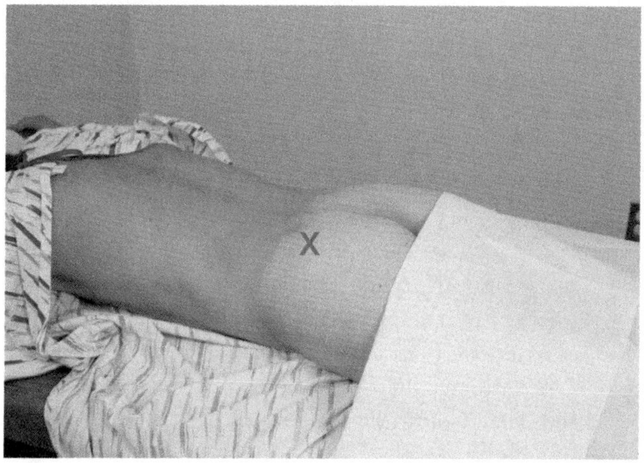

Figure 24-19 The dorsogluteal intramuscular injection site. Locate the superior posterior iliac spine and the greater trochanter. Draw an imaginary line between the two locations. The area above and outside this line is the injection site. (See also Figure 24-23A).

Ventrogluteal Site. The ventrogluteal site (gluteus medius muscle) can generally accommodate the majority of medications ordered for intramuscular injection. It may be used for individuals from infancy to adulthood. The ventrogluteal site is relatively free of major nerves and vessels, thereby making it a choice site for intramuscular injections. To locate the ventrogluteal injection site, palpate to find the greater trochanter, the anterior superior iliac spine, and the bony ridge of the iliac crest (Figure 24-20). With these three locations identified, place the palm of your hand against the greater trochanter with the tip of your index finger on the anterior superior iliac spine. Then spread your middle finger as far from the index finger as possible. Place an *x* in the center of

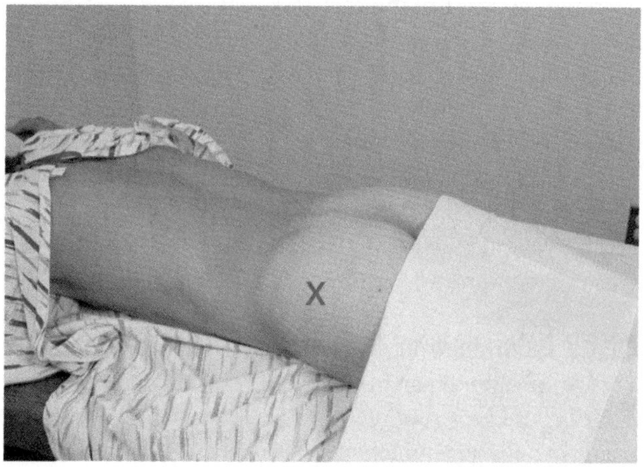

Figure 24-20 The ventrogluteal intramuscular injection site. Palpate the greater trochanter, iliac crest, and anterior superior iliac spine. If given into the patient's left buttock, the palm of the right hand is placed on the greater trochanter and the index finger on the anterior superior iliac spine. The middle finger is spread along the iliac crest posteriorly as far as possible. A V shape is formed. Give the injection in the middle of the V. (See also Figure 24-23B).

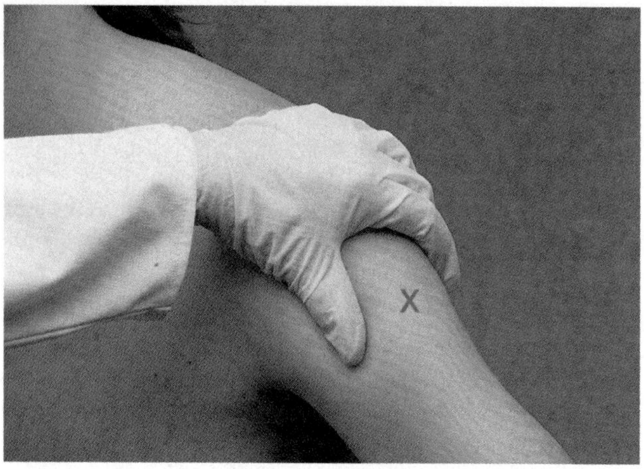

Figure 24-21 The deltoid intramuscular injection site is located on the upper outer aspect of the arm, below the lower edge of the acromion. (See also Figure 24-23C.)

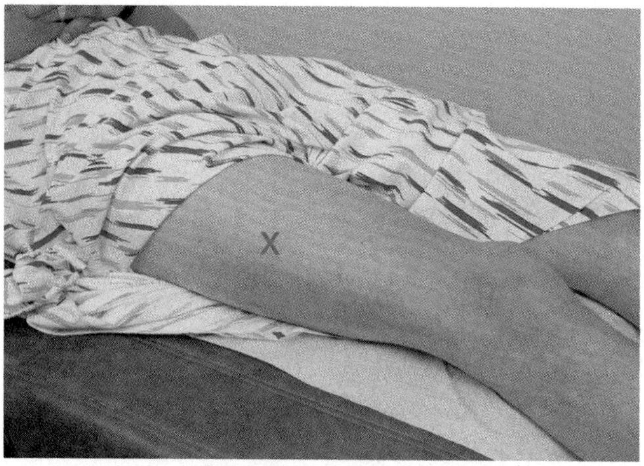

Figure 24-22 The vastus lateralis intramuscular injection site is located by dividing the leg into thirds by palpating the greater trochanter and the patella. The injection is given into the middle third of the area. (See also Figure 24-23D.)

the triangle formed by the middle and index fingers to mark the correct injection site (see Figure 24-23B).

Deltoid Muscle. The deltoid muscle is a small but adequate site for certain intramuscular injections. These intramuscular preparations include vaccines, narcotics, sedatives, and vitamin preparations. The site should not be used for an infant. To locate the deltoid injection site, place your fingers on the shoulder and find the acromion (lateral triangular projection of the spine of the scapula forming the point of the shoulder) and the deltoid tuberosity that lies lateral to the side of the arm, opposite the axilla (Figure 24-21 and 24-23C). The correct injection site is 1 to 2 inches (about the width of three fingers) below the acromion.

CAUTION: Do not inject medicine into the upper and lower aspects of the deltoid muscle. Care should be taken to avoid brachial and axillary nerves and blood vessels, the radial nerve, acromion, and the humerus.

Vastus Lateralis Site. The vastus lateralis is the preferred site for intramuscular injections in infants and children. It is also used for intramuscular injections in adults. This site generally accommodates the majority of intramuscular injections ordered and is a relatively safe site because the nerves and vessels supplying the area are not generally endangered. The vastus lateralis is a part of the quadriceps femoris. The muscle is located on the anterolateral aspect of the patient. For infants and children, the site lies below the greater trochanter of the femur and within the upper lateral quadrant of the thigh (Figure 24-22 and 24-23D).

For the adult patient, the correct injection site is within the middle third of the muscle.

BASIC GUIDELINES FOR ADMINISTRATION OF INJECTIONS

Regardless of the type of injection, there are basic guidelines that one must follow to safeguard the patient. These guidelines are presented according to the sequence of the events to which they relate:

1. Adhere to the "Six Rights" of proper drug administration.
2. Always evaluate each patient as an individual.
3. Select a needle-syringe unit that is the appropriate size for the proper administration of a parenteral medication.
4. Correctly prepare the appropriate parenteral equipment and supplies for use. Wash hands and put on gloves. Always use OSHA guidelines and follow standard precautions.
5. Select the correct site for the intended injection.
6. Prepare the patient properly for the injection.
7. For subcutaneous and intramuscular injections, use a smooth, quick, dartlike motion to insert the needle into the patient's skin. Use the correct angle of insertion (45 or 90 degrees) for the injection.
8. Once the needle is inserted, gently pull back on the plunger (aspirate) to ensure that the needle is not in a blood vessel.
   CAUTION: If blood appears in the syringe on aspiration, smoothly withdraw the needle, properly discard the used unit, and prepare another injection for administration. Repeat the preceding steps.
9. Slowly inject the medication into the patient.

- Volume of drug administered:
  Usual 1.0 mL to 2.0 mL
  Maximum 3.0 mL
- Needle sizes frequently used:
  18G to 23G. 1¼ in. to 2 in.
  (greater length needed for very obese individuals)
- Acceptable patient position:
  Prone
- Angle of injection:
  90° angle to flat surface upon which prone patient is lying
- Advantages of site:
  Large muscle mass accommodates deep IM/Z-track injections.
  Injection not visible to patient.
- Disadvantages of site:
  Boundaries of the upper, outer quadrant are often arbitrarily selected and may exceed margin of safety.
  Danger of injury to major nerves and vascular structures if incorrect site or technique is used.
  Subcutaneous fat in area is often very thick; an injection intended for muscle may in fact be subcutaneous.
  Difficult area in which to maintain proper asepsis.
  Should abscesses develop, incision and drainage are complicated by proximity of large nerves and vascular structures.
- Additional considerations:
  IM injection using the dorsogluteal site requires strict adherence to proper anatomical site location and injection technique.

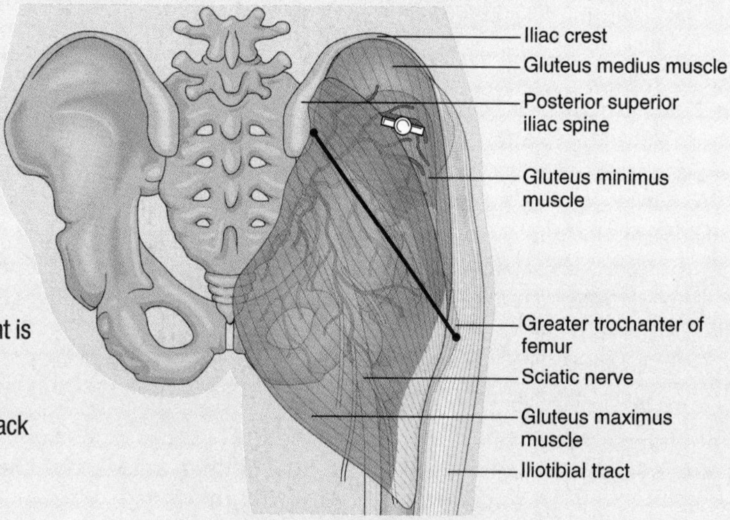

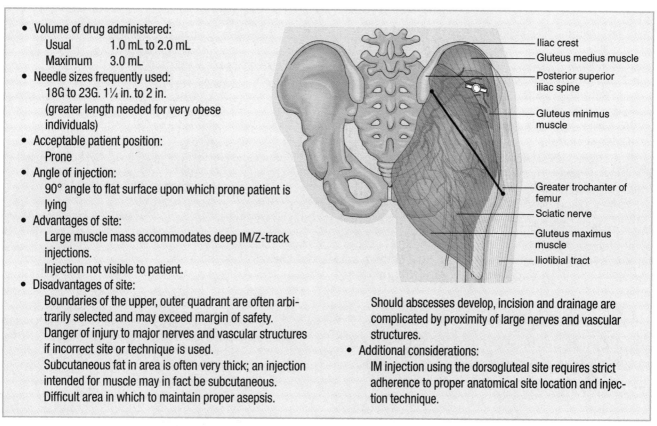

Figure 24-23A Injection technique for dorsogluteal site, adult and pediatric (2 years and older).

- Volume of drug administered:
  Usual 1.0 mL to 2.0 mL
  Maximum 3.0 mL
- Needle sizes frequently used:
  18G to 23G. 1¼ in. to 2 in.
- Acceptable patient positions:
  Supine, lateral
- Angle of injection:
  Angle the needle slightly toward the iliac crest
- Advantages of site:
  Relatively free of major nerves and vascular branches.
  Well localized by bony anatomical landmarks.
  Thinner layer of subcutaneous fat than dorsogluteal site.
  Sufficient muscle mass for deep IM/Z-track injections.
  Readily accessible from several patient positions.
- Disadvantages of site:
  Health professional's unfamiliarity with site.
- Additional considerations:
  Serves as alternative to dorsogluteal and vastus lateralis for deep IM/Z-track injections.

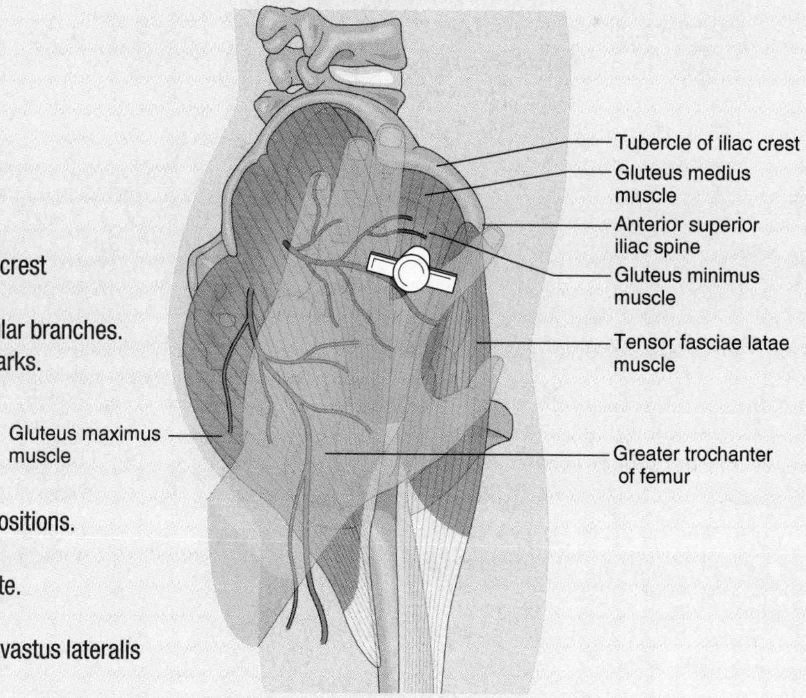

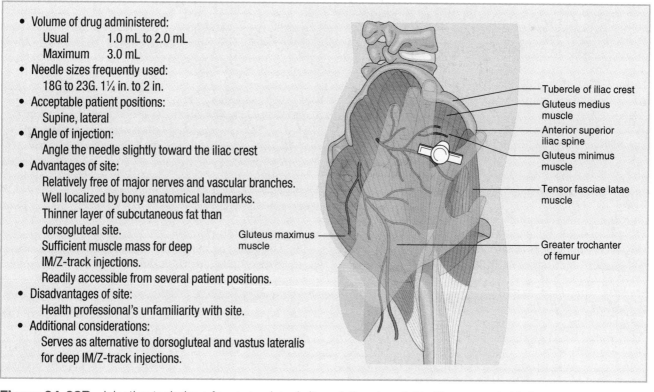

Figure 24-23B Injection technique for ventrogluteal site, adult and pediatric (2 years and older).

- Volume of drug administered:
  Usual 0.5 mL
  Maximum 2.0 mL
- Needle sizes frequently used:
  23G to 25G. ⅝ in. to 1½ in.
- Acceptable patient positions:
  Sitting, prone, supine, lateral
- Angle of injection:
  90° angle to the skin surface (or angled very slightly upward toward acromion)
- Advantages of site:
  Easily accessible.
  General patient acceptance of site.

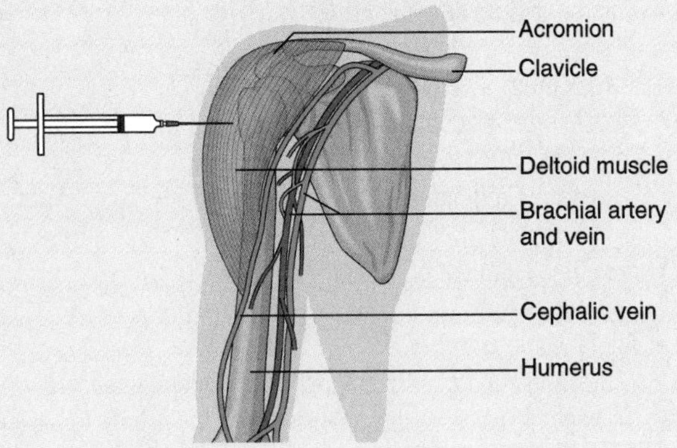

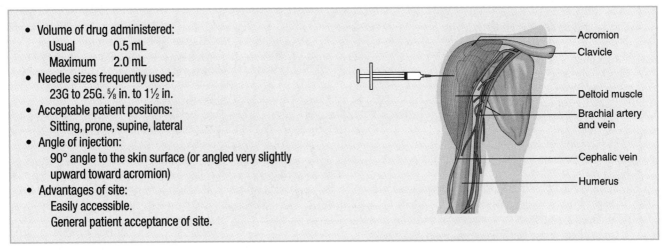

Figure 24-23C Injection technique for deltoid site, adult and pediatric (15 months and older).

- Volume of drug administered:
  Usual 1.0 mL
  Maximum 5.0 mL
- Needle sizes frequently used:
  20G to 23G. 1¼ in. to 1½ in.
- Acceptable patient positions:
  Supine, sitting
- Angle of injection:
  90° angle to the skin surface (for small or thin adults the technique used for pediatric injections may be preferable)
- Advantages of site:
  Large muscle mass can tolerate relatively large quantities of medication.
  Surface area provides sufficient space for several injections.
  Free of major nerves and vascular branches.

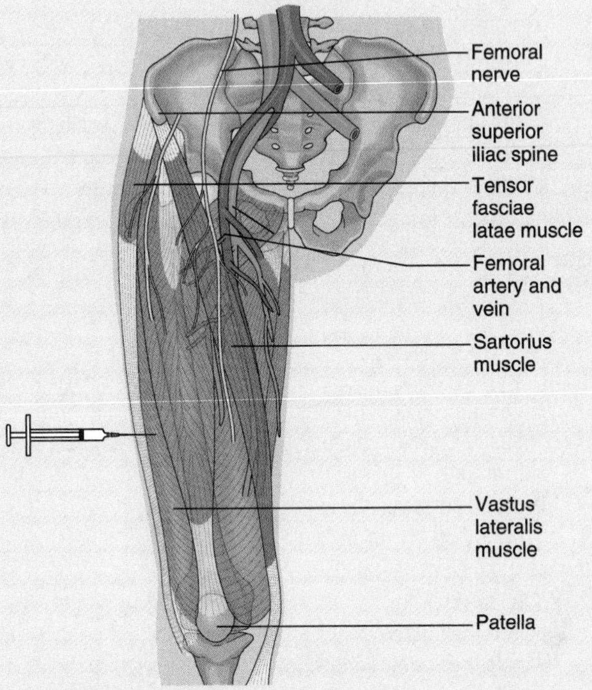

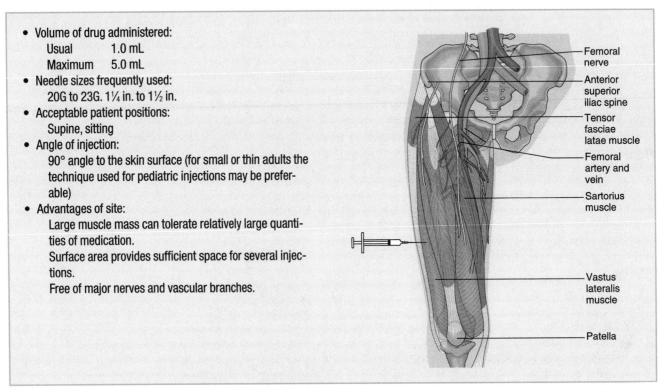

Figure 24-23D Injection technique for vastus lateralis site, adult and pediatric (2 years and older).

10. With a quick, smooth motion, remove the needle from the injection site. Immediately activate the safety mechanism and discard the syringe needle unit in a puncture-proof container. Cover the injection site with a dry, sterile cotton swab and gently massage the site.
    CAUTION: Do not massage the site when administering insulin, Imferon, or heparin.
11. Remove the cotton swab and check for bleeding. If bleeding occurs after applying pressure for 30 seconds, apply a sterile adhesive strip to the injection site.
12. Remove gloves.
13. Observe the patient for any signs of hypersensitivity. Take precautions to ensure the patient's safety.
14. Properly discard the used equipment and supplies. This should be done immediately.
15. Wash hands.
16. Follow documentation procedures to record the administration of the medication.
17. Before releasing the patient, wait the appropriate amount of time, and make sure the patient is given proper instructions and is not experiencing any unusual effects.
18. Return medications to shelf/storage.

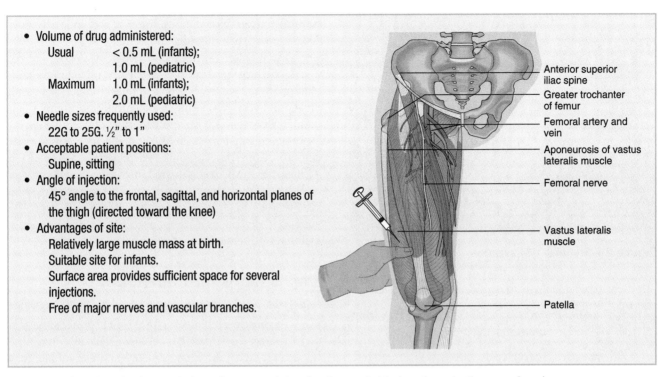

- Volume of drug administered:
  - Usual < 0.5 mL (infants); 1.0 mL (pediatric)
  - Maximum 1.0 mL (infants); 2.0 mL (pediatric)
- Needle sizes frequently used:
  22G to 25G. ½" to 1"
- Acceptable patient positions:
  Supine, sitting
- Angle of injection:
  45° angle to the frontal, sagittal, and horizontal planes of the thigh (directed toward the knee)
- Advantages of site:
  Relatively large muscle mass at birth.
  Suitable site for infants.
  Surface area provides sufficient space for several injections.
  Free of major nerves and vascular branches.

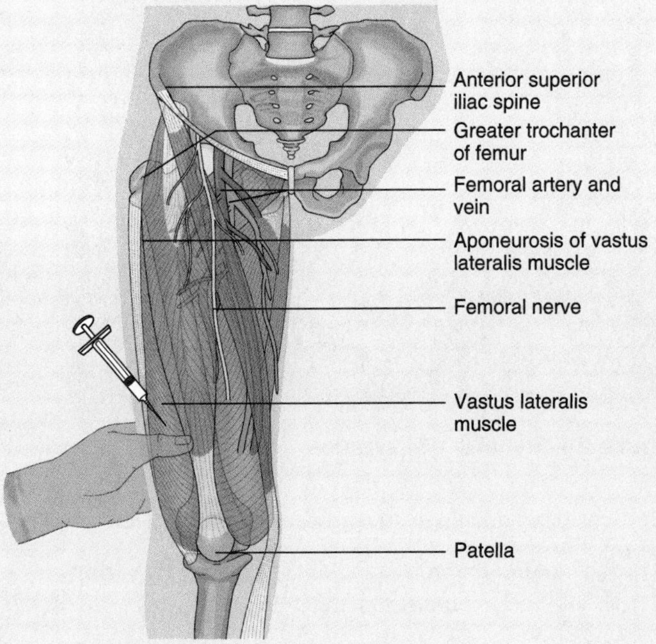

Figure 24-23E Injection technique for vastus lateralis site, pediatric (newborn to 2 years of age).

Procedures 24-1 through 24-9 include:

- Procedure 24-1: Administration of Oral Medications
- Procedure 24-2: Withdrawing Medication from a Vial
- Procedure 24-3: Withdrawing Medication from an Ampule
- Procedure 24-4: Administration of Subcutaneous, Intramuscular, and Intradermal Injections
- Procedure 24-5: Administering a Subcutaneous Injection
- Procedure 24-6: Administering an Intramuscular Injection
- Procedure 24-7: Administering an Intradermal Injection of Purified Protein Derivative (PPD).
- Procedure 24-8: Reconstituting a Powder Medication for Administration
- Procedure 24-9: Z-Track Intramuscular Injection Technique

Z-TRACK METHOD OF INTRAMUSCULAR INJECTION

Imferon is an example of a medication that must be administered by using the Z-track method. This medication and others that are irritating to the subcutaneous tissues and may discolor the skin are given in this manner. (The *Physician's Desk Reference* is a good reference source for help in determining the correct route technique for injections.)

The Z-track technique is similar to an intramuscular injection, except that the skin is pulled to the side before needle insertion. This causes a displacement of the tissues and the medication enters in a manner that will not allow it to seep back into the subcutaneous tissues and up to the skin's surface. Because the medications are irritating, for the comfort of the patient, change the needle on the syringe after aspirating the medication from the ampule or vial before injecting the patient with the medication. See Procedure 24-9.

ADMINISTRATION OF ALLERGENIC EXTRACTS

It may be the responsibility of the medical assistant to administer allergenic extracts. It is important to observe the following:

- Allergic extracts are *always* given in subcutaneous tissue, *never* in the muscle.
- Use a tuberculin syringe with a 25G, ⅝-inch needle, or a 26G, ⅜-inch needle, or a 27G, ½-inch needle or 1 cubic centimeter allergist syringes (Figure 24-24).
- Use a site rotation system for each injected extract.

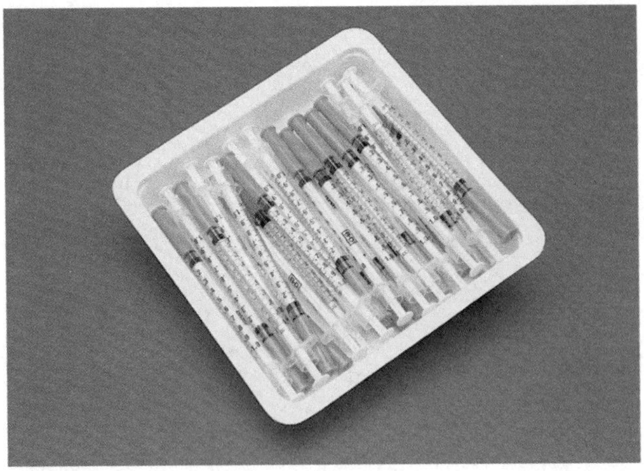

Figure 24-24 Allergist syringes.

- Correctly document the procedure and dosage.
- Allergenic extracts should be refrigerated; they should retain potency for 10 to 12 weeks.
- Adverse reactions such as itching, swelling, and redness should be reported immediately to the physician.
- Severe reactions such as anaphylactic shock have occurred; therefore, emergency equipment and supplies must be available for use (see Chapters 9 and 23 for emergency supplies).
- Allergy testing should only be done when physician is present.
- Patient should wait 20 to 30 minutes after injection to be certain there has been no reaction.

Example:
Patient's Name:

Date	Dose	Site
6/24/XX	1st 0.01 mL s.c.	Lt. arm
6/27/XX	2nd 0.02 mL s.c.	Rt. arm
6/30/XX	3rd 0.03 mL s.c.	Lt. arm

The patient should be observed for 20 to 30 minutes after the injection of an allergenic extract.

Susceptible individuals can experience development of allergic reactions to many foreign substances. It is prudent that the allergic patient be totally aware of those substances and things that are known allergens.

INHALATION METHODS OF MEDICATION ADMINISTRATION

The act of drawing breath, vapor, or gas into the lungs is known as inhalation. Inhalation therapy may involve the administration of medicines, water vapor, and such gases as oxygen, carbon dioxide, and helium.

An inhaler may be used to deliver medications to the lungs. Medications that use an inhaler include bronchodilators, mucolytic agents, and steroids. Inhalers are useful in the delivery of treatment for chronic obstructive pulmonary disease (COPD) and reversible obstructive airway disease. An inhaler is a small, handheld apparatus, usually an aerosol unit, that contains a microcrystalline suspension of medication. When activated, it produces a fine mist or spray containing the medication. This suspension is then drawn into the respiratory tract, settling deep into the lungs and alveoli. See Chapter 18 for information about pulmonary diseases and procedures.

Implications for Patient Care

- Patients should be instructed to follow the prescribed medication regimen. The prescribed medicine and the type of inhaler to be used will determine the method of administration. A handheld inhaler may be used for oral or nasal inhalation, depending on the type ordered by the physician.

Patient Education

- Patients should be advised to avoid overuse of the inhaler. Tolerance, rebound bronchospasm, and adverse cardiac effects can occur from overuse. Instruct the patient to notify the physician should the prescribed dose of medication fail to produce the desired effect.
- Instruct the patient to perform good oral hygiene, including rinsing of the mouth and mouthpiece of equipment, after the inhalation treatment (to prevent the possible growth of fungi).
- Caution the patient against the continued use of a metered-dose canister after the stated number of actuations. If the medication contains adrenaline, fatalities can occur if heart rate and blood pressure increase.

Inhalation therapy may be contraindicated in patients with delicate fluid balance, cardiac arrhythmias, **status asthmaticus**, and hypersensitivity to the medication. As with any medication, the physician will determine the treatment regimen for each patient. See Chapter 18 for information about pulmonary diseases and procedures.

Administration of Oxygen

Oxygen is a colorless, odorless, tasteless gas that is essential for life. When the body does not have an adequate supply of oxygen, a state of **hypoxemia** (lack of oxygen in the blood) develops, and the irreversible damage to vital organs is possible. When a lack of oxygen threatens a person's survival, supplemental oxygen must be prescribed and administered immediately, and arterial blood gas analysis will have to be made after oxygen administration has been started. If it is not an emergency or life-threatening situation, an arterial blood gas analysis will be made before the physician prescribes the dosage and method of administration. The normal range for oxygen in the arterial blood is 80 to 100 mm Hg (millimeters mercury). Oxygen is supplied in tanks (Figure 24-25) for use in the ambulatory care setting, but in a hospital setting, oxygen is piped in through a wall pipe system.

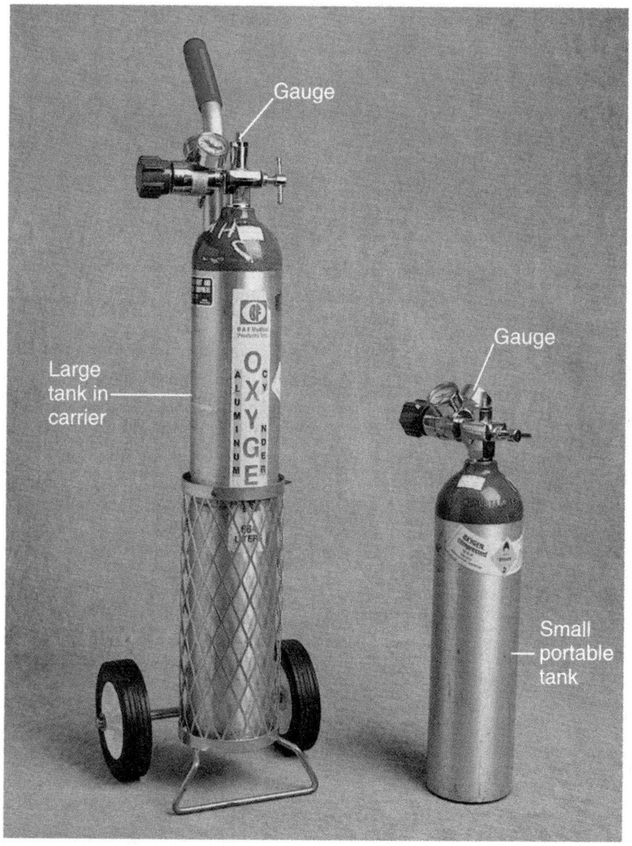

Figure 24-25 Oxygen tanks. Note gauge at top of tanks.

Dosage. When oxygen is to be administered, dosage is based on individual needs. Because oxygen is a drug, the physician will prescribe the flow rate, concentration, method of delivery, and length of time for administration. Oxygen is ordered as liters per minute (LPM) or L/min and as percentage of oxygen concentration (%).

It is the medical assistant's responsibility to follow physician orders and adhere to the guidelines for proper drug administration. Always assess the patient as an individual, explain the procedure, and carefully observe the patient for signs of improvement or symptoms of oxygen toxicity.

CAUTION: Oxygen toxicity may develop when 100% oxygen is breathed for a prolonged period. As with any other drug, toxicity depends on dose, time, and the patient's response. The higher the dose, the shorter the time required to develop toxicity. Symptoms of oxygen toxicity are substernal pain, nausea, vomiting, malaise, fatigue, numbness, and a tingling of the extremities.

High concentrations of inhaled oxygen cause alveolar collapse, intraalveolar hemorrhage, hyaline membrane formation, disturbance of the central nervous system, and **retrolental fibroplasia** in newborns.

NOTE: **Apnea** (absence of breathing) can result when giving oxygen at a flow-rate greater than 2 liters per minute to patients with COPD, especially those with emphysema.

Methods of Oxygen Delivery. Many methods are available today for the delivery of oxygen. The more commonly prescribed methods include the use of nasal cannulas, nasal catheters, and masks. Other methods of delivery involve the use of isolettes, hoods, and tents.

Nasal Cannula. When a low concentration of oxygen is desired, the nasal cannula (Figure 24-26) is the simplest and most convenient method for the administration of oxygen. Made of plastic, the nasal cannula consists of two hollow prongs through which oxygen passes, and a strap or other device to secure it to the patient's head (Figure 24-27). Do not place the direct flow of oxygen against the patient's nasal mucosa, because this causes tissue dehydration. Flow rates greater than 2 to 4 L/min require humidification.

Nasal Catheter. The nasal catheter is a disposable plastic tube that has small holes at the inserted end. These holes diffuse the flow of oxygen for better distribution to lung tissue with minimum dehydration. The nasal catheter is seldom used today, because it causes mucus

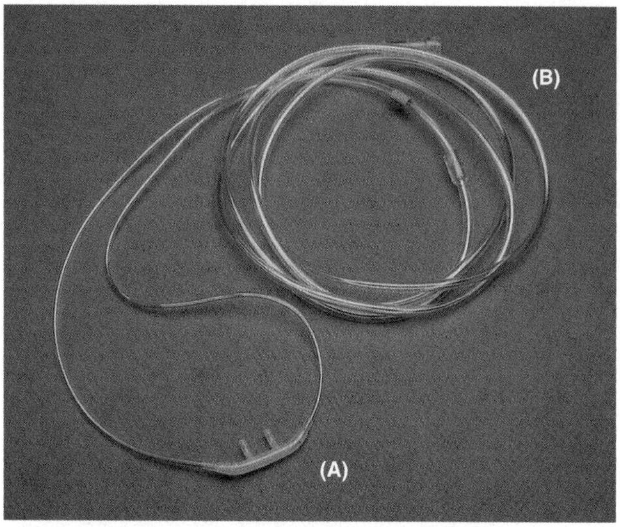

Figure 24-26 (A) Oxygen cannula. (B) Tubing.

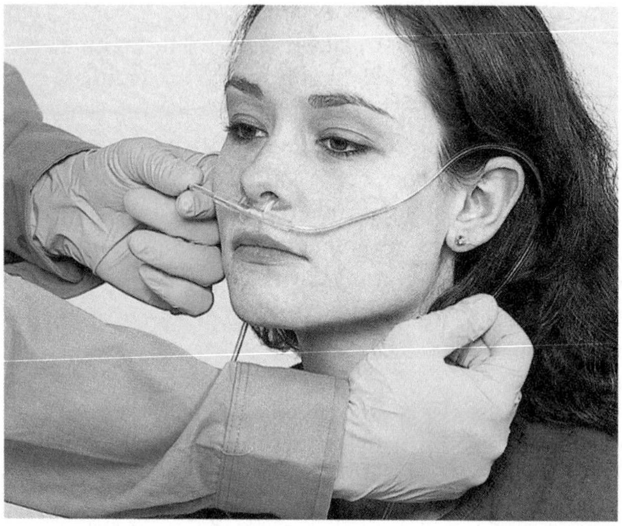

Figure 24-27 Medical assistant adjusts nasal cannula around patient's head for oxygen administration.

Patient Education

Explain safety measures to the patient who uses oxygen at home. Cigarettes, lighters, candles, and other smoking materials should not be used in the room where oxygen is used. Instruct the patient to wear nonstatic-producing clothing, such as cotton.

membrane irritation and has to be changed every eight hours. Because of the discomfort caused to the patient by the catheter, the nasal cannula is the preferred method for the delivery of oxygen.

Mask. The common types of masks used for inhalation therapy include plastic disposable, partial rebreather, nonrebreather, and Venturi (Figure 24-28). These devices are used when the patient requires high humidity and a precise amount of oxygen. To be effective, the mask must be fitted snugly to the patient (Figure 24-29).

CAUTION: Oxygen must be humidified before delivery to the patient to prevent drying of the respiratory mucosa.

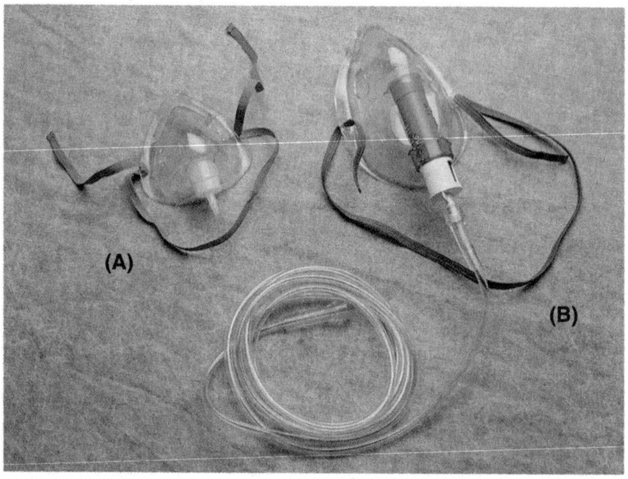

Figure 24-28 Oxygen masks: (A) without tubing; (B) with tubing.

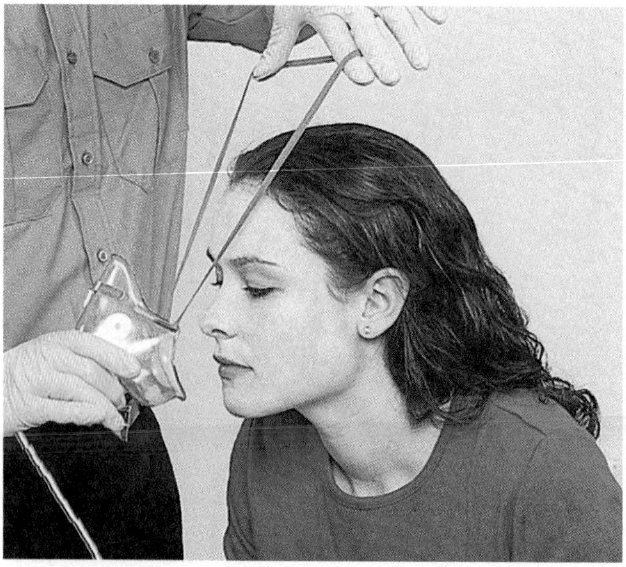

Figure 24-29 Medical assistant adjusts oxygen mask around patient's head.

Oxygen Safety Precautions. Oxygen supports combustion; thus, there is the danger of a fire being started when oxygen is in use. Extreme caution should be exercised because ignition can be caused by friction, static electricity, or a lighted cigar or cigarette when oxygen is being administered. In the physician's office, oxygen is generally stored in tanks. These tanks must be checked on a regular basis and replaced as necessary. See Chapter 18 for information about pulmonary diseases and procedures.

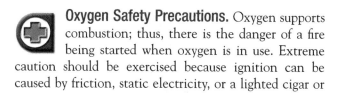

Procedure 24-1 Administration of Oral Medications

STANDARD PRECAUTIONS:

PURPOSE:

Correctly administer an oral medication after receiving a physician's order and assembling the necessary equipment and supplies.

EQUIPMENT/SUPPLIES:

Proper medication
Medication note
Medicine cup
Water, milk, or juice for patient

PROCEDURE STEPS:

1. Verify the physician's order.
2. Follow the "Six Rights" (Figure 24-30A).
3. Perform medical asepsis handwash.
4. Work in a well-lighted, quiet, clean area.
5. Assemble equipment and supplies. RATIONALE: A well-lighted area for preparing medications is important because you must be able to see well to accurately pour medications. A quiet area is free from distractions, and medical asepsis helps fight transmission of microorganisms.
6. Obtain the correct medication using the medicine note.
7. Compare the medication label with the medication note (first time). RATIONALE: Reading from a medicine note helps prevent errors while pouring the medication.
8. Check the expiration date. RATIONALE: Outdated medication may be deteriorated or altered in some way and be harmful to the patient.
9. Calculate dosage if necessary.
10. Correctly prepare (a, b, or c) (Figure 24-30B).
    a. Multiple-dose solid medication
    b. Unit dose medication
    c. Liquid medication
11. Compare medicine label with medication note (second time).
12. Properly transport the medicine.

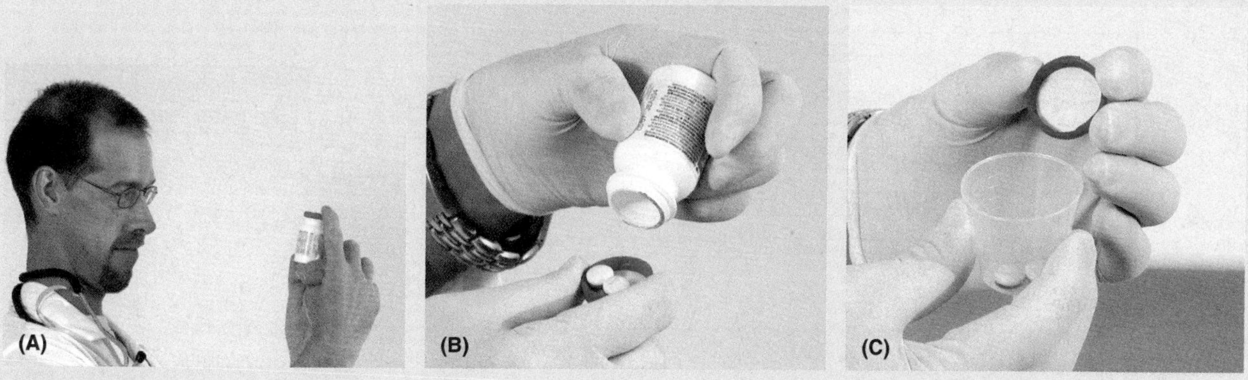

Figure 24-30 (A) Medical assistant checks for right drug, right dose, right route, and expiration date before pouring medication. (B) Medical assistant pours capsules from the cover of the medicine container into a medicine cup before administering medicine to the patient. The medication is poured into cover to avoid contamination of medicine. (C) Medical assistant administers the medication, being certain that patient takes the medicine.

(continues)

(continues)

Procedure 24-1 (continued)

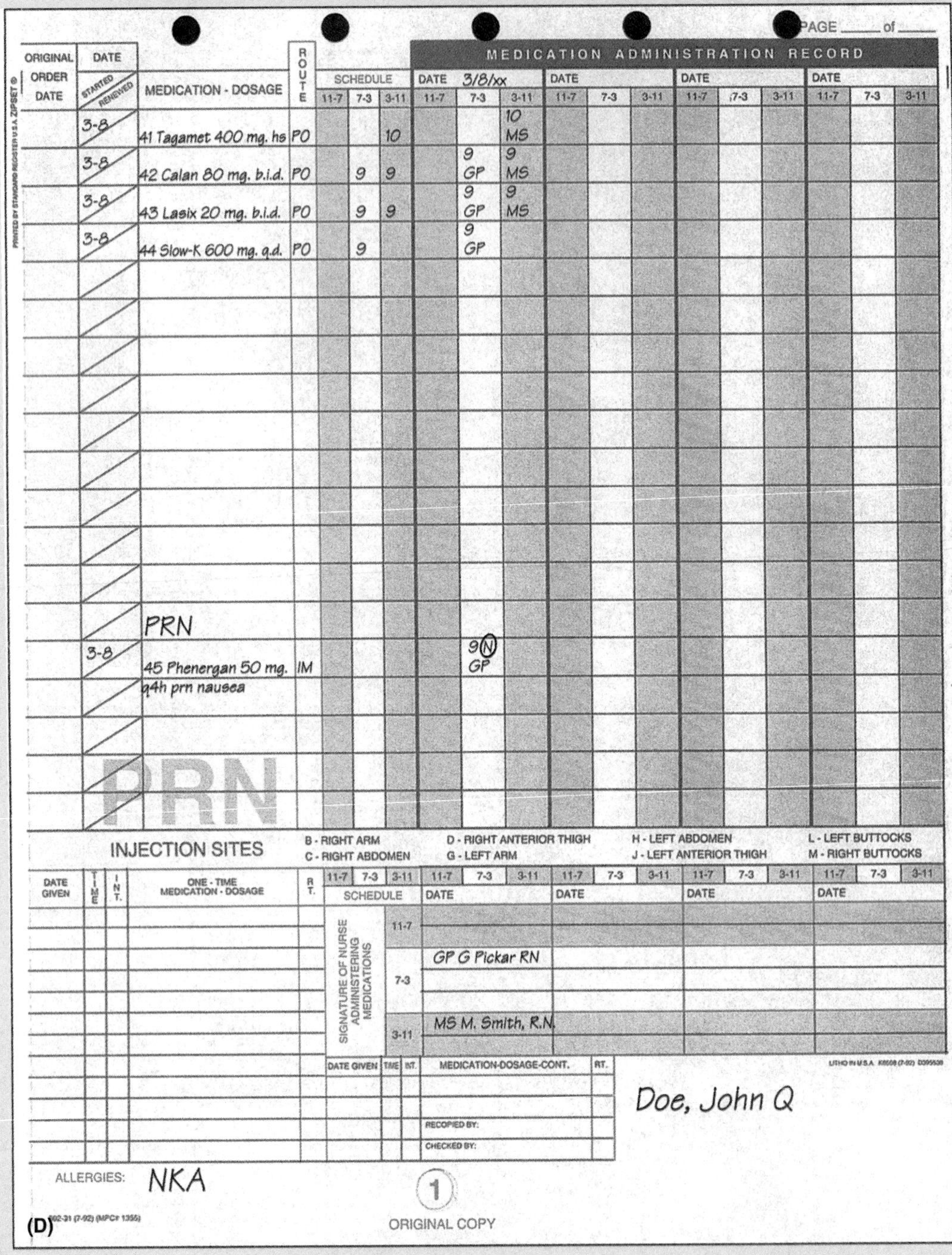

PAGE ____ of ____

MEDICATION ADMINISTRATION RECORD

PRINTED BY STANDARD REGISTER U.S.A. ZIPSET ®

ORIGINAL ORDER DATE	DATE STARTED / RENEWED	MEDICATION - DOSAGE	ROUTE	SCHEDULE 11-7	SCHEDULE 7-3	SCHEDULE 3-11	DATE 3/8/xx 11-7	7-3	3-11	DATE 11-7	7-3	3-11	DATE 11-7	7-3	3-11	DATE 11-7	7-3	3-11
	3-8	41 Tagamet 400 mg. hs	PO			10			10 MS									
	3-8	42 Calan 80 mg. b.i.d.	PO		9	9		9 GP	9 MS									
	3-8	43 Lasix 20 mg. b.i.d.	PO		9	9		9 GP	9 MS									
	3-8	44 Slow-K 600 mg. q.d.	PO		9			9 GP										
		PRN																
	3-8	45 Phenergan 50 mg. q4h prn nausea	IM					9 (N) GP										

PRN

INJECTION SITES: B - RIGHT ARM; C - RIGHT ABDOMEN; D - RIGHT ANTERIOR THIGH; G - LEFT ARM; H - LEFT ABDOMEN; J - LEFT ANTERIOR THIGH; L - LEFT BUTTOCKS; M - RIGHT BUTTOCKS

DATE GIVEN	TIME	INT.	ONE - TIME MEDICATION - DOSAGE	RT.

SIGNATURE OF NURSE ADMINISTERING MEDICATIONS

SCHEDULE	DATE	DATE	DATE	DATE
11-7				
7-3	GP G Pickar RN			
3-11	MS M. Smith, R.N.			

DATE GIVEN	TIME	INT.	MEDICATION-DOSAGE-CONT.	RT.
			RECOPIED BY:	
			CHECKED BY:	

Doe, John Q

ALLERGIES: NKA

1

ORIGINAL COPY

(D)

Figure 24-30 *(continued)* (D) Example of a medication administration record for patient's chart.

(continues)

Procedure 24-1 (continued)

13. Identify the patient. Explain the procedure.
14. Assess patient. Take vital signs if indicated. RATIONALE: Always assess the patient for body size, physical condition, age, and gender to be certain the dose and route are appropriate prior to administration of certain medications. BP or pulse must be taken to ascertain if the vital signs are within normal limits.
15. Assist patient to a comfortable position.
16. Check medication label a third time.
17. Administer the medication. Provide water. Be certain that the patient takes the medicine (Figure 24-30C). RATIONALE: Some patients, for various reasons, may deliberately not swallow their medication.
18. Provide for the patient's safety: Observe the patient for any adverse reactions.
19. Care for equipment and supplies according to OSHA guidelines.
20. Document that you administered the medication either in the patient's record or on the medication administration record of the patient's chart (see Figure 24-30 and 24-6D).
21. Return the medication to the shelf/storage area.

Procedure 24-2 Withdrawing Medication from a Vial

STANDARD PRECAUTIONS:

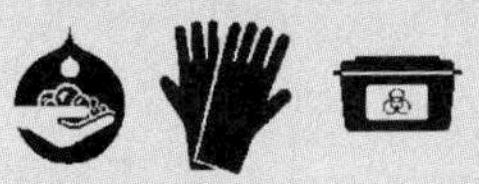

PURPOSE:

Medication is supplied in a variety of packaging. Medication from a vial must be drawn into a syringe for parenteral injection.

EQUIPMENT/SUPPLIES:

Medication order	Vial of medication
Medication note	Alcohol wipes
Appropriate syringe and needle with cover	Disposable gloves
	Sharps container

PROCEDURE STEPS:

1. Read the medication order and assemble equipment. Check for the "Six Rights." Read the vial label by holding it next to the medicine card (first time).
2. Wash hands. Apply gloves.
3. Select the proper size needle and syringe for the medication and the route (e.g., for subcutaneous injection of insulin, 100-U insulin syringe and 25G, $\frac{5}{8}$-inch needle). If necessary, attach the needle to the syringe.
4. Check the vial label against the medication note (second time).
5. Remove the metal or plastic cap from the vial. If the vial has been opened previously, clean the rubber stopper by applying an alcohol wipe in a circular motion (Figure 24-31A).
6. Remove the needle cover—pull it straight off.
7. Inject air into the vial as follows:
   a. Hold the syringe pointed upward at eye level. Pull back the plunger to take in a quantity of air that is exactly equal to the ordered dose of medication.
   b. Leave vial on tabletop/countertop.
   c. Insert the needle through center of the rubber stopper of the vial. Inject the air by pushing in the plunger (Figure 24-31B).
8. Invert the vial. Hold the vial and the syringe steady. Pull back on the plunger to withdraw the measured dose of medication. Measure accurately. Keep the tip of the needle below the surface of the liquid; otherwise, air will enter the syringe. Keep syringe at eye level (Figure 24-31C).
9. Check the syringe for air bubbles. Remove them by tapping sharply on the syringe. Push the air bubbles back into the vial (Figure 24-31D).

(continues)

Procedure 24-2 (continued)

Check measurement for accuracy, draw more medication if needed.

10. Remove the needle from the vial. Replace the sterile needle cover (Figure 24-31E) using "scoop" method.
11. Check the vial label against the medication note (third time).
12. Place the filled syringe and medication vial on a medicine tray with an alcohol wipe and the medication note. The dose is now ready for injection.

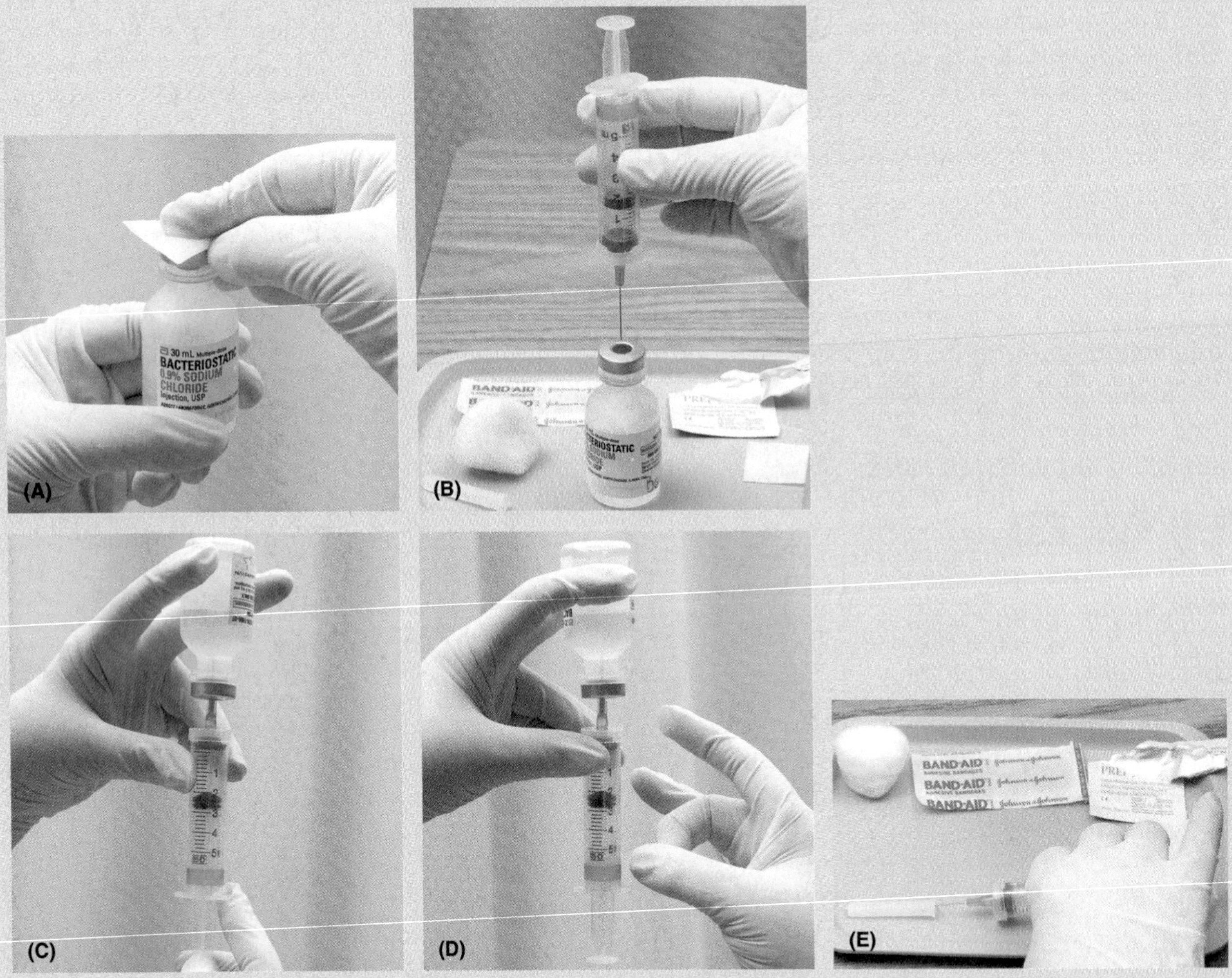

Figure 24-31 (A) Disinfect the rubber stopper on the medication vial with an alcohol wipe. (B) Keeping the bevel of the needle above the fluid level, inject an amount of air equal to medication quantity to be withdrawn. (C) Hold syringe pointed upward at eye level and with the bevel of the needle in the medication. Pull back plunger and aspirate the quantity of medication ordered. (D) Tap syringe to eliminate air bubbles. Hand should hold syringe while tapping it. (E) After the correct dose has been withdrawn, recover the sterile needle using "scoop" method. Place medicine on a tray with medication note, the medication vial, and an alcohol wipe and safely transport to the patient.

(continues)

Procedure 24-2 (continued)

13. If medication is a tissue irritant, change to another sterile needle. RATIONALE: Tissue irritants can cause tissue necrosis. Activate safety mechanism.
14. Immediately after the injection, activate the safety mechanism. Discard the syringe-needle unit into a sharps container.
15. Remove gloves and dispose in biohazard waste container.
16. Wash hands.
17. Document the procedure.
18. Return the vial to the proper storage area. Destroy medication note.

DOCUMENTATION

8/9/20XX 2:30 PM Vitamin B_{12} (Cyanocobalamin) 100 mcg IM (R) deltoid area. W. Slawson, CMA

Procedure 24-3 Withdrawing Medication from an Ampule

STANDARD PRECAUTIONS:

PURPOSE:

Medication is supplied in a variety of packaging. An ampule is a sterile, glass, single-dose container of liquid medication. It is aspirated into a syringe for injection.

EQUIPMENT/SUPPLIES:

Medicine tray and medication note
Ampule of medication
Alcohol wipes
Sterile gauze sponges
Sharps container
Sterile filter needle and syringe
Gloves

PROCEDURE STEPS:

1. Check the physician's order. Write out medication note.
2. Wash hands and gather equipment. Put on gloves.
3. Select ampule of medication. Read label and check medication note for correct medication, dose, route, and time (first time). Check medication expiration date.
4. Flick ampule of medication (medication will often get "trapped" above the neck of the ampule). A sharp flick of the wrist will help force all of the medication down below the neck of the ampule into the body of the ampule (Figure 24-32A). RATIONALE: This is important to ensure all medication is available in the body of the ampule to calculate the correct dose. If some of the medication remains trapped above the neck in the top of the ampule, some medication will not be available for use and it is possible to give an incorrect dose, especially if the patient is to receive the entire contents of the ampule.
5. Thoroughly disinfect the neck with an alcohol swab. Check label (second time). RATIONALE: The needle will enter the opening of the ampule and wiping the neck of the ampule before removal of the top ensures disinfection of the neck or opening of the ampule.

(continues)

Procedure 24-3 (continued)

6. With a sterile gauze, wipe dry the neck of the ampule. Completely surround the ampule with the gauze and forcefully snap off the top of the ampule by pulling the top toward you (Figure 24-32B). RATIONALE: Ensure medical assistant safety from possible injury from broken glass. Discard top in sharps container.
7. Place opened ampule down on medicine tray. Check label (third time).
8. With a prepared sterile syringe-needle unit that has a filter on the needle, aspirate the required dose into the syringe (Figure 24-32C). Cover needle with sheath using scoop method and transport with medication ampule to patient on the medicine tray. RATIONALE: Filtered needles prevent glass particles from being aspirated with medication.
9. Change needles. RATIONALE: The filter needle may contain glass particles.
10. Identify the patient.
11. Administer medication.
12. Discard syringe-needle unit into sharps container. Cotton balls are discarded in biohazard waste container if there is any blood on them.
13. Remove gloves and dispose in biohazard waste container. Dispose of ampule into sharps container.
14. Wash hands.
15. Document the procedure. Destroy medication note.

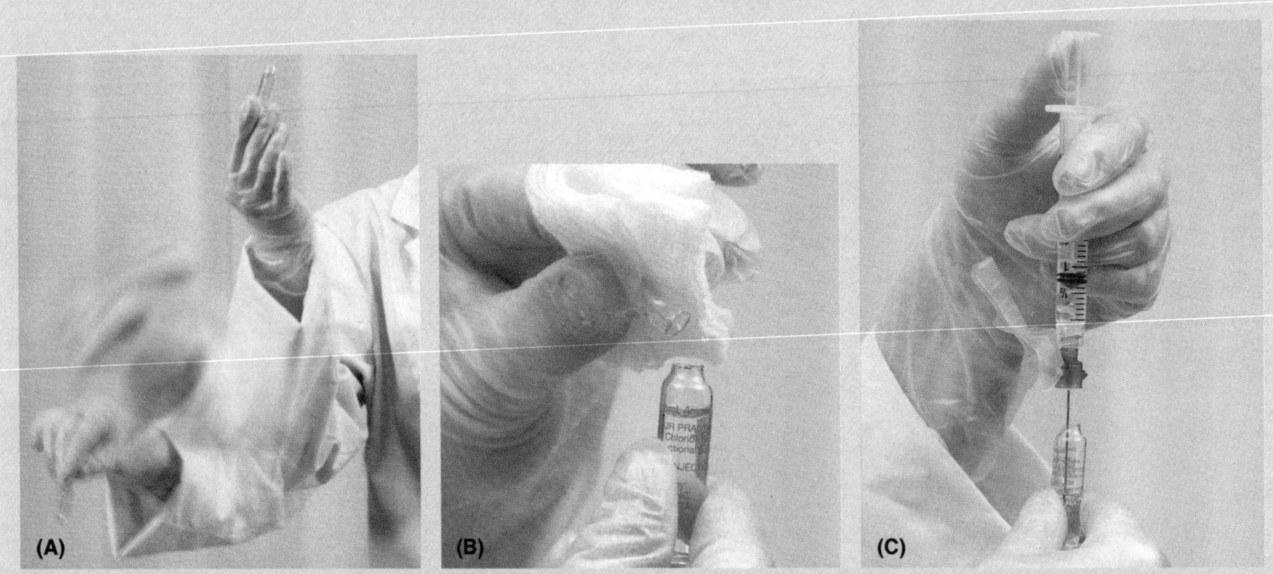

Figure 24-32 (A) Hold ampule by the top and force all the medication into the bottom of the ampule by a snap of the arm and wrist. (B) Remove top from ampule. Snap away from you by pulling top toward you. (C) Draw the required dose into syringe.

DOCUMENTATION

5/12/20XX 11:20 AM Phenergan 25 mg IM (R) dorsogluteal area. B. Abbott, RMA

Procedure 24-4 Administration of Subcutaneous, Intramuscular, and Intradermal Injections

STANDARD PRECAUTIONS:

PURPOSE:

To properly administer subcutaneous, intramuscular, and intradermal injections.

EQUIPMENT/SUPPLIES:

Medicine tray
Medication as ordered by the physician and medication note
Appropriately sized needle and syringe
Alcohol wipes
Disposable gloves
Sharps container
Cotton ball

PROCEDURE STEPS:

1. Verify the physician's order. Make out medication note taking information from physician's order sheet from patient record.
2. Follow the "Six Rights."
3. Perform medical asepsis hand cleansing. Adhere to OSHA guidelines.
4. Work in a well-lighted, quiet, clean area.
5. Select the appropriate syringe and needle and alcohol wipe.
6. Select the correct medication.
7. Compare the medication label with the medication note (first time).
8. Check expiration date on medicine.
9. Calculate dosage, if necessary.
10. Prepare syringe and needle for use (Figure 24-33A–C).
11. Withdraw medication from vial.
12. Compare medicine label with the medication note (second time).
13. Place filled syringe and needle on the medicine tray with medication note and vial. Check the medication label with the medicine note (third time).
14. Transport the medicine to the patient.
15. Identify the patient. Explain the procedure.
16. Assess the patient. Put on gloves.
17. Prepare the patient for the injection (drape, position, allay apprehension).
18. Select an appropriate injection site. Follow a rotating schedule if appropriate.
19. Cleanse the injection site with a sterile alcohol wipe. Use a circular motion, working from the center out to about 2 inches beyond the planned injection site.

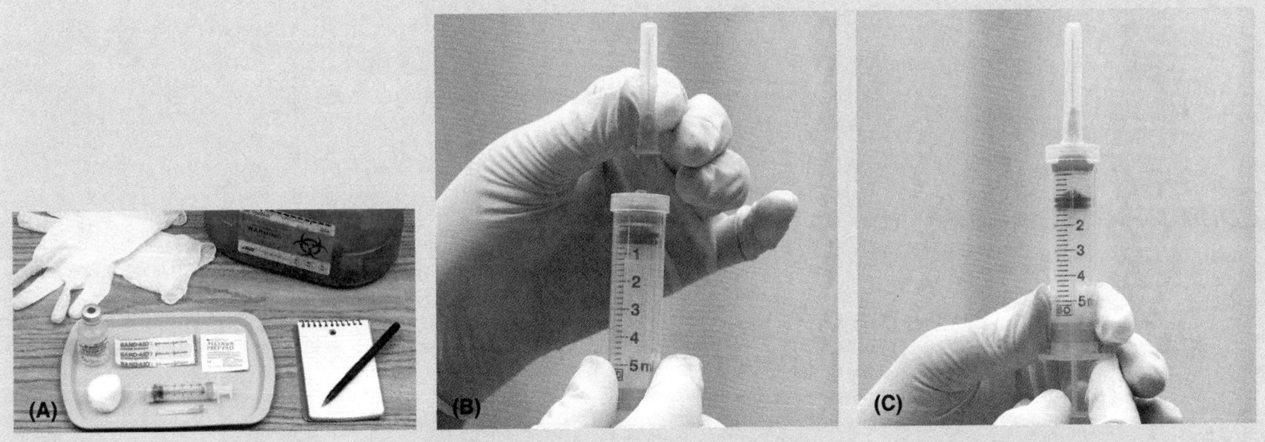

Figure 24-33 Preparing the syringe-needle unit for use: (A) Assemble the equipment and supplies needed to draw up medication from a vial. (B) Secure the needle by twisting it clockwise. (C) Pull the plunger to check for ease of gliding operation.

(continues)

Procedure 24-4 (continued)

20. Allow the skin to dry.
21. Administer the injection. Aspirate to be certain needle is not in a blood vessel (except for intradermal injection). Immediately activate safety mechanism and dispose of syringe and needle in a puncture-proof container.
22. Massage injection site with a cotton ball unless contraindicated (such as insulin, Imferon, heparin).
23. Observe the patient for signs of difficulty.
24. Inspect the injection site for bleeding, apply adhesive strip if necessary.
25. Properly dispose of used equipment and supplies. Remove gloves.
26. Perform medical asepsis handwash.
27. Correctly document the procedure. Return the vial to storage. Destroy medication note.

Procedure to follow should the medical assistant sustain an accidental needlestick after the injection:

- Thoroughly wash the site where the stick occurred.
- Cleanse the skin with an antiseptic.
- Report the incident to your supervisor and manager.
- Document the incident and retain a copy for yourself.
- Obtain medical attention. Be tested for hepatitis B and C viruses and HIV.
- Fill out appropriate OSHA paperwork (200 form).

Procedure 24-5 Administering a Subcutaneous Injection

STANDARD PRECAUTIONS:

PURPOSE:
Correctly administer a subcutaneous injection after receiving a physician's order and assembling the necessary equipment and supplies.

EQUIPMENT/SUPPLIES:

Medication ordered by physician	Alcohol wipes
Medication note	Gloves
Appropriately sized needle and syringe	Sharps container
	Adhesive strip
	Medicine tray

PROCEDURE STEPS:
1. Verify the physician's order. Make out a medication note.
2. Follow the "Six Rights."
3. Perform medical asepsis handwash. Adhere to OSHA guidelines.
4. Work in a well-lighted, quiet, clean area.
5. Select the appropriate equipment and supplies.
6. Select the correct medication.
7. Compare the medication label with the medication note (first time).
8. Check expiration date on medicine.
9. Calculate dosage, if necessary.
10. Correctly prepare the parenteral medication.
11. Compare medication label with the medication note (second time).
12. Correctly transport the medicine to the patient on the tray, with the vial.
13. Identify the patient. Explain the procedure.
14. Assess the patient. Put on gloves.
15. Prepare the patient for the injection (drape, position, allay apprehension).
16. Check syringe with the medication note (third time).
17. Select an appropriate injection site.
18. Correctly cleanse the site with alcohol using a circular motion starting with the injection site

(continues)

Procedure 24-5 (continued)

and moving outward to a 2-inch diameter. Allow skin to dry.

19. Remove needle guard.
20. Grasp skin to form a 1-inch fold.
21. Insert needle quickly at a 45-degree angle (Figure 24-34).
22. Aspirate to be certain needle is not in a blood vessel.
23. Slowly inject the medicine.
24. Quickly remove the needle and syringe and activate the safety mechanism. Release the skin.
25. Immediately dispose of needle and syringe in a sharps container.
26. Cover site. Massage (unless contraindicated as with insulin, Imferon, and heparin).
27. Provide for patient's safety.
28. Properly dispose of used supplies. Remove gloves and wash hands. Return medication vial to storage.
29. Document the procedure. Destroy the medication note.

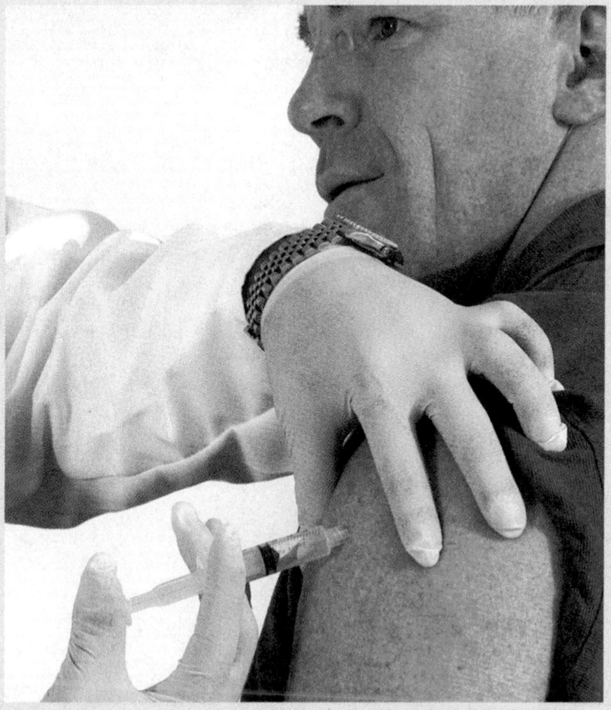

Figure 24-34 Insert needle at 45-degree angle into upper arm.

DOCUMENTATION

12/16/20XX 10:00 AM NPH insulin 8 units subcutaneously (L) upper arm area. S. Jones, CMA

Procedure 24-6 Administering an Intramuscular Injection

STANDARD PRECAUTIONS:

PURPOSE:

Correctly administer an intramuscular injection after receiving a physician's order and assembling the necessary equipment and supplies.

EQUIPMENT/SUPPLIES:

Medication ordered by physician with medication note
Appropriately sized needle and syringe
Alcohol wipes
Gloves
Sharps container
Medicine tray
Adhesive strip

(continues)

Procedure 24-6 (continued)

PROCEDURE STEPS:

1. Verify the physician's order. Make out a medication note.
2. Follow the "Six Rights."
3. Perform medical asepsis handwash. Adhere to OSHA guidelines.
4. Work in a well-lighted, quiet, clean area.
5. Obtain the appropriate equipment and supplies.
6. Obtain the correct medication.
7. Compare the medication label with the medication note (first time).
8. Check expiration date.
9. Calculate dosage, if necessary.
10. Correctly prepare the parenteral medication.
11. Compare medicine label with the medication note (second time).
12. Transport the medicine to the patient on tray, with the vial.
13. Identify the patient. Explain the procedure.
14. Assess the patient. Put on gloves.
15. Prepare the patient for the injection (drape, position, allay apprehension).
16. Compare the medication note with the syringe (third time).
17. Select an appropriate injection site.
18. Correctly cleanse the site with alcohol using a circular motion and covering a 2-inch diameter. Allow the skin to dry.
19. Remove needle guard.
20. Stretch the skin **taut,** pulling it tight.
21. Using a dartlike motion, insert needle to the hub at a 90-degree angle (Figure 24-35).
22. Release the skin.
23. Aspirate to check for blood.
24. Slowly inject the medicine.
25. Quickly remove the needle and syringe and activate safety mechanism.
26. Immediately dispose of needle and syringe in a sharps container.
27. Cover site. Massage (unless contraindicated as with insulin, Imferon, and heparin).
28. Dispose of equipment. Remove gloves.
29. Wash hands.
30. Observe the patient for signs of difficulty.
31. Provide for patient's safety. Return medication vial to storage.
32. Document the procedure. Destroy the medication note.

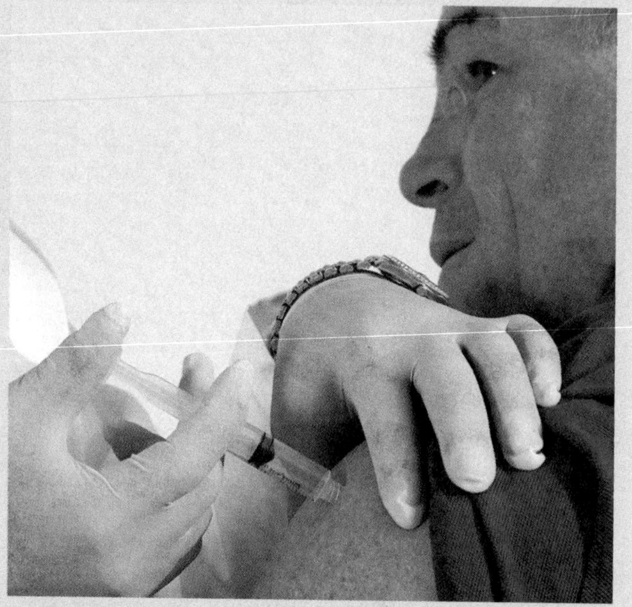

Figure 24-35 Using deltoid muscle, insert needle to the hub at a 90-degree angle.

DOCUMENTATION

12/16/20XX 10:00 AM Demerol 75 mg IM (L) deltoid. S. Jones, CMA

Procedure 24-7 Administering an Intradermal Injection of Purified Protein Derivative (PPD)

STANDARD PRECAUTIONS:

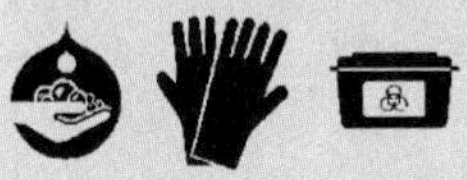

PURPOSE:

Correctly administer an intradermal injection of PPD after receiving a physician's order and assembling the necessary equipment and supplies.

EQUIPMENT/SUPPLIES:

Medication as ordered by physician with medication note
Appropriately sized needle and syringe
Alcohol wipes
Disposable gloves
Sharps container
Medicine tray
Adhesive strip

PROCEDURE STEPS:

1. Verify the physician's order. Make out a medication note.
2. Follow the "Six Rights."
3. Perform medical asepsis handwash. Adhere to OSHA guidelines.
4. Work in a well-lighted, quiet, clean area.
5. Organize the appropriate equipment and supplies.
6. Select the correct medication (PPD).
7. Compare the medication label with the medication note (first time).
8. Check expiration date.
9. Calculate dosage, if necessary.
10. Correctly prepare the parenteral medication.
11. Compare medication label with the medication note (second time).
12. Correctly transport the medicine to the patient on tray with medication vial.
13. Identify the patient. Explain the procedure.
14. Assess the patient. Put on gloves.
15. Prepare the patient for the injection (drape, position, allay apprehension).
16. Check medication note with syringe (third time).
17. Select an appropriate injection site (Figure 24-36A). For other sites, refer back to Figure 24-18B.
18. Correctly cleanse the site with alcohol using a circular motion and covering a 2-inch diameter. Allow the skin to dry.
19. Remove needle guard.
20. Pull the skin tissue taut.
21. Carefully insert the needle at a 5- to 10-degree angle, bevel upward to about $\frac{1}{8}$ inch. Do not aspirate. Release skin.
22. Steadily inject PPD to form a wheal (Figure 24-36B).

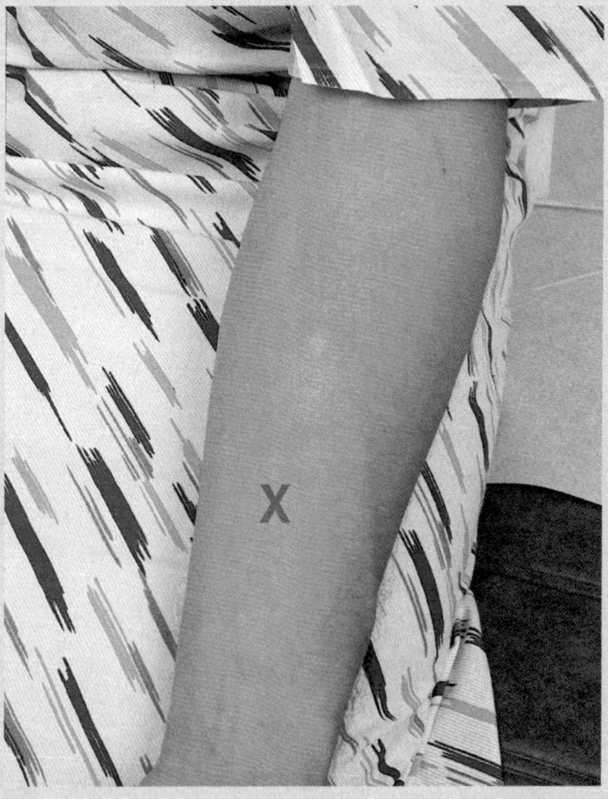

Figure 24-36A One site for administering an intradermal injection is near the center of the forearm.

(continues)

Procedure 24-7 (continued)

23. Correctly remove the needle after a brief delay.
    RATIONALE: Minimizes leakage.
24. Activate safety mechanism.
25. Immediately dispose of needle and syringe in a sharps container.
26. Blot site. Do not massage. Remove gloves.
27. Wash hands.
28. Observe the patient for signs of difficulty.
29. Provide for patient's safety.
30. Caution patient not to rub wheal.
31. Return vial to storage and document the procedure. Destroy the medication note.
32. The injected area should be read in 48 to 72 hours for the amount of induration (hardness) to determine tuberculosis exposure. Measure the induration. If injection area is hardened and elevated 10 mm or larger, the test is positive and the doctor should be notified.

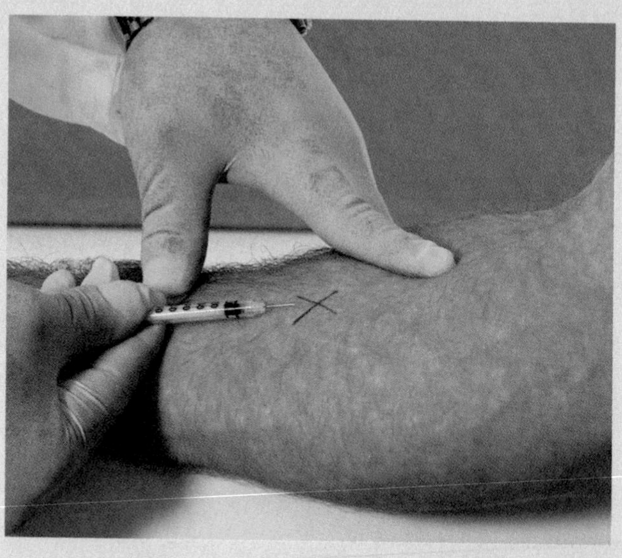

Figure 24-36B Steadily inject the medicine.

DOCUMENTATION

10/14/20XX 10:00 AM 0.1 ml PPD ID (L) forearm. S. Jones, CMA

Procedure 24-8 Reconstituting a Powder Medication for Administration

STANDARD PRECAUTIONS:

PURPOSE:

Drugs for injection may be supplied in a powdered (dry) form and must be reconstituted to a liquid for injection. A diluent (usually sterile water) is added to the powder, mixed well, and the appropriate dose is drawn up to be administered.

EQUIPMENT/SUPPLIES:

Medication as ordered by the physician and medication note
Diluent
Two appropriately sized needles and syringes
Alcohol wipes
Disposable gloves
Sharps container

(continues)

Procedure 24-8 (continued)

PROCEDURE STEPS:

1. Prepare the needle-syringe unit in preparation for reconstituting powder medication (Figure 24-37A).
2. Remove tops from diluent and powder medication containers and wipe with alcohol swabs (Figure 24-37B).
3. Insert the needle through the rubber stopper on the vial of diluent. The syringe should have an amount of air in it equal to the amount of diluent to be withdrawn (Figures 24-37C).

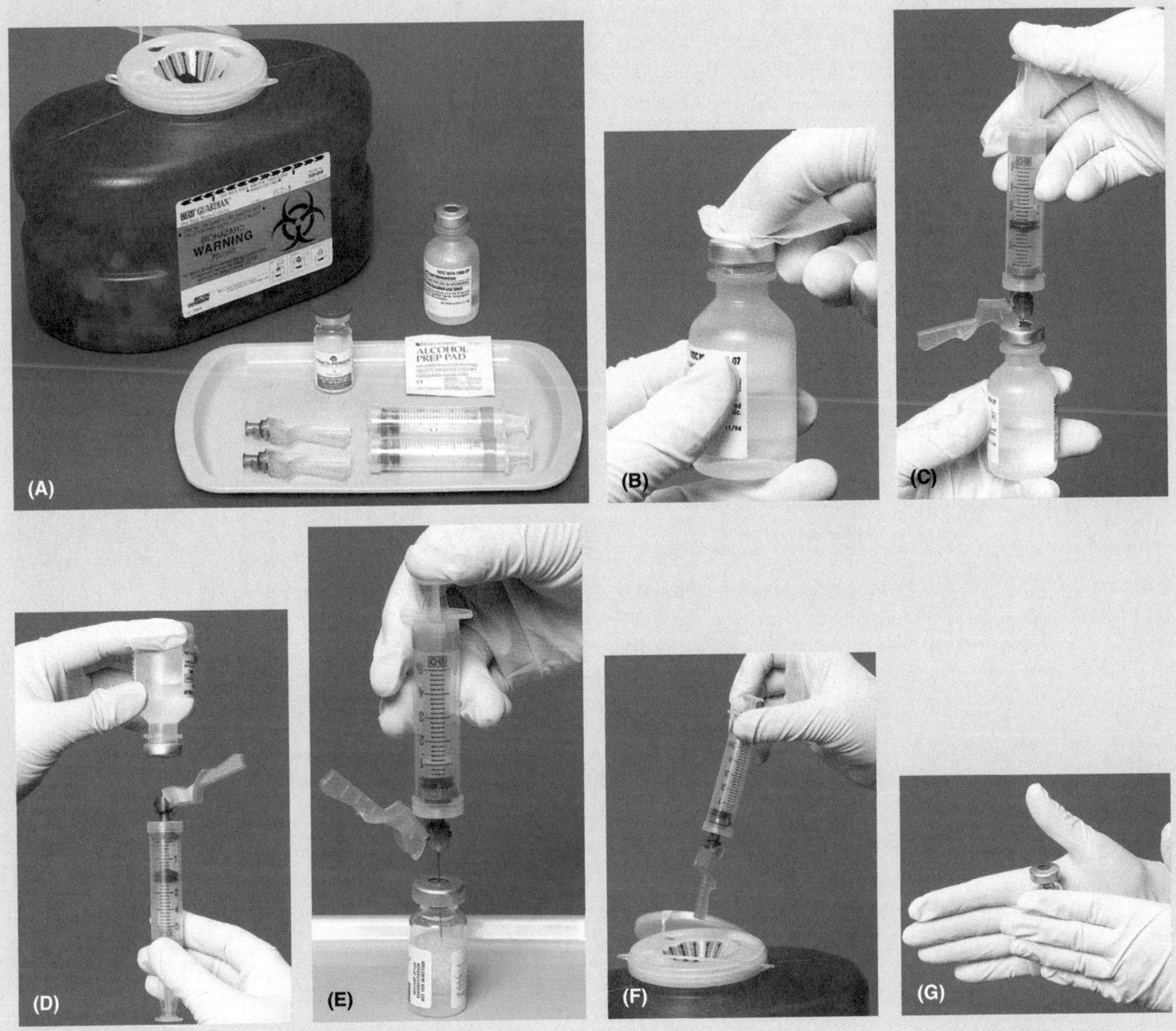

Figure 24-37 (A) Supplies for reconstituting powder medication. (B) Remove top from diluent and powdered medication. Wipe top of each with an alcohol wipe. (C) Inject air in an equal amount to diluent being removed from the vial. (D) Prepare to remove the needle from the vial after withdrawing diluent. (E) Inject diluent into vial containing powdered medication. (F) Discard safety needle-syringe unit. (G) Roll vial of solution medication between palms of hands to mix well. Label vial with date, amount of diluent added, strength of dilution, time mixed, and your initials.

(continues)

Procedure 24-8 (continued)

4. Withdraw the appropriate amount of diluent to be added to the powder medication (Figures 24-37D).
5. Inject the diluent into the powder medication vial (Figure 24-37E).
6. Remove needle from vial and discard into sharps container (Figure 24-37F).
7. Roll the vial between the palms of the hands to completely mix together the powder and diluent (Figure 24-37G). Label the multiple-dose vial with the dilution or strength of the medication prepared, the date and time, your initials, and the expiration date.
8. With a second sterile needle and syringe, withdraw the desired amount of medication (Figure 24-37H).
9. Flick away any air bubbles that cling to side of syringe (Figure 24-37I).
10. The medicine tray with reconstituted medication and vial is ready for transport to the patient (Figure 24-37J).
11. Proceed as in Steps 11 to 32 of Procedure 24-6, Administering an Intramuscular Injection.

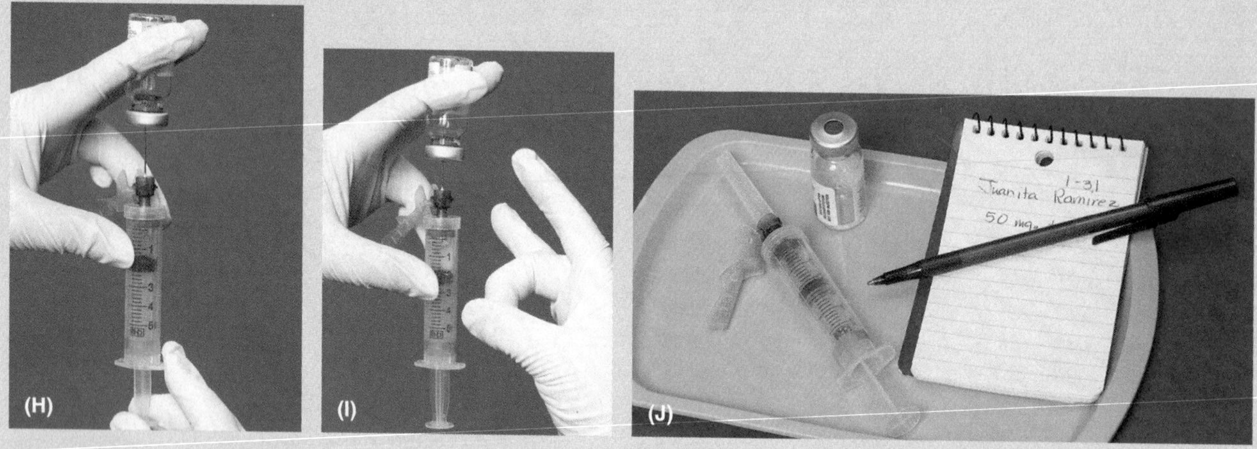

Figure 24-37 *(continued)* (H) Use a second sterile needle-syringe unit to draw the prescribed dose of medication ordered by the physician. (I) Flick away any air bubbles that cling to the side of the syringe. Withdraw more medication if needed. (J) Medicine tray shows prepared injection ready for transport to patient. Labeled, reconstituted medication will be taken to the room with the syringe and placed on the shelf or in the refrigerator according to the manufacturer's instructions after the injection is given.

Procedure 24-9 Z-Track Intramuscular Injection Technique

STANDARD PRECAUTIONS:

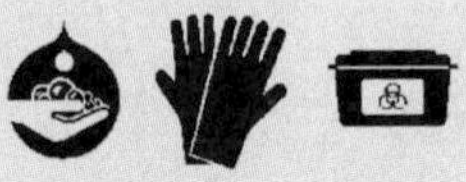

PURPOSE:

Correctly administer a Z-track intramuscular injection after receiving a physician's order and assembling the necessary equipment and supplies.

EQUIPMENT/SUPPLIES:

Medication ordered by physician and medication note
Appropriately sized needle and syringe
Alcohol wipes
Disposable gloves
Sharps container
Medicine tray
Adhesive strip

PROCEDURE STEPS:

1. Verify the physician's order. Make out a medication note.
2. Follow the "Six Rights."
3. Perform medical asepsis hand cleansing. Adhere to OSHA guidelines.
4. Work in a well-lighted, quiet, clean area.
5. Organize the appropriate equipment and supplies.
6. Select the correct medication.
7. Compare the medication label with the medication note (first time).
8. Check expiration date.
9. Calculate dosage, if necessary.
10. Correctly prepare the parenteral medication.
11. Compare medicine label with the medication note (second time).
12. Correctly transport the medicine to the patient.
13. Identify the patient. Explain the procedure.
14. Assess the patient. Put on gloves.
15. Prepare the patient for the injection (drape, position, allay apprehension).
16. Recheck medication note with the order and the syringe (third time).
17. Select an appropriate injection site.
18. Correctly cleanse the site with alcohol using a circular motion and covering a 6-inch diameter. Allow the skin to dry.
19. Remove needle guard.
20. Pull the skin laterally 1½ inch away from the injection site.
21. Insert needle quickly, using a dartlike motion at a 90-degree angle. Maintain Z position (Figure 24-38).
22. Aspirate to check for blood.
23. Slowly inject medication.

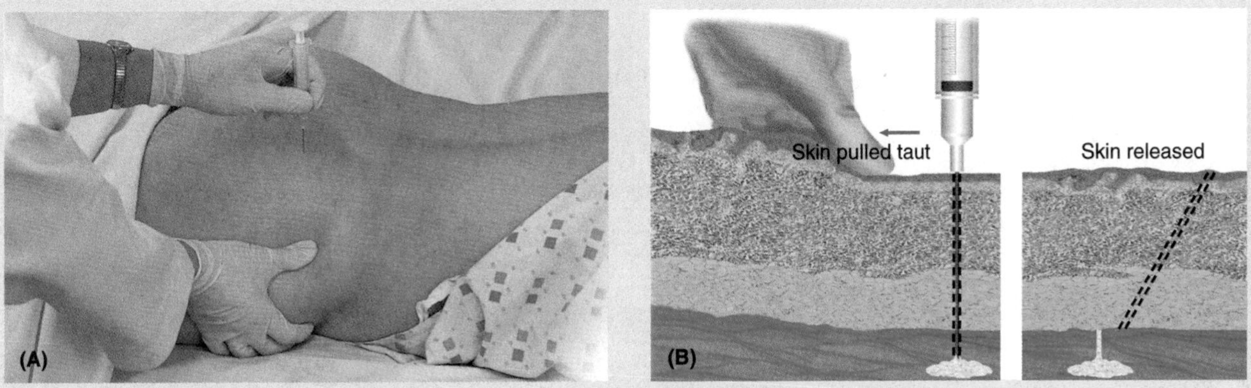

Figure 24-38 Z-track technique for intramuscular injection. (A) With client supine, grasp and pull the muscle laterally before injecting medication. (B) Inject medication. Keep skin pulled taut for 10 seconds. Quickly withdraw the needle and release the skin to seal the site.

(continues)

Procedure 24-9 (continued)

24. Wait 10 seconds before removing needle to allow medication to begin to be absorbed.
25. Remove needle and syringe at same angle of insertion.
26. Immediately release traction of the Z position to seal off the needle track. This prevents medication from reaching the subcutaneous tissues and the surface of the skin.
27. Immediately activate safety mechanism and dispose of needle-syringe unit in a sharps container.
28. Cover site. Do not massage.
29. Remove gloves. Wash hands.
30. Observe patient for signs of difficulty.
31. Provide for patient safety.
32. Return medication vial to storage.
33. Document the procedure.

DOCUMENTATION

12/01/20XX 2:00 PM Interferon 30 mcg IM (R) Dorsogluteal muscle using Z-track technique. J. Guerro, CMA

Case Study 24-1

Abigail Johnson, a patient of Dr. Lewis, has been unable to keep her Type II noninsulin-dependent diabetes mellitus under control with oral hypoglycemics, and Dr. Lewis has decided that Abigail needs to begin to take insulin injections. Today in the clinic, her fasting blood glucose level is 190 mg/ml. Dr. Lewis prescribes Humulin® insulin 10 units subcutaneously stat.

CASE STUDY REVIEW

1. What size insulin syringe should be used?
2. What does the medication label state are the number of units per milliliter? Show how to calculate the correct dosage.
3. Discuss the route of administration and the specifics about insulin administration that require it to be given slightly differently from other subcutaneous injections.
4. Describe several topics of discussion in which you would engage Abigail to help her learn how to better control her disease.

Case Study 24-2

Alice Chambers weighs 28 pounds and is 33 inches tall. The adult dose is erythromycin 400 mg every 6 hours by mouth.

CASE STUDY REVIEW

1. Calculate the dose of erythromycin Alice needs.
2. If the physician ordered erythromycin by injection rather than by mouth, how would the dose be calculated if the erythromycin adult dose is 400 mg/ml?
3. What size needle and syringe are appropriate for giving Alice the injection?

SUMMARY

Administering medications is one of the most important and essential responsibilities that the medical assistant performs. This chapter has presented a review of some of the fundamental elements of pharmacology, dosage calculations, and medication administration.

Each state has enacted laws governing the practice of medicine, nursing, and pharmacy. These laws vary from state to state; therefore, it is essential that one become familiar with the laws of the state in which one is employed before administering any medication.

Under the law, those administering medications are expected to be knowledgeable about the drugs that they administer and the effects the drug may or will have on the patient. They are responsible for their own actions.

STUDY FOR SUCCESS

To reinforce your knowledge and skills of information presented in this chapter:

- ❑ Review the Key Terms
- ❑ Practice the Procedures
- ❑ Consider the Case Studies and discuss your conclusions
- ❑ Answer the Review Questions
  - ❑ Multiple Choice
  - ❑ Critical Thinking
- ❑ Navigate the Internet by completing the Web Activities
- ❑ Practice the StudyWARE activities on your student CD
- ❑ Apply your knowledge in the Student Workbook activities
- ❑ Complete the Web Tutor sections
- ❑ View and discuss the DVD situations

REVIEW QUESTIONS

Multiple Choice

1. A written legal document that gives directions for compounding, dispensing, and administering medication to a patient is a:
   a. medication note
   b. prescription
   c. medication order
   d. subscription
2. An abbreviation symbol that means nothing by mouth is:
   a. non rep
   b. NPO
   c. IM
   d. mm
3. Insulin-dependent diabetes mellitus is:
   a. Type I
   b. Type II
   c. Type III
   d. Type IV
4. Body surface area is used:
   a. when calculating children's dosages
   b. when calculating adult dosages
   c. when determining an injection site
   d. when selecting an appropriately sized needle
5. An injection given just below the surface of the skin at a 15-degree angle is called a(n):
   a. intramuscular injection
   b. intradermal injection
   c. subcutaneous injection
   d. parenteral injection

Critical Thinking

1. Describe the process to follow to determine the state law regarding a medical assistant administering medications.
2. What is a medication order? Describe its purpose.
3. List nine parts of a prescription and define each part.
4. Name and describe factors that can affect medication dosage. Explain why and how the dosage is affected.
5. List the fundamental units of the metric system.
6. Name two methods used to calculate children's dosages of medication.
7. List and describe the "Six Rights."
8. A fellow student tells you that she accidentally gave a patient the incorrect dose of medication. Explain in detail what should be done.
9. You accidentally stick yourself with a used needle. What are the steps to take?
10. Discuss allergenic extracts. What are they? What safeguards are needed after administration?
11. List two reasons for the physician to prescribe oxygen for a patient. Describe how oxygen is administered and oxygen safety.

Calculation Problems

1. Calculate the following dosages according to body surface area (BSA):

   If the adult dose of E.E.S. tabs is 400 mg every 6 hours, what is the dosage for a child who is 35 inches tall and weighs 28 pounds (BSA 0.57)?

   If the adult dose of penicillin V potassium, USP, is 250 mg every 6 to 8 hours, what is the dosage for a child who is 24 inches tall and weighs 35 pounds (BSA 0.56)?
2. Calculate the following dosages according to kilogram of body weight:

   The physician orders Augmentin 20 mg/kg/day for Sally Whitney, who weighs 72 pounds. The dose is to be divided and given every 8 hours. What is the total dose? What is the amount to be given every 8 hours?

   The physician orders Cefadyl 40 mg/kg for George Kipperley, who weighs 78 pounds. The dose is to be divided into four equal doses. What is the total dose? What is the amount to be given in four equal doses?

   The physician orders Garamycin 2.0 mg/kg every 8 hours for a child who weighs 86 pounds. What is the correct dosage?
3. The physician ordered 64 units of U-100 Humulin insulin. Shade the correct dosage on the U-100 syringe pictured.

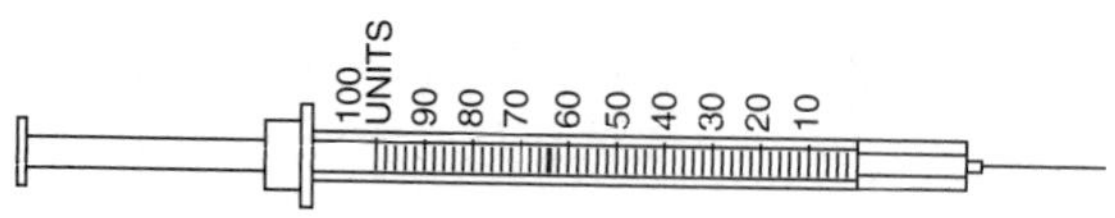

Using the proportional or formula method, calculate the following dosages.

4. The physician orders 125 mg of Diamox. On hand you have 250 mg tablets. You will give ____ tablets to your patient.
5. The physician orders 250 mg of Tagamet liquid. On hand you have 300 mg/5 ml. How many milliliters will you give?

WEB ACTIVITIES

1. Search for a Web site to explore the various types of safety needles available for injection and venipuncture. What is the most recent ruling by OSHA in regard to these types of needles?
2. Check the Web site http://www.mederrors.com and search for the following:
   a. What is the most common medication error?
   b. Which group of medical professionals makes the most medication errors?
   c. How can medication errors be prevented?

REFERENCES/BIBLIOGRAPHY

Centers for Disease Control and Prevention, Division of Health Care Quality Promotion (2004, February). *Workbook for designing, implementing, and evaluating a sharps injury prevention program*. Retrieved from http://cdc.gov/sharpsafety/wk_info.html. Accessed August 9, 2004.

Josephson, D. (2004). *Intravenous infusion therapy for nurses principle and practice*. (2nd ed.). Clifton Park, NY: Thomson Delmar Learning.

Prescription for drug safety. (2003, March). *Consumer Reports on Health*, *15*(3), 1, 4–6.

Taber's cyclopedic medical dictionary. (22nd ed.). (2003). Philadelphia: FA Davis.

To the point. (2004, August 2). *Advance for nursing serving RN's in New England*, *4*(17), 30–31.

THE DVD HOOK-UP

DVD Series	Program Number
Skills Based Series	9
Skills Based Series	10

Chapter/Scene Reference
- *Entire program*

This chapter discussed the medical assistant's role in prescription writing, administering nonparenteral medications, and administering parenteral medications.

In one of the first scenes in Program 9, the physician gave Tyrah verbal medication orders for two separate patients. In cases where the physician dictates his or her notes, he or she may not have anything written in the chart so he or she may give a verbal order to save time.

1. What did Tyrah do as soon as the doctor gave her the verbal orders?
2. You will notice that the doctor used common prescription abbreviations when talking to Tyrah. Do you think that was wise? What are some of the abbreviations that the doctor used that are no longer considered acceptable with certain governmental agencies?
3. What did you think of Tyrah's nails when she demonstrated the inhaler?
4. Do you think there was a more sanitary way of demonstrating the inhaler instead of using the patient's inhaler? Should Tyrah have observed Mrs. Edmonson when she practiced her inhaler?

You will notice that the book illustrates the medical assistant wearing gloves when withdrawing medications; however, Program 10 of the DVD program showed the medical assistant without gloves drawing up medication?

1. Why might it be a bit more sanitary to wear gloves when drawing up medications?
2. The medical assistant in the DVD program allowed the alcohol to dry before administering the injection. Is this acceptable with your teacher? What is the purpose of allowing the alcohol to dry before injecting the patient?

DVD Journal Summary

Write a paragraph that summarizes what you learned from watching today's DVD programs. Making a medication error could result in a negative reaction or even death to the patient. Write a paragraph that will reassure your instructors that you will be cautious when drawing up and administering medications.

CHAPTER 25

Electrocardiography

OUTLINE

Anatomy of the Heart
Electrical Conduction System of the Heart
The Cardiac Cycle and the ECG Cycle
- Calculation of Heart Rate on ECG Graph Paper

Types of Electrocardiographs
- Single-Channel Electrocardiograph
- Multichannel Electrocardiograph
- Automatic Electrocardiograph Machines
- Electrocardiograph Telephone Transmissions
- Facsimile Electrocardiograph
- Interpretive Electrocardiograph

ECG Equipment
- Electrocardiograph Paper
- Electrolyte
- Sensors or Electrodes
- Lead Wires
- Electrocardiograph Machine
- Care of Equipment

Lead Coding
The Electrocardiograph and Sensor Placement
- Standard Limb or Bipolar Leads
- Augmented Leads
- Chest Leads or Precordial Leads

Standardization and Adjustment of the Electrocardiograph
Standard Resting Electrocardiography
Mounting the ECG Tracing
Interference or Artifacts
- Somatic Tremor Artifacts
- AC Interference
- Wandering Baseline Artifacts
- Interrupted Baseline Artifacts
- Patients with Unique Problems

Myocardial Infarctions (Heart Attacks)
Cardiac Arrhythmias
- Atrial Arrhythmias
- Ventricular Arrhythmias

Defibrillation
Other Cardiac Diagnostic Tests
- Holter Monitor (Portable Ambulatory Electrocardiograph)
- Treadmill Stress Test or Exercise Tolerance ECG
- Thallium Stress Test
- Echocardiography/Ultrasonography

KEY TERMS

Amplified
Amplitude
Angiogram
Arrhythmia
Artifact
Augment
Baseline
Bipolar
Bradycardia, Sinus
Calibration
Cardiac Catheterization
Cardiac Cycle
Cardioversion
Countershock
Defibrillation
Defibrillator
Deoxygenated
Depolarization
Diastole
Electrocardiogram
Electrocardiograph
Electrocardiography
Electrodes
Electrolyte
Galvanometer
Infarction
Ischemia
Isoelectric
Lead Wires
Mounting
Noninvasive
Normal Sinus Rhythm
Oscilloscope
Precordial
Repolarization
Rhythm Strip
Sensor
Sonographer
Stylus
Syncope

(continues)

KEY TERMS (continued)

Systole
Tachycardia, Sinus
Test Cable
Thallium Scan
Tracing
Transducer
Ultrasonography
Unipolar

FEATURED COMPETENCIES

CAAHEP—ENTRY-LEVEL COMPETENCIES

Diagnostic Testing

- Perform electrocardiography

Patient Care

- Obtain vital signs
- Prepare and maintain examination and treatment areas
- Prepare patient for and assist with routine and specialty examinations
- Prepare patient for and assist with procedures, treatments, and minor office surgeries
- Screen and follow-up test results

Patient Instruction

- Provide instruction for health maintenance and disease prevention

ABHES—ENTRY-LEVEL COMPETENCIES

Clinical Duties

- Prepare patients for procedures
- Take vital signs
- Recognize emergencies
- Prepare and maintain examination and treatment area

(continues)

OBJECTIVES

The student should strive to meet the following performance objectives and demonstrate an understanding of the facts and principles presented in this chapter through written and oral communication.

1. Define the key terms as presented in the glossary.
2. Follow the circulation of blood through the heart starting at the vena cavae.
3. Describe the electrical conduction system of the heart.
4. State three reasons why patients may need an electrocardiogram (ECG).
5. Identify the various positive and negative deflections and describe what each represents in the cardiac cycle.
6. Explain the purpose of standardization of the electrocardiogram.
7. Identify the 12 leads of an ECG and describe what area of the heart each lead represents.
8. State the function of ECG graph paper, electrodes (sensors), and electrolyte.
9. Describe various types of ECGs and their capabilities.
10. Explain each type of artifact and how each can be eliminated.
11. Name and describe the purposes of the various cardiac diagnostic tests as outlined in this chapter.
12. Identify the placement of Holter monitor electrodes.
13. Describe the reason for a patient activity diary during ambulatory electrocardiography.
14. Identify six arrhythmias and explain the cause of each.
15. Explain how to calculate heart rates from an ECG tracing.
16. Identify a common coding system used to code each lead on an ECG tracing.
17. Describe the procedure for mounting and ECG tracing.

SCENARIO

Wanda Slawson, CMA, clinical medical assistant at Inner City Health Care, recently had her own physical examination that included her first electrocardiogram (ECG). This is now Wanda's baseline ECG, which provides a basis for future ECG readings to be compared. Because Wanda currently has no heart problems, future tests will indicate differences from her normal baseline ECG. It was different for Wanda to be the patient versus the person performing the ECG. Having the test performed on her, Wanda can now relate to feelings many of her patients must have felt when having an ECG. These included feelings of fear that the test may be abnormal; a cold feeling because even though the room temperature was normal, she was partially uncovered and the pads were cold when applied; and anxiousness because she found it difficult to stay completely still through the entire tracing. Wanda could empathize more with her patients after she had the test than she did before her test. Wanda now makes a more concerted effort to allay patient fears and make patients comfortable during ECGs.

FEATURED COMPETENCIES (continued)

- Assist physician with examinations and treatments
- Use quality control
- Perform selected tests that assist with diagnosis and treatment
- Screen and follow up patient test results
- Perform electrocardiograms

Instruction

- Teach patients methods of health promotion and disease prevention

Spotlight on Certification

RMA Content Outline

- Electrocardiography

CMA Content Outline

- Systems, including structure, function, related conditions and diseases
- Principles of operation
- Quality control
- Performing selected tests

INTRODUCTION

Many physicians include an ***electrocardiogram*** *(ECG or EKG) as part of a complete physical examination, especially for patients who are 40 years or older, for patients with a family history of cardiac disease, or for patients who have experienced chest pain. It is a noninvasive, safe, and painless procedure that can provide the physician with valuable information about the health of the patient's heart or suspected cardiac symptoms. A graphic representation of the heart's electrical activity, an ECG measures the amount of the electrical activity produced by the heart and the time necessary for the electrical impulses to travel through the heart during each heartbeat.*

Some reasons for ***electrocardiography*** *are to: (1) detect myocardial* ***ischemia,*** *(2) estimate damage to the myocardium caused by a myocardial* ***infarction,*** *(3) detect and evaluate cardiac* ***arrhythmia,*** *(4) assess effects of cardiac medication on the heart, and (5) determine if electrolyte imbalance is present. An ECG cannot always detect impending heart disease or cardiovascular disease. The ECG is used in conjunction with other laboratory and diagnostic tests to assess total cardiac health. An ECG alone cannot diagnose disease.*

In a medical office or ambulatory care setting, it is the medical assistant who records the ECG; therefore, special knowledge and skills are necessary and include these aspects of the correct electrocardiography procedures: patient preparation; operation of the ***electrocardiograph;*** *elimination of* ***artifacts, mounting,*** *and labeling the ECG; and maintenance and care of the instrument.*

ANATOMY OF THE HEART

The heart has four chambers: two upper chambers known as atria, and two lower chambers known as ventricles. **Deoxygenated** blood enters the right atrium from the superior and inferior vena cavae and passes through the tricuspid valve into the right ventricle. In a healthy heart, the blood between right and left sides cannot mix together. It then travels to the lungs via the pulmonary arteries. The deoxygenated blood gives off the carbon dioxide and picks up oxygen in the capillary bed of the lungs. Oxygenated blood is pumped through the pulmonary vein into the left atrium, through the mitral valve, into the left ventricle. The oxygenated blood then passes through the aortic valve into the aorta and from the aorta to all cells, tissues, and organs of the body (Figure 25-1). The cycle begins with each heartbeat.

On its external surface, the heart is surrounded by coronary arteries that supply the myocardium with its blood supply from which oxygen and nutrients are obtained. See the section on the circulatory system in Chapter 18.

ELECTRICAL CONDUCTION SYSTEM OF THE HEART

There are basically two kinds of cardiac cells: electrical cardiac cells and myocardial cells. The electrical cells, which are located in distinct pathways around and through the heart, are sensitive to electrical impulses. Their pathways are referred to as the conduction system of the heart and have specific names.

The body's natural pacemaker, the sinoatrial (SA) node, is located in the upper part of the right atrium.

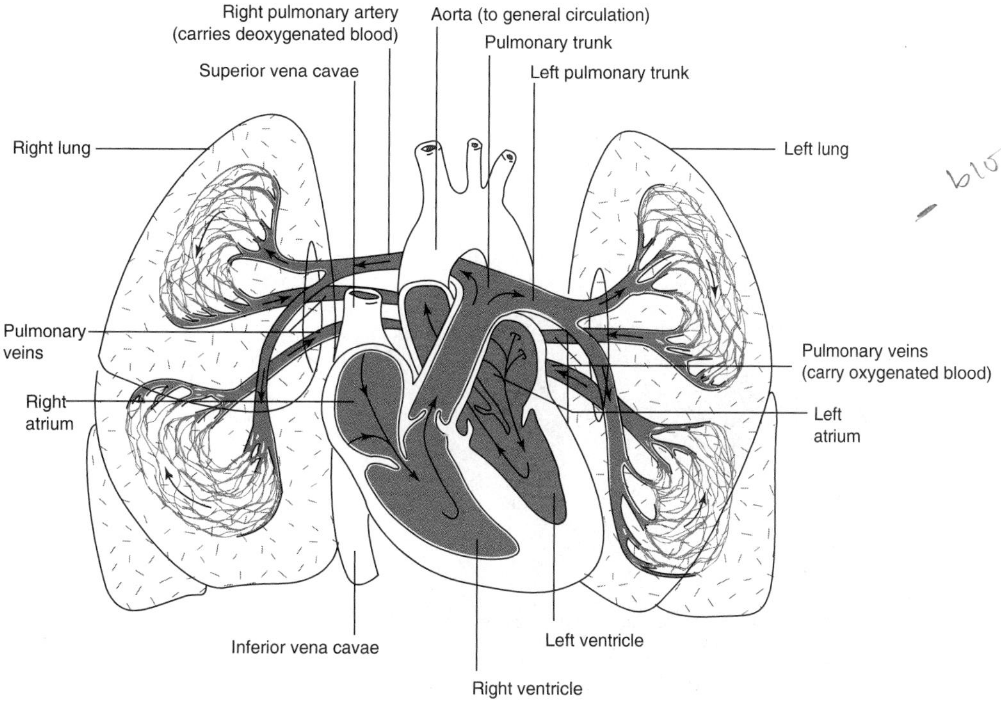

Figure 25-1 Oxygenated blood passing through the heart and onto the rest of the body.

It sends out an electrical impulse that begins and regulates the heartbeat. When the electrical impulses are sent along the pathways or conduction system of the heart (via the electrical cells), the myocardial cells contract, causing the heart muscle to pump the blood from chamber to chamber and through the lungs. The contraction of the cardiac cells is called **depolarization** (from the electrical "discharge"). The first chambers affected (contracted) by the electrical discharge from the SA node are the atria. From the atria, the electrical impulses travel along the conduction system toward the ventricles, to the atrioventricular (AV) node, located at the base of the right atrium. From here, the electrical impulses are transmitted to the bundle of His. The bundle of His divides into right and left bundle branches that continue the electrical impulses on to the Purkinje fibers. These fibers disperse the electrical impulses to the right and left ventricles, causing them to contract. The heart recovers electrically **(repolarization),** then relaxes briefly (polarization), and then a new impulse is begun by the SA node and the cycle begins again (Figure 25-2). This cycle is known as the **cardiac cycle** and it represents one heartbeat. The electrocardiograph records the electrical activity that causes the contraction **(systole)** and the relaxation **(diastole)** of the atria and ventricles. The ECG cycle is the recording or the graphic representation of the cardiac cycle. These electrical impulses can be recorded on special ECG paper or displayed on an **oscilloscope.**

THE CARDIAC CYCLE AND THE ECG CYCLE

The **baseline,** or **isoelectric,** line is the flat line that separates the various waves. It is present when there is no current flowing in the heart. The waves are either deflecting upward, known as positive deflection, or deflecting downward, known as negative deflection from the baseline.

The P, QRS, and T waves, recorded during the ECG, represent the depolarization (contraction) and repolarization (recovery) of the myocardial cells. The P wave represents atrial depolarization and is recorded as a positive deflection. The QRS complex represents ventricular depolarization and is measured from the beginning of the first wave of the QRS to the end of the last wave of the QRS complex (refer back to Figure 25-2). The T wave represents ventricular repolarization and is a positive deflection. The recovery of the atria is so slight, it is lost behind the QRS complex.

Each complete cardiac cycle takes about 0.8 second with each wave taking an appropriate amount of time if the heart is healthy. By observing and measuring the size, shape, and location of each wave on an ECG recording, the physician can analyze and interpret the conduction

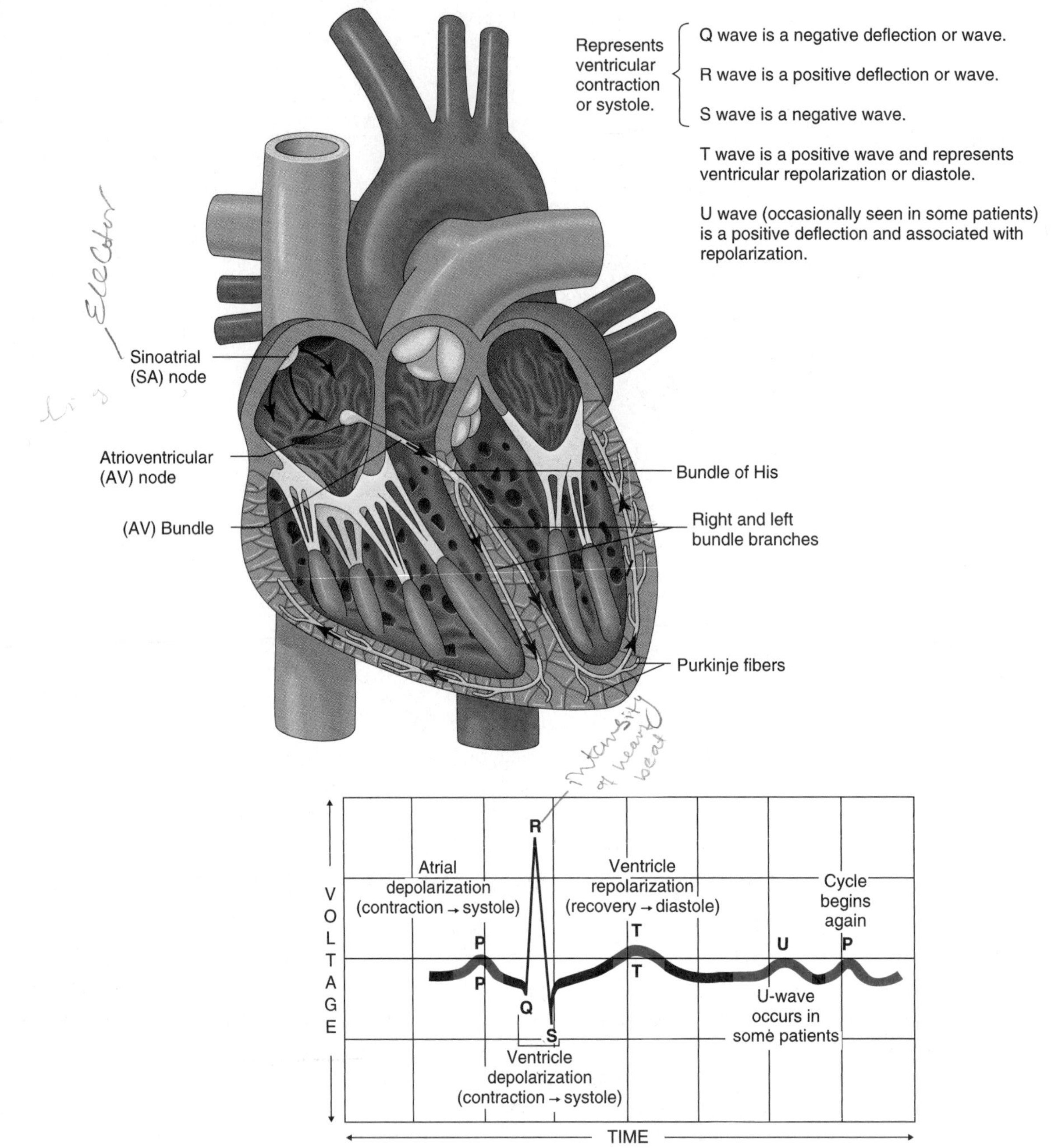

Figure 25-2 The heartbeat is controlled by electrical impulses that comprise the continuous cardiac cycle.

of electricity through the cardiac cells, the heart's rhythm and rate, and the health of the heart in general.

Calculation of Heart Rate on ECG Graph Paper

ECG graph paper is divided into 1-mm squares (small squares) and 5-mm squares (large squares). Each large square is 25 small squares and is 5 mm high and 5 mm wide. On the horizontal line, one small square represents 0.04 second. On the vertical line, one small square represents 1 mm of voltage. Because a large square is five small squares wide and five deep, each small square represents 0.2 second horizontal and 5 mm vertical. **NOTE:** Every fifth line, both horizontally and vertically, is darker than the other lines, making squares that are 5 × 5 mm (Figure 25-3). These measurements are accepted worldwide and enable the physician to interpret the time of each deflection on the horizontal line and cardiac electrical activity (voltage) on the vertical line to help determine cardiac health.

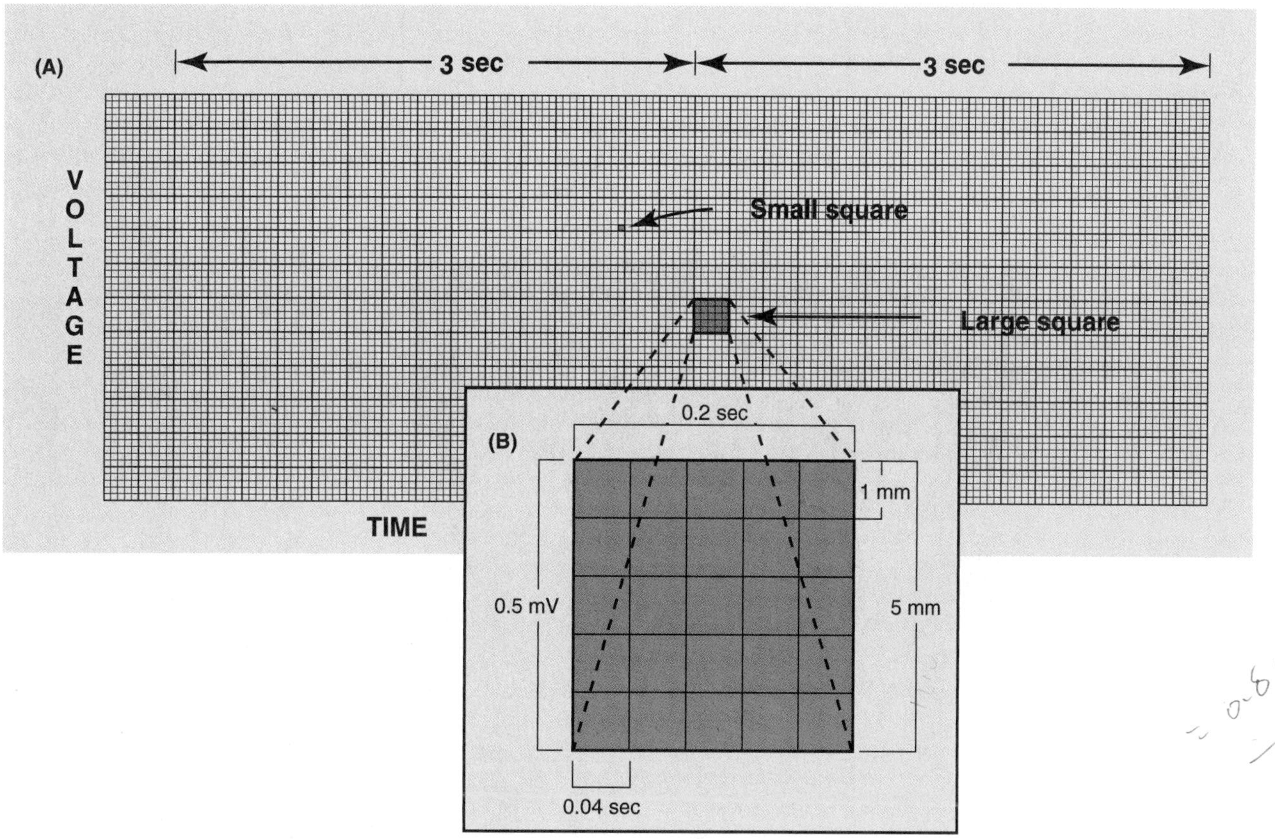

Figure 25-3 Electrocardiogram graph paper measurements allow medical professionals to determine the time and voltage of heartbeats. (A) The small square is 1 mm wide and 1 mm high. One small square = 0.04 second. (B) The large square consists of 25 small squares and measures 5 mm wide and 5 mm high. One large square = 0.04 × 5 or 0.2 second.

Because all cardiac complexes consist of P, QRS, and T, and the electrocardiograph paper measures time on the horizontal line, it is possible to calculate heart rate. Count the number of 5-mm boxes (number within the dark lines) between two R waves. Divide this number into 300. The result will be the heart rate per minute.

Example: One small square (1 mm) = 0.04 second in time
One large square (5 mm) = 0.04 × 5 = 0.2 second
Divide 60 seconds (1 minute) by 0.2 second
60 ÷ 0.2 = 300

Critical Thinking

Explain the significance of the small and large boxes on ECG paper. There are 2.5 large boxes between each cardiac cycle. What is the heartbeat per minute?

Example: There are three large squares between two R waves.

300 ÷ 3 = 100

The heartbeat is 100 beats per minute.

TYPES OF ELECTROCARDIOGRAPHS

Single-Channel Electrocardiograph

A conventional 12-lead single-channel electrocardiograph can be used in either manual mode or automatic mode. When using automatic mode, the 12-lead ECG tracing is complete in less than 40 seconds. With a single-channel machine, only one lead can be recorded at a time. If not automatic, the single-channel ECG requires manually turning the lead selector on and off between each of the 12 leads. It may also require the leads to be coded so that they can be identified later and properly mounted. Lead coding and mounting are explained more fully later in this chapter. The ECG tracing from a single-channel machine will need to be cut and mounted onto special forms for filing into the patient record. See Figure 25-4 for a sample of a single-channel electrocardiograph machine and tracing.

Multichannel Electrocardiograph

An electrocardiograph that can simultaneously record several different leads is known as a multichannel electrocardiograph. The conventional electrocardiograph records one lead at a time. A three-channel machine,

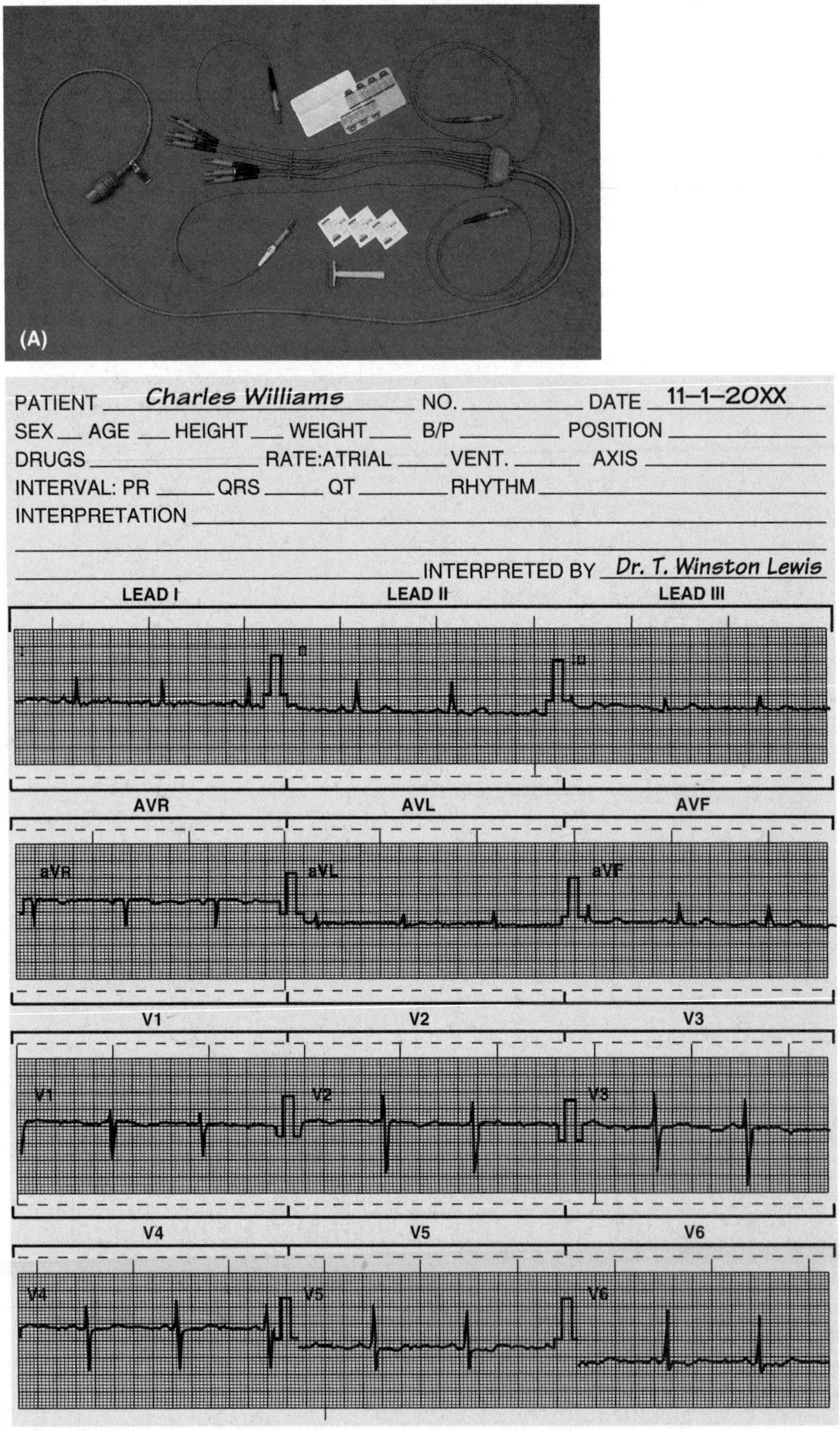

(B)

Figure 25-4 (A) Supplies for single-channel 12 lead electrocardiograph. (B) Mounted single ECG tracing or recording.

one type of multichannel electrocardiograph, records three channels at one time. It records Lead I, II, and III, followed by aVR, aVL, and aVF, followed by V_1, V_2, and V_3, followed by V_4, V_5, and V_6. The advantage of the multichannel machine is its speed. The most common multichannel machine used in the physician's office is the three-channel machine. This type of machine requires three-channel recording paper that is 8½ × 11 inches and fits into the patient record with no cutting or mounting. Refer to Figure 25-5 for an example of multichannel tracing. Other multichannel electrocardiograph machines are available. In addition to the 3-channel, there are 6- and 12-channel machines. Some have a built-in rechargeable battery, an interpretation software program, a spirometery module, and transmission capability.

Automatic Electrocardiograph Machines

When using an automatic electrocardiograph, the lead length and switching of leads are done automatically by the electrocardiograph and there is no need to advance the control knob. For these reasons, both time and paper can be saved with the automatic machine. The automatic machine also comes equipped with a manual control that can be used if a longer tracing is necessary.

Electrocardiograph Telephone Transmissions

An electrocardiogram can be transmitted via a telephone line to an ECG interpretation site when using an

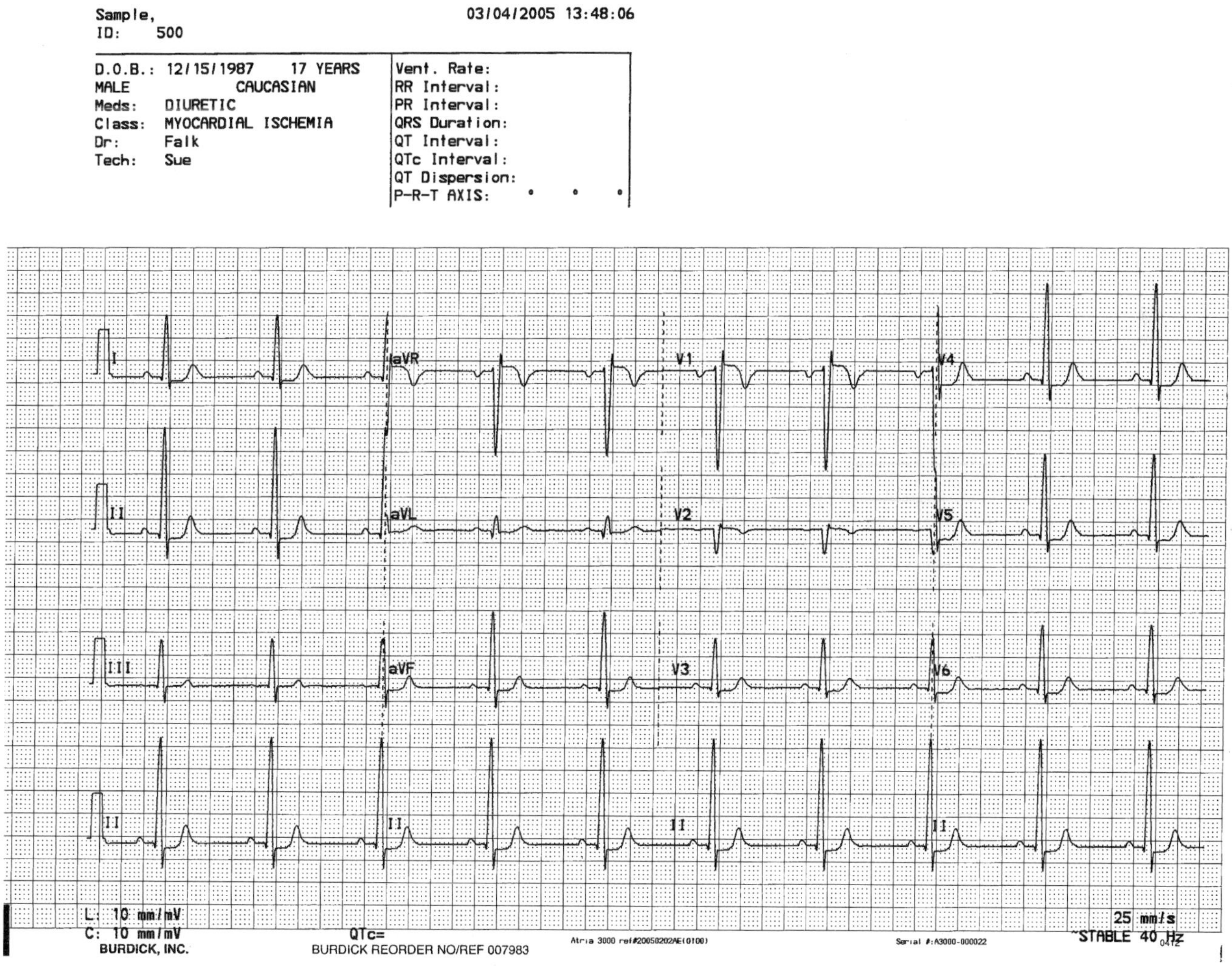

Figure 25-5 Example of three-channel electrocardiogram recording where three leads are recorded simultaneously. (Courtesy of Quinton Cardiology, Inc.)

electrocardiograph with such capabilities. A recording printout and interpretation (many times interpretation is done by a cardiologist or by a computer) are transmitted automatically on the electrocardiograph. Results of the ECG can be transmitted verbally as well.

Facsimile Electrocardiograph

The physician may need a rapid, expert ECG interpretation from an off-site diagnostician. Direct ECG fax transmits from the electrocardiograph to a fax machine and a high-quality facsimile is produced and sent to a diagnostic physician who calls back with a reading. This saves time by eliminating the step of copying the report and sending it via the traditional fax machine.

Interpretive Electrocardiograph

The interpretive electrocardiograph has a built-in computer program that interprets the ECG tracing while it is being recorded, allowing for faster diagnosis and treatment. The physician in charge will review the tracing before a diagnosis is confirmed and treatment is begun.

ECG EQUIPMENT

Electrocardiograph Paper

ECG paper can be either black or dark blue and is wax or plastic coated with a white or pink background and color lines. The paper is heat and pressure sensitive. As the heated **stylus** of the electrocardiograph moves across the paper, the background coating is melted away revealing the black or blue color of the paper and the ECG cycles are recorded or traced. The heat of the stylus can be adjusted to obtain a sharp, clear recording, or **tracing**. Medical assistants should learn how to adjust the proper control using the specific manual or instructions that accompany the electrocardiograph in their facility.

Electrolyte

Because the skin is a poor conductor of electricity, there are various types of conductive **electrolyte** substances applied with each electrode to pick up the electrical current. The impulses are transmitted to the electrocardiograph by metal tips on the patient lead wires or cables that are attached to the sensors. Because electrolyte substances must contain moisture to properly conduct impulses, they are manufactured in the forms of gels, lotions, pastes, presaturated pads, or, more commonly, are contained within adhesive sensors. For our purposes here, we use the disposable self-adhesive electropads/sensors.

Sensors or Electrodes

There are various types of **sensors** or **electrodes** made of metal or other conductive material. The sensors detect the electrical impulses on the body surface and relay them through cables, or leads wires to the ECG machine.

Disposable Electrodes. Disposable sensors contain a layer of electrolyte gel on their adhesive surface and can be used on both the limbs and chest. They do not require additional electrolytes. These sensors are applied to the skin of the limbs and chest and held in place by the adhesive. The self-adhesive electrodes are discarded after use.

Lead Wires

Once the self-adhesive sensors are placed, a series of lead wires coming from the machine will be connected to them. Small clips, sometimes referred to as alligator clips, will grasp the tabs on the sensors (Figure 25-6). This completes the circuit from the patient to the machine.

THE PROCESS OF RECORDING CARDIAC ELECTRICITY

Skin—Poor conductor
Electrolyte—Must contain moisture to conduct current
Electrodes—Must contain metal to conduct current
Metal clips or tips—To connect the electrodes to the lead wires
Lead wires—To conduct the current from the patient to the machine
Amplifier in the machine—To amplify the electricity enough to measure it
Stylus—An instrument to record the electrical pattern
ECG paper—On which the stylus can record the pattern

Older electrocardiographs may have plain lead wire tips for use with the older metal plates and suction cups. They can easily and inexpensively be converted to use the current self-adhesive sensor electrodes. The only conversion equipment necessary is a set of "alligator" clips that will fit over the end of the lead wire tips. Contact the manufacturer or a medical supplier for conversion sets.

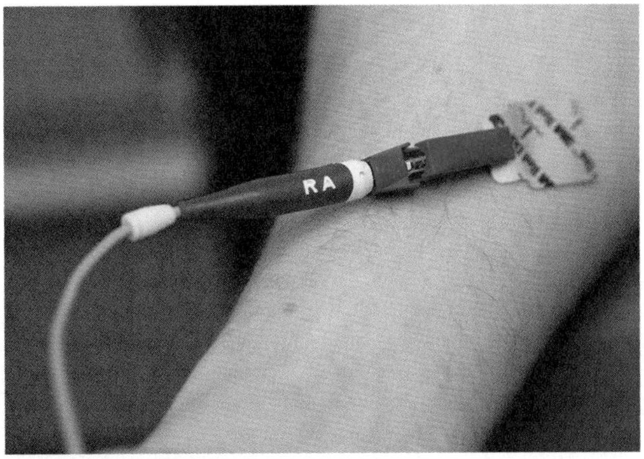

Figure 25-6 Alligator clip and disposable sensor.

Electrocardiograph Machine

Because the electrical activity that comes from the body is small, it is made larger, or amplified, by the **amplifier** of the electrocardiograph machine. The voltage is changed into a mechanical motion by the **galvanometer** and recorded on the paper by the heated stylus.

Care of Equipment

Once the ECG tracing is complete, remove the lead wires from the sensors, then remove the sensors from the patient. Dispose of the sensors. Check supplies on machine so it is ready for next use. Neatly and loosely place the lead wires on top of or beside the machine. Change the ECG paper when necessary according to manufacturer's suggestions.

LEAD CODING

There are a number of codes used to identify each lead recorded on the ECG reading. There are 12 leads recorded using the 10 lead wires. These codes are necessary for later identification and for mounting purposes. Newer electrocardiographs will automatically mark (code) each lead in the upper margin of the ECG paper during the recording. Older electrocardiographs must be manually coded by depressing the lead marker button. See Figure 25-7 for an example of a common coding system.

THE ELECTROCARDIOGRAPH AND SENSOR PLACEMENT

The standard electrocardiogram consists of 10 sensors that record 12 leads of the heart's electrical activity from different angles, allowing for a thorough three-dimensional interpretation of its activity. The electrical impulses given off by the heart are picked up by the electrodes and conducted into the machine through **lead wires.**

The electrodes are placed on the patient's four limbs and chest. The four limb leads are right arm (RA), left arm (LA), right leg (RL), and left leg (LL). The right leg electrode is not used as part of the recording. It is an electrical reference point only. The limb leads are placed on the fleshy, nonmuscular area of upper arms and lower legs. The chest leads are known as precordial leads, V leads, or C leads, and use an electrode for each of six areas on the chest wall or one electrode that is moved to six different positions on the chest wall. (This depends on the type of electrocardiograph being used.)

Standard Limb or Bipolar Leads

The first three leads that are recorded on a standard ECG are called Leads I, II, and III (Figure 25-8A). These are known as **bipolar** leads because each of them uses two limb electrodes that record simultaneously. Lead I records electrical activity between the right arm (RA) and left arm (LA); lead II records electrical activity between the right arm (RA) and left leg (LL); lead III records activity between the left arm (LA) and left leg (LL). Lead II is used as a **rhythm strip** because it portrays the heart's rhythm better than the other leads. The rhythm strip is usually a separate longer recording approximately 6 to 12 inches.

Augmented Leads

The next three leads are **augmented** (added to) leads and are designated aVR, aVL, and aVF (Figure 25-8B). The aV stands for augmented voltage; the R, L, and F stand for right, left, and foot (or leg). These are **unipolar** leads. Lead aVR records electrical activity from the midpoint between the left arm added to the left leg, directed to the right arm. Lead aVL records electrical activity from the midpoint between the right arm added to the left leg, directed to the left arm. Lead aVF records electrical activity from the midpoint between the right arm added to the left arm, directed to the left leg. Because these three leads produce such small electrical impulses, the electrocardiograph machine augments, or increases, their size to record them. Figure 25-8B will help you visualize the augmented process.

Chest Leads or Precordial Leads

The remaining six leads of the standard 12-lead ECG are the chest leads or **precordial** leads (Figure 25-8C). These are unipolar leads and are designated V_1, V_2, V_3, V_4, V_5, and V_6. These leads record the heart's electrical impulse

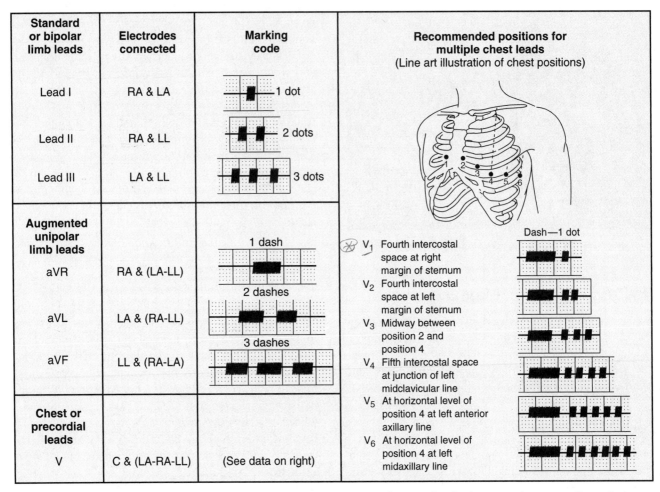

Standard or bipolar limb leads	Electrodes connected	Marking code	Recommended positions for multiple chest leads (Line art illustration of chest positions)
Lead I	RA & LA	1 dot	
Lead II	RA & LL	2 dots	
Lead III	LA & LL	3 dots	
Augmented unipolar limb leads			
aVR	RA & (LA-LL)	1 dash	
aVL	LA & (RA-LL)	2 dashes	
aVF	LL & (RA-LA)	3 dashes	
Chest or precordial leads			
V	C & (LA-RA-LL)	(See data on right)	

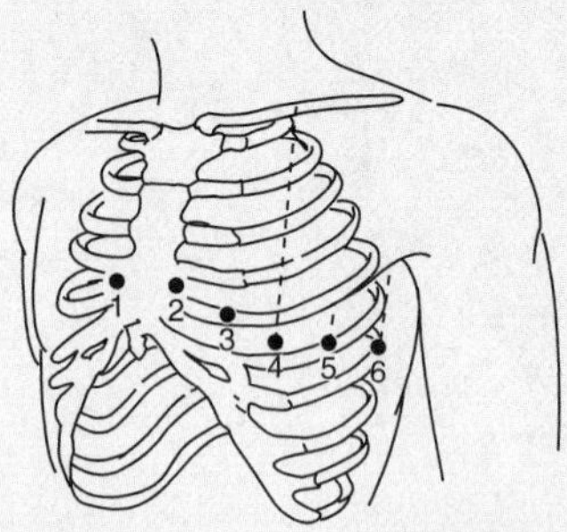

Lead	Position	Marking code
V_1	Fourth intercostal space at right margin of sternum	Dash—1 dot
V_2	Fourth intercostal space at left margin of sternum	
V_3	Midway between position 2 and position 4	
V_4	Fifth intercostal space at junction of left midclavicular line	
V_5	At horizontal level of position 4 at left anterior axillary line	
V_6	At horizontal level of position 4 at left midaxillary line	

Figure 25-7 Example of a common coding system for electrocardiogram leads that must be manually coded on older electrocardiographs. Accurate coding is accomplished by pressing the lead marker button appropriately. (Courtesy of Quinton Cardiology, Inc.)

from a central point within the heart to one of six predesignated positions on the chest wall where an electrode is attached. The correct position *must* be used for each lead recording.

The anatomical positions for placement of the chest or precordial leads are:

V_1—fourth intercostal space at right margin of sternum
V_2—fourth intercostal space at left margin of sternum
V_4—fifth intercostal space on left midclavicular line
V_3—midway between V2 and V4 (**NOTE:** This is correct order, V3 after V4.)
V_5—horizontal to V4 at left anterior axillary line
V_6—horizontal to V4 at left midaxillary line

When using an electrocardiograph with one chest wire, the chest electrode must be moved manually one by one to each of the six chest lead positions. This necessitates stopping the instrument between each chest lead to move the electrode to the next appropriate position on the chest wall. Some electrocardiographs have six lead wires allowing all six chest leads to be applied at one time; therefore, there is no interruption between chest lead recordings. (See Figure 25-18 in Procedure 25-1).

STANDARDIZATION AND ADJUSTMENT OF THE ELECTROCARDIOGRAPH

The value of an ECG recording depends on it being performed accurately. To ensure a precise and reliable recording, you must standardize the ECG instrument before every ECG performed. The standardization of the machine is a quality-assurance check to determine if the machine is set and working properly. Standardization measurements have been adopted internationally as a means of accurate **calibration** according to universal measurements. The universal standard is that 1 mV (millivolt) of cardiac electrical activity will deflect the stylus exactly 10 mm high. This is the equivalent of 10 small squares on the ECG paper. Figure 25-9 shows an example of the 10-mm standardization at the beginning of each row.

(A) Standard limb or bipolar leads

	Electrodes Connected
Lead I	LA and RA
Lead II*	LL and RA
Lead III	LL and LA

* Also used for rhythm strip

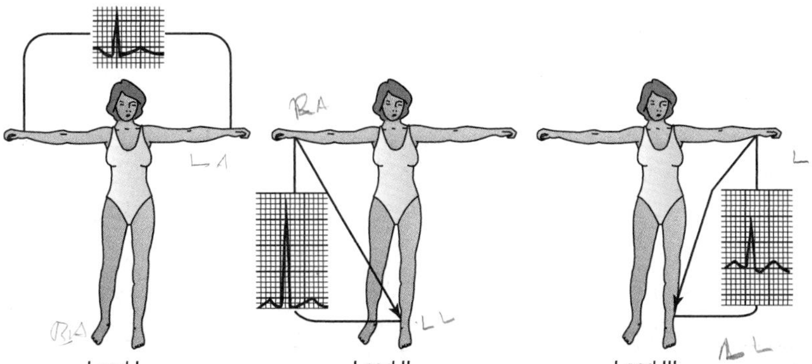

(B) Augmented limb leads

aVR	RA and (LA-LL)
aVL	LA and (RA-LL)
aVF	LL and (RA-LA)

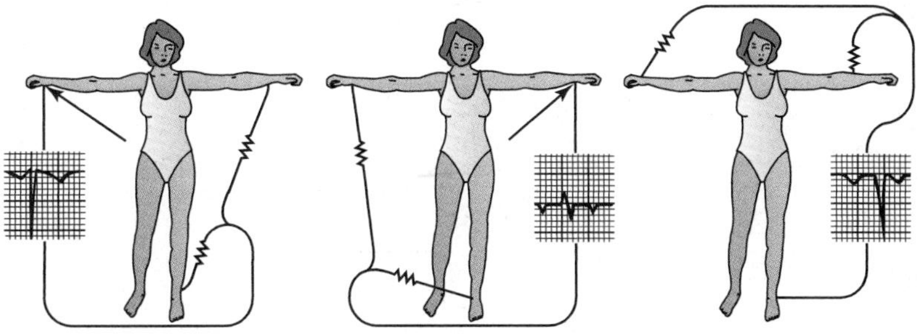

(C) Precordial or chest leads	Electrodes connected	Placement
V_1	V_1 and (LA-RA-LL)	Fourth intercostal space at right margin of sternum
V_2	V_2 and (LA-RA-LL)	Fourth intercostal space at left margin of sternum
V_4	V_4 and (LA-RA-LL)	Fifth intercostal space at junction of left midclavicular line
V_3	V_3 and (LA-RA-LL)	Midway between position 2 and position 4
V_5	V_5 and (LA-RA-LL)	At horizontal level of position 4 at left anterior axillary line
V_6	V_6 and (LA-RA-LL)	At horizontal level of position 4 at left midaxillary line

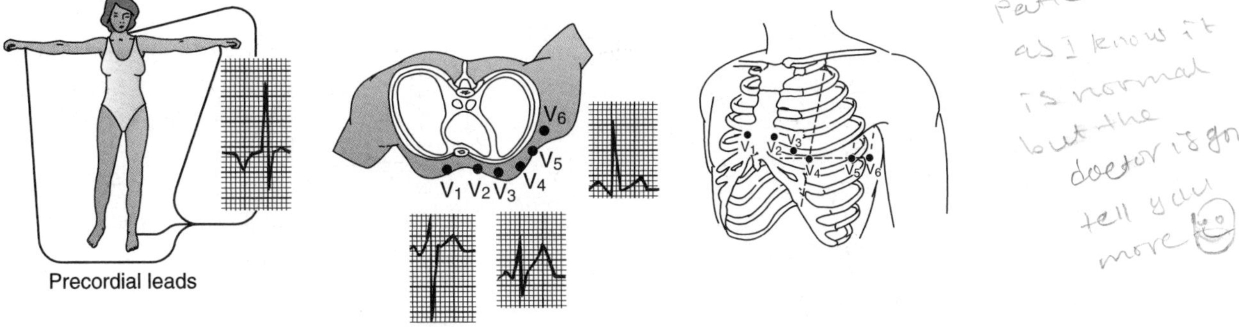

Figure 25-8 Lead types, connections, and placement. (A) Standard limb or bipolar leads. (B) Augmented limb leads. (C) Precordial or chest leads.

On occasion, R waves may be large and go off the paper. Repositioning the stylus may not correct the situation. In such instances, the medical assistant can record the lead(s) in which the R wave is large at one-half sensitivity. This action will record all ECG cycles at half their normal **amplitude.**

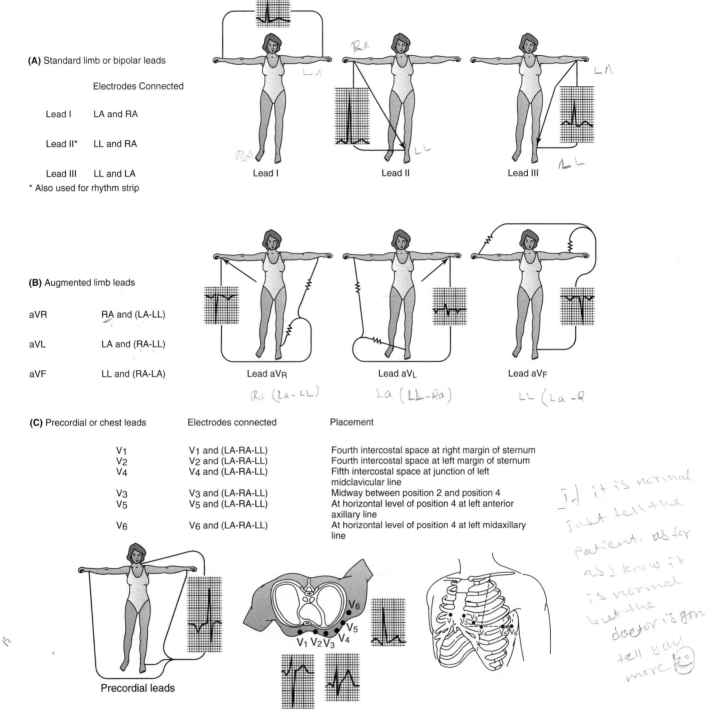

Conversely, the waves of the ECG cycles may be small, making it difficult to interpret. In this circumstance, the medical assistant can record the ECG cycles at twice the normal standard. This action will record ECG cycles at twice their normal amplitude. Whenever a change is made from a normal standardization (10 mm

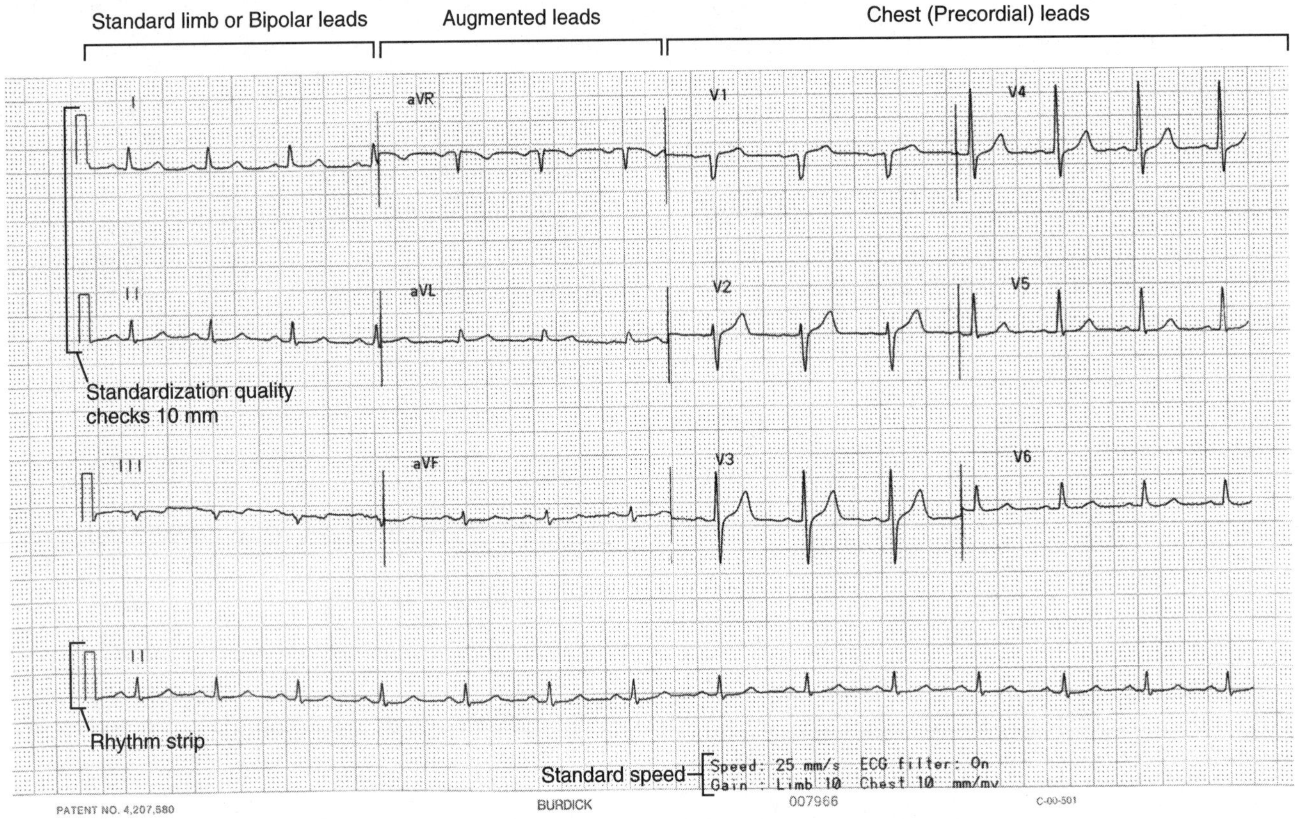

Figure 25-9 An electrocardiogram showing all 12 leads recorded in minutes at one time with no interruption. (Courtesy of Quinton Cardiology, Inc.)

high) to either a one-half standardization (5 mm high) or a double standardization (20 mm high), the medical assistant must include the adjusted standardization mark with that particular lead to alert the physician to the change in standard. The standard must be returned to normal to prevent accidentally running the next lead at a standard other than normal. The paper is usually run at a speed of 25 mm/second. If cycles are too close together, the paper speed can be adjusted to 50 mm/second. Make a note on the ECG paper if paper speed or amplitude is changed.

STANDARD RESTING ELECTROCARDIOGRAPHY

Regardless of the type of electrocardiograph used, the basic components of the standard electrocardiography procedure remain the same. Patient preparation, placement of limb and chest leads, attachment of lead wires, and elimination of artifacts vary little from one electrocardiograph to another. Procedure 25-1 explains a 12-lead ECG using a multiple-lead channel electrocardiograph. Medical assistants must be familiar with the electrocardiograph machine in their facility and should thoroughly review the manufacturer's instruction manual that accompanies the machine before performing the procedure. Knowledge of the basic procedures included here can be adapted for all other electrocardiographs.

MOUNTING THE ECG TRACING

Commercially prepared mounting forms are available and the medical assistant should mount the completed tracing after the physician has reviewed the entire recording. The mounting of the ECG recording will depend on the machine. Some machines will produce a strip already printed on a durable paper record. Some machines will produce a long strip that will need to be cut apart and adhered to a mounting paper or card. There are many options within these two varieties. Included with any ECG recording, though, should be the patient's name, date, address, age, sex, blood pressure, height and weight, and cardiac medications on the mounting form.

INTERFERENCE OR ARTIFACTS

The ECG is a valuable diagnostic aid to the physician and must be performed accurately. The medical assistant is responsible for obtaining a recording that can be easily read and interpreted by the physician.

There can be unusual and unwanted activity in the tracing not caused by the electrical activity of the heart. These defects in the ECG tracing are known as artifacts; and their appearance can make the ECG tracing difficult to read and interpret. Four of the more common artifacts are somatic tremor, alternating current (AC) interference, wandering baseline, and interrupted baseline. The medical assistant should understand the causes of each type of artifact and know how to eliminate them. The newer machines have filters, which will automatically filter out the artifact.

Somatic Tremor Artifacts

Somatic tremor artifact is also known as muscle tremor. It is characterized by unnatural baseline deflections such as jagged peaks or irregularity of spacing and height. The tracing appears fuzzy (Figure 25-10A). Somatic tremor occurs when the patient is apprehensive or uncomfortable and can result in involuntary muscle movement. Voluntary muscle movement occurs when the patient moves, talks, coughs, and so on. Parkinson's disease, a nervous system disorder, is an example of involuntary somatic tremor. It is not possible for the patient to control the muscle tremors. (Often, involuntary somatic tremor can be minimized somewhat by having the patient slide the hands under the buttocks during the recording.)

It is natural for the patient to feel apprehensive before and during the ECG tracing. Reassurance and an explanation of the procedure will allay apprehension and relax muscles. Be certain the patient is comfortable. Use pillows for the head and under the knees; be sure the temperature of the room is comfortable. These simple techniques will help to minimize somatic tremor.

AC Interference

The AC interference artifact is caused by electrical interference and appears as a series of small regular peaks (Figure 25-10B). Electricity present in medical equipment or wires in the area can leak a small amount of energy into the room in which the ECG is being recorded. The current can be picked up by the patient's body and it will be detected by the ECG tracing as an AC artifact.

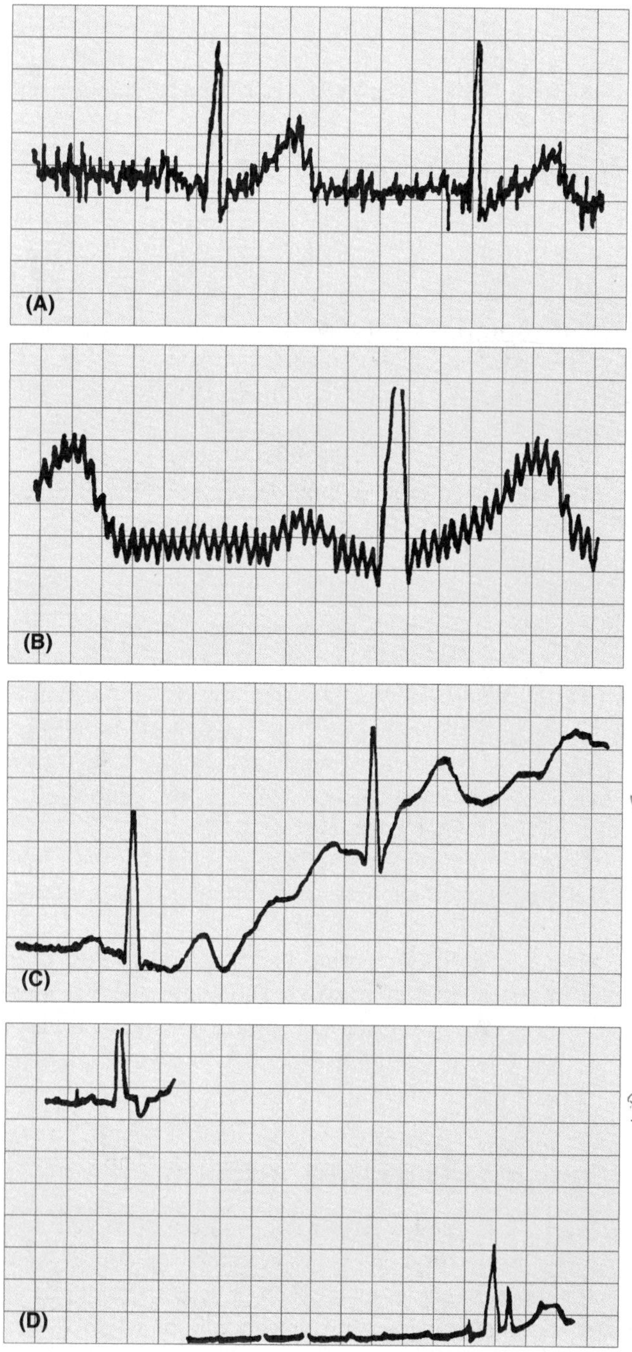

Figure 25-10 Electrocardiogram artifacts. (A) Somatic tremor. (B) Alternating current. (C) Wandering baseline. (D) Interrupted baseline. (Courtesy of Quinton Cardiology, Inc.)

Common Causes of AC Interference Artifacts. Some common causes of AC interferences are:

1. Improper grounding of electrocardiograph. There are three-pronged plugs in the newer electrocardiographs that are inserted into a properly grounded three-receptacle outlet. This reduces AC interference from improper grounding.
2. Presence of other electrical equipment in the room. Unplug other electrical equipment in the room (electrical examination tables, lamps, autoclaves, and so on).
3. Electrical wiring in the floor, ceiling, or walls. Move the ECG table away from walls.

4. Crossed lead wires and lead wires not following body contour. Straighten lead wires and be sure they are positioned to follow the patient's body contour.

Wandering Baseline Artifacts

A wandering baseline occurs when the stylus moves from the center of the ECG paper resulting in the complexes "wandering" across the ECG paper; for example, from the top of the paper to the bottom, or bottom to top (Figure 25-10C). This makes it difficult to follow the complexes when the physician reads the recording and interprets it.

Common Causes of Wandering Baseline Artifacts.

Wandering baseline artifacts can be caused by the following conditions:

1. Electrodes applied too loosely or too tightly. There should be equal tension on all four limb leads, metal tips should be firmly attached to the electrodes, and the patient cable should not have tension on it nor be dangling to cause pulling on the electrode.
2. Corroded or dirty electrodes or metal tips of the lead wires. Clean and rinse after each use.
3. Inappropriate amount or poor-quality electrolyte gel or paste. Each electrode should have the same amount of electrolyte gel or paste on it.
4. Lotions, oils, or creams on the patient's skin that interfere with the adhesive sticking well. Remove any of these substances before applying the electrode by vigorously rubbing the area with rubbing alcohol.

Interrupted Baseline Artifacts

On occasion, the baseline will become interrupted and there will be a break between waves (Figure 25-10D). A probable cause could be a broken patient cable or a lead wire that may have become detached from an electrode, or an electrode that has come completely off.

Patients with Unique Problems

On occasion, the medical assistant will perform an ECG on a patient who has unique medical problems. An obese woman, a woman with large breasts, or a patient with thick chest muscles will make it difficult to palpate the intercostal spaces. Place the chest leads on the chest as accurately as you can.

A limb amputation or a cast will require the medical assistant to apply the sensors as close to the preferred site as possible, higher on the limb. Place the sensor in a similar position on the other limb.

Do not place sensors on wounds, open areas, sutures, or staples. Try to situate the sensors as close to the preferred site as possible.

If the patient has dyspnea, the ECG can be taken with the patient in semi-Fowler's position. (See Chapter 13 for positions).

If you have difficulty performing an ECG on patients with certain medical problems or conditions, ask for assistance from your supervisor/delegator.

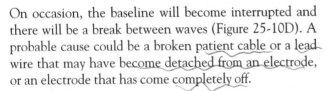

> **Critical Thinking**
>
> Mr. Williams has a diagnosis of Parkinson's disease. The physician requests an ECG. What strategies can you use to ensure an adequate tracing?

MYOCARDIAL INFARCTIONS (HEART ATTACKS)

Myocardial infarctions (heart attacks) are the number one cause of death in the United States today. With the approval of your employer–physician, medical assistants are in an excellent position to offer healthy tips and suggestions from which patients can benefit. For instance, they can offer patient health tips regarding diet and exercise while applying the ECG equipment and provide handouts and Web sites for them to research (Table 25-1).

TABLE 25-1 BEHAVIORS TO ADOPT FOR A HEALTHY HEART
The physician may want the medical assistant to remind patients of the following healthy behaviors:
1. Avoid tobacco.
2. Take medications as prescribed.
3. Report any unusual symptoms or problems to the physician.
4. Eat a low-fat, low-cholesterol, low-sodium diet.
5. Exercise regularly with physician's permission.
6. Get adequate rest.
7. Keep weight under control and at an acceptable level.
8. Practice stress reduction behaviors.

Patient Education

Atherosclerosis is the buildup of fatty deposits on the lining of coronary arteries causing narrowing and obstruction of the arteries. Blood flow to the heart muscle is diminished particularly when the heart is called on to work harder; for example, during increased physical activity, emotional stress, exposure to cold temperatures, and after a heavy meal. The heart's muscle tissue responds to these conditions by symptoms of pain or discomfort beneath the sternum, into the neck, jaw, left arm and shoulder, and throat. Rest usually relieves the pain. This condition is known as angina pectoris.

Treatment for angina consists of rest and medication. Nitroglycerin may be prescribed in tablet or patch form. Change in lifestyle and other suggestions as noted in Table 25-1 may be recommended. Tests that the physician may order include a 12-lead ECG, a stress ECG (stress test), blood tests, chest radiograph, and coronary angiogram.

Pain that does not subside after rest may indicate a more serious condition: a complete obstruction of the coronary arteries and no blood flow to the heart muscle, a myocardial infarction, or heart attack. Seek immediate medical attention if pain persists.

CARDIAC ARRHYTHMIAS

The medical assistant should recognize cardiac arrhythmias that occur during the ECG recording and without alarming the patient make the physician aware of them as soon as they are noticed. The normal, healthy ECG cycle consists of P, QRS, and T in a regularly appearing sequence or pattern. The term **normal sinus rhythm** refers to an ECG that is within normal limits (WNL). The normal adult heart rate is 60 to 100 beats/min. A rate less than 60 beats/min is known as **sinus bradycardia** (Figure 25-11A); a rate greater than 100 beats/min is known as **sinus tachycardia** (Figure 25-11B). These two heart rates, although regular in rhythm, are still considered to be cardiac arrhythmias.

Atrial Arrhythmias

Premature Atrial Contractions (PACs). Healthy individuals can experience PACs. They are seen in patients who use tobacco and stimulants such as caffeine, but can forewarn of more serious cardiac problems. This type of arrhythmia is characterized by a cardiac cycle that occurs before the next cycle is due. The P wave is shaped differently from the P wave of the normal cycle (Figure 25-12A).

Paroxysmal Atrial Tachycardia (PAT). This arrhythmia also can be seen in healthy individuals; however, it can appear in persons with cardiac disease. PAT is characterized by its unprovoked sudden onset and abrupt termination. The heart rate is regular and ranges between 160 to 250 beats/min. The episode usually lasts only a few seconds; the heart rate then returns to its original rate (Figure 25-12B). The patient may describe a fluttering in the chest, apprehension, shortness of breath, and on occasion, dizziness.

Atrial Fibrillation. This arrhythmia can be seen in healthy individuals or those with cardiac disease. In younger patients, common causes can be congenital heart disease and mitral valve damage caused by rheumatic heart disease. In older patients, the arrhythmia can be caused by hypertension, coronary artery disease, or mitral valve prolapse. It is characterized by extremely rapid, incomplete contractions 400 to 500 beats/min resulting in small, irregular, and uncoordinated complexes that are difficult to measure accurately because the P waves cannot be distinguished (Figure 25-12C).

Ventricular Arrhythmias

Premature Ventricular Contractions (PVCs). This arrhythmia can be seen in healthy individuals and patients with hypertension, coronary artery disease, and lung disease. In healthy individuals, PVCs can be caused by tobacco, anxiety, alcohol, and medications that contain epinephrine (Figure 25-13A). PVCs are seen on ECG tracings fairly frequently and are considered common disturbances in the rhythm. They are characterized

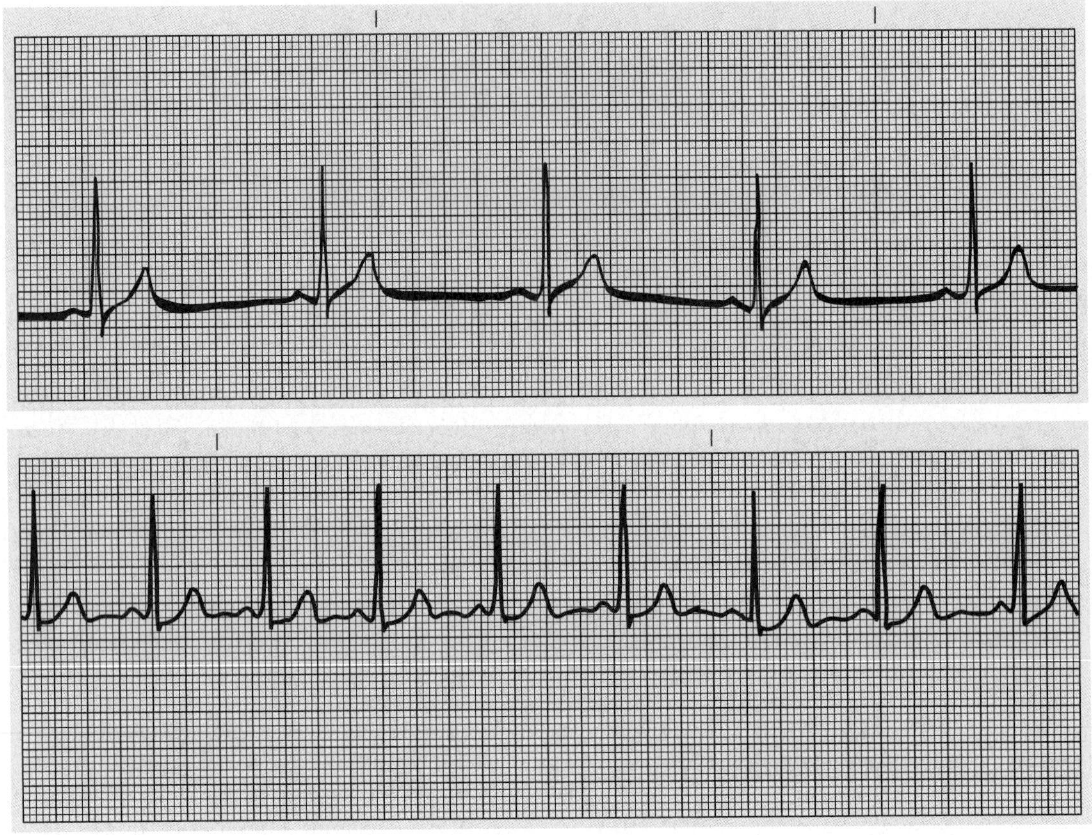

(A) (B)

Figure 25-11 (A) Heart rate shown is 50 beats/min, known as sinus bradycardia because it is less than 60 beats/min. One large square = 0.2 second; one minute (60 seconds) ÷ 0.2 = 300. There are six large squares between R waves: 300 ÷ 6 = 50 beats/min. (B) Sinus tachycardia is a heart rate faster than 100 beats/min. There are three large squares between R waves: 300 ÷ 3 = 100 beats/min.

by a beat that comes early in the cycle, has no P wave, a wide QRS complex, and a different T wave. The PVC is followed by a pause before the occurrence of the next normal cycle.

Ventricular Tachycardia. This arrhythmia is seen in patients with cardiac disease, both acute and chronic. It is common in coronary artery disease, and frequently the patient experiencing a myocardial infarction will have ventricular tachycardia as a result of the infarction (Figure 25-13B). The arrhythmia is manifested by three or more PVCs that occur at a rate ranging from 150 to 250 beats/min. There are no P waves and the QRS complexes are distorted. Ventricular tachycardia is life threatening and can rapidly deteriorate into fibrillation and cardiac standstill.

Ventricular Fibrillation. This arrhythmia is seen in patients experiencing a myocardial infarction or in patients with existing cardiac disease. It may be preceded by PVCs or ventricular tachycardia or may begin as ventricular fibrillation. It is a life-threatening arrhythmia (Figure 25-13C).

DEFIBRILLATION

A **defibrillator** is an electrical device that applies **countershocks** to the heart through electrodes or pads placed on the chest wall (Figure 25-14). The purpose is to convert cardiac arrhythmia into normal sinus rhythm. This is known as **defibrillation** or **cardioversion.** In some offices and clinics, a defibrillator is kept on a crash cart for quick access in emergency situations. The medical assistant should regularly check the equipment for proper operation and preparedness, and assist the physician as needed.

Automated external defibrillators (AEDs) are widely used and are found in many places where many people congregate such as an airport, the workplace, and in private homes for individuals at risk for cardiac arrest.

The devices are portable, small, and battery operated. Emergency medical technicians, police, and fire-

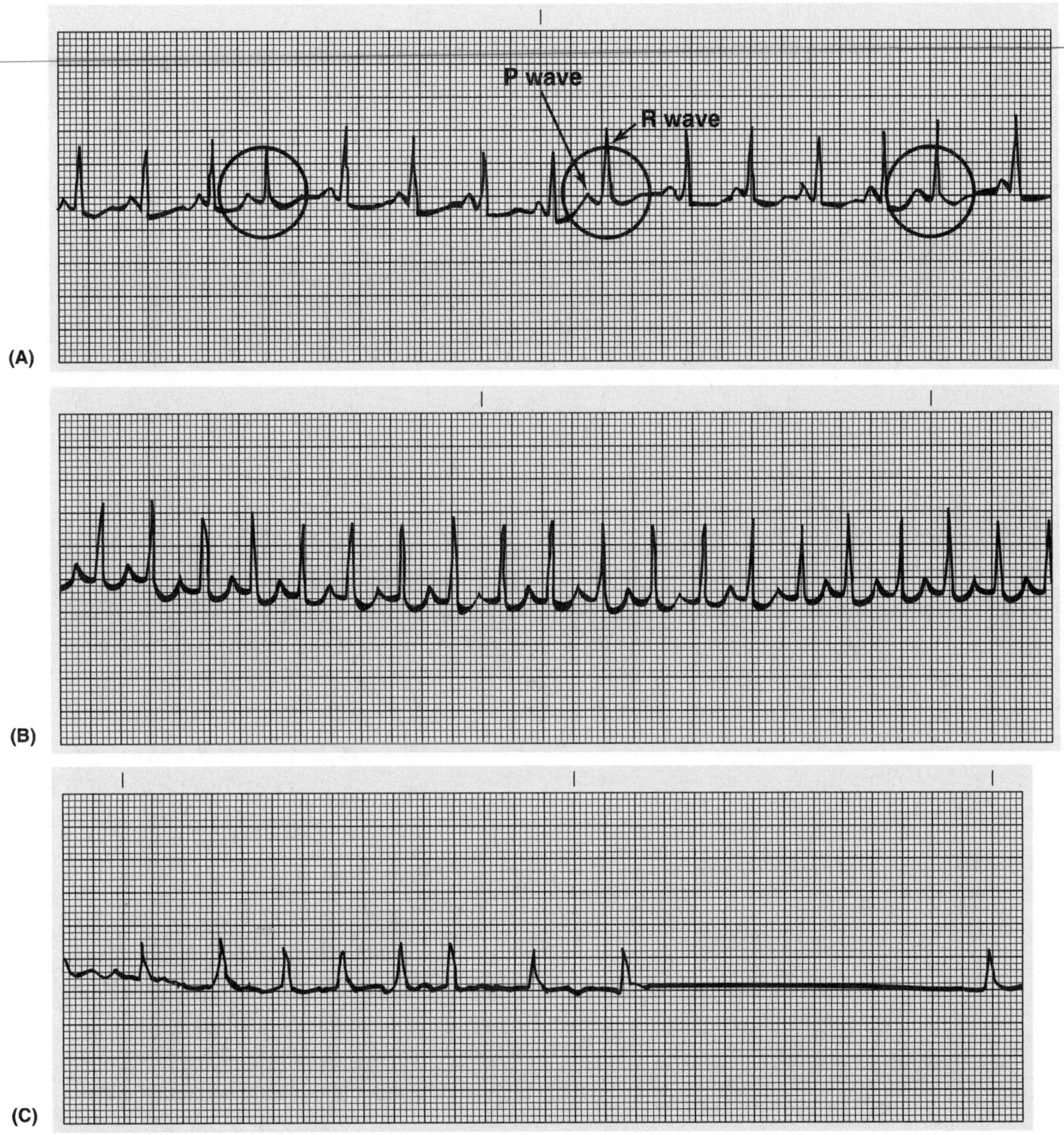

Figure 25-12 Atrial arrhythmias. (A) Premature atrial contractions. (B) Paroxysmal atrial tachycardia. (C) Atrial fibrillation.

fighters trained in defibrillation techniques and who are the first to respond in an emergency were primarily the individuals who used these devices. Now, many citizens are certified to use AEDs.

If an individual experiences a myocardial infarction, it is not uncommon for ventricular fibrillation to occur. If the fibrillation can be stopped within the first five minutes, using a defibrillator, the life can be saved. (See Chapter 9 for more about AEDs).

OTHER CARDIAC DIAGNOSTIC TESTS

Holter Monitor (Portable Ambulatory Electrocardiograph)

The Holter monitor is a portable continuous recording of cardiac activity for a 24-hour period (Figure 25-15). The patient is monitored while going about the usual daily activities with no restrictions. This **noninvasive** test

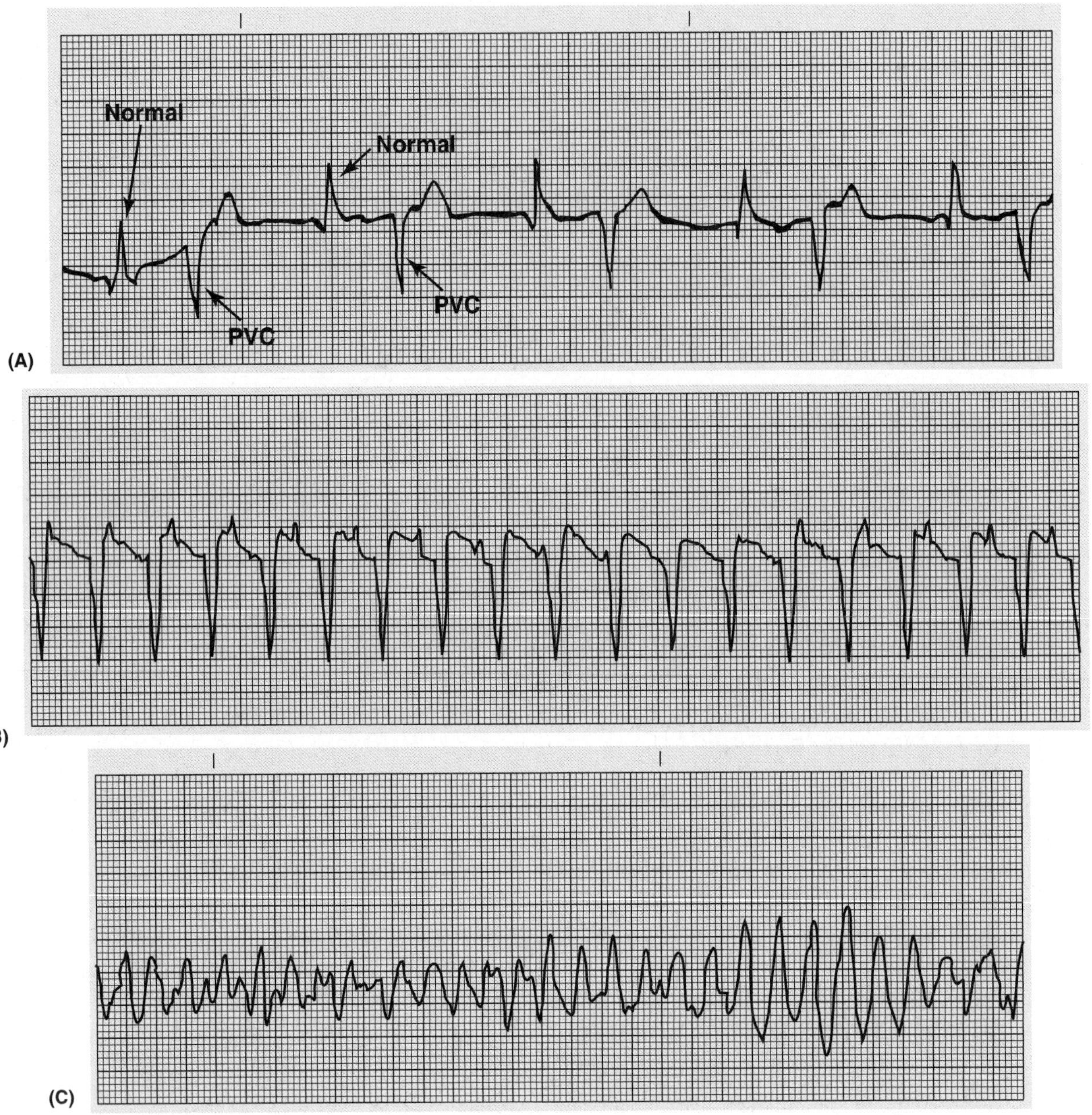

Figure 25-13 Ventricular arrhythmias. (A) Premature ventricular contractions (PVCs). (B) Ventricular tachycardia. (C) Ventricular fibrillation.

helps to diagnose cardiac arrhythmias by correlating them with the patient's symptoms. Some symptoms are **syncope,** fatigue, chest pain, and vertigo. This type of monitoring is useful for patients whose arrhythmias are sporadic in nature and whose arrhythmia is not able to be found on a 12-lead ECG tracing. Also, ambulatory monitoring helps assess the function of an artificial pacemaker and the effectiveness of antiarrhythmic medications.

Special electrodes attached to lead wires are placed in the appropriate areas of the patient's chest. A special portable tape recorder, computer or magnetic, will continually record the heart's electrical activity for a 24-hour period. The monitor is a battery-operated recorder that is placed in a leather pouch or bag and is worn by the patient either on a belt around the waist or by a strap over the patient's shoulder. See Table 25-2 for placement.

Other computerized continuous cardiac monitoring devices are available and are prescribed for patients according to the patient's symptoms and the practitioner's preference. The tracing can be read over the telephone or is computerized.

Some cardiac monitoring devices are sent directly to the patient from the supplier complete with printed or telephone directions for the patient. When the specific

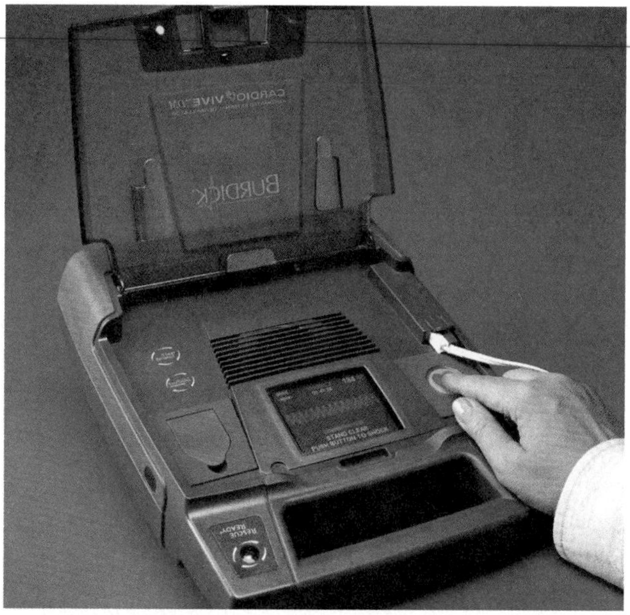

Figure 25-14 The CardioVive DM AED. (Courtesy of Quinton Cardiology, Inc.)

time period has elapsed for the particular monitor being used, the patient is responsible for returning the device to the supplier.

Medical Assistant's Role. The medical assistant is responsible for preparing the patient, instructing the patient, checking and replacing the battery, and applying and removing the monitor.

Holter Monitor Electrode Placement. Special disposable electrodes, which are round plastic and have a strong adhesive backing, are available for the Holter monitor. These disposable electrodes contain an electrolyte gel. There may be either four or five electrodes depending on whether the monitor has a built-in ground. Notice that the leads for the Holter monitor are applied to different locations than the electrodes of a resting ECG. Table 25-2 explains the lead placement.

Holter Monitor Attachment. Once the Holter monitor has been attached to the patient, the monitor should be

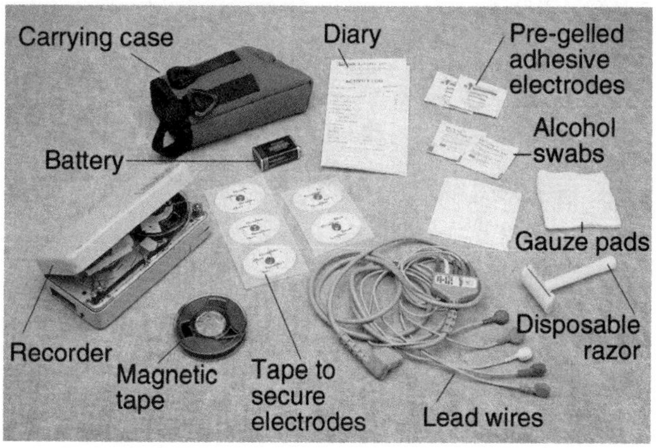

Figure 25-15 Holter monitor and supplies needed for application.

Patient Education

When preparing patients to wear a 24-hour Holter monitor instruct them in the following:

1. Keep a diary of daily activities, symptoms, and emotions, and note the time of occurrence.
2. Depress the event marker only briefly and when experiencing a significant symptom. Overuse of the marker can mask the ECG tracing.
3. Do not shower, bathe, or swim while wearing the monitor because the recording could be interrupted or the monitor could be damaged.
4. Do not handle the electrodes. Doing so could cause artifacts.
5. Do not remove the recorder from its case.
6. Do not use an electric blanket. This can cause interference.

TABLE 25-2 HOLTER MONITOR ELECTRODE PLACEMENT

Electrode	Lead	Location
A (black)	mV_1	Fourth intercostal space at right of the sternal edge
B (white)	mV_5	Right clavicle, just lateral to sternum
C (brown)	mV_1	Left clavicle, just lateral to the sternum
D (red)	mV_5	Fifth intercostal space at left axillary line
E (green)	Ground	Lower right chest wall

Following are examples of some of the daily activities that should be recorded by the patient in the patient activity diary:

- Eating meals
- Ascending and descending stairs
- Sexual activity
- Medications taken
- Times of sleep
- Smoking
- Bowel movements
- Physical exercise

checked for effectiveness by attaching the **test cable** to the monitor and the other end to an ECG instrument. A baseline strip can be recorded to verify the correct wave activity and lack of artifact. If there are inaccurate readings, the monitor may not have been applied properly. The medical assistant can reconnect the leads to the electrodes or reposition the electrodes and reconnect the leads (see Procedure 25-2). The skin should be cleaned with the alcohol and rubbed with gauze to roughen it. Males should be shaved so that the electrodes adhere well.

Patient Activity Diary. The patient activity diary is an important component of the monitoring procedures. As noted in the Patient Education box, all activities and emotional states, and the time of their occurrence, should be noted during the 24-hour monitoring time. Symptoms such as chest pain, shortness of breath, dizziness, palpitations, and so on, and the time the event occurred should also be noted. Patient symptoms recorded while being monitored can be compared with the patient's notations in the activity diary and correlated to the heart's activity. Symptoms can be further noted by the patient briefly depressing an event marker button located at one end of the monitor. This places an electronic "tag" on the tape. This signal can alert the person interpreting the ECG to look for a significant event or abnormality on the tape.

Holter Monitor Removal. The patient is instructed to return to the office or ambulatory care center 24 hours later to have the monitor removed. Usually no appointment is necessary. The tape is analyzed by a Holter monitor scanner or by a computer. This is usually done in the ECG department of a nearby hospital. The physician will receive a written report with samples of any abnormalities that were picked up during the monitoring period. A follow-up appointment is scheduled with the physician to discuss the results.

Critical Thinking

State three purposes for a Holter monitor to be used and give the instructions that the patient will need to know while wearing the monitor.

Treadmill Stress Test or Exercise Tolerance ECG

On occasion patients have symptoms of cardiac problems that do not appear as abnormalities on a resting ECG. The physician may prescribe a treadmill stress test or exercise tolerance test to aid in the determination of the patient's diagnosis and prognosis. The test is done to diagnose heart disorders, to diagnose the probable cause of the patient's chest pain, and to assess the patient's cardiac ability after cardiac surgery. The treadmill stress test is a noninvasive ECG tracing taken under controlled conditions while the patient is closely monitored by the medical assistant and the physician. Frequent blood pressure readings are taken. The patient wears comfortable clothing and flat shoes such as sneakers with rubber soles and exercises on a treadmill at prescribed rates of speed (Figure 25-16). Electrodes are applied to the chest only.

As with the Holter monitor, the patient's skin should be cleaned with alcohol and rubbed with gauze to

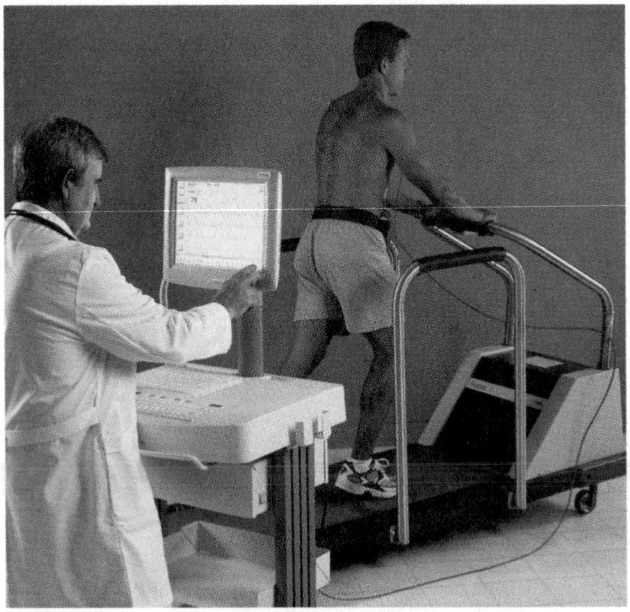

Figure 25-16 The Quest Exercise Stress System. (Courtesy of Quinton Cardiology, Inc.)

roughen it. Male patients should be shaved at the site of the electrodes to ensure electrode adherence.

The myocardium requires extra oxygen during exercise and in the presence of narrowed or obstructed coronary arteries; the additional workload on the myocardium will often be demonstrated as an abnormality on the ECG recording. There should be no pain, shortness of breath, or excess fatigue. If any of these or other unusual symptoms occur, the physician may terminate the test because this could indicate cardiac disease.

At the conclusion of the test, the patient is told to rest. Monitoring continues until the vital signs and heart rate return to normal. Prior to the patient leaving the office, the patient should be instructed to rest, refrain from a hot bath or shower, avoid stimulants such as caffeine, and avoid extreme temperature changes for several hours.

Complications such as a myocardial infarction or a serious arrhythmia can occur during testing. Although these events are unusual, appropriate emergency equipment must be readily available and the medical assistant should check them frequently for proper functioning. Some equipment to have on hand in a crash cart for cardiac emergencies include oxygen, antiarrhythmic drugs, an Ambu-bag™, a defibrillator, an airway, an endotracheal tube, and a laryngoscope. The medical assistant is responsible for checking the supplies and plugging in the defibrillator.

Further diagnostic tests such as **cardiac catheterization** may be necessary to diagnose the extent of the atherosclerosis buildup and obstruction of the coronary arteries.

Thallium Stress Test

Thallium stress test is similar to a treadmill stress test in that the patient has an ECG tracing while exercising on the treadmill after having been given an injection of a radioactive substance such as thallium. The thallium stress test is performed in the outpatient department of the hospital or in a cardiology office or clinic.

Echocardiography/Ultrasonography

Echocardiography is a noninvasive, diagnostic test that uses ultrasound (ultrahigh-frequency sound waves) to image the internal structures of the heart. X-rays are not useful. General anatomy, myocardial function, valve function, and heart chamber size can be evaluated. Echocardiography may be performed in a cardiologist's office.

During **ultrasonography,** a handheld **transducer** acts as a transmitter and receiver of the high-frequency sound waves as it is held against the chest wall and moved over the heart area. As the sound waves go through the skin and hit internal structures, echoes are sent back to the transducer. A machine converts the images when the various structures provide different echoes. The images can then be examined by a computer and converted into photographs and films of structures and blood flow.

There is little patient preparation other than to have the patient lie on the examination table with the four-limb leads of a 12-lead electrocardiograph attached. The test is usually performed by a **sonographer.** The physician will view the results later and inform the patient.

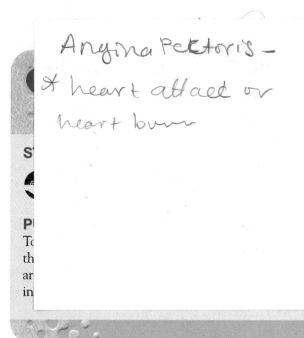

Angina Pektoris -
* heart attack or
heart burn

...erform Single-Channel ...r Multichannel Electrocardiogram

S...

P...
To ... of
th ... fy
ar ... al
in ... er-

mine if electrolyte imbalance is present, identify cardiac ischemia, and determine the effects of hypertension or other disorders on the heart.

EQUIPMENT/SUPPLIES:

Examination or ECG table with pillow and sheet or blanket
Patient gown (open in front)
Automated electrocardiograph with patient cable wires
Alligator clips

(continues)

Procedure 25-1 (continued)

Electropads (sensors)
ECG paper
Alcohol
Gauze squares
Mounting form/card
Razor

PROCEDURE STEPS:

1. Perform tracing in a quiet, warm, and comfortable room away from electrical equipment that may cause artifacts. RATIONALE: Patient is less apprehensive in a quiet atmosphere. AC interference is minimized when ECG is performed away from electrical equipment.
2. Wash hands, gather equipment, identify the patient, and explain the procedure to the patient. RATIONALE: Following these universal steps minimizes transmission of microorganisms and reassures patient.
3. Have the patient remove clothing from the waist up and uncover lower legs; nylon stockings must be removed; socks can be worn. RATIONALE: Electropads must be placed on bare skin for optimum conductivity of electricity. Provide a sheet or blanket for privacy and warmth. Place the patient in supine position on the examination table with arms and legs supported. Pillows may be used under the knees and head. RATIONALE: All four limbs and chest must be uncovered for proper electrode placement.
4. Explain that the procedure is painless and why it is necessary not to move or talk during the procedure. RATIONALE: Patient cooperation ensures good quality tracing.
5. Place the electrocardiograph with the power cord pointing away from the patient. Do not allow the cable to go underneath the table. RATIONALE: This helps reduce AC interference.
6. Apply the limb electropads (sensors) first. Apply the sensors to the fleshy parts of the four limbs. If the sensor does not adhere well, use an alcohol wipe on the skin, let it dry, and apply a new sensor. Shave sites if necessary. RATIONALE: Skin oils can be removed by alcohol, thus improving the adherence of the sensor. By removing excess hair on the chest, the sensor will adhere better. Place sensors on a nonbony, nonmuscular (fleshy) area of the upper arms and lower legs. Arm sensors should have tab pointing down, leg sensors point upward. RATIONALE: Artifact can be reduced if sensors are placed on nonbony, nonmuscular areas of the limbs. Directing tabs properly reduces tension on the electrodes.
7. Place the sensors on the chest wall on the appropriate intercostal spaces with sensors pointing downward. Shave chest sites if necessary.
8. Attach lead wires from the ECG machine to each sensor using alligator clips, special clips applied to the ends of the lead wires (Figure 25-17 A–C). Be sure to connect lead wires to the correct sensors. Lead wires are labeled with abbreviations (RA,

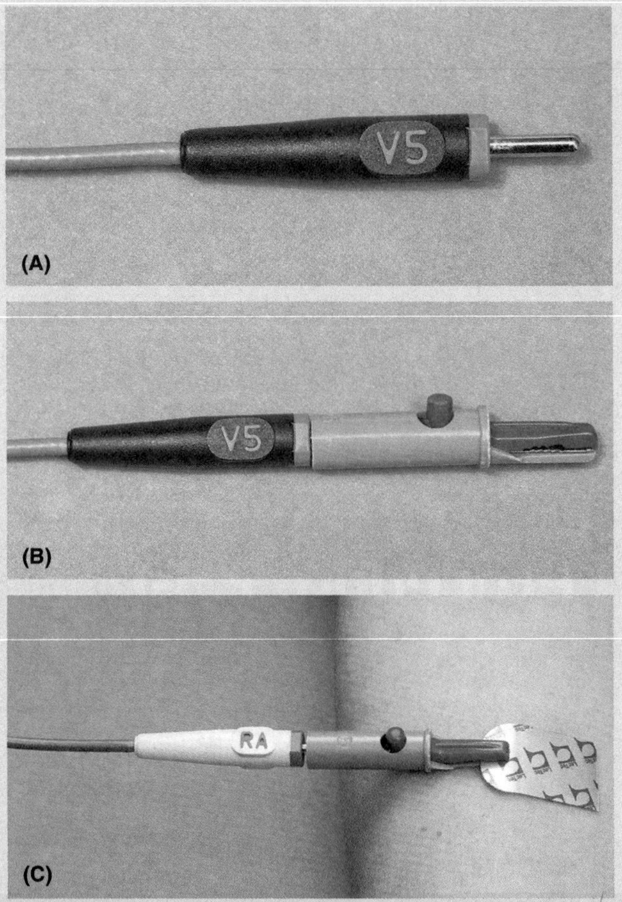

Figure 25-17 (A) Lead wires with nothing attached. (B) Alligator clip attached to top of lead wires. (C) Alligator clip attached to sensor on patient's arm.

(continues)

Procedure 25-1 (continued)

LA, RL, LL, and V or C) and are color-coded as follows: RA = white; LA = black; RL = green; LL = red, V or C = (chest) = brown or multicolored depending on machine model. The lead wires should follow the patient's body contour. RATIONALE: Following body contour prevents sensors from being pulled off.

9. The patient cable is supported either on the table or on the patient's abdomen. Plug the patient cable into the electrocardiograph.
10. Turn the instrument to ON.
11. Enter information (patient name, date of birth, age, height, weight, sex, identification number, and cardiac medications the patient is presently taking). RATIONALE: The ECG machine automatically prints the information entered onto the ECG printout.
12. Remind the patient not to talk and to try not to move. (If the patient has a neuromuscular condition such as Parkinson's disease and cannot remain still, try having the patient slide his or her hands under the buttocks.) RATIONALE: Somatic tremor artifact may be lessened when the patient's hands are slid under the buttocks.
13. Press AUTO and the machine will automatically record and standardize the tracing. RATIONALE: Standardization ensures a dependable and accurate ECG.
14. The single-channel machine prints each lead sequentially on a strip of ECG paper. A multichannel machine prints the tracing on an 8 1/2- × 11-inch sheet of paper.
15. Check the quality of the tracing (artifacts, low voltage) before disconnecting lead wires. If it is necessary to repeat the tracing, first correct the problem that is causing a poor quality tracing. RATIONALE: Checking the tracing before removing the electropad sensors will save your time if you must repeat the ECG.
16. Disconnect lead wires and remove the electropad sensor from the patient.
17. Assist patient as needed.
18. Be certain the patient information is on the tracing before giving it to the physician to read.
19. If the tracing is a single-channel tracing, cut and mount it remembering to handle carefully. Place in patient's record.
20. Document procedure.

DOCUMENTATION

4/19/20XX 2:00 PM Twelve-lead ECG completed. Tracing given to Dr. Woo. Patient cooperative and seemed comfortable throughout procedure and says she "feels fine" after tracing. W. Slawson, CMA

Procedure 25-2 Perform Holter Monitor Application

STANDARD PRECAUTIONS:

PURPOSE:

To detect sporadic cardiac arrhythmias, to determine correlation of symptoms with activity, and to evaluate chest pain and cardiac status after pacemaker implantation or after acute myocardial infarction.

EQUIPMENT/SUPPLIES:

Holter monitor	Alcohol swabs
Patient activity diary	Gauze
Blank magnetic tape	Carrying case
Disposable electrodes	Belt or shoulder strap
Razor	

PROCEDURE STEPS:

1. Wash hands and assemble equipment.
2. Prepare the equipment by removing old (used) battery from the monitor and replacing it with a new battery. Insert a blank magnetic tape into the monitor. RATIONALE: Installing a new battery each 24-hour period will ensure the monitor will function because it will have sufficient power.
3. Wash hands.
4. Identify the patient and explain the procedure. RATIONALE: Adherence to patient guidelines helps ensure an accurate tracing.
5. Have patient remove clothing from the waist up.
6. Have patient sit on the examination table or chair. RATIONALE: This allows for patient comfort and relaxation and for the medical assistant to place the electrodes appropriately.
7. Locate the correct electrode placement sites. The skin must be prepared in the following way:
   a. Dry shave patient's chest at each electrode site if chest is hairy.
   b. Rub the shaved area with alcohol. Let area dry.
   c. Abrade the skin slightly with a dry 4 × 4 gauze. Areas should be red. RATIONALE: Shaved site and abraded skin help the electrodes to adhere better to the skin and facilitate easier removal.
8. Take the electrodes from the package and peel away the backing from one of them (electrode should be moist). Continue to remove electrodes one by one and attach as in Step 9.
9. Apply adhesive-backed electrode to the appropriate sites by applying firm pressure at the center of the electrode and moving outward toward the edges. Starting at the center of the electrode, apply pressure firmly and move outward on the electrode. Run your fingers along the outer rim to ensure firm attachment. Avoid moving from one side of electrode to the other. Gel could be forced out and could cause interference. RATIONALE: Firmly attached electrodes ensure a good quality tracing.
10. Attach the lead wires to the electrodes. Connect them to the patient cable.

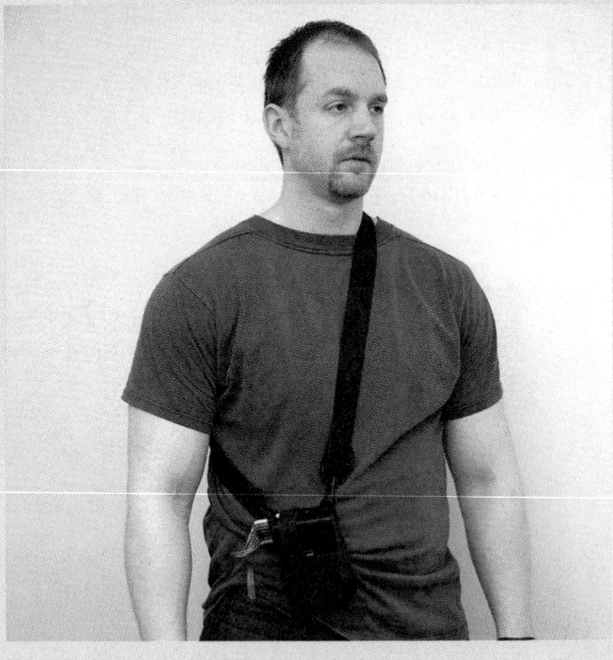

Figure 25-18 Holter monitor in its carrying case and secured by a shoulder strap. The monitor can also be attached to a belt and worn around the patient's waist.

(continues)

Procedure 25-2 (continued)

11. Plug the monitor into an electrocardiograph with the test cable. Run a baseline tracing. RATIONALE: Running a baseline tracing will validate proper setup of electrodes and confirm there is no malfunction of the leads or cable.
12. Place the electrode cable so that it extends from between the buttons of the patient's shirt or from below the bottom of the shirt.
13. Place the recorder into its carrying case and either attach it to the patient's belt or over the patient's shoulder. Be certain there is no pulling on the lead wires (Figure 25-18). RATIONALE: Pulling on electrodes could cause them to become detached.
14. Plug the electrode cable into the monitor. Record the starting time in the patient activity log (diary). RATIONALE: The beginning time is noted to correlate cardiac activity with the patient activity log.
15. Give the activity log to the patient, being certain that the patient information is completed. RATIONALE: The activity log helps correlate cardiac activity with patient symptoms.
16. Inform patient what time the following day the monitor will be removed. Remind the patient to bring along the activity log/diary.
18. Wash hands.
19. Document procedure in the patient's record.

DOCUMENTATION

3/2/20XX 10:00 AM Holter monitor applied. Patient given complete written instructions and restrictions and seems to understand them well. Time and date noted on activity log. Patient reminded to return to cardiac clinic at the same time tomorrow (10:15 AM) to have monitor removed and also to bring the activity diary. Patient given after-hours number if he needs assistance. J. Guerro, CMA

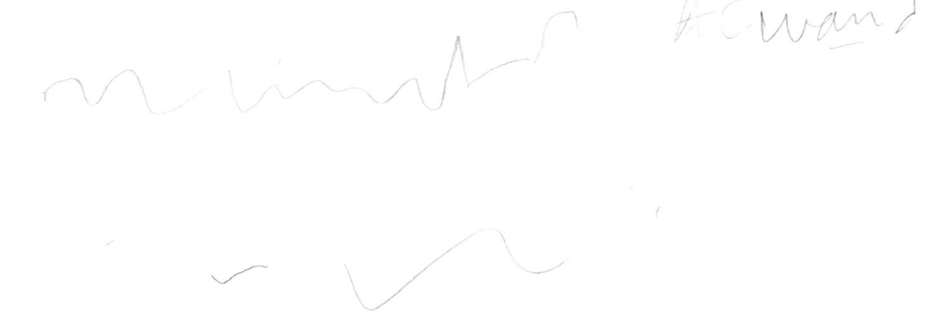

Case Study 25-1

Abigail Johnson, who is in her mid-70s, arrives at the urgent care center reporting chest pain. She has been seen on two other occasions for similar pain and has a history of diabetes, hypertension, arteriosclerotic heart disease, and angina pectoris. Medical assistant Wanda Slawson immediately alerts Dr. Rice of Mrs. Johnson's chest pain, and then takes her into the cardiac examination and treatment room. Dr. Rice tells Wanda to have Mrs. Johnson take one of her nitroglycerin tablets and to perform an ECG on her. Mrs. Johnson is restless and anxious as Wanda prepares for the ECG and while the tracing is in progress. There is significant somatic tremor. Wanda attempts to allay Mrs. Johnson's apprehension to obtain a good quality ECG. The patient's pain subsides within a few minutes and she begins to feel better.

CASE STUDY REVIEW

1. What immediate action could Wanda have taken if Mrs. Johnson's pain had not subsided?
2. Mrs. Johnson tells Wanda that Dr. Rice explained arteriosclerotic heart disease and angina pectoris to her, but that she was nervous and understood little and that she is embarrassed to admit that to Dr. Rice. How can Wanda explain, in language that the patient can comprehend, what causes arteriosclerotic heart disease and angina, and what Mrs. Johnson experiences during an attack of angina? What strategies can Wanda teach Mrs. Johnson to promote healthier habits and prevent more serious heart problems?
3. Research community resources are available for persons with Mrs. Johnson's heart condition. Explain how Mrs. Johnson could benefit from them.

Case Study 25-2

George Matthews, a 79-year-old patient of Dr. Abbott, has a history of cardiovascular heart disease. He tells Dr. Abbott that today he has been experiencing "palpitations and slow and fast heartbeats and sometimes dizziness." Dr. Abbott orders a resting ECG that shows no evidence of arrhythmia and decides that a Holter monitor electrocardiograph for Mr. Matthews might be helpful in diagnosing a cardiac arrhythmia.

CASE STUDY REVIEW

1. Describe why Dr. Abbott ordered a Holter monitor electrocardiography for Mr. Matthews.
2. What instructions will you give to Mr. Matthews about wearing the monitor?
3. Mr. Matthews says he is not certain what activities should be recorded in the patient activity diary. Explain what they are and the reason for their importance.

SUMMARY

Electrocardiography is a noninvasive, painless procedure that is helpful in diagnosing heart arrhythmias, ischemia, and effects of cardiac medications. Wires with sensors are attached to the patient's arms, legs, and chest. The electrocardiograph amplifies the electrical currents generated by the electrical cells of the heart. A series of deflections (waves) is recorded on special ECG paper when a heated stylus on the electrocardiograph moves across the paper. The cardiac cycles that appear are then interpreted by the physician. The recording or tracing, known as an ECG, represents the heart's rate, rhythm, and other myocardial actions. Each of the 12 leads of the recording becomes part of the patient's permanent record.

In addition to a resting ECG, other types of electrocardiography can be done. Cardiac stress testing is done while the patient is physically challenged to perform increasingly strenuous exercises. The heart's tolerance to the increased demands placed on it during exercise can be observed and recorded while the patient is being closely monitored. This type of electrocardiography helps determine cardiac health and arrhythmias that would not be evident if a resting ECG were done.

Holter electrocardiography or ambulatory cardiac monitoring is an ECG test done as the patient goes about normal daily activities. The patient wears chest leads and carries a small recording device on a belt or on a strap over the shoulder for a period of 24 hours and documents activities in the patient activity diary. This type of electrocardiography helps diagnose cardiac arrhythmias that occur sporadically and may be difficult to capture on a resting ECG because of their unpredictability. Echocardiography is a diagnostic test that uses ultrasound to image the internal structures of the heart. Myocardial function, valvular function or defects, and chamber size can be determined.

In most instances, the medical assistant is responsible for patient preparation, patient education, operation of the electrocardiograph, elimination of artifacts, mounting, labeling, and placing ECG readings into the patient's file, and maintenance and care of the equipment. The diagnostic value of the test depends on the medical assistant's accuracy and skill.

STUDY FOR SUCCESS

To reinforce your knowledge and skills of information presented in this chapter:

- ❑ Review the Key Terms
- ❑ Practice the Procedures
- ❑ Consider the Case Studies and discuss your conclusions
- ❑ Answer the Review Questions
  - ❑ Multiple Choice
  - ❑ Critical Thinking
- ❑ Navigate the Internet by completing the Web Activities
- ❑ Practice the StudyWARE activities on your student CD
- ❑ Apply your knowledge in the Student Workbook activities
- ❑ Complete the Web Tutor sections
- ❑ View and discuss the DVD situations

REVIEW QUESTIONS

Multiple Choice

1. Which of the following is the most common type of artifact?
   a. somatic tremor
   b. AC interference
   c. wandering baseline
   d. interrupted baseline
2. Which of the following may cause somatic tremor?
   a. too much electrolyte
   b. cable across patient's lap
   c. corroded sensors
   d. Parkinson's disease
3. One cardiac cycle (heartbeat) takes approximately how long?
   a. 0.2 second
   b. 0.4 second
   c. 0.6 second
   d. 0.8 second
4. Which of the following indicates ventricular depolarization?
   a. QRS complex
   b. P wave
   c. T wave
   d. S-T segment
5. Another name for V leads is:
   a. precordial
   b. augmented
   c. standard
   d. limb

Critical Thinking

1. The physician wants you to explain to Mrs. Johnson (see Case Study 1) what behaviors she can adopt to have a healthy heart. With a partner, role-play medical assistant and patient and explain to the patient what she can do to improve her heart's health.
2. During the ECG, the equipment malfunctions. What options are available to the medical assistant?
3. Name four cardiac abnormalities that can be detected on an ECG.
4. Identify the placement of the 12 leads of the ECG.
5. The patient coughs and moves during the ECG. How can this affect the ECG tracing?
6. Explain standardization and why it is important.
7. What causes AC interference, wandering baseline, and interrupted baseline and how can they be eliminated?

WEB ACTIVITIES

Search on the Internet for a national organization that focuses on heart and blood vessel disorders such as the American Heart Association or American College of Cardiology.

1. Print information about risk factors for cardiovascular heart disease.
2. What is the mortality rate for first-time myocardial infarctions for men versus women? Is there any difference in the mortality rate?
3. Are the symptoms identical in male and female patients when they are experiencing a myocardial infarction? Explain the similarities/differences between them.
4. Determine if there are newer types of 24-hour cardiac monitoring devices. How are they the same as or different from the Holter monitor?

REFERENCES/BIBLIOGRAPHY

Delaune, S. C., & Ladner, P. (2002). *Fundamentals of nursing standards and practice* (2nd ed.). Clifton Park, NY: Thomson Delmar Learning.

Passanisi, C. (2001). *Electrocardiology essentials*. Clifton Park, NY: Thomson Delmar Learning.

Taber's cyclopedic medical dictionary. (20th ed.). (2005). Philadelphia: FA Davis.

THE DVD HOOK-UP

DVD Series
Skills Based Series

Program Number
13

Chapter/Scene Reference
- *Entire program*

This chapter discusses the proper techniques for performing electrocardiographic procedures.

In the first scene, the student extern prepared Mr. Byrne for his ECG. Typically, men do not wear gowns when exposing only the chest. Mr. Byrne, however, has a little more breast tissue than most men.

1. Do you think that the extern should have offered him a gown for modesty purposes?

Things do not always go as planned. In the majority of cases, the patient is placed in a supine position for an ECG. In today's program, the patient was unable to lie down for the ECG because of a neck and back injury.

1. What are some other obstacles that may interfere with the way you would normally attach or run an ECG?

DVD Journal Summary
Write a paragraph that summarizes what you learned from watching today's DVD program. What steps could you take to help a patient relax who is anxious about having an ECG?

UNIT 7
Laboratory Procedures

CHAPTER 26

Safety and Regulatory Guidelines in the Medical Laboratory

OUTLINE

Clinical Laboratory Improvement Amendments of 1988
- The Intention of CLIA '88
- General Program Description
- Categories of Testing
- Contents of the Law
- CLIA '88 Regulation for Quality Control in Automated Hematology
- Aftermath of CLIA '88
- Impact of CLIA on Medical Assistants
- Where to Find More Information Regarding CLIA '88

OSHA Regulations
- The Standard for Occupational Exposure to Hazardous Chemicals in the Laboratory
- Chemical Hygiene Plan

OSHA Regulations and Students
- Avoiding Exposure to Chemicals

Cumulative Trauma Disorders

OBJECTIVES

The student should strive to meet the following performance objectives and demonstrate an understanding of the facts and principles presented in this chapter through written and oral communication.

1. Define the key terms as presented in the glossary.
2. Identify the governmental agency that regulates procedures performed on patients, and describe the agency's main concerns.
3. List the types of human specimens that CLIA regulates.
4. Name two performance requirements CLIA imposes on all laboratories.
5. Describe how CLIA '88 regulates the use of quality control in automated hematology instruments.
6. Recall the three categories of testing and list several from the waived category.

(continues)

KEY TERMS

- Acetone
- Aegis
- Body Fluid
- Calibration
- Chemotherapeutic Agents
- Communicable
- Ethyl Alcohol
- Excretion
- Federal Register
- Forensic
- Formaldehyde
- Fume Hood
- Mandate
- Medical Asepsis
- Microscopy
- Proficiency Testing
- Provider Performed Microscopy (PPM)
- Pulmonary Edema
- Quality Assurance
- Quality Control
- Reimbursement
- Requisition
- Secretion
- Suppressed Immune System
- Waived

FEATURED COMPETENCIES

CAAHEP—ENTRY-LEVEL COMPETENCIES

Clinical Competencies

Fundamental procedures

- Dispose of biohazard materials
- Practice Standard Precautions

Legal Concepts

- Perform within legal and ethical boundaries
- Document appropriately

Operational Functions

- Use methods of quality control

ABHES—ENTRY-LEVEL COMPETENCIES

Clinical Duties

- Apply principles of aseptic techniques and infection control
- Recognize emergencies
- Use quality control
- Dispose of biohazard materials
- Practice Standard Precautions

Legal Concepts

- Determine needs for documentation and reporting
- Document accurately
- Maintain licenses and accreditation
- Monitor legislation related to current healthcare issues and practices
- Perform risk management procedures

Office Management

- Evaluate and recommend equipment and supplies for practice

Instruction

- Orient and train personnel

OBJECTIVES (continued)

7. Discuss the importance of CLIA to the medical assistant.
8. Identify and discuss the contents of the law of CLIA '88.
9. Describe HCFA form 116 and explain its purpose.
10. Identify two OSHA standards that seek to safeguard employees.
11. Describe MSDS manuals and their purpose. Differentiate among the four colors and five numbers of the National Fire Protection Association

SCENARIO

At Inner City Health Care, Dr. Susan Rice ordered a complete urinalysis for patient May Pankey. Dr. Rice's medical assistant, Wanda Slawson, CMA, has obtained the specimen from the patient and performed the physical examination and the chemical examination of the urine and has documented her findings on the lab report form. She has also spun a test tube of urine in the centrifuge and has prepared a slide of the sediment for Dr. Rice to examine under the microscope. While Wanda is waiting for the doctor, she examines the slide to see if she can identify any abnormalities. She will compare her findings with Dr. Rice's findings to see how closely she comes to correctly identifying the cellular components in the urine sediment. This is one way for Wanda to continue her education on a daily basis while performing her clinical duties.

INTRODUCTION

Laboratory safety is a concern for all—management, staff, and patients. An unsafe work environment and work practices can threaten the emotional and physical health of the health care worker, as well as the patient. Injuries are costly on many levels: personally to the injured individual, lost work days, workers' compensation, medical treatment, potential legal action, and potential fines from regulatory agencies. These situations have a direct effect on the individuals involved, but they also have an indirect effect by lowering staff morale, ultimately resulting in less productivity. Management's response to safety is the key. Appropriate orientation, annual reviews, periodic drills, and consistent enforcement of staff adherence to policy are all part of a successful laboratory safety program.

All health care providers continually come into contact with patients who are ill. Some patients have ***communicable*** *or contagious diseases; others may have a* ***suppressed immune system*** *that does not protect them from infection. In the course of performing your duties as a medical assistant, you will be in contact with blood and* ***body fluids*** *that may be highly infectious. It is of extreme importance that your health and safety, as well as the health and safety of your patients, be protected.*

There are a number of infection control measures that can be used to reduce the transmission of bloodborne and other pathogens. ***Medical asepsis,*** *also known as infection control, consists of procedures and practices that health care professionals use to prevent the spread of infection (see Chapter 10). State and federal agencies also have established policies, procedures, and guidelines for health care providers and employers to follow to reduce the risk for transmission of infectious diseases. This chapter, as well as Chapter 10, examines the major guidelines.*

The Centers for Disease Control and Prevention (CDC) in Atlanta, Georgia, a division of the United States Public Health Department, is an agency that investigates various diseases in an attempt to control them and makes recommendations on how to prevent the spread of disease. The CDC issued the system of seven isolation categories for patients with infectious diseases; it recommended the guidelines known as Universal Precautions; and, in 1996, it released Standard Precautions, which represent the most current and comprehensive approach to infection control. The CDC Guidelines for Standard Precautions and Universal Precautions are covered thoroughly in Chapter 10. This chapter focuses on the federal regulations of the Clinical Laboratory Improvement Amendments of 1988 (CLIA '88) and the Occupational Safety and Health Administration (OSHA) in relation to the physicians' office laboratory (POL).

CLIA '88 and OSHA, together with the CDC, regulate the safety of patients and health care workers. CLIA '88 comes under the ***aegis,*** *or protection, of the Health Care Financing Administration (HCFA) of the U.S. Department of Health and Human Services (DHHS) of the federal government. OSHA comes under the U.S. Department of Labor. Both agencies require that health care settings, including clinical laboratories, adhere to the strict regulations that they set forth.*

The purpose of CLIA '88 is to safeguard the public by regulating all testing of specimens taken from the human body. The purpose of OSHA is to require employers to ensure employee safety in regard to occupational exposure to potentially harmful substances.

CLIA '88 and OSHA guidelines are discussed separately in this chapter. Keep in mind as you go through this chapter that CLIA '88 is designed to protect patients and OSHA regulations are designed to protect workers. Table 26-1 summarizes the guidelines and purposes of CDC, CLIA '88, and OSHA.

CLINICAL LABORATORY IMPROVEMENT AMENDMENTS OF 1988

CLIA '88 was designed to set safety policies and procedures that protect patients.

In 1988, there was a public outcry as a result of articles published in the *Washington Post* and the *Wall Street Journal* and televised reports of deaths that were

Spotlight on Certification

RMA Content Outline
- Medical law
- Asepsis
- Laboratory procedures (safety)
- First aid

CMA Content Outline
- Medicolegal guidelines & requirements
- Principles of infection control
- Processing specimens
- Quality control
- Preplanned action

CMAS Content Outline
- Legal and Ethical Considerations
- Asepsis in the Medical Office
- Medical Office Emergencies
- Safety
- Supplies and Equipment

TABLE 26-1 FEDERAL HEALTH AND SAFETY GUIDELINES

Guidelines	Issuing Agency	Purpose
Standard Precautions	Centers for Disease Control and Prevention (CDC), U.S. Public Health Department, Atlanta, Georgia	Issued in 1996 to augment and synthesize Universal Precautions and techniques known as body substance isolation (BSI). Standard Precautions contain measures intended to protect all health care providers, patients, and visitors from infectious diseases.
Transmission-based Precautions	CDC	Designed to reduce the risk for airborne, droplet, and contact transmission of pathogens. These are used in addition to Standard Precautions and are intended for specific categories of patients.
Universal Blood and Body Fluid Precautions (Universal Precautions)	CDC	Released in 1985 to assist health care providers to greatly reduce the risk for contracting or transmitting infectious diseases, particularly AIDS and hepatitis B.
Clinical Laboratory Improvement Amendments of 1988 (CLIA '88)	Health Care Financing Administration (HCFA), U.S. Department of Health and Human Services (DHHS)	Safeguards the public by regulating all testing of specimens taken from the body
Occupational Safety and Health Administration (OSHA) Guidelines	OSHA, U.S. Department of Labor	Requires employers to ensure employee safety in regard to occupational exposure to potentially harmful substances

TABLE 26-2 APPROVED ACCREDITING ORGANIZATIONS UNDER CLINICAL LABORATORY IMPROVEMENT AMENDMENTS OF 1988

American Association of Blood Banks
8101 Glenbrook Road
Bethesda, MD 20814-2749
Government Relations
(301) 907-6977

American Osteopathic Association
142 East Ontario Street
Chicago, IL 60611
(312) 202-8070

American Society of Histocompatibility and Immunogenetics
17000 Commerce Parkway, Suite C
Mt. Laurel, NJ 08054
(856) 642-4415

College of American Pathologists
325 Waukegan Road
Northfield, IL 60093-2750
Laboratory Accreditation Program
(800) 323-4040

Commission on Office Laboratory Accreditation (COLA)
9881 Broken Land Parkway, Suite 200
Columbia, MD 21046-1195
(410) 381-6581

Joint Commission on Accreditation of Healthcare Organizations
One Renaissance Boulevard
Oakbrook Terrace, IL 60181
(630) 792-5000

Revised June, 2005.

attributed to misread Pap smears. The public wanted action taken to ensure its safety, particularly in regard to laboratory testing. The outcry prompted the federal government to become more involved in regulating laboratories.

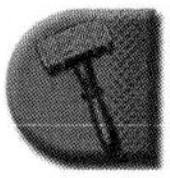

Although CLIA had been enacted into law in 1967, the issue of the misread Pap smears caused Congress to reexamine the regulations it had set forth in 1967. Thus, CLIA '88 was passed and included amendments to the original law. The amended regulations took effect on September 1, 1992.

States can seek exemptions from the CLIA standards if they have regulations that are comparable to those imposed by CLIA. If the federal government grants the state an exemption, laboratories in these states are under the control of state standards and applicable fees, not federal standards and fees. As of July 2002, only Washington and New York have Exempt State Status.

Some accrediting bodies have revised their rules in an effort to meet HCFA's CLIA '88 requirements. HCFA can then give deemed status (equivalency) to these accrediting bodies. Laboratories accredited by these deemed status bodies are considered to meet HCFA's requirements. To date, HCFA has granted deemed status to the organizations listed in Table 26-2.

The Intention of CLIA '88

The intent of CLIA '88 is to protect the public by regulating all laboratory tests performed on specimens taken from the human body; that is, blood and body **secre-**

tions and **excretions.** The specimens are those used in the diagnosis, treatment, and prevention of disease. Previous regulations (Medicare, Medicaid, and CLIA '67) were based on the site and scope of the laboratory testing. CLIA '88 regulates laboratory testing regardless of site, scope, volume, or frequency. As of July 2000, registered CLIA laboratories total more than 145,000 with physicians' office laboratories making up more than 65% of the total. The regulations require that all laboratories in the United States and its territories meet performance requirements that are based on how complex a test is and the risk factors that are associated with incorrect test results. Laboratories must comply with the requirements to be certified by the DHHS. The following laboratories are exempt from the regulations: laboratories that perform only tests for **forensic,** or legal, purposes; research laboratories that do not produce results used in patient treatment; facilities certified by the National Institute on Drug Abuse to perform only urine drug testing; and states, territories, and municipalities with licensure. (Currently, California, Florida, Georgia, Hawaii, Nevada, North Dakota, Rhode Island, Tennessee, Virginia, the Commonwealth of Puerto Rico, and the municipality of New York City are licensed.)

It is necessary to understand what the CLIA '88 regulations encompass and how they impact medical assistants and other health care workers who participate in testing human specimens. It is important because all laboratories, including POLs, must abide by the CLIA law.

CLIA '88 regulations are based on the complexity of tests performed and they affect all aspects of the laboratory. They specify the type of test performed, personnel involved in testing, and **quality control.**

General Program Description

Congress passed CLIA in 1988, establishing quality standards for all laboratory testing to ensure the accuracy, reliability, and timeliness of patient test results regardless of where the test was performed. A laboratory is defined as any facility that performs laboratory testing on specimens derived from humans for the purpose of providing information for the diagnosis, prevention, or treatment of disease, or impairment or assessment of health. CLIA is user-fee funded; therefore, all costs of administering the program must be covered by the regulated facilities.

The final CLIA regulations were published on February 28, 1992, and are based on the complexity of the test method; thus, the more complicated the test, the more stringent the requirements. Three categories of tests have been established: waived; moderate complexity, including the subcategory of **provider-performed microscopy** (PPM); and high complexity. CLIA specifies quality standards for proficiency testing (PT), patient test management, quality control, personnel qualifications, and quality assurance as applicable. Because problems in cytology laboratories were the impetus for CLIA, there are also specific cytology requirements.

The HCFA is charged with the implementation of CLIA, including laboratory registration, fee collection, surveys, surveyor guidelines and training, enforcement, approvals of PT providers, accrediting organizations, and exempt states. The CDC is responsible for test categorization and CLIA studies.

To enroll in the CLIA program, laboratories must first register by completing an application, pay fees, be surveyed if applicable, and become certified. CLIA fees are based on the certificate requested by the laboratory (i.e., waived, PPM, accreditation, or compliance) and the annual volume and types of testing performed (Table 26-3). Waived and PPM laboratories may apply directly for their certificate because they are not subject to routine inspections. Those laboratories that must be surveyed routinely—that is, those performing moderate- or high-complexity testing—can choose whether they wish to be surveyed by HCFA or by a private accrediting organization. The HCFA survey process is outcome-oriented and uses a quality assurance focus and an educational approach to assess compliance.

Data indicate that CLIA has helped to improve the quality of testing in the United States. The total number of quality deficiencies has decreased approximately 40% from the first laboratory survey to the second. Similar findings were demonstrated in the review of PT data. The educational value of PT in laboratories was known before CLIA existed. Initial PT failures are also addressed with an educational, rather than punitive, approach by CLIA.

Work is currently in progress with the CDC and HCFA to develop a final CLIA rule that will reflect all comments received and new technologies.

TABLE 26-3 CLINICAL LABORATORY IMPROVEMENT AMENDMENTS FEES ARE BASED ON VOLUME (AS OF AUGUST 2004)

Fee Category	Volume	Fee
Waived	NA	$150
PPM	NA	$200
Low volume A	Less than 2,000 tests	$150
Schedule A	2,000–10,000 tests	$150
Schedules B–J	10,000–1,000,000 tests	$200 to $7,940

NA, not applicable; PPM, provider-performed microscopy.

Categories of Testing

CLIA '88 is under the aegis of the HCFA of the DHHS. HCFA has designated three categories of testing:

1. Waived tests
2. Moderate-complexity tests, including PPM
3. High-complexity tests

Each of these categories has different requirements for personnel and quality control.

Waived tests are simple, unvarying, and require a minimum of judgment and interpretation. Test error carries minimal hazard to the patient. Waived tests represent the lowest percentage of the total number of tests performed (Table 26-4).

PPM tests are moderate-complexity tests but represent a subcategory that was added at the request of physicians.

To categorize moderate- and high-complexity tests, the following criteria are used:

- The degree of operator intervention needed
- The necessary knowledge and experience the operator possesses
- The degree of maintenance and troubleshooting needed to perform the tests

Even though most of the tests medical assistants perform fall into the waived category, POLs will often perform moderate tests, including the PPM tests. POLs are not limited to any category as long as they have sufficiently trained and credentialed personnel, equipment, and approval.

The waived list in Table 26-4 is a general list. Every manufacturer of the self-contained test kits has applied for and received Food and Drug Administration (FDA) approval for their particular test to be on the CLIA waived list. To find out if your particular brand of a self-contained test kit is on the CLIA waived list, you can view an entire up-to-date listing at the FDA Web site http://www.fda.gov (be forewarned, though, the list is very long). You can obtain a list of categories and the complete CLIA'88 guidelines from the **Federal Register** or from the CDC Web site (http://www.phppo.cdc.gov; use key term "CLIA").

Contents of the Law

1. All laboratories are required to register with CLIA '88 even if just one test is performed, regardless of whether there is Medicare and Medicaid **reimbursement** and regardless in which of the categories the test is found.
2. The regulations apply to all laboratories.
3. The regulations are specific to the complexity of the test. The waived tests are the simplest with the least

TABLE 26-4 LIST OF ANALYTES CURRENTLY ON THE CLINICAL LABORATORY IMPROVEMENT AMENDMENTS OF 1988 WAIVED LIST

Amines	Gastric occult blood	Opiates	Urine qualitative dipstick ketone
Amphetamines	Glucose or glucose monitoring device	Ovulation test by visual color comparison	Urine qualitative dipstick leukocytes
Bladder tumor-associated antigen	Glycosylated hemoglobin (HbA1C)	Phencyclidine (PCP)	Urine qualitative dipstick nitrite
Cannabinoids (THC)	hCG, urine	Prothrombin time	Urine qualitative dipstick pH
Catalase, urine	*Helicobacter pylori* antibodies	Spun microhematocrit	Urine qualitative dipstick protein
Cholesterol, high-density lipoprotein	*Helicobacter pylori* (bacteriology)	Streptococcus group A	Urine qualitative dipstick specific gravity
Cholesterol, total	Hematocrit	Triglyceride	Urine qualitative dipstick urobilinogen
Cocaine metabolites	Hemoglobin	Urine dipstick or tablet analytes, nonautomated	Vaginal pH
Creatinine	Infectious mononucleosis antibodies	Urine qualitative dipstick bilirubin	
Erythrocyte sedimentation rate	Ketones, blood	Urine qualitative dipstick blood and hemoglobin	
Ethanol	Methamphetamines	Urine qualitative dipstick glucose	
Fecal occult blood	Microalbumin		
Fructosamine	Nicotine and metabolites		

Source: Clara Sliva, Acting CLIA Coordinator

Note: Tests waived by Food and Drug Administration; Centers for Disease Control and Prevention (CDC) through August, 2004. There are more than 500 Test Systems (products) approved for the analytes listed above. For an up-to-date list, visit the CDC Web site at: http://www.phppo.cdc.gov

amount of regulations. Standards become more stringent as the complexity of the test increases.

4. A laboratory must obtain a certificate to perform tests. An initial filing for a certificate is made on form 116 with HCFA of the DHHS. One of five certificates can be obtained. (There can be a state exemption as previously mentioned.)
   a. *Certificate of Waiver*. This certificate is issued to a laboratory to perform only waived tests.
   b. *Certificate for PPM Procedures*. This certificate is issued to a laboratory in which a physician, midlevel practitioner, or dentist performs no moderate complexity tests other than the PPM procedures (Table 26-5). This certificate permits the laboratory to also perform waived tests.
   c. *Certificate of Registration*. This certificate enables the entity to conduct moderate- and high-complexity laboratory testing until the entity is determined by survey to be in compliance with CLIA regulations.
   d. *Certificate of Compliance*. This certificate is issued to a laboratory after an inspection finds the laboratory to be in compliance with all applicable CLIA requirements.
   e. *Certificate of Accreditation*. This is a certificate that is issued to a laboratory on the basis of the laboratory's accreditation by an organization approved by HCFA.

   To date, more than 150,000 CLIA certifications have been issued, more than half being Certificates of Waiver or PPM.
5. All five certificates require renewal every two years.
6. After a laboratory has been certified, it must notify HCFA within six months if it changes the type of tests it performs. Changing the tests performed may change the laboratory's classification.

TABLE 26-5 PROVIDER-PERFORMED MICROSCOPY PROCEDURES

- All direct wet-mount preparations for the presence or absence of bacteria, fungi, parasites, and human cellular elements
- All potassium hydroxide (KOH) preparations
- Pinworm examinations
- Fern tests
- Postcoital direct, qualitative examinations of vaginal or cervical mucus
- Urine sediment examinations
- Nasal smears for granulocytes
- Fecal leukocyte examinations
- Qualitative semen analysis (limited to the presence or absence of sperm and detection of motility)

HCFA Form 116

HCFA form 116 for the clinical laboratory application for CLIA, HCFA-116, must be completed and returned to the HCFA of the DHHS within 30 days of receipt. The form collects information regarding a laboratory's operation and is needed to evaluate fees, to determine baseline data, to update existing data, and to fulfill legal requirements. The information obtained from the application will give the surveyor of the laboratory a perspective of the laboratory's operation and if it will be subject to an on-site inspection.

7. Some examples of sanctions or penalties imposed by HCFA for noncompliance with CLIA law follow:

Infraction	*Penalty*
Failure to enroll with HCFA	Denial or revocation of certificate
Nonparticipation in proficiency testing	A score of zero (a score of 80% is required)
Failure to return the proficiency testing result	A score of zero

   In addition, Medicare and Medicaid payments may be suspended or terminated and civil penalties of up to a $10,000 fine per violation or per day of noncompliance may be imposed.

   For CLIA '88 conditions other than proficiency testing, newly regulated laboratories will not be subjected to penalties during the first inspection cycle unless it is determined that the laboratories' inadequacies pose immediate patient danger.
8. The law **mandates quality assurance** for nonwaived tests. Laboratories are required to establish policies and procedures through programs that assess test quality; identify problems and correct them; assure precise, dependable, and punctual reporting of test results; and guarantee sufficient competent staff. In addition, laboratories must assure that all quality-control data are studied, and if there is a complaint, an investigation must be undertaken and appropriate action taken and recorded. It is a requirement that quality-assurance records be maintained.
9. The law mandates quality control for nonwaived tests. Laboratories are required to have an adequate supply of equipment to perform the number and types of tests that they offer. A procedures manual must be available in the testing area and must include complete testing instructions. Documentation of maintenance programs for instruments, equipment, and test systems must be evident.

10. The law establishes requirements for the correct collection, transportation, and storage of specimens and the reporting of results. (See No. 16, Patient Test Management.)
11. The law mandates maintenance of records, equipment, and facilities of laboratories performing nonwaived tests. (See No. 17, Documentation.)
12. The law mandates personnel standards. There are requirements for personnel who perform nonwaived tests and they spell out the necessary qualifications and responsibilities required of them. Each person who does the tests must be licensed by the state if required, have a high school diploma or equivalent, have adequate training, and be able to demonstrate an understanding of laboratory procedures; **calibration,** or standardization of instruments; specimen collection; and quality control. Personnel must report test results accurately and with dependability. All high-complexity tests must be done by technologists and technicians except for cytology, which requires more stringent qualifications.
13. The law mandates **proficiency testing** for nonwaived tests. The procedures and tests found in the waived category are exempt from proficiency testing, regardless of the type of laboratory in which the tests are performed. Moderate- and high-complexity test laboratories must enroll in proficiency testing programs that are approved by the DHHS. The proficiency testing samples are checked in the same manner as patient specimens. Unsatisfactory performance on a proficiency testing check can result in various penalties ranging from termination of the laboratory's license to operate to the termination of reimbursement from Medicare and Medicaid.
14. The law mandates unannounced on-site inspection. All laboratories in the moderate- and high-complexity category are subject to unannounced inspections by DHHS or an agency assigned to the task by DHHS. Laboratories that perform only waived tests must prove that tests are being done according to the manufacturer's directions. Inspections can involve interviewing employees, observation of employees performing tests, analysis of data, and documentation of results. Violations of requirements by any laboratory can result in penalties. The cost of inspection will be billed to the laboratory.
15. The law mandates an annual listing of laboratories that have had action taken against them.
16. The law mandates patient test management. All laboratories must have a strategy for properly receiving and processing specimens and for the precise reporting of the results. Written instructions regarding collection, safeguarding of specimens, and labeling of specimens must be available for patients. There must be a specific procedure for the reporting of life-threatening results and a follow-through to the person requesting the test. Test records must be kept for two years after the reporting of results.
17. The law mandates documentation. The following documentation must be done and be available:
    - Specimen
      - Patient preparation
      - Specimen collection procedure
      - Proper labeling technique
      - Preservation of specimen if applicable
    - Proficiency testing
      - Corrective action taken
    - Quality control and quality assurance
      - Any corrective action taken
    - Problem and complaint log
    - **Requisitions** or written requests
      - Patient name
      - Name and address of laboratory
      - Date and time of collection
      - Name of test requested
      - Diagnosis
    - Results
      - Name and address of laboratory where test is done
      - Test name
      - Test results, including normal ranges listed on test results
      - Disposition of unacceptable specimens must be released to authorized person
    - Log of Results
      - Printouts from instruments report must be kept
      - Identification of person performing test
      - Patient identification number
      - Specimen identification
      - Date
      - Time specimen is received in laboratory
      - Specimen rejection log maintained
      - Records and dates of all tests done

Criteria. To be categorized as a PPM procedure, the procedure must meet the following criteria:

1. The examination must be personally performed by one of the following practitioners:
   a. A physician during the patient's visit on a specimen obtained from his or her own patient or from a patient of a group medical practice of which the physician is a member or an employee

   b. A midlevel practitioner, under the supervision of a physician or in independent practice only if authorized by the state, during the patient's visit on a specimen obtained from his or her own patient or from a patient of a clinic, group medical practice, or other health care provider of which the midlevel practitioner is a member or an employee
   c. A dentist during the patient's visit on a specimen obtained from his or her own patient or from a patient of a group dental practice of which the dentist is a member or an employee
2. The procedure must be categorized as moderately complex.
3. The primary instrument for performing the test is the microscope, limited to bright-field or phase-contrast microscopy.
4. The specimen is labile, or a delay in performing the test could compromise the accuracy of the test result.
5. Control materials are not available to monitor the entire testing process.
6. Limited specimen handling or processing is required.

To be categorized as a laboratory performing waived tests, the procedures must meet the following criteria:

1. The tests must be simple laboratory examinations and procedures that are cleared by the FDA for home use, use methods that are simple and accurate so errors are negligible, or pose no reasonable risk for harm to the patient if performed incorrectly.
2. The tests performed must be on CLIA's waived test list.
3. The manufacturer's instructions for performing the tests must be followed.
4. Minimal scientific and technical knowledge is required to perform the test, or knowledge required to perform the test may be obtained through on-the-job instruction.
5. Minimal training is required for preanalytic, analytic, and postanalytic phases of the testing process, or limited experience is required to perform the test.
6. Reagents and materials are generally stable and reliable, or reagents and materials are prepackaged; premeasured; or require no special handling, precautions, or storage conditions.
7. Operational steps are either automatically executed (such as pipetting, temperature monitoring, or timing of steps) or are easily controlled.
8. Calibration quality-control materials are stable and readily available, and external proficiency testing materials, when available, are stable.
9. Test system troubleshooting is automatic or self-correcting, clearly described, or requires minimal judgment, and equipment maintenance is provided by the manufacturer, is seldom needed, or can be performed easily.
10. Minimal interpretation and judgment are required to perfom preanalytic, analytic, and postanalytic processes, and resolution of problems requires limited independent interpretation and judgment.

CLIA '88 Regulation for Quality Control in Automated Hematology

CLIA '88 regulations require that three different procedures be performed in the quality-control protocol for automated hematology instruments. The procedures include calibration, control samples, and proficiency testing. CLIA's regulations require that the automated hematology instrument be calibrated at regularly scheduled intervals with either a calibrator sample or a normal control sample. Many manufacturers of automated

The recent findings of errors in processes at Certificate of Waiver (COW) laboratories and PPM procedure certificate laboratories are of concern. Both COW and PPM procedure laboratories currently have virtually no oversight. Results of studies indicate that, even though COW laboratories have the least amount of complexity to their tests, there are huge gaps in quality of the tests performed. It was discovered that POLs are lacking in the areas of following instructions, quality assurance, and quality control. PPM procedure laboratories were lacking in the areas of inappropriate certificates, not documenting personnel competency, and not evaluating test accuracy. Although these findings are of concern to the CLIA program, no patient harm has been documented due to these errors. Personnel performing the tests at the COW laboratories surveyed were mostly nurses and physicians. Centers for Medicare and Medicaid Services (CMS) confirmed that lack of routine oversight in COW and PPMP laboratories continues to be a significant challenge to ensuring quality testing. They recommend the following:

- Institute educational programs for COW and PPMP laboratories
- Validate the effectiveness of this educational program
- Survey a percentage of COW and PMP laboratories annually
- Develop a self-assessment for PPMP laboratories
- Provide educational material as part of the CLIA enrollment process
- Have State Survey Agencies contact COW and PPM procedure laboratories to verify test menus

hematology instruments recommend or may require that the instrument be recalibrated at shorter intervals than are required by CLIA '88. CLIA '88 mandates that two levels of control samples be tested first each day on any parameter that will be performed on a patient's sample. These quality-control checks must be performed before the patient's sample is tested. The results for quality-control samples must fall within two standard deviations of the expected mean value for that sample.

In addition to calibrations and control sample testing, an ambulatory care setting that uses automated hematology instruments must enroll in a proficiency testing program with a reference laboratory that is CLIA '88 approved.

Aftermath of CLIA '88

There are many individuals who have serious concerns about whether CLIA has led to improved testing as was intended, or if the law has just produced an overload of paperwork and problems. Some question if the law will be fully implemented or even eliminated altogether.

Important developments help to put the law into perspective. HCFA has postponed the date that Medicare payments would be cut off for failure to register. The deadline has been postponed at least three times. The American Medical Association (AMA) complained that unannounced inspections of POLs would disrupt patient office visits. As a result, the Secretary of DHHS declared that POL inspections would be announced.

The category of PPM was added as another certificate and testing category because physicians argued that the microscopic tests were essential to their practice. Already the PPM has expanded to include midlevel practitioners such as nurse practitioners, nurse midwives, and physician assistants.

The law states that CLIA must be self-supporting. There are far fewer laboratories registered than was originally anticipated, and the result is a significantly lower amount of revenue than had been expected.

It is interesting to note that the CDC has proposed easing CLIA regulations by adding another category of testing. It would fall between the waived tests and the moderately complex tests. The tests within this new category would be subject to minimal regulation. This proposal is under consideration. Many question whether CLIA will have any value if this event occurs.

Impact of CLIA on Medical Assistants

CLIA '88 requires every facility that tests human specimens for diagnosis, treatment, and prevention of disease to meet specific federal requirements. The law applies to any facility that performs tests for the preceding purposes. This includes any POLs and ambulatory care setting, two typical areas where medical assistants are employed. The law covers all facilities even if only one test or a few basic tests are done and even if there is no charge for the testing.

Medical assistants may be responsible not only for performing the tests, but also for maintaining personnel records including such information as workers' college diplomas, state licenses, national certifications, employees' continuing education, and recredentialing. Employee hepatitis B status must also be on file. Medical assistants may be involved with compiling a procedures manual on how to perform every test done; these must be reviewed every year. An instrument log must be available on each piece of equipment. Systems must be in place for calibration, quality control, quality assurance test recording, and proficiency testing (if higher than waived category tests are performed). Documentation by medical assistants is of utmost importance; for instance, there may be a quality-control plan in action, but it may not be written down in detail.

Medical assistants are the only health care professionals trained specifically for the ambulatory setting, including the POL procedures. Lacking a medical laboratory technician or medical technologist in the POL, the burden of quality performance of the waived tests falls to the person specifically trained in that area, the medical assistant. Because the laboratory training of the medical assistant focuses primarily on the CLIA waived tests, it is of major concern that medical assisting programs offer the best training possible in the areas of quality assurance, quality control, and following manufacturer's instructions. Keep in mind that the medical assistant may be the only health care professional in the POL who has had formal training in the performance of the waived laboratory tests. Add that to the recent findings of the errors in processes at COW and PPM procedure laboratories and medical assistants are definitely on the front lines of assuring the best quality for test results performed in the POLs.

Because HCFA has received only a fraction of the money that they expected to collect from application fees, there is little money to carry the CLIA '88 program forward. Medical assistants must realize that CLIA '88 is the law even though a number of laboratories have not seen inspectors nor felt any impact from the CLIA '88 regulations. Some laboratories are delaying concern about CLIA '88 rules and do not understand the law and, therefore, have not fully implemented the regulations. Medical assistants must know and comply with the law and be prepared for a CLIA inspection. Penalties are imposed on laboratories that are not in compliance with the law.

Medical assistants who perform clinical laboratory procedures need to be aware that they must keep up with government changes.

Where to Find More Information Regarding CLIA '88

The original CLIA '88 guidelines and updates are available from the Federal Register for a fee. See the appendices for ordering information or visit the HCFA Web site (http://www.cms.hhs.gov; then click on CLIA).

OSHA REGULATIONS

OSHA regulations are intended to ensure employers have a safe and healthy work environment for their employees. There are two OSHA standards that have the greatest impact: *The Occupational Exposure to Hazardous Chemicals* (revised from *The Hazard Communication Standard*) and *The Bloodborne Pathogen Standard. The Bloodborne Pathogen Standards* is reviewed in Chapter 10. This chapter discusses the standard for *Occupational Exposure to Hazardous Chemicals*. It is important to note that states have their own worker safety standards. Those state standards are required to be as strict or greater than the federal OSHA standards. Recently, a state became aware that its standards did not meet the federal levels in regard to cardiopulmonary resuscitation and first-aid training and is currently undergoing some "standard revisions" to comply.

The Standard for Occupational Exposure to Hazardous Chemicals in the Laboratory

In an effort to reduce the number of chemically related illnesses and injuries in the workplace, OSHA published its *Hazard Communications Standard* in 1983. This led many states to develop *right-to-know* laws. In 1992, OSHA expanded the *Hazard Communications Standard*, and published *The Occupational Exposure to Hazardous Chemicals in the Laboratory Standard*, which specifically addressed clinical laboratories.

Critical Thinking

Compare who CLIA protects with who OSHA protects. Do they have similar missions?

The intention of this law is to heighten employee awareness of risks linked with chemical dangers. It serves to improve work practices through employee training and identification of hazardous chemicals that exist in the workplace. The use of protective equipment is utilized to protect employees from harmful chemicals.

Chemical Hygiene Plan

The Chemical Hygiene Plan (CHP) on hazardous chemicals is the core of the OSHA safety standard on hazardous chemicals. A written plan must specify the training and information requirements of the standard. Certain specific control measures such as **fume hoods** and glove boxes must be included in the plan. A designated employee is the chemical hygiene or safety officer. Provisions for housekeeping and maintenance of the facility are included. OSHA standards are not optional and penalties are imposed for noncompliance with the standard. Employers must take the time to meet the requirements not only to be in compliance with the law, but to protect employees as well.

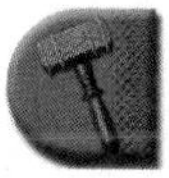

All laboratories and ambulatory care settings, including physicians' offices, must comply with a chemical hygiene plan to meet the OSHA regulations. The only laboratories exempt from compliance are those that exclusively use methods that do not place employees at risk for exposure to chemicals that are hazardous. For example, there may be POLs that perform only dipstick tests or use other commercially prepared kits in which reagents are not exposed and as a result they are exempt from compliance. The primary component of the OSHA standard is that a written chemical hygiene plan and program must be operational if chemicals are stored in a facility and handled by employees. Some examples of chemicals include, but are not limited to, stains, **ethyl alcohol,** sodium hypochlorite (household bleach), **formaldehyde,** fixatives, preservatives, injectables such as **chemotherapeutic agents, acetone,** and so on. Many laboratory accidents result in chemical-related illnesses ranging from eye irritations to **pulmonary edema.**

There are three primary goals that an employer must accomplish to be in compliance with the OSHA standard for chemical exposure. The first is that there must be an inventory undertaken and a list compiled of all chemicals considered hazardous. The following information must be documented (Figure 26-1): the quantity of chemical stored per month or year; whether the substance is gas, liquid, or solid; the manufacturer's name and address; and the chemical hazard classification.

Second, a Material Safety Data Sheet (MSDS) (Figure 26-2) manual must be assembled. The MSDS

SAMPLE

CHEMICAL INVENTORY FORM

Office of ____________________

Date ____________________

Chemical Name	Catalog #	Quantity Stores L./gm. (monthly)	Physical State	Hazard Class				Manufacturer	Comments
				H	F	R	P		

(H) Health
0 - Minimal
1 - Slightly
2 - Moderate
3 - Serious
4 - Extreme

(F) Fire Hazard
0 - Will not burn
1 - Slight
2 - Moderate
3 - Serious
4 - Extreme

(R) Reactivity
0 - Stable is not reactive with water
1 - Slight
2 - Moderate
3 - Serious
4 - Extreme

(P) Protection
A. - Goggles
B. - Goggles/Gloves
C. - Goggles/Gloves/Apron
D. - Face Shield/Gloves/Apron
E. - Goggles/Gloves/Mask
F. - Goggles/Gloves/Apron/Mask
X. - Gloves

Figure 26-1 Sample chemical inventory form for listing chemicals on the premises, including quantity, physical state, hazard class, manufacturer, and comments. (Courtesy of POL Consultants)

statements are provided by the manufacturer when the chemicals are purchased and will give detailed information about the chemical and whether it is a health hazard. The MSDS statements are to be organized into a notebook for employee use and should be located in an area of immediate access by employees. Every employee who is exposed or works with chemicals needs to read the MSDS about those chemicals and know where the manual is kept. The various chemicals are labeled using the National Fire Protection Association's color and number method (Figure 26-3). There are four colors, each signifying a warning to the person handling the chemical(s). They are:

- Blue signifies a health hazard
- Red signifies a fire hazard

BLUE: HEALTH HAZARD

4 = Danger: May be fatal
3 = Warning: Corrosive or toxic
2 = Warning: Harmful if inhaled
1 = Caution: May cause irritation
0 = No unusual hazard

RED: FIRE HAZARD

4 = Danger: Flammable gas or extremely flammable liquid
3 = Warning: Flammable liquid
2 = Caution: Combustible liquid
1 = Caution: Combustible if heated
0 = Noncombustible

MATERIAL SAFETY DATA SHEET

I – PRODUCT IDENTIFICATION

COMPANY NAME: We Wash Inc.

ADDRESS: 5035 Manchester Avenue
Freedom, Texas 79430

Tel No: (314) 621-1818
Nights: (314) 621-1399
CHEMTREC: (800) 424-9343

PRODUCT NAME: Spotfree

Product No.: 2190

Synonyms: Warewashing Detergent

II – HAZARDOUS INGREDIENTS OF MIXTURES

MATERIAL:	(CAS#)	% By Wt.	TLV	PEL
According to the OSHA Hazard Communication Standard, 29CFR 1910.1200, this product contains no hazardous ingredients.		N/A	N/A	NA

III – PHYSICAL DATA

Vapor Pressure, mm Hg: N/A
Evaporation Rate (ether=1): N/A
Solubility in H_2O: Complete
Freezing Point F: N/A
Boiling Point F: N/A
Specific Gravity H_2O=1 @25C: N/A

Vapor Density (Air=1) 60–90F: N/A
% Volatile by wt N/A
pH @ 1% Solution 9.3–9.8
pH as Distributed: N/A
Appearance: Off-White granular powder
Odor: Mild Chemical Odor

IV – FIRE AND EXPLOSION

Flash Point F: N/AV

Flammable Limits: N/A

Extinguishing Media: The product is not flammable or combustible. Use media appropriate for the primary source of fire.

Special Fire Fighting Procedures: Use caution when fighting any fire involving chemicals. A self-contained breathing apparatus is essential.

Unusual Fire and Explosion Hazards: None Known

V – REACTIVITY DATA

Stability - Conditions to avoid: None Known

Incompatibility: Contact of carbonates or bicarbonates with acids can release large quantities of carbon dioxide and heat.

Hazardous Decomposition Products: In fire situations heat decomposition may result in the release of sulfur oxides.

Conditions Contributing to Hazardous Polymerization: N/A

Figure 26-2 Example of a Material Safety Data Sheet (MSDS) listing product name, hazardous ingredients, physical data, fire, explosion, reactivity, health hazard data, emergency and first-aid procedures, spill or leak procedures, protection/control measures, and special precautions. (Courtesy of POL Consultants, 2 Russ Farm Way, Delanco, NJ 08075, (856) 824-0800.)

Spotfree

VI – HEALTH HAZARD DATA

EFFECTS OF OVEREXPOSURE (Medical Conditions Aggravated/Target Organ Effects)

A. ACUTE (Primary Route of Exposure) EYES: Product granules may cause mechanical irritation to eyes.
SKIN (Primary Route of Exposure): Prolonged repeated contact with skin may result in drying of skin.
INGESTION: Not expected to be toxic if swallowed, however, gastrointestinal discomfort may occur.

B. SUBCHRONIC, CHRONIC, OTHER: None known.

VII – EMERGENCY AND FIRST AID PROCEDURES

EYES: In case of contact, flush thoroughly with water for 15 minutes. Get medical attention if irritation persists.
SKIN: Flush any dry Spotfree from skin with flowing water. Always wash hands after use.
INGESTION: If swallowed, drink large quantities of water and call a physician.

VIII – SPILL OR LEAK PROCEDURES

Spill Management: Sweep up material and repackage if possible.
Spill residue may be flushed to the sewer with water.

Waste Disposal Methods: Dispose of in accordance with federal, state and local regulations.

IX – PROTECTION INFORMATION/CONTROL MEASURES

Respiratory: None needed

Eye: Safety glasses

Glove: Not required

Other Clothing and Equipment: None required

Ventilation: Normal

X – SPECIAL PRECAUTIONS

Precautions to be taken in Handling and Storing: Avoid contact with eyes. Avoid prolonged or repeated contact with skin. Wash thoroughly after handling. Keep container closed when not in use.
Additional Information: Store away from acids.

Prepared by: D. Martinez

Revision Date: 04/11/XX

Seller makes no warranty, expressed or implied, concerning the use of this product other than indicated on the label. Buyer assumes all risk of use and/or handling of this material when such use and/or handling is contrary to label instructions.

While Seller believes that the information contained herein is accurate, such information is offered solely for its customers' consideration and verification under their specific use conditions. This information is not to be deemed a warranty or representation of any kind for which Seller assumes legal responsibility.

Figure 26-2 (continued)

CHEMICAL WARNING LABEL DETERMINATION

The Hazard Communication Act contains specific labeling requirements. Labels must be on all hazardous chemicals that are shipped to and used in the workplace. Labels must not be removed. Material safety data sheets for all chemicals will be available to employees.

Manufacturer Requirements: Chemical manufacturers are required to evaluate chemicals, determine status as hazards, provide material safety data sheets (MSDS), and label all shipped chemicals properly. Manufacturer labels must never be removed. The best way to determine the hazards of the chemical is to read the MSDS, obtain an OSHA designated list or State Hazardous Substance list. For most mixed chemicals, it is necessary to contact the manufacturer for MSDS.

Office Chemicals: Search through your office and write down all chemicals you have in the office. Most pharmaceuticals and common household products do not come under this standard. Ingredients can then be compared to a list of regulated substances or MSDS sheets will provide necessary information.

Employer's Responsibility: Any hazardous chemical used in the workplace that is not in its original container must be labeled with the identity of the chemical and hazards. "Target Organ" chemical labels may be used. The label must include the chemical and common name, warnings about physical and health hazards, and the name and address of the manufacturer. The employer is to compile a chemical inventory list that is to be updated as needed. MSDS information should be located in a place where it is accessible to all employees. Label and MSDS information should be provided during the safety training program.

Identity: The term identity can refer to any chemical or common name designation for the individual chemical or mixture, as long as the term used is also used on the list of hazardous chemicals and the MSDS.

NOTE: If a chemical is poured into another container for immediate use, it does not need to be labeled.

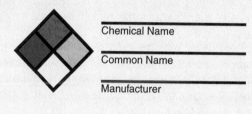

Chemical Name

Common Name

Manufacturer

Figure 26-3 Chemical warning label determination indicates necessary information for labels, including manufacturer's requirements, office chemicals, employer's responsibility, and identity of chemical or its common name. (Courtesy of POL Consultants, 2 Russ Farm Way, Delanco, NJ 08075, (856) 824-0800.)

- Yellow signifies an instability hazard
- White signifies use of personal protective equipment (PPE)

The numbers 0 to 4 are used in conjunction with the colors to indicate the level of risk for each product and are assigned by the manufacturer using the rating system. The numbers can be found on the MSDS. See Figure 26-4.

Third, the employer is required to provide a hazard communication educational program to the employee within 30 days of employment and before the employee handles any hazardous chemicals (Figure 26-5A). The training program should consist of the location and identification of hazardous chemicals, how to read and understand the labels on the chemicals, where the MSDS manual is kept, when to use PPE, and procedures to follow for chemical spills. The training sessions must be documented, signed by the employer, and

YELLOW: REACTIVITY

4 = Danger: Explosive at room temperature
3 = Danger: May be explosive if spark occurs or if heated under confinement
2 = Warning: Unstable or may react if mixed with water
1 = Caution: May react if heated or mixed with water
0 = Stable: Nonreactive when mixed with water

WHITE: PPE

A Goggles
B Goggles, gloves
C Goggles, gloves, apron
D Face shields, gloves, apron
E Goggles, gloves, mask
F Goggles, gloves, apron, mask
X Gloves

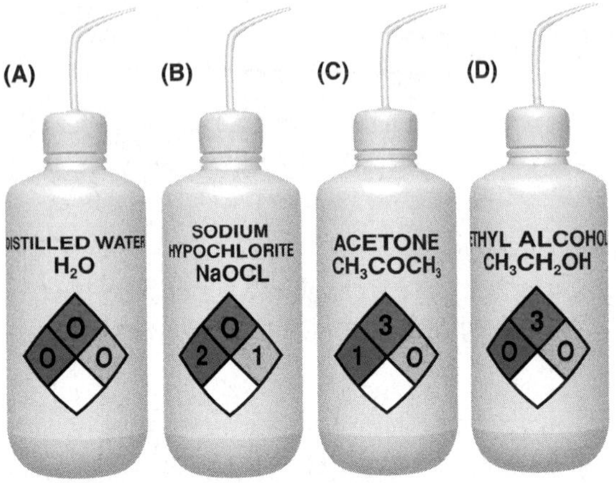

Figure 26-4 Four containers are marked using the National Fire Association's color and number method for identifying and warning of chemical hazards: (A) distilled water: presents no health, fire, or reactivity hazard and requires no personal protective equipment when used (all areas represented by zeros); (B) sodium hypochlorite: does not promote a fire hazard (red/0), is harmful if inhaled (blue/2), and it may react if heated or mixed with water (yellow/1); (C) acetone: a flammable liquid (red/3), may cause irritation (blue/1), stable and non-reactive when mixed with water (yellow/0); (D) ethyl alcohol: a flammable liquid (red/3), no unusual health hazard (blue/0), and stable and non-reactive when mixed with water (yellow/0). (Courtesy of POL Consultants, 2 Russ Farm Way, Delanco, NJ 08075, (856) 824-0800.)

permanently retained in the employee record (Figure 26-5B).

Requirements of Chemical Hygiene Plan (CHP). The requirements for a CHP include:

- Employers must have an operational written plan (a manual) relevant to the safety and health of employees.
- Written instructions on the use of PPE must be available.
- Fume hoods or biohazard hoods must be checked regularly.
- Training sessions must be held for employees regarding their right to know what hazardous chemicals are in their work environment.
- It is the employer's legal responsibility to provide medical attention for an employee should an accidental chemical spill occur.
- The responsibility for executing training sessions, keeping manuals current, and documentation is designated to an employer.

SAFETY TRAINING FORM

Safety training will be offered to all employees within 30 days of employment or before the employee assumes responsibilities that involve exposure to body fluids or chemicals.

Items to be covered in training session:

- General explanation of OSHA laws
- General explanation of the epidemiology and symptoms of HBV and HIV
- Who is at risk in office
- Modes of transmission of HBV and HIV
- Method of control in workplace
- Universal Precautions
- Handwashing
- Personal protective equipment
- How to clean up spills
- What to do after a needlestick injury
- Medical follow-up after an exposure
- Cleaning protocol for office
- Hazardous Communication Standard
- Types of chemical labels
- How to read MSDS and NFPA signs
- Warning signs
- How to get MSDS
- Location of MSDS
- How to store chemicals
- How to record chemical inventory
- Hazardous Waste laws
- How to comply with laws
- How to use and label bio-bins and sharps containers
- How to keep records
- Who keeps the records
- Medical consent forms
- HBV forms
- Safety training certificate
- Engineering control records

Figure 26-5A Safety Training Form is an example of items to be covered by employer during training session regarding Occupational Safety and Health Administration (OSHA) laws and exposure to chemicals, blood, body fluids, or other potentially infectious material. (Courtesy of POL Consultants, 2 Russ Farm Way, Delanco, NJ 08075, (856) 824-0800.)

- Instruction must be provided regarding disposal of hazardous waste produced in the workplace. (Usually a hazardous waste company is contracted by the employer.)
- Each employee's record must have a written statement, signed by the employer, stating the employer's responsibility to arrange for employee training and a safe work environment.

SAMPLE

CERTIFICATE OF TRAINING

First Name Middle Initial Last Name

has completed the

OSHA HAZARD COMMUNICATION
INFORMATION TRAINING PROGRAM

This certificate indicates your successful participation in a program instructing you of your rights as a worker and the proper handling of hazardous substances in the workplace.

Date Employee Signature

Instructor's Signature

Employer's Signature

Figure 26-5B Sample Certificate of Training shows employee has completed OSHA hazard communication information training program. (Courtesy of POL Consultants, 2 Russ Farm Way, Delanco, NJ 08075, (856) 824-0800.)

Critical Thinking

Name three other professions beside health care that should abide by OSHA regulations? For each profession, list four rules that should be in place. Do you think they are in place?

Importance of Chemical Standard to Medical Assistants. Meeting the requirements set forth by OSHA is not optional. All must comply or face penalties. All employees, including medical assistants, have the right to know and be given information and be educated regarding chemical hazards that they are exposed to in their place of employment. Medical assistants can be exposed to hazardous chemicals through skin contact, injection, or inhalation. Because many laboratory accidents result in chemical-related illnesses, it is important for medical assistants to understand how the law affects them, their place of employment, and their employer. Medical assistants and other health care providers should know what hazards they face, and know the proper technique for handling, storing, and disposing of hazardous chemicals. Medical assistants in administrative positions must use their knowledge and skills to provide a safe work environment for themselves and their staff.

OSHA REGULATIONS AND STUDENTS

With the passage of the OSHA laws, all students with potential exposure to chemicals and bloodborne pathogens should follow all safety procedures as outlined by OSHA. Because students are not considered employees of a health care facility and are attending an educational institution, they do not fall under the OSHA guidelines. They should, however, take precautions to avoid contact with potentially infectious materials and toxic chemicals wherever learning is taking place.

Avoiding Exposure to Chemicals

Students may come into contact with harmful chemicals when doing procedures that can cause such problems as burns to the skin and eyes. Students will be made aware of these through information packaged with kits and the MSDS. As a general rule, if the chemical comes in contact with the skin, it must be flushed with water immediately and continued for five minutes. Chemicals that get into the eye must be flushed for 15 minutes (unless contradicted on the label). Refer to the MSDS for specific postexposure procotol. Eyewash stations and showers should be available in case of accidental exposure to hazardous chemicals with a follow-up in the emergency department.

Chemical spills should be carefully cleaned following the procedure for the particular chemical. The same chemical biohazard spill cleanup kits used in POLs can be used in school laboratories. Students should familiarize themselves with the contents of the kits and the instructions for use before an actual spill occurs.

Toxic fumes can occur with certain chemicals and certain tests can cause lung irritation and damage. This type of chemical should be handled under a fume hood that will take the fumes away by means of a ventilation mechanism.

A student safety laboratory manual outlining an exposure control plan with emphasis on Standard Precautions, PPE, work practice controls, lists of hazardous chemicals, and MSDS should be compiled and accessible. Students should be thoroughly familiar with its contents. In addition, students should be educated as to the location and identification of hazardous chemicals just as employees are.

It is of utmost importance that students learn about and understand the OSHA standards and comply with them. In so doing, they will safeguard themselves from harmful chemicals and bloodborne pathogens.

CUMULATIVE TRAUMA DISORDERS

Recently, OHSA has been focusing its attention on a new threat to the workplace: ergonomic hazards. Ergonomics is the study of the workplace. OSHA published its first standard, *Ergonomic Hazards*, in 1991. At the heart of these guidelines is the prevention of cumulative trauma disorders. Cumulative trauma disorders are injuries involving the musculoskeletal or nervous system, such as carpal tunnel syndrome and trigger finger. They are the result of long-term, repetitive work actions, such as gripping, keyboard use, pipetting, and microscopy. Limiting or preventing repetitive work actions is the key to minimizing cumulative trauma disorders. Use of ergonomically correct equipment and supplies, proper work site design, staff training, and job rotation are essential in creating an ergonomically sound workplace.

Case Study 26-1

Marie Tyndall is a student in the Jackson Heights Community College Medical Assisting Program. She and two other classmates have been assigned the project of creating a plan for cleaning up spills that might occur in the classroom laboratory and assuring that all students using the laboratory have been trained in the proper procedure.

CASE STUDY REVIEW

1. What materials would your group need?
2. How would your group go about learning the proper steps in the clean-up process?
3. How would your group assure that all other students in the laboratory also have the proper training?

SUMMARY

Infectious diseases and accidents occur through lack of education and carelessness. Medical assistants must understand the importance of the regulations and guidelines set forth by the federal government and follow through by helping employers implement them. In doing so, the health and safety of patients and health care workers will be protected, the spread of infectious diseases can be kept under control, and the risk for contracting an infectious disease such as AIDS or hepatitis B will be greatly minimized.

Every medical office and ambulatory care setting must, by law, have clearly written and readily available manuals containing information about Standard Precautions, CLIA '88, and OSHA for the safe handling, storage, and disposal of blood, body fluids, and chemicals.

(continues)

SUMMARY (continued)

Through consistent use of Standard Precautions and adherence to the CLIA and OSHA laws, health care providers can acquire the behaviors and techniques needed to safeguard themselves and their patients.

Because of frequent changes in the laws, it is necessary for medical assistants and all other health care providers to keep abreast of the government mandates.

STUDY FOR SUCCESS

To reinforce your knowledge and skills of information presented in this chapter:

- ❑ Review the Key Terms
- ❑ Consider the Case Study and discuss your conclusions
- ❑ Answer the Review Questions
  - ❑ Multiple Choice
  - ❑ Critical Thinking
- ❑ Navigate the Internet by completing the Web Activities
- ❑ Practice the StudyWARE activities on the CD
- ❑ Apply your knowledge in the Student Workbook activities
- ❑ Complete the Web Tutor sections
- ❑ View and discuss the DVD situations

REVIEW QUESTIONS

Multiple Choice

1. Standard precautions were issued by:
   a. DHHS
   b. CDC
   c. HCFA
   d. OSHA
2. CLIA '88 was made law to regulate:
   a. the disposal of infectious waste
   b. the use of chemicals in the workplace
   c. laboratory tests performed on specimens taken from the human body
   d. the transmission of the HIV virus
3. The core of the OSHA safety standard for chemical exposure is:
   a. the dipstick test
   b. the chemical hygiene plan
   c. the quantity of chemical stored per month
   d. the MSDS manual
4. The agency that requires employers to ensure employee safety concerning occupational exposure to potentially harmful substances is:
   a. CDC
   b. U.S. Public Health Department
   c. HCFA
   d. OSHA
5. Successful laboratory safety programs include:
   a. threats to the emotional and physical health of health care workers
   b. lost workdays and increased workers' compensation claims
   c. orientation, periodic drills, and consistent enforcement of policy
   d. potential fines from regulatory agencies
6. CLIA regulations specify all the following except:
   a. the type of test performed
   b. the personnel involved in testing
   c. quality control
   d. the methods used in testing
7. The agency charged with implementing CLIA is:
   a. CDC
   b. United States Public Health Department
   c. HCFA
   d. OSHA
8. Which is not an approved provider for PPM procedures?
   a. a physician
   b. a nurse practitioner
   c. a dentist
   d. a medical assistant

9. The standard published by OSHA to prevent cumulative trauma disorders is:
   a. *Workplace Standard*
   b. *Standard for Prevention of Cumulative Trauma*
   c. *Ergonomic Hazards*
   d. *Ergonomic Standard*
10. Match the chemical warning color with the hazard represented.

1. Blue	a. Reactivity or instability
2. Red	b. Use PPE
3. Yellow	c. Health
4. White	d. Fire
	e. Disaster

Critical Thinking

1. Explain the purpose of CLIA '88 and tell why the law was amended.
2. Name three categories of testing and explain each category.
3. Discuss the 17 major components of CLIA '88.
4. Describe quality control and quality assurance. Why are they important?
5. What is HCFA Form 116? Explain its use.
6. You have been asked to develop a manual for your physician–employer. The manual is to detail a chemical hygiene plan (CHP) for all employees in the office. How would you proceed? What should be included in the plan? In the CHP include three major goals that will ensure the physician–employer's compliance with the hazard standard. You have been asked to compile a manual of the MSDSs. What must be included in the manual and from where does the information come?

WEB ACTIVITIES

1. Using the Internet, go to http://www.cms.hhs.gov and search for the list of CLIA waived tests. Is this test extensive/brand specific or general?
2. Go into the FDA's Web site at http://www.fda.gov and see if the list of CLIA waived tests on that site differs. What do you think is the reason for the lists to be different or the same?
3. While you are searching those two Web sites, find out what language(s) is acceptable for labels on hazardous chemicals.

REFERENCES/BIBLIOGRAPHY

Centers for Medicare & Medicaid Services. Retrieved from http://www.cms.hhs.gov. Accessed May 9, 2005.

U.S. Food and Drug Administration. (2004). *Databases on the FDA Web site*. Retrieved from http://www.fda.gov/search/databases.html. Accessed June 16, 2005.

THE DVD HOOK-UP

DVD Series: Skills Based Series | **Program Number:** 11

Chapter/Scene Reference
- *Introduction to Venipuncture, Hematology, and Immunology Procedures*

This chapter discusses safety and regulatory guidelines for the medical office.

Both the chapter and selected DVD scene discuss the three major categories for testing.

1. What is the most common category that medical offices fall into for laboratory testing? Why?
2. In a waived laboratory, which personnel have the authority to perform microscopy?
3. What does CLIA stand for and who oversees CLIA?

DVD Journal Summary
Write a paragraph that summarizes what you learned from watching the selected scene from today's DVD program. What would you do if you found out that your employer was running tests that he should not, based on the office's CLIA classification?

CHAPTER 27

Introduction to the Medical Laboratory

OUTLINE

The Laboratory
- Purposes of Laboratory Testing
- Types of Laboratories
- Laboratory Personnel
- Laboratory Departments
- Panels of Laboratory Tests

Quality Controls/Assurances in the Laboratory
- Control Tests
- Proficiency Testing
- Preventative Maintenance
- Instrument Validations
- The Medical Assistant's Role

Laboratory Requisitions and Reports

Specimen Collection
- Proper Procurement, Storage, and Handling
- Processing and Sending Specimens to a Laboratory

Microscopes
- Types of Microscopes
- How to Use a Microscope
- How to Care for a Microscope

OBJECTIVES

The student should strive to meet the following performance objectives and demonstrate an understanding of the facts and principles presented in this chapter through written and oral communication.

1. Define the key terms as presented in the glossary.
2. Explain the purposes of laboratory testing.
3. Describe the main similarities and differences between independent laboratories and physicians' office laboratories.
4. Explain the levels of laboratory personnel in relation to their education, skills, and duties.
5. List eight different departments within the medical laboratory and list at least two types of testing performed within each of those departments.
6. Name nine of the most common laboratory profiles and explain the body system or function being surveyed.

(continues)

KEY TERMS

Assay
Asymptomatic
Baseline Values
Biopsy
Clinical Chemistry
Clinical Diagnosis
Condenser
Control Test
Culture and Sensitivity (C & S)
Cytology
Diagnosis
Diaphragm
Differential Diagnosis
DNA
Electrolyte
Glucose
Hematology
Histology
Hormone Replacement Therapy (HRT)
Hospital-Based Laboratories
Immunohematology
Immunology
Invasive
Microbiology
Mycology
Objective
Panel
Parasitology
Patient Service Centers
Peak
Physician Office Laboratory (POL)
Qualitative Test
Quantitative Test
Reagent
Reference Laboratories
Reference Values

(continues)

KEY TERMS (continued)

Requisition
Serum
Therapeutic Drug Monitoring (TDM)
Toxicology
Trough
Urinalysis
Virology

FEATURED COMPETENCIES

CAAHEP—ENTRY-LEVEL COMPETENCIES

Fundamental Procedures

- Practice Standard Precautions

Legal Concepts

- Identify and respond to issues of confidentiality
- Perform within legal and ethical boundaries
- Document appropriately
- Demonstrate knowledge of federal and state health care legislation and regulations

Patient Instruction

- Explain general office policies
- Instruct individuals according to their needs

Operational Functions

- Use methods of quality control

ABHES—ENTRY-LEVEL COMPETENCIES

Professionalism

- Project a positive attitude
- Evidence a responsible attitude
- Conduct work within scope of education, training, and ability

(continues)

OBJECTIVES (continued)

7. Explain the concepts of quality control and quality assurance in the medical laboratory.
8. Describe at least three methods of assuring quality in the medical laboratory.
9. Demonstrate how to correctly complete a laboratory requisition.
10. List 10 pieces of information required on a written laboratory requisition.
11. Explain the rationale behind proper patient preparation before laboratory testing.
12. Explain where accurate and reliable information might be obtained about proper procurement, storage, and handling of laboratory specimens.
13. On a diagram, label the parts of a compound microscope.
14. Explain the function of a compound microscope.
15. Demonstrate the proper use of a compound microscope.
16. List six rules to assure proper care of a compound microscope.

SCENARIO

At Inner City Health Care, Dr. Susan Rice has ordered urine tests for Annette Samuels, who came to the clinic reporting stomach cramps. Wanda Slawson, CMA, will obtain the necessary specimen and send it to an independent laboratory for testing. Wanda gives Annette specific instructions on how to prepare for the urine test and how to collect the urine. She asks Annette if she has any questions and she has Annette repeat the instructions to be sure she understands them. When Annette returns with the specimen, Wanda immediately labels it and prepares it to be sent to the laboratory. With a reassuring smile, she tells Annette when to call the clinic for the results.

FEATURED COMPETENCIES (continued)

Communication

- Serve as liaison between Physician and others
- Application of electronic technology

Clinical duties

- Apply principles of aseptic techniques and infection control
- Use quality control
- Collect and process specimens
- Dispose of biohazardous materials
- Practice standard precautions

Legal Concepts

- Determine needs for documentation and reporting
- Document accurately

Spotlight on Certification

RMA Content Outline
- Medical law
- Laboratory procedures

CMA Content Outline
- Medicolegal guidelines and requirements
- Principles of infection control
- Principles of operation
- Processing specimens
- Quality control

CMAS Content Outline
- Legal and Ethical Considerations
- Asepsis in the Medical Office
- Supplies and Equipment

INTRODUCTION

Physicians use laboratory tests to diagnose illnesses, assess patients' health, and manage chronic diseases such as diabetes and arthritis. Medical assistants in physicians' offices, clinics, and laboratories may be responsible for patient preparation, obtaining specimens, and testing or sending specimens to an independent laboratory. It is important for medical assistants to be aware of laboratory procedures to ensure accurate testing.

THE LABORATORY

The current health care environment offers numerous options in the methods used to process laboratory tests.

- The specimen may be obtained and the test performed within the **physician office laboratory (POL).**
- The specimen may be procured and packaged for transport to a separate laboratory.
- The patient may be referred to a separate laboratory for collection and testing of the specimen.

Each laboratory setting has specific requirements for the training and qualifications of the health care personnel who work in that setting. The equipment, supplies, and paperwork, as well as the instructions given to the patient are also determined by the type of laboratory. Whichever laboratory setting is selected, the focus should be on the safety of the public, the patient, and the health care personnel, while always maintaining quality testing to ensure accurate results.

Purposes of Laboratory Testing

Physicians (and other health care providers) depend on the ability of medical laboratories to help in determining a patient's state of health or disease in some of the following ways.

To Record an Individual's State of Health. Blood tests may be performed periodically, usually during a routine physical examination, to be assured of healthy normal ranges, also known as **reference values.** Then in the future, if illness occurs, the **baseline values** are available for comparison.

To Satisfy Employment, Insurance, or Legal Requirements. If an accident occurs, quite often blood is tested for the presence of drugs and alcohol. Such a determination can prove a person guilty or innocent of a crime. Sometimes, places of employment or life insurance companies request laboratory tests to be assured that their employees or clients are free of illegal or dangerous drugs. Employment-required drug and alcohol testing is a classic example of this reason for testing.

To Gain Statistics for Research and Clinical Trials. Laboratory tests are sometimes a part of the data gathered for research and for clinical trials information. When we read about the relation between osteoporosis and **hormone replacement therapy (HRT),** the information is gathered through research. Clinical trials might address the efficacy of certain medications, vitamins, and minerals on osteoporosis in women on HRT.

To Detect Asymptomatic Conditions or Diseases. Occasionally, a patient will have no complaints of illness and will be **asymptomatic**—that is, exhibit no symptoms that might be associated with a disease process—but during routine screening or testing in another, perhaps unrelated, area, a disorder may be discovered. An example is a young man presenting at the office for an athletic physical. During routine urinalysis, it is discovered he is harboring a mild bladder infection.

To Confirm a Clinical Diagnosis. When a patient reports specific symptoms and describes a particular condition (subjective information), and data are compiled through a clinical examination (objective information), the physician may be able to determine a **diagnosis** without the aid of laboratory tests. This is referred to as a **clinical diagnosis.** To confirm a clinical diagnosis, the physician will order laboratory tests. For example, a child has symptoms of a strep throat infection such as sudden onset of sore throat, fever, headache, and upset stomach. On visual examination, the physician discovers small abscesses on the child's tonsils. The physician is almost certain that the diagnosis will be strep throat, but a quick and simple strep test is performed to confirm the clinical diagnosis.

To Differentiate between Two or More Diseases. Sometimes, a patient presents with a combination of symptoms that can be related to more than one condition. For the physician to diagnose accurately, a laboratory test is performed. In situations such as these, the physician chooses to perform the simplest and least **invasive** laboratory test to rule out a particular disease before requiring more extensive testing. This is known as a **differential diagnosis.** For example, if the child in the preceding case had a negative strep test but perhaps exhibited other more systemic symptoms, a blood test might confirm mononucleosis or another condition. The physician is then able to differentiate between the two diagnoses—strep throat and mononucleosis.

To Diagnose. If symptoms are vague, thereby making the clinical diagnosis difficult for the physician, a series of laboratory tests may be required. Sometimes a **panel,** or group of related tests, is ordered. This helps narrow the field for diagnosis. An example is if a patient presents with reports of severe fatigue, but preliminary testing does not indicate a diagnosis. Further testing will eventually either lead the physician in a specific direction or at least eliminate a wide variety of conditions.

To Determine the Effectiveness of Treatments. After a patient has been diagnosed and has begun treatment, the physician monitors the patient's health to be sure that the treatment is therapeutic. For example, a patient diagnosed with epilepsy must take an effective amount of antiseizure medication. A blood test is used to check the level of medication in the patient's system. Sometimes the physician wants to know the highest and lowest ranges of medication in the patient's blood to determine if the levels are within a therapeutic range, called **therapeutic drug monitoring (TDM),** and to check for drug toxicity (if the drug level is too high). To measure the highest level of medication in the patient's blood serum (called the **peak**), we will take the specimen about a half hour after the patient has taken his or her regular dose of medicine. If we want to measure the lowest level (called the **trough**), we will take the specimen just before the patient takes his or her next scheduled dose of medicine. A periodic blood test can also be used to determine the effectiveness of dietary and lifestyle changes in reducing blood cholesterol levels.

To Prevent Diseases/Disorders. Protection of the public, families, and coworkers can warrant laboratory tests. An example is protecting an unborn child from contracting genital herpes through the birthing process. A culture of the mother's cervical and vaginal mucosa helps to determine if the child is at risk. If the culture is positive, performing a caesarean section is the treatment of choice to protect the newborn from contracting herpes.

To Prevent the Exacerbation of Diseases. Patients with chronic conditions require regular blood tests to prevent exacerbation of the disease. When the results of the blood test are obtained, the physician or patient determines whether it is necessary to adjust the diet or medication. For example, a patient with diabetes tests his or her blood regularly to measure the blood sugar, or **glucose,** level. If the blood sugar level is too high or too low, the patient may adjust her insulin dosage or have something to eat to return her blood sugar level to normal.

Types of Laboratories

There are many different types and locations of medical laboratories. They are identified by their size, capabilities, and affiliations. Independent laboratories may be located within medical centers or large clinics. They often have small satellite **patient service centers** located near more isolated medical facilities or in areas of convenience to patients. Satellite laboratories facilitate patients' specimens being obtained closer to their neighborhoods and ambulatory care settings. The specimens are usually couriered back to the independent central laboratory for processing.

Hospital-based laboratories perform most of the tests required by that hospital area, but even large hospitals use reference laboratories for specialized testing. **Reference laboratories** are independent, regionally located laboratories that service larger areas. Reference laboratories are used by hospitals and physicians for complex, expensive, or specialized tests.

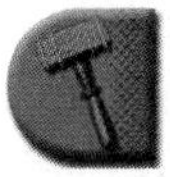

In a business sense, medical laboratories are quickly becoming more and more competitive. Growth and profitability depend on community relations and service, convenience, efficiency, cost, location, and even reputation. Competition often places the medical assistant and other medical personnel in a position of being asked to recommend a particular medical laboratory over another. Unless the physician–employer has a strong preference for using a particular laboratory, or not referring to a particular laboratory, the patient should choose the laboratory. The patient's insurance plan may also be a factor in determining which laboratory is used. Many insurance plans require the patient to use a particular laboratory or to choose a laboratory from those participating in the plan to guarantee payment for the tests. The medical assistant is then a resource for options rather than a referral service. The law is clear that a physician may not have a financial interest in the laboratory to which he or she refers patients.

Point-of-Care Testing (POCT). With the many changes in health care delivery and managed care, the clinical laboratory is also experiencing changes to improve clinical services in the laboratory area. On the forefront of change in the laboratory is POCT, also referred to as near-patient testing or bedside testing. Medical conditions, location of the patient, and treatment methods often require laboratory results as quickly as possible so proper medical care can be administered without delay. POCT uses small instruments that provide rapid, accurate results when used correctly.

Medical personnel can be trained to do laboratory tests of moderate complexity (as defined by CLIA '88) during POCT. The laboratory staff, because of their education, knowledge, and experience in this area, are responsible for advice and management of the quality control and various aspects of this new area of testing. The extension of this laboratory service demands cooperation and cross-departmental efforts from all nontraditional personnel in the health care facility. POCT also has provided new career tracks for the laboratorian, together with multiple skills for several disciplines of health care providers.

POLs. POLs are those laboratories physically set within the office. Some of the more commonly performed medical laboratory tests can easily and inexpensively be performed in the office by the medical assistant. With a simple fingerstick and a few readily available medical supplies, a patient's blood glucose levels can be determined. Another commonly performed test in the ambulatory care setting is the **urinalysis** in which urine is physically, chemically, and microscopically examined for irregularities. With the availability of the many varieties of self-contained kits, tests for strep throat, pregnancy, blood sugar (serum glucose) levels, and hidden (occult) blood in stool can be performed quickly. Other kits are being developed daily. Patients may use a kit that can be purchased without a prescription at home. Some of the home kits available to the general public are "just as accurate" as the kits used in medical offices. The major difference is that the person performing the test may not be trained, which may affect the accuracy of the test results. Consistent quality-control measures might not be used by the non-medical person (see Quality Control/Assurances in the laboratory section). For example, a pregnancy test kit may be exposed to extreme temperatures either in the patient's care, while on a grocer's shelf, or in the patient's home. These extreme temperatures may invalidate the chemical reaction in the test kit. More training, education, and credentialing are required as the complexity of the testing and equipment increases. If the results are not within normal limits, the physician needs to be consulted for confirmation and diagnosis/treatment. (See CLIA '88 in Chapter 26 for specific testing parameters.)

Laboratory Personnel

All independent medical laboratories must be managed by a pathologist, a physician who specializes in disease processes. Additional staffing consists of clinical laboratory scientists, technicians, clinical laboratory assistants, phlebotomists, and medical assistants. Many agencies certify laboratory personnel.

Clinical Laboratory Scientists/Medical Technologists. Certified clinical laboratory scientists and medical technologists are qualified to perform analysis testing in all departments of the laboratory. They often are department supervisors and have leadership roles within the laboratory personnel structure. Clinical laboratory scientists and medical technologists have earned a bachelor's degree and completed a minimum of one year of internship training. Certification is then obtained by passing a national certification examination issued by one of the following agencies:

- MT (ASCP)—Medical Technologist
  American Society for Clinical Pathology
- MT (AMT)—Medical Technologist
  American Medical Technologists
- CLS (NCA)—Clinical Laboratory Scientist
  National Credentialing Agency for Medical Laboratory Personnel
- RMT (ISCLT)—Registered Medical Technologist
  International Society for Clinical Laboratory Technology
- CLT (DHHS)—Clinical Laboratory Technologist
  Department of Health and Human Services

Clinical Laboratory Technician (CLT)/Medical Laboratory Technician (MLT). Certified CLTs are qualified to perform qualitative and quantitative testing under supervision. CLTs have completed two years of formal education and training. Certification is then obtained by passing a national certification examination issued by one of the following agencies:

- MLT (ASCP)—Medical Laboratory Technician
  American Society for Clinical Pathology
- MLT (AMT)—Medical Laboratory Technician
  American Medical Technologists
- CLT (NCA)—Clinical Laboratory Technician
  National Credentialing Agency for Medical Laboratory Personnel
- RLT (ISCLT)—Registered Laboratory Technician
  International Society for Clinical Laboratory Technology

Phlebotomist/Phlebotomy Technician. Certified phlebotomists and phlebotomy technicians require training programs with additional on-the-job experience. Phlebotomists and phlebotomy technicians are required to take a certification examination and/or register with a governing body, depending on state laws. Certification examinations are issued by the following organizations:

- PBT (ASCP)—Phlebotomy Technician
  American Society for Clinical Pathology
- RPT (AMT)—Registered Phlebotomy Technician
  American Medical Technologists
- CPT (ASPT)—Certified Phlebotomy Technician
  American Society for Phlebotomy Technicians
- CLP (NCA)—Clinical Laboratory Phlebotomist
  National Credentialing Agency for Medical Laboratory Personnel

Medical Assistant. Medical assistants are multiskilled professionals dedicated to assisting in patient-care management. Medical assistants work in medical offices, clinics, and ambulatory care centers. They perform administrative duties and clinical procedures, including basic waived laboratory tests. Formal education, training, and externship are obtained through community colleges, vocational-technical schools, and proprietary (private) institutions. Certification is obtained through a national certification examination issued by the following organizations (see Chapters 1 and 35 for additional information regarding certification):

- CMA (AAMA)—Certified Medical Assistant
  American Association of Medical Assistants
- CMAS (AMT)—Certified Medical Administrative Specialist
  American Medical Technologists
- RMA (AMT)—Registered Medical Assistant
  American Medical Technologists

Laboratory Departments

Laboratories are usually divided into departments and may even be subdivided, depending on the size and specialties within the laboratory (Figure 27-1). The various departments perform special tests within their expertise (Table 27-1). Categorization becomes evident when test results are requested over the telephone or whenever there is a need to converse with laboratory personnel. Through knowledge of the various departments within the laboratory, information can be more readily obtained.

Hematology Department. The **hematology** department tests the formed (cellular) elements of the blood. These tests may be quantitative or qualitative. The **quantitative tests** involve actual number counts such as counting the number of white blood cells (WBC), red blood cells (RBC), or platelets. The **qualitative tests** focus on the quality or characteristics of the components, such as the size, shape, and maturity of the cells. In addition, the hematology department tests the ability of the blood

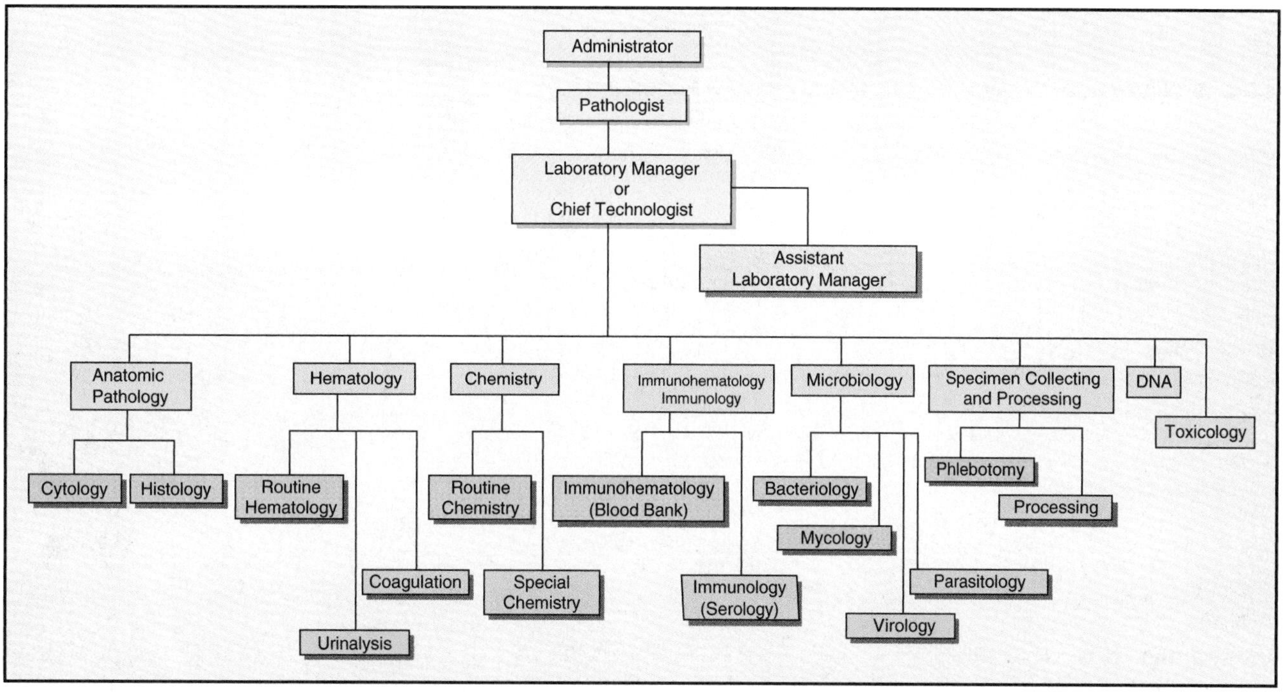

Figure 27-1 Departments in a typical medical laboratory.

components to perform their individual tasks correctly. An example of this is testing the coagulation ability of clotting factors in blood.

Urinalysis Department. Urinalysis is the physical, chemical, and microscopic examination of urine. Required cultures are sent to the microbiology or bacteriology department. In a large laboratory, the urinalysis department is often located under hematology because of the microscopic examinations performed on urine (Figure 27-2).

Clinical Chemistry Department. The **clinical chemistry** department analyzes the chemical composition of blood, cerebrospinal fluid, and joint fluid. Some of the procedures within this department include **assay** of enzymes in the **serum,** serum glucose, or **electrolyte** levels. Toxicology, including TDM and identification of drugs of abuse, is also performed in this department.

Immunohematology (Blood Bank) Department. **Immunohematology** is a special area that deals with

TABLE 27-1 CATEGORIES OF LABORATORY TESTS

HEMATOLOGY	
White blood cell (WBC) count	Hematocrit (Hct)
Red blood cell (RBC) count	Prothrombin time (PT)
Differential white blood cell count (Diff)	Erythrocyte sedimentation rate (ESR)
Hemoglobin (Hgb)	Platelet count
CLINICAL CHEMISTRY	
Glucose	Potassium
Blood urea nitrogen (BUN)	Bilirubin
Creatinine	Cholesterol
Total protein	Triglycerides
Albumin	Uric acid
Globulin	Lactate dehydrogenase, LD (LDH)
Calcium	Aspartate aminotransferase, AST (SGOT)
Inorganic phosphorus	Alanine aminotransferase, ALT (SGPT)
Chloride	Alkaline phosphatase
Sodium	Phospholipids

(continues)

TABLE 27-1 (continued)

SEROLOGY (IMMUNOLOGY/IMMUNOHEMATOLOGY) AND BLOOD BANKING	
Syphilis detection tests (VDRL, RPR)	Rheumatoid factor (RA factor)
C-reactive protein test (CRP)	Mono test
ABO blood typing	Heterophil antibody titer test
Rh typing	Hepatitis tests
Rh antibody titer test	HIV tests: ELISA and Western blot
Cross-match	Antistreptolysin O (ASO) titer
Direct Coombs' test	Pregnancy tests
Cold agglutinins	
URINALYSIS	
Physical analysis of urine:	Bilirubin
Color	Urobilinogen
Clarity	Nitrite
Specific gravity	Leukocyte esterase
Chemical analysis of urine:	Microscopic analysis of urine:
pH	Red blood cells
Glucose	White blood cells
Protein	Epithelial cells
Ketones	Casts
Blood	Crystals
MICROBIOLOGY	
Candidiasis	Pneumonia
Chlamydia	Streptococcal sore throat
Diphtheria	Tetanus
Gonorrhea	Tonsillitis
Meningitis	Tuberculosis
Pertussis	Urinary tract infection
Pharyngitis	
PARASITOLOGY	
Amebiasis	Scabies
Ascariasis	Tapeworm disease (cestodiasis)
Hookworm disease	Toxoplasmosis
Malaria	Trichinosis
Pinworm disease (enterobiasis)	Trichomoniasis
CYTOLOGY	
Chromosome studies	
Pap test	
HISTOLOGY	
Tissue analysis	
Biopsy studies	
DNA	
DNA testing compares individuals according to their individual genotype.	
TOXICOLOGY	
The toxicology department tests for chemicals, specifically for drugs and other toxins in blood.	

blood typing procedures, cross-matching, and the separation and storage of blood components for transfusion, as well as antibody–antigen reactions.

Serology (Immunology) Department. The serology **(immunology)** department is the area of the laboratory that performs tests to evaluate the body's immune response, both production of antibodies and the cellular immune response. Procedures in this area include the detection of antibodies to bacteria and viruses, as well as antibodies produced against one's own body (autoimmune), as in rheumatic diseases such as rheumatoid arthritis and lupus erythematosus. Diseases such as AIDS have helped move laboratory evaluation of the cellular immune system out of the research setting and into the diagnostic setting of the medical laboratory. Molecular biology and flow cytometry

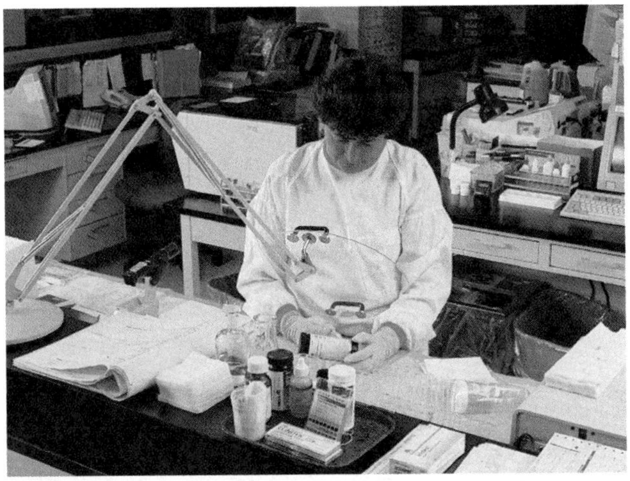

Figure 27-2 Clinical reference laboratories may have a separate urinalysis department where the laboratory professional tests urine for physical, chemical, or microbiologic properties.

are becoming commonplace in today's medical laboratory. Traditionally, serology has been an area within the microbiology department, but with the introduction of many new immunologic techniques, most medical laboratories now include a separate immunology department.

Toxicology. The **toxicology** department tests for toxic substances in a person's blood and monitors any drug usage, therapeutic levels of medication prescribed, or toxicity to the drugs being used. Medications commonly monitored for toxicity are digoxin, phenobarbital, lithium, and pain management drugs. Blood tests also determine levels of occupational exposure to metals and chemicals in the course of one's employment. Testing for drug usage/toxicity is now required in a growing number of pre-employment physical examinations. Toxicity levels for chemicals and metals include lead, zinc, iron, copper, arsenic, and carbon dioxide. The Department of Social and Health Services requires toxicology tests in child protection cases. Drug testing is often required for special assistance in low-income housing and other public financial assistance programs. The reasons are wide and varied for drug testing and growing every year, making this department larger than in the past.

DNA. The second area within the medical laboratory growing larger each year is the **DNA** department. With the advent of DNA tests for proving paternity and maternity of children and the growing use of DNA testing for criminal cases, DNA testing is quickly becoming a major focus in many laboratories.

Microbiology Department. The **microbiology** department is the area in the laboratory where microorganisms such as bacteria and fungi are grown in an appropriate medium, cultured, and then identified. Sensitivity tests are then performed to identify which antibiotics can effectively eradicate the pathogenic organisms. The combination of culturing and identifying the best antibiotic is called a **Culture and Sensitivity (C & S). Mycology** is an area within the microbiology department where fungi are studied. **Virology** is an area within the microbiology department where viruses are studied.

Parasitology Department. Parasitology is a subdivision of the microbiology department where ova and parasite (O & P) tests are performed on specimens such as feces. The specimens are examined for the presence of parasites or their eggs.

Cytology Department. The **cytology** department is the area in which microscopic examinations of cells are performed to detect early signs of cancer and other diseases. The Papanicolaou test, known as the Pap smear, for irregular cervical cells is an example of a test performed in the cytology department.

Histology Department. Histology is the study of tissue sample biopsies for the determination of disease. Frozen samples or **biopsies** are sliced/stained and then microscopically examined for cancer and other anomalies.

Panels of Laboratory Tests

Laboratory tests are often categorized into related groups to provide information about a particular body system or related bodily function. The groups are usually referred to as panels. In addition, laboratory tests are organized into panels for ease of ordering. For a current list of HCFA-approved organ- and disease-oriented panels, refer to Table 27-2.

Medicare requires that providers order tests under their approved panels. Providers may not refer to panels under other names such as the previously named Chem Screen, SMAC, Chem 7, and so on. The panels listed in Table 27-2 are the only panels allowed. If a provider would like a specific series or combinations of tests under a special panel, he or she must apply to the Health Care Financing Administration (HCFA) for the approval to design their own panel.

QUALITY CONTROLS/ ASSURANCES IN THE LABORATORY

The accuracy of any laboratory test result depends on all safeguards being followed. These standards ensure the quality of the testing equipment, supplies, personnel,

TABLE 27-2 HEALTH CARE AND FINANCE ADMINISTRATION (HCFA)–APPROVED ORGAN- AND DISEASE-ORIENTED PANELS (WITH CURRENT PROCEDURAL TERMINOLOGY [CPT] CODES) EFFECTIVE APRIL 1, 2000

Basic Metabolic Panel (CPT code 80048)
BUN (84520)
Calcium, total (82310)
Carbon dioxide (82374)
Chloride (82435)
Creatinine (82565)
Glucose (82947)
Potassium (84132)
Sodium (84295)

General Health Panel (CPT code 80050)
Comprehensive metabolic panel (CPT code 80053)
CBC w/manual differential (80054) or CBC w/automated differential (85025)
TSH (84443)

Electrolyte Panel (CPT code 80051)
Carbon dioxide (82374)
Chloride (82435)
Potassium (84132)
Sodium (84295)

Comprehensive Metabolic Panel (CPT code 80053)
Albumin (82040)
Alkaline phosphatase (84075)
Bilirubin, total (82247)
BUN (84520)
Calcium, total (82310)
Carbon dioxide (82374)
Chloride (82435)
Creatinine (82565)
Glucose (82947)
Potassium (84132)
Protein, total (84155)
Sodium (84295)
SGOT (AST) (84450)
SGPT (ALT) (84460)

Obstetric Panel (CPT code 80055)
CBC w/manual differential (80054) or CBC w/automated differential (85025)
Hepatitis B surface antigen (87340)
Rubella antibody (86762)
Syphilis test, qualitative (e.g., VDRL, RPR) (86592)
Antibody screen, RBC (86850)
Blood typing, ABO (86900) and Rh (D) (86901)

Lipid Panel (CPT code 80061)
Cholesterol (82465)
HDL cholesterol (83718) and LDL cholesterol, calculated
Triglyceride (84478)

Renal Function Panel (CPT code 80069)
Albumin (82040)
BUN (84520)
Calcium, total (82310)
Carbon dioxide (82374)
Chloride (82435)
Creatinine (82565)
Glucose (82947)
Phosphorous (84100)
Potassium (84132)
Sodium (84295)

Arthritis Panel (CPT code 80072)
Uric acid (84550)
ESR, erythrocyte sedimentation rate (85651)
Fluorescent noninfectious agent, screen (86255)
Rheumatoid factor, qualitative (86430)

Acute Hepatitis Panel (CPT code 80074)
Hepatitis A antibody, IgM (86709)
Hepatitis B core antibody, IgM (86705)
Hepatitis B surface antigen (87340)
Hepatitis C antibody (86803)

Hepatic Function Panel (CPT code 80076)
Albumin (82040)
Alkaline phosphatase (84075)
Bilirubin, direct (82248)
Bilirubin, total (82247)
Protein, total (84155)
SGOT (AST) (84450)
SGPT (ALT) (84460)

TORCH Antibody Panel (CPT code 80090)
Cytomegalovirus antibody, IgG (86644)
Herpes simplex (1 & 2) antibody, IgG (86694/86695)
Rubella antibody, IgG (86762)
Toxoplasmosis antibody (86677)

and the accuracy of the test results. There are many factors that can compromise the accuracy of laboratory test results. Among these factors are collection of specimen, temperature, amount or age of specimen, time limits of test, and using chemicals or reagents past their expiration dates. Even when laboratory guidelines are strictly followed, inaccurate results may be obtained by using test kits that have been exposed to extreme heat or cold, or using chemicals or reagents after their expiration. It is important to follow all laboratory guidelines, but the medical assistant must also confirm that the specimen, chemicals, and test kits are handled and processed properly.

Control Tests

To further ensure accurate test results, **control test** samples are tested together with the patient's sample. The control samples have a known value, negative or positive result, or abnormal or normal result, which is compared with the results of the patient's test. One of the purposes of this control measure is to minimize human error. By being able to compare a sample of known value or positive (or negative) test result with the patient's test, the health care worker performing the test can accurately determine the result. An error in the testing method may be discovered if the control sample does not test accurately.

Another purpose of the control test is to check the **reagents** or chemicals. If the control sample is not showing accurate results, it may be determined that the chemicals (reagents) are faulty or have expired. On receiving any test in the POL, the person responsible for quality assurance and quality control (probably the medical assistant performing the tests) should perform the calibration or control test provided by and as directed by the manufacturer. This ensures proper test function.

Proficiency Testing

CLIA '88 requires laboratories to participate in an accredited proficiency program for certain identified tests (see Chapter 26 for CLIA '88 requirements). Proficiency testing is similar to quality control in that "known" proficiency samples are tested the same as patient samples. The difference is an approved outside agency evaluates the accuracy of the testing and submits the performance records to HCFA for CLIA '88 compliance.

Preventative Maintenance

Preventative maintenance helps identify potential problems before they actually occur. Procedures include manufacturer-recommended maintenance on equipment; daily temperature checks on refrigerators, freezers, and incubators; daily checks on expiration dates of reagents and supplies; and instrument log and centrifuge checks.

Instrument Validations

The quality of test results can be ensured by consistently checking the calibration and linear range of the instruments and machines. If the equipment is not maintained or is functioning improperly, accurate test results cannot be assured.

The Medical Assistant's Role

Medical assistants are educated to perform administrative office duties, prepare patients, collect specimens, and perform waived tests in such a manner that patients and health care personnel are safe from contamination, the patient is not harmed, the sample is reliable, and the test is accurate. These four aspects of quality laboratory testing are critical for accuracy. When the patient is prepared properly, the specimen is obtained as expertly as possible, the reagents and equipment are in the best condition and calibration possible, and the test is performed by a trained professional, the test results will be accurate.

LABORATORY REQUISITIONS AND REPORTS

A written **requisition** for laboratory work must be sent to the laboratory with the patient or with the specimen (Figure 27-3). These forms are preprinted with the most commonly requested tests separated into logical categories. Additional space is provided for writing special requests. The laboratories that patients use will be happy to provide your medical agency with these forms. Laboratory requisition forms are now computer generated, and the physician–employer's name, address, and other information necessary for proper reporting and recordkeeping are often preprinted on the forms. If the requisitions are

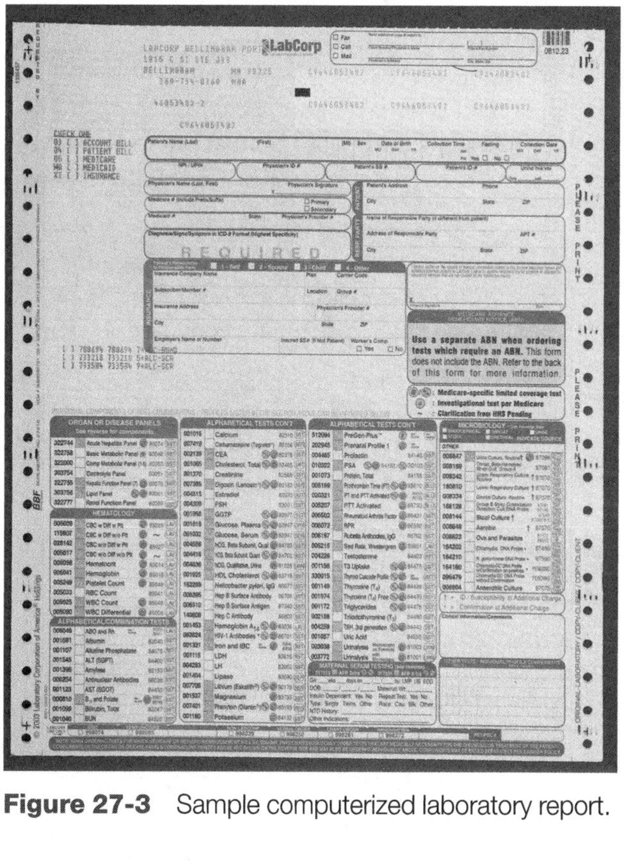

Figure 27-3 Sample computerized laboratory report.

not preprinted, spaces are provided for the information to be written in. If the facility does not have computer-generated laboratory requisitions, or in the event of a computer malfunction, the medical assistant must know what information is required on a handwritten requisition. Regardless of whether the requisition is handwritten or computer generated, the information must be complete, accurate, and clearly legible. A properly completed requisition contains the following data:

- Physician's name, account number, address, and telephone number. This information is necessary to contact the office for any clarification or further information, and to report the results.
- Patient's name, address, and telephone number. Be sure the name is complete and spelled correctly. Avoid using alternate versions of the patient's name without also including the proper, legal name. Make certain to include apartment numbers and zip codes. This information will be used for billing purposes, as well as medical records. Social Security numbers and middle initials are helpful when it is necessary to differentiate between patients.
- Patient's billing information, insurance, and identification number. Because the patient is often not the person who is the subscriber to the insurance, the subscriber's name, address, telephone number, and insurance identification numbers are extremely important, especially if the patient does not live with the subscriber. Some patients have secondary insurance coverage. Be sure to include that data also. The laboratory would prefer to receive an additional sheet of information than to have incomplete insurance records in its business office.
- Unique patient identifier. This can be an identification number that is hospital or laboratory generated. In the outpatient setting, this can be the patient's Social Security number or date of birth.
- Patient's age/date of birth and sex. Age and sex both influence the results of some tests and should not be assumed.
- Source of specimen. This information is especially important when dealing with tests such as cultures and biopsies. In the case of cultures, knowing the source of the specimen aids the laboratory in determining whether the specimen contains normal flora or is abnormal for that area of the body.
- Time and date of the specimen collection. Some tests require that the specimen be tested fairly quickly after leaving the body; other tests must be performed after a certain period has elapsed. The time and date of the specimen collection are important because accuracy can be compromised if the specimen is not sent to the laboratory in a reasonable amount of time.
- Test requested. This is usually a matter of putting a check mark in the appropriate box on the requisition, but it is surprising how often laboratories receive specimens with nicely completed requisitions and no indication of the test desired.
- Medications the patient is taking. Because medication can influence some test results, it is important that the laboratory be provided this information. Patients are often asked to refrain from taking certain medications before testing. Be sure to consult with the physician to verify orders. If a medication is not discontinued before testing, the type of medication, the dosage amount, and the time of the last dose must be included on the requisition.
- Clinical diagnosis. The physician's tentative diagnosis is useful to the laboratory in helping to differentiate between diagnoses or confirm a diagnosis. The clinical diagnosis may also alert the laboratory personnel to any possible special considerations of which to be aware. For example, if diabetes is suspected, the laboratory will give special consideration to the glucose value. The diagnosis or preferably the ICD-9 code is also necessary for billing.
- Urgency of results. Sometimes the physician needs a test to be performed immediately (STAT) or would like a result as soon as possible (ASAP). The physician's orders need to be clearly stated on the requisition. Additional space is also provided for other special instructions if necessary.
- Special collection/patient instructions. Examples include fasting specimens, timed collections, and "do not collect from a specific area" instructions.
- If copies of the results are to be sent to a second physician, the medical assistant must include the physician's full name, address, and fax number. Be careful to print the fax number clearly so the patient's results are not sent to the wrong place in error.

> Many offices choose to copy both sides of the patient's insurance card and clip it to the laboratory requisition. This assures the laboratory will have all insurance information they need to bill for their services.

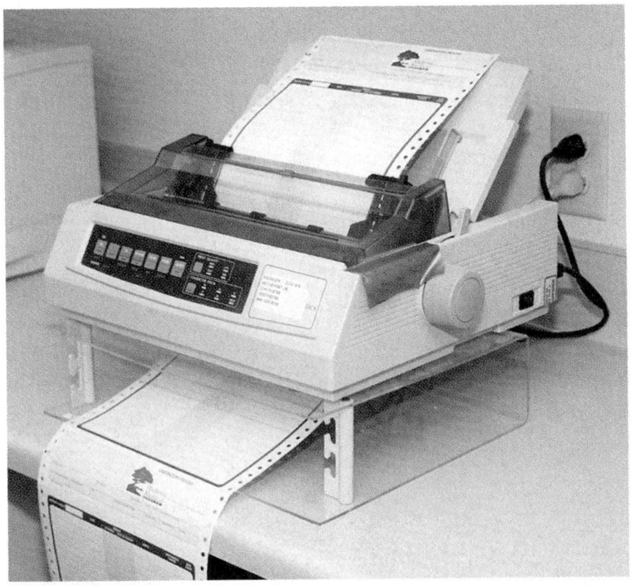

Figure 27-4 Computerized laboratory report transmitted directly from the reference lab to the physician's office.

The laboratory will send back a written report (Figure 27-4) that will contain the following information:

- Name, address, and telephone number of the laboratory
- Referring physician's name, address, and identification numbers
- Patient's name, identification number, age, and sex
- Date the specimen was received by the laboratory
- Date and time the specimen was collected
- Date the laboratory reported the results
- The test name, results, and normal reference ranges if applicable

Reports are often sent electronically by fax or are made available through electronic medical records, together with the written report. Abnormal test results are always flagged in some way, either in a different color, a different column, or perhaps designated by a star or simply by *H* (for high) or *L* (for low). Critical values (results that may indicate serious medical conditions) are alerted to the physician by a phone call from the laboratory.

When the results are received, the medical assistant should attach them to the patient's chart for the physician to review and initial before filing them. The physician should be alerted to any abnormal test results as soon as possible. Laboratories often send results via computer-generated reports directly to the physician's office or hospital.

If patients want a copy of the results for their own records, their physician must send permission or the patient will need to sign a release form. This is required by HIPAA.

SPECIMEN COLLECTION

Proper Procurement, Storage, and Handling

Instructions for procuring, storing, and handling and transporting laboratory specimens properly may be obtained from the independent laboratories. Most laboratories will provide the office/clinic with a step-by-step instruction manual, sometimes called a Compendium, a laboratory manual, or a user manual and will also be available to answer any additional questions by telephone.

Obtaining the specimen in the proper manner and using the right equipment will assure that a high-quality specimen is submitted to the laboratory. Some guidelines for specimen collection are as follows:

- Check the physician's orders and identify the patient.
- Refer to the laboratory instruction manual or consult the laboratory for specific collection instructions.
- Instruct the patient in any necessary dietary restriction.
- Instruct the patient to ingest special food or take other substances if required.
- Select or provide to the patient appropriate containers with the proper preservatives in them, if required.
- Be certain to label the specimen with the patient's name, identification number, date, type of specimen, time of collection, and physician's name. Label the container, not the lid, because the lid will be removed during testing. Label the container, not the wrapping, because the wrapping will be separated from the container when testing is performed, for example, throat swabs.
- Obtain the specimen or instruct the patient to provide the specimen according to the directions given by the laboratory.
- Follow applicable OSHA bloodborne pathogens guidelines (refer to Chapter 10) when packaging the specimen for transport so it will not leak or

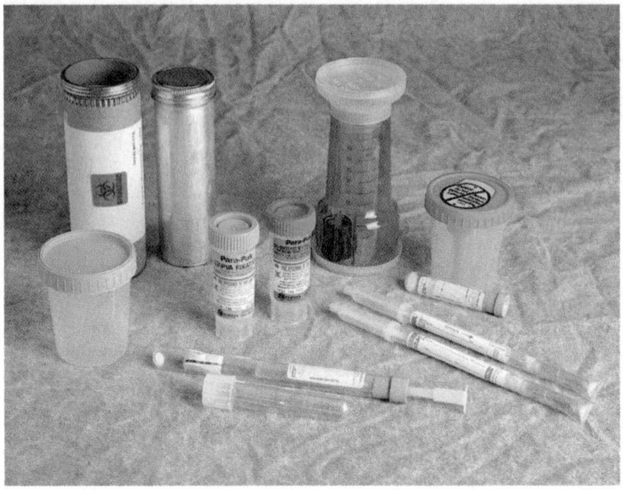

Figure 27-5 Various types of collection and transportation containers for laboratory specimens.

contaminate the courier or other office staff and so that it will safely arrive at the laboratory without being damaged or destroyed (see Figure 27-5).

- Document in the patient's chart the type of specimen collected, the tests ordered, which laboratory the specimen is being sent to (even if it is being tested in your POL), how the patient tolerated the procedure (including any complications), and other pertinent information according to your office policy. Many offices also keep a copy of the laboratory requisition in the patient's chart for later reference. If the testing is performed in your POL, the results of the test should be recorded on a laboratory report form and, after the physician has initialed it, filed in the laboratory section of the chart.

Processing and Sending Specimens to a Laboratory

Specimens collected by the medical assistant are often sent from the office to a laboratory many miles away or are picked up by a courier representing the outside laboratory. These are often large commercial laboratories that are not associated with a local hospital laboratory. The patient's insurance often dictates the laboratory contracted to perform the patient's testing. It is not unusual for several different laboratories to pick up at one location. A situation could be that the blood work from patient Jones would go to laboratory A, the blood work from patient Smith would go to laboratory B, and a urine sample from patient Doe would be tested in the laboratory within the building. It sometimes can be confusing as to where to send the specimen.

Patient Education

The patient will often need to be instructed on a specific preparation before a specimen is taken. Because food and medication can greatly influence test results, a patient may need to be instructed not to eat for several hours before having the specimen taken or drawn. Fasting means the patient may not have anything except water for the 12 hours before the test. NPO means the patient may not have even water. The patient may need to refrain from taking a routine dosage of medication before the test is performed. Sometimes the patient preparation instructions will include a special diet for a few days. Regardless of how simple instructions may seem, it is important to give the patient clear, written directions. Take the time to go over any instructions with the patient (and sometimes other family members). Your patients will welcome the opportunity to ask questions and to have a written set of instructions to take home.

All these laboratory test results are dependent on the quality of the specimen submitted. The quality of the specimen depends on the patient preparation, proper collection, correct patient identification, and transportation of the specimen. If there is any doubt or question regarding the type of specimen to be collected, it is imperative that the appropriate laboratory be called to clarify the specimen needed. There are often differences between laboratories; the type of specimen acceptable for one laboratory is not necessarily the acceptable specimen for another laboratory.

MICROSCOPES

One of the most used pieces of equipment in the medical laboratory is the microscope. Consisting of a light source, eyepieces, objectives, **condenser,** and **diaphragm,** the microscope enables us to see bacteria and other microorganisms that are much too small to be seen without magnification.

Types of Microscopes

The most commonly used microscope in the clinic is the compound microscope (Figure 27-6). As the name indicates, the image is compounded by the use of two different lenses. One lens compounds or increases the magnification produced by the other lens. The first lens system is located in the **objectives,** and the second lens system is in the eyepiece (ocular). The light source is a bulb in the base. The light is directed up through the specimen on the slide and into the objective lenses. The light, or image, is then reflected by the condenser onto the specimen to the ocular lenses for visualization.

The eyepiece may have a single (monocular) lens, or there may be two (binocular) lenses. This lens is not adjustable or changeable. The magnification in the eyepiece is usually 10 times (10×) the normal size of the object being viewed.

The objective lenses are adjustable between low power, high power, and oil immersion. When we are viewing through the microscope under low power, we are able to see more of the slide but with less detail than when using high power. When we view under high power, we are able to see a smaller portion of the field but with greater detail. The low-power objective lens allows the item being viewed to be magnified 10 times larger than life. This magnification combined with the 10 times magnification of the ocular lens allows us to see microscopically 100 times the normal size (10× × 10× = 100×).

By combining the 10-power (10×) ocular lens with the high-power objective lens, which has the magnification power of forty times life (40×), we are able to increase our magnification vision to 400 times the normal size (10× × 40× = 400×). This is enough magnification to see large microorganisms, but it is still not enough to see smaller organisms, such as bacteria, clearly. An oil-immersion lens is needed to view bacteria closely.

The oil-immersion lens enables us to multiply the ocular lens magnification (10×) by one hundred (100×) to reach a possible total magnification of one thousand times normal life size (10× × 100× = 1,000×). Because more light is needed to actually see this amount of magnification, the lens is immersed in oil. This prevents the scattering and loss of light rays, which naturally occurs when light travels through air, consequently increasing the efficiency of the magnification.

Other types of microscopes have been developed especially for specific uses. One is the phase-contrast microscope specifically designed for viewing specimens that are transparent and unstained. Some microscopic specimens must be stained with a fluorescent dye to be examined in detail (e.g., when detecting specific bacteria). A fluorescent microscope is the instrument best suited for viewing those specimens. In dark-field microscopy, the light is reflected from an angle, which causes the specimen to appear as a bright object on a dark field.

Another type of microscope is the electron microscope (Figure 27-7). Special training is required to operate this sophisticated instrument. The electron microscope is large (several feet tall) and expensive; therefore, it is only found in larger regional and hospital laboratories. An electronic beam, rather than light, is passed through the specimen. The image is projected onto a fluorescent screen and may then be photographed and enlarged. Using the electron microscope enables us to view extremely small organisms, such as viruses, in great detail and in three dimensions. Figure 27-8 illustrates blood cells seen using an electron microscope.

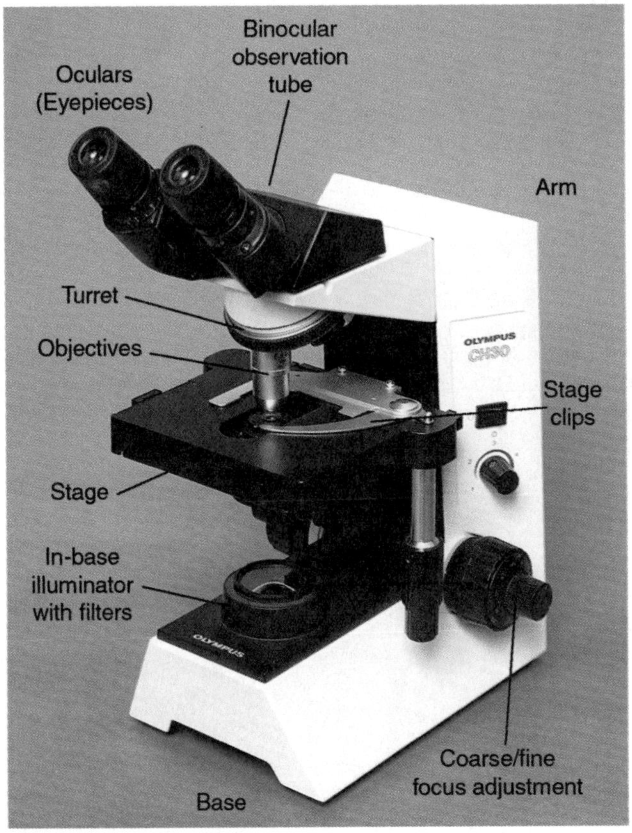

Figure 27-6 Basic compound microscope.

How to Use a Microscope

Besides being able to adjust a microscope's magnification, it may be necessary to adjust focus. The microscope contains a coarse adjustment and a fine adjustment. The coarse adjustment is to be used with the low-power (short) objective only. The coarse adjustment is used to bring the object into view. The fine adjustment may then be used to sharpen the image. Depending on the individual microscope, the

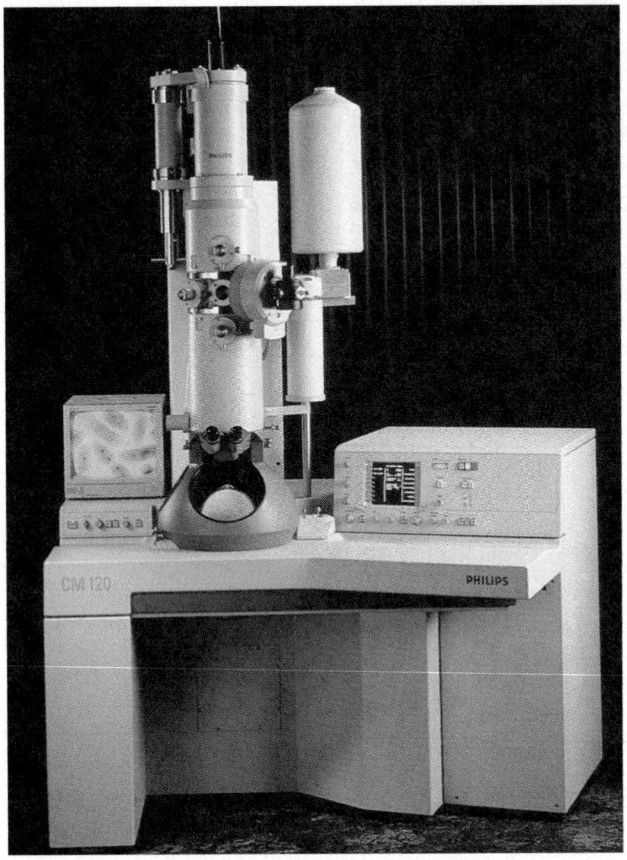

Figure 27-7 S440 scanning electron microscope.

coarse and fine adjustments may raise and lower the nosepiece, which houses the objectives, or they may raise and lower the stage, or platform, on which the slide rests.

It is important always to remember to raise the platform of the lower objectives using the coarse adjustment and the low-power objective *while viewing the slide from the side*. This allows the lens to come close to the slide without actually touching it. If the slide is not viewed from the side for the coarse adjustment, there is the possibility of running the objective through the slide and seriously damaging the lens and the microscope, or of breaking the slide. After bringing the slide and objective together, the adjustments may be made through the ocular, always moving away from the slide. Once the item is in view, the fine adjustment may be used for clarity.

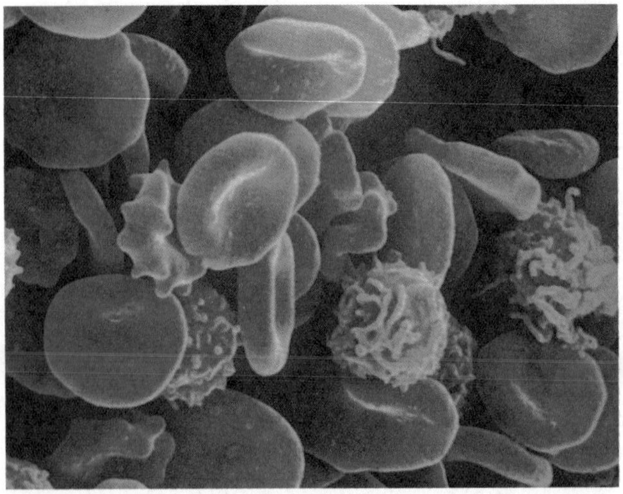

Figure 27-8 Blood cells as seen under an electron microscope.

The bulb in the base, which directs light through the slide, first goes through a condenser and then through an iris diaphragm. The condenser is used to control the intensity of the light, and the iris diaphragm may be adjusted to control the amount of light.

To use the oil-immersion lens, place a drop of cedar or mineral oil on top of the coverslip directly over the specimen on the slide. Then carefully lower the oil-immersion lens into the oil, making sure that the lens never actually touches the slide.

How to Care for a Microscope

Microscopes can be expensive and, like any precision instrument, should be treated with care. Some practices that will extend the life of a microscope and maintain the quality of its performance are:

- Always follow the manufacturer's and clinic's rules for the care and maintenance of the microscopes.

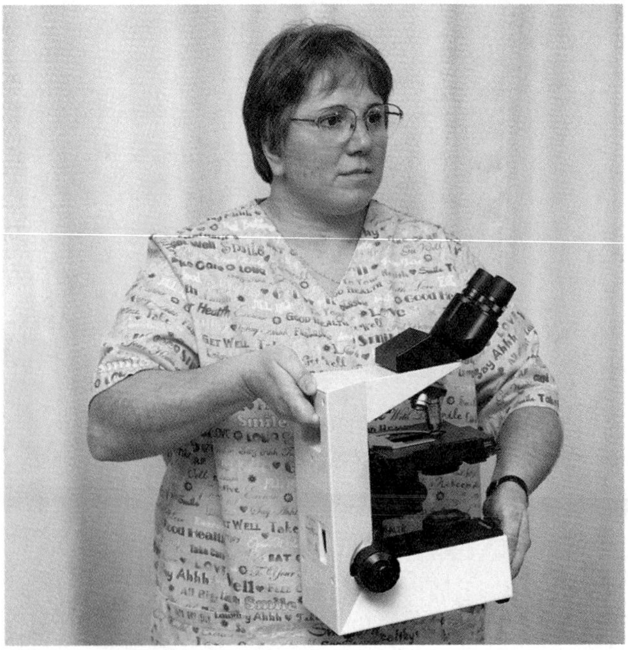

Figure 27-9 The proper way to carry a microscope.

- Carry the microscope with one hand securely supporting the base and the other hand holding the arm (Figure 27-9).
- Keep the microscope covered when it is not being used.
- Clean the lenses with special lens paper and lens cleaner after each use. Using standard tissue can scratch the lenses.
- When looking through the eyepiece and focusing, always move the platform away from, never toward, the eyepiece to prevent the objective from coming into contact with the slide. If you are actually looking at the platform, then you can move it closer to the eyepiece without coming into contact with the slide.
- Use oil only with the oil-immersion lens.

Procedure 27-1 Using the Microscope

STANDARD PRECAUTIONS:

PURPOSE:

To properly use a microscope to view microscopic organisms using the coarse and fine adjustments, as well as the low- and high-power and oil-immersion objectives.

EQUIPMENT/SUPPLIES:

Hand disinfectant
Microscope (monocular or binocular)
Lens paper
Lens cleaner
Prepared slides (commercially available)
Immersion oil
Surface disinfectant
NOTE: Procedure will vary slightly according to microscope design. Consult the operating procedure in the microscope manual for specific instructions.

PROCEDURE STEPS:

1. Wash hands.
2. Assemble equipment and materials.
3. Clean the ocular(s) and objectives with lens paper.
4. Use the coarse adjustment to raise the eyepiece or lens unit.
5. Rotate the 10×, or low-power, objective into position, so that it is directly over the opening in the stage.
6. Turn on the microscope light.
7. Open the diaphragm until maximum light comes up through the condenser.
8. Place the slide on the stage (specimen side up).
9. Locate the coarse adjustment.
10. Look directly at the stage and 10× objective and turn the coarse adjustment until the objective is as close to the slide as it will go.
    NOTE: Do not lower any objective toward a slide while looking through the ocular(s).
11. Look into the ocular(s) and slowly turn the coarse adjustment in the opposite direction (as in Step 10) to raise the objective (or lower the stage) until the object on the slide comes into view.
12. Locate the fine adjustment.
13. Turn the fine adjustment to sharpen the image.
    NOTE: If a binocular microscope is used, the oculars must be adjusted for each individual's eyes.
    a. Adjust the distance between the oculars so that one image is seen (as when using binoculars).
    b. Use the coarse and fine adjustments to bring the object into focus while looking through the right ocular with the right eye.
    c. Close the right eye, look into the left ocular with the left eye, and *use the knurled collar on the left ocular* to bring the object into sharp focus. (Do not turn the coarse or fine adjustment at this time.)
    d. Look into the oculars with both eyes to observe that the object is in clear focus. If it is not, repeat the procedure.
14. Scan the slide by either method:
    a. Use the stage knobs to move the slide left and right and backward and forward while looking through the ocular(s),

(continues)

Procedure 27-1 (continued)

or

b. Move the slide with the fingers while looking through the ocular(s) (for microscope without movable stage).

15. Rotate the high-power (40×) objective into position while observing the objective and the slide to see that the objective does not strike the slide.
16. Look through the ocular(s) to view the object on the slide; it should be almost in focus.
17. Locate the fine adjustment.
18. Look through the ocular(s) and turn the fine adjustment until the object is in focus. Do not use the coarse adjustment.
19. Adjust the amount of light. This can be done by closing the diaphragm, lowering the condenser, or adjusting the light at the source.
20. Scan the slide as in Step 14, using the fine adjustment if necessary to keep the object in focus.
21. Rotate the oil-immersion objective to the side slightly (so that no objective is in position).
22. Place one drop of immersion oil on the portion of the slide that is directly over the condenser.
23. Rotate the oil-immersion objective into position, being careful not to rotate the 40× objective through the oil.
24. Look to see that the oil-immersion objective is touching the drop of oil.
25. Look through the ocular(s) and slowly turn the fine adjustment until the image is clear. Use only the fine adjustment to focus the oil-immersion objective.
26. Adjust the amount of light using the procedure in Step 19.
27. Scan the slide using the procedure in Step 14.
28. Rotate the 10× objective into position (do not allow the 40× objective to touch the oil).
29. Remove the slide from the microscope stage and gently clean the oil from the slide with lens paper. A copeland jar containing a solvent cleaner, such as xylene, can be used to remove excess oil from the slide.
30. Clean the oculars, 10× objective, and 40× objective with clean lens paper and lens cleaner.
31. Clean the 100× objective with lens paper and lens cleaner to remove all oil.
32. Clean any oil from the microscope stage and condenser.
33. Turn off the microscope light and disconnect.
34. Position the eyepiece in the lowest position using the coarse adjustment.
35. Center the stage so that it does not project from either side of the microscope.
36. Cover the microscope and return it to storage.
37. Clean the work area; return slides to storage.
38. Wash hands.

Case Study 27-1

Edith Leonard came to Inner City Health Care because she was experiencing sight disturbances, constant thirst, and fainting spells. After examining Edith, Dr. Ray Reynolds ordered a glucose tolerance test. Certified medical assistant Wanda Slawson gave Edith a special diet that she was to follow for the three days preceding the test and instructions regarding fasting before the test.

Edith has returned to the clinic to have the test. "Did you follow the diet I gave you, Mrs. Leonard?" Wanda asks. "Yes, I did." "Did you have anything to eat this morning?" "No, but I did have a cup of coffee. I thought it would be all right because I drink it black. I can't start the day without my coffee."

CASE STUDY REVIEW

1. Should Wanda perform the test? Explain your answer.
2. How can Wanda emphasize the importance of following the diet, fasting, and test instructions?
3. What can Wanda do to try to ensure Edith's cooperation?

SUMMARY

If disease did not exist, we would have little need for clinical laboratories. If we were not susceptible to viral illnesses, if bacteria never infected our bodies, if our bodies always operated in their healthiest state regardless of what we did to them, and, perhaps most important of all, if we chose our parents wisely, there would be little that a clinical laboratory would be asked to do. The fact that our bodies are susceptible to disease necessitates the existence of clinical laboratories.

Together with clinical laboratory personnel, medical assistants play an important role in laboratory testing. They prepare patients for tests, obtain specimens, and perform simple, routine tests or send specimens to the appropriate laboratory. Medical assistants are educated to perform these tasks in a manner that ensures the accuracy of the test and safeguards the health of patients and health care personnel.

STUDY FOR SUCCESS

To reinforce your knowledge and skills of information presented in this chapter:

- ❑ Review the Key Terms
- ❑ Practice the Procedure
- ❑ Consider the Case Study and discuss your conclusions
- ❑ Answer the Review Questions
  - ❑ Multiple Choice
  - ❑ Critical Thinking
- ❑ Navigate the Internet by completing the Web Activities
- ❑ Practice the StudyWARE activities on the textbook CD
- ❑ Apply your knowledge in the Student Workbook activities
- ❑ Complete the Web Tutor sections

REVIEW QUESTIONS

Multiple Choice

1. All of the following statements concerning point-of-care testing are true *except:*
   a. performed at the patient's bedside
   b. must be performed by certified laboratory professionals
   c. provides for rapid, accurate results
   d. the medical laboratory's role includes training and management of quality control
2. Independent medical laboratories must be managed by a:
   a. clinical laboratory technologist
   b. pathologist
   c. clinical laboratory technician
   d. medical assistant
3. The hematology department of a laboratory:
   a. studies microorganisms and their activities
   b. studies blood and blood-forming tissues
   c. detects the presence of disease-producing human parasites or eggs present in specimens taken from the body
   d. detects the presence of abnormal cells
4. The quality of patient test results is maintained by:
   a. instrument calibration procedures
   b. preventative maintenance procedures
   c. quality control testing
   d. all of the above
5. When a patient or specimen is sent to a laboratory for testing, the medical assistant also sends:
   a. a written requisition
   b. a report
   c. the patient's file
   d. an insurance form

6. The most commonly used microscope in the clinic is the:
   a. fluorescent microscope
   b. electron microscope
   c. phase-contrast microscope
   d. compound microscope

Critical Thinking

1. A patient asks you to recommend a laboratory for the tests ordered by the physician. How will you respond to the request? What are some factors that will influence your response?
2. A patient performed a pregnancy test at home, but the physician has requested a pregnancy test in the office. Explain to the patient why the home test may not be as accurate as the test performed in the office.
3. The physician has ordered a metabolic panel for a patient. What is a panel, and how will it help the physician to diagnose the patient's condition?
4. Explain why it is important to handle and process specimens, test kits, and chemicals properly.
5. The time and date of specimen collection were not included on the requisition form. Why are these data always important to the laboratory?
6. Explain how a compound microscope is able to magnify.

WEB ACTIVITIES

1. For each group of laboratory personnel discussed in this chapter, search the Internet for a Web site that pertains to it. What kind of information does it offer?
2. Locate a local hospital's Web site. Does it outline all the specialty departments described in this chapter? What unique services do they offer?
3. Visit your insurance company's Web site. Does it specify which laboratories must be used?

REFERENCES/BIBLIOGRAPHY

American Medical Technologists. (2004). Retrieved from http://www.amt1.com. Accessed May 9, 2005.

American Society for Clinical Laboratory Science. (2004). Retrieved from http://www.ascls.org. Accessed May 9, 2005.

American Society for Clinical Pathology. (2004). Retrieved from http://www.ascp.org. Accessed May 9, 2005.

National Accrediting Agency for Clinical Laboratory Sciences. Retrieved from http://www.naacls.org. Accessed May 9, 2005.

National Credentialing Agency for Medical Laboratory Personnel. Retrieved from http://www.nca-info.org. Accessed May 9, 2005.

CHAPTER 28

Phlebotomy: Venipuncture and Capillary Puncture

OUTLINE

Why Collect Blood?
The Medical Assistant's Role in Phlebotomy
Anatomy and Physiology of the Circulatory System
- Collection of Blood Specimens

Venipuncture Equipment
- Syringes and Needles
- Safety Needles and Blood Collection Systems
- Vacuum Tubes and Adapters/Holders
- Anticoagulants, Additives, and Gels
- Order of Draw
- Tourniquets
- Specimen Collection Trays

Venipuncture Technique
- Approaching the Patient
- Preparing Supplies and Greeting the Patient
- Patient and Specimen Identification
- Positioning the Patient
- Selecting the Appropriate Venipuncture Site
- Applying the Tourniquet
- Performing a Safe Venipuncture
- Specimen Collection
- The Syringe Technique
- Vacuum Tube Specimen Collection
- Butterfly Needle Collection System
- Patient Reactions
- The Unsuccessful Venipuncture
- Criteria for Rejection of a Specimen
- Factors Affecting Laboratory Values

Capillary Puncture
- Composition of Capillary Blood
- Capillary Puncture Sites
- Preparing the Capillary Puncture Site
- Performing the Puncture
- Collecting the Blood Sample

KEY TERMS

Additive
Aliquot
Anticoagulant
Buffy Coat
Cannula
Centrifuge
Constrict
Dilate
Edematous
Erythrocyte
Hematoma
Hemoconcentration
Hemolysis
Hypoglycemia
Leukocyte
Lipemia
Oxygenated
Palpate
Phlebotomy
Plasma
Primary Container
Serum
Thixotrophic Separator Gel
Thrombocyte
Tourniquet
Venipuncture
Viscosity

FEATURED COMPETENCIES

CAAHEP—ENTRY-LEVEL COMPETENCIES

Clinical Competencies

Fundamental Procedures

- Perform handwashing
- Dispose of biohazard materials
- Practice Standard Precautions

Specimen Collection

- Perform venipuncture
- Perform capillary puncture

General Competencies

Professional Communications

- Recognize and respond to verbal communication
- Recognize and respond to nonverbal communication

Legal Concepts

- Identify and respond to issues of confidentiality
- Perform within legal and ethical boundaries
- Establish and maintain the medical record
- Document appropriately

Patient Instructions

- Instruct individuals according to their needs

Operational Functions

- Use methods of quality control

ABHES—ENTRY-LEVEL COMPETENCIES

Professionalism

- Maintain confidentiality at all times
- Conduct work within scope of education, training, and ability

(continues)

OBJECTIVES

The student should strive to meet the following performance objectives and demonstrate an understanding of the facts and principles presented in this chapter through written and oral communication.

1. Define the key terms as presented in the glossary.
2. Explain the medical assistant's responsibility to the patient in terms of quality of care and respect of the patient as a human being.
3. Explain why the medical assistant has a special responsibility to present a neat, pleasant, and competent demeanor.
4. Differentiate between serum and plasma.
5. State the relationship between diameter and the gauge of the needle.
6. Explain the principle of the vacuum tube system.
7. State the manner in which anticoagulants prevent coagulation.
8. Name the anticoagulant associated with the various color-coded vacuum tubes.
9. State the purpose of additives to vacuum tubes.
10. Explain the three skills used in collecting blood specimen.
11. Explain the importance of correct patient identification, complete specimen labeling, and proper handling, storage, and delivery.
12. Describe the step-by-step procedure for drawing blood with a syringe, vacuum tube system, butterfly, or capillary puncture.
13. Explain how to handle the various reactions a patient might have to venipuncture.
14. List two items commonly used in phlebotomy that may cause a problem with a patient who has a latex sensitivity or allergy.

SCENARIO

At Inner City Health Care, medical assistant Bruce Goldman often performs venipunctures. Bruce is personable and has an easy-going manner that makes patients feel comfortable with him. He takes time to talk to patients before performing a venipuncture to determine their feelings about the procedure and to learn about their previous experiences. Bruce is confident and professional in his interactions with patients. He is always well-groomed, and he treats patients with respect. Using his social, technical, and administrative skills, Bruce is usually able to collect the necessary blood samples while providing a positive experience for patients.

FEATURED COMPETENCIES (continued)

Clinical Duties

- Prepare patients for procedures
- Apply principles of aseptic techniques and infection control
- Use quality control
- Collect and process specimens
- Dispose of biohazard materials
- Practice standard precautions
- Perform venipuncture
- Perform capillary puncture

Legal Concepts

- Document accurately

Spotlight on Certification

RMA Content Outline

- Anatomy and physiology
- Human relations
- Asepsis
- Laboratory procedures

CMA Content Outline

- Systems, including structure, function related conditions and diseases
- Maintaining confidentiality
- Medical records
- Principles of infection control
- Equipment preparation and operation
- Safety precautions
- Collecting and processing specimens; diagnostic testing

CMAS Content Outline

- Anatomy and physiology
- Professionalism
- Asepsis in the medical office
- Communication

INTRODUCTION

The task of collecting blood samples from patients for diagnostic testing is known as phlebotomy. The health care professional who performs this duty varies at each health care setting. The task of phlebotomy is not restricted to one individual. A variety of individuals are cross trained to do phlebotomy and other tasks. Many health care settings do not have enough patients to justify having a phlebotomist available at all times. Therefore, the medical assistant may be designated to perform phlebotomy procedures.

WHY COLLECT BLOOD?

Phlebotomy is the process of collecting blood for diagnostic purposes or bloodletting as a therapeutic measure. The history of bloodletting dates back to the early Egyptians and continues into modern times. Phlebotomy in the past was a method to cure individuals with "bad" blood. The blood was drained out of individuals as a treatment, thereby alleviating the patient's symptoms. Phlebotomy is now used to help determine the disease process taking place and to determine the method of treatment. Without the collection of blood samples, physicians would have few means available to assist them in making diagnoses.

THE MEDICAL ASSISTANT'S ROLE IN PHLEBOTOMY

A phlebotomist is a person trained to obtain blood specimens by venipuncture and capillary puncture techniques. The phlebotomist's primary role is to collect blood as efficiently as possible for accurate and reliable test results. How the medical assistant will be involved in phlebotomy will vary greatly from one health care environment to another. The medical assistant performing venipuncture will have direct contact with the patient and perform tasks that are critical to the patient's diagnosis and care. During the direct contact with the patient, the medical assistant will leave an impression with the patient. It can be positive or negative depending on the skill with which the medical assistant performs the venipuncture.

It is the medical assistant's responsibility to provide high-quality care to patients. The medical assistant must act professionally when working with patients. Professionalism is displayed by performing tasks in an efficient, competent manner; wearing clean, neat attire; and showing concern for patients and their feelings.

Patients will not tell family and friends that their blood was run through expensive state-of-the-art instruments but rather that the person drawing their blood sample was friendly and skilled. A smile and a kind word can allay a patient's fear and do a lot to win a permanent customer and patient to the physician's office.

ANATOMY AND PHYSIOLOGY OF THE CIRCULATORY SYSTEM

To be prepared to collect blood, the medical assistant must understand the system that carries the blood and the composition of the blood. The system in which the blood is transported is the circulatory system. Blood forms in the organs of the body. The bone marrow is the primary factory for production of blood cells. The lymph nodes, thymus, and spleen are also sites for the production of blood cells. The function of blood is to carry oxygen to body tissues and to remove the waste product, carbon dioxide. The blood also carries nutrients to all parts of the body and moves the waste products to the lungs, kidneys, liver, and skin for elimination.

The circulatory system consists of the heart, which pumps blood through the body by way of tubing called arteries, veins, and capillaries. When blood flows away from the heart, it flows in arteries; blood flowing back to the heart flows through the veins. Connecting most of the arteries and veins are the capillaries (Figure 28-1).

ARTERIES TO VEINS	
Arteries	**Veins**
1. Carry blood from the heart, carry oxygenated blood (except pulmonary artery)	1. Carry blood to the heart, carry deoxygenated blood (except pulmonary vein)
2. Normally bright red in color	2. Normally dark red in color
3. Elastic walls that expand with surge of blood	3. Thin walls/less elastic
4. No valves	4. Valves
5. Can feel a pulse	5. No pulse

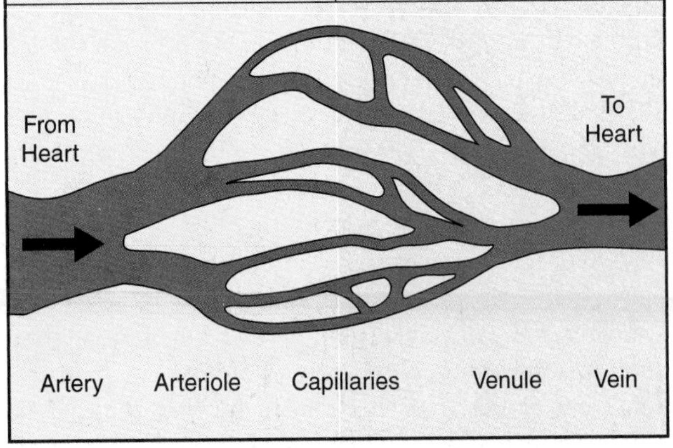

Figure 28-1 Blood flows from the heart through the arteries and back to the heart through the veins.

Arteries have a thick wall that helps them withstand the pressure of the pumping action of the heart. The arteries branch to form arterioles, which branch again to become capillaries. The capillaries then begin coming together to form venules, and the venules then become veins. As blood flows through the body, it follows this path of artery-arteriole-capillary-venule-vein. **Oxygenated** arterial blood, which contains a high level of oxygen, leaves the heart and carries the oxygen to the tissue by releasing the oxygen through the cell walls of the capillaries. At the same time, carbon dioxide is being absorbed by the blood, and then is transported to the lungs to be exhaled as a waste product. The flow of the blood also regulates body temperature. When the body gets warm, the capillaries in the extremities **dilate** and let off heat. This process then cools the body. If the body becomes cold, the capillaries **constrict** and less blood flows through, thereby conserving heat for the rest of the body.

The body contains approximately 6 liters (L) of blood, 45% of which is formed elements. The formed cellular elements consist of **erythrocytes, leukocytes,** and **thrombocytes** (Figure 28-2). The remaining 55% of the blood is liquid. Generally 2.5 milliliters (ml) blood will yield about 1 ml serum. The liquid portion of uncoagulated blood is known as **plasma.** Plasma is the fluid that provides a matrix for blood cells, electrolytes, proteins, and chemicals to travel throughout the body via the blood vessels. Blood flowing through the body contains a substance called fibrinogen. The clotting process converts the fibrinogen into fibrin. The fibrin is like a sticky spider web that traps the formed elements into the fibrin mass called a clot. The clot then contracts and the liquid **(serum)** portion is extracted. The serum is a clear, straw-colored liquid that is used for many of the tests done in the laboratory. The main difference between serum and plasma is that plasma contains fibrinogen, and serum does not.

The formed elements and the liquid portion of the blood are often separated for laboratory testing. To speed the removal of the serum from a tube of blood, an instrument called a **centrifuge** spins the blood. A carrier holds the tubes of blood, and when the centrifuge is activated, the carrier spins. The spinning action of the carrier pushes the blood cells to the bottom of the tube. The blood separates according to weight. The clot goes to the bottom of the tube and the serum goes to the top.

To produce a plasma specimen, the blood must be prevented from clotting by the use of a chemical **anticoagulant.** Blood collected in a tube containing an anticoagulant can be centrifuged to separate the formed elements (cells) from the plasma. The bottom layer will contain the erythrocytes, then there will be a thin layer called the **buffy coat.** The buffy coat contains a mixture

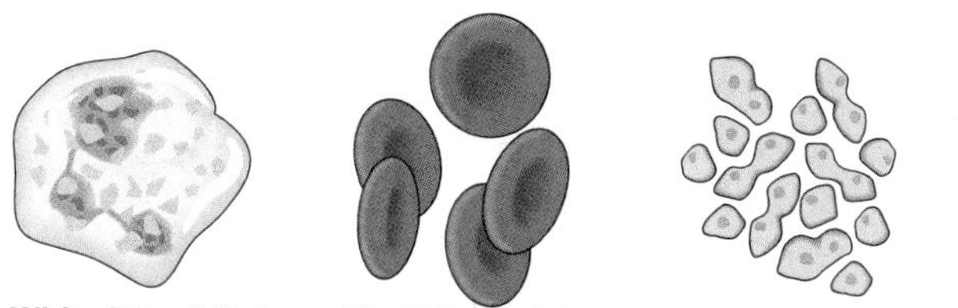

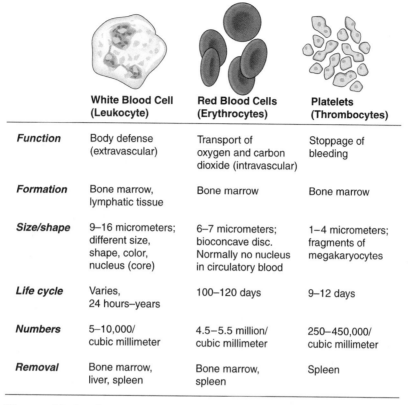

	White Blood Cell (Leukocyte)	Red Blood Cells (Erythrocytes)	Platelets (Thrombocytes)
Function	Body defense (extravascular)	Transport of oxygen and carbon dioxide (intravascular)	Stoppage of bleeding
Formation	Bone marrow, lymphatic tissue	Bone marrow	Bone marrow
Size/shape	9–16 micrometers; different size, shape, color, nucleus (core)	6–7 micrometers; bioconcave disc. Normally no nucleus in circulatory blood	1–4 micrometers; fragments of megakaryocytes
Life cycle	Varies, 24 hours–years	100–120 days	9–12 days
Numbers	5–10,000/ cubic millimeter	4.5–5.5 million/ cubic millimeter	250–450,000/ cubic millimeter
Removal	Bone marrow, liver, spleen	Bone marrow, spleen	Spleen

Figure 28-2 Cellular elements of blood.

of leukocytes and thrombocytes, which are lighter and less numerous than the red blood cells (RBCs). On top of all these layers is the plasma layer. The plasma will contain fibrinogen and usually is slightly hazy (Figure 28-3).

Serum Blood Collection. Most laboratory tests are performed on serum, plasma, or whole blood. Generally, when a serum sample is needed, a serum separator vacuum tube with thixotropic gel is used. The purpose of the thixotropic gel is to create a barrier between the clotted cells and the serum during centrifugation. This protects the serum from contamination from any hemolysed RBCs. There will be certain restrictions in some cases; refer to the laboratory user manual to verify tube requirements. When a serum separator tube is used, several steps must be followed:

1. Perform venipuncture by the preferred method.
2. Invert the tube five times to activate the clotting.
3. Allow the specimen to clot with the tube in the upright position in a rack for at least 30 minutes but no longer than an hour.
4. Centrifuge the tube at 2,500 *g* for 15 minutes.
5. Store the tube upright or transfer the serum to a plastic transport vial for pickup by the laboratory.

These are usually frozen specimens and require a stat pickup. Check the manual to see indications.

There will be different requirements for different laboratories. *Note:* Do not use serum separator tubes for therapeutic drug monitoring (TDM) or toxicology studies. The gel has a tendency to absorb the drugs, thereby decreasing the accuracy of the test results. Collect these samples in a plain

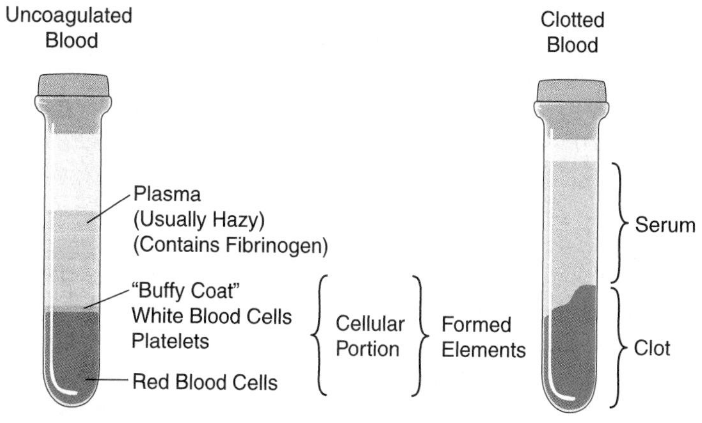

Figure 28-3 Vacuum collection tubes showing serum and plasma.

red-top vacuum tube. Remove the serum immediately (if indicated in the test requirements) after centrifugation and place it in a plastic transport vial. Indicate if the specimen is a serum specimen or for type and cross match.

Plasma and Whole-Blood Collection. Tubes containing anticoagulants are used to collect plasma and whole-blood samples. There are a variety of different anticoagulant tubes that can be used. The anticoagulant needed in the tube will be specified by the laboratory or testing requirements. Preparing the plasma specimen for transport or testing is similar to serum preparation:

1. Perform venipuncture by the preferred method.
2. Invert the tube 8 to 10 times to mix the blood with the anticoagulant.
3. Centrifuge the tube at 2,500 *g* for 10 minutes.
4. Transfer the plasma to a plastic transport vial for pickup by the laboratory. Do not allow any blood cells to mix with the plasma specimen. Indicate the specimen as a plasma specimen and what type of anticoagulant was used. There will be different requirements for different laboratories. Refer to your laboratory user manual for the appropriate test requirements.

To prepare whole blood specimens for transport or testing:

1. Perform venipuncture by the preferred method.
2. Invert the tube 8 to 10 times to mix the blood with the anticoagulant.
3. Maintain the tube at room temperature unless otherwise instructed. Never freeze a whole-blood sample unless specifically instructed to do so.

Collection of Blood Specimens

The most commonly used method for blood collection is **venipuncture.** To obtain a blood sample, the medical assistant must locate a vein that is acceptable for blood collection. The preferred site for venipuncture is the antecubital space, which is located anterior to the elbow on the inside of the arm. The veins are near the surface and are large enough to give access to the blood (Figure 28-4). The median cubital vein is the vein that is used the majority of the time. When this vein is not available, any of the other veins that can be felt may be used. These veins include the basilic, cephalic, and median veins. When necessary, veins on the dorsal surface of the hand or wrist may be used for venipuncture, but they are more painful for the patient and may require a smaller needle or the use of a butterfly apparatus.

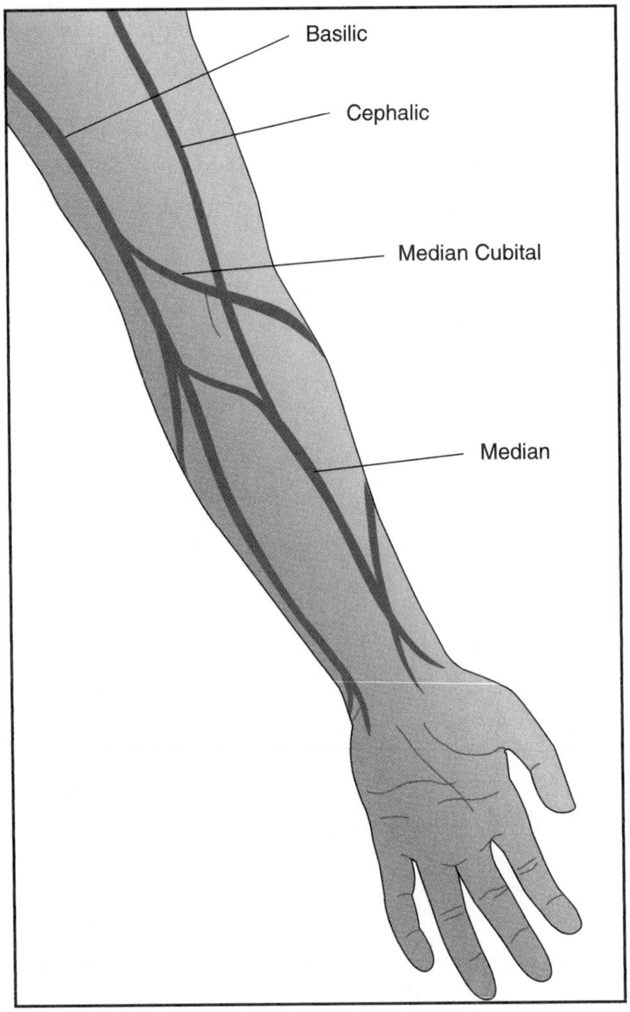

Figure 28-4 Superficial veins of the arm.

The veins of the feet are an alternative when the arms are not available. A physician's permission is needed before drawing blood from the veins of the legs and feet. The physician may not want the patient's leg or foot veins punctured because the act of drawing blood may cause clots to form. These clots then have the possibility of dislodging and causing a blockage elsewhere in the body. It would be extremely rare for a medical assistant to use this location. The physician should be consulted before a foot puncture is considered. And the person performing a foot draw must be specially trained for that procedure.

The arteries in the arm consist of the brachial artery in the brachial region of the arm and the radial and ulnar arteries in the wrist (Figure 28-5). Special techniques are necessary to puncture arteries to obtain a blood specimen for the examination of gases absorbed by the blood. Arterial punctures and the techniques used to draw blood from these locations for blood gas testing are not generally done by a medical assistant. Refer to individual state

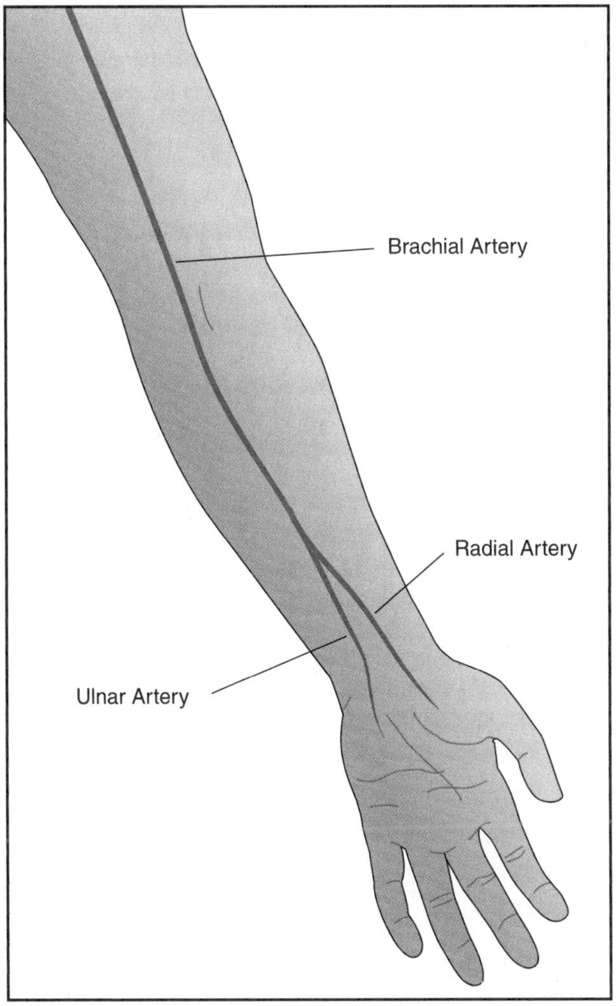

Figure 28-5 Arteries of the arm.

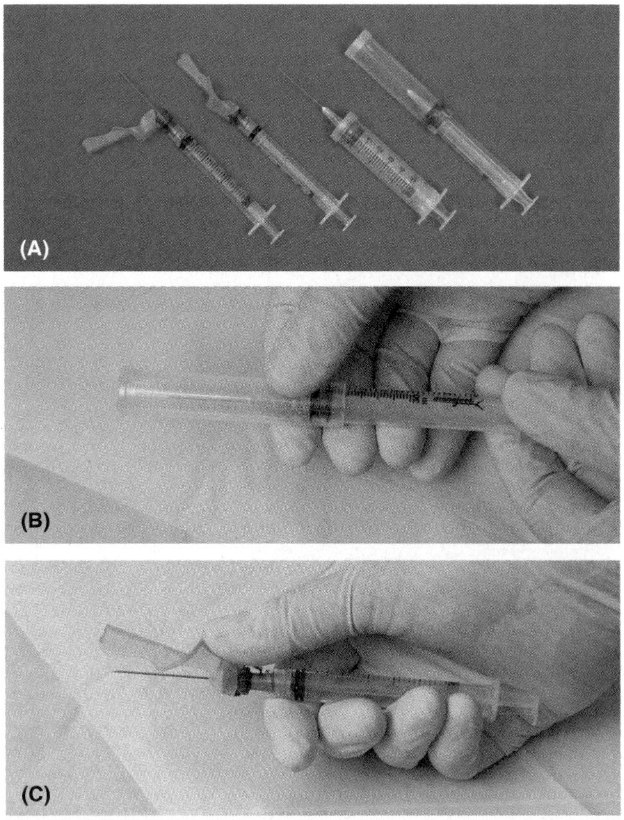

Figure 28-6 (A) Safety syringes with needles, before and after safety mechanisms are engaged. (B) Pull entire casing over the needle to engage this type of safety mechanism. Once engaged, it is locked into place. (C) With the thumb or forefinger, press the safety mechanism over the needle or press against a hard surface. Once engaged, it is locked into place.

laws for specific training and certification/registration requirements.

VENIPUNCTURE EQUIPMENT

All methods of venipuncture require the invasive procedure of punturing into a vein to obtain a blood sample. The three methods we use to perform venipuncture are the syringe method, the vacuum tube method, and the butterfly method. Each method has advantages and disadvantages (Table 28-1). It is important that the well-trained medical assistant have options when attempting to draw blood from a wide range of patients in a variety of situations. There will be times in one's career when one method will be preferred over another. Regardless of which method is chosen to perform the blood draw, the blood will probably be transferred into a vacuum tube eventually. This is because vacuum tubes contain the chemicals and substances necessary for the blood tests to be performed.

Syringes and Needles

Syringes used in venipuncture are usually made of plastic (Figure 28-6). They come in a variety of sizes. Each manufacturer has their own packaging and coloring, thus there is really no significance related to the color and design of syringes. Most syringes used in venipuncture will be 5 and 10 ml in size.

Needles attached to syringes and used for venipuncture do not necessarily differ in function and design from needles used for injections (Figure 28-6). They come in a wide variety of lengths and gauges. Most common sizes for venipuncture are 20, 21, and 22 gauges and about 1 or 1.5 inches in length (Table 28-2). Sixteen gauge needles are often used for blood banking procedures. Remember, the larger the number, the smaller the gauge.

Another type of needle used in venipuncture is the special needle, designed for use with the vacuum tube method. This needle has a double end—the longer needle to puncture the vein and the shorter needle to puncture

TABLE 28-1 COMPARISON OF BLOOD COLLECTION METHODS

Method	Indications for Use	Advantages	Disadvantages
Vacuum tube	Routine collection Multiple tubes are needed Whenever possible	Fast Relatively safe Best specimen quality Large collection amount possible	May not work with: Small veins Fragile veins Difficult draws Small children Hand or feet draws
Butterfly assembly	Small or fragile veins Difficult draws Small children or older adult patients	Least likely to collapse vein Less painful to patient Can attach syringe Can attach tube adapter Least likely to pass through small veins Good specimen quality	Syringe not as safe since tube transfer is necessary Specimen may be hemolyzed Not good for large amounts of blood
Syringe	Children Infants Older adult patients Onocology patients Severely burned patients Obese patients Inaccessible veins Extremely fragile veins Home testing by patient Procedure requires capillary specimen	Easy to perform Requires small amount of specimen	Not good for dehydrated patients Not good for patient with poor circulation Cannot collect for: Blood cultures Erythrocyte sedimentation rate

Source: Courtesy of Sheri R. Greimes, CMA, PBT (ASCP).

TABLE 28-2 NEEDLE GAUGES USED IN PHLEBOTOMY

Gauge Size	Comments
23	Often considered too small, can cause hemolysis of blood cells; used sometimes with butterfly system
22	Preferred for pediatric phlebotomy or very small veins of the hands or feet
21	Most common size used with vacuum tubes
20	Appropriate, but large for common phlebotomy
18	Not used for phlebotomy, but sometimes used in blood banking/donations
16	Most commonly used in blood banking/donations

into the vacuum tube (Figure 28-7). These needles also come in a variety of gauges and lengths, the most common is the same as the standard needle described previously: 20, 21, and 22 gauge, 1 to 1.5 inches in length. When selecting a double-ended needle for use with the vacuum tube, you will use a multidraw needle, which enables drawing of more than one tube of blood. The multidraw needles come with a rubber sheath over the shorter needle, which goes into the vacuum tube. This rubber sheath prevents blood from leaking out of the needle during tube changes. Multidraw needles are sometimes referred to as multisample or multiple sample needles.

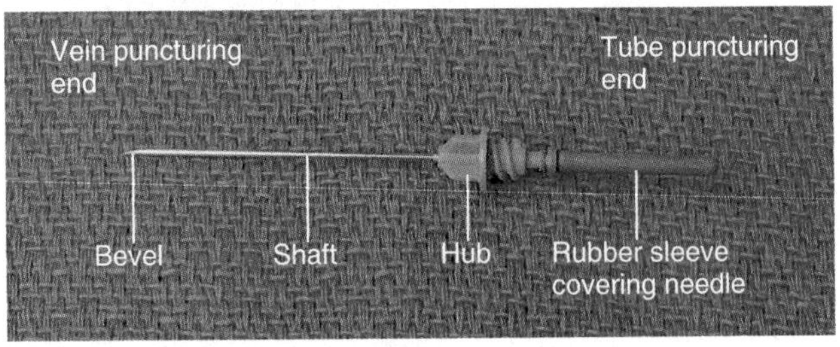

Figure 28-7 Multidraw needle for vacuum tube blood collection system.

Another type of needle used in venipuncture is on a "winged" infusion set called the butterfly collection system (Figure 28-8). Because of the reasons we use the butterfly collection system, the needles are, of course, smaller, usually 21, 23, or 25 gauge.

More details about each collection method are discussed later in this chapter.

Safety Needles and Blood Collection Systems

Occupational Safety and Health Administration (OSHA) requires that safety needles be made available to employees to prevent on-the-job needlestick injuries. The huge variety of safety needles and blood collection systems currently available greatly reduces the risks for accidental needlesticks. The main issue is decid-

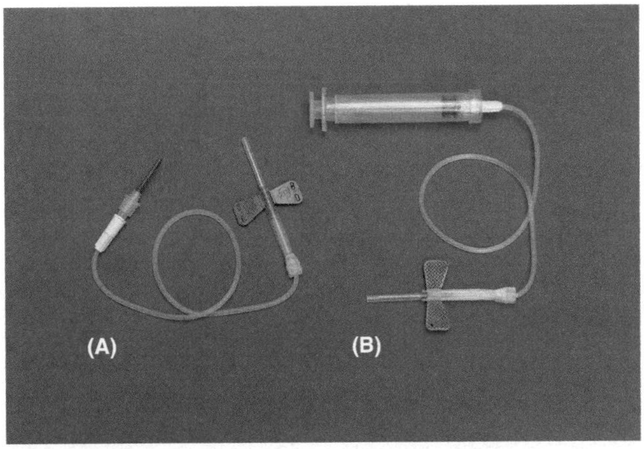

Figure 28-8 (A) Winged infusion set (butterfly) with safety needle. (B) Butterfly attached to syringe.

ing which to select for use in your clinic based on personal preferences. OSHA requires that employers make purchasing decisions based on formal feedback from front-line employees rather than costs and administrative contracts. This means that you have a great deal of choice about what systems you choose to use. It is recommended that you examine a variety of safety system on a regular basis to determine which one gives you the greatest protection from accidental needlestick injury. These systems are often referred to as needlestick prevention devices (NPDs). Among the available systems are passive systems in which the needle is automatically covered when withdrawn and systems that require the medical assistant to activate a mechanism of covering the needle. Within each type are many options and brands. This chapter discusses and shows a few currently available options in no particular order. The first is the Plexus Puncture Guard system as shown in Figure 28-9. Before withdrawing the needle from the patient's vein, a **cannula** is clicked into place. The cannula fills the inside of the needle virtually blunting the tip. Another option shown in Figure 28-10 is the Eclipse system by Becton-Dickinson (Rutherford, NJ), which requires the medical assistant to snap a cover over the needle after it is removed from the vein. A third option, called the Safety-Lok, also manufactured by Becton-Dickinson, requires the medical assistant to slide the cover over the needle until it locks into place. Whichever system you choose, always combine the safest equipment with the safest practices for the best all-around benefit for you, your coworkers, and your patients. Many accidents occur when we become distracted or hurried in our tasks.

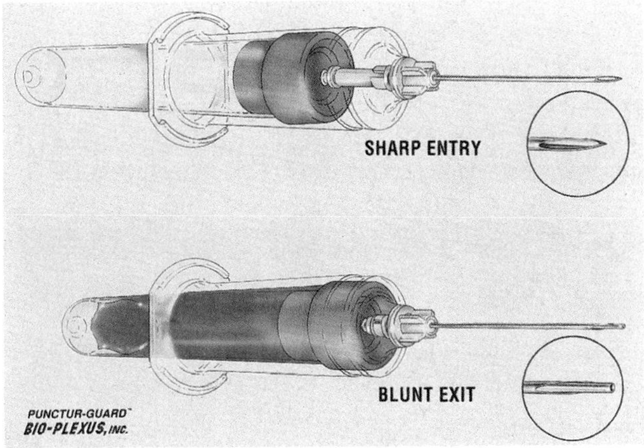

Figure 28-9 Puncture Guard is one type of safety needle. (Courtesy of BioPlexus, Inc., Tolland, CT.)

Vacuum Tubes and Adapters/Holders

The vacuum tube system is often called the Vacutainer system. Vacutainer can be a misnomer because the term *Vacutainer*® is a brand name for the vacuum tube system manufactured by Becton-Dickinson. Medical assistants often say Vacutainer when they are using another company's product.

Vacuum tubes are vacuum-packed test tubes with rubber stoppers. The safest ones are made of plastic and have screw-on caps. They are available in a variety of sizes for a variety of uses (Figure 28-11). Vacuum tubes come plain or with added chemical or substances necessary for the appropriate test to be run. The color of the rubber stopper designates the additive inside the tube. Although most colors are universal regardless of manufacturer, the shades may vary and can be confusing to beginners. It is always best to read the label to determine the additive if the shade is different.

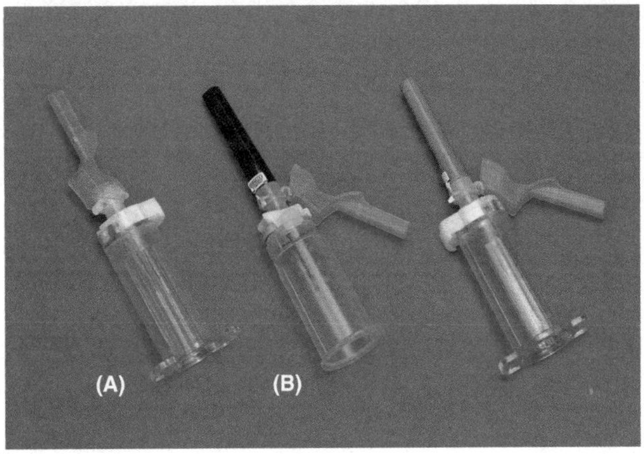

Figure 28-10 Eclipse safety needles for use with vacuum tubes, (A) after the safety mechanism has been engaged and (B) before the safety mechanisms have been engaged. On the left with the needle cap still attached, on the right with the needle exposed.

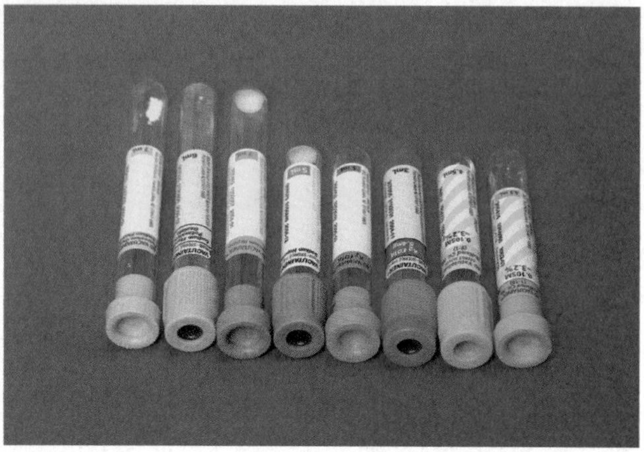

Figure 28-11 An assortment of vacuum tubes. Vacuum tubes come in a variety of sizes for a variety of uses.

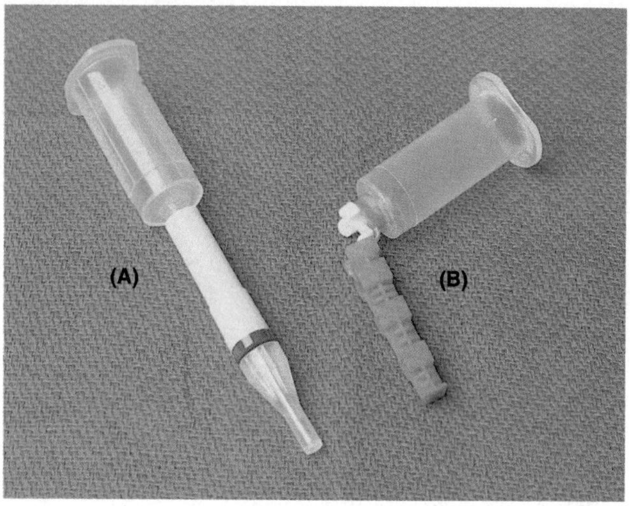

Figure 28-13 Safety tube holders. (A) Safety needle and holder. (B) Locking cover.

Plastic holders or tube adapters, as shown in Figure 28-12, are used in conjunction with the vacuum tubes. Figure 28-13 shows safety holders developed to minimize the risk for accidental needlesticks. Some plastic holders are reusable, but there is much debate about the appropriateness of reusing them, even after disinfection. They are fairly inexpensive and the inner threads will eventually wear out, therefore replacing them frequently is always good practice. The holders with the safety mechanisms shown in Figure 28-13 are not reusable.

Anticoagulants, Additives, and Gels

Different tests require different types of blood specimens. Some specimens require a serum sample and need to be drawn in a tube that allows the blood to clot. Others require a whole-blood or plasma specimen and need to be drawn in a tube that does not allow the blood to clot.

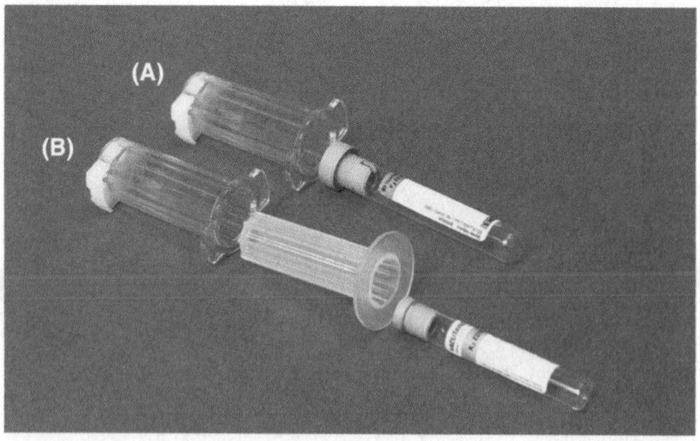

Figure 28-12 Holders for the vacuum tube system. (A) Regular size holder. (B) An adapter for use with smaller tubes. Both have safety release mechanisms.

To prevent the clotting of the blood, the tube contains an anticoagulant. An anticoagulant is a chemical substance that prevents the clotting by removing calcium in the form of calcium salts or by inhibiting the conversion of prothrombin to thrombin. Coagulation occurs naturally according to the steps in Table 28-3. If a step is prevented, the blood does not clot.

The process of clotting can be prevented in the vacuum tube. A tube containing an anticoagulant removes one of the steps in the process, preventing the blood from clotting. The step removed depends on the anticoagulant used. The basic anticoagulants used consist of oxalates, citrates, ethylenediaminetetraacetic acid (EDTA), or heparin (Figure 28-14). Anticoagulants are identified by tube color. It is important to use the correct anticoagulant for the test because the improper anticoagulant can alter test results (Table 28-4).

Various **additives** are used to improve the quality of the specimen. These additives are not anticoagulants or preservatives but are used to improve specimen quality or accelerate specimen processing. Some serum tubes have a clot activator that speeds the clotting process. The clot activator consists of silica (small glass) particles on the sides of the tubes that initiate the clotting process. The silica particles work as a catalyst for the clotting process by

TABLE 28-3 STEPS TO BLOOD CLOTTING
1. Uncoagulated blood
2. Calcium utilized
3. Prothrombin converts to thrombin
4. Fibrinogen converts to fibrin
5. Clot forms

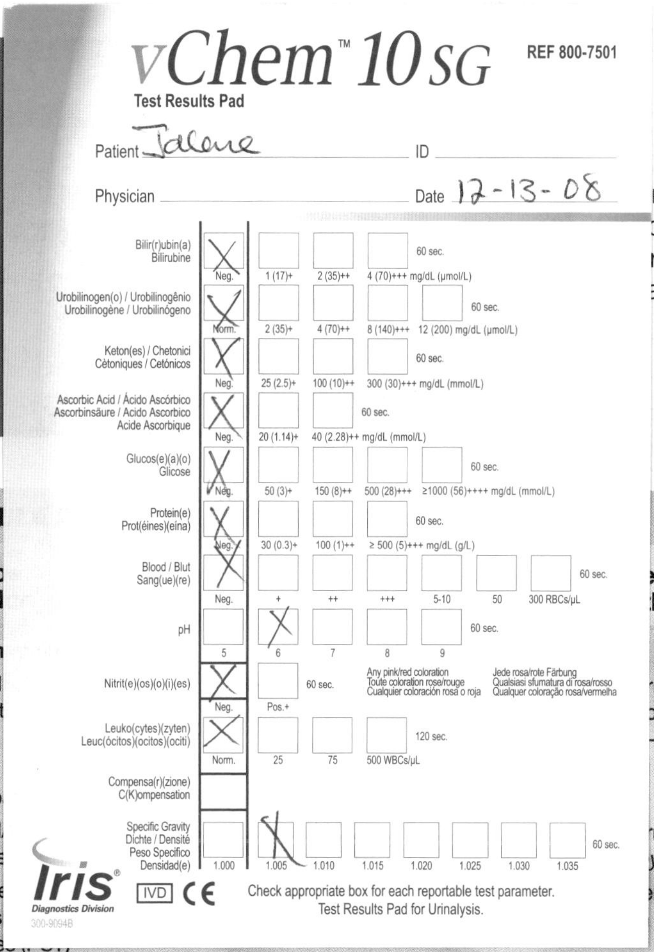
vChem™ 10 SG REF 800-7501
Test Results Pad

Patient Jalene ID

Physician Date 12-13-08

Bilir(r)ubin(a) / Bilirubine	X Neg.	1 (17)+	2 (35)++	4 (70)+++ mg/dL (µmol/L)	60 sec.			
Urobilinogen(o) / Urobilinogênio / Urobilinogène / Urobilinógeno	X Norm.	2 (35)+	4 (70)++	8 (140)+++	12 (200) mg/dL (µmol/L)	60 sec.		
Keton(es) / Chetonici / Cètoniques / Cetónicos	X Neg.	25 (2.5)+	100 (10)++	300 (30)+++ mg/dL (mmol/L)	60 sec.			
Ascorbic Acid / Ácido Ascórbico / Ascorbinsäure / Acido Ascorbico / Acide Ascorbique	X Neg.	20 (1.14)+	40 (2.28)++ mg/dL (mmol/L)	60 sec.				
Glucos(e)(a)(o) / Glicose	X Neg.	50 (3)+	150 (8)++	500 (28)+++	≥1000 (56)++++ mg/dL (mmol/L)	60 sec.		
Protein(e) / Prot(éines)(eína)	X Neg.	30 (0.3)+	100 (1)++	≥ 500 (5)+++ mg/dL (g/L)	60 sec.			
Blood / Blut / Sang(ue)(re)	X Neg.	+	++	+++	5-10	50	300 RBCs/µL	60 sec.
pH	5	X 6	7	8	9	60 sec.		
Nitrit(e)(os)(o)(i)(es)	X Neg.	Pos.+	60 sec.	Any pink/red coloration / Toute coloration rose/rouge / Cualquier coloración rosa o roja	Jede rosa/rote Färbung / Qualsiasi sfumatura di rosa/rosso / Qualquer coloração rosa/vermelha			
Leuko(cytes)(zyten) / Leuc(ócitos)(ocitos)(ociti)	X Norm.	25	75	500 WBCs/µL	120 sec.			
Compensa(r)(zione) / C(K)ompensation								
Specific Gravity / Dichte / Densité / Peso Specifico / Densidad(e)	1.000	X 1.005	1.010	1.015	1.020	1.025	1.030	1.035 — 60 sec.

Iris® Diagnostics Division 300-9094B IVD CE

Check appropriate box for each reportable test parameter.
Test Results Pad for Urinalysis.

…re 28-14 Standard anticoagulant tubes with con…onal stoppers (left) and with Hemogard closures (right). …ray top: antiglycocytic agent. (B) Green top: heparin. …avender top: EDTA. (D) Light blue top: citrate.

TA…

Tub… Col…		**…ent for Testing …he Tests Performed**
Non…		
Red… clott…		…rminations …oss match—blood bank —chemistry HIV testing—serology/immunology
Sep…		
Red… "tige…		…rminations: BMPs, panels (lipids, thyroid, etc.), FSH, PSA, …ylori, etc.—chemistry
Gre… plas… tube…		…rminations—chemistry studies—coagulation
Additive Tubes		
Light blue: anticoagulant	Sodium citrate	Coagulation studies—all go to Coagulation Department Fibrinogen, platelet aggregation, prothrombin time (PT)—Coumadin therapy Partial thromboplastin time (PTT)—heparin therapy
Green: anticoagulant	Sodium heparin Ammonium heparin Lithium heparin	Electrolytes—chemistry Coagulation studies, platelet counts—coagulation STAT chemistry panels—chemistry
Lavender: anticoagulant	Ethylenediaminetetraacetic acid (EDTA)	Whole-blood specimen—hematology CBC, WBC, differentials, sedimentation rates, hemoglobins, glycohemoglobins, hematocrits
Gray: antiglycolitic	Sodium fluoride or potassium oxalate	Blood glucose levels—chemistry Blood alcohol levels (ETOH)
Special Tubes		
Yellow	Sodium polyanetholesulfonate (SPS) Acid dextrose citrate (ACD)	Blood cultures—microbiology DNA or paternity testing—hematology Viral loads (cell morphology)—cytology/serology
Royal blue	Trace-element free May contain heparin in some tubes—check label	Toxicology studies—chemistry (lead levels, copper, iron, etc.)

Standard Order of Draw—NCCLS Guidelines as of December 2004

First—Blood culture tubes or vials: yellow top or culture bottles
Second—Sodium citrate: light blue top
Third—Serum tubes: red tops and red/gray tops (SST)
Fourth—Heparin tubes: green top
Fifth—EDTA tubes: lavender top
Sixth—Glycolitic inhibiter: gray top

Source: Courtesy of Sheri R. Greimes, CMA, PBT (ASCP).

BMP = basic metabolic panel; CBC = complete blood count; ETOH = ethyl alcohol; FSH = follicle-stimulating hormone; HIV = human immunodeficiency virus; PSA = prostate-specific antigen; RPR = rapid plasma reagin; SST = strains specific typing; WBC = white blood cell count.

Actions of Additives

Potassium oxalate	Binds calcium
Flouride	Inhibits glycolysis
Sodium citrate	Binds calcium
EDTA	Binds calcium
Lithium heparin	Inhibits prothrombin to thrombin
Thrombin	Promotes speedy clot formation
No additive	Clot naturally forms
Sodium polyanetholesulfonate (SPS)	Binds calcium
Glass particles	Promotes clotting
Ammonium heparin	Inhibits prothrombin to thrombin

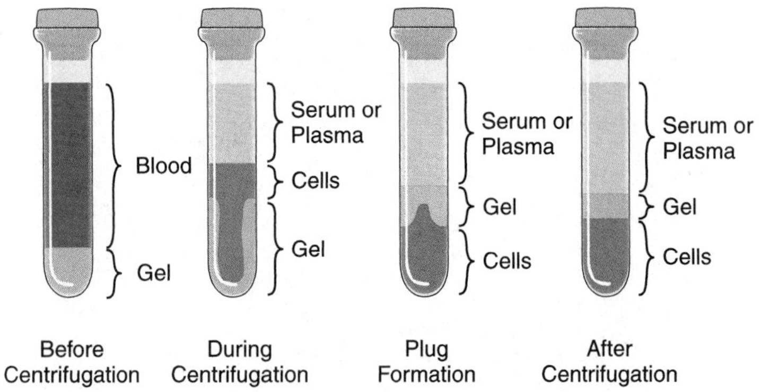

Figure 28-16 Separator gel tube: centrifugation process.

Critical Thinking

Which vacuum tube would you use to draw a serum specimen: lavender or red top? Why did you choose that tube? What differentiates the two tubes?

helping the clotting process to start. The plastic vacuum tubes with the red tops have clot activators (glass particles) in them. The glass red top vacuum tubes do not.

A type of clot activator that is used for STAT (emergency) testing is thrombin. The thrombin is in the tube to chemically increase the speed of the clotting process and to hasten the complete formation of the clot.

Serum and plasma tubes can also be purchased with a **thixotropic separator gel** (Figure 28-15). The gel is an inert material that undergoes a temporary change in **viscosity** during centrifugation. When centrifuged, the gel changes to a liquid and moves up the sides of the tube to create a barrier between the blood cells or clot and the liquid portion of the blood. The gel then forms a solid plug and separates the cells/clot from the plasma/serum (Figure 28-16).

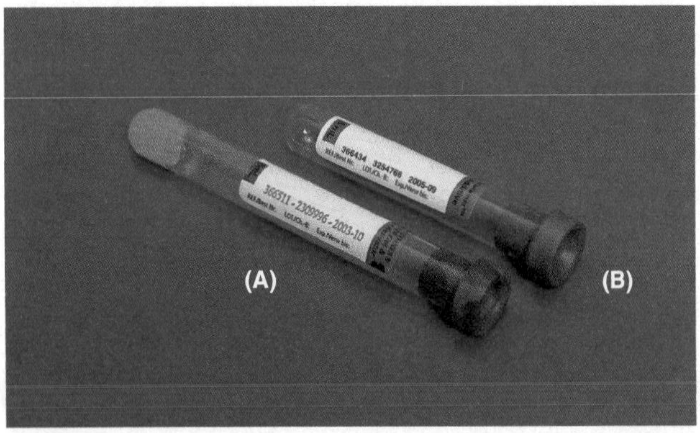

Figure 28-15 Standard vacuum tubes. (A) Red/gray top (glass) tube contains clot activators and thixotrophic gel. (B) Plain red top tube contains no anticoagulant or additives. The plastic red top contains glass particles to promote clotting.

Order of Draw

The order in which blood is drawn or mixed with the additives is important. Sterile collection bottles (for blood cultures) need to be filled first to prevent any contamination. After the sterile bottles are filled, the order of mixing with the additive depends on the method used to obtain the specimen. Later in this chapter is discussed the methods of obtaining the specimen: the syringe, the butterfly needle assembly, and the direct vacuum tube draws. Whichever method used to obtain the blood, it will eventually be transferred to either a vacuum tube or a blood culture bottle. The order in which it is transferred is listed in each of those sections. Table 28-4 also lists the order of draw into vacuum tubes.

Tourniquets

The **tourniquet,** when applied to the arm, constricts the flow of blood in the arm and makes the veins more prominent. The tourniquet is a soft, pliable, rubber or elastic strip approximately 1 inch wide by 15 to 18 inches long (Figure 28-17). The rubber strip serves as the best tourniquet for all conditions. Velcro strips are also available. The Velcro strip cannot be cleaned easily and is too expensive to dispose of after each use. The rubber strip can easily be released with one hand. Being about 1 inch wide, it does not cut into the patient's arm but distributes the pressure. The tourniquet can easily be disinfected and is inexpensive enough that it can be

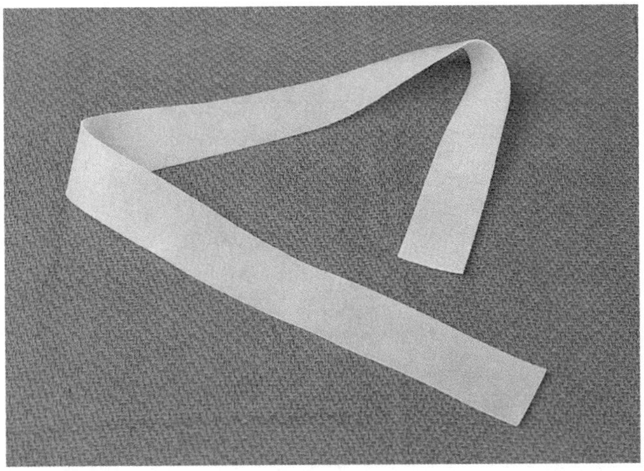

Figure 28-17 Soft rubber tourniquet.

replaced often. If the tourniquet is obviously contaminated, it should be discarded into biohazard waste. If a patient has been identified as having a latex hypersensitivity, you must use a nonlatex tourniquet.

A blood pressure cuff can also be used as a tourniquet. Its use is primarily for veins that are difficult to locate using a standard tourniquet. The blood pressure should be taken first, and then the cuff should be maintained slightly below the diastolic pressure (40 mm/Hg average).

Specimen Collection Trays

The medical assistant may need a specimen collection tray to hold all the equipment necessary for proper specimen collection. The tray can be taken to the patient in the examination room so that whatever procedure is performed the phlebotomy can be conducted without searching for the proper equipment. The trays vary depending on the type of collections done. Because the tray is also used to transport blood specimens, the OSHA *Bloodborne Pathogen Standard* requires the tray be all red or prominently labeled with an approved biohazard symbol. The tray is usually preferred because it is more portable and can easily be taken to the patient. The trays come in a variety of sizes and shapes to better fit the preference and needs of the individual collecting the blood sample (Figure 28-18). Sometimes the equipment is stored in a special drawer for venipuncture equipment in each examination room or in a central laboratory area.

VENIPUNCTURE TECHNIQUE

Venipuncture is a detailed process that consists of many steps (Table 28-5).

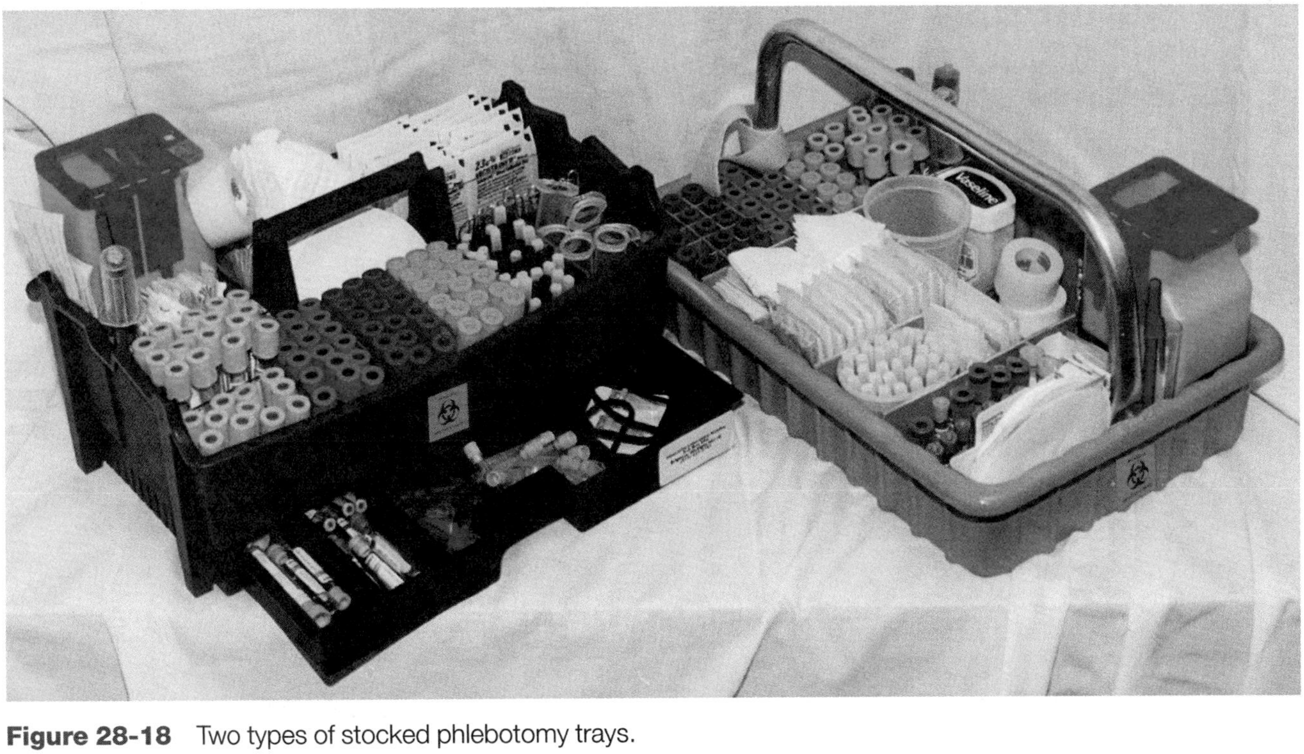

Figure 28-18 Two types of stocked phlebotomy trays.

TABLE 28-5 STEPS IN VENIPUNCTURE
1. Identify the patient.
2. Verify test ordered.
3. Verify diet/drug restrictions; e.g., fasting vs. nonfasting.
4. Wash hands. Put on gloves, as well as safety glasses and mask, if there is a potential for blood splatter.
5. Assemble supplies and inspect equipment.
6. Reassure the patient and explain the procedure.
7. Position the patient.
8. Verify paperwork and tubes.
9. Perform venipuncture.
10. Fill the tubes.
11. Bandage the patient's arm.
12. Dispose of sharps in the proper container.
13. Label the tubes.
14. Remove gloves and other PPE. Dispose of properly. Wash hands.
15. Chill specimen (only for certain tests).
16. Process paperwork. Complete laboratory requisition.
17. Send correctly labeled tubes to the office laboratory or prepare them to be sent to a reference laboratory.
18. Document procedure.

Greeting the Patient

1. Reassure the patient that the procedure is going to be simple and there will only be a slight inconvenience.
2. Be friendly, outgoing, and talk to the patient, explaining the procedure. Polite conversation with all patients gives them the feeling someone cares about them.
3. Do not tell the patient that the procedure will not be painful. Explain that the procedure can be slightly uncomfortable but you will take care to cause the least discomfort possible. If the patient seems overly concerned about pain, check frequently with him or her to see how he or she is doing. If the patient seems extremely apprehensive, ask if he or she would prefer to lie down during the procedure. This may prevent further problems if the patient faints.
4. Exhibit concern for patients, because this will result in happier patients who will return in the future for care from the same physician.

Approaching the Patient

The first step to a successful venipuncture is to put the patient at ease. The medical assistant uses many skills when interacting with patients during phlebotomy. Three of the skills used are:

1. Social skills
2. Technical skills
3. Administrative skills

Social skills are used by the medical assistant to obtain cooperation from the patient. Some patients will be calm, whereas others may be extremely frightened. The nicest patient may be irritable and may even become physically or emotionally abusive when placed in the unfamiliar health care setting. The medical assistant uses social skills to put the patient at ease, allay the patient's fears, and persuade the patient to allow blood to be drawn.

After calming the patient and explaining the procedure, the medical assistant uses technical skills to perform the phlebotomy with a minimum of pain to the patient. As important as it is to obtain a good specimen, it is equally important to treat the patient with empathy. Using social and technical skills, the medical assistant can provide a positive experience for the patient. A patient who has had a positive experience will talk with friends and neighbors about that experience, which could result in new patients for the physician's office, the clinic, or the laboratory.

For the medical assistant, administrative skills involve drawing the correct patient's blood and correctly labeling the specimen. Incorrect labeling constitutes the greatest number of errors in phlebotomy. All patient specimens must be positively identified on the **primary container,** the container that holds the specimen, to avoid any errors in reporting of results, thereby affecting patient diagnosis or treatment.

Preparing Supplies and Greeting the Patient

Prepare all supplies and equipment before the venipuncture. Place all tubes within easy reach to avoid crossing over the patient and possibly moving the needle after it is in the patient. Remember that occasionally a tube will not fill completely; therefore, it is best to keep a few spare tubes or have the phlebotomy tray within reach.

Patient and Specimen Identification

Proper patient and specimen identification is essential to accurate patient testing. The results of specimen testing will be incorrect if the specimen is not accurately identified. When entering the room, do not say, "Mr. Jones, I'm here to draw your blood," assuming if the patient says "Yes" this is Mr. Jones. The patient may not have been paying attention and may answer yes even if it is not his name. Ask the patient to state his or her full name. If the patient is unable to communicate with you, or if you are in an inpatient environment such as a hospital or extended care facility, always check the patient's identification wristband or check with the caretaker. In the ambulatory setting, a good policy is to ask for picture identification from non–English-speaking patients.

Once the medical assistant has identified the patient and the blood is drawn, the specimen needs proper identification. The patient's first and last name, middle initial, any assigned identification number, the date, the time, and the initials of the person collecting the specimen must be written on the tube immediately after drawing the patient's blood. Label the tubes clearly, using a permanent marker, before leaving the patient's presence. By doing so, if the tubes are taken to the physician's office laboratory or an outside reference laboratory, the specimens will be properly identified. Any paperwork or forms accompanying the specimens must be checked with the blood tubes to verify that names and numbers match.

Many offices are using various types of computer systems for test ordering and result reporting. The computer label has several advantages in that it lists the specific tests that are ordered and the required specimen and specimen requirements. The label can also be adhesive so it can be attached directly to the tube. Smaller labels can also be printed at the same time for smaller aliquot specimens. An **aliquot** specimen is a portion of a specimen that has been taken for use or storage. The computer has multiple advantages in timing the printing of orders, sorting lists of orders for one patient at one time, and speeding entry of draw times and test results. The computer labels print off in a roll with one label following the other. Two attached labels (Figure 28-19) require special attention. One label must be checked carefully with the other to assure that each label is for the same person, date, and time. Labels may also contain bar codes to assist in electronic patient and specimen identification. With computerized systems, the medical assistant will verify by entering information into the computer when the blood is drawn.

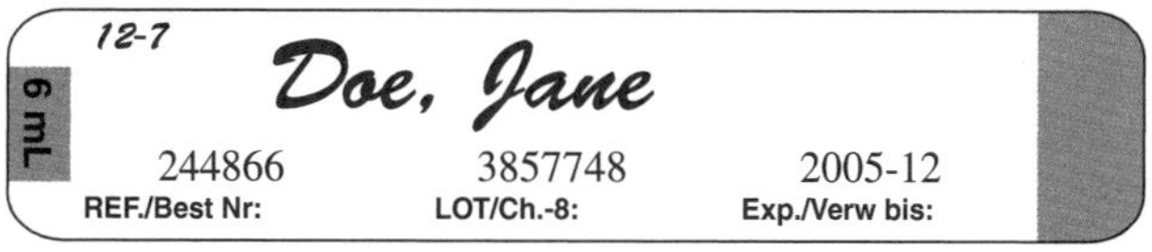

Figure 28-19 Adhesive computer-generated labels for identifying specimen tubes from one patient.

Positioning the Patient

The position of the patient is critical for proper patient blood collection. The best position is the position that is comfortable for the patient and the health care professional. Proper positioning of the patient will make the patient feel more at ease and facilitate the performance of the venipuncture.

Selecting the Appropriate Venipuncture Site

The appropriate venipuncture site can vary depending on the patient. The usual site that is first checked is the antecubital region of the arm. The primary vein used in the

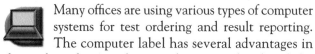

Positioning the Patient

Before a patient's blood is drawn, discuss with the patient any previous problems with blood being taken. Usually one of two situations must be addressed:

1. Patients who do not have a problem with having blood drawn.
   a. The patient must be in a seated or reclining position before any attempt is made to draw blood.
   b. Do not allow the patient to sit on a tall stool or stand while drawing blood. There is always the possibility that the patient will faint (syncope) and be injured.
   c. The sitting position requires a chair with adequate arm supports that are adjustable for the best venipuncture position.
2. Patients who will faint (syncope).
   a. Apprehensive patients and patients who indicate they have fainted in the past when having blood drawn should be instructed to lie down.
   b. The reclining position is the ideal position from which to draw a blood sample from the patient.
   c. A pillow may be required to help support the patient's arm by keeping it straight for easier venous access.

Patient Safety

- Question the patient about his or her past experiences with venipuncture.
- Position the patient properly to avoid injury.
- Do not attempt to draw blood on a combative patient.
- Restrain uncooperative children.
- Note allergies or sensitivities to latex, alcohol, and tape adhesives.

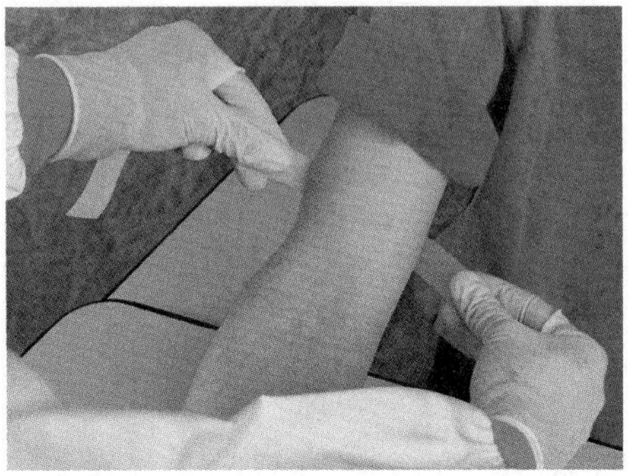

Figure 28-20A Wrap the tourniquet around the arm 3 to 4 inches above the venipuncture site. Keeping the tourniquet flat to the skin will help minimize the discomfort felt by the patient.

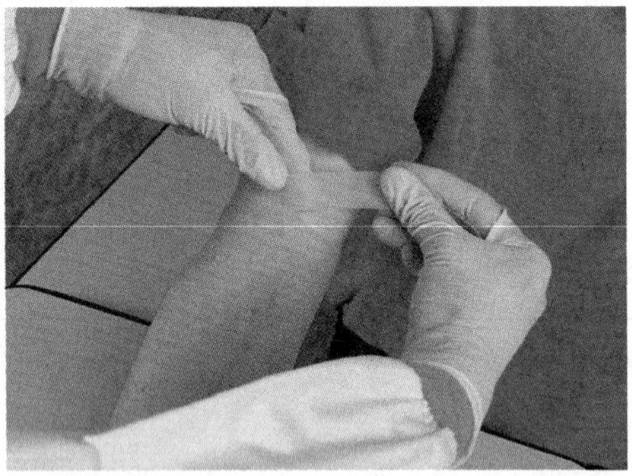

Figure 28-20B Stretch the tourniquet tight and cross the ends.

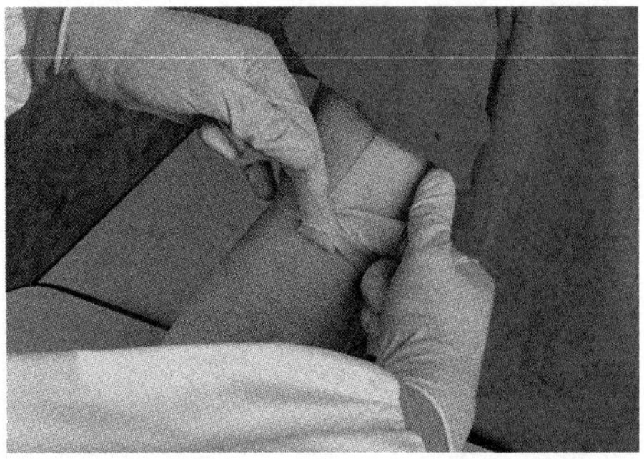

Figure 28-20C While holding the ends tight, tuck one portion of the tourniquet under the other.

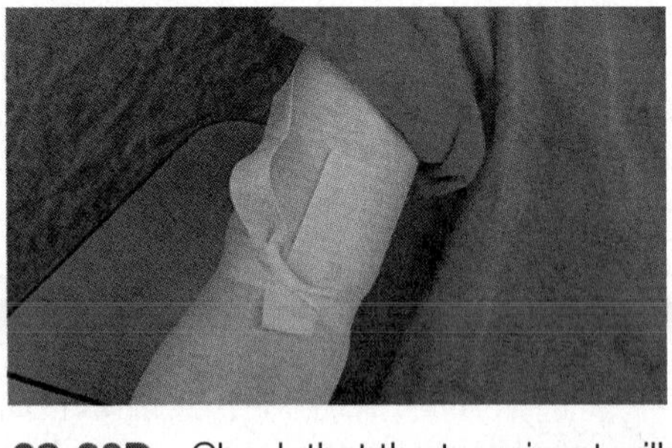

Figure 28-20D Check that the tourniquet will not come loose. The ends of the tourniquet should be pointed upward and not hanging into the intended venipuncture site.

antecubital region of the arm is the median cubital vein. This is usually the prominent vein in the middle of the bend of the arm. Refer back to Figure 28-4. The basilic or cephalic vein can be used as an alternative. These veins may not be accessible or may not be prominent enough to obtain a blood sample. The next step is to go to the back of the hand to determine other possibilities. The veins in the back of the hand have the tendency to "roll" more than the arm veins because they are not supported by as much tissue and are closer to the surface. To avoid this, the vein will have to be held in place securely while a smaller gauge needle or a butterfly is used. The hand veins are ideal for a 3- to 5-cc syringe with a 22 gauge needle. Careful, slow pulling on the syringe will obtain the blood sample without collapsing the vein or hemolyzing the blood. The veins at the back of the wrist are also an alternative, but they are generally much more painful than the other sites. The foot and ankle veins may also be used if the patient's physician gives permission to use them and the medical assistant is properly trained to perform venipuncture on the lower extremities. The veins in the foot or ankle will also have the tendency to "roll." The medical assistant will in all likelihood never draw from the foot or ankle, but this is an area that will give an acceptable blood sample when all other attempts have failed.

The order for checking for the best available site is: (1) antecubital region of the arm, (2) back of hand, (3) back of wrist, and (4) ankle or foot. The next alternative is to have a more experienced medical assistant check. If venous access is not possible, draw the sample by capillary puncture if the test can be performed on a capillary specimen. Check the laboratory manual for criteria.

Applying the Tourniquet

A tourniquet must be used to assist the medical assistant in feeling a vein. The tourniquet is applied 3 to 4 inches above the intended puncture site. It is applied tightly enough to slow the flow of blood in the veins but not so tightly as to prevent the flow of blood in the arteries (Figures 28-20A–D). This is similar to damming a small stream. When a stream is dammed, the water forms a pond in front of the dam. With the tourniquet applied, the veins fill with blood, pooling in the veins below the tourniquet. This pooling of blood makes the veins more prominent. The veins can then be **palpated** (examined with the fingertips) to determine their direction, depth, and size. The tourniquet should be on the arm no longer than one minute. A stream will become stagnant when it no longer flows. A tourniquet that is left on too long will cause **hemoconcentration** of the blood, an increased concentration of constituents in the blood sample that may lead

Critical Thinking

You are having a difficult time getting the needle to cooperate when putting together a butterfly system and you accidentally contaminate it. The patient has the tourniquet already on her arm. What do you do? Why? Is there something else you could have done?

to inaccurate test results. If the patient has sensitive skin or a skin problem, the tourniquet should be applied over the patient's upper arm clothing or a piece of gauze pad. This will minimize the discomfort felt by the patient.

The tourniquet often causes greater discomfort for patients than the venipuncture itself. The tourniquet should ideally be removed as soon as blood flow is established. This is not practical for the novice medical assistant. The act of removing the tourniquet may move the needle or vein just enough so that no more blood can be obtained and a second venipuncture must be performed. It is recommended to wait until just before the needle is removed from the patient to remove the tourniquet. If the tourniquet is not removed before the needle is removed, the patient will bleed heavily. Blood will be forced out of the needle hole and into the surrounding tissue, resulting in a **hematoma** (an accumulation of blood around the venipuncture site).

Performing a Safe Venipuncture

The first step in actual collection of a venous blood specimen is to find the site that will give the best blood return. The vein must be palpated with the tip of the index finger. Feel for and trace the path of the vein several times. Avoid using the thumb because it has a pulse and is not as sensitive as the rest of the fingers. The vein will feel soft and bouncy to the touch. The roundness of the vein and the direction it follows may be determined. All veins are not straight up and down the arm. If no veins become prominent, retie the tourniquet tighter but not so tightly as to stop the flow of arterial blood into the arm. If the tourniquet is tied tightly enough to stop arterial blood flow, the patient will no longer have a pulse in the wrist. If this occurs, immediately remove the tourniquet because this indicates that blood has ceased flowing below the tourniquet.

If the "vein" that is felt has a pulsing action to it, it is an artery, not a vein, and the vessel should not be punctured. Tendons can be deceptive and give the appearance of veins. They do not have the soft, bouncy feel and will be hard to the touch. Puncturing a tendon will give no blood return and will be painful to the patient. Nerves also run the length of the arm. The nerves cannot be seen or felt, but by avoiding deep, probing venipunctures, the chance of puncturing a nerve will be diminished. If the patient complains that the venipuncture is extremely painful, it is best to stop and try another site.

Veins of **edematous** arms, which are swollen because of fluid in the tissue, will not be prominent and the tourniquet will not be effective because of the swelling. Using the tourniquet in this instance may cause tissue damage. It leaves a temporary indentation in the arm. Areas of scarring should also be avoided because of possible injury or excessive pain to the patient. Specimens collected from an area of a hematoma may cause erroneous test results. If another vein site is not available, the specimen is collected distal from the hematoma. Because of the potential for harm to the patient due to lymphostasis (the stoppage of the flow of lymph), the arm on the side of a mastectomy or any lymphatic compromise should be avoided. If the patient has had a double mastectomy, a physician should be consulted before drawing the blood.

Specimen Collection

The patient has been identified, paperwork and tubes have been verified, equipment has been assembled, and the patient is in a comfortable position. Hand washing is the most critical step to preventing the spread of infection. Before touching the patient, medical assistants should wash their hands. It is good practice to wash your hands in view of the patient to give the patient confidence in your technique. The next step is to tie the tourniquet. Have the patient close the hand, and then select a vein. If possible, place the patient's arm in a downward position. After locating an acceptable vein, mentally map the location. Set mental sites on the vein by visualizing the puncture site as the target for an accurate puncture. Cleanse the site with a gauze pad wet with 70% isopropyl alcohol solution. A commercially prepared alcohol pad or one with 0.5% chlorhexidine in alcohol may also be used. Wipe the skin firmly with an alcohol pad. This removes any oil, sweat, perfume, lotions, and skin contaminations. This process is often referred to as "defatting" the skin. Allow the area to air dry, or you may dry it with a clean cotton ball or gauze pad. Puncturing the skin through wet alcohol can cause hemolysis of the specimen and give the patient a stinging sensation. Residual alcohol can also contaminate the specimen.

Some authorities suggest putting on gloves first and then palpating for the vein. This technique is required for the patient who is isolated because of a communicable disease and is good practice for all patients. Standard Precautions require that personal protective equipment be

Correct Hand Position to Hold a Syringe

1. The needle is attached to the syringe.
2. Hold the syringe and needle system in your dominant hand, cradling it on your four fingers. A right-handed person would hold the syringe in the right hand, leaving the left hand to pull on the plunger. A left-handed person would do the opposite.
3. Place the thumb on top of the syringe (Figure 28-21).
4. With the syringe held in this position, turn it slightly so the bevel of the needle is facing up.
5. Hold the hand in such a position that by tilting the point of the needle down slightly the needle will enter the skin at a 15-degree angle and about 0.5 cm below the point where the vein was felt.

Correct Needle Position

The patient will experience the least amount of pain if the bevel of the needle is facing upward when the needle is inserted into the vein. The bevel of the needle is upward when the opening in the needle is visible when you look straight down on the needle as it is inserted. This position also helps prevent the suction from causing the inside wall of the vein to adhere to the needle bevel, thus occluding the needle.

The needle should be inserted at a 15- to 30-degree angle to the surface of the skin (Figure 28-22).

The skin should be held taut until the needle has been inserted. This technique allows the point of the needle to enter the skin with little drag or bunching of the skin, thereby reducing the discomfort of the puncture.

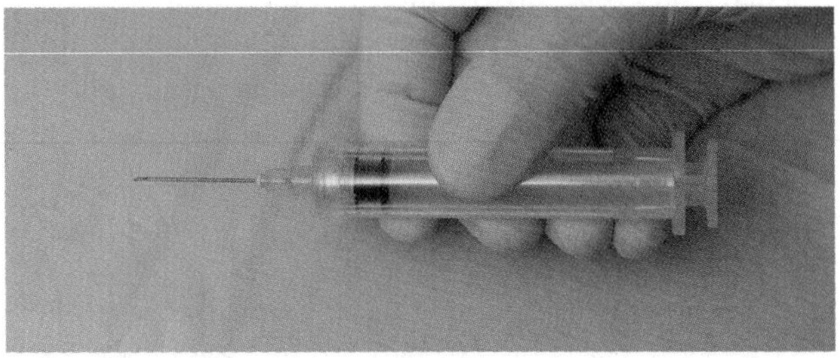

Figure 28-21 Proper hand position to hold a syringe for blood collection.

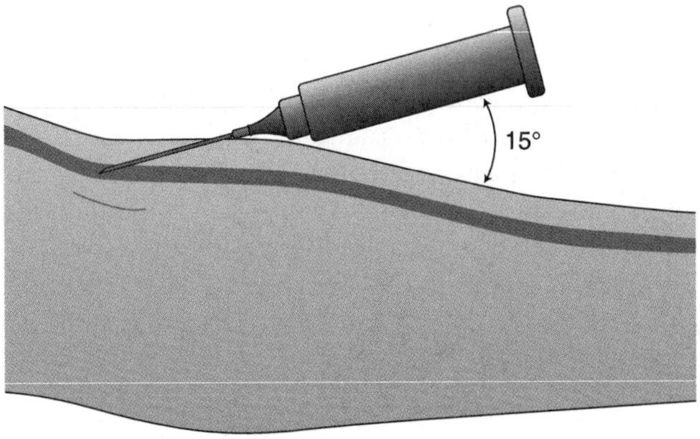

Figure 28-22 Proper angle of needle insertion for venipuncture.

worn when there is a chance of coming in contact with blood and body fluid. If the patient has veins that are difficult to palpate, the gloves may be put on after the site has been palpated and before the cleansing. To avoid forgetting where the collection site is, palpate the vein 1 to 2 inches above and below the intended puncture site. It helps the medical assistant feel that the vein is located in a straight line and these points can be used to "reset" the mental crosshairs without contaminating the venipuncture site. Safety glasses and a mask must be worn if there is a potential for blood spatter.

The Syringe Technique

The syringe technique is used less often than the vacuum tube method. The syringe is ideal for collecting small volumes of blood from fragile, thin, or "rolling" veins or veins on the back of the hand or from the foot. Pulling on the plunger of the syringe creates suction; the larger the syringe, the greater the suction that can be obtained. Too great a suction might cause the vein to collapse. Vein collapse can be avoided by pulling the plunger slowly and by resting between pulls to allow the vein to refill. Because pediatric and geriatric patients often have thin and fragile veins, the syringe is the preferred method of venipuncture for them. The use of a syringe larger than 15 ml is not recommended. If more than 12 ml is needed, the butterfly collection method should be considered. Syringe draws are also ideal in special procedures when the blood must be transferred to a different container. Procedure 28-2 gives detailed instructions for venipuncture with syringe.

When a syringe is used, the blood obtained must be placed in appropriate containers. The order of filling the tubes is important.

The use of a needle to transfer blood from a syringe to a vacuum tube or culture bottle is unsafe and prohibited by OSHA. The use of a safety system such as the BD Vacutainer Blood Transfer Device is recommended (Figure 28-23). After drawing the blood into the syringe, activate the needle's safety mechanism, then remove the

When transferring blood from a syringe to a vacuum tube, keep these safety features in mind:

- Never transfer to a vacuum tube using a needle. When transferring from a syringe to a vacuum tube, use a needleless transfer device.
- Never push the blood into the vacuum tube. It will fill on its own.
- Always wear gloves, goggles, and face guard when performing this procedure.

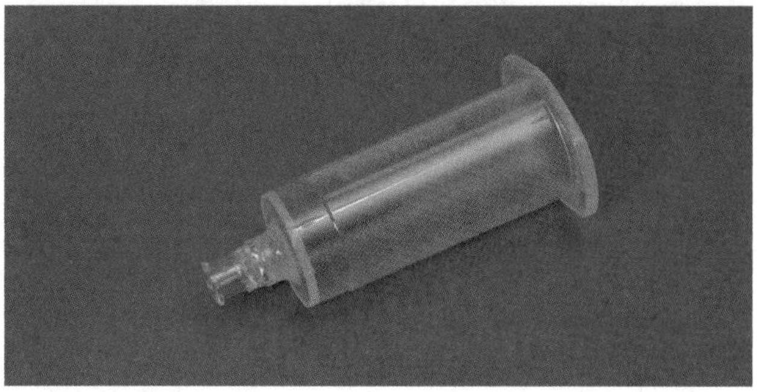

Figure 28-23 BD Vacutainer Blood Transfer Device.

needle and dispose of it. Connect the needleless syringe to the transfer device. Insert a vacuum tube to the device and allow the blood to transfer from the syringe to the tube using the tube's vacuum. Never push on the syringe plunger or force the blood into the tube. This could cause the tube's stopper to pop off. When the appropriate tubes have been filled, dispose of the entire syringe and transfer assembly as one unit according to your clinic policies.

Immediately on filling, mix any tubes containing additives.

The order of transferring from the syringe to the vacuum tube is important. If a syringe is used and the blood is then transferred into the vacuum tubes, the blood has the potential to start clotting in the syringe. Knowing that, it is important to get the blood into anticoagulant as soon as possible. If the syringe is the method of drawing, transfer to the anticoagulant tubes first. Because the additives in some of the tubes will interfere with the actions of the additives in other tubes if accidentally cross-transferred, there is an order to which anticoagulant tubes should be filled. Refer to the box titled "Order of Filling Tubes from a Syringe."

Order of Filling Tubes from a Syringe

1. Blood culture tubes or bottles (sterile procedures)
2. Coagulation "citrate" tube (blue tube)
3. Heparin tube (green tube)
4. EDTA tube (lavender tube)
5. Oxalate/fluoride tube (gray tube)
6. Nonadditive "clot" tubes (red stoppered or gel tubes)

Vacuum Tube Specimen Collection

The vacuum tube system is an improvement over the syringe method yet maintains many similarities. When the syringe method is used, a vacuum is created as the medical assistant pulls on the syringe plunger. The vacuum tube method has the vacuum already in the tube. Another advantage of the vacuum tube system is that with multiple blood samples, syringes do not need to be changed; only the tubes need to be changed.

The similarity between the vacuum tube system and the syringe system is that the holder and needle are held in the same manner (Figure 28-24). The syringe is held in a manner that allows the medical assistant access to pull on the plunger. Access must be left in the vacuum tube system for one tube to be pulled out and another inserted. The hand that pulled on the plunger of the syringe is the hand that changes tubes with the vacuum tube system.

The procedure for venipuncture with the vacuum tube system follows the same steps as the syringe method with only slight variations.

With multiple tube draws, the order of drawing the tubes is very important. Traditionally, glass vacuum tubes have been used, and the red top tube was always drawn first (after sterile culture tubes) because the red top tubes contained no chemicals or other additive that would interfere with the actions of the other colored tubes. We need to always be concerned with "cross contamination" of additives and chemicals. The former glass vacuum tubes have now been replaced with safer plastic vacuum tubes with screw-on lids. Blood collected in the safer plastic red top vacuum tubes does not clot as well with the glass red

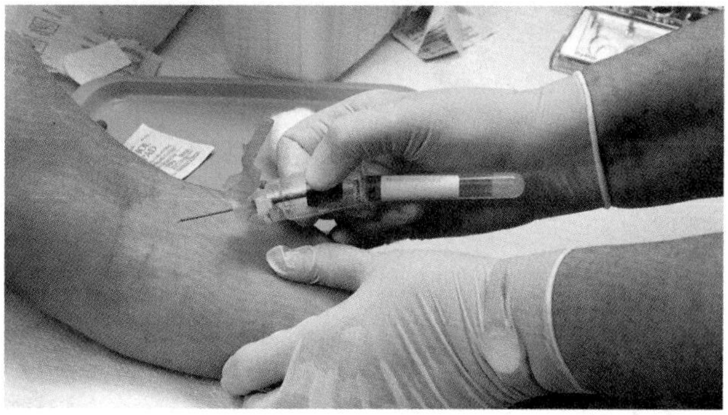

Figure 28-24 Proper hand position to hold a vacuum tube system.

top vacuum tubes, so glass particles have been added to the interior of the plastic red top tubes to promote clotting. This addition changes the "order of draw." When using the safer plastic vacuum tubes, the order becomes: sterile, blue (citrate), red top and/or SST, green, lavender, and gray. The only change is that when using the plastic tubes the red top is now drawn after the citrate blue top. Evidently the glass particles in the plastic tube can become transferred to the blue citrate tube and cause clotting within the citrate tube. Good advice is to check with the tube manufacturer for the recommended order of draw. The National Committee for Clinical Laboratory Standards (NCCLS) recommends a specific order of draw using the vacuum tube system (see Table 28-4).

Butterfly Needle Collection System

A system that combines benefits of the syringe system and the vacuum tube system is the butterfly collection system. The butterfly collection system has on one end a 21 or 23 gauge needle with attached plastic wings. Six or 12 inches of tubing leads from the needle. On the other end of this tubing is a hub that can attach to a syringe. A needle covered by a rubber sleeve can also be attached to the tubing. The covered needle screws into an evacuated tube holder (Figure 28-25).

The butterfly system is used for small veins that are difficult to puncture with the vacuum tube system and standard vacuum tube system needle. The system also facilitates drawing from veins that have a tendency to collapse. The winged needle of the butterfly needle will slide into a small surface vein in the back of the hand, wrist, or foot. Instead of entering the vein at the usual 15-degree angle, the winged needle is inserted at a 5- to 10-degree angle, and then threaded into the vein. This procedure anchors the needle in the center of a small vein that is inaccessible by other methods. If the patient moves, the tubing gives flexibility so the needle will stay anchored and not pull out of the vein. The butterfly collection set works well on children who have small veins and the tendency to move while blood is being collected.

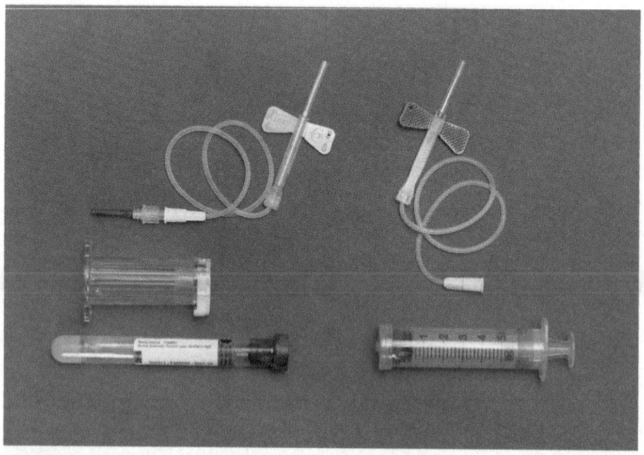

Figure 28-25 Butterfly needle sets with connections for either a (left) vacuum tube or (right) syringe.

Critical Thinking

You are preparing to perform a venipuncture on a geriatric patient who has fragile veins. Which system would you use: a syringe or a vacuum tube system? What makes one technique more successful in this case?

The system also gives the adaptability of initiating a draw with a syringe and then finishing it with the evacuated tube system. A syringe can be filled for procedures that require a syringe sample. It can then be removed, and the vacuum tube system can be attached for multiple tube collection. Remember to draw into or transfer into the vacuum tubes in the proper order. See text box "Order of Filling Tubes from a Syringe" and Table 28-4. Although the butterfly collection system has many benefits, it is not used for all collections. It is more expensive than the needle system. The additional expense is unnecessary for the majority of venipunctures.

Patient Reactions

Patients can have a variety of reactions to having their blood drawn. The medical assistant must anticipate these reactions and respond appropriately as quickly as possible. The most common patient reaction is pain. The patient will indicate that the venipuncture is painful. Slightly reposition the needle, and then loosen the tourniquet. Loosening the tourniquet often helps because the tourniquet may be pinching the arm and causing discomfort rather than the needle. Avoid deep, probing venipunctures because they may go deeply into the arm and get too close to the nerves. If the pain persists, discontinue the venipuncture.

Other possible patient reactions and the medical assistant's appropriate responses are listed in Table 28-6.

The Unsuccessful Venipuncture

Methods of vein stimulation are shown in Table 28-7. When a blood sample cannot be obtained, it may be necessary to change the position of the needle. Rotate the needle half a turn. The bevel of the needle may be against the wall of the vein. If the needle has not penetrated the vein far enough, advance it further into the vein. Advance it only slightly; a small change may mean the difference between a failed and a successful venipuncture. If the

TABLE 28-6 PATIENT REACTIONS TO BLOOD DRAWS

Patient Reaction	Medical Assistant Response
1. Syncope (fainting)	Immediately remove the tourniquet, then the needle, and stop the patient from falling. Lower the patient's head and arms. Wipe the patient's forehead and back of the neck with a cold compress if necessary. If the patient does not respond, notify a physician, move the patient to the floor, and place a pillow under the patient's legs.
2. Nausea	If a patient becomes nauseated, apply cold compresses to the patient's forehead. Give the patient an emesis basin, and have facial tissues ready if the nausea does not diminish. Deep, slow breathing through the mouth may help.
3. Insulin shock/ **hypoglycemia**	The first signs of insulin shock are a cold sweat and pallor similar to the signs of syncope. The patient becomes weak and shaky, sudden mental confusion may follow, and it appears as though the patient's personality changes instantly. Call the physician if the patient loses consciousness. This can happen especially to patients having a fasting blood sugar test.
4. Convulsions	The patient loses consciousness and exhibits violent or mild convulsive motions. Do not try to restrain the patient. Move objects or furniture out of the way to prevent the patient from striking objects and being hurt. Help the patient to the floor and into a reclining position. The patient usually recovers within a few minutes. Notify the physician about the patient's reaction. The physician will determine when to release the patient.

needle has penetrated too far into the vein, pull back a little. Always withdraw the needle slowly when the venipuncture has been unsuccessful. The blood often may start coming just as it seems the needle is ready to come out of the skin. The tube used may not have sufficient vacuum. Try another tube before withdrawing the needle.

Probing the site is not recommended. Probing is painful to the patient and may cause a hematoma. Never attempt a venipuncture more than two times. If a blood sample cannot be obtained after two attempts, have another person attempt the draw. Notify the patient's physician if two medical assistants have been unsuccessful.

Criteria for Rejection of a Specimen

The primary goal of the medical assistant is to provide an acceptable specimen for laboratory testing as required by the physician. There are certain general criteria that must be met for a specimen to be acceptable. If the criteria are not met, the specimen is rejected and another venipuncture of the patient must be performed.

Table 28-8 lists quality-assurance controls for specimen collection and processing. The list is not all inclusive. The type of specimen that is acceptable and the volume required are determined by the procedure ordered. The quality-control checks done by the

TABLE 28-7 METHODS OF VEIN STIMULATION

1. Position the patient's arm lower than his or her heart.
2. Reapply the tourniquet; it may not be tight enough.
3. Massage the arm from the wrist to the elbow to encourage venous return.
4. Tap sharply at the venipuncture site with your fingertips. This can cause the veins to dilate.
5. Use a blood pressure cuff in place of the tourniquet. Pump it to about 40–60 mm Hg.
6. Warm the venipuncture site with a warming device or a warm washcloth (not hotter than 100°F.)
7. Have the patient make a fist. Do not have the patient pump his or her fist; that can cause a false high level of potassium in the specimen.

TABLE 28-8 QUALITY ASSURANCE FOR SPECIMEN COLLECTION AND PROCESSING

1. Each specimen must have its own label attached to the specimen's primary container.
2. Each specimen must have a laboratory requisition label.
3. Labels must have the patient's complete name and identification number, date of birth, date and time, and your signature.
4. Specimens in syringes with needles still attached are unacceptable.
5. All specimens must be in the appropriate anticoagulant.
6. Blood collection tubes with anticoagulant must be at least 75% full. All blood collection tubes for coagulation testing must be at least 90% full.
7. Uncoagulated blood specimens must be free of clots.
8. Certain tests require specimens to be free of hemolysis and **lipemia**, a milky appearance due to lipids.
9. The specimen may need to be recollected if the results do not agree with what the physician believes is the diagnosis of the patient.
10. Do not combine partially filled tubes.
11. Do not mix tubes of different additives.
12. As soon as possible, invert tubes 8 to 10 times to prevent microclots from forming.
13. Mix tubes gently to prevent **hemolysis** of specimen.

laboratory may indicate the results are valid. If the results do not agree with what the physician believes is the patient's diagnosis, the blood specimen may need to be redrawn to confirm the results. This is accomplished by either retesting the specimen or collecting another sample. This will either reconfirm that blood was drawn from the correct patient or that the patient's test results changed significantly.

Factors Affecting Laboratory Values

There are numerous variables that can affect laboratory test results. The specimens are tested by analytic instruments that give accurate and precise results. These results will accurately reflect what is wrong with the patient only if the specimen is collected correctly. The medical assistant is responsible for collecting and caring for the specimen properly. When in doubt of how to care for a specimen, refer to the manual supplied by your laboratory or contact the laboratory for specific instructions. It is always better to ask the question and perform the proper procedure than not to ask and have to repeat the venipuncture. In addition, if you ever do need to repeat a venipuncture because of improper collection or handling of the specimen, the patient should not be billed for the second collection. Patient physiologic factors may also contribute to inaccurate results. Other factors that can alter results are listed in Table 28-9.

Occasionally, a specimen will require protection from light, incubation, refrigeration, or chilling immediately after collection. Any delay in these requirements will alter the results. Your laboratory manual will direct you as to which specimens need to be chilled. See Table 28-10 for examples of special handling requirements.

The medical assistant is not the only person who can affect test results. The patient can knowingly or unknowingly alter the results by certain actions. An example of this occurs when a patient has had a cup of coffee but claims not to have had anything to eat or drink. The patient is often under the misconception that black coffee without sugar will not be a problem. Caffeine and smoking affect the metabolism and can affect the test results.

TABLE 28-9 FACTORS AFFECTING LABORATORY RESULTS

Factor	Effect
Blood alcohol	When drawing a specimen for blood alcohol testing, a nonalcohol-based antiseptic should be used to clean the venipuncture site. The cleansing alcohol may falsely elevate the test result.
Diurnal rhythm	Some specimens must be drawn at timed intervals because of medication or diurnal (daily) rhythm. The exact time of collection must be noted on the specimen.
Exercise	Strenuous short-term exercise can make the heart work harder and increase the heart enzymes. Long-term exercise such as that performed by highly trained runners can cause erroneous results due to runner's anemia.
Fasting	Patient not in fasting state when fasting is required. Results of tests will not be accurate.
Hemolysis	Destruction of red blood cell membrane and release of intercellular contents into serum/plasma can be caused by not allowing alcohol to air-dry at venipuncture site, using a needle that is too small (less than 22 gauge), forcing the blood into a vacutainer tube from a syringe, or shaking the vacutainer tube instead of mixing by gentle inversion when mixing tubes with additives.
Heparin	Incorrect heparin used that interferes with tests being run on patient.
Stress	In children, violent crying before a specimen is collected can increase the white blood cell count.
Tourniquet on too long	Hemoconcentration, change in chemical concentration.
Volume	Not enough blood will cause a dilution factor, which can change the size of the cells and therefore produce a variation in test results.

CAPILLARY PUNCTURE

Venipuncture is the most frequently performed phlebotomy procedure, but it is not the procedure of choice in all circumstances. An alternative to venipuncture is capillary puncture, also known as dermal puncture or skin puncture.

Capillary puncture is a method of obtaining one to several drops of blood for a variety of tests. With proper instruments, tests such as a complete blood count, RBC count, white blood cell (WBC) count, hemoglobin, and hematocrit can be run. One drop of blood can be used to test glucose blood levels, a few drops of blood can fill capillary tubes, and several drops can complete a phenylketonuria (PKU) test card. Tests that cannot be run on capillary blood specimens are sedimentation rates, blood cultures, coagulation studies, and any other tests requiring large amounts of serum or plasma.

Capillary puncture is the method of choice with two types of patients: when patient blood volume is a concern, such as with infants, and when vein access is difficult, such as with burned or scarred patients. Capillary puncture should not be used when a patient is edematous, dehydrated, or has poor peripheral circulation.

Composition of Capillary Blood

Blood obtained via capillary puncture is a mixture of blood from arterioles, venules, capillaries, and interstitial fluid.

TABLE 28-10 COMMON LABORATORY TESTS THAT REQUIRE SPECIAL HANDLING

Laboratory Test	Special Handling
A, vitamin	Protect from light by wrapping tube in foil.
Acid phosphatase	Deliver to laboratory within hour. Separate, freeze serum after clotting.
Adrenocorticotropic hormone (ACTH)	Place in ice slurry.
Alcohol, blood	Do **NOT** use alcohol pad to clean site.
Ammonia	Place in ice slurry.
B_6, vitamin	Protect from light by wrapping tube in foil.
B_{12}, vitamin	Protect from light by wrapping tube in foil.
Beta-carotene	Protect from light by wrapping tube in foil.
Bilirubin, total or direct	Protect from light by wrapping tube in foil.
Catecholamines	Place in ice slurry.
Clot retraction	Incubate in 37°C until clotted.
Cold agglutinins	Warm tube, incubate in 37°C.
Complement C4	Separate and freeze serum after clotting.
Complement, total (CH50)	Let clot in refrigerator, separate immediately and freeze immediately.
Complement, total (CH100)	Let clot in refrigerator, separate immediately and freeze immediately.
Cryofibrinogen	Warm tube, incubate in 37°C.
Gastrin	Place in ice slurry.
Gentamicin	Label peak or trough and time of last medication.
Glucose tolerance	Label tubes with time intervals of draw specimens.
Human leukocyte antigen (HLA-B27)	Do **NOT** refrigerate or freeze, record date and time collected.
Lactic acid	Place in ice slurry.
Parathyroid hormone (PTH)	Place in ice slurry.
pH / blood gas	Place in ice slurry.
Porphyrins	Protect from light by wrapping tube in foil.
Prostate-specific antigen	Deliver to laboratory within one hour, separate, freeze serum after clotting.
Prostatic acid phosphatase	Deliver to laboratory within one hour, separate, freeze serum after clotting.
Prothrombin time (PT)	Refrigerate.
Partial thromboplastin time (PTT)	Refrigerate, test within four hours of drawing specimen.
Pyruvate	Place in ice slurry.
Red cell folate	Protect from light by wrapping tube in foil.
Renin	Place in ice slurry.
Thioridazine (Mellaril)	Protect from light by wrapping tube in foil.
Tobramycin	Label peak or trough and time of last medication.

Source: Courtesy of Sheri R. Greimes, CMA, PBT (ASCP).

In most instances, a capillary puncture specimen most resembles arterial blood. There may be significant differences between specimens obtained by capillary puncture and those collected by venipuncture. For example, the glucose level may be increased in capillary blood, whereas the potassium, calcium, and total protein levels may be decreased. It is therefore important to always note on the specimen when capillary blood has been obtained.

Capillary Puncture Sites

The usual site for capillary puncture in adults and children is the fingertip (Figure 28-26). In adults, the ring finger is often selected because it usually is not callused. In infants, the lateral or medial plantar surface of the heel pad is usually used, and the procedure is often called a heelstick. The heelstick is most often performed when testing for PKU, which is covered in detail in Chapter 32.

Preparing the Capillary Puncture Site

The area selected for a capillary puncture must be carefully prepared. The puncture site will be warm if blood circulation is adequate. Coolness of the skin indicates decreased circulation. To increase circulation, the site may be gently massaged, or a warm, moist towel, face cloth, or warm pack (at a temperature not higher than 100°F) may be placed on the site for three to five minutes.

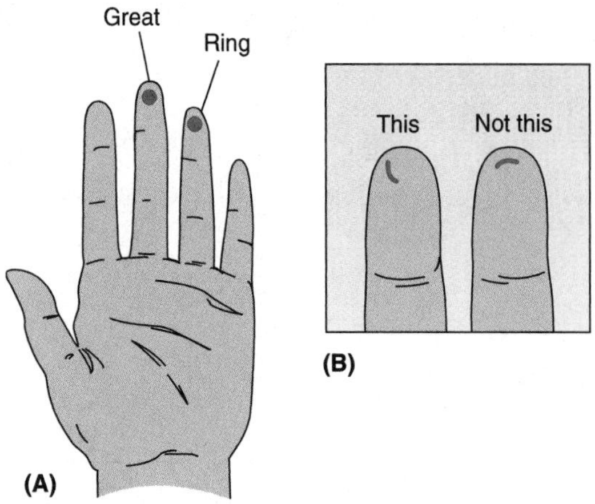

Figure 28-26 (A) Capillary blood collection sites. (B) Correct direction of capillary puncture.

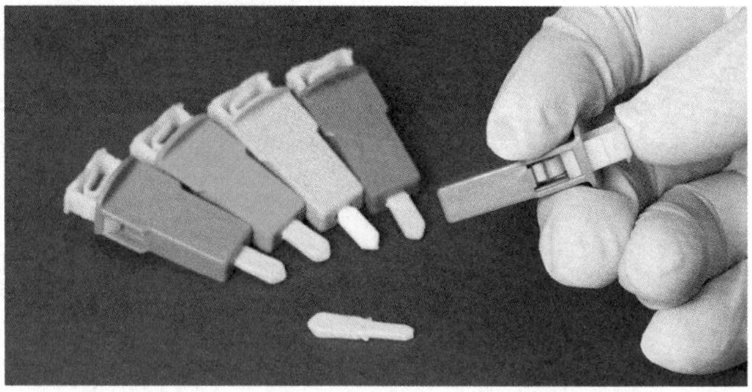

Figure 28-27 Microtainer® Genie brand lancets are available in different types for various purposes. They are color coded and have specific information on their packaging.

Alcohol-soaked gauze or cotton should be used to cleanse and disinfect the puncture site. The site should then be allowed to air-dry, or dry with a gauze pad. A cotton ball is not recommended because the tiny cotton fibers can stay on the puncture site, assisting in clotting, which is not desirable at this point. When the puncture is complete, a cotton ball may be used as a compress. Residual alcohol at the puncture site results in hemolysis of the specimen, which may affect test results, as well as cause a burning sensation to the patient. Betadine® (povidone iodine) should not be used to clean the puncture site. Blood contaminated with iodine may falsely increase certain blood chemistries.

Performing the Puncture

Safety glasses, a mask, and gloves should be worn by the medical assistant while performing capillary puncture. Some patients bleed quite readily from the puncture so be sure to have extra gauze on hand. The patient's hand and finger should be held so the puncture site is readily accessible. The puncture is made at the tip of the fleshy pad and slightly to the side (see Figure 28-26). The skin near the chosen site should be pulled taut. If the tips of the fingers are heavily callused or thickened, a lancet with a longer point may be used. Capillary punctures are performed using semiautomated devices such as the disposable Microtainer® Brand Safety Flow Lancet®.

The BD Microtainer® Genie Lancet is shown in Figure 28-27. After cleaning the puncture site, twist off the indicator as directed on the tab. Press the safety lancet firmly against the puncture site. Hold the lancet between your fingers and press the white button with your thumb. The lancet should not bounce off the skin. The puncture should be performed in one quick, steady movement. Once you have depressed the plunger, the button will lock into housing and the needle will be permanently encapsulated. Practice working the lancet until you are comfortable with the action.

Collecting the Blood Sample

The first drop of blood is wiped away with dry, sterile gauze because it contains tissue fluid, which dilutes the blood drop and can also activate clotting. The second and following drops of blood are used for test samples. Depending on the tests to be performed, the blood may be collected in capillary tubes or other capillary collecting devices. Capillary tubes are small-diameter glass or plastic tubes that are open at both ends. Capillary tubes are extremely fragile and care should be taken to prevent breakage. The tubes have a colored line around one end. A red or black line indicates that the tube contains heparin, an anticoagulant, and will yield a nonclotted specimen. A blue line indicates that the tube contains no anticoagulant and will yield a clotted specimen. When taking the blood sample directly from the puncture site, a capillary tube that contains anticoagulant would be used; when taking blood from a vacuum tube that already has anticoagulant in it, the plain capillary tube would be used. Capillary tubes are used for many tests, depending on the equipment available. Chapter 29 explains how to use capillary tubes to check hematocrit levels. When capillary tubes are used for hematocrit tests, they are called microhematocrit tubes.

It may be necessary to massage the finger to increase the blood flow. It is best to massage the whole hand, taking care not to apply direct pressure near the puncture site. Squeezing the fingertip should be avoided; this forces tissue fluid into the blood sample and dilutes it or may cause hemolysis. Do not use a scooping technique when collecting blood from the puncture site. Scooping can break the RBC membranes, leading to hemolysis.

Figure 28-28 shows the basic steps to follow when filling a capillary tube. Allow well-rounded drops of blood

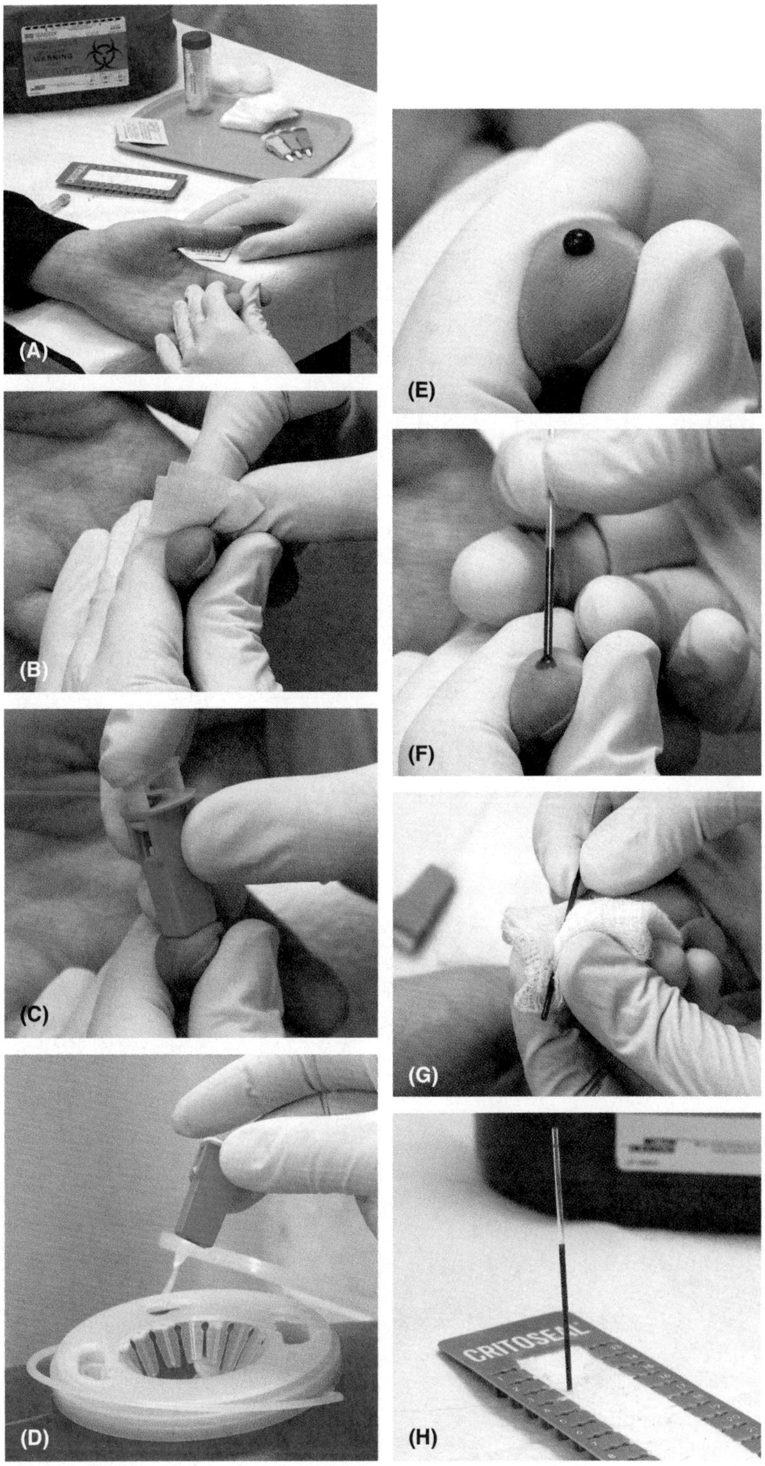

Figure 28-28 Collecting a specimen into a capillary tube through capillary puncture. (A) Assemble the equipment and supplies needed to perform a capillary puncture for microhematocrit testing and select the best site. (B) Clean the site with alcohol. (C) Perform the puncture. (D) Discard the lancet into the sharps container. (E) Wipe off the first drop and allow a well-rounded drop to form. (F) Holding the capillary tube horizontally, touch the end to the drop and allow the tube to fill. (G) Carefully wipe blood off the outside of the tube. (H) Gently place the end of the tube into the sealing clay. Draw one other tube (some laboratories recommend a total of three tubes in the event that one breaks).

to form at the puncture site. Holding the capillary tube at a horizontal position, gently touch the tip of tube to the top of the blood drop. The blood will enter the tube through "capillary action" caused by surface tension. Take care to not tilt the tube downward, which can cause air to enter the tube, nor upward, which can cause blood to come out of the tube. Continue to fill the tube until it is two-thirds to three-quarters full. When the tube is sufficiently filled, remove it from the drop and, at the same time, place your gloved finger over the opposite end of the tube. This will prevent the blood from flowing out of the tube. Keep your gloved finger over the end of the tube and, using your other hand, wipe off any residue blood from the outside of the tube with a gauze pad. Gently place the end of the tube into the sealing clay. Sealing clay trays are specially made for this purpose. They have numbered sections to help identify the samples. Some capillary tubes have plastic caps. Carefully follow the manufacturer's instructions for the type of tube you are using.

During the filling of the tubes, if the flow of blood begins to slow, rewipe the puncture site firmly with dry gauze (not a cotton ball). This action will dislodge the platelet plug and allow the blood to flow freely. Be sure the patient is relaxed. Have the patient take a deep breath. After filling the required number of tubes, apply a cotton ball compress to the puncture site. The patient can usually help hold the compress. The compression should be held in place for one to three minutes, depending on the patient. If the patient is taking aspirin, Coumadin therapy, or other anticoagulants, compression should be for at least five minutes.

In many ways the procedure for capillary puncture is similar to the other collection procedures discussed in this chapter (e.g., patient identification, safety precautions, specimen labeling). Procedure 28-5 provides a detailed description of capillary puncture.

Order of Draw for Capillary Puncture

The order of draw for microcollection differs from that used in venipuncture. If multiple specimens are collected, EDTA specimens (lavendar caps) are collected first, then other additive specimens (green, gray caps), and lastly specimens that clot (red or gel caps).

Procedure 28-1 Palpating a Vein for Venipuncture

STANDARD PRECAUTIONS:

PURPOSE:

To obtain venous blood with limited discomfort to the patient.

EQUIPMENT/SUPPLIES:

Gloves	Gown or laboratory coat
Goggles and mask, if necessary	Tube holder
Gauze	Alcohol swab
Tourniquet	Tubes
Needle	Bandage
	Sharps container

PROCEDURE STEPS:

1. Identify the patient. Ask the patient's name and verify it with the computer label or identification number. If a fasting specimen is required, verify that the patient has not had anything to eat or drink except water for 12 hours. RATIONALE: Proper identification of the patient and specimen and assuring that the patient has properly prepared for the blood tests are quality-control and quality-assurance measures.
2. Wash hands. Put on gloves, as well as safety glasses and mask if there is a potential for blood splatter.
3. Apply tourniquet 3 to 4 inches above the venipuncture site. Apply tightly enough to slow venous blood flow but not so tight that blood flow in arteries is stopped. Refer to Figure 28-20. RATIONALE: Applying the tourniquet too tightly can lead to excessive engorgement of the veins, causing blood to enter the tissues during puncture, further causing a hematoma.

(continues)

Procedure 28-1 (continued)

4. Have the patient close the hand and place the patient's arm in a downward position. Do not allow the patient to pump his or her hand. RATIONALE: Having the patient close his or her hand and positioning the arm below the heart causes enlargement of the vein, allowing for an easier, more successful puncture. Pumping of the hand can lead to excessive engorgement of the vein, causing blood to leak into surrounding tissue during the puncture, which will cause a hematoma to occur.
5. Palpate the antecubital space of the arm, feeling for the basilic or cephalic vein with the tip of your index finger. RATIONALE: The tip of your finger is less callused and more sensitive.
6. Feel for a soft bounce and a roundness to the vein. Follow the direction of the vein. RATIONALE: Following the direction of the vein gives you the correct direction for the puncture.
7. After locating an acceptable vein, mentally map the location. Visualize the puncture site. RATIONALE: Mentally mapping the location and visualizing the puncture site will help in planning a successful draw.
8. If a vein cannot be found in the antecubital space of the arm, then the hand veins must be checked following the same procedure. Venipuncture is more successful when a butterfly is used for hand vein collection. RATIONALE: Butterfly is more successful because the hand veins have a greater tendency to roll.

Procedure 28-2 Venipuncture by Syringe

STANDARD PRECAUTIONS:

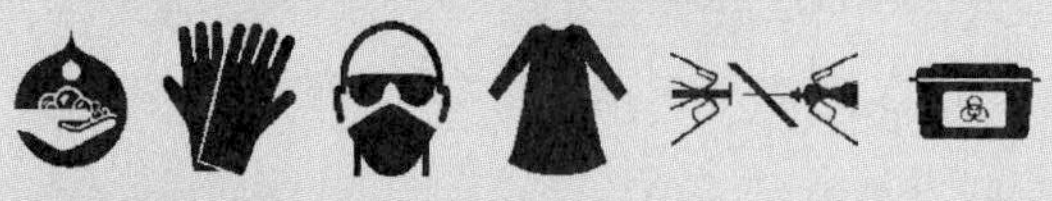

PURPOSE:

To obtain venous blood acceptable for laboratory testing as required by a physician.

SPECIMEN:

Venous blood collected by syringe and aliquoted into vacuum or special collection containers

EQUIPMENT/SUPPLIES:

Gloves	Tourniquet
Safety glasses and mask (optional)	70% isopropyl alcohol swab
10-cc syringe, 21 gauge needle	Cotton balls
Vacuum tube(s) or special collection tube(s)	Adhesive bandage or tape
	Sharps container
	Test tube rack

PROCEDURE STEPS:

1. Position and identify the patient. Ask the patient's name and verify it with the tests ordered and the computer label or identification number. If a fasting specimen is required, verify that the patient has not had anything to eat or drink except water for 12 hours. RATIONALE: Proper identification of the patient and the tests ordered and assuring that the patient is properly prepared for the blood tests are all quality-control and quality-assurance measures.
2. Wash hands and apply gloves and goggles/face shield. RATIONALE: Clean hands further protect the patient. Gloves protect you. Goggles/face shield should always be worn if there is a possibility of blood splatter.
3. Open the sterile needle and sterile syringe packages and assemble if necessary. Pull the plunger halfway out and push it all the way in again. RATIONALE: Preparing the equipment ahead

(continues)

Procedure 28-2 (continued)

of time assures a smoother process. Syringes can stick when new, so pulling once on the plunger prevents it from sticking during the venipuncture.

4. Select the proper vacuum tubes for later transfer of the specimen; tap all tubes containing anticoagulants and check the expiration dates. Arrange them in a holding rack. RATIONALE: Having the supplies ready and in the rack saves confusion later. The rack is a safety item so you are not holding the tube while transferring the specimen. Tapping the tubes ensures that all the additive is dislodged from the stopper and wall of the tubes. Checking expiration dates is a quality-assurance measure.
5. Select a site and apply the tourniquet. See Procedure 28-1. RATIONALE: Applying the tourniquet causes the vein to enlarge for easier venipuncture.
6. Ask the patient to close the hand. The patient must not pump the hand. Place the hand in a downward position. RATIONALE: Closing the hand and placing the arm in a downward position further enlarges the vein, allowing for easier venipuncture. Pumping the hand can damage the quality of the specimen collected.
7. Select a vein, noting the location and direction of the vein. RATIONALE: This allows you to prepare mentally for the venipuncture (Figure 28-29A).
8. Clean the site with an alcohol swab with one firm swipe. RATIONALE: Alcohol removes body oils and contamination (Figure 28-29B).
9. Avoid touching the site after cleansing. RATIONALE: The site should stay as clean as possible.
10. Draw the skin taut with your thumb by placing it 1 to 2 inches below the puncture site. RATIONALE: This will anchor the vein.
11. With the bevel up, line up the needle with the direction of the vein and perform the puncture. The point of the needle should enter the skin about ¼ inch below where the vein was palpated. With experience, a sensation of entering the vein can be felt. Once the vein has been entered, do not move the needle. RATIONALE: Lining up the needle with the vein is a mental exercise to help enter the vein in the proper

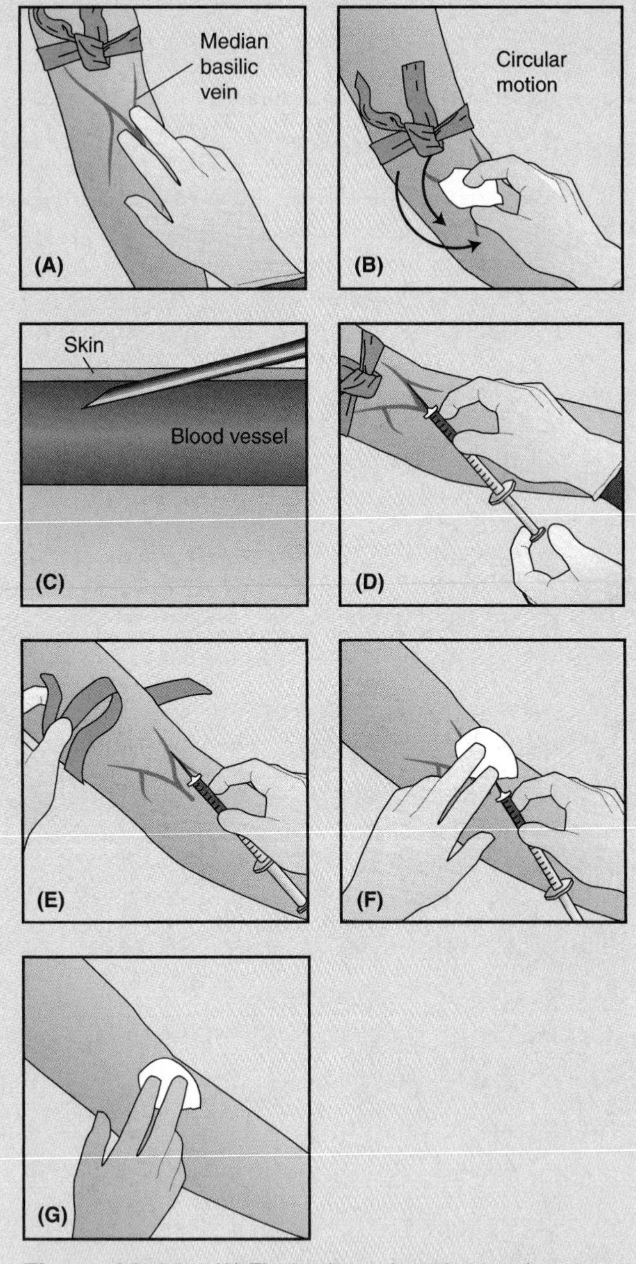

Figure 28-29 (A) Find vein and apply tourniquet. (B) Apply alcohol and allow to air dry. (C) Needle entering the blood vessel. (D) Withdraw blood slowly. (E) Release tourniquet. (F) Apply sterile pad before withdrawing needle. (G) Have patient apply pressure to the site until clot forms.

(continues)

Procedure 28-2 (continued)

direction. Entering the skin a fraction of an inch below the palpated site will aid in entering the vein at the palpated site (Figure 28-29C).

12. Let go of the skin and use that hand to pull back on the plunger. Pull gently and only as fast as the syringe fills. If the vein collapses, stop pulling on the plunger and let the vein refill. RATIONALE: Pulling too rapidly or too hard can cause the vein to collapse (Figure 28-29D).
13. When the syringe if full, have the patient open the hand. Remove the tourniquet. RATIONALE: Opening the hand and removing the tourniquet releases the pressure so the needle can be removed (Figure 28-29E).
14. Lightly place a cotton ball above the puncture site and remove the needle in the same direction as inserted. RATIONALE: Holding the cotton ball above the site allows for immediate pressure to be applied once the needle is removed (Figure 28-29F).
15. Apply pressure to the site for two to three minutes. Let the patient assist by holding the pressure if desired. The patient may elevate the arm but should be instructed not to bend the elbow. RATIONALE: Two to three minutes is usually time enough for the bleeding to stop. Elevating the arm while holding pressure aids in the clotting. Bending the elbow can cause a hematoma to form (Figure 28-29G).
16. Aliquot blood into the appropriate tubes in the rack in the proper order. Refer to the "Order of Draw" instructions in this chapter (see Table 28-4). During transfer, you may hold each tube at the base only. RATIONALE: Having the tubes in the rack and holding the tubes at the base protects your hand from accidental needlestick during the transfer process.
17. Puncture the vacuum tube through the rubber stopper with the syringe needle and allow the blood to enter the tube until the flow stops. Never push on the plunger or force blood into the tube. RATIONALE: Pushing on the plunger and forcing blood into the vacuum tube can cause the rubber stopper to pop off, splashing blood.
18. Implement safety mechanism or devices on the needle immediately. RATIONALE: Immediate implementation of safety mechanisms will protect from accidental needlesticks.
19. Mix any anticoagulant tubes immediately. RATIONALE: Mixing the anticoagulants right away minimizes the chance of miniclots forming.
20. Discard the syringe and needle into a sharps container and the contaminated cotton ball and other contaminated waste into a red bag. RATIONALE: Proper disposal of sharps and biohazard waste protects all of us.
21. Label all tubes before leaving the room. If any special treatment is required for the specimens, institute the handling protocol right away. RATIONALE: Labeling the tubes right away lessens the chances of a mix-up error. Proper handling of specimens ensures an accurate test result.
22. Check the patient. Observe him or her for signs of stress. RATIONALE: Venipuncture can be stressful for some patients.
23. When sufficient pressure has been applied to stop the bleeding, apply a small pressure bandage by pulling a cotton ball in half, applying it to the puncture site, and placing an adhesive bandage or tape over it (Figure 28-29H). Instruct the patient to remove the bandage in 20 minutes. If the patient is sensitive or allergic to latex, be sure to use nonlatex paper tape. If the bleeding has not stopped after two to three minutes, have the patient continue to hold direct pressure on

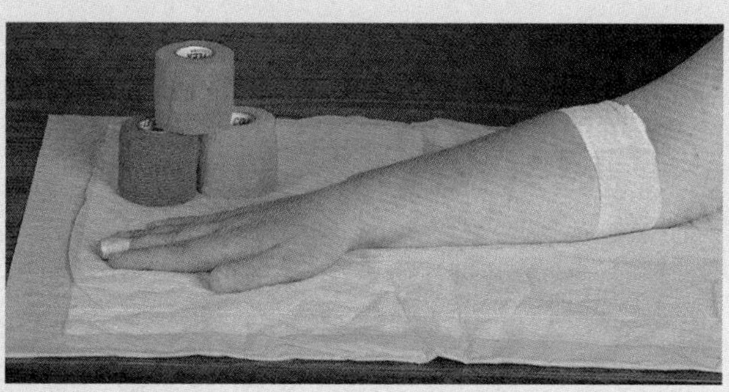

Figure 28-29 (continued) (H) Adhesive bandages for venipuncture come in a variety of colors.

(continues)

Procedure 28-2 (continued)

the site for another five minutes with his or her arm elevated above the heart. He or she can do this by lying down with his or her arm on a pillow. Recheck after five minutes. RATIONALE: The patient should not leave your care until the bleeding has stopped.

24. Disinfect tray and supplies and dispose of all contaminated items properly. Remove gloves using proper technique. RATIONALE: Proper disposal and disinfection of all contaminated supplies and equipment protects all of us from exposure to biohazardous substances.
25. Wash hand, record the procedure, and complete the laboratory requisition. RATIONALE: Washing hands after removing gloves further protects from biohazardous substances and lessens the chance of cross contamination to the patient's chart and the laboratory requisition. Completing the documentation and requisition as soon as possible after the procedure improves accuracy.

DOCUMENTATION

11/13/XX 2:54 PM Venipuncture performed right arm for CBC and sed rate. Specimen sent to Inner City Lab. Identification #987654321. Patient tolerated the procedure well and will call back tomorrow for the test results. Joe Guerrero, CMA

Procedure 28-3 Venipuncture by Vacuum Tube System

STANDARD PRECAUTIONS:

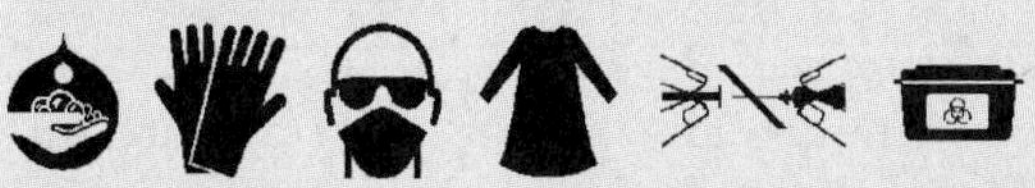

PURPOSE:

To obtain venous blood acceptable for laboratory testing as required by a physician.

SPECIMEN

Venous blood collected by vacuum tubes. Volume of blood dependent on size of tube and test requirements.

EQUIPMENT/SUPPLIES:

Gloves
Goggles and mask, if necessary
Vacuum tube adapter/holder
21 gauge multidraw needle
Vacuum tube(s) or special collection tube(s)
Tourniquet
70% isopropyl alcohol swab
Cotton balls
Adhesive bandage or tape
Sharps container

PROCEDURE STEPS:

1. Position and identify the patient. Ask the patient's name and verify it with the tests ordered and the computer label or identification number. If a fasting specimen is required, verify that the patient has not had anything to eat or drink except water for 12 hours. RATIONALE: Proper identification of the patient and the tests ordered and assuring that the patient is properly prepared for the blood tests are all quality-control and quality-assurance measures.
2. Wash hands and apply gloves and goggles/face shield. RATIONALE: Clean hands further protect the patient. Gloves protect you. Goggles/face

(continues)

Procedure 28-3 (continued)

shield should always be worn if there is a possibility of blood splatter.

3. Break the seal on the shorter needle, thread the shorter needle into the holder/adapter. RATIONALE: Preparing the equipment ahead of time assures a smoother process.
4. Tap all tubes containing anticoagulants and check the expiration dates. RATIONALE: Tapping the tubes ensures that all the additive is dislodged from the stopper and wall of the tubes. Checking expiration dates is a quality-assurance measure.
5. Insert the first tube into the holder/adapter without penetrating the stopper. Reference the "Order of Draw" chart (see Table 28-4) to select the first tube. RATIONALE: The stopper should not be penetrated to avoid losing the vacuum. The order of draw is important to avoid contaminating a nonadditive tube with additive.
6. Select a site and apply the tourniquet. See Procedure 28-1. RATIONALE: Applying the tourniquet causes the vein to enlarge for easier venipuncture.
7. Ask the patient to close the hand. The patient must not pump the hand. Place the hand in a downward position. RATIONALE: Closing the hand and placing the arm in a downward position further enlarges the vein allowing for easier venipuncture. Pumping the hand can damage the quality of the specimen collected.
8. Select a vein, noting the location and direction of the vein. RATIONALE: This allows you to prepare mentally for the venipuncture (Figure 28-30A).
9. Clean the site with an alcohol swab with one firm swipe. RATIONALE: Alcohol removes body oils and contamination (Figure 28-30B).
10. Avoid touching the site after cleansing. RATIONALE: The site should stay as clean as possible.
11. Draw the skin taut with your thumb by placing it 1 to 2 inches below the puncture site. RATIONALE: This will anchor the vein.
12. With the bevel up, line up the needle with the direction of the vein and perform the puncture. The point of the needle should enter the skin about ¼ inch below where the vein was palpated. With experience, a sensation of entering the vein can be felt. Once the vein has been entered, do not move the needle. RATIONALE: Lining up the needle with the vein is a mental exercise to help enter the vein in the proper direction. Entering the skin a fraction of an inch below the palpated site will aid in entering the vein at the palpated site (Figure 28-30C).
13. Let go of the skin and use that hand to grasp the flange of the vacuum tube holder and push the tube forward until the needle has completely entered the tube (Figure 28-30D). Do not change hands while performing venipuncture. The hand performing the venipuncture is the hand that is holding the vacuum tube holder. The other hand is free for tube insertion and removal. RATIONALE: Using the flange of the adapter helps you hold the needle steady while changing tubes. Changing hands while performing venipuncture could cause the needle to move.
14. Fill the tube until the vacuum is exhausted and the blood flow stops. Rotate tubes so the label is down. RATIONALE: Letting the tubes completely fill will assure the right ratio of blood to additive. Positioning the label down enables you to see the tube filling.
15. When the blood ceases, gently remove the vacuum tube from the needle and holder. Do this by grasping the tube with the fingers and palm of your spare hand and using your thumb to push off from the flange of the holder. RATIONALE: Using the flange will help steady the needle.
16. Immediately mix the blood in the anticoagulant tubes by gently inverting them several times. RATIONALE: Mixing the anticoagulant tubes right away minimizes the chance of miniclots forming (Figure 28-30E).
17. Insert the second tube onto the needle by using the same motion as the first tube (Figure 28-30F). Let it fill; then remove it with the same motion as the first tube. Invert it several times if it contains anticoagulants. RATIONALE: Mixing the additives prevents the blood from coagulating (Figure 28-30G).

(continues)

Procedure 28-3 (continued)

18. When the last tube has filled, remove it from the needle. Ask the patient to open his hand and release the tourniquet. RATIONALE: Removing the last tube from the needle prevents any residual suction from drawing blood through the tissues when the needle is removed from the vein. Opening the hand and removing the tourniquet relieves pressure so the needle can be removed without causing excessive blood loss through the puncture site.
19. Lightly place the cotton ball above the puncture site and smoothly remove the needle from the arm in the same direction of insertion. RATIONALE: Holding the cotton ball above the site allows for immediate pressure to be applies once the needle is removed.
20. Immediately activate the safety device. RATIONALE: Activating the safety device protects you from accidental needlesticks (Figure 28-30H).
21. Apply pressure on the site for two to three minutes. Let the patient assist by holding the pressure. Ask him or her not the bend his or her arm, but he or she may elevate his or her arm while applying pressure. RATIONALE: Two to three minutes is usually time enough for bleeding to stop. Elevating the arm while holding pressure aids in the clotting. Bending the elbow can cause a hematoma to form.

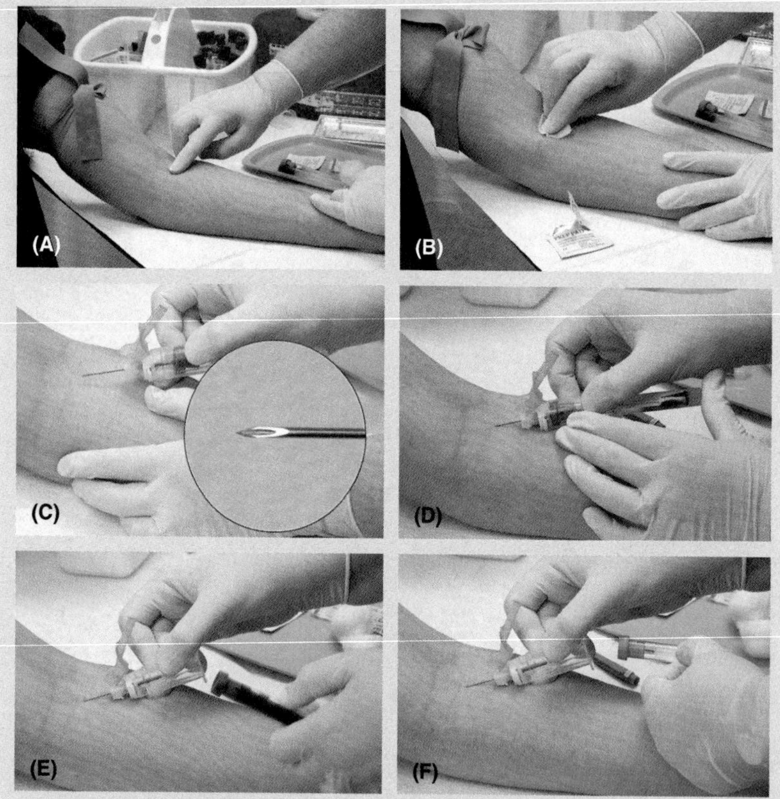

Figure 28-30 Performing a venipuncture with a vacuum tube assembly. (A) After tying the tourniquet, palpate the vein. (B) Cleanse the site with alcohol. (C) While holding the skin taut, hold needle with bevel up and penetrate the vein with a smooth, rapid movement. (D) Grasp the flange of the vacuum tube holder and push the tube forward until the needle has completely entered the tube. (E) When the tube has stopped filling, remove it gently from the needle and holder. Invert it several times to mix the additives. (F) Place another tube onto the needle and let it fill.

(continues)

Procedure 28-3 (continued)

22. Dispose of the needle into a sharps container and the contaminated cotton ball and other contaminated waste into a biohazard red bag. RATIONALE: Proper disposal of sharps and biohazard waste protects all of us.
23. Label all the tubes before leaving the patient. If any special treatment is required for the specimens, institute the handling protocol right away. RATIONALE: Labeling the tubes right away lessens the chances of a mix-up error. Proper handling of the specimens ensures accurate test results (Figure 28-30I, J).
24. Check the patient. Observe him or her for signs of stress. He or she should stop bleeding within two to three minutes. If the bleeding has stopped, apply a small pressure bandage by pulling a cotton ball in half, applying it to the site, and placing an adhesive bandage or tape over it. The patient

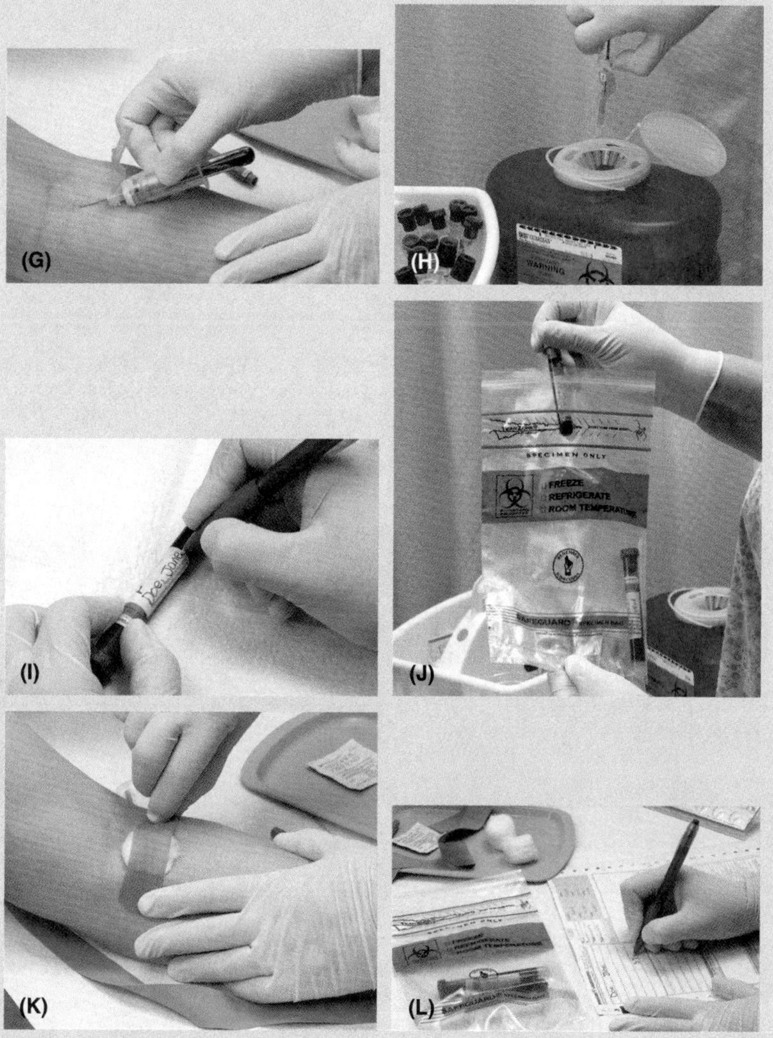

Figure 28-30 (continued) (G) Allow the second (last) tube to fill, then remove it and invert it several times to mix the additive. (H) As you smoothly remove the needle from the vein, apply pressure with the cotton ball. After removing the needle from the vein, activate the safety device immediately and dispose of the needle into the sharps container. (I) Properly label the tubes. (J) Package the specimens for transport. (K) Check the patient; apply a bandage. (L) Complete the laboratory requisition.

(continues)

Procedure 28-3 (continued)

should be instructed to remove the bandage in about 20 minutes. If the patient is sensitive to latex, be sure to use a nonlatex paper tape. If the bleeding has not stopped, have the patient continue to hold direct pressure another five minutes with his or her arm elevated about his or her heart level. Have him or her lie down with his or her arm up on a pillow. Recheck the site after five minutes of additional direct pressure. RATIONALE: Check the patient for signs of distress because venipuncture can be stressful for some people. The patient should not leave your care until the bleeding has stopped (Figure 28-30K).

25. Disinfect all surfaces and supplies/equipment. Remove gloves using proper technique. Dispose of contaminated items appropriately. RATIONALE: Proper disposal and disinfection of all contaminated supplies and equipment protects us all from exposure to dangerous biohazard substances.
26. Wash hands, record the procedure, and complete the laboratory requisition. RATIONALE: Washing hands after removing gloves further protects from biohazard substances and lessens the chance of cross contamination to the patient's chart and the laboratory requisition. Completing the documentation and requisition as soon as possible after the procedure improves accuracy (Figure 28-30L).

DOCUMENTATION

4/27/XX 8:36 AM Venipuncture performed left arm for CBC, Hgb & Hct, and thyroid panel. Specimen sent to Inner City Lab. Patient ID # 56776523. Patient tolerated the procedure well and will return on Monday the 30th for a recheck. Joe Guerrero, CMA

Procedure 28-4 Venipuncture by Butterfly Needle System

STANDARD PRECAUTIONS:

PURPOSE:
To obtain venous blood acceptable for laboratory testing as required by a physician.

SPECIMEN
Venous blood collected by butterfly needle system. Volume of blood dependent on size of tube and test requirements. The butterfly tubing can be either connected to a syringe or to a vacuum tube holder. This procedure covers both options. If the syringe collection is used, the specimen will be transferred into vacuum tubes after the collection.

EQUIPMENT/SUPPLIES:
Gloves
Goggles and mask, if necessary
Vacuum tube holder if using a vacuum tube connection
A 10- to 15-ml/cc syringe if using a syringe connection
Butterfly needle system with 21 gauge needle (use a multisample needle system with a luer adapter for attaching to the vacuum tube and a hypodermic needle for syringe attachment)
Vacuum tubes
Tourniquet
70% isopropyl alcohol swab
Gauze or cotton balls
Adhesive bandage or tape
Sharps container

(continues)

Procedure 28-4 (continued)

PROCEDURE STEPS:

1. Position and identify the patient. Ask the patient's name and verify it with the computer label or identification number.
2. If a fasting specimen is required, verify that the patient has not had anything to eat or drink except water for 12 hours.
3. Wash hands.
4. Put on gloves, as well as safety glasses and mask if there is a potential for blood splatter.
5. Assemble equipment.
6. Open the package of butterfly needle system. If using the multisample needle, connect the needle to the vacuum tube holder/adapter. If using the hypodermic needle and syringe, connect the needle to the syringe. If using a syringe, set the vacuum tubes in a rack for later use. RATIONALE: The more organized you are before the venipuncture; the smoother the procedure will go.
7. Tap the vacuum tubes to be sure any additive is dislodged from the stopper and sides of the tube. Check the expiration dates. RATIONALE: Dislodging the additive will assure proper ratio in the specimen. The tubes should not be older than their expiration date.
8. Apply the tourniquet. RATIONALE: Applying a tourniquet enlarges the vein, making it more accessible.
9. Ask the patient to close his or her hand. The patient should not pump his or her hand. If possible, place the arm in a downward position. RATIONALE: Pumping of hand can lead to excessive engorgement of the vein, which can cause blood to enter the tissues during the puncture, causing a hematoma.
10. Select the vein noting the direction and location of the vein. RATIONALE: You will want to enter the vein in the same direction it is going.
11. Clean the site with an alcohol swab using one swift firm swipe and allow to dry. RATIONALE: Alcohol removes body oils and other contaminations. Puncturing the skin through wet alcohol can cause stinging and hemolysis of the specimen and will contaminate the specimen.
12. Avoid touching the site after cleansing. RATIONALE: Touching the skin will recontaminate it.
13. Draw the skin taut by placing your thumb 1 to 2 inches below the site and pulling down firmly. RATIONALE: This will anchor the vein.
14. Hold the wings of the butterfly together with the bevel up, line up the needle with the vein, and smoothly insert it into the vein at about a 5- to 10-degree angle. RATIONALE: This process will cause the least amount of discomfort and provide the greatest success.
15. Remove your hand from holding the skin taut. RATIONALE: You will need one hand free to handle the other equipment.
16. If you are connected to a vacuum tube holder, grasp the flange of the vacuum tube holder and push the tube forward until the needle has completely entered the tube. RATIONALE: Using the flange when inserting and removing vacuum tubes will help the needle stay in position.
17. If you are connected to a syringe, pull gently on the syringe. RATIONALE: Pulling too rapidly can cause the vein to collapse.
18. Do not change hands while performing venipuncture. The hand performing the venipuncture is the hand that is holding the vacuum tube holder. The other hand is for inserting and removing the vacuum tubes. RATIONALE: Changing hands can cause the needle to change position.
19. If you are collecting directly into vacuum tubes, remove and replace the vacuum tubes as explained in Procedure 28-3 until you have drawn the necessary amounts. If you are drawing into a syringe, you will be limited to the size of the syringe being used. RATIONALE: You do not have the option of removing and replacing the syringe during a draw.
20. When the syringe is filled, ask the patient to open his or her hand and release the tourniquet. RATIONALE: Opening of the hand and releasing the tourniquet takes the pressure off the vein and allows the blood to flow freely through the arm.
21. Lightly place a cotton ball above the puncture site and smoothly remove the needle from the arm in the same direction of insertion. RATIONALE: You are getting the cotton ball ready so you can apply pressure on the puncture site immediately on removing the needle.

(continues)

Procedure 28-4 (continued)

22. Activate the safety device of the butterfly needle immediately. RATIONALE: The safety devices are better able to protect if activated immediately.
23. Apply pressure on the site. Let the patient assist by holding the pressure. Ask him or her not the bend his or her arm. He or she may elevate his or her arm while applying pressure though. RATIONALE: Applying pressure and elevating the arm lessens the chance of bruising, whereas bending the elbow increases the chance of the patient forming a hematoma.
24. If using a syringe, aliquot blood into the appropriate tubes as outlined in Procedure 28-2. RATIONALE: Following proper procedure when transferring blood from the syringe into the vacuum tubes ensure the best specimens for testing.
25. Dispose of the needle into a sharps container. RATIONALE: Immediate disposal of contaminated needles is the safest practice.
26. Label all the tubes. RATIONALE: Not labeling the tubes right away increases the likelihood of a mix-up error.
27. Check the patient. Observe him or her for signs of stress. RATIONALE: Patient safety is a primary concern. Venipuncture can be difficult for some patients.
28. The patient should stop bleeding within two to three minutes. If the bleeding has stopped, apply a small pressure bandage by pulling a cotton ball in half, applying it to the site, and placing an adhesive bandage or tape over it. The patient should be instructed to remove the bandage in about 20 minutes. If the patient is sensitive to latex, be sure to use a nonlatex paper tape. If the bleeding has not stopped, have the patient continue to hold pressure another five minutes with his or her arm elevated about his or her heart level, then recheck. RATIONALE: The patient should not be released from your care until the bleeding has stopped.
29. Clean up tray and supplies; dispose of contaminated cotton ball. Remove gloves using proper technique. Discard gloves into biohazard container and disinfect goggles. RATIONALE: Proper disposal and disinfection of contaminated supplies and equipment protects from exposure to biohazard substances.
30. Wash hands, record the procedure and complete the laboratory requisition. RATIONALE: Washing hands after removing the gloves further protects from biohazard substances and lessen the chance of cross contamination to the patient's chart and laboratory requisition. Completing the documentation and requisition as soon as possible after the procedure improves accuracy.

DOCUMENTATION

11/13/XX 2:54 PM Venipuncture performed right arm for CBC and sed rate. Specimen sent to Inner City Lab. Identification #987654321. Patient tolerated the procedure well and will call back tomorrow for the test results. Joe Guerrero, CMA

Procedure 28-5 Capillary Puncture

STANDARD PRECAUTIONS:

PURPOSE:
To obtain capillary blood acceptable for laboratory testing as required by a physician.

SPECIMEN:
Capillary blood collected by finger puncture. Volume of blood dependent on size of microcollection devices and test requirements.

EQUIPMENT/SUPPLIES:
Gloves
Goggles and mask, if necessary
70% isopropyl alcohol swab or pad
Microcollection tubes or capillary tubes
Safety lancet
Gauze
Adhesive bandage or tape
Sharps container
Cotton balls
Biohazard red bag

PROCEDURE STEPS:

1. Assemble the supplies. RATIONALE: Organizing the supplies before the procedure assures a more timely and professional test.
2. Identify the patient, introduce yourself, explain the procedure, and recheck the physician's orders. RATIONALE: Introducing yourself and explaining the procedure will establish a professional relationship with the patient and might help put him or her at ease. Identifying the patient and rechecking the physician's orders will assure the proper tests will be performed on the right patient.
3. Wash hands and apply gloves. RATIONALE: Washing your hands protects the patient, and applying gloves protects you.
4. Assemble the equipment and supplies. RATIONALE: Assembling the equipment assures a smoother, more organized procedure.
5. Select the puncture site on the fleshy part of the ring or middle finger, avoiding the very tip and the sides. RATIONALE: The ring and middle fingers generally will have less calluses and scarring. The tip and sides are more sensitive than the fleshy part.
6. Have the patient wash his or her hands in very warm water; if necessary, apply a warming pack to the fingertip, encourage the patient to relax, and provide a comfortable, professional atmosphere. RATIONALE: The patient washing his or her hands in very warm water provides two benefits: his or her hands will be cleaner and warmer, which encourages better blood to the area. Appling a warming pack to the fingertips will further encourage blood flow. A relaxed patient in a comfortable, professional atmosphere is more likely to provide a better sample.
7. Clean the selected puncture site with alcohol and allow it to air-dry or dry it with a gauze pad. RATIONALE: Alcohol will remove any residue soap or debris. Allowing the alcohol to dry will prevent irritation and stinging. If the site is wiped dry, the irritation of the gauze pad will further encourage blood to the area.
8. Holding the distal phalange firmly, perform the puncture across the lines of the fingerprint rather than along the lines. RATIONALE: Holding the distal phalange firmly will add support to the finger and prevent the patient from pulling back on the finger during the puncture. Puncturing across the fingerprint will assist the blood to form a drop rather than flow across the fingertip.
9. Using a gauze pad, wipe away the first drop. RATIONALE: The first drop usually contains contamination from the alcohol and tissue fluid and would not be a good representation of the blood sample needed. Using gauze rather than cotton to wipe it away lessens the likelihood of it clotting too quickly.
10. Collect the specimen according to the test being performed (see Chapter 29 for hemoglobin and hematocrit; see Chapter 32 for PKU, glucose, and other specialty tests performed on capillary blood).
11. Check the patient. He or she should hold firm, direct pressure on the site for at least two minutes. If the bleeding has stopped, an adhesive

(continues)

Procedure 28-5 (continued)

strip may be applied. If the bleeding has not stopped yet, hold firm, direct pressure on the site for another five minutes and then recheck. Adhesive strips are not recommended for patients younger than 2 years. RATIONALE: The bleeding should be stopped before the patient leaves your care. Adhesive strips for children younger than 2 years are not recommended because they are a choking hazard.

12. Disinfect the area and equipment, remove your gloves, and dispose of them into a biohazard waste container. Wash hands. RATIONALE: Biohazard waste should be controlled for everyone's protection. Hand washing after removing gloves further protects you.
13. Record the procedure and complete the laboratory requisition or test. The laboratory requisition is completed in the presence of the patient if possible. RATIONALE: Documentation is critical for good patient records. Completing the laboratory requisition in the presence of the patient provides accurate insurance and personal information if needed for the insurance forms and for your medical records.

DOCUMENTATION

4/27/XX 8:15 AM Capillary puncture performed left ring finger for Hgb A1c. Patient tolerated the procedure well. Dr. Lewis is scheduled to see the patient today to discuss progress. Joe Guerrero, CMA

Procedure 28-6 Obtaining a Capillary Specimen for Transport Using a Microtainer Transport Unit

STANDARD PRECAUTIONS:

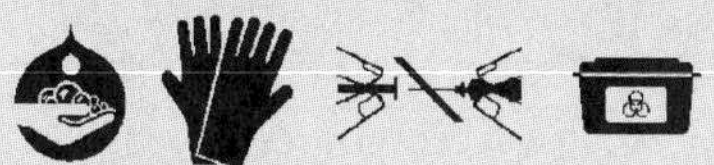

PURPOSE:

To obtain a specimen of capillary blood for transport to a laboratory for testing, using a Microtainer.

SPECIMEN:

Capillary blood collected by fingerstick method. Volume of specimen sufficient to fill the Microtainer to the fill line.

EQUIPMENT/SUPPLIES:

Capillary puncture supplies:
- Gloves
- Alcohol swab
- Gauze
- Safety lancet
- Cotton balls
- Adhesive bandage
- Sharps container and biohazard waste receptacle

Microtainer transport unit
Laboratory requisition

(continues)

Procedure 28-6 (continued)

Small sturdy container with a tightly fitting lid (such as a urine specimen cup)
Pen
Biohazard specimen transport bag

PROCEDURE STEPS:

1. Determine the appropriateness of submitting a capillary specimen for the specific test you are performing. RATIONALE: Not all tests can be performed on capillary specimens.
2. Assemble the supplies. RATIONALE: Organizing the supplies before the procedure assures a more timely and professional test.
3. Identify the patient, introduce yourself, explain the procedure, and recheck the physician's orders. RATIONALE: Introducing yourself and explaining the procedure will establish a professional relationship with the patient and might help put him or her at ease. Identifying the patient and rechecking the physician's orders will assure the proper tests will be performed on the right patient.
4. Wash hands, apply gloves, and perform the capillary puncture according to Procedure 28-5. RATIONALE: Washing your hands protects the patient, and applying gloves protects you.
5. Discard the first drop of blood. Wipe it away with a gauze square. RATIONALE: The first drop can contain mostly alcohol residue and tissue fluid and would not be a good representation of the blood sample needed. Using gauze rather than cotton to wipe it away lessens the likelihood of it clotting too quickly.
6. Allow a good size drop to form. RATIONALE: Allowing a good size drop to form is a good idea with any capillary specimen; the blood is more likely to stay in a drop and not flow over the finger.
7. Scoop the drop into the Microtainer (Figure 28-31A). RATIONALE: This is the method used to get the specimen into the tip of the Microtainer.
8. Tip the Microtainer, allowing the drop to slide into the tube (Figure 28-31B). RATIONALE: As soon as a drop is obtained on the scoop it should be moved into the tube where it can mix with the additive.
9. Gently agitate the tube. RATIONALE: Agitating the tube allows the additive to mix with the blood.
10. Continue collection of blood until the tube is filled (Figure 28-31C). RATIONALE: The tube must be filled to the fill line to ensure the proper ratio of blood to additive.
11. Provide the patient with a cotton ball and ask him or her to hold pressure on the puncture site. RATIONALE: The pressure with a cotton ball will encourage the wound to clot.
12. Remove the scoop from the Microtainer and discard the scoop into the sharps container (Figure 28-31D). RATIONALE: The scoop is contaminated with blood and therefore is considered to be biohazard waste. Being hard plastic, it is capable of scratching someone, so the sharps container is safer than the red bag waste receptacle.
13. Remove the colored cap from the back of the Microtainer and place it securely onto the opening. RATIONALE: Placing the cap securely onto the Microtainer will ensure the specimen will stay in the Microtainer during handling and transport.
14. Place the capped Microtainer into a small sturdy container with a tight-fitting lid. RATIONALE: Placing the Microtainer in another container protects it from being uncapped and (because of its small size) lost in transport. The Microtainer is also not large enough for adequate labeling.
15. Label the container. RATIONALE: Proper labeling assure the proper tests on the right specimen.
16. Fill out the laboratory requisition while the patient is present. RATIONALE: Any questions

(continues)

Procedure 28-6 (continued)

about the patient's address and insurance can be answered immediately if the patient is present while you complete the form.

17. Check the patient's puncture site. If bleeding has stopped, apply an adhesive strip, answer any questions the patient has, and release the patient. RATIONALE: Caring for the patient both physically and emotionally shows a professional dedication to your job.
18. Document the procedure in the patient's chart/medical record. RATIONALE: Documentation assure that the proper information is recorded into the patient's chart/medical record.

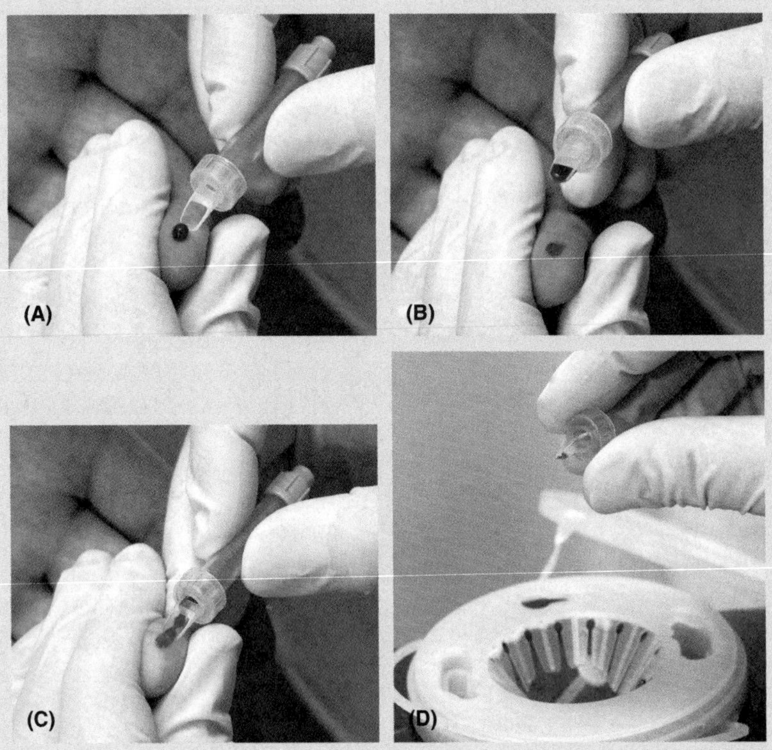

Figure 28-31 Collecting a capillary specimen for transport. (A) Allow drop to form. Touch the scoop on Microtainer to the blood drop. (B) Tip the Microtainer up so the blood flows in to the tube. Agitate it gently to mix the anticoagulant with the blood. (C) Continue gathering blood until the tube is filled to the marked level. (D) Remove the scoop from the Microtainer and dispose of the scoop into the sharps container.

DOCUMENTATION

3/3/XX 4:15 PM Capillary puncture was performed for a CBC. Specimen (Microtainer) sent to Inner City Laboratory. Patient tolerated the procedure well and will call in on Friday (3/6/XX) for the results. No return appointment scheduled. W. Slawson, CMA

Case Study 28-1

Inner City Health Care is short-staffed today, and medical assistant Liz Corbin is feeling pressed for time. She has many tasks to complete, but first she must perform a venipuncture. She greets the patient, Wayne Elder, in a perfunctory manner, discouraging time-wasting conversation. Although Wayne appears apprehensive, he is not resistant, so Liz quickly assembles the necessary supplies, applies the tourniquet, and inserts the needle. While she is drawing his blood, Wayne faints.

CASE STUDY REVIEW

1. What should Liz do now?
2. What could Liz have done to prevent this situation from occurring?
3. In the future, what are some steps Liz can take to provide a positive experience for venipuncture patients?

SUMMARY

With a little practice, the medical assistant will become an expert at phlebotomy. The skills of phlebotomy cannot be learned primarily from a textbook; continuous practice will develop the skill to perfection. It may take months before the medical assistant feels comfortable and is able to obtain a sample without difficulty.

In all phlebotomy, safety is of the utmost consideration. Dispose of all sharps properly and separately from the noncontaminated trash. Proper hand cleansing between patients and wearing gloves, goggles, and masks with each phlebotomy will assure safety for both the patient and the medical assistant.

Proper specimen collection and handling of the specimen after collection by the medical assistant will assure that the patient obtains the most accurate result. The specimen must be treated in such a way that the integrity of the specimen is maintained. The quality of the sample must be the same when collected as when tested. Correct method of draw, order of draw, and the correct handling of the sample after collection will reduce the number of factors affecting the sample and give the most accurate result possible.

STUDY FOR SUCCESS

To reinforce your knowledge and skills of information presented in this chapter:

- ❑ Review the Key Terms
- ❑ Practice the Procedures
- ❑ Consider the Case Study and discuss your conclusions
- ❑ Answer the Review Questions
  - ❑ Multiple Choice
  - ❑ Critical Thinking
- ❑ Navigate the Internet by completing the Web Activities
- ❑ Practice the StudyWARE activities on the CD
- ❑ Apply your knowledge in the Student Workbook activities
- ❑ Complete the Web Tutor sections
- ❑ View and discuss the DVD situations

REVIEW QUESTIONS

Multiple Choice

1. Drawing blood with a 25-gauge needle increases the chance for:
   a. vein collapse
   b. hematomas
   c. hemoconcentration
   d. hemolysis
2. An anticoagulant is an additive placed in vacuum tubes to:
   a. dilute the blood before testing
   b. ensure the sterility of the tube
   c. make the blood clot faster
   d. prevent the blood from clotting
3. When collecting a blood sample with a vacuum tube system, the last tube drawn is withdrawn from the holder before removing the needle from the patient to:
   a. avoid hematoma at the venipuncture site
   b. avoid dripping blood out the end of the needle
   c. prevent clotting of the blood
   d. cause the blood to clot
4. Leaving the tourniquet on a patient's arm for an extended length of time before drawing blood may cause:
   a. hemoconcentration
   b. specimen hemolysis
   c. stress
   d. bruising
5. The single most important way to prevent the spread of infection from patient to patient is:
   a. gowning and gloving
   b. hand washing
   c. always wearing masks
   d. avoid breathing on clients
6. Under Standard Precautions, all used needles are to be disposed of in the following manner:
   a. recapped
   b. discarded intact in a sharps container
   c. bent
   d. broken or cut off
7. When drawing multiple specimens in vacuum tubes, it is important to fill which of the following color-stoppered tubes first?
   a. light blue
   b. green
   c. lavender
   d. red
8. The anticoagulant of choice when drawing coagulation studies such as PT and APTT is:
   a. (red) no anticoagulant
   b. (light blue) sodium citrate
   c. (lavender) EDTA
   d. (green) heparin
9. When the medical assistant cannot perform a venipuncture successfully after two attempts, the medical assistant should:
   a. try at least two more times
   b. notify the physician
   c. ask another medical assistant to try
   d. request the test for the next day
10. If the blood is drawn too quickly from a small vein, the vein has a tendency to:
    a. collapse
    b. bruise
    c. disintegrate
    d. roll
11. What is OSHA's policy about choosing the safest needle systems to prevent accidental needlestick injuries?
    a. The clinic administrators can choose whatever is most cost effective.
    b. The clinic administrators should carefully choose the safest system for their staff.
    c. The clinic administrators must select the safest equipment based on feedback from the people who are using the needles.
    d. OSHA is not interfering with the clinics' rights to use any system they choose.

Critical Thinking

1. A frightened patient begins crying when you enter the room to perform a venipuncture. How will you handle the situation? What is your responsibility to the patient? Why are your demeanor and appearance important in this type of situation?
2. Explain the difference between serum and plasma. Describe how serum and plasma samples are collected.
3. How can vein collapse be avoided on a geriatric patient?
4. Discuss how clots are formed and what can be done to stop the clotting process.
5. You have calmed the crying patient and successfully drawn the patient's blood. What will you do next? Why is this step important? Describe the skills you have used.
6. The patient cries out in pain when you insert the needle into the vein. What will you do to make the patient more comfortable? If you decide to try another site, how will you locate it?

WEB ACTIVITIES

1. Visit the CDC and other government Web sites for the most current information on Standard Precautions and proper protection during blood draws.
2. Search the keywords "phlebotomy" and "puncture" on the Web. What organizations can you find that offer information for medical assistants?
3. Search the Internet for the laws in your state governing phlebotomy training.

REFERENCES/BIBLIOGRAPHY

Walters, N. J., Estridge, B. H., & Reynold, A. P. (2000). *Basic medical laboratory techniques* (4th ed.). Clifton Park, NY: Thomson Delmar Learning.

Wedding, M. E., & Toenjes, S. A. (1998). *Medical laboratory procedures* (2nd ed.). Philadelphia: FA Davis.

THE DVD HOOK-UP

DVD Series	Program Number
Skills Based Series	**11**

Chapter/Scene Reference
- *Administer Venipuncture, Vacuum Tube, and Syringe Method*
- *Preparing Slides for a Differential*
- *Administering Capillary Puncture and Performing Hematocrit Testing*

This chapter discusses the various techniques for obtaining blood specimens from patients.

Today's designated scenes illustrate three various methods that are used to collect blood samples. The first method was the vacuum tube system. There was a special order for filling the blood tubes. The order of draw was slightly different between the DVD program and the text in this chapter. This is because both projects were written at different time intervals and the tube order changed between the projects. The information in this chapter has the latest information for the correct order of draw.

1. What is the order of draw according to this chapter? Does the order change when using a syringe? How about the capillary method? What will you do to make certain that you stay up to date with the latest information regarding tube orders and other important laboratory information once you graduate?
2. This chapter states that you should label the tubes immediately after the blood draw, but the DVD program states that you should label the tube before drawing the blood. Which technique does your instructor want you to follow?
3. Why is it important to determine if the patient followed all the fasting instructions before taking the patient's blood?

DVD Journal Summary

Write a paragraph that summarizes what you learned from watching the selected scenes from today's DVD program. Lori, the medical assistant, spoke about a patient who had a syncope episode while performing a phlebotomy. The patient fell back hitting his head on the floor, and he immediately went into convulsions. The convulsions eventually stopped and the patient underwent X-rays. Fortunately, the patient had no damage as a result of the fall. How will you ascertain that your patients are safe during and after a blood draw? What are some signs that could indicate that the patient may faint? How would you feel if the patient did injure himself or herself while under your care?

CHAPTER 29

Hematology

OUTLINE

OBJECTIVES

The student should strive to meet the following performance objectives and demonstrate an understanding of the facts and principles presented in this chapter through written and oral communication.

1. Define the key terms as presented in the glossary.
2. Describe the process of hematopoiesis.
3. Discuss how the clinical science of hematology and the complete blood count (CBC) are used in the diagnosis and treatment of disease.
4. Compare the normal versus abnormal values of the CBC parameters.
5. Describe which blood tests and methods are within the scope of the medical assistant performing under a CLIA Waived Test Certificate.
6. Discuss how the hemoglobin and hematocrit are used to diagnose anemia.
7. Describe how the erythrocyte indices are used in the differential diagnosis of anemias.
8. Perform the calculations necessary to derive the erythrocyte indices mean corpuscular cell volume, mean corpuscular hemoglobin, and mean corpuscular hemoglobin concentration.
9. List the five types of normal white blood cells and give the identifying characteristics of each.

(continues)

KEY TERMS

Anisocytosis
Basophil
Complete Blood Count (CBC)
Eosinophil
Erythrocyte
Erythrocyte Indices
Erythrocyte Sedimentation Rate
Erythropoietin
Hematocrit
Hematology
Hematopoiesis
Hemoglobin
Hemoglobinopathy
Hypochromic
Leukocyte
Lymphocyte
Macrocytic
Microcytic
Monocyte
Neutrophil
Normochromic
Normocytic
Thrombocyte

FEATURED COMPETENCIES

CAAHEP—ENTRY-LEVEL COMPETENCIES

Clinical Competencies

Fundamental Procedures

- Perform handwashing
- Dispose of biohazard materials
- Practice Standard Precautions

Specimen Collection

- Perform capillary puncture

Diagnostic Testing

- Perform hematology testing

General Competencies

Legal Concepts

- Identify and respond to issues of confidentiality
- Perform within legal and ethical boundaries
- Establish and maintain the medical record
- Document appropriately
- Demonstrate knowledge of federal and state health care legislation and regulations

Operational Functions

- Use methods of quality control

ABHES—ENTRY-LEVEL COMPETENCIES

Clinical Duties

- Apply principles of aseptic techniques and infection control
- Use quality control
- Collect and process specimens
- Perform selected tests that assist with diagnosis and treatment

(continues)

OBJECTIVES (continued)

10. Describe the differences in the procedures for the Wintrobe and Westergren erythrocyte sedimentation rates.
11. Recognize the physiologic reasons why the erythrocyte sedimentation rate varies with different states of health and disease.
12. List the two general types of automated hematology instruments used in the ambulatory care setting and describe their technology.
13. Perform the laboratory procedures included in this chapter in a manner acceptable for entry-level employment.

SCENARIO

The physicians in the office of Drs. Lewis and King often order hematologic tests to assist them in diagnosing and treating patients. As she performs the tests in the physician's office laboratory, medical assistant Audrey Jones uses her knowledge of hematology every day. Audrey is comfortable using an automated hematology analyzer or performing tests manually because she understands the purposes and procedures of the tests. She always follows all safety and quality-control guidelines to protect herself and others and to ensure the accuracy of test results.

FEATURED COMPETENCIES (continued)

- Dispose of biohazard materials
- Practice Standard Precautions
- Perform hematology

Legal Concepts

- Document Accurately

INTRODUCTION

Hematology *is the study of the blood cells and coagulation in both normal and diseased states. The two main components of the blood are plasma (the liquid portion) and cells. Cells of the blood are also known as the formed elements of the blood. The study of hematology is usually limited to the cellular components of the blood and does not include the chemistry of the blood. See Chapter 32 for the chemistry of blood and test related to blood chemistry.*

The cellular components of blood include ***erythrocytes*** *(red blood cells [RBCs]),* ***leukocytes*** *(white blood cells [WBCs]), and* ***thrombocytes*** *(platelets). Blood has many different functions. RBCs are responsible for supplying oxygen to all the cells of the body and removing the waste products of the cells: carbon dioxide. WBCs are involved in fighting infection, as well as producing antibodies for the immune system to defend against foreign antigens. There are five basic types of WBCs and they all have specific disease-fighting functions. Platelets are involved in homeostasis, the control of bleeding. Figure 28-2 shows the cellular elements of blood.*

Hematopoiesis *is defined as the formation of blood cells (Figure 29-1). The process of hematopoiesis, as well as the blood-forming tissues of the body, is included in the study of hematology. In the embryo, hematopoiesis occurs in the yolk sac, liver, and spleen. After we are born, the primary site for the production of erythrocytes, granulocytes, and platelets is the bone marrow. Lymphocytes are also produced in the bone marrow, as well as in the lymph nodes. At birth, most of the bone marrow in the body is capable of producing blood cells. This process is confined to the bone marrow of the ribs, vertebrae, sternum, and iliac crest by the age of 20 years. Bone marrow that is producing cells is known as red marrow. As the area for hematopoiesis is reduced, the red bone marrow is replaced by yellow marrow, which is stored fat. When a physician collects a bone marrow sample in an adult, the site chosen for sampling is the sternum or the iliac crest because this is where the blood cells are still being produced.*

Spotlight on Certification

RMA Content Outline
- Asepsis
- Laboratory procedures

CMA Content Outline
- Principles of infection control
- Processing specimens
- Quality control
- Performing selected tests

CMAS Content Outline
- Asepsis in the medical office

Critical Thinking

What do you think would happen if you did not have any leukocytes? What would your symptoms be?

HEMATOLOGIC TESTS

Hematologic tests are the second most common tests performed in the physicians' office laboratory (POL). The most common test is the urinalysis. The cellular components of the blood may be affected by changes in either the blood-forming organs or in other tissues of the body. The study of these changes forms the basis of hematologic tests performed in the POL.

Hematologic tests performed in the clinical laboratory include:

- Hemoglobin
- Hematocrit
- WBC count
- Differential WBC count
- RBC count
- RBC indices
- Platelet count
- Erythrocyte sedimentation rate (ESR)
- Prothrombin time (PT)

The results of these hematologic tests provide valuable information used by the physician in making a

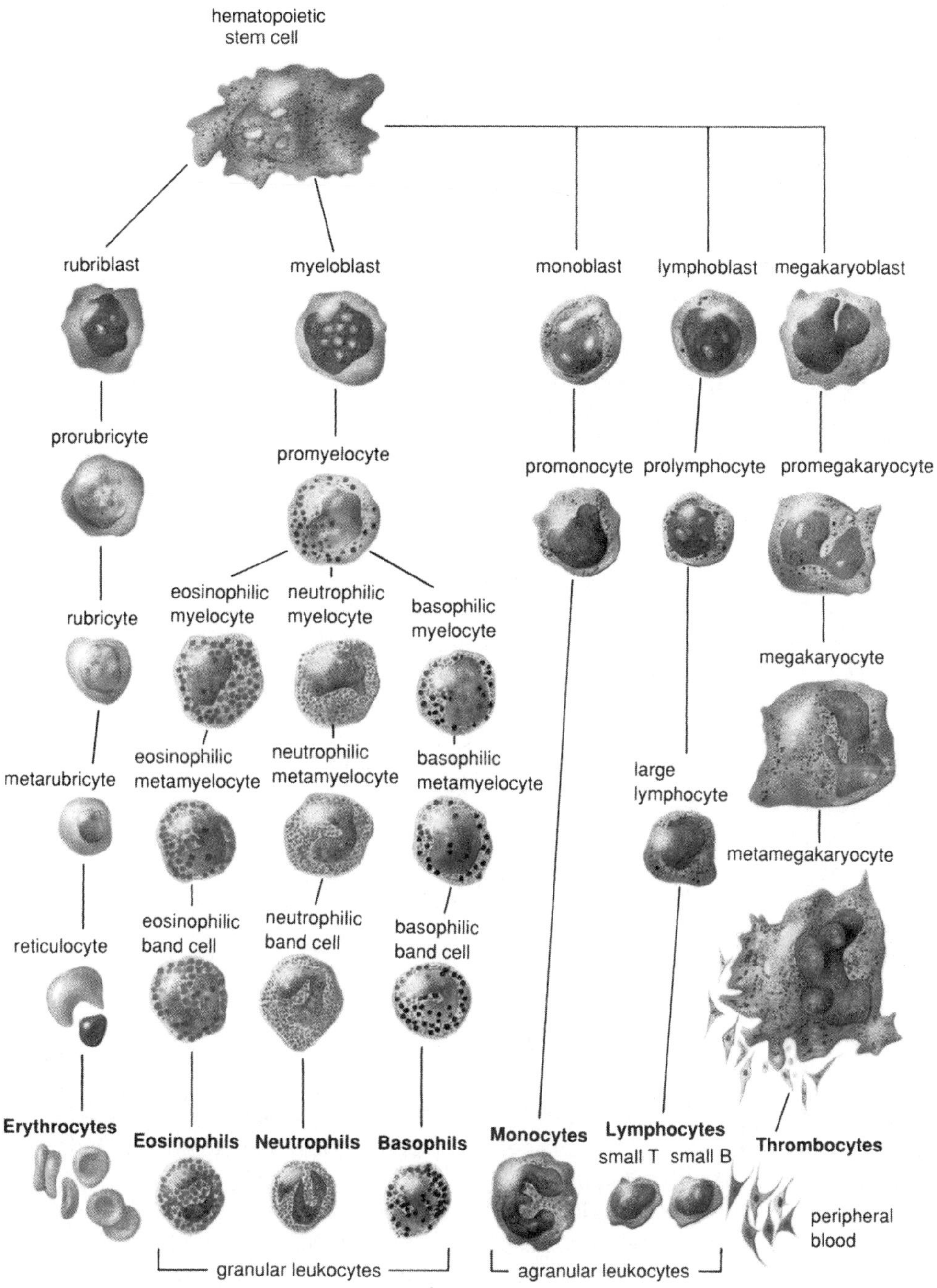

Figure 29-1 Hematopoiesis showing blood cells and platelet formation starting with hematopoietic stem cell.

diagnosis, evaluating a patient's progress, and regulating further treatment.

The laboratory test ordered most frequently on blood in the ambulatory care setting is the **complete blood count (CBC).** The exact number of parameters included in the CBC will vary from laboratory to laboratory (Figure 29-2). The CBC generally includes:

- Hemoglobin determination
- Hematocrit determination
- RBC count
- WBC count
- Erythrocyte indices (often included in CBC)
- Differential WBC count

All these tests can be performed by manual testing procedures or with an automated hematology analyzer. Manual blood cell counts are considered by the Clinical

Pat Name: Page: 1
Unit #/Acct #:
Loc:
Phys-Service:

****

In: 11/12/XX 0843
Out: 11/12/XX 1002
Coll Time: 11/12/XX 0840
Order Phys:

| CBC WITH DIFFERENTIAL |

Spec: Blood
Techs: V185 T180*
[A9331600017/4590]

Result Name	Result	Reference Range
WBC(10*3/ul):	7.4	4.8-10.8
RBC(10*6/ul):	4.51	4.2-5.4
Hgb(gm/dl):	12.8	12.0-16.0
Hct(%):	37.9	37.0-47.0
MCV(fl):	84.1	81.0-99.0
MCH(pg):	28.4	27.0-31.0
MCHC(gm/dl):	33.8	32.0-36.0
RDW(%):	13.6	11.5-14.5
Plt Cnt(X(10)3):	303	130-450
Neutrophil(%):	62.0	43-75
Lymph(%):	29.7	20-51
Mono (%):	5.9	2-11
Eos(%):	2.0	0-7.5
Basos(%):	0.4	0-2
Neutrophil(X(10)3):	4.7	1.5-6.6
Lymph (X(10)3):	2.2	1.5-3.5
Mono(X(10)3):	0.4	0-1.0
Eos (X(10)3):	0.1	0-0.7
Baso(X(10)3):	0.0	0-0.1

End of Report - 03/09/XX 15:34

Single Test Report-HEMATOLOGY

Figure 29-2 Hematology report form.

Laboratory Improvement Act (CLIA) to be of moderate to high complexity; whereas the automated tests are considered to be moderately complex; therefore, neither are within the medical assistant's scope of practice. The manual blood cell counts are performed only at reference laboratories by medical technicians. The automated analyzers may be located in the POL, but the testing and interpretation of the tests, the maintenance of the analyzers, as well as training and supervision of laboratory personnel is performed by the medical technician.

HEMOGLOBIN AND HEMATOCRIT TESTS

Hemoglobin and **hematocrit** tests are part of the CBC, however, they are frequently individually ordered by the physician rather than a CBC. The abbreviations for hemoglobin and hematocrit are Hgb and Hct, respectively. Although they are separate tests, they have a unique relationship with each other but may be performed individually. Both the hemoglobin and the hematocrit are performed to obtain similar information about RBCs in relation to the rest of the blood sample, but they also give decidedly different information. In normal results, the hemoglobin often will be about one third the number of the hematocrit.

Hemoglobin is the major component of the RBC and serves to transport oxygen and carbon dioxide through the body. Hemoglobin, which is responsible for about 85% of the dry weight of the RBC, is a conjugated protein composed of heme and globin. A single hemoglobin molecule consists of four globin chains with a heme group attached to each globin (Figure 29-3). The central component of each heme group is an iron molecule. One oxygen molecule can be transported to each heme group; therefore, each RBC can carry four oxygen molecules.

Synthesis of the heme portion of the hemoglobin molecule requires iron, which is usually obtained though our diets. The daily iron requirement for an adult man is

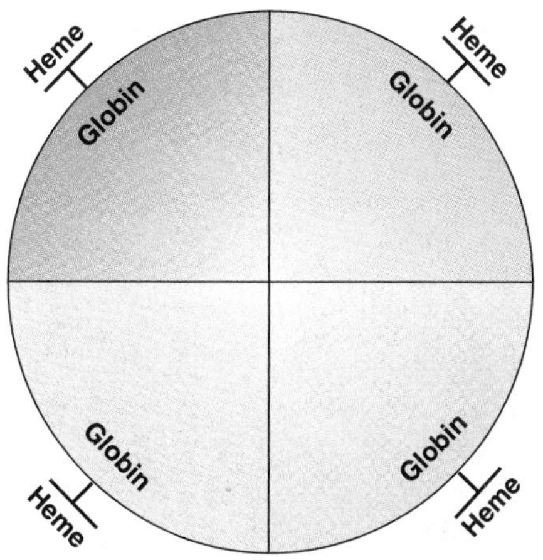

Figure 29-3 A normal hemoglobin molecule containing four globin chains with a heme group attached to each globin. One oxygen molecule can be transported by each heme group.

about 0.5 mg/day, whereas a menstruating woman requires about four times that much, or 2 mg/day.

Hemoglobin carries about 95% of the oxygen to the body cells and carries away about 27% of the carbon dioxide. The RBCs pick up the oxygen in the lungs from when we breathe in, and they drop off the carbon dioxide in the lungs to be expelled when we breathe out. The rest of the carbon dioxide is removed through other processes. Oxygenated hemoglobin is bright red, and hemoglobin unbound to oxygen is darker. This explains the bright red color of arterial blood (going from the lungs and to the cells) and the darker color of venous blood (going back to the lungs).

A second function of hemoglobin is as a blood buffer; that is, hemoglobin helps maintain the proper pH balance of the blood as it picks up and drops off oxygen and carbon dioxide.

The production of new RBCs and consequently the formation of new hemoglobin is triggered by a hormone called **erythropoietin,** which is produced in the kidney. The erythropoietin process is activated when the body cells sense a low oxygen level.

There are several forms of hemoglobin. Hemoglobin A (Hgb A) is the most common form found in adults. The other hemoglobin types are abnormal and are responsible for a group of diseases known as **hemoglobinopathies.** These abnormal forms of hemoglobin include hemoglobin S (Hgb S), hemoglobin C, and hemoglobin E. Hgb S is the most common abnormal form of hemoglobin observed in the laboratory. It is the form of hemoglobin that causes sickle cell anemia. When Hgb S molecules are subjected to certain conditions, they alter the physical structure of the RBCs. The RBCs assume a sickle shape, which makes it difficult, if not impossible, for the cell to pass through a capillary bed.

The most frequent hemoglobin disease seen in the ambulatory care setting is anemia, with iron deficiency anemia being the most common type. A decrease of available iron in the body is the most common cause of this type of anemia. Lack of available iron can be caused by insufficient intake through the diet (called nutritional anemia); losing iron because of a bleeding problem (called hemorrhagic anemia); or less common, congenital defects, industrial toxins, diseases of bone marrow (aplastic anemia), and a variety of other disorders. In nutritional anemia, the laboratory finding will usually show a normal or near-normal hematocrit (because these patients will have the right percentage of RBCs) but a low hemoglobin. Their RBCs will be hypochromic (pale) because they lack oxygen. The main symptom of anemia, fatigue, is also caused by lack of oxygen.

Hemoglobin is measured in the POL using an automated device called the HemoCue (see Figure 29-6). The HemoCue is an infrared analyzer that measures the density of the hemoglobin pigment by light refraction. The more hemoglobin present in the sample, the more light is refracted. This is a quick method, uses only a small drop of blood, and gives immediate results (see Procedure 29-1).

CAUTION: The solution within the HemoCue is poisonous. Precautions to observe when working with any reagents includes wearing gloves, working in a well-ventilated area, properly disposing of used reagents, wiping up all spills, and hand washing.

The normal reference values for hemoglobin vary according to both the age and sex of the individual (Table 29-1).

The hematocrit (packed RBC volume) is the ratio of the volume of packed RBCs to that of the whole-blood specimen. Packed RBC volume is expressed as a percentage of the whole specimen. This is achieved manually or by automated methods. Most medical assistants working in ambulatory care settings use the manual microhematocrit method (see Procedure 29-2) It requires only a few drops of blood either directly into a microhematocrit tube obtained by capillary draw, or the sample can be taken from a vacuum tube containing ethylenediaminetetraacetic acid

TABLE 29-1 NORMAL HEMOGLOBIN VALUES OR REFERENCE RANGES BY AGE AND/OR SEX

Newborn	15–20 g/dl
Age three months	9–14 g/dl
Age ten months	12–14.5 g/dl
Adult woman	12–16 g/dl
Adult man	13–18 g/dl

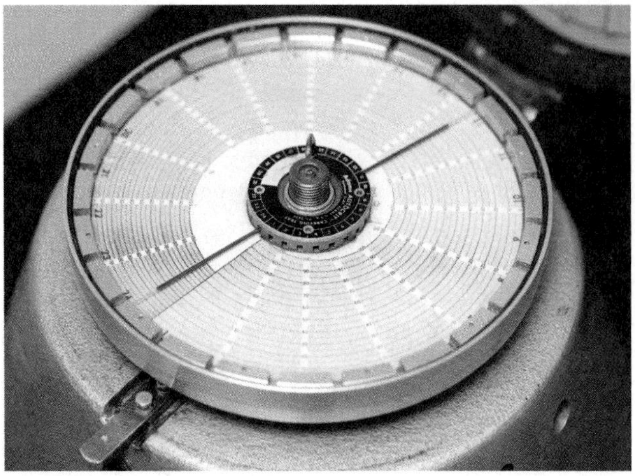

Figure 29-4 Microhematocrit centrifuge.

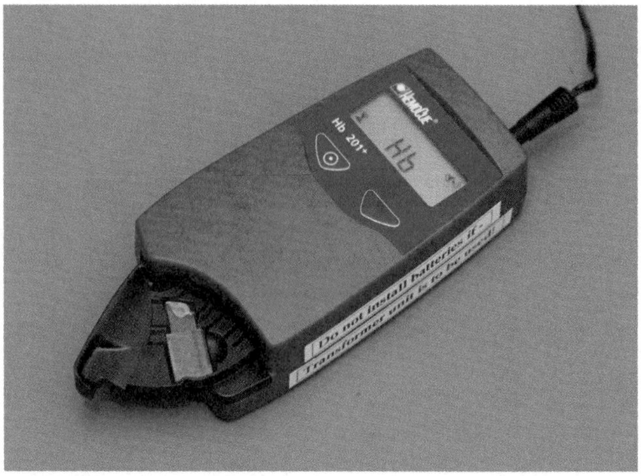

Figure 29-6 HemoCue instrument used for automated test.

(EDTA) after a venipuncture. Chapter 28 explains both capillary draw and venipuncture.

The cellular components of the blood sample separate into layers when they are centrifuged at high speeds (Figures 29-4 and 29-5). The cellular layers arrange themselves with the RBCs at the bottom of the tube. RBCs are the most numerous and the heaviest of the cellular components. WBCs and platelets form a thin layer called the buffy coat on top of the erythrocytes. The buffy coat has a whitish tan appearance. The plasma often is so clear it is difficult to see.

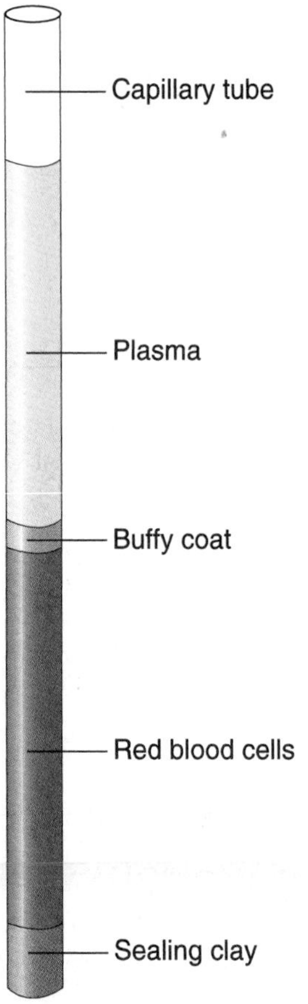

Figure 29-5 Diagram of packed cell column in the hematocrit tube showing separation of cellular components after centrifugation.

The WBC count of the sample can be estimated by measuring the buffy coat thickness. Each 0.1 mm of the buffy coat equals approximately 1,000 WBC/mm^3. Therefore, a buffy coat of 1 mm would equal a leukocyte count of approximately 10,000 WBCs/mm^3, and a 0.5 mm reading would equal 5,000 WBCs/mm^3. The cell counts may be reported in units of microliters (μl), which are equivalent to cubic millimeters.

The normal values of hematocrit will vary according to the age and sex of the individual (Table 29-2).

Sources of error associated with the microhematocrit method include improper centrifugation, resulting in increased trapped plasma, and improper reading of the packed RBC volume, such as including the buffy coat layer.

Procedure 29-2 explains the microhematocrit method of determining blood hematocrit levels. Review Chapter 28 sections on capillary tubes and capillary draw together with Procedure 29-5.

TABLE 29-2 NORMAL HEMATOCRIT VALUES OR REFERENCE RANGES BY AGE AND/OR SEX

Newborn	45–60%
1-year-old child	27–44%
Adult female	36–46%
Adult male	40–55%

WHITE AND RED BLOOD CELL COUNTS

WBC and RBC counts can be performed using either a manual or automated method. Because neither method is considered CLIA waived, neither is within the scope of practice for the medical assistant. The Introduction discusses the functions of blood cells, and you will learn much more in your anatomy and physiology course. The formation of blood cells is shown in Figure 29-1. Because blood cell counts are not performed by medical assistants, this section does not discuss the test process itself but rather the diagnostic implications of the leukocyte count with the differential.

White Blood Cells and Differential

WBCs do not necessarily remain within the blood vessels like RBCs do. They leave the blood vessels and travel to the tissues of the body to find and destroy pathogens. When a "bacterial battle" is fought in an area and many WBCs have died, the "battlefield" may be too large for the body to clean up. In these cases, pus can occur. A localized accumulation of pus is called an abscess and often must be incised (lanced) to aid in the removal of the pus. Chapter 19 includes an incision and drainage surgery for the very purpose of incising and draining an abscess. Antibiotics are also useful in some cases to help the leukocytes fight off the bacteria and remove the infection. When leukocytes travel into the tissues, most of them do not return to the bloodstream. The lymphocyte is the only type that does; it travels to the lymphatic system where it is specialized and matured (hence, its name), then returns to the bloodstream to await a mission. The normal values for white blood cells vary with age. Babies need more, because they do not have antibody protections built up yet (see Table 29-3).

WBCs or leukocytes can be divided into two basic groups; granulocytes, which contain granules within their cytoplasm, and agranulocytes, which do not contain granules. The presence of granules can be visualized by the trained eye after a staining process during the manual WBC count. Even during the automated method, the leukocyte is identified by the contents of the cytoplasm and the shape of their nuclei. The granulocytes are the **neutrophils, basophils,** and **eosinophils** (notice they all end in *-phil,* which will help you remember their cytoplasm is "filled" with granules). The agranulocytes are the lymphocytes and the monocytes.

The nuclei of the leukocytes differ from each other, as well as the cytoplasm. All three of the granulocytes contain nuclei that are multilobed or segmented (sometimes they are even called segs). They are described as being polymorphonuclear cells (*poly* means "many," *morpho* means "shape," and *nuclear* means "nucleus"). The immature neutrophil has a nucleus that has not yet formed lobes and is called a band cell (or stab cell) because its nucleus looks sort of like a comma. The agranulocytes do not form lobed nuclei; their nuclei are rounded in a single mass. Because of their single nuclei, the aganulocytes are sometimes called mononuclear (meaning one nucleus). Because so many different names can be confusing, this chapter provides an identification guide and pictures for you (see Tables 29-4 and 29-5 and Figure 29-7).

Each of the five types provide specialized protection. Some of their methods include phagocytosis, detoxification, inflammation, and immune response.

Phagocytosis is an engulfing process performed by all leukocytes, but especially the neutrophils and the monocytes. Once the bacteria or particles are engulfed, the material is destroyed by enzymes present in the leukocyte. Phagocytosis is so important as a means of

TABLE 29-3 NORMAL LEUKOCYTE COUNTS

Leukocyte Count (cells/mm³)

Age	Average	Reference Range
Newborn	18,000	9,000–30,000
1-year-old toddler	11,000	6,000–14,000
6-year-old child	8,000	4,500–12,000
Adult	7,000	4,500–11,000

TABLE 29-4 NORMAL VALUES FOR A DIFFERENTIAL LEUKOCYTE COUNT IN ADULTS

Neutrophil Bands: 3–5%
Neutrophil bands increase in appendicitis and many other diseases.

Neutrophil Segs: 54–62%
Segmented neutrophils increase in appendicitis and many other diseases. An elevation in neutrophils usually is indicative of an infectious disease.

Lymphocytes: 25–33%
Lymphocytes increase with infectious mononucleosis, lymphocytic leukemia, and many diseases of viral origin.

Monocytes: 3–7%
Monocytes increase in tuberculosis and monocytic leukemia.

Eosinophils: 1–3%
Eosinophils increase with allergic reactions, hay fever, and parasitic infections.

Basophils: 0–1%
Basophils increase in polycythemia vera, chicken pox, and ulcerative colitis.

TABLE 29-5 LEUKOCYTE IDENTIFICATION GUIDE

Cell Types	Functions
Granulocytes	
Neutrophils Mature are segmented cells/segs Immature are bands or stabs	Phagocytosis of bacteria Destruction by enzymes
Eosinophils	Detoxification of toxins and harmful substances Neutralize histamine Destroy parasitic worms
Basophils	Mediate inflammation Release histamine to increase inflammation Release heparin to inhibit blood clotting
Agranulocytes	
Monocytes	Phagocytosis to clean up
Lymphocytes	Destruction of viruses Immune response

protection; we would die if our leukocytes lost their ability to perform this process.

Detoxification is a neutralizing process that is effective against poisons and other harmful substances. Eosinophils use detoxification to control allergic reactions and histamine production.

Inflammation is a general process that occurs as a sequence of events. Chapter 10 explains the inflammatory process in more detail. The leukocyte most actively involved in inflammation is the basophil, which releases histamine into injured tissue to increase inflammation (antihistamines work to reduce inflammation). Basophils also contain the anticoagulant heparin. The basophil synchronizes the entire inflammatory process, thus the poison is rendered harmless, the offending agents are eliminated, and the area is cleaned-up of all the necrotic tissue and is ready for repair.

Immune response is a series of complicated and involved specific antigen–antibody reactions. Simply stated, when a harmful substance enters the human body,

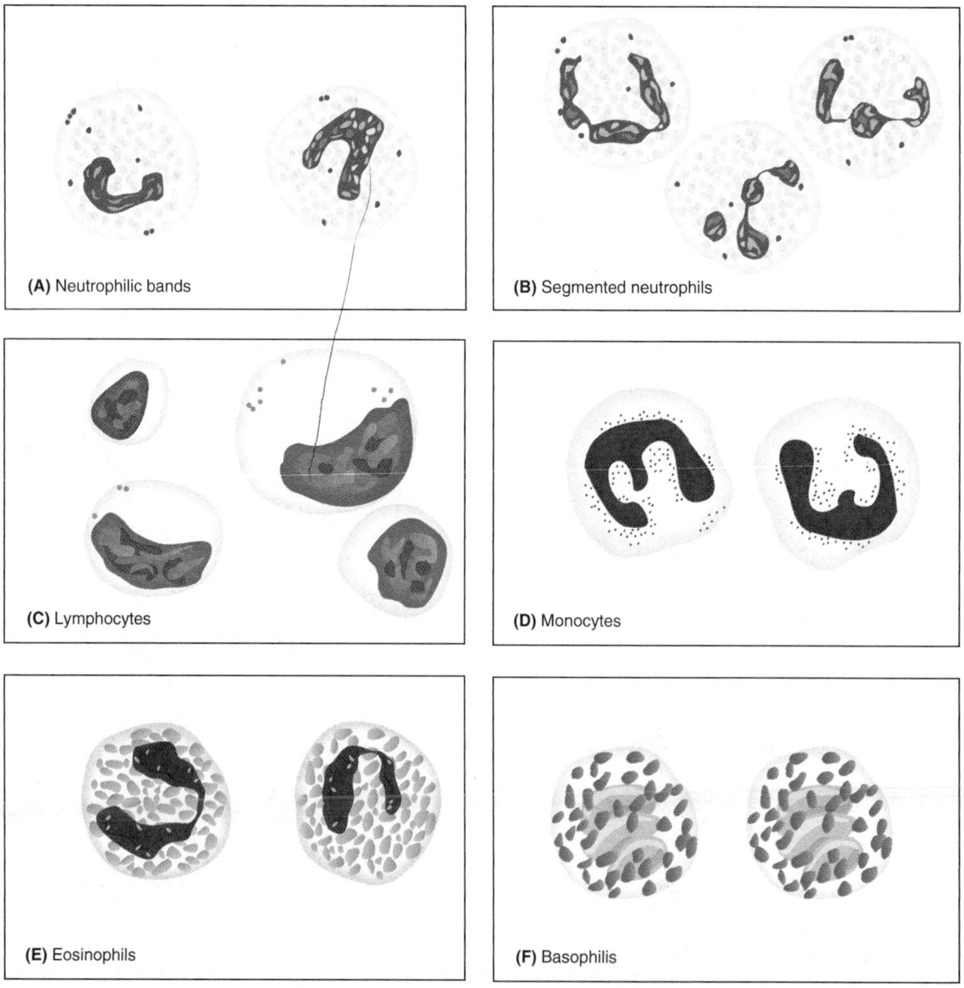

Figure 29-7 Various types of leukocytes from a stained blood smear.

the adaptive immune response provided by the lymphocyte destroys the harmful substance. A "memory" is created so the next time the body is exposed, it recognizes the intruder and is better able to avoid the illness again. This is called immunity. Immunity can be permanent or temporary, passively acquired or actively acquired. Passively acquired immunity is gifted to us either in utero (congenital or natural) or through an injection (artificial). Actively acquired immunity requires us to actively fight off a disease, and because we take active part in creating the immunity, it is usually permanent. Passively acquired immunities do not make us sick, but they usually do not last longer than six months, either.

Not only do the leukocytes fight off pathogens/toxins in a variety of ways, they also are fairly specific in the types of pathogens they do battle with (see Table 29-4). Neutrophils are our most numerous of all leukocytes and for good reason. They are there to destroy bacteria, which is our most common enemy. The second largest group is the lymphocytes, and they fight our second most common enemy: viruses. Lymphocytes are also involved in immune responses, which explains why we have immunity to viruses and not to other substances or microbes. Basophils release histamine to increase inflammation into injured tissues. Inflammation usually is our friend, but sometimes the inflammation is too severe.

This is what can happen in an allergic reaction. Eosinophils are especially well suited to battle the inflammation accompanying allergic-type reactions because they neutralize the histamines. Monocytes could be likened to the "cleanup crew" because these "big eaters" come in later to clean up the battlefield of the cellular debris and other substances.

Some examples of blood cell changes associated with disease states are:

1. When a patient is experiencing an acute appendicitis, the white blood cell count will increase rapidly with a high percentage of neutrophils. There will also be an increase in the number of early or younger forms of these cells.
2. Patients who are suffering from a virus infection, especially adults, will frequently experience a reduction in white blood cells and the percentage of lymphocytes will increase. Patients with infectious mononucleosis will have increased numbers of lymphocytes, many of which will be atypical.
3. When patients have iron deficiency anemia, their indices will demonstrate red blood cells that show marked reduction in hemoglobin content. Their erythrocytes will appear hypochromic, lacking or low in color, because they lack the normal amount of hemoglobin in the red blood cell.

TABLE 29-6 NORMAL ERYTHROCYTE COUNTS

Age	Reference Range
Newborn	$5.0–6.5 \times 10^6/mm^3$
1-year-old child	$4.0–5.0 \times 10^6/mm^3$
Adult woman	$4.0–5.5 \times 10^6/mm^3$
Adult man	$4.5–6.0 \times 10^6/mm^3$

Red Blood Cells

RBCs (erythrocytes) are very different from WBCs, in composition, function, and in numbers (See Table 29-6). Remember from the Introduction that erythrocytes are responsible for carrying oxygen to the body's cells and bringing back the carbon dioxide. To have room to carry the oxygen and carbon dioxide molecules, the erythrocyte leaves its nucleus in the bone marrow where it is formed. The nucleus is used again and again to create other erythrocytes. Our bodies are efficient at recycling our raw materials. If an erythrocyte is released from the bone marrow before it is mature, it may retain some of its nucleus material. It is then called a reticulocyte (retic). About 1% of the circulating erythrocytes are reticulocytes, but showing an increase in the number of circulating reticulocytes is an indication that the body needs more erythrocytes. This can occur in cases of hemorrhage and anemia. Erythrocytes can be of varying sizes also. When an erythrocyte is of normal size, it is called **normocytic.** Those that are larger are called **macrocytic,** and those that are smaller are called **microcytic.** When the erythrocytes show marked variation in size, this condition is called **anisocytosis.** The normal erythrocyte has a round or slightly oval shape. If the shape of the erythrocytes show marked variation, this is a condition known as poikilocytosis.

The RBC should contain hemoglobin that fills about half of the cell. The RBC is biconcave, so most of the hemoglobin is seen around the outer part of the cell. The central area of the RBC is pale. RBCs with the proper amount of hemoglobin are called **normochromic.** Those that do not have enough hemoglobin, that demonstrate too large of a pale central area, are called **hypochromic.**

PLATELETS

The normal number of platelets (thrombocytes) is 140,000 to 400,000/cm μl. Thrombocytes are actually fragments of cytoplasm. Like mature erythrocytes, thrombocytes have no nuclei. Thrombocytes are involved in the

Clinical Laboratory Improvement Amendment, 1988 (CLIA '88) Regulation Regarding WBC Differential Counts

- Laboratories that are certified for waiver-level testing only are not permitted to perform manual WBC differential counts.
- Laboratories with a moderate-complexity certification can perform a manual differential WBC count but may only identify and report normal cells.
- Laboratories certified to perform tests of high complexity can perform a manual differential WBC count and are permitted to identify and report both abnormal and normal cells.
- Laboratories with moderate to complex certification can perform automated WBC counts including the reporting of abnormal results. Only qualified medical technicians and higher personnel may use and maintain the machines.

See Chapter 26 for details on CLIA '88 regulations.

clotting of blood, or coagulation. Coagulation is a complex series of events that contains 13 distinct steps. A brief overview is provided here. When the body is physically injured, chemicals are released. Included in these chemicals are thromboplastin from injured tissues and plasma proteins and factors released from platelets. These chemicals form prothrombin activator. Prothrombin activator (with calcium) converts (activates) a blood protein called prothrombin into thrombin. Thrombin converts another blood protein called fibrinogen into fibrin. Fibrin is stringy and traps the sticky blood cells in a web at the site of injury, forming a plug of sorts. Eventually, the plug starts drying up, shrinks (pulling the edges of a wound together), and forms a scab.

What is really fascinating about the clotting of blood is why it does not normally clot inside the blood vessels. There are two chemicals made in the human body that prevent that from happening. One is heparin, which is released from basophils and endothelial cells, and the other chemical is antithrombin, which is released by the liver. The body needs blood to clot to stop bleeding, but it is important that it not clot inside the body where it can cause problems and even death.

ERYTHROCYTE INDICES

The **erythrocyte indices** include the mean corpuscular (cell) volume (MCV), the mean corpuscular hemoglobin (MCH), and the mean corpuscular hemoglobin concentration (MCHC). These indices (plural for index) are calculations that provide information about the size of the RBCs and the hemoglobin content. The blood parameters needed to calculate all three indices are the RBC count, the hematocrit, and the hemoglobin. The erythrocyte indices values are important in the diagnosis or classification and treatment of different types of anemia. Table 29-7 shows normal values for the erythrocyte indices.

TABLE 29-7 NORMAL VALUES FOR THE ERYTHROCYTE INDICES

MCV	80–100 fl
MCH	27–33 pg
MCHC	32–36 g/dl

Before the automated hematology instrument became commonly used in the ambulatory care setting, the erythrocyte indices were not included as a part of the CBC because the RBC count was not an accurate measurement.

The following formulas are used to calculate the erythrocyte indices:

$$\text{MCV} = \frac{\text{Hematocrit}}{\text{RBC (in millions)}} \times 10$$

The result is reported in femtoliters (fl), a unit of volume 10^{-15} L, formerly reported in cubic microns (μm^3). This index gives the average volume of an RBC in the sample.

$$\text{MCH} = \frac{\text{Hemoglobin (in grams)}}{\text{RBC (in millions)}} \times 10$$

The result is expressed in picograms (pg), a micro microgram, or 1×10^{-12} g. This index estimates the weight of hemoglobin in a RBC of the sample.

$$\text{MCHC} = \frac{\text{Hemoglobin (in grams)}}{\text{Hematocrit}} \times 10$$

This result is expressed in grams/deciliter (g/dl). The MCHC is the average concentration of hemoglobin in a given volume of packed RBCs (hematocrit).

Critical Thinking

If the patient's hematocrit is 37 and the RBC count is 5 million, what would the MCV be?

Using Erythrocyte Indices to Diagnose

The MCH and MCV will be increased in megaloblastic anemias such as vitamin B_{12} and folate deficiency anemias. They will also be increased in acute blood loss anemia, chronic hemolytic anemias, aplastic anemias, hypothyroidism, and liver disease. The MCH and MCV will be decreased in hypochromic and microcytic anemias, including iron deficiency anemia, thalassemias, and occasionally in hyperthyroidism.

The MCHC will be increased in hereditary spherocytosis. It will be normal in macrocytosis. The MCHC will be decreased in iron deficiency anemia. The stained blood smear of a person with iron deficiency anemia will demonstrate RBCs that are both hypochromic and microcytic.

ERYTHROCYTE SEDIMENTATION RATES (ESR OR SED RATE)

The **erythrocyte sedimentation rate** (ESR), as the name implies, is a measurement of the rate at which the RBCs in a well-mixed, anticoagulated blood sample will fall, or settle, toward the bottom when it is placed in a vertical tube. This test is commonly referred to in the laboratory as a "sed rate." See Procedure 29-3. The ESR has been used for many years in the diagnosis and treatment of many disease states of the body. It is an inexpensive, accurate, and easy test to perform. Two factors that influence the sedimentation rate are the condition of the surface membrane of the RBC and changes in the level of fibrinogen in the plasma of the blood. During disease conditions in the body, the surface membrane of the RBC is altered, and this affects the rate at which the RBCs fall in the tube. RBCs will demonstrate this change even after the disease has subsided because RBCs have an average life of 120 days. For this reason, the ESR is a more accurate tool in diagnosing the onset of a disease than in checking the progress of treatment.

Fibrinogen is a plasma protein. The level, or concentration, of fibrinogen is altered during various disease states of the body.

Two ways to perform an ESR test are the Wintrobe method and the Westergren method. Both methods will provide the same information. Because of the simplicity in setting up the Westergren ESR, it has become the more widely used method in the ambulatory care setting's POL.

Wintrobe Method

An EDTA venous blood sample is thoroughly mixed. With the use of a Pasteur pipette, the blood is transferred to a Wintrobe tube. The blood is added to the left zero mark at the top of the tube. It is important that no air bubbles are present in the blood column. The tube is placed exactly vertical in a rack and allowed to stand for exactly 60 minutes. The test is read by determining the number of millimeters (mm) the red cells have settled. The tube has a total capacity of 100 mm. The test is reported in millimeters per hour (Figure 29-8). Table 29-8 shows normal values for the Wintrobe method of ESR.

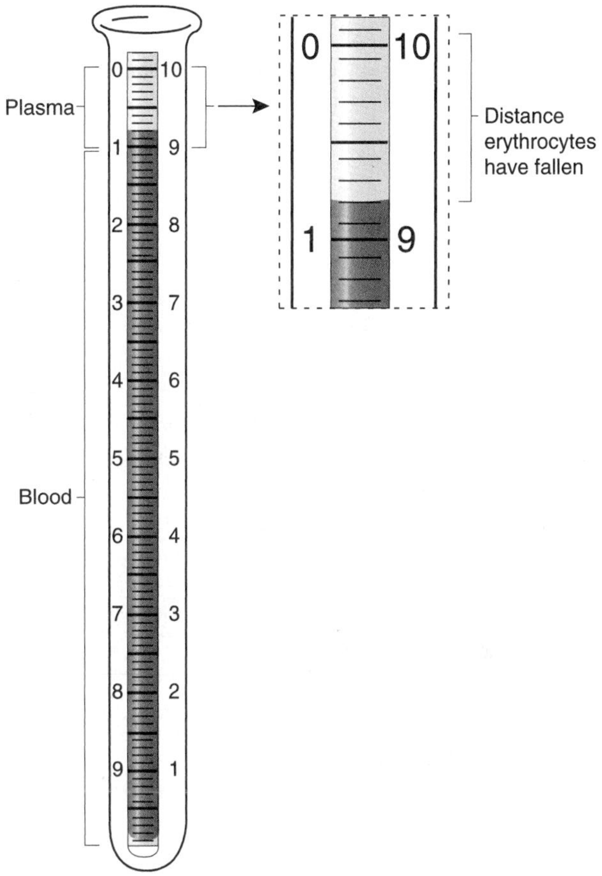

Figure 29-8 Wintrobe sedimentation tube showing settling of cells. The example shown illustrates a sedimentation of 8 mm.

Westergren Method

The Westergren method differs from the Wintrobe method in that the blood sample is mixed with 3.8% sodium citrate solution before the tube is filled. The blood and sodium citrate are mixed and the tube is filled to the zero mark and placed exactly vertical in a rack. The tube

TABLE 29-8	NORMAL VALUES FOR THE WINTROBE METHOD OF ESR
Male patients	0–9 mm/hr
Female patients	0–20 mm/hr

TABLE 29-9 NORMAL VALUES FOR THE WESTERGREN METHOD OF ESR

Male patients younger than 50 years	0–15 mm/hr
Male patients older than 50 years	0–20 mm/hr
Female patients younger than 50 years	0–20 mm/hr
Female patients older than 50 years	0–30 mm/hr

is read after exactly 60 minutes, and the test is reported in millimeters per hour. Table 29-9 shows normal values for the Westergren method of ESR.

The Polymedco company has produced a Sediplast® system to perform a Westergren ESR that is self-filling. It is a completely closed system that protects laboratory personnel from the risks associated with blood handling. The Sediplast® ESR System is shown in Figure 29-9.

The following guidelines should be followed when performing Wintrobe and Westergren ESR procedures to ensure accurate test results:

1. The tube must remain exactly vertical during the one-hour test time.
2. The test must be read at exactly 60 minutes (1 hour).

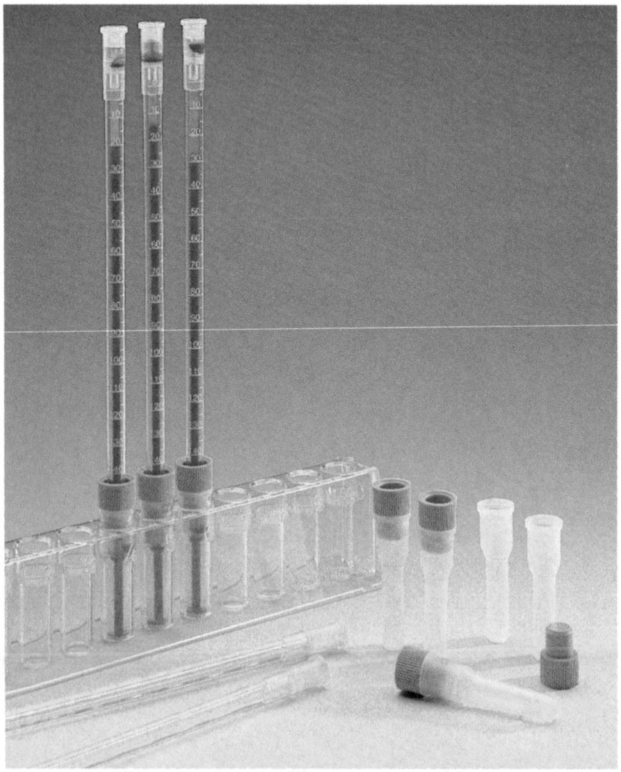

Figure 29-9 Westergren method using Sediplast® ESR System. The picture shows three filled tubes standing in the rack. Note the diluting vials with sodium citrate solution (right). (Courtesy of POLY-MEDCO Inc.)

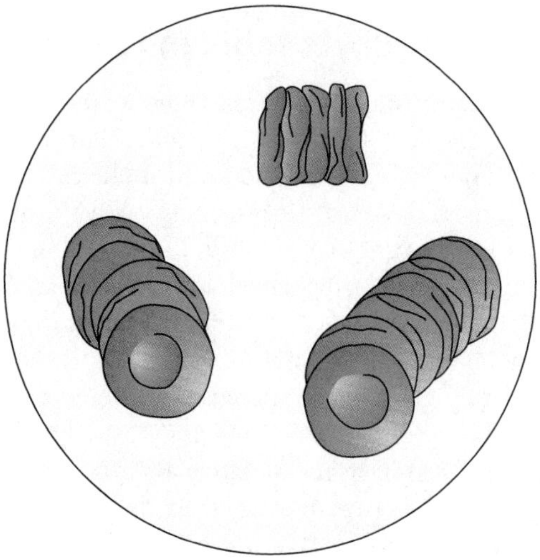

Figure 29-10 Erythrocytes forming rouleaux.

3. The counter on which the rack is placed must be free of vibrations.
4. The test should be set up within two hours after the blood is drawn.
5. The test should be conducted at room temperature.
6. The tube should not be placed in a draft, and it should not be exposed to direct sunlight.
7. The column of blood must be free of bubbles.

The erythrocytes in normal, nondiseased blood tend to remain suspended in the plasma. They do not aggregate (clump) together to form rouleaux. Rouleaux is a phenomenon where RBCs form aggregates that look like rolls or stacks of coins (Figure 29-10).

This aggregate form causes the rate of sedimentation to increase. RBCs have membrane properties that tend to make them remain separated in the plasma. During certain diseased states, this repelling property is lost and the RBCs tend to aggregate.

Using the ESR to Diagnose

ESRs are increased in infections and inflammatory diseases, tissue destruction, and other conditions that lead to an increase in plasma fibrinogen. They are also increased with menstruation, pregnancy, malignant neoplasms, and multiple myeloma. With anemia, the ESR increases according to the severity of the condition.

The ESR may be normal in osteoarthritis and in some cases of cirrhosis and malaria. The ESR values are decreased in polycythemia, spherocytosis, and sickle cell anemia.

AUTOMATED HEMATOLOGY

Use of the automated or semiautomated hematology instruments are not categorized as waived testing under

CLIA, and therefore are not within the medical assistant's scope of practice. All procedures performed with automated instrumentation are modifications of manual methods. Automated hematology procedures have many advantages over the manual methods. They are faster, less expensive, simple to operate, and accurate. The instruments can be calibrated and lend themselves to control testings. Most are equipped with printers that produce printed results. Many can store quality-control results and print out quality-control data summary sheets.

In addition to performing a wide variety of hematologic tests, many automated hematology instruments also calculate part or all of the RBC indices and print the results. Some automated hematology instruments can be connected to other computers in the medical facility.

The hematologic parameters that are available on different automated office hematology instruments are:

- RBC count
- WBC count
- Hemoglobin
- Hematocrit
- Platelet count
- MCV
- MCHC
- MCH
- Percentage of granulocytes
- Granulocyte count (neutrophils, eosinophils, basophils)
- Percentage of lymphocytes/monocytes
- Nongranulocyte count (lymphocytes and monocytes)
- Mid-cell count (monocytes and band neutrophils)
- Percentage of mid-cells
- Lymphocyte count
- Percentage of lymphocytes
- RBC distribution width (RDW)

Procedure 29-1 Hemoglobin Determination (HemoCue®)

STANDARD PRECAUTIONS:

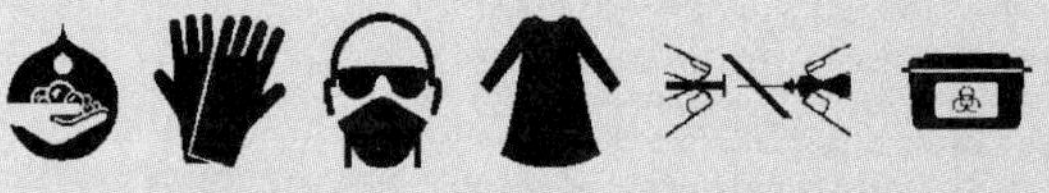

PURPOSE:

Properly and safely perform an automated hemoglobin determination to evaluate the oxygen capacity of the blood.

EQUIPMENT/SUPPLIES:

Gloves
Disinfectant
Capillary puncture equipment or blood samples collected in EDTA
HemoCue® System, or other waived hemoglobin analyzer with supplies appropriate for the analyzer
Biohazard red bag
Sharps container
NOTE: Consult manufacturer's instructions for specific procedure.

PROCEDURE STEPS:

1. Wash hands and put on gloves.
2. Assemble equipment and materials.
3. Turn on instrument to warm up. Calibrate or standardize the instrument according to the manufacturer's directions.
4. Perform a capillary puncture (see Chapter 28) observing the *Bloodborne Pathogen Standard.* Wipe away the first drop of blood.
5. Collect blood from the puncture using a capillary or cuvette appropriate for the analyzer to be used. Avoid trapping air bubbles in the collection device.
6. Wipe excess blood from the outside of the collection device (if appropriate) being careful not to touch the open end of the device.
7. Insert the filled cuvette into the HemoCue® photometer within 10 minutes of filling the cuvette. Read the hemoglobin value from the display and record.

(continues)

Procedure 29-1 (continued)

8. Discard all contaminated materials into biohazard containers.
9. Return all equipment to proper storage.
10. Wipe counters with disinfectant.
11. Remove and discard gloves into biohazard container.
12. Wash hands.
13. Document the results.

Procedure 29-2 Microhematocrit

STANDARD PRECAUTIONS:

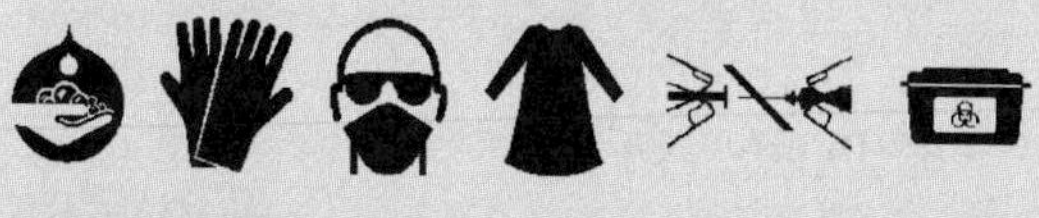

PURPOSE:

Properly and safely perform the microhematocrit procedure using a few microliters of blood in a capillary tube to separate the cellular elements of the blood from the plasma by centrifugation.

EQUIPMENT/SUPPLIES:

Gloves
Capillary tubes, plain and with heparin
Acrylic safety shield
Sealing clay
Microhematocrit centrifuge and reader
Tube of anticoagulated venous blood (or commercially available simulated blood)
70% alcohol or alcohol swabs
Gauze and cotton balls, sterile
Safety lancets
Surface disinfectant or 10% chlorine bleach solution
Biohazard container
Puncture-proof sharps container
NOTE: Consult the instruction manual for the centrifuge being used. Refer to the specific procedure being performed.

PROCEDURE STEPS:

1. Wash hands and put on gloves.
2. Assemble equipment and materials for capillary puncture and microhematocrit.

For direct specimen method, complete Steps 3a–g. When using a sample from a blood specimen tube, go to Step 4.

3. Fill two capillary tubes from a capillary puncture.
   a. Perform a capillary puncture (see Chapter 28). Dispose of lancet into sharps container.
   b. Wipe away the first drop of blood and dispose of gauze into biohazard container.
   c. Touch one end of a heparinized capillary tube to the second drop of blood.
   d. Allow the tube to fill three-quarters full by capillary action. Hold tube level. Fill tubes about three-fourths full.
   e. Fill a second tube in the same manner.
   f. Wipe the outside of the filled capillary tube with gauze to remove excess blood.
   g. Seal the capillary tube by placing it into the tray of sealing clay (see Figure 29-11). Proceed to Step 5.
4. If using venous blood, fill two capillary tubes using a tube of EDTA anticoagulated blood (if not available, proceed to Step 5):
   a. Mix the tube of blood thoroughly by gently rocking the tube from end to end a minimum of two minutes by mechanical mixer or 50 to 60 times by hand.
   b. Remove cap from the tube (with an acrylic safety shield placed between worker and tube).
   c. Tilt the tube so that blood is near the top edge of the tube.

(continues)

Procedure 29-2 (continued)

d. Insert the tip of a plain capillary tube into the blood and fill three-quarters full by capillary action. NOTE: Wipe the outside of the filled capillary tube with gauze to remove excess blood.
e. Seal the tube by placing the end into the tray of sealing clay.
f. Fill a second tube in the same manner.

5. Check to see if the interior sealing clay edge appears level in the tubes.
6. Place tubes into the microhematocrit centrifuge with *sealed* ends securely against the gasket (balance the centrifuge by placing the tubes opposite each other). Make a note of which patient sample is in which slot # (Figure 29-12).
7. Fasten lids securely.
8. Set the timer and adjust the speed if necessary.
9. Centrifuge for the prescribed time.

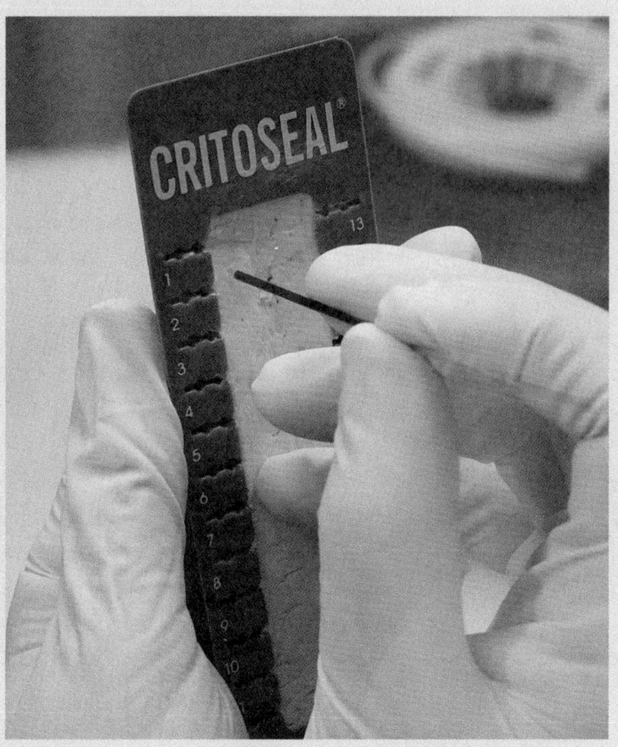

Figure 29-11 Sealing the microhematocrit tube with sealing clay.

10. Allow the centrifuge to come to a complete stop before unlocking the lid(s).
11. Determine the microhematocrit values using one of the following methods:
    a. A centrifuge that requires calibrated tubes and has a built-in scale:
       (1) Position the tubes as directed by the manufacturer's instructions.
       (2) Read the microhematocrit value.
    b. A centrifuge without a built-in reader:
       (1) Carefully remove capillary tubes from centrifuge.
       (2) Place tube on the microhematocrit reader card provided.
       (3) Follow instructions on the reader to obtain the microhematocrit value.
12. Average the values from the two tubes and record the microhematocrit as a percentage.
13. Discard the capillary tubes into the sharps container.
14. Clean and return equipment to proper storage.
15. Clean the work area with disinfectant.
16. Remove and discard gloves into biohazard container and wash hands.
17. Document the results.

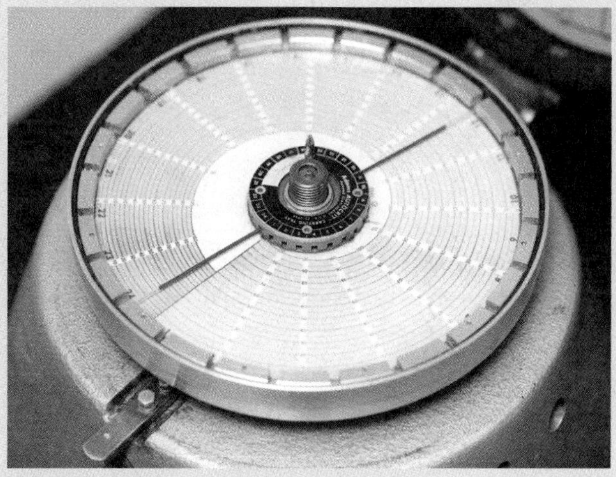

Figure 29-12 Setting the microhematocrit tubes properly into the centrifuge.

Procedure 29-3 Erythrocyte Sedimentation Rate

STANDARD PRECAUTIONS:

PURPOSE:

Properly and safely examine a blood sample by using either the Sediplast® (Westergren) or Wintrobe method to record the ESR.

EQUIPMENT/SUPPLIES:

Gloves
Sample of venous blood collected in EDTA
Sediplast® kit (or other ESR kit):
- Sedivial and sedirack
- Sediplast® autozeroing pipette
- Pipette capable of delivering up to 1.0 ml

Wintrobe method:
- Wintrobe sedimentation tube (disposable or reusable)
- Wintrobe sedimentation rack
- Long-stem Pasteur-type pipette with rubber bulb

Timer
Disinfectant
Biohazard disposal container
Acrylic face shield or goggles and mask
Sharps container
NOTE: Consult the manufacturer's package insert for specific instructions for the ESR kit being used.

PROCEDURE STEPS:

1. Wash hands and put on gloves.
2. Assemble equipment and materials.
3. Gently mix blood sample for two minutes.
4. Perform either method a (Sediplast® ESR) or method b (Wintrobe):
   a. Sediplast® ESR (modified Westergren) method:
      (1) Remove stopper on sedivial and fill to the indicated mark with 0.8 ml blood. Replace stopper and invert vial several times to mix (or mix using pipette).
      (2) Place sedivial in Sediplast® rack on a level surface.
      (3) Gently insert the disposable Sediplast® pipette through the pierceable stopper with a twisting motion and push down until the pipette rests on the bottom of the vial. The pipette will autozero the blood and any excess will flow into the sealed reservoir compartment.
      (4) Set timer for one hour.
      (5) Return blood sample to proper storage. (If no laboratory work will be performed during the incubation, remove gloves, discard appropriately, and wash hands. Reglove before handling test materials.)
      (6) Let the pipette stand undisturbed for exactly one hour, and then read the results of the ESR: Use the scale on the tube to measure the distance from the top of the plasma to the top of the RBCs.
      (7) Record the sedimentation rate:
      ESR (Mod. Westergren, 1 hr) = ___ mm
      (8) Dispose of tube and vial in appropriate biohazard container.
   b. Wintrobe method:
      (1) Place tube in Wintrobe sedimentation rack.
      (2) Check the leveling bubble to ensure that the Wintrobe rack is level.
      (3) Fill Wintrobe tube to the zero mark with well-mixed blood using the Pasteur pipette and being careful not to overfill.
      NOTE: Tube must be filled from the bottom to avoid getting air bubbles in the tube.
      (4) Set timer for one hour. Be certain the tube is vertical and left undisturbed for the entire hour.
      (5) Return blood sample to proper storage. (If no other laboratory work is scheduled, remove gloves, discard appropriately, and wash hands. Reglove before handling test materials.)
      (6) Measure the distance the erythrocytes have fallen (in mm): after exactly one hour, use the scale on the tube to measure the distance from the top of the plasma to the top of the RBCs.
      (7) Record the sedimentation rate:
      ESR (Wintrobe, 1 hr) = ___ mm
      (8) Disinfect and clean equipment and return to storage.
      NOTE: If disposable equipment is used, dispose of in biohazard container.
5. Clean work area with surface disinfectant.
6. Remove gloves and discard into biohazard container.
7. Wash hands.
8. Document the results.

Procedure 29-4 Obtaining Blood for Blood Culture

STANDARD PRECAUTIONS:

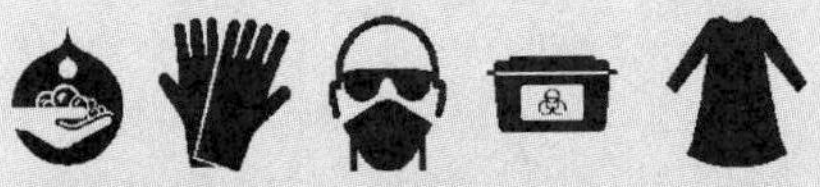

PURPOSE:

While performing venipuncture from two separate sites, prepare two culture bottles of blood from each site for culture (four total).

EQUIPMENT/SUPPLIES:

Nonsterile glove for use with povidone-iodine solution
Sterile gloves
Laboratory requisition
Blood culture bottles, anaerobic and aerobic (usually four: two bottles each for two sets of cultures)
70% isopropyl alcohol
Povidone-iodine solution swabs or towelettes
Venipuncture supplies (according to method used) for two separate sites
Biohazard red bag
Sharps container
Labeling pen

PROCEDURE STEPS:

1. Identify the patient, introduce yourself, and explain the procedure.
2. Assure that the patient has not initiated antimicrobial therapy. RATIONALE: Antibiotic therapy can interfere with the culture results. If the patient has started antibiotics, the name and strength of the antibiotic, dosage, duration, and last dose must be documented clearly on the laboratory report.
3. Wash hands and put on gloves. RATIONALE: Washing hands before any laboratory process prevents contamination of the specimen. Gloving provides personal protection.
4. Assemble equipment and supplies according to the venipuncture procedure being used and the laboratory requirements. Check expiration dates on all collection and culture supplies. RATIONALE: Organizing your work area prevents confusion and error due to missing supplies. Usually two separate sites are used for collection, with two bottles (one aerobe and one anaerobe) from each site. Occasionally, three sites will be necessary. Expired supplies and culture bottles must not be used.
5. Place the culture bottles on a flat surface within reach during the procedure. Mark the correct fill line on both bottles at 10 ml per bottle (1–3 ml per bottle for pediatric patients). RATIONALE: Marking the fill line helps in viewing the proper amount during the procedure.
6. Prepare the venipuncture site with isopropyl alcohol and allow to dry, then apply povidone-iodine in progressively larger concentric circular circles from the inside outward. The iodine must remain on the skin for one full minute and be allowed to dry naturally. The venipuncture site should not be touched after the skin is disinfected. RATIONALE: Alcohol removes oils and other debris, the povidone-iodine is a more thorough antiseptic. One full minute is required to ensure antisepsis. Touching the site may recontaminate it.
7. Cleanse the bottle tops with alcohol and povidone-iodine solution. RATIONALE: The bottle tops need to be disinfected to remove contamination. NOTE: Some laboratory guidelines state that iodine can disintegrate the rubber stopper and therefore should not be used. Follow your laboratory guidelines as stated in your laboratory manual.
8. Remove the preparation glove and apply the sterile gloves using sterile procedure. RATIONALE: Sterile gloves will assure the procedure will be as sterile as possible.
9. Perform venipuncture according to method used. Insert the aerobic culture bottle onto the needle. Fill to the appropriate line, usually 10 ml per bottle (1–3 for pediatric patients). Remove the first bottle, invert 8 to 10 times, and apply the second (anaerobic) bottle. Fill. Remove the second bottle and invert 8 to 10 times. Complete the venipuncture procedure according to the method used. RATIONALE: Follow your laboratory manual guidelines. The aerobic bottle should be filled first because there will be some residual air in the needle. The anaerobic bottle will then collect only blood. Inverting the bottles assures the culture media will be well mixed with the blood.
10. Complete the venipuncture procedure as determined by the method used. Remove the remaining iodine from the skin with isopropyl alcohol.

(continues)

Procedure 29-4 (continued)

RATIONALE: The next two bottles will be filled from a different site. The iodine solution can irritate the skin and should be removed.

11. Perform venipuncture at the second site, repeating the process as stated above. The second and subsequent culture bottles must be collected within 30 minutes of the first. RATIONALE: The 30-minute time frame rules out the possibility of transient bacteria coming into the blood (such as through teeth brushing or scratching a skin lesion, and so on).
12. The culture bottles should be stored at room temperature and *not* refrigerated. RATIONALE: Room temperature is ideal for the cultures so organisms are not destroyed.
13. Label the bottles with the patient's name, date, time, and other required information. RATIONALE: Labeling with the required information prevents mix-ups of specimens and assures a quality timeline. Specimens will be rejected if not labeled properly.
14. Dispose of all contaminated supplies, disinfect all surfaces, remove gloves, and wash hands. RATIONALE: Using appropriate disposal techniques and disinfecting all surfaces according to Standard Precautions safely control biohazard substances.
15. Complete the laboratory requisition including the date and time of each specimen collected, any antibiotic therapy the patient is on, the name and strength of the antibiotic, as well as the dosage, duration, and the last dose taken. Include the clinical diagnosis and any special organisms suspected or to rule out. The laboratory requisition must indicate if the culture is for *brucella* or *francisella*. The information on the laboratory requisition should match exactly the information given on the bottles. RATIONALE: Labeling with the required information prevents mix-ups of specimens, assures a quality timeline, and assure the laboratory will have the necessary information. Specimens will be rejected if there is a discrepancy between the information on the bottle and the information on the laboratory requisition.
16. Document the procedure in the laboratory section of the patient's chart/medical record. RATIONALE: Necessary information and the patient's medical record will be accurate and complete.

Case Study 29-1

Today is busier than usual at Drs. Lewis and King. While she is performing an ESR for Jim Marshal, a patient in his late 30s, medical assistant Audrey Jones is called on to help with another patient. She hurriedly places the sedimentation rack on top of an incubator in the sunlight by an open window and leaves to assist Dr. King.

CASE STUDY REVIEW

1. List two ways in which the test results may be affected.
2. What are the normal Westergren ESR values for male and female patients younger than 50 years?
3. What are the best conditions for an accurate test?

SUMMARY

Hematology tests are the second most frequently performed tests in the ambulatory care setting. Only the urinalysis is performed more frequently. Medical assistants must have a knowledge of hematology to accurately and efficiently perform the tests. The study of hematology includes hematopoiesis, which is the formation of the blood elements, as well as the hematologic tests and their relation to the pathology of the body.

This chapter has introduced the more common hematologic tests that are performed in the ambulatory care setting, including all the parts of the CBC, the ESR methods, and the erythrocyte indices. All of these tests are used by the physician in the diagnosis and treatment of disease.

Most of the hematology procedures performed in today's ambulatory care setting use some type of automated instrumentation. Some automated hematology instruments require a diluted blood sample, whereas others do not. Both methods of automated instrumentation are discussed in this chapter.

Blood specimens used in the sampling of hematologic procedures are biohazardous material. Be sure to follow Universal and Standard Precautions when you work with these specimens. See Chapter 10.

STUDY FOR SUCCESS

To reinforce your knowledge and skills of information presented in this chapter:

- ❑ Review the Key Terms
- ❑ Practice the Procedures
- ❑ Consider the Case Study and discuss your conclusions
- ❑ Answer the Review Questions
  - ❑ Multiple Choice
  - ❑ Critical Thinking
- ❑ Navigate the Internet by completing the Web Activities
- ❑ Practice the StudyWARE activities on the CD
- ❑ Apply your knowledge in the Student Workbook activities
- ❑ Complete the Web Tutor sections
- ❑ View and discuss the DVD situations

REVIEW QUESTIONS

Multiple Choice

1. Which of the following is *not* a cellular component of blood?
   a. erythrocytes
   b. leukocytes
   c. thrombocytes
   d. erythropoietin
2. The formation of blood is defined as:
   a. erythropoietin
   b. hematopoiesis
   c. mean corpuscular volume
   d. hemoglobinopathy
3. Sickle cell anemia, a hereditary disease, has which type of hemoglobin?
   a. hemoglobin S
   b. hemoglobin A
   c. hemoglobin E
   d. hemoglobin C
4. The volume of packed red cells compared with the total volume of the sample is calculated for which test?
   a. hematocrit
   b. hemoglobin
   c. MCH
   d. MCV

5. The most common white cell type found in the granulocytic series is the:
   a. lymphocyte
   b. monocyte
   c. neutrophil
   d. basophil
6. The erythrocyte indices are used for the diagnosis, classification, and treatment of different:
   a. infections
   b. anemias
   c. inflammatory diseases
   d. neoplasms
7. Which hematologic test result shows an increase with infections, inflammatory disease, pregnancy, and tissue destruction?
   a. hemoglobin
   b. MCV
   c. hematocrit
   d. ESR
8. The most frequent hemoglobin disease seen in the ambulatory care setting is:
   a. iron deficiency anemia
   b. sickle cell anemia
   c. leukemia
   d. anisocytosis
9. Which test within a CBC is within the scope of practice of a medical assistant under CLIA's waived test category?
   a. Using a HemoCue® to determine a hemoglobin level
   b. Using a hemacytometer to count WBCs manually
   c. Using the Unopette system to count RBCs manually
   d. Using an automated blood analyzer that requires calculations and mixing of reagents

Critical Thinking

1. What hematologic factors do the erythrocyte indices provide information about? List one example for each index in which a disease causes an elevation or decrease.
2. You are serving your externship in a local clinic. A physician has made a tentative diagnosis of appendicitis for a patient. In addition to the urinalysis, what single hematologic test is most likely to confirm the diagnosis?
3. List the guidelines that must be followed to assure accurate sed rate results.
4. How does aspirin interfere with clotting?
5. What test would have elevated results if a patient had systemic arthritis? Why?

WEB ACTIVITIES

1. Visit the CDC's Web site to review Standard Precautions required during blood collection.
2. Does the American Heart Association's Web site offer parameters for different blood counts and hematology values? Are guidelines and tips on specimen collection outlined?

REFERENCES/BIBLIOGRAPHY

Palko, T., & Palko, H. (1996). *Laboratory procedures for the medical office*. Columbus, OH: Glencoe/McGraw-Hill.

Walters, N. J., Estridge, B. H., & Reynolds, A. P. (2000). *Basic medical laboratory techniques* (4th ed.). Clifton Park, NY: Thomson Delmar Learning.

THE DVD HOOK-UP

DVD Series: **Skills Based Series** | Program Number: **11**

Chapter/Scene Reference
- *Administering Capillary Puncture and Performing Hematocrit Test*
- *Performing Automated Hemoglobin*
- *Performing ESR Test*

This chapter discusses common hematologic procedures that are performed in the medical office.

The selected scenes in this program taught you how to perform a hematocrit, hemoglobin, and ESR test. Procedures will vary depending on the equipment used.

1. The selected clip for performing a hematocrit test stated that you may test one or two tubes, depending on equipment used and the policy of your office. Why is it best to run two tubes when measuring a patient's hematocrit?
2. How can you make certain that you are performing waived tests when working in a waived laboratory?
3. What tube color should you use for hematologic testing? Is the ESR considered a hematologic test?

DVD Journal Summary
Write a paragraph that summarizes what you learned from watching the selected scenes from today's DVD program. It is important to make certain that test results are accurate. What would you do if your controls do not match what is listed on the control bottle and the office supervisor tells you to ignore the control values?

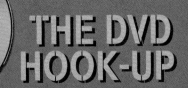

CHAPTER 30

Urinalysis

OUTLINE

OBJECTIVES

The student should strive to meet the following performance objectives and demonstrate an understanding of the facts and principles presented in this chapter through written and oral communication.

1. Define the key terms as presented in the glossary.
2. Explain the process of urine formation.
3. Discuss the importance of safety procedures and quality control when working with urine.
4. Describe the importance of proper collection and preservation of the 24-hour urine specimens.
5. Identify the proper technique for examining the physical characteristics of a urine specimen.
6. Explain pathologic and nonpathologic causes of abnormal physical characteristics of urine.
7. Describe methods for chemical examination of a urine specimen.
8. Explain the need to confirm abnormal results.
9. Describe the confirmatory tests for ketones, glucose, protein, and bilirubin.
10. Identify the proper method of preparing urine sediment for microscopic examination.
11. Identify normal and abnormal structures found during the microscopic examination of urine sediment.

KEY TERMS

Acetest®
Acid/Base Balance
Amorphous
Bilirubin
Bilirubinuria
Casts
Circadian Rhythm
Clinitest®
Creatinine
Critical Values
Crystals
Culture and Sensitivity (C&S)
Cultures
Glucose
Glucosuria
Hematuria
Hyaline
Ictotest®
Ketoacidosis
Ketone
Ketonuria
Ketosis
Leukocyte Esterase
Midstream Collection
pH
Quality Control
Reagent
Reagent Test Strip
Refractometer
Screening
Sediment
Specific Gravity
Supernatant
Turbid
Urea
Urinalysis
Urinary Tract Infection (UTI)
Urobilinogen

FEATURED COMPETENCIES

CAAHEP—ENTRY-LEVEL COMPETENCIES

Clinical Competencies

Fundamental Procedures

- Perform handwashing
- Dispose of biohazard materials
- Practice Standard Precautions

Specimen Collection

- Inform patients in the collection of a clean-catch mid-stream urine specimen
- Perform urinalysis

General Competencies

Legal Concepts

- Perform within legal and ethical boundaries
- Document appropriately

Patient Instructions

- Instruct individuals according to their needs

Operational Functions

- Use methods of quality control

ABHES—ENTRY-LEVEL COMPETENCIES

Professionalism

- Conduct work within scope of education, training, and ability

Clinical Duties

- Prepare patients for procedures
- Apply principles of aseptic techniques and infection control
- Use quality control
- Collect and process specimens

(continues)

SCENARIO

At Inner City Health Care, clinical medical assistant Wanda Slawson performs many urinalyses. Although urinalysis is a routine procedure, Wanda recognizes its importance as a diagnostic tool, and she performs each test carefully to ensure accurate results. Wanda takes time to instruct patients in the proper collection procedures. She encourages patients to ask questions before collecting the urine sample, and she provides written instructions for easy reference. When she performs the urinalysis, Wanda follows safety and quality-control guidelines. By paying attention to the details of the procedure, Wanda does her best to ensure the quality of the urinalysis results.

FEATURED COMPETENCIES (continued)

- Perform selected tests that assist with diagnosis and treatment
- Dispose of biohazard materials
- Practice Standard Precautions
- Instruct patients in the collection of a clean-catch mid-stream urine specimen
- Perform urinalysis

Legal Concepts

- Document accurately

Spotlight on Certification

RMA Content Outline

- Anatomy and physiology
- Patient education
- Asepsis
- Laboratory procedures

CMA Content Outline

- Systems, including structure, function, related conditions and diseases
- Patient instruction
- Legislation
- Principles of infection control
- Collecting and processing specimens; diagnostic testing

CMAS Content Outline

- Asepsis in the medical office
- Communication

INTRODUCTION

Examination of the urine ***(urinalysis)*** *as a diagnostic tool for many diseases has been performed for centuries by medical practitioners. Urinalysis refers to the study of urine as an aid in patient diagnosis or to follow the course of disease. The urine examination is a routine part of most physical examinations.*

The routine urinalysis is one of the most frequently performed procedures in the medical office laboratory. Many tests can be performed on one urine sample. This procedure is often ordered because urine is easily obtained, and much information about the body's metabolism may be gained from the results of this testing.

When physicians order a "routine urinalysis," they expect timely and accurate results. Results can indicate a systemic disease process or renal (kidney) or urinary tract disease.

Practice, experience, and attention to detail are the most important tools in achieving quality results. Following Standard Precautions when working with any body fluid is mandatory.

URINE FORMATION

Before discussing the analysis of urine, it is helpful to understand how urine is formed in the human body. The formation and excretion of urine is the principal way the body excretes water and gets rid of waste. These waste products, if not removed, rapidly can become toxic.

The kidney is a highly specialized organ that eliminates soluble (dissolved in water) waste products of metabolism. Urine is formed in the kidney and is excreted from the body by way of the urinary tract system (Figure 30-1). The kidney also regulates the fluid outside the cells of the body by eliminating certain fluids and returning other fluids, maintaining a careful balance (homeostasis). In this manner, the body is protected from dramatic changes in

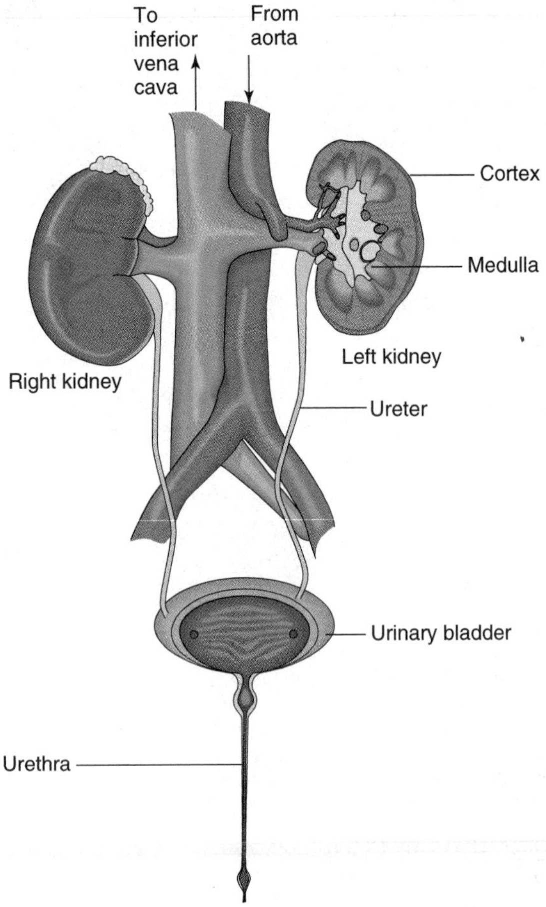

Figure 30-1 The urinary system.

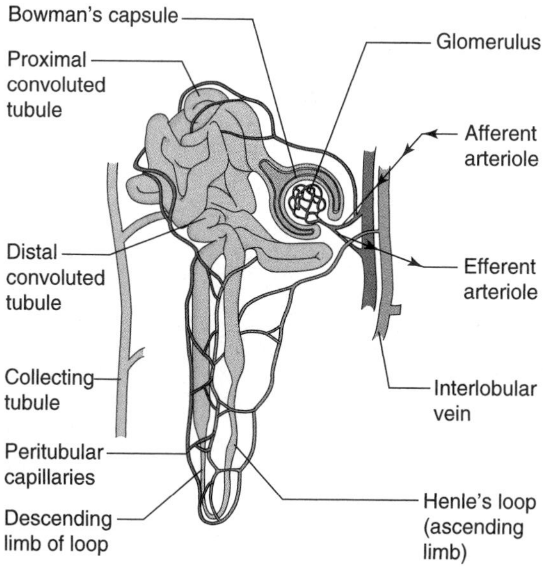

Figure 30-2 Parts of the nephron including the glomerulus.

fluid volume, acidity and alkalinity **(acid/base balance),** composition, and pressure.

There are two kidneys, one on each side of the body. They are about 11 to 12 cm long and 5 to 6 cm wide. Kidneys are shaped like a lima bean with their concave border directed toward the midline of the body. The left kidney is slightly higher than the right.

Filtration

The kidney filters waste products, salts, and excess fluid from the blood. The filtering unit of the kidney is called the glomerulus. The part of the kidney that concentrates the filtered material is called the tubule. Together, the glomerulus and the tubule combine to form the nephron (Figure 30-2).

Most of the work of the kidney is done by the nephrons. There are approximately one million nephrons in each kidney. Each minute, more than 1,000 ml of blood flow through the kidney to be cleansed. In the glomerulus, certain substances are filtered out of the blood. The remaining filtrate then passes into the tubule where various changes occur. Substances filtered out from the body can include water, ammonia, electrolytes, **glucose,** amino acids, **creatinine,** and **urea.** These wastes leave the body in the eliminated urine.

For example, when diabetics have excess sugar in their blood, the body attempts to eliminate the excess glucose through the urine. Routine urinalysis testing will reveal the excess glucose, alerting the physician to the presence of too much glucose. Diabetes can be diagnosed in this manner, as well as determining that a patient with diabetes is not taking enough insulin to control the glucose in the blood.

Reabsorption

While passing through the kidney, some substances may need to be reabsorbed by the blood. Approximately 180 L of filtrate are produced daily by the body, but only 1 to 2 L of urine are eliminated from the normally functioning human body. Therefore, much of the filtrate, including water, sodium, chloride, potassium, bicarbonate, glucose, calcium, and amino acids, is reabsorbed into the body.

Under normal conditions, blood cells and most proteins stay in the blood plasma because they are too large to pass through the walls of the capillaries of the glomerulus. If blood cells and excess protein are found in the urine, the physician is alerted that the kidney is not filtering properly due to an irregular condition affecting the urinary tract.

As long as the concentration of glucose in the blood is less than 180 mg/dl (milligrams per deciliter), the glucose will be completely reabsorbed. If the level increases to more than 180 mg/dl, the glucose is not reabsorbed. Substances such as glucose that are reabsorbed in relation to their concentration in the blood are known as threshold substances. The needs of homeostasis call for sugar and protein to be almost completely reabsorbed, whereas other threshold substances such as creatinine, amino acids, potassium, sodium, and chloride are only partially reabsorbed.

Secretion

Near the end of the blood's journey through the kidney, specifically in the distal convoluted tubule, other substances that have not already been filtered are secreted into the urine. Such substances as hydrogen and ammonium ions may be secreted into the urine in exchange for sodium. Certain drugs in the blood at this point may also be secreted into the urine.

URINE COMPOSITION

After urine progresses through a healthy kidney, it is approximately 96% water and 4% dissolved substances, most of which come from either dietary intake or metabolic waste products. These substances are primarily urea,

Critical Thinking

1. What are the three actions that take place in the formation of urine?
2. Why do you suppose we test for sugar in urine but not salt/sodium?

TABLE 30-1 NORMAL AND ABNORMAL SUBSTANCES IN URINE

Normal	Abnormal
Urea	Bile
Uric acid	Blood
Creatinine	Fat
Sodium	Glucose
Potassium	Protein
Ammonium	White blood cells
Sulfate	Urobilinogen
Chloride	Microorganisms (bacteria, parasites)

salt, sulfates, and phosphates. Abnormal constituents of urine include red and white blood cells, fat, glucose, casts, bile, acetone, and hemoglobin (Table 30-1).

When certain disease processes occur in the human body, the following changes in urine production and composition can occur:

- The amount of urine excreted can increase or decrease
- Urine color can change
- Urine appearance can vary
- Urine odor can change
- Cells can be present in urine
- Chemical constituents in urine can change
- Urine concentration (specific gravity) may vary

SAFETY

Chapter 26 of this textbook covers the guidelines set up by government agencies to ensure the safety of everyone working in the health care field and for the protection of our environment. These guidelines are now referred to as Standard Precautions. Other terms used to describe care when handling infectious materials are Transmission-Based Precautions and biohazard precautions.

QUALITY CONTROL

As in every area of the laboratory, every effort must be made by health care professionals to produce test results free from error. Much pressure is placed by regulatory agencies on facilities that perform laboratory tests such as urinalysis to maintain standards that will ensure reliable results. **Quality-control** (QC) programs are an important part of urine testing to ensure accurate and reliable results for the patient. QC programs must be incorporated into every urine testing procedure. Because many of the tests are interpreted by visual examination, the QC procedures are dependent on the expertise of the person performing the examination.

Testing protocols must be written out and available to personnel. Records of testing must be maintained. Equipment and instruments used for urine testing must be maintained and checked daily for proper calibration. If the instrument should require recalibration, the manufacturer's instructions are provided with the instrument.

Always be careful to perform the QC procedures *exactly* as you perform the procedures on actual patient samples. Documentation of the performance of daily control testing must be kept for at least three years. With the advent of computer storage, the data can now be stored indefinitely. Commercially available urine control samples can be purchased from a number of manufacturers. Positive and negative controls should be run each day on all tests to be performed. Control results should be recorded on a daily log for easy access. The control samples should be stored as directed by the manufacturer.

Precautions To Use When Handling Urine Specimens

- Treat all specimens as if they were infectious, handling them with gloved hands.
- Avoid splashes or creation of aerosols when handling or disposing of urine specimens. Wearing face shields will prevent splashes from getting into the eyes, nose, or mouth.
- Process urine specimens as soon as possible.
- Store urine specimens appropriately in a designated refrigerator that contains no food or drink items.
- Dispose of urine appropriately, possibly in a designated sink (run water to wash the specimen into the drain) or toilet.

CLINICAL LABORATORY IMPROVEMENT AMENDMENTS OF 1988 (CLIA '88)

The regulations under the new CLIA are discussed in Chapter 26. Several CLIA '88 regulations apply to the medical assistant performing urine testing. They include:

- Appropriate training in the methodology of the test being performed
- Understanding of urine-testing QC procedures

Critical Thinking

1. What criteria does CLIA use to determine which tests are in each category?
2. In a urinalysis, which part is not in CLIA's waived category?

- Proficiency in the use of instrumentation, being able to troubleshoot problems
- Knowledge of the stability and proper storage of **reagents** (substances involved in urine testing)
- Awareness of factors that influence test results
- Knowledge of how to verify test results
- The microscopic examination of urine is designated by CLIA to be a PPMP (physician-performed microscopy procedure), and therefore must be performed by a physician. The medical assistant is trained and able to prepare the slide for viewing and reading by the physician. The medical assistant should always take the opportunity to view the slide and discuss the finding with the physician as part of professional development and continued education.

URINE CONTAINERS

The first step toward achieving proper results during laboratory testing is proper collection of the specimen to be tested. There are a variety of containers (Figure 30-3) used for urine collection, including nonsterile containers for random specimens (urinalysis), sterile containers for **cultures** (testing specimens for growth of bacteria), and 24-hour collection containers with added preservatives.

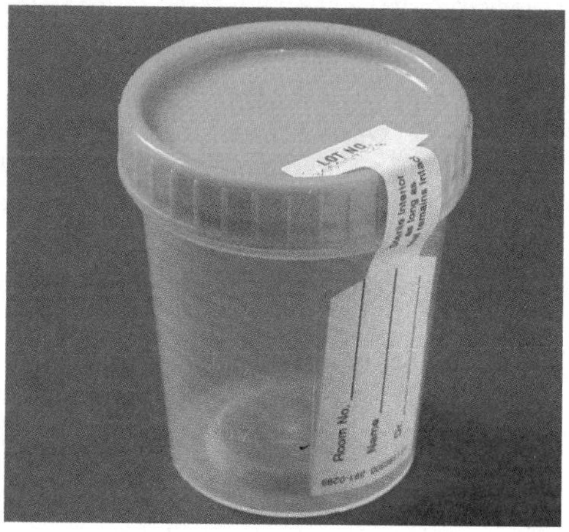

Figure 30-3 Urine collection containers should be calibrated, clear enough to see through, and have a secure lid.

Just before handing the urine specimen cup to the patient, label the cup with the patient's name, the date, and the time. Some facilities require more information, so follow the protocol of your facility. Always use a permanent marker so the information stays clear. Always label the cup, not the lid. This practice assures that the specimen will not be separated from the label if the lid is removed. If the patient is unable to procure a specimen, discard the cup and give the patient a new cup if the patient is later able to give a specimen.

Occasionally, a patient will bring a sample with him or her in a generic container from home. The medical assistant must determine if the container is appropriate for a laboratory specimen and if the urine has been handled properly to assure the best test results. General recommendations are to provide the patient with a new urine specimen cup and request a fresh sample. The exception to this rule would be if the patient has brought a "first morning void" specimen in an appropriate container.

Most laboratories have containers made specifically for urine collection, but any container can be used for urinalysis testing as long as it is very clean and dry. However, if the sample is to be cultured (tested for microorganisms), it must be collected in a sterile container. In some cases, catheterization (see later in this chapter) also is used.

URINE COLLECTION

Urine Specimen Types

Patients may have questions about how a specimen should be collected. The medical assistant must be able to give proper instructions using common terms that the patient will be able to understand. Following are common types of urine specimens that might be ordered frequently by physicians.

Random (Spot) Specimen. Random (spot) urine samples are specimens that can be obtained at any time and

Critical Thinking

1. Is there any test that can be performed on urine that is not in a sterile container?
2. If a patient brings in a urine specimen from home in a clean baby food jar, can it be used for any testing or any part of a urinalysis?

are the most commonly collected specimens. Any random urine specimen can be used for routine urinalysis. However, a concentrated specimen is preferable to one that is dilute.

First Morning Void Specimen. The first morning void is typically the most concentrated specimen and is usually the specimen of choice for many urine tests.

Fasting/Timed Specimens. A fasting (going without food and drink except water) urine specimen is ordered less often than a random specimen. The physician may want to measure a urinary substance without interference from food intake. Some physicians may require an overnight fast. Others may ask the patient to have a meal and then urinate four hours later.

It is up to the medical assistant to give the patient proper instruction as to how to collect a fasting, or timed, specimen. Written directions given to the patient in addition to oral instructions are best. A regular urinalysis container can be used for a fasting specimen. It does not require a sterile container.

Twenty-Four-Hour Specimen. Urine varies in its concentration of certain substances at different times during any 24-hour period because of **circadian rhythm** and the intake of food and water. For instance, the amount of water excreted is greatest from 10 AM to noon and 4 to 6 PM. Chloride is in its highest concentration from noon to 2 PM. Therefore, a 24-hour specimen is sometimes requested when quantitative tests (measuring the amount) for different substances are desired. The results of this type of collection then will be expressed in *units per 24 hours*. Some commonly tested substances include sodium, potassium, calcium, and creatinine.

The container used to collect this amount of urine should be of adequate size. Usually a one-gallon, dark-colored plastic bottle is used. For measuring some urine constituents, preservatives need to be added to the bottle before the collection begins. Without the preservative, these substances may break down and be impossible to quantify. Preservatives include thymol, toluene, and certain acids.

Urine collected over a 24-hour period is refrigerated between collections. After the collection is complete, it must be returned to the medical laboratory as soon as possible.

Many 24-hour urine bottles contain preservatives. Some preservatives are strong acids or bases. As with all laboratory chemicals, the medical assistant and the patient should avoid contact between the preservative and the skin. Vapors must not be inhaled when adding the specimen to the container. In the patient's written instructions, there should be a warning about avoiding contact with preservatives.

Physicians sometimes choose to have a 2-hour or a 12-hour specimen instead of the usual 24-hour collection. All of the collection steps for a 24-hour specimen apply. Recording the time of day is important (a 2-hour specimen is usually collected in the afternoon).

Collection Methods

In addition to ordering what type of urine specimen is desired (random, fasting, 24-hour), the physician might also order a certain type of collection method to collect the specific sample. These methods include random, clean-catch, midstream, and catheterization.

Random Collection. Random collection is the most common collection performed in an outpatient setting. It simply means there is no particular time placed on the collection (as opposed to first morning void or 24-hour specimen). Patients are requested to give the specimen whenever they are present for their appointment. If a patient has already voided, not knowing a specimen was necessary, the medical assistant may offer him or her several glasses of water in an attempt to procure another specimen. Because the kidneys are constantly producing urine, the patient should be able to offer a specimen within 15 to 20 minutes if he or she drinks several glasses of water.

Clean-Catch Midstream Collection. To avoid as much contamination as possible when collecting a specimen, physicians prefer that the patient cleanse the genital area before collection. The clean-catch order means that cleansing towelettes are provided in addition to a urine container. Male patients are directed to cleanse the urethral opening twice with cleansing towelettes, and female patients are directed to cleanse the urethral area with three swipes, using three separate towelettes. (Refer to Patient Education box and to Procedure 30-7 for the complete instructions.) Female patients should also be instructed to notify the medical assistant if they are menstruating during the collection.

After cleansing, the patient should begin to urinate into the toilet. The patient begins urinating, pulls the cup into the urine stream, and collects the sample, then removes the cup from the stream and voids the rest of the urine into the toilet. This is called a midstream specimen. The midstream urine should be as free of contamination as possible.

Catheterized Collection. Urinary catheterization involves insertion of a sterile flexible tube into the uri-

Patient Education

24-Hour Urine Collection

1. When giving a patient any type of instructions, make sure that the patient understands the importance of each step. Always provide written instructions as well. Emphasize that failing to follow the instructions will cause the results to be invalid, requiring another collection.
2. The patient begins a 24-hour collection by emptying the bladder and not keeping the specimen. The container is then labeled with the time of bladder emptying. Patients generally start the collection between 6 and 8 PM, but any 24-hour period is acceptable.
3. Explain that each time the patient urinates within the 24-hour period, the urine is placed into the collection bottle.
4. Instruct the patient to refrigerate the bottle between urinations.
5. Explain to the patient that at the end of the 24-hour period, the patient should urinate and place the urine in the bottle. The exact time should be written on the label as the "ended" or "completed" time.
6. The most common errors in the 24-hour urine specimen collection are the inclusion of the first voided specimen and the discarding of one or more of the voided specimens during the 24-hour period. Be sure the patient understands these steps.

nary bladder through the urethra. Although urinary catheterization is performed for many reasons, this section discusses only the use of catheterization as a way to obtain a urinary sample. See Chapter 18 for the complete procedure for performing a urinary catheterization (see Procedures 18-2 and 18-3).

Obtaining a urine specimen by catheterization is performed when a completely sterile specimen is needed or when the patient is unable to follow cleansing instructions. It may be that the patient does not understand the language, is mentally unable to comprehend the instructions, or is physically unable to perform the process. It is the medical assistant's responsibility to determine if the patient understands the instructions for obtaining a clean-catch midstream urine sample and is able to perform the process.

Catheterization is a sterile procedure and is only performed under a physician's order and only by health care professionals who have been adequately trained. Because the urinary bladder is considered a sterile environment, if the catheterization is not performed properly, bacteria may be introduced into the patient's bladder causing a bladder infection.

Culture and Sensitivity of Urine. Occasionally, the physician will order a **culture and sensitivity (C&S)** of a urine specimen. The medical assistant is responsible for preparing the sample for transport. Currently, the most commonly used system is the Urine Culture and Sensitivity Transport kit (see Procedure 30-6).

EXAMINATION OF URINE

Urine should be examined in a fresh state, preferably while still warm if possible. However, occasionally the urine sample cannot be tested immediately. If immediate testing is not possible, the urine should be refrigerated at about 4°C or stored on ice. The urinalysis should be performed as soon as possible, preferably within 2 hours. **Crystals** and **casts** begin to break down after 2 hours. Any time delay allows bacteria to multiply and can lead to inaccurate microbiology results.

The routine urinalysis procedure is composed of three parts:

- *Physical* examination of the urine
- *Chemical* examination of the urine
- *Microscopic* examination of urine sediment

The medical assistant should remember to wash hands, put on gloves, and follow all of the safety guidelines when performing any of the following procedures. Some facilities require eye protection when pouring urine or performing any procedure where splashing urine into the eye could occur. All surface areas in the

Patient Education

When instructing the patient in collecting a clean-catch, midstream urine specimen for laboratory analysis:

1. The patient should be provided with a clean or sterile covered urine cup, a pair of gloves, and adequate cleansing towelettes (three for female patients, two for male patients). The cup should be labeled with the patient's name and the date. Caution the patient not to contaminate the inside of the cup. A shelf near the toilet is extremely helpful for patients, allowing them to have the towelettes and cup within reach during collection of the specimen.
2. Instruct the patient in proper cleansing of the genital area. It is best to give the patient written instructions as well. Men and women should have separate instructions. The written instructions should be posted next to the toilet for reference by the patient during the procedure. Logically, the female instructions should be posted on the wall beside the toilet at reading level while she is sitting, and the male instructions should be posted on the wall behind the toilet at reading level while he is standing. Laminating the instruction documents protects the writing from any sprays or splashes.
   - *Men:* After thoroughly washing his hands, the male patient should retract the foreskin on the penis (if not circumcised). A cleansing towelette should be used to cleanse the urethral opening with a single stroke directed from the tip of the penis toward the ring of the glans. The cleansing procedure should be repeated again using a new towelette.
   - *Women:* After thoroughly washing her hands, the female patient should position herself comfortably on the toilet seat and spread her knees as far apart as she can. She should spread the outer vulval folds and hold them open with one hand. With the other hand, using the first towelette, the patient should cleanse on one side from front to back with one swipe, disposing of the towelette into the toilet. With the second towelette, she should wipe on the other side front to back with one swipe, disposing of that towelette into the toilet. While still holding the vulval folds open, she should use the third towelette to wipe the urethral opening front to back with one swipe. She may dispose of that towelette into the toilet, too. She should continue to hold the vulval folds open until she has completed the collection of the urine specimen.
3. Instruct the patient also about the midstream collection technique. Explain why it is necessary. These instructions should also be written and included with the clean-catch written directions.
   - After cleansing the area using the clean-catch directions, the patient should begin to void into the toilet. The specimen cup should then be held into the stream until it is about half full, then the cup should be removed from the stream. Assure the patient that urinalysis can be performed on a small amount of urine if they are unable to give half a cup. The patient may finish urinating into the toilet. Only the middle portion of the urine flow is included in the sample. After the specimen has been collected, the container should be capped. After securely capping the urine cup, the patient may cleanse the outside of the cup if desired. The patient should always avoid touching the inside of both the container and the lid.
4. The patient should be instructed on where/how to return the specimen to the medical assistant. Some physicians' office laboratories (POLs) have a special shelf with a small door opening into the laboratory, whereas other offices prefer the patient actually hand the specimen to the medical assistant directly. Either way, the specimen should be taken immediately into the laboratory by the medical assistant.
5. All surface areas in the restroom should be immediately decontaminated in preparation for the next patient.

restroom should be decontaminated immediately after procuring or testing urine specimens.

Physical Examination of Urine

When the medical assistant begins the process of performing a urinalysis, the first step is performing the physical examination. This examination consists of:

- Assessing the volume of the urine specimen, making sure that the specimen is sufficient for testing
- Observing and recording the color, appearance, and transparency of the specimen
- Noting any unusual urine odor
- Measuring the specific gravity of the specimen

Procedure 30-1 illustrates how to assess the volume, color, appearance, transparency, and odor of urine. Procedure 30-2 illustrates testing for the specific gravity.

Specimen Volume. The first step in performing a urinalysis is to determine if the sample's volume is adequate for testing.

The medical assistant must have enough urine to fill a test tube with at least 10 ml (about two teaspoons) of urine with enough leftover in the specimen cup to completely insert and wet a chemical reagent strip and to culture if ordered.

The volume we usually request of the patient is a half cup, but patients should be assured that samples of much less volume can be tested. If the patient is only able to submit a small volume of urine, we would determine which tests we can perform, depending on the priority for the physician according to the patient's suspected diagnosis. For example, if we only need to test for protein and glucose, we would only need enough urine for the chemical reagent strip portion and would not need to fill the test tube. If we needed to test for a microscopic examination of the urine, such as to diagnose a bladder infection, we would need a full test tube, as well as some extra urine for a culture. These tests are thoroughly discussed later in this chapter.

The physician should be consulted for further direction if the amount of urine submitted is less than needed for the complete urinalysis. The urinalysis report should reflect that the quantity was not sufficient for complete testing. The medical assistant should write "QNS" (for quantity not sufficient) where applicable or follow clinic protocol.

If the patient is able to give less than 10 ml of urine for the test tube, the medical assistant should make a note of the amount of urine used. For example, if the patient provides 5 ml, the medical assistant may go ahead with the microscopic examination of urine but should note on the report that the specimen was only 5 ml. The rationale for this notation becomes clear when you understand that the amount of a substance found in 10 ml of urine will be less in a smaller sample. In other words, if the patient has five white blood cells in 10 ml of urine, he or she might only have two to three white blood cells in 5 ml of urine. Unless the notation is made that the sample was smaller, the physician may diagnose incorrectly.

Most clinics/POLs do not require that the urine volume be noted unless it is less than adequate for a complete urinalysis.

Urine Color. There is a wide range of color in normal urine, usually ranging from a pale yellow to a dark yellow or amber. The range of color usually is because of the concentration of the urine. A darker color generally indicates a more concentrated urine. The color of urine comes from normal metabolic processes, the end products of which are deposited in the urine.

After assessing the adequacy of the urine volume, the medical assistant then observes and records the color of the urine, as in Procedure 30-1.

The diet and certain drugs can add substances to the urine that give it a specific color. The medical assistant should be familiar with common reasons for abnormally colored urine and whether they are pathologic (due to a disease process) or nonpathologic abnormalities. For example, the most common pathologic cause of red urine is the presence of red blood cells, known as **hematuria**. Red blood cells in urine may indicate bleeding in the urinary tract either because of a bladder infection or a kidney stone. A nonpathologic example of abnormally colored urine is the medication Pyridium, which can turn the urine bright orange. Table 30-2 lists several urine color variations and possible causes.

TABLE 30-2 URINE COLORS AND POSSIBLE CAUSES

Color	Possible Cause
Straw to yellow	Normal
Orange to amber	Concentrated urine
Colorless	Dilute urine
Deep yellow	Vitamin intake
Bright orange	Drugs, usually Pyridium
Orange-brown	Urobilin
Greenish orange	Bilirubin
Smokey	Red blood cells
Wine red/reddish brown	Hemoglobin pigments
Green or blue	Methylene blue

Urine Transparency. Urine transparency normally is not significant by itself. However, it may be helpful when included with the rest of the urinalysis information. Transparency of urine usually is recorded as clear, cloudy, hazy, or **turbid** (opaque), as in Procedure 30-1. These descriptive terms may vary in different facilities.

There are many causes of cloudy urine, most of which are considered normal. Cloudiness could be contributed to contamination from vaginal discharges, white blood cells, bacteria, or yeast. As urine cools, sometimes crystals form that also may give urine a cloudy appearance.

Urine Odor. With experience, the medical assistant will recognize certain odors in the urine that can indicate specific conditions. Odors, though not recorded on the final laboratory urinalysis report, should not be disregarded. For example, the urine of a diabetic patient who may have a condition known as **ketoacidosis** may have a sweet odor. Urine full of bacteria will have a foul odor that is easily recognized.

Urine Specific Gravity. **Specific gravity** is defined as the ratio of the weight of a given volume of a substance to the weight of the same volume of distilled water at the same temperature. Distilled water used as the reference point has been given the specific gravity value of 1.000. The specific gravity of urine indicates the concentrations of solids such as phosphates, chlorides, proteins, sugars, and urea that are dissolved in urine.

Variations in urine specific gravity can give the physician diagnostic information. In uncontrolled diabetes, glucose in released into the patient's urine. Glucose molecules are dense and may give the urine a high specific gravity. Another reason for high specific gravity readings is dehydration, because there is less fluid being released by the body in relation to whatever chemicals are in the urine. The color of this urine will also probably be darker. In a well-hydrated patient, the specific gravity is low, meaning that the urine is mostly water. The normal range of specific gravity for urine is from 1.003 to 1.035. Specific gravity is highest in the first morning samples because the urine is more concentrated.

Specific gravity is often tested by using either a test strip, urinometer or a refractometer. A urinometer is a calibrated, floating device. A **refractometer** measures the amount of light that is bent by particles suspended in a liquid. A specific gravity reading is also available in conjunction with chemical testing on some reagent strips. The urinometer is the least accurate method and perhaps the most difficult; it is therefore being replaced by the refractometer or reagent dip strips in most POLs.

Urinometer. A urinometer is made from a small glass tube weighted to float in a sample of urine (usually 15 ml). The glass tube has been calibrated, and the stem of the tube has been marked accordingly to read 1.000 at the bottom of the meniscus in distilled water at room temperature. The meniscus is the curvature that appears in a liquid's upper surface when the liquid is placed in a container. The medical assistant reads the specific gravity of the urine from the stem at the meniscus. However, the temperature of the urine must be taken into account if it differs from 70°F, which is normal room temperature. The buoyancy of a liquid changes with the temperature. If the urine is allowed to come to room temperature, the medical assistant risks the physical and chemical changes that can occur to urine when left for more than 20 minutes. It is because of these and other conflicting processes (such as human error) that the urinometer is not recommended as the best option for measuring the weight (specific gravity) of urine.

Refractometer. The most common tool for determining the specific gravity of liquids is the refractometer (Figures 30-4 and 30-5). This instrument measures the refractive index of urine, which is the speed at which light travels through the air as compared with the speed at which it passes through urine. Light is slowed, and therefore bent, as it encounters particles—the more particles, the more bend. The bend can be used to determine the total number of particles and is not affected by the weight of the particles.

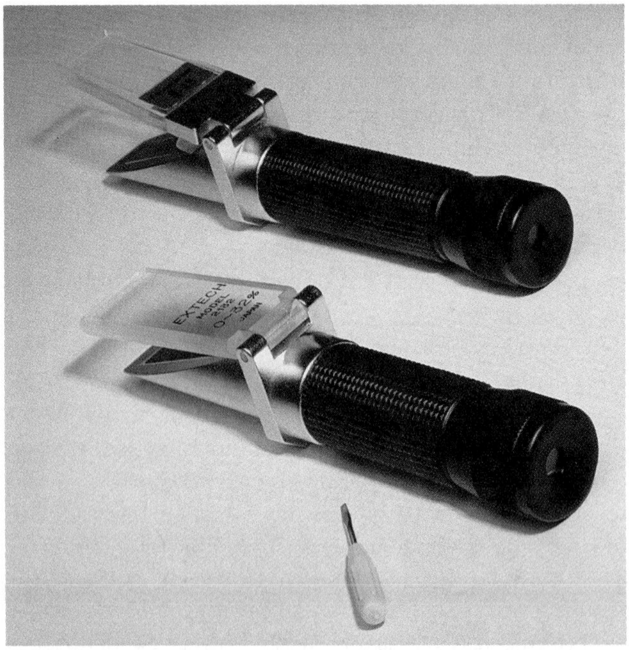

Figure 30-4 Refractometers.

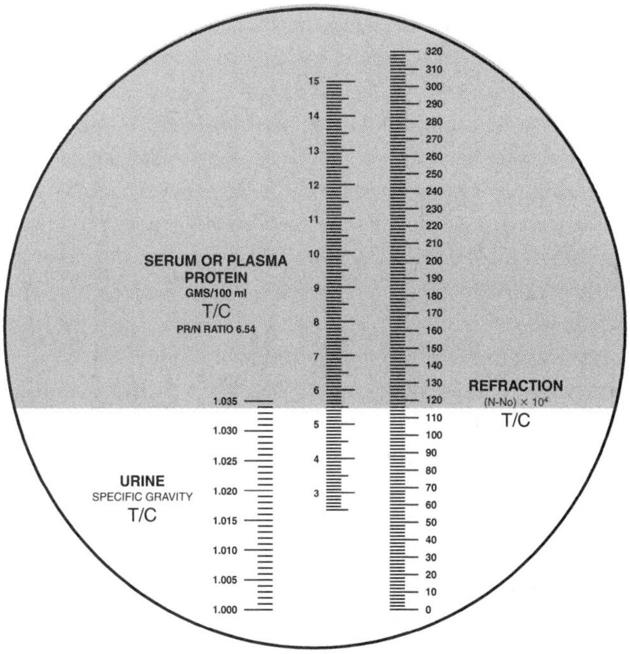

Figure 30-5 Specific gravity as viewed through a refractometer.

The refractometer reading is about 0.002 less than that of the true specific gravity. This slight difference is more than made up for by the ease of using the instrument and the instrument's reliability. This instrument only needs a drop or two of urine, and the result does not have to be adjusted for temperature as long as the temperature is between 60° and 100°F. See Procedure 30-2.

Reagent Dip Strips. Reagent dip strips that include specific gravity are available through a variety of many medical laboratory supply companies. Look for SG in the name, such as brands MultiStix 10 SG or Chemstrip 10 SG (the "10" designates there are 10 tests included on those particular dip strips). Keep in mind that the more tests available on the reagent dip strips, the more expensive the product will be.

Chemical Examination of Urine

After the physical testing of a urine specimen, the next step in urinalysis testing is chemical testing. This procedure once was complex, but today many manufacturers have made the task simple through a wide range of ready-to-use reagents and the reagent test strip, or dipstick (Figure 30-6), as it is more commonly known.

A **reagent test strip,** or dipstick, is a narrow strip of plastic on which pads containing reagents for different reactions are attached. The pads have reagents to test for many metabolic processes, including kidney and

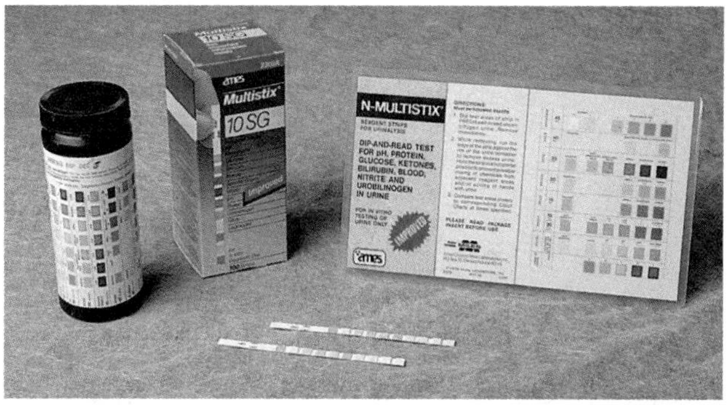

Figure 30-6 Chemical reagent dip strips with color-coded chart.

liver functions, **urinary tract infection (UTI),** and **pH** balance. The reagent test strip is the primary tool used for chemical examination of urine. Specific confirmatory tests or methods may be necessary based on the result of the reagent test strip. Table 30-3 lists some tests available on urine reagent strips.

Specific Reagent Dip Strip Tests. *Glucose* is the sugar most commonly found in urine. Glycosuria and **Glucosuria** are both terms to describe the condition of having glucose in urine. Sugar is normally filtered out of urine in the glomerulus of the kidney and is reabsorbed in the renal tubules. If the body has too much glucose in the blood, the extra will not be reabsorbed and instead will "spill" into the urine. Reagent Dip Strips are embedded with an enzyme called glucose oxidase, which detects glucose. Of course the first pathological condition we think of for glucosuria is diabetes, but other nonpathological conditions can cause some glucose to spill into the urine. Glucose is stored by the liver and used for energy. Although unusual, conditions such as extreme physical or emotional stress can cause the liver to put a lot of glucose into the blood. Eating an unusual amount of sugar can also cause high amounts of glucose in the blood and either of these conditions can cause excess glucose to be lost in the urine. These nonpathological causes are some of the reasons further testing is required before a diagnosis of diabetes can be made.

TABLE 30-3 CHEMICAL TESTING AVAILABLE ON URINE REAGENT TEST STRIPS

pH	Blood
Protein	**Urobilinogen**
Glucose	Nitrite
Ketones	**Leukocyte esterase**
Bilirubin	Specific gravity

Bilirubin is a yellow-orange substance that comes from the breakdown of hemoglobin. Hemoglobin is contained within our red blood cells. Because individual RBCs only live for 120 days, they are constantly breaking down and being replaced. When the RBCs "die," the "heme" part of the hemoglobin circulates in the blood until the liver filters it out. The liver is responsible for changing the heme into a water-soluble substance called bilirubin. Before it gets to the liver, it is called "indirect" or "free" bilirubin. After it leaves the liver, it is called direct or conjugated bilirubin. The liver sends the conjugated bilirubin to the gall bladder where it is released with bile into the small intestine. When there is a blockage in the liver or gall bladder ducts or when there is a disorder or disease of the liver, the bilirubin cannot get past the gall bladder to the small intestine, so it continues to circulate in the blood. This excess of bilirubin in the blood can lead to yellow-orange skin called *jaundice*. The body will try to get rid of extra bilirubin through the urine. Hence, any detection of bilirubin in the urine **(bilirubinuria)** can be indicative of a problem in the liver and/or gall bladder. Newborn babies can be jaundiced because their systems are not mature enough to rid the bile. Because bilirubin breaks down in sunlight, we treat jaundiced babies with special "bili-lights" to help them break down the bilirubin in their skin. Knowing that bilirubin is so unstable, we need to protect it from light in our urine samples, another good reason to test urine samples immediately. Keep in mind that further testing is required before a diagnosis can be made, because bilirubinuria is a symptom, not a disease.

Ketones are formed whenever the body uses fat/fatty acids for energy rather than carbohydrates/sugars. This can happen whenever there is a low intake of carbohydrates/sugars such as in dieting and in certain metabolic disorders such as diabetes. In diabetes, the body lacks insulin or is unable to use sugar properly for energy, so it uses fatty acids. Insulin is a chemical that helps us use sugar for energy, so some diabetics replace their insulin. As fats are broken down, ketone bodies form and "spill" into the urine. The presence of ketones in urine is called **ketonuria.** The burning of fats for energy is called *ketosis* or sometimes *lipolysis*. Persons on carbohydrate-careful diets often use chemical reagent dip strips to check if their urine contains ketones; thus indicating that their bodies are burning fats. **Ketosis** should not be confused with ketoacidosis, which is a dangerous condition for diabetics and alcoholics.

Specific gravity (SG) has been discussed previously in this chapter and is available as a test option on many brands of chemical reagent dip strips. The normal SG for urine is between 1.000 (very dilute urine) to 1.030 (concentrated urine).

Blood in urine is called *hematuria*. If the blood in the urine is not from a nonpathogenic source, such as a contaminate from menstruation, it is indicative of either a bladder infection (often called a *urinary tract infection* [UTI]) or irritation of the urinary tract from a kidney stone or, rarely, a neoplasm. Many chemical reagent dip strips differentiate between hemoglobin and intact red blood cells. Hemoglobin in urine is called *hemoglobinuria* and can indicate pathogenic conditions such as severe infectious diseases, transfusion reactions, and hemolytic anemias. A nonpathogenic cause of hemoglobinuria occurs when the urine is allowed to sit too long, so any RBCs present start breaking down, thus releasing their hemoglobin. Sometimes the chemical reagent dip strips will indicate that blood is present in the urine, but no blood cells are seen during the microscopic examination. This is an example of hemoglobin being present rather than the intact RBCs. The presence of blood in urine is combined with the patient symptoms and other tests to arrive at a diagnosis.

pH is the abbreviation for potential hydrogen ion concentration. The pH test determines if the urine is alkaline or acidic. The scale for pH runs from 0 for the most acidic to 14 for the most alkaline or base. Neutral pH, of course, is 7. The pH of urine varies from 4.5 to 8. The kidneys and lungs are responsible for helping the blood stay at its perfect pH (7.35 to 7.45). The kidneys do this by adjusting the substances they secrete. A person can die if their blood is too acidic (acidosis) or too alkaline (alkalosis). Because there is so little room for deviation in the pH of our blood, our kidneys and lungs are constantly adjusting our secretions. Many things affect the pH of the urine, from medication and diets to pathological conditions. Diets high in protein, some medications, renal tuberculosis, high fevers, and uncontrolled diabetes can cause acidic urine whereas alkaline urine can be caused by diets high in vegetables, citrus fruits, dairy products, some medications, and UTIs. We can also cause a false high-pH reading by letting a urine specimen sit at room temperature for too long.

Protein (albumin) may be secreted in very small (trace) amounts by the kidneys. The present of protein in urine (proteinuria) occasionally may have a nonpathological basis such as excessive exercise, exposure to extreme heat or cold, or extreme emotional stress. Any substantial and/or consistent presence of protein in urine is of concern for renal disease. Protein is a fairly large molecule and for it to be allowed through the filtering glomerulus of the kidney usually damages the glomerulus, or the filtering pressure is too high. Conditions such as high blood pressure and diabetes can cause damage to the filtering glomerulus. A false high-protein reading can occur when large amounts of WBCs, RBCs, epithelial cells, or bacteria are present in the urine. When these four types of cells rupture in urine, they can release protein, causing a false-positive reading. It is important to note, too, that any protein reading in dilute urine is of concern because a normal SG in the same patient would show a much higher level of proteinuria. Thus, it is important to look at the SG of the specimen whenever finding protein in urine.

Urobilinogen is a substance formed when bacteria in the digestive tract breaks down bilirubin. A very small percentage is excreted in the urine and is increased in liver disease. Urobilinogen gives color to feces.

Nitrite forms in urine when certain pathogenic bacteria are present. These specific bacteria convert normal nitrate in urine to abnormal nitrite, thus the presence of nitrite in urine is always indicative of these pathogenic bacteria being present in sufficient quantities to cause a bladder infection. Whenever nitrite is positive in a urine sample, we will also see the presence of white blood cells, bacteria, and often red blood cells. A urine culture is often ordered by the physician to determine the type of bacteria and the best medication to eradicate it.

Leukocytes are white blood cells. They may either be granulocytes or agranulocytes. Either type can fight urinary tract infectious bacteria, or either type may be present in infected urine. You will learn more about specific WBCs in another chapter. The chemical reagent dip strips will only detect esterase from granulocytes and will not detect the presence of agranulocytes, so a microscopic examination is still important as well as a urine culture and sensitivity. These results along with the patient's symptoms will help the physician diagnose and treat the UTI.

Reagent Test Strip Quality Control. Reagent test strips are easy to use, but the complexity of the chemical testing should not be overlooked. As with any chemical reaction, each test involves multiple steps that are sensitive to temperature, time, dilution, and other factors. Outdated strips or reagents should never be used, so be sure to check the expiration date every time. To get optimum results, a certain amount of care must be taken when handling and storing the reagent strips. They must not be exposed to moisture, volatile substances, direct sunlight, or excess heat. The strips should not be removed from their original container except at the time of use. Always follow the manufacturer's instructions for storage. Test results are represented by a color change. The test result is compared with a color chart on the label of the reagent test strip container. Employees performing this test should be tested for color blindness as many of the color changes are subtle.

Reagent test strips are ready to use directly from their container. Correct QC procedures should be followed as required by CLIA '88 and the facility where the testing is performed. This usually includes using a QC urine sample (with predetermined results). All that is needed for this testing are the strips, QC specimen, and patient specimens. Procedure 30-5 explains how to perform a urinalysis chemical examination.

There are also automated urine analyzers (Figure 30-7A and B) capable of timing and reading the test strip. These instruments can be quite expensive and are

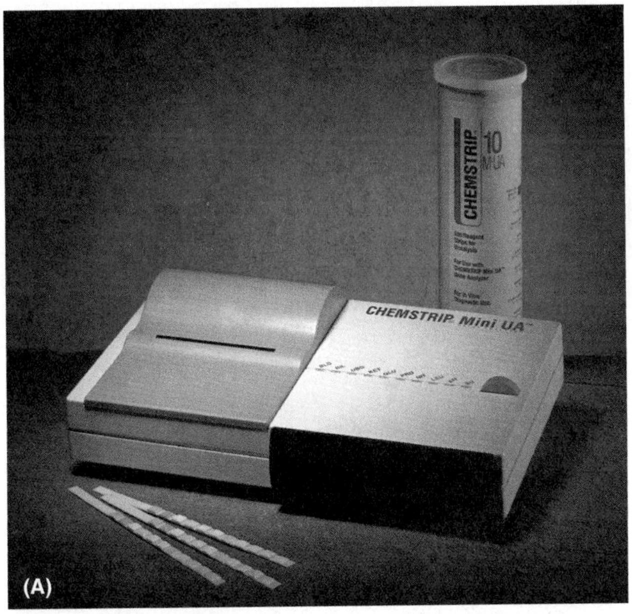

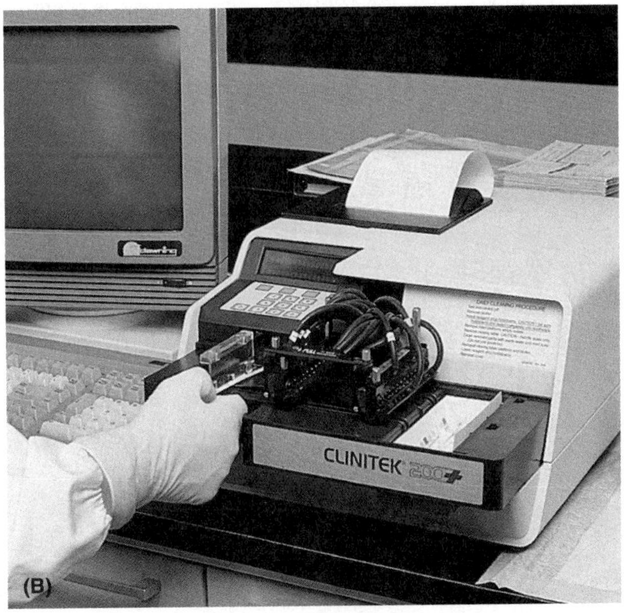

Figure 30-7 (A) The Chemstrip Mini UA Urine Analyzer is a semiautomated analyzer that provides accuracy and consistency of results when properly used. It is often used in laboratories where the volume of tests analyzed is less than 40 strips per hour. (Courtesy of Boehringer Mannheim.) (B) The Clinitek 200 semiautomated urine analyzer may be used in larger laboratories where there is a moderate to high volume of tests. Results are printed on a paper printout.

Critical Thinking

If a medical assistant is color blind, does that mean she/he cannot perform the chemical testing of urine? What (if any) accommodations can be made for her/him?

not available in small laboratories. Currently, automated urine analyzers are used more frequently because they are more accurate and cut down on human error.

When reporting results, it is important to use the proper units and terms as directed by your laboratory. An example of the sensitivity of the reagent strips is shown in Table 30-4 (there is variation in sensitivity among manufacturers).

Confirmatory Testing. Because the reagent test strips are actually **screening** tests, some positive results must be confirmed with more sensitive or specific methods. These tests include but are not limited to protein, ketones, bilirubin, and reducing sugars (to use when the glucose result is positive). Each laboratory will have a specific procedure for performing these confirmatory tests.

Protein. The most common confirmatory test for protein is the sulfosalicylic acid (SSA) test. It relies on the precipitation of protein, causing turbidity (cloudiness) in the test tube when added to a sample of urine. Urine samples should be centrifuged and a clear supernatant used. The amount of precipitate found is roughly proportional to the protein concentration present. A negative test has no cloudiness; a trace amount is barely perceptible; a 1+ result is cloudy but not granular; a 2+ result is cloudy and granular; a 3+ result is heavy cloudiness with clumping; and a 4+ result is dense with large clumps. This is a qualitative method. A semiquantitative method is available by using a set of commercially available standards and comparing the turbidity of the patient sample to that of the standards.

Ketones. The **Acetest®** is a test for ketones that is available in tablet form. **Ketones** are produced during increased metabolism of fat. If ketones are present in urine, a drop of urine added to the tablet will produce a purple color (Figure 30-8).

Bilirubin. The **Ictotest®** is a specific test for **bilirubin.** It is approximately four times as sensitive as the reagent strip method. The test includes a tablet and an absorbent mat. If bilirubin is present, a purple color will develop when a urine drop is placed on the tablet.

Reducing sugars. The **Clinitest®** uses a prepared tablet and a color reaction comparison chart to help determine the quantity of sugar in the urine. The Clinitest® is used to detect any number of sugars and other components in urine such as lactose, galactose, sucrose, fructose, and pentose, as well as uric acid, creatinine, and ascorbic acid. The chemical reagent test strips only detect glucose and are not able to detect all these reducing sugars. Screening for reducing substances is especially important in pediatric populations. Newborn babies who show a positive Clinitest® may have a serious condition called galactosemia in which they lack the enzyme necessary to convert galactose to glucose. These babies can suffer from anorexia, vomiting, and diarrhea. This condition can cause permanent brain damage and even death. The tablet used in the test contains copper sulfate, citric acid, sodium hydroxide, and sodium carbonate. The test is based on a copper reduction reaction known as the Benedict's test.

TABLE 30-4 REAGENT STRIP SENSITIVITY

Test	Range	Normal Value
pH	5–9	5–8
Protein	Negative to positive*	Negative
Glucose	Negative to >1,000 mg/dl	Negative
Ketone	Negative to >80 mg/dl	Negative
Bilirubin	Negative to large	Negative
Blood	Negative to large	Negative
Leukocyte Esterase	Negative to large	Negative
Nitrites	Negative to positive	Negative
Urobilinogen	0.2–8.0 mg/dl	2.0 mg/dl

*Note that positive results in a newborn for glucose, ketone, and protein are considered **critical values** and should be reported to the physician immediately.

Microscopic Examination of Urine Sediment

In addition to the physical and chemical examination of urine, the medical assistant should also be familiar with the microscopic examination of urine. CLIA '88 considers the microscopic examination of urine to be a PPMP and not within the category of waived tests. Neverthe-

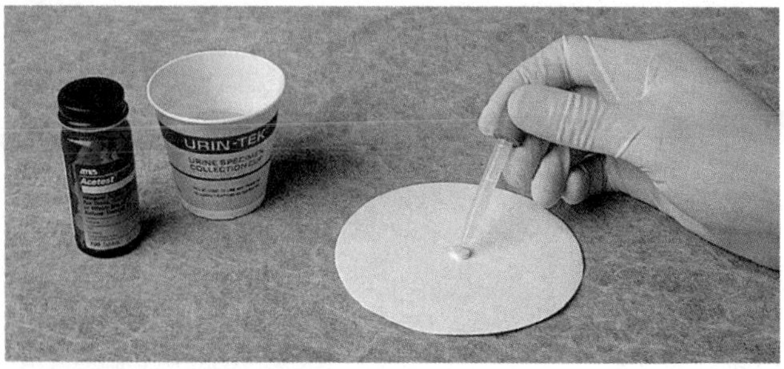

Figure 30-8 The Acetest® is a common test used to confirm the presence of ketones in urine.

less, the medical assistant must be able to properly centrifuge the specimen and set up a slide of the urine sediment for the physician to examine. It is recommended that the medical assistant have a working knowledge of all urine sediment, the pathologic significance of the components, and how to report the presence of sediment components. The **sediment** (insoluble material) at the bottom of the centrifuge tube is used for the microscopic examination (see Chapter 27 for proper use of the microscope). The microscopic examination is helpful in determining kidney disease, disorders of the urinary tract, and systemic disease. It is particularly important that urine be freshly voided and examined as soon as possible to prevent deterioration of sediment components.

One of the most important items to have on hand when performing a microscopic urine examination is a urine color atlas. It takes years to be able to correctly identify abnormal components of urine. A color atlas should always be available to the medical assistant to help with identification.

Some laboratories make use of urine stains to add color to certain structures in the urine sediment. Sedistain® is an example of such a stain. Refer to Procedure 30-5.

Sediment Components. Sediment is obtained by centrifugation of 10 to 15 ml of urine. The solid substances, such as cells and crystals, will be forced to the bottom of the test tube, leaving clear fluid called supernatant on the top. The **supernatant** urine is carefully poured off. Most urine test tubes are specifically formed to assist in the process of pouring off all but 1 ml of the supernatant fluid. This is accomplished by quickly inverting the tube completely upside down (do not shake the tube in this position). When returned to the upright position, the 1 ml of fluid will be present in the bottom of the tube, together with the urine sediment. This is the perfect amount of supernatant fluid needed to resuspend the sediment. Try the inversion process first with plain water until you are able to perform it easily. After the supernatant has been poured off, the sediment needs to be resuspended or mixed back into the 1 ml of fluid. This mixing can be accomplished by gently tapping the tube on the counter or flicking it with your finger until the sediment and cellular components have all been mixed and resupended in the fluid. A drop of sediment is then placed on a slide and examined microscopically.

When viewing a normal urine specimen, the medical assistant may see very little under the microscope. Squamous epithelial cells (Figure 30-9) may be seen, especially in women. These cells have no medical significance because they are skin cells continuously sloughed off into the urine. They are generally reported as few, moderate, or many. If the physician sees many epithelial cells in the urine specimen, it is indicative that the specimen is contaminated with skin cells. Better education of the patient of the reasons for and the technique of a clean-catch midstream collection should result in a less contaminated specimen.

Abnormal Urine Sediment Cells and Microorganisms. The methods of reporting abnormal urine sediment may vary among health facilities. Microscopic examination of the urine sediment may indicate one or more of the following cells and microorganisms:

Red blood cells. Red blood cells appear as pale, light-refractive disks when seen under high power. Large amounts of red blood cells in urine (hematuria) indicate disease or trauma. These cells are counted in a microscopic field (high-power field, or HPF) and reported as cells counted per HPF (e.g., 10/HPF).

White blood cells. A few white blood cells can appear in normal urine. More than four white blood cells in urine often indicate a UTI. White blood cells are slightly larger than red blood cells, may appear granular, and have a visible nucleus (the red blood cell has no nucleus). Figure 30-10 shows both red and white blood cells in urine.

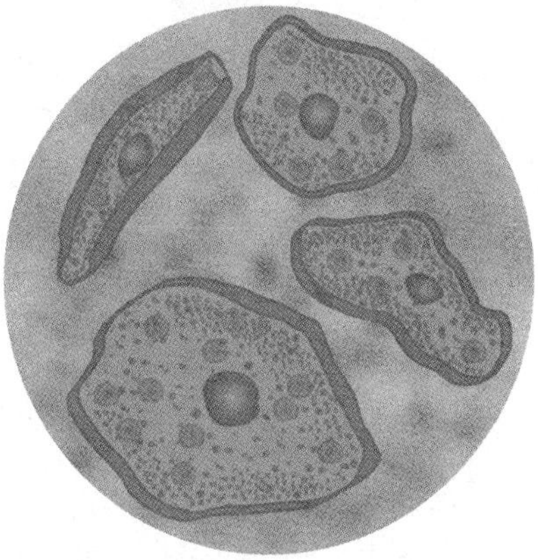

Figure 30-9 Squamous epithelial cells.

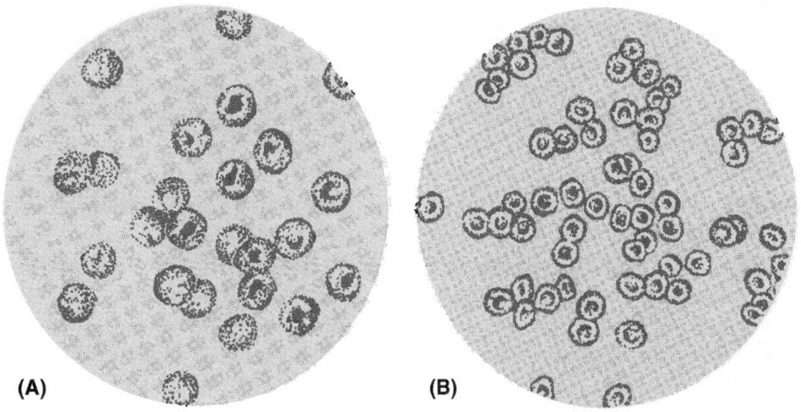

(A) (B)

Figure 30-10 (A) White blood cells in urine. (B) Red blood cells in urine.

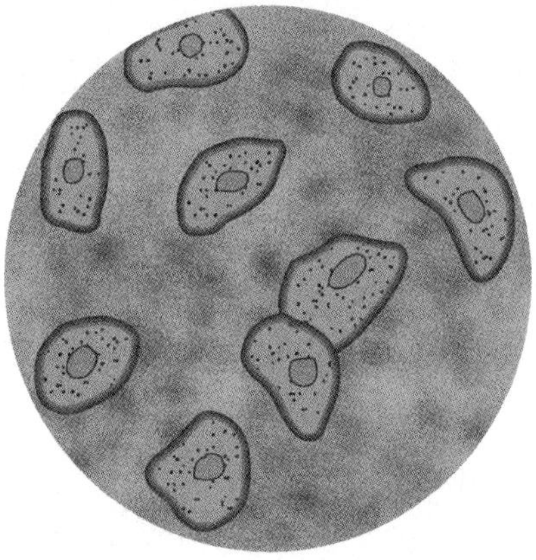

Figure 30-11 Renal epithelial cells.

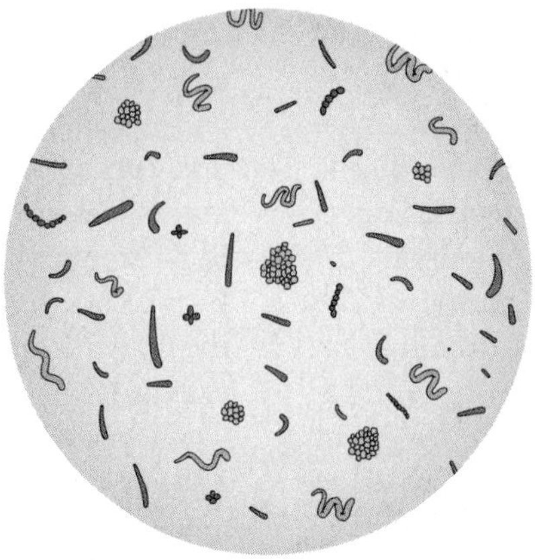

Figure 30-12 Mixed bacteria in urine.

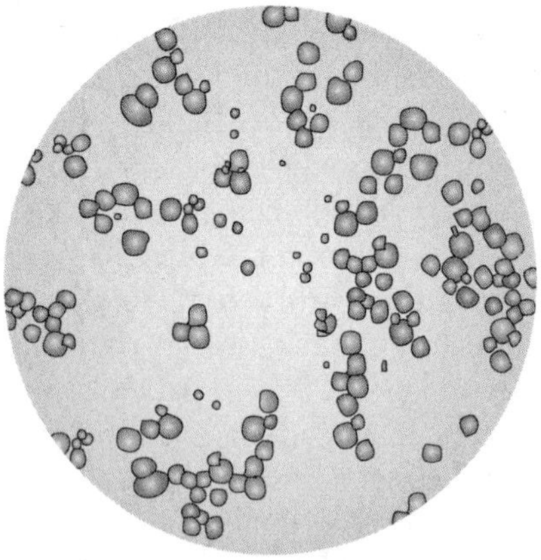

Figure 30-13 Yeast in urine.

White blood cells are reported in the same manner as red blood cells.

Renal epithelial cells. Renal epithelial cells (Figure 30-11) can indicate kidney disease if they are present in large numbers. They can be confused with both white blood cells and other epithelial cells. They are also reported in the same manner as white and red blood cells.

Bacteria. Bacteria can appear as tiny round or rod-shaped objects (Figure 30-12). Rod-shaped bacteria are generally easier to see because round bacteria may appear as **amorphous,** or shapeless, material. Bacteria often seem to be shaking or vibrating. This is called Brownian Movement and is caused by the molecules of water bumping against the bacteria. Bacteria can be active, actually moving across the microscopic field. If a lot of bacteria are seen, and the specimen is not an obviously contaminated specimen, the indication is usually a UTI. The physician will consider the presence of leukocytes and patient symptoms to make a diagnosis and will often order a C&S of the urine. Bacteria can be reported as few, moderate, many, and loaded. If both rod-shaped and round bacteria are seen in the same specimen, they may be reported as mixed bacteria.

Yeast. Yeast cells (Figure 30-13) may be present in urine, possibly indicating a yeast infection in the urinary tract. Yeast cells are smaller than red blood cells but may appear similar to them. Yeasts are round and can be observed budding. To distinguish between yeast and red blood cells if there is a question, a drop of dilute acetic acid is added to the urine sediment. The red blood cells will lyse, but the yeast will not. The most common yeast found is *Candida albicans*. Yeasts are reported as the amount per HPF.

Parasites. The most frequently seen parasite in urine is *Trichomonas vaginalis* (Figure 30-14). *Trichomonas* is a parasite that can infect the urinary tract. It is often recognized by the movement of its tail (flagella). Always check with a physician or someone more familiar with these organisms before reporting this organism.

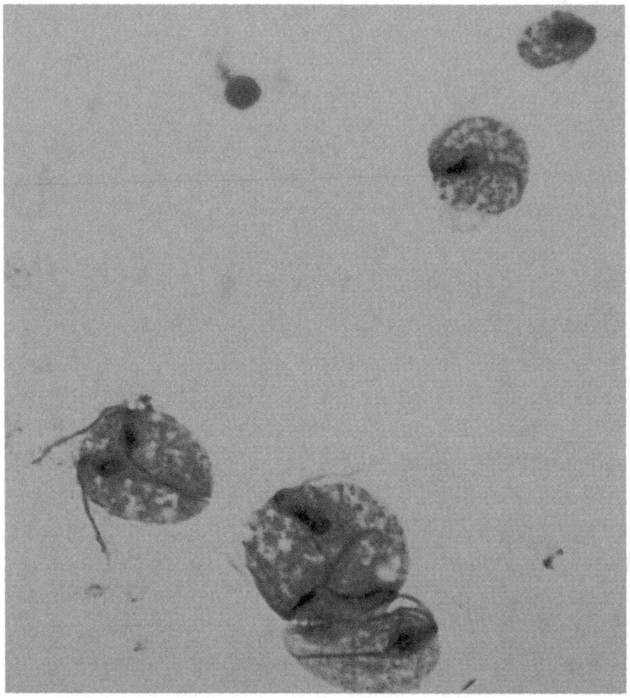

Figure 30-14 *Trichomonas* in stained urine sediment.

Sperm. Sperm is reported when seen in male and female urine. Sperm have oval bodies with one long, thin flagella (Figure 30-15A).

Artifacts. Hair, fibers, powder, and oil are among the substances that may appear in urine sediment as a result of contamination during collection or later. If a structure cannot be identified using a good urine atlas, it probably is an artifact. A urine atlas will also show illustrations of artifacts. If in doubt, get an expert opinion (see Figure 30-15B).

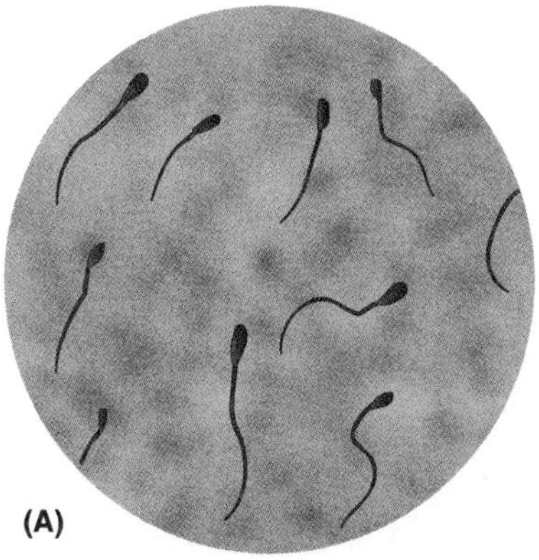

Spermatozoa in urine sediment

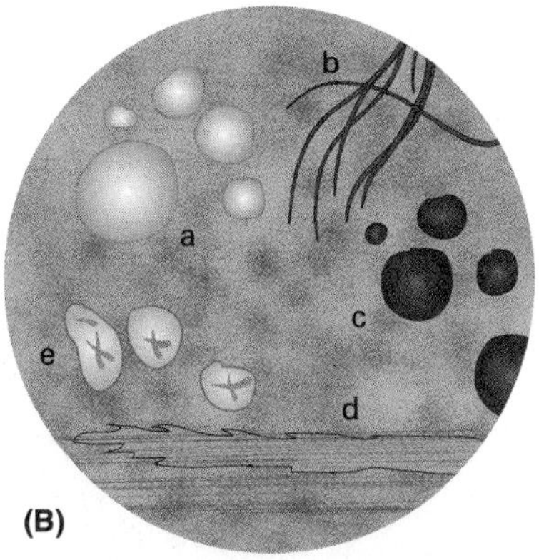

Examples of artifacts which may be seen in urine sediment: (a) air bubbles, (b) fibers, (c) oil droplets, (d) hair, (e) starch or powder granules

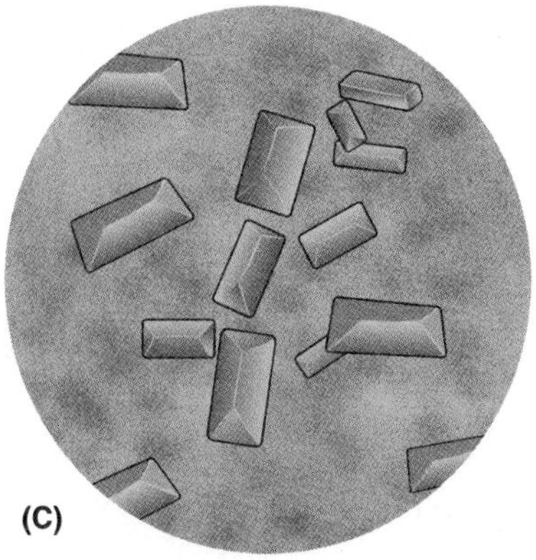

Triple phosphate crystals in urine sediment

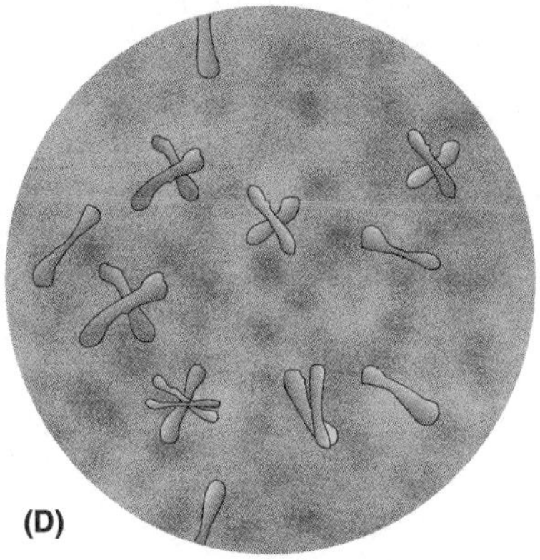

Calcium carbonate crystals in urine sediment

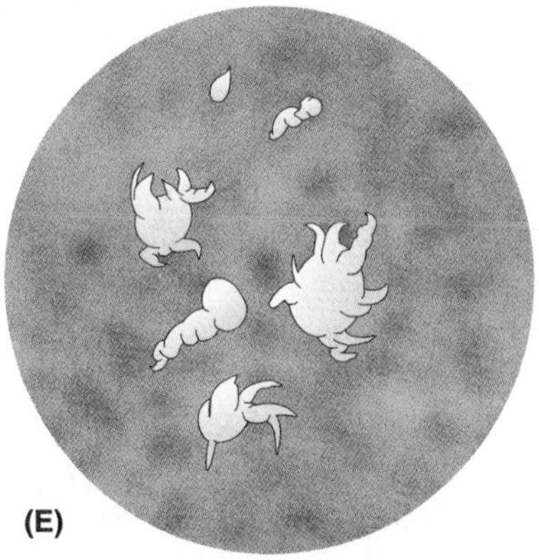

Ammonium biurate in urine sediment

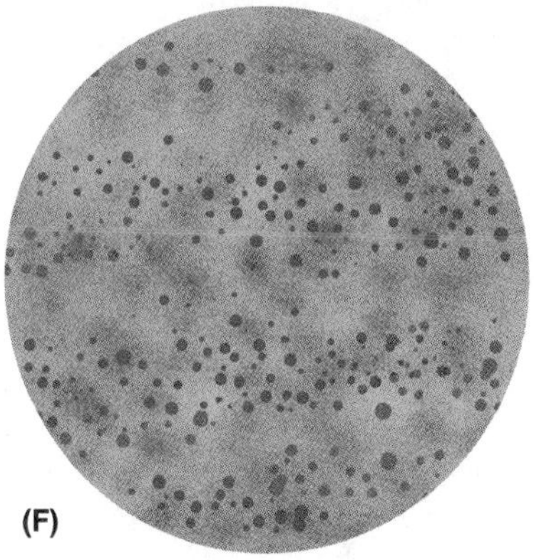

Amorphous phosphates in urine sediment

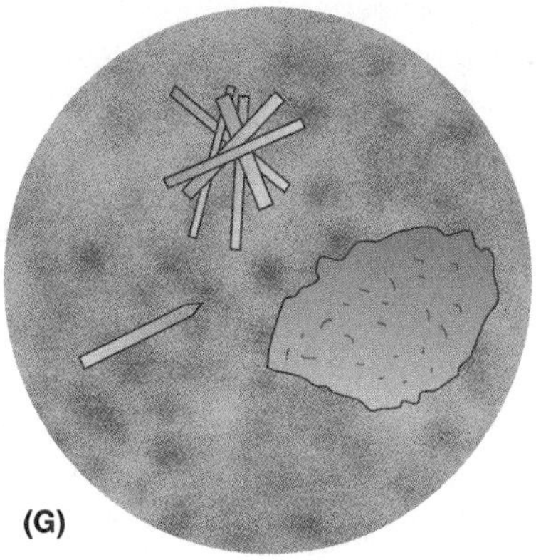

Calcium phosphate in urine sediment

Figure 30-15 Crystals and miscellaneous structures that can appear in urine.

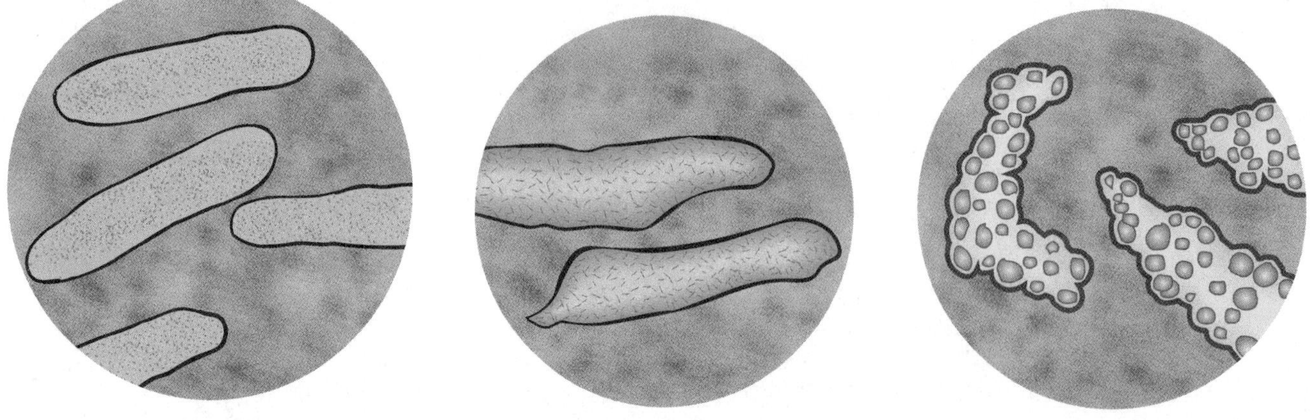

(A) Hyaline (B) Granular (C) Cellular

Figure 30-16 Casts in urine sediment. (A) Hyaline. (B) Granular. (C) Cellular.

Crystals in Urinary Sediment. Crystals make up unorganized urine sediment. Because crystals are big, the tendency of the medical assistant is to pay attention to them. However, they are the most insignificant part of the urinary sediment; thus, they require little attention. These crystals include calcium phosphate, triple phosphate, calcium oxalate, amorphous phosphates and urates, and calcium carbonate. These crystals generally form as urine specimens stand, especially when refrigerated. Many laboratories do report these crystals. Refer to a urine color atlas to identify crystals. Figure 30-15 (panels C–G) illustrates several kinds of crystals that can be found in urine.

A few crystals in urine should be particularly noted if seen because they may indicate disease states. Uric acid, cystine, and sulfa drug crystals can indicate disease states. Refer to a urine atlas to observe the shape of these crystals.

Casts in Urinary Sediment. Casts are important to see and identify in urine sediment. It takes a great deal of experience and expertise to recognize the many different kinds of casts that can be in sediment.

Casts are formed when protein accumulates and precipitates in the kidney tubules. The casts are then washed into the urine. Most casts are made from a particular type of protein called Tamm-Horsfall mucoprotein. Other proteins can also form casts. Serum proteins can form waxy casts. The presence of casts in the urine may indicate kidney disease.

Casts are cylindrical with rounded or flat ends. They are classified according to the substances observed inside them. Some casts may include debris as they are forming and may appear cellular or granular.

The most common cast seen in urine sediment is the **hyaline** cast. Rare hyaline casts can be seen in normal urine but increase with any kidney disease. They can also be seen as a result of fever, emotional stress, or strenuous exercise. Hyaline casts are nearly transparent and can be difficult to see under the microscope without some light adjustment.

Other types of casts include granular casts, containing remnants of disintegrated cells that appear as fine or coarse granules. Cellular casts may contain epithelial cells, red blood cells, or white blood cells. Figure 30-16 illustrates hyaline, granular, and cellular casts.

As mentioned before, identification of casts in urine takes an experienced eye. The medical assistant should always ask for assistance when identifying casts in urine sediment. See Procedures 30-4 and 30-5.

Patient: May Pankey | Chart # 567-89 | MA: B. Goldman CMA | **URINALYSIS** | City Health Care

Req. by: Dr. Woo | Date/Time Spec. Rec'd: 3-3-XX 10:15 AM | Date Test Completed: 3-3-XX 10:18 AM

	TEST	NORM	RESULT	TEST	NORM	RESULT
☐ VOID	Color	Yellow	lt yellow	Protein	Neg	neg.
☒ CC	Glucose	Neg	neg.	Nitrite	Neg	neg.
☐ CATH	Ketone	Neg	neg.	Leuk	Neg	neg.
☐ TURBID	Sp. Gr.	1.001-1.030	1.010			
☐ HAZY	Blood	Neg	neg.			
☒ CLEAR	Ph	5 – 8	6.0			

MICRO

TEST	NORM	RESULT	TEST	NORM	RESULT
WBC	0 – 2	–0–	Bact.	Trace	tr.
RBC	0 – 2	–0–	Mucus	None	–0–
Epith.	Few	rare	Casts	Occ	–0–
Cryst.	None	–0–			

OTHER: J. Woo

Figure 30-17 A sample of a completed urinalysis report.

Urinalysis Report

When reporting the results of a urinalysis, you may use a ready-made form, or your clinic may create a form specifically for your practice. The report should contain the patient's name, the type of urine specimen (voided or catheterized and if it was a clean-catch, midstream specimen), the doctor who ordered the urinalysis, the medical assistant performing the physical and chemical portions of the urinalysis, the date and time the specimen was obtained and the date and time it was tested, and the findings (see Figure 30-17 for an example of a urinalysis report).

Procedure 30-1 Assessing Urine Volume, Color, and Clarity

STANDARD PRECAUTIONS:

PURPOSE:

Determine and document the volume of a urine sample.

EQUIPMENT/SUPPLIES:

Gloves	Biohazard container
Urine container	Disinfectant cleaner
Laboratory report form	

PROCEDURE STEPS:

1. Wash hands and put on gloves. RATIONALE: Washing hands before any laboratory process prevents contamination of the specimen. Gloving provides personal protection.
2. Assemble equipment and supplies. RATIONALE: Organizing your work area prevents confusion and error caused by missing supplies.
3. Follow all safety guidelines, being careful not to splash the urine specimen. Wipe up all spills immediately with disinfectant cleaner. RATIONALE: Preventing splashes and spill will prevent exposure to biohazardous substances. Cleaning any spill immediately prevents further contamination and risk for exposure.
4. Examine the specimen for proper labeling. Any unlabeled specimen is not to be tested. If the missing, unlabeled specimen cannot be identified, the patient should be notified to submit a new specimen. The physician ordering the test should be notified of the delay. The specimen should be labeled on the cup, not the lid. RATIONALE: An unlabeled specimen cannot be proven to come from any particular patient and we should never guess or assume whose specimen it is. The physician should be notified so he or she is kept informed about the processing of laboratory tests he or she orders. The specimen should be labeled on the cup rather than the lid, because the lid can be removed from the specimen and mixed up with other lids.
5. Assure the lid is securely tightened and mix the urine thoroughly. RATIONALE: Securing the lid will prevent leaking of urine while mixing. Mixing the specimen will suspend all particles and cellular components in the specimen so the urine that is poured into the centrifuge tube contains a good sampling of the specimen.
6. Measure and note the amount of urine in the specimen if it is less than 10 ml. The amount of the specimen does not have to be noted if it is more than 10 ml. RATIONALE: If the sample is less than 10 ml, the sample is considered an inadequate amount. If unable to obtain an adequate amount, the testing may still be run on the sample, but the exact amount of the specimen should be well noted on the laboratory report form, and the test should be run according to the priority set by the physician. For example, he or she may request only a C&S be performed or only chemical testing using chemical reagent dip strips rather than a complete urinalysis. Samples that are not of adequate quantity to perform the test ordered should be marked as QNS (quantity not sufficient).
7. Next, the urine color should be assessed and noted. Many medical assistants find it helpful to assess the color against a white background. Be sure to have good lighting. In the practice

(continues)

Procedure 30-1 (continued)

setting, comparing a variety of urine specimens with each other will help with learning about color assessment. Refer to Table 30-2 for appropriate urine color descriptors. RATIONALE: The color of urine is helpful in predicting the concentration of the specimen. The white background helps with assessment of the color, and good lighting also is helpful. Urine color names should come only from accepted color descriptors, not from arbitrary names.

8. After the volume and color have been assessed and recorded, the clarity of the urine is assessed. Holding the urine against a white background with good lighting, observe it for cloudiness. If you can clearly see print through the urine, it is said to be clear. If the urine appears cloudy, it is said to be slightly cloudy, cloudy, or very cloudy/turbid. Record the description on the report form. RATIONALE: The clarity of the urine is useful in predicting the presence of contaminants such as skin cells, mucus, and other debris.
9. Dispose of the specimen into the toilet or designated sink and all supplies into appropriate biohazard containers. Disinfect all reusable equipment and all surfaces. RATIONALE: Using appropriate disposal techniques and disinfecting all surfaces according to Standard Precautions safely controls all biohazard substances.
10. Remove gloves. Wash hands.
11. Document the procedure.

Procedure 30-2 Using the Refractometer to Measure Specific Gravity

STANDARD PRECAUTIONS:

PURPOSE:

Measure and record the specific gravity of a urine specimen.

EQUIPMENT/SUPPLIES:

Refractometer	Lint-free tissues
Urine sample	Biohazard container
Gloves	Disinfectant cleaners
Pipettes	Laboratory report form
Distilled water	

PROCEDURE STEPS:

1. Wash hands and put on gloves. RATIONALE: Washing hands before any laboratory process prevents contamination of the specimen. Gloving provides personal protection.
2. Assemble equipment and supplies. RATIONALE: Organizing your work area prevents confusion and error caused by missing supplies.
3. Follow all safety guidelines, being careful not to splash the urine specimen. Wipe up all spills immediately with disinfectant cleaner. RATIONALE: Preventing splashes and spills will prevent exposure to biohazardous substances. Cleaning any spill immediately prevents further contamination and risk for exposure.
4. QC must be performed on the refractometer before every use. This is accomplished by checking the specific gravity of a drop of distilled water:
   a. Clean the surface of the prism and the cover with lint-free tissue and distilled water. Wipe dry.
   b. Depending on the type of refractometer used, you may either apply the drop and then close the cover, or close the cover and apply the

(continues)

Procedure 30-2 (continued)

drop of distilled water to the notched portion of the cover so it flows over the prism. (Figure 30-18).

c. With the instrument tilted to allow light to enter, view the scale and read the specific gravity number (Figure 30-19). It should be exactly 1.000.

d. If the QC test shows the refractometer to be calibrated properly, you may record the results on your QC sheet and proceed to test the urine specimen (Step 5). If the QC test shows the refractometer to be inaccurate. If the refractometer does not measure the second sample of distilled water accurately, the instrument is not calibrated properly. Use the small screwdriver to adjust the calibration. Do this adjustment using distilled water until the gauge reads 1.000.

5. Test the urine specimen exactly as the distilled water was tested and record the specific gravity on the urinalysis report form.
6. Dispose of the specimen into the toilet or designated sink and all supplies into appropriate biohazard containers. Disinfect all reusable equipment and all surfaces. RATIONALE: Using appropriate disposal techniques and disinfecting all surfaces according to Standard Precautions safely controls all biohazard substances.

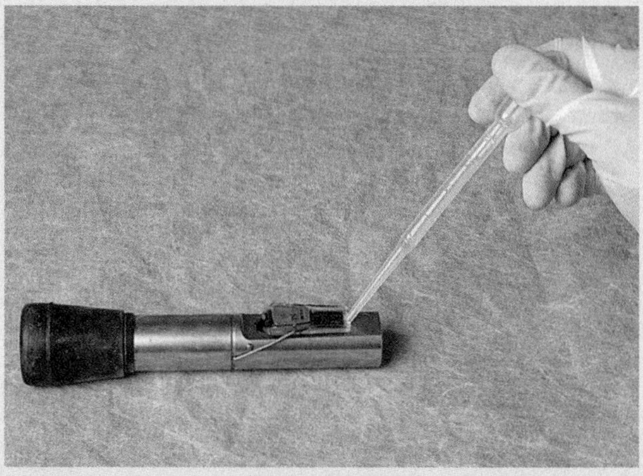

Figure 30-18 A pipette or dropper may be used to fill the refractometer with urine.

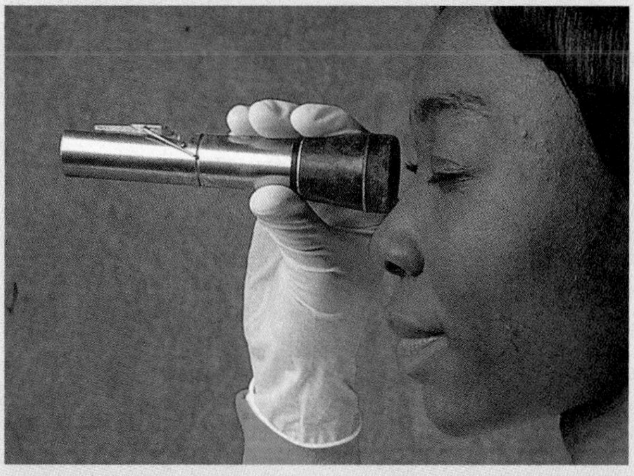

Figure 30-19 The medical assistant looks through the refractometer. The instrument is held toward a light source.

Procedure 30-3 Performing a Urinalysis Chemical Examination

STANDARD PRECAUTIONS:

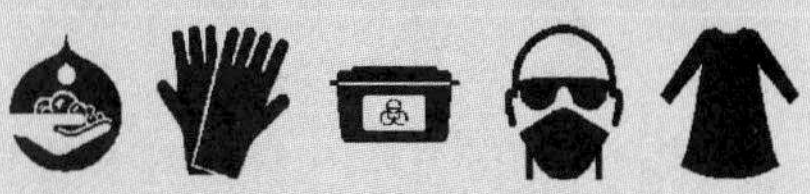

PURPOSE:

Detect any abnormal chemical constituents of a urine specimen.

EQUIPMENT/SUPPLIES:

Gloves
Urine test strips
Urine specimen
Biohazard container
Disinfectant cleaner
Laboratory report form

PROCEDURE STEPS:

1. Wash hands and put on gloves. RATIONALE: Washing hands before any laboratory process prevents contamination of the specimen. Gloving provides personal protection.
2. Assemble equipment and supplies. RATIONALE: Organizing your work area prevents confusion and error caused by missing supplies.
3. Follow all safety guidelines, being careful not to splash the urine specimen. Wipe up all spills immediately with disinfectant cleaner. RATIONALE: Preventing splashes and spills will prevent exposure to biohazardous substances. Cleaning any spill immediately prevents further contamination and risk for exposure.
4. Examine the specimen for proper labeling. Any unlabeled specimen is not to be tested. If the missing, unlabeled specimen cannot be identified, the patient should be notified to submit a new specimen. The physician ordering the test should be notified of the delay. The specimen should be labeled on the cup, not the lid. RATIONALE: An unlabeled specimen cannot be proven to come from any particular patient and we should never guess or assume whose specimen it is. The physician should be notified so he or she is kept informed about the processing of laboratory tests he or she orders. The cup should be labeled on the cup rather than the lid, because the lid can be removed from the specimen and mixed up with other lids.
5. Assure the lid is securely tightened and mix the urine thoroughly. RATIONALE: Securing the lid will prevent leaking of urine while mixing. Mixing the specimen will suspend all particles and cellular components in the specimen so the urine that is poured into the centrifuge tube contains a good sampling of the specimen.
6. If you are planning to perform a complete urinalysis, label a urine centrifuge tube with the patient's name and pour 10 ml into the tube for the microscopic examination. Set aside in the centrifuge. RATIONALE: Setting this portion of the sample aside assures that it is not contaminated by the chemicals of the test strips or the process of the chemical examination.
7. Read and follow the manufacturer's instructions exactly. The following procedure is a basic guideline. RATIONALE: Each manufacturer will provide specific instructions related to their product. Even manufacturers whose test strips you are already familiar with could change their instructions. The package insert should be read carefully every time a new package is used.
8. Remove a test strip from the container and replace the cap tightly. RATIONALE: Strips are adversely affected by light and moisture and should always be kept sterile in the original container with the lid securely on.
9. Immerse the test strip completely in the well-mixed urine and remove it immediately (Figure 30-20A). While removing the test strip from the cup, tap it gently onto a paper towel to remove excess urine (Figure 30-20B). RATIONALE: Removing the excess urine prevents the specimen from cross contamination of adjacent chemical pads on the strip, which can cause inaccurate results.
10. Properly time the test for each test pad. RATIONALE: Proper timing is essential for accurate results. The manufacturer's instructions will clearly list the proper time for each test.
11. Holding the test strip close to the container (or chart), but not touching it, compare the color of

(continues)

Procedure 30-3 (continued)

the pads on the test strip with the color guides on the container (or chart) (Figure 30-20C). RATIONALE: Touching the chart or container with the wet test strip will contaminate the chart/container with urine. If this accidentally happens, be sure to disinfect the surface well.

12. Record the results on the laboratory report form.
13. Dispose of the specimen into the toilet or designated sink and all supplies into appropriate biohazard containers. Disinfect all reusable equipment and all surfaces. RATIONALE: Using appropriate disposal techniques and disinfecting all surfaces according to Standard Precautions safely controls all biohazard substances.
14. Remove gloves. Wash hands.
15. Document the procedure.

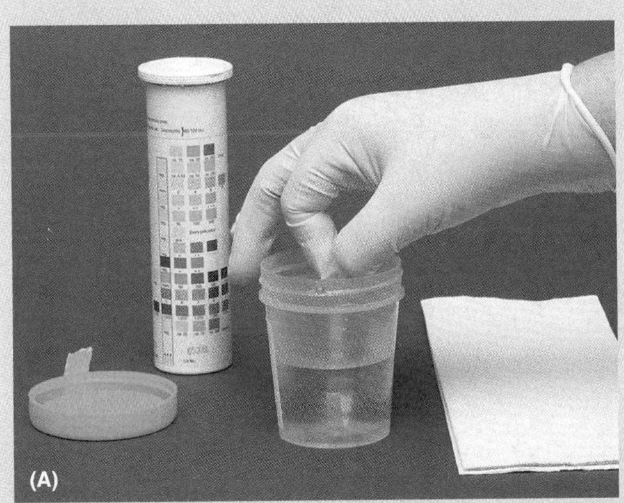
(A)

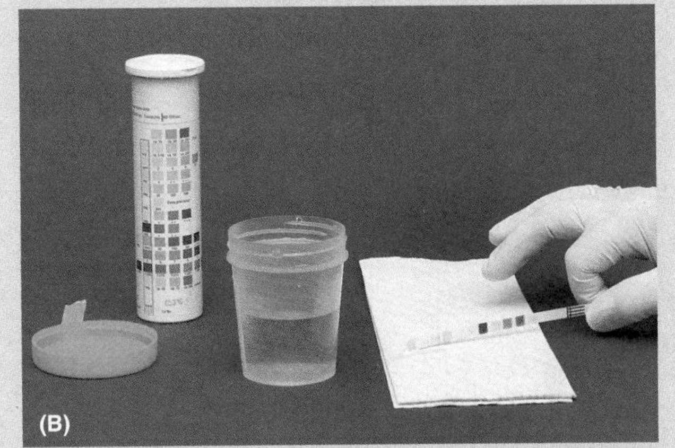
(B)

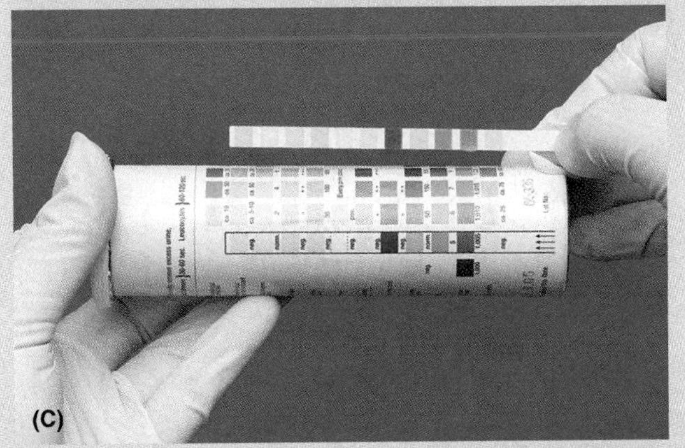
(C)

Figure 30-20 Performing a chemical examination of urine. (A) Immerse the reagent strip into the urine. (B) Remove the strip, tap it lightly on a paper towel to remove excess urine. (C) Read the strip by matching the color on the strip to the color chart. Take care not to touch the strip onto the color chart.

Procedure 30-4 Preparing Slide for Microscopic Examination of Urine Sediment

STANDARD PRECAUTIONS:

PURPOSE:

Prepare slide for a microscopic examination of urine sediment.

EQUIPMENT/SUPPLIES:

Gloves	Sharps container
Microscope	Centrifuge tubes and holder
Centrifuge	Urine atlas guide
Microscope slides	Disinfectant cleaner
Coverslips	Biohazard container
Disposable pipettes	SediStain (optional)

PROCEDURE STEPS:

1. Wash hands and put on gloves. RATIONALE: Washing hands before any laboratory process prevents contamination of the specimen. Gloving provides personal protection.
2. Assemble equipment and supplies. RATIONALE: Organizing your work area prevents confusion and error caused by missing supplies.
3. Follow all safety guidelines, being careful not to splash the urine specimen. Wipe up all spills immediately with disinfectant cleaner. RATIONALE: Preventing splashes and spills will prevent exposure to biohazardous substances. Cleaning any spill immediately prevents further contamination and risk for exposure.
4. Examine the specimen for proper labeling. Any unlabeled specimen is not to be tested. If the missing, unlabeled specimen cannot be identified, the patient should be notified to submit a new specimen. The physician ordering the test should be notified of the delay. The specimen should be labeled on the cup, not the lid. RATIONALE: An unlabeled specimen cannot be proven to come from any particular patient and we should never guess or assume whose specimen it is. The physician should be notified so he or she is kept informed about the processing of laboratory tests she or he orders. The cup should be labeled on the cup rather than the lid, because the lid can be removed from the specimen and mixed up with other lids.
5. Assure the lid is securely tightened and mix the urine thoroughly. RATIONALE: Securing the lid will prevent leaking of urine while mixing. Mixing the specimen will suspend all particles and cellular components in the specimen so that the urine poured into the centrifuge tube contains a good sampling of the specimen.
6. Label a urine centrifuge tube with the patient's name and pour 10 ml into the tube. Set into the centrifuge. Balance the centrifuge, securely close and lock the lid, and spin at 1,500 *g* (revolutions per minute) for five minutes. RATIONALE: The urine sediment will be forced to the bottom of the test tube and then will be placed on a slide for microscopic examination.
7. After centrifugation, pour off the supernatant, leaving about 1 ml in the bottom of the tube. Add two drops of SediStain if desired. Remix the sediment by tapping gently on the counter or with your fingernail. RATIONALE: The test will be performed on the sediment only so the excess supernatant is not needed. SediStain colors the cells and other elements for easier viewing.
8. Place a drop of the well-mixed sediment onto a clean microscope slide. Cover with a coverslip by holding the coverslip at an angle to the drop, bringing the edge close to the drop until the urine spreads along the edge of the coverslip, and then gently lower the coverslip onto the drop. Keep the tube. RATIONALE: Using this technique to place the coverslip onto the specimen will prevent air pockets from forming. Keep the tube in the event that a fresh slide needs to be prepared.
9. Place the slide onto the microscope stage but do not leave the light on. RATIONALE: Do not leave the light on because this will heat the slide and destroy the specimen.
10. Alert the physician that the slide is ready for viewing. RATIONALE: The microscopic examination is considered by CLIA to be in the moderately complex test category of PPM Procedures. You are encouraged to view and discuss the microscopic examination with the physician as part of your professional development and continuing education. If you do view the slide before the physician views it, do not leave on

(continues)

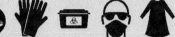

Procedure 30-4 (continued)

the light. If the slide dries before the physician can view it, prepare a fresh slide.

11. NOTE: The following steps are included so the medical assistant can learn to examine urine microscopically even though the physician must perform the actual assessment.
    a. When examining urine sediment, it is important to keep the light subdued by lowering the condenser and to constantly vary the fine focus adjustment to view the structures that are faint. Proper lighting and focus adjustments take a great deal of practice.
    b. Scan the sediment using a 100× (low-power) magnification. A 100× magnification is achieved by using the 10× objective lens (10× × 10× = 100×).
    c. View 10 to 15 fields and around the edges of the slide for casts. Casts are often forced to the edges. It may be necessary to use the 40× objective (400× magnification) to identify the casts.
    d. Scan the slide using the 40× objective (400× 5 high magnification) for other cells and formed elements. The count is obtained by averaging the number of each formed element or cell in 10 to 15 visualized fields.
12. After the physician is finished with the specimen and the patient has left the clinic, dispose of the specimen into the toilet or designated sink and all used supplies into appropriate biohazard containers. Disinfect all reusable equipment and all surfaces. RATIONALE: Using appropriate disposal techniques and disinfecting all surfaces according to Standard Precautions safely controls all biohazard substances. Remember that microscopic slides and coverslips are glass and should be placed into an appropriate biohazard sharps container.

Procedure 30-5 Performing a Complete Urinalysis

STANDARD PRECAUTIONS:

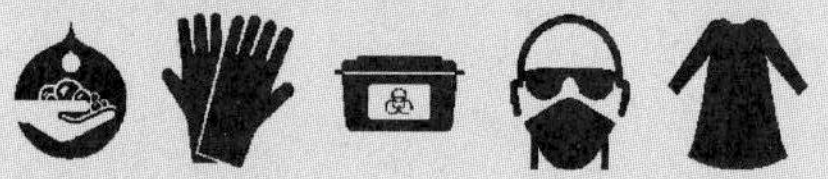

PURPOSE:

Perform a complete urinalysis, including the physical, chemical, and microscopic examination within 30 minutes of obtaining the specimen.

EQUIPMENT/SUPPLIES:

- Gloves
- Urine specimen
- Pipettes
- Centrifuge tube
- Centrifuge
- Microscope
- Microscope slides
- Coverslip
- Permanent marker
- SediStain (optional)
- Reagent test strips (dipsticks)
- Urine atlas
- Refractometer
- Distilled water
- Lint-free tissues
- Biohazard container
- Sharps container
- Disinfectant cleaner
- Laboratory report form

PROCEDURE STEPS:

NOTE: The following procedure is a compilation and summary of the physical, chemical, and microscopic examination of urine (see Procedures 30-1, 30-2, 30-3, and 30-4). For details within each step, refer to the specific procedure as referenced.

1. Wash hands and put on gloves.
2. Assemble equipment and supplies.
3. Follow all safety guidelines.
4. Examine the specimen for proper labeling.
5. Assure the lid is securely tightened and mix the urine thoroughly.
6. Label a urine centrifuge tube with the patient's name, pour 10 ml into the tube and set it into the centrifuge. Balance the centrifuge, securely close and lock the lid, and spin at 1,500 g (revolutions per minute) for five minutes.
7. While the sample is being centrifuged, assess and record the color and clarity.

(continues)

Procedure 30-5 (continued)

8. Perform the specific gravity test using a refractometer if specific gravity is not included in the chemical test strip.
9. Perform the chemical examination following the manufacturer's instructions. Record the results.
10. After centrifugation, pour off the supernatant, leaving about 1 ml in the bottom of the tube. Add two drops of SediStain if desired. Remix the sediment by tapping gently on the counter or with your fingernail.
11. Place a drop of the well-mixed sediment onto a clean microscope slide. Cover with a coverslip.
12. Place the slide onto the microscope stage and alert the physician that the slide is ready for viewing.
13. Dispose of the specimen into the toilet or designated sink and all supplies into appropriate biohazard containers. Disinfect all reusable equipment and all surfaces. Remember that microscopic slides and coverslips are glass and should be placed into an appropriate biohazard sharps container.
14. File the completed laboratory report form into the laboratory section of the patient's medical record/chart and document the procedure.

DOCUMENTATION

11/13/XX 4:15 PM Complete urinalysis performed on random voided specimen. Report filed. Joe Guerrero, CMA

Procedure 30-6 Utilizing a Urine Transport System for C&S

STANDARD PRECAUTIONS:

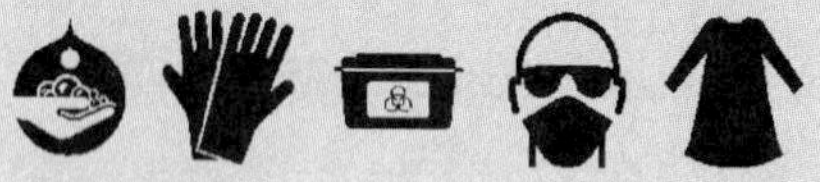

PURPOSE:

Prepare a urine specimen for transport using a Culture and Sensitivity Transport Kit.

EQUIPMENT/SUPPLIES:

Gloves
Sterile urine cup and specimen
Urine Culture and Sensitivity Transport kit
Laboratory requisition
Paper towel

PROCEDURE STEPS:

1. Wash hands and put on gloves. RATIONALE: Washing hands before any laboratory process prevents contamination of the specimen. Gloving provides personal protection.
2. Assemble equipment and supplies (Figure 30-21A shows one type of system). RATIONALE: Organizing your work area prevents confusion and error caused by missing supplies.
3. Follow all safety guidelines, being careful not to splash the urine specimen. Wipe up all spills immediately with disinfectant cleaner. RATIONALE: Preventing splashes and spills will prevent exposure to biohazardous substances. Cleaning any spill immediately prevents further contamination and risk for exposure.
4. Examine the specimen for proper labeling. RATIONALE: The specimen cup must be properly labeled to assure QC.

(continues)

Procedure 30-6 (continued)

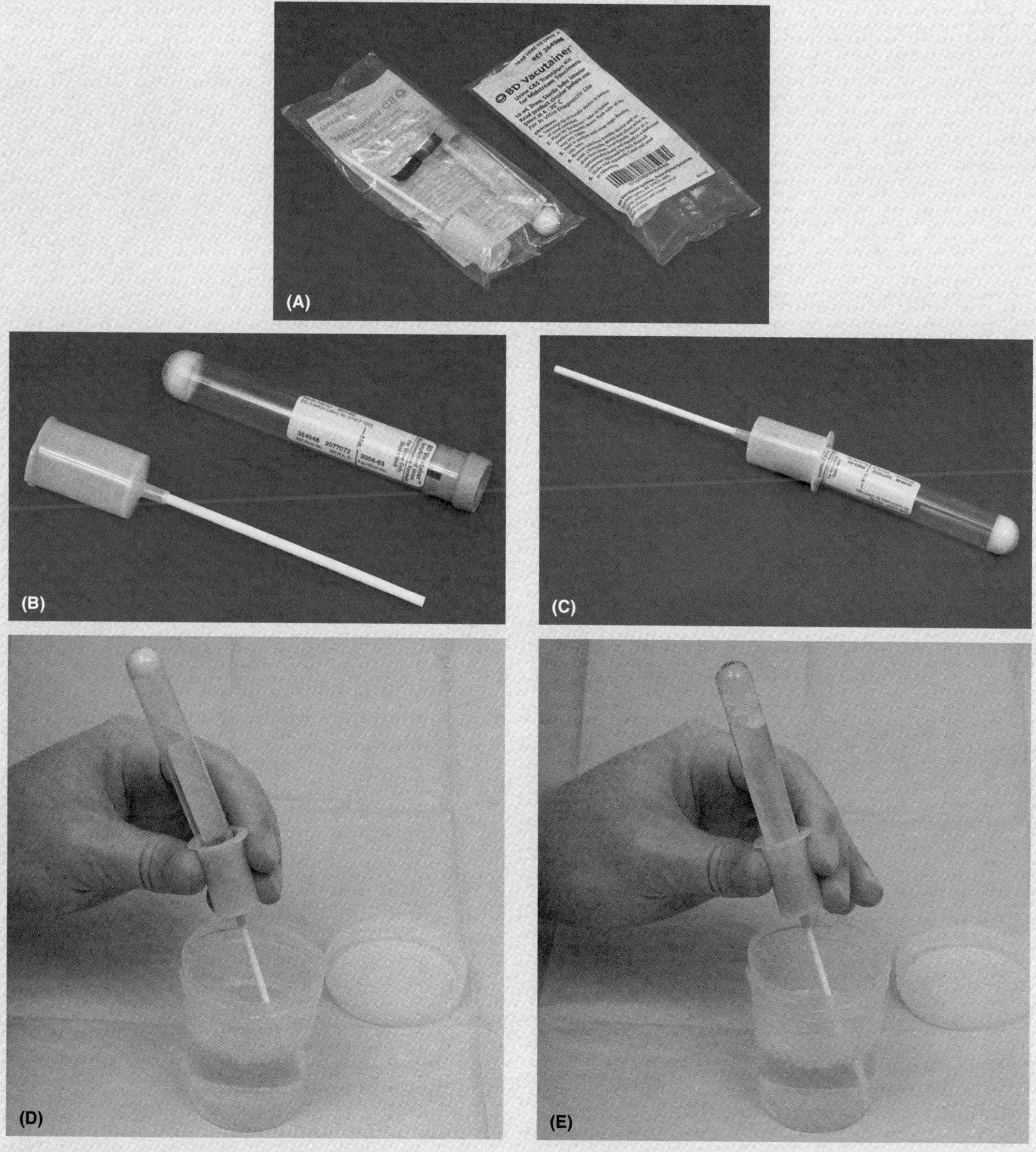

Figure 30-21 The urine transport kit for culture and sensitivity (C&S). (A) Packaged as a kit. (B) The components of the kit. (C) The tube is connected to the straw and adaptor. (D) The end of the straw is placed in the urine (the vacuum tube is not pushed completely onto the adaptor until the straw is submerged in the urine). (E) The vacuum in the tube draws up the urine.

Procedure 30-6 (continued)

5. Check the urine C&S Transport kit expiration date. RATIONALE: If the kit has expired, the contents cannot be guaranteed sterile.
6. Open the urine C&S Transport kit package (Figure 30-21B). Remove the cap from the specimen cup, placing the lid upside down on the paper towel. RATIONALE: The cap must be placed upside down to maintain the sterile inner surface.
7. Follow the manufacturer's instructions exactly:
   a. Place the urine tube in the tube adapter (Figure 30-21C) and the specimen straw into the urine within the specimen cup (Figure 30-21D).
   b. Advance urine tube into the adapter, pushing the tube onto the needle while keeping the specimen straw submerged in the urine.
   c. Allow the vacuum in the urine tube to draw up the urine. Fill to the exhaustion of the vacuum within the tube (Figure 30-21E).
   d. Remove the tube and the specimen straw/adapter unit and dispose of it into a biohazard container.
   e. Gently invert the tube 8 to 10 times to mix the preservative within the tube.
8. Label the tube with patient's name, date, time, and other required information. RATIONALE: labeling with the required information prevents mix-ups of specimens and assures a quality timeline.
9. Dispose of all contaminated supplies, disinfect all surfaces, remove gloves, and wash hands. RATIONALE: Using appropriate disposal techniques and disinfecting all surfaces according to Standard Precautions safely controls biohazard substances.
10. Complete the laboratory requisition and document the procedure in the patient's chart/medical record. RATIONALE: Proper documentation assures the laboratory will have the necessary information and the patient's medical record will be accurate and complete.

Procedure 30-7 Instructing a Patient in the Collection of a Clean-Catch, Midstream Urine Specimen

PURPOSE:

To instruct a patient in the proper technique of collecting a urine specimen suitable for urinalysis testing.

EQUIPMENT AND SUPPLIES:

Gloves
Urine cup with a secure lid
Cleansing towelettes (2 for males, 3 for females)
Marking pen

PROCEDURE STEPS:

1. Wash hands and assemble the supplies. RATIONALE: Always wash hands before working with each patient as a means of preventing disease transmission. Being organized assures that the procedure will be performed in a professional manner.
2. Identify the patient, introduce yourself, and provide for a private area free from distractions. RATIONALE: Identifying the patient assures that the right patient will have the right procedure. Intoducing yourself provides for a professional rapport with the patient. Providing for a private area assures that the patient will have the freedom to ask questions and that confidentiality will be maintained. Being in an area that is free from distractions allows you to use a moderate

(continues)

Procedure 30-7 (continued)

voice volume and still be heard and understood by the patient.

3. Provide the patient with a capped urine cup labeled with his/her name, a pair of gloves, and the cleansing towelettes. RATIONALE: The cup should be labeled (not the cap) prior to giving it to the patient so there is not a chance of a mixup. Gloves will protect the patient's hand from containimation from the urine and from the genital area, the towelettes will be used for cleansing the area prior to obtaining the sample.
4. Show the patient the written instructions posted in the bathroom. RATIONALE: The patient should always have written instructions in case he or she forgets a step and the instructions should be posted at a level that can be read by the female patient while sitting and the male patient while standing.
5. Explain to the patient why the urine sample should be a midstream clean-catch sample and what that means. RATIONALE: When the patient understands the reasons behind the instructions, he or she is much more likely to follow the steps completely.
6. Ask the patient to first wash his or her hands and apply the gloves. RATIONALE: Gloves are worn to protect the patient's hands from contamination.
7. Explain the cleansing process for a clean-catch: For the male patient, explain that he is to cleanse the urethral opening twice, using two separate towelettes before he begins to urinate. For the female patient, explain that she will need to spread her labia and cleanse from front to back first on one side, then the other, and lastly, in the middle. Explain that she is to hold her labia apart until the urine sample is obtained. RATIONALE: Cleansing the urethral opening assures that the sample will have no or few epithelial cells from the skin. Epithelial cells are quite large and can make the urine difficult to evaluate microscopically because the bacteria and other cells can be hidden behind them.
8. Explain the process of obtaining the midstream specimen: For both the male and the female patients, he or she is to bring the cup into the stream and obtain about half a cup before removing the cup from the stream. RATIONALE: The mid-stream catch is used to further prevent epithelial cells from entering the sample. If the patient were to stop and start the urine flow, the chances of epithelial contamination increases.
9. Explain to the patient that he or she should then secure the cap onto the cup. RATIONALE: The secure lid will prevent spillage.
10. The patient may rinse the outside of the capped cup if needed and towel dry it. RATIONALE: Rinsing and drying the outside of the cup will remove any urine that may be present.
11. The patient is to then remove the gloves, dispose of them into the red bag waste recepticle, and wash his or her hands. RATIONALE: Contaminated waste should always go into red bag recepticles. Hands should be washed to remove any residual powder from the gloves and/or contamination that may have touched the hands.
12. Using a paper towel as a barrier, the cup may be returned to the medical assistant or placed in the lab recepticle as directed. RATIONALE: The POL often has a shelf or designated area for the patient to place the urine sample onto. If not, the sample may be handed to the medical assistant. The paper towel creates a barrier between the specimen and the hand.

Case Study 30-1

Annette Samuels came to Inner City Health Care today because she is experiencing frequent urination, itching, and burning when urinating. Dr. Rice ordered a urinalysis, which clinical medical assistant Wanda Slawson is performing. Wanda notes that the urine has a cloudy appearance and the dipstick tests positive for nitrites. Wanda confers with Dr. Rice, who instructs her to prepare a slide for a microscopic examination of the specimen.

CASE STUDY REVIEW

1. Why does Dr. Rice want this specimen examined microscopically?
2. What should Wanda expect to find if she examines the specimen?
3. How would the findings be reported?

SUMMARY

This chapter summarizes the basics of the urinalysis. Physicians order a variety of tests on urine to help them determine or rule out certain abnormalities to make a correct diagnosis and prescribe treatment.

Urine is formed as blood is filtered through the kidney. Substances such as by-products of metabolism, mineral excesses, cells, bacteria, parasites, crystals, and casts can be found in the urine during examination.

It is important for the medical assistant to:

- Understand the proper collection techniques for urine specimens. Medical assistants often are called on to instruct patients in the proper collection procedures.
- Understand the safety guidelines involved with collecting and handling specimens, preservatives, and reagents. These guidelines must *always* be observed.
- Understand the importance of and the procedures for maintaining a consistent quality-control program.
- Understand how to properly perform the urinalysis, following up with proper confirmatory tests when necessary.
- Understand and be constantly aware of factors that may interfere with the accuracy of a urinalysis.

STUDY FOR SUCCESS

To reinforce your knowledge and skills of information presented in this chapter:

- ❑ Review the Key Terms
- ❑ Practice the Procedures
- ❑ Consider the Case Study and discuss your conclusions
- ❑ Answer the Review Questions
  - ❑ Multiple Choice
  - ❑ Critical Thinking
- ❑ Navigate the Internet by completing the Web Activities
- ❑ Practice the StudyWARE activities on the CD
- ❑ Apply your knowledge in the Student Workbook activities
- ❑ Complete the Web Tutor sections
- ❑ View and discuss the DVD situations

REVIEW QUESTIONS

Multiple Choice

1. What safety guideline is important to follow during a routine urinalysis?
   a. use the same pipette for all patients' urine samples
   b. allow urine to sit at room temperature to ferment the urine properties
   c. once tested, urine can be disposed of by the janitorial service
   d. treat all specimens as if they were infectious
2. What are the three basic parts of a typical urine examination?
   a. volumetric, chemical, and macroscopic
   b. pathologic, chemical, and confirmatory
   c. physical, chemical, and microscopic
   d. random, 24-hour, and catheterized
3. What is the specimen of choice for routine urinalysis?
   a. sterile
   b. clean-catch
   c. catheterized
   d. timed
4. A diabetic patient will normally have an excess of what substance in the urine?
   a. hemoglobin
   b. glucose
   c. insulin
   d. sodium
5. What is the most common way of doing a chemical analysis of urine in a physician's office?
   a. reagent strip test
   b. Clinitest®
   c. culture test
   d. Acetest®
6. Positive results for the following during chemical testing of newborn urine should be immediately reported to the physician:
   a. blood, pH, nitrates
   b. bilirubin, blood, leukocyte esterase
   c. pH, urobilinogen, specific gravity
   d. glucose, ketone, and protein
7. Confirmatory tests are done to:
   a. confirm negative results from initial testing
   b. confirm positive results from initial testing
   c. confirm urine volume
   d. confirm urine turbidity
8. What confirmatory urine test is done to test for evidence of incomplete fat metabolism?
   a. Clinitest®
   b. sulfosalicylic acid test
   c. Ictotest®
   d. Acetest®
9. Which substance or structure is automatically considered abnormal when found in urine?
   a. phosphates
   b. urea
   c. blood
   d. salt

Critical Thinking

1. What is the importance of proper urine collection?
2. When is a urine preservative necessary?
3. Why is the first morning specimen preferred for routine urinalysis?
4. What would give a urine sample a cloudy appearance?
5. If urine were kept at a temperature of 16°C and specific gravity were performed, what adjustment, if any, would have to be made to the results?

WEB ACTIVITIES

1. Search for CLIA information on the Internet. Are guidelines posted for specimen collection? When were these guidelines last updated?
2. According to CLIA, which tests are waived in regard to urinalysis and which tests are not?
3. Visit the CDC's Web site and review the Standard Precautions that apply to urine collection and analysis.

REFERENCES/BIBLIOGRAPHY

Walters, N. J., Estridge, B. H., & Reynold, A. P. (2000). *Basic medical laboratory techniques* (4th ed.). Clifton Park, NY: Thomson Delmar Learning.

Wedding, M. E. & Toenjes, S. A. (1998). *Medical laboratory procedures* (2nd ed.). Philadelphia: FA Davis.

THE DVD HOOK-UP

DVD Series: **Skills Based Series**
Program Number: **12**

Chapter/Scene Reference

- *Introduction to Specimen Collection and Processing Procedures*
- *Administering and Performing Urinalysis*
- *Administering 24-Hour Urine Test*

This chapter discusses common urologic procedures that are performed in the medical office.

In one of the first scenes, Dr. Rao's medical assistant Shannon explains to Mr. Bean how to collect a clean-catch urine sample.

1. What do you think about the chemistry between Shannon and Mr. Bean?
2. This chapter states that you should not touch the dipstick against the bottle when performing a chemical analysis of the urine. Did Shannon follow those guidelines? What should you do if you accidentally touch the bottle with the contaminated dipstick?
3. Today's program stated that you should not insert the dipstick into the original specimen container. Why?

DVD Journal Summary

Write a paragraph that summarizes what you learned from watching the selected scenes from today's DVD program. Mr. Bean and Shannon really struggled to connect. What could Shannon have done differently to improve her encounter with Mr. Bean? Do you think that Mr. Bean was trying to hide something?

CHAPTER 31

Basic Microbiology

OUTLINE

OBJECTIVES

The student should strive to meet the following performance objectives and demonstrate an understanding of the facts and principles presented in this chapter through written and oral communication.

1. Define the key terms as presented in the glossary.
2. Define microbiology, discussing classifications and nomenclature relevant to the microbiology laboratory.
3. Describe bacterial cell structure.

(continues)

KEY TERMS

Aerobic
Aerosols
Agar
Anaerobic
Biochemical Tests
Broth Tubes
Culture
Dermatophytes
DNA
Expectorate
Genus
Gram Stain
Holding Media
Immunosuppressed
Inoculate
Lumbar Puncture
Microbiology
Mordant
Morphology
Mycology
Nematode
Normal Flora
Nosocomial
Ova
Parasitology
Pathogen
Petri Dish
Potassium Hydroxide (KOH)
Protozoa
Quality Control
Reagents
Sensitivity
Species
Spores
Stab Culture
Taxonomy
Virology
Wet Mount
Wood's Lamp

FEATURED COMPETENCIES

CAAHEP—ENTRY-LEVEL COMPETENCIES

Clinical Competencies

Fundamental Procedures

- Dispose of biohazard materials
- Practice Standard Precautions

Specimen Collection

- Obtain specimens for microbiological testing

Diagnostic Testing

- Perform microbiology testing

General Competencies

Legal Concepts

- Perform within legal and ethical boundaries
- Document appropriately
- Demonstrate knowledge of federal and state health care legislation and regulations

Patient Instructions

- Instruct individuals according to their needs

Operational Functions

- Use methods of quality control

ABHES—ENTRY-LEVEL COMPETENCIES

Professionalism

- Conduct work within scope of education, training, and ability

Clinical Duties

- Apply principles of aseptic techniques and infection control
- Use quality control
- Collect and process specimens

(continues)

OBJECTIVES (continued)

4. List and describe the equipment used in the physicians' office laboratory (POL).
5. Explain how to safely handle microbiology specimens.
6. Describe the importance of and steps involved in quality control in the POL.
7. Explain the types of microbiology specimens collected in the POL and how they are collected.
8. List different types of stains used to microscopically observe microorganisms.
9. List the different classifications of media used in the POL and microbiology laboratory.
10. Describe how organisms are inoculated onto various media.
11. Describe the significance of sensitivity testing.
12. List two parasites and two fungi that can be observed in the POL.

SCENARIO

To aid in diagnosing and treating patients, the physicians at Drs. Lewis and King's office order tests to identify disease-causing bacteria, fungi, viruses, and parasites. Some of these tests, such as the quick tests for Group A Streptococcus, are performed in the office laboratory, whereas other tests are sent to a reference laboratory. Regardless of where the test will be performed, medical assistant Joe Guerrero follows all Safety Precautions when handling specimens. He checks the test manufacturer's or laboratory's procedures and carefully completes each step. By following all safety guidelines and test procedures, Joe ensures his and others' safety. He also obtains a high-quality specimen for testing.

FEATURED COMPETENCIES (continued)

- Perform selected tests that assist with diagnosis and treatment
- Dispose of biohazard materials
- Practice Standard Precautions
- Obtain throat culture for microbiological testing
- Perform microbiological testing

Legal Concepts

- Document accurately

Spotlight on Certification

RMA Content Outline

- Medical law
- Asepsis
- Laboratory procedures

CMA Content Outline

- Equipment preparation and operation
- Principles of operation
- Principles of infection control
- Collecting and Processing Specimens and Diagnostic Testing

CMAS Content Outline

- Legal considerations
- Aspepsis in the medical office

INTRODUCTION

The field of ***microbiology*** *encompasses the study of all microorganisms, living structures that can be seen only with the powerful magnification of a microscope. The word* microbiology *comes from the Greek words* micro *(small) and* bios *(living). The field of microbiology includes the study of such organisms as bacteria, fungi, viruses, parasites, and algae (Table 31-1).*

Many medical textbooks in microbiology include extensive study of all of the preceding organisms, including lesser known species in each category. It is the goal of this chapter to introduce the student to the field of microbiology with emphasis on bacteria, fungi, and parasites. Safety while working with microorganisms in the laboratory is emphasized. The relation of bacteria to diseases also is explored.

THE MEDICAL ASSISTANT'S ROLE IN THE MICROBIOLOGY LABORATORY

The role of the medical assistant in microbiology within the physicians' office laboratory (POL) is to obtain specimens, test specimens within the Clinical Laboratory Improvement Act (CLIA) waived categories, and prepare slides and **cultures** for microscopic examination by the physician or for transport to an outside laboratory.

This chapter discusses cultures in detail. Simply put, a culture is a sample of a body secretion that is placed on special media to allow the bacteria to grow. Some samples of cultures discussed in this chapter are throat cultures, sputum cultures, urine, blood, vaginal and penile, and wound cultures. Cultures are usually allowed to grow in optimum temperatures and environments for at least 12 hours before they are examined for identification.

In certain situations, a physician may request a **sensitivity** in addition to the culture. This is a test that will identify which antibiotic or antibiotics will effectively kill the microorganism identified as causing the infection.

In healthy individuals, several types of bacteria are found naturally in various parts of the body. These natural bacteria are called **normal flora.** These organisms are always present and help with the body's immune system. In disease, the causative microorganism is called a **pathogen** because it causes harm to the body.

The medical assistant's technique must be exact to avoid laboratory error. The medical assistant also must assure that the specimen for culture was taken with sterile supplies and delivered to the laboratory in a reasonable amount of time. Delivery time of the specimen or culture may vary depending on the type of specimen collected for culture. Some specimens may be refrigerated without harm. Some may be kept in **holding media**—media that will keep a specimen on a swab moist until it is cultured. These variations are discussed later in specimen processing.

By doing the smear, culture, and identification through biochemical tests, the microbiologist can identify the organism and aid the physician in diagnosing and treating the patient. Most identification of organisms can be done successfully within 12 to 24 hours. Some organisms may take longer to grow.

TABLE 31-1 BIOLOGIC SCIENCES

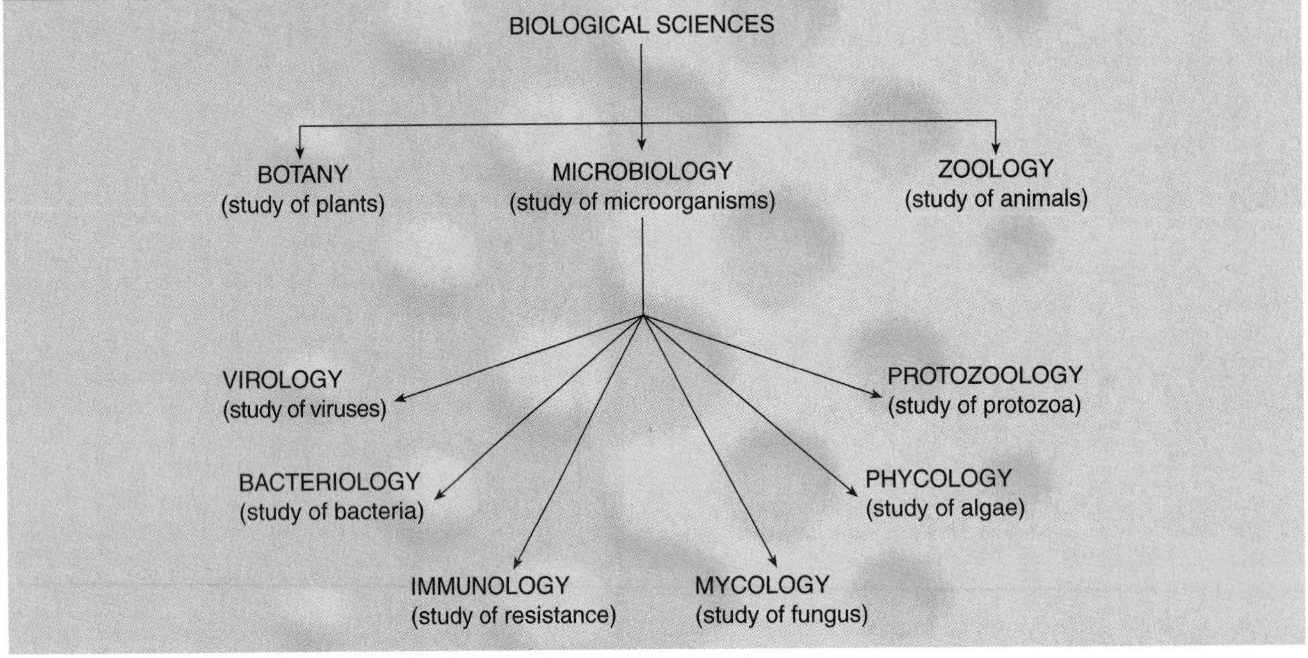

Many test kits are currently available to test for microbiologic pathogens; these kits are quick and fairly simple to perform. CLIA has identified which test kits are within their waived category and therefore appropriate for the medical assistant and other nonlaboratory medical personnel to perform. (See Table 31-7 for specific strep test kits that are CLIA waived.) What used to take days and required the expertise of a laboratory technologist now takes minutes and can be performed within the POL and sometimes even within patients' homes. The at-home pregnancy tests were probably the first test kits available over the counter, but now there are literally hundreds. The test kits range from urine testing for cocaine and other drugs to cholesterol and cancer screening tests.

MICROBIOLOGY

Classification

Taxonomy deals with the classification of living organisms.

A common system divides living organisms into kingdoms. Before the discovery of the microscope in the sixteenth century, there were two known kingdoms, animal and plant. A new kingdom of microscopic organisms, the *Protista,* was developed because most microbes are neither plant nor animal. The members of this kingdom are called *protists* and are one-celled organisms (Table 31-2).

The microorganisms of importance in medical microbiology are divided into two groups: the lower protists, or *prokaryotes* (including blue–green algae and bacteria), and the higher protists, or *eukaryotes* (including **protozoa,** algae, and fungi).

Nomenclature

The system used for naming bacteria is a two-part system of names. Two Greek or Latin names are used, the first name being a **genus,** which is capitalized. The second name is the **species** name, which is not capitalized. These names may reflect a characteristic of a bacterium or names of places or persons associated with the discovery of the microorganism. For example, *Salmonella typhi*

TABLE 31-2 KINGDOM PROTISTA

I. Lower protists
  1. Prokaryotic—nuclear material not organized
    A. Bacteria
    B. Blue-green algae
II. Higher protists
  1. Eukaryotic—true nucleus
    A. Algae
    B. Slime molds
    C. Fungus
    D. Protozoa

was discovered by an American microbiologist named Salmon. The bacterium causes typhoid fever.

Individuals who study bacteria are referred to as bacteriologists or microbiologists. These individuals have taken extensive courses in the field of microbiology. In most laboratories, clinical laboratory scientists or assistants help perform microbiology procedures. The job of these individuals is to quickly and efficiently identify the organism in a given culture that has been properly obtained and brought to the laboratory within a reasonable time frame.

Together with routine bacteriologic cultures, many microbiology departments, especially in larger health care facilities, perform **parasitology** procedures for the identification of parasites; **virology** procedures for the identification of viruses; and **mycology** procedures for the identification of fungi. If an institution such as a clinic or POL is too small to properly identify many microorganisms, cultures often are sent to a reference laboratory. These laboratories are specialized laboratories with up-to-date equipment to handle large amounts of complex tests. In today's health care environment, it is cost-effective to centralize expensive and complex procedures. Instead of 10 small laboratories each having their own specialized equipment, one laboratory buys the equipment and runs the specialized test for all 10 laboratories.

The microbiology department works closely with the infection control department of a hospital to determine if certain organisms are causing infections throughout the hospital. These infections can be acquired by an **immunosuppressed** patient and become a serious problem. Infections acquired in hospitals are referred to as **nosocomial** infections and should be closely monitored. Some common nosocomial infections are caused by bacteria such as Staphylococcus, Serratia, and monilia (a yeast).

Certain types of bacteria and yeasts that are identified and grown in the laboratory must be reported to the Department of Public Health in your county or state because they are communicable diseases. These diseases vary from city to city and state to state. Some of the common bacteria that are reported are Salmonella, Shigella, and those organisms that cause sexually transmitted diseases (STDs), such as gonorrhea, syphilis, chlamydia, and herpes. The state and county you work in will have a list of reportable diseases that the clinic or POL will have posted.

Cell Structure

All living forms are alike in that their cells contain a nuclear material referred to as **DNA** (deoxyribonucleic acid), which carries special genetic information. The main structural difference of eukaryotes and prokaryotes is the arrangement of the nucleus. A eukaryote has a well-defined or true nucleus and is a higher form of microorganism. The prokaryote is a lower form of microorganism and has a simple nucleus that is not well-defined.

The bacterial cell, classified as a lower protist, is a single-celled organism with a cytoplasmic cell membrane, cell wall, and nucleus. The nucleus is not well-defined. The cell grows by taking in materials from the environment. After a certain amount of growth, the bacteria reproduce by division of the cell. Certain conditions are required for this reproduction to take place.

Figure 31-1 illustrates a basic bacterial cell. Not all bacteria possess flagella for motility, as some are not motile. Some bacteria can encapsulate themselves in protein, providing protection from antibiotic penetration and white blood cell attack. Once encapsulated they are called **spores,** an inactive state that can help bacteria resist chemicals, freezing, drying, radiation, and heating. Bacterial spores are so resistant they can live 150,000 years and can survive in dust. Tetanus is an example of bacteria that create spores.

EQUIPMENT

Basic equipment needed in a microbiology department of a clinic or a POL varies depending on the size of the

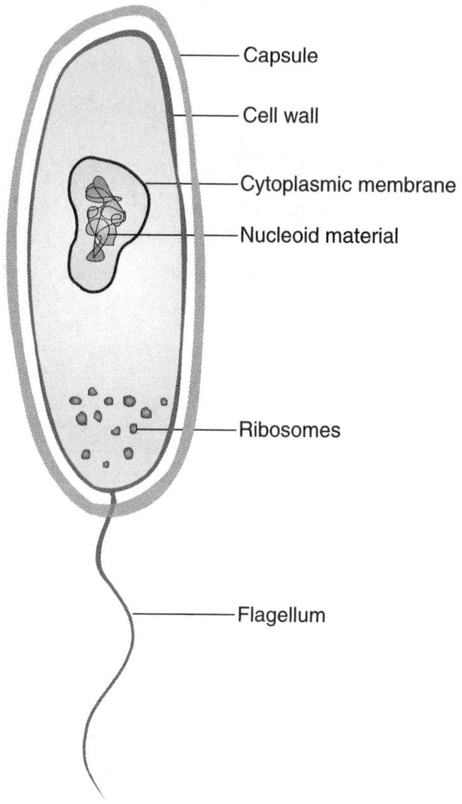

Figure 31-1 Basic bacterial cell.

facility. Most laboratories have some of the following equipment.

Autoclave

An autoclave (Figure 31-2) is used in the laboratory to sterilize equipment that may have been contaminated while processing specimens. It can be used to sterilize contaminated materials as well. The setting of 15 pounds per square inch and a temperature of 121°C for 15 to 20 minutes is sufficient to kill infectious agents, spores, viruses, and contaminants. Many laboratories no longer use autoclaves because of the use of presterilized and disposable equipment. Waste products are put into biohazardous bags and are disposed of by a service outside the health care facility.

Microscope

An important piece of equipment for the POL or clinic is the microscope. This instrument is used to view organisms that cannot be seen with the naked eye on a prepared slide. Skill in using the microscope is necessary to gain information from studying the slide. The microscope is a delicate instrument and should be cared for properly as stated by the manufacturer. (See Chapter 27 for more information on the microscope.)

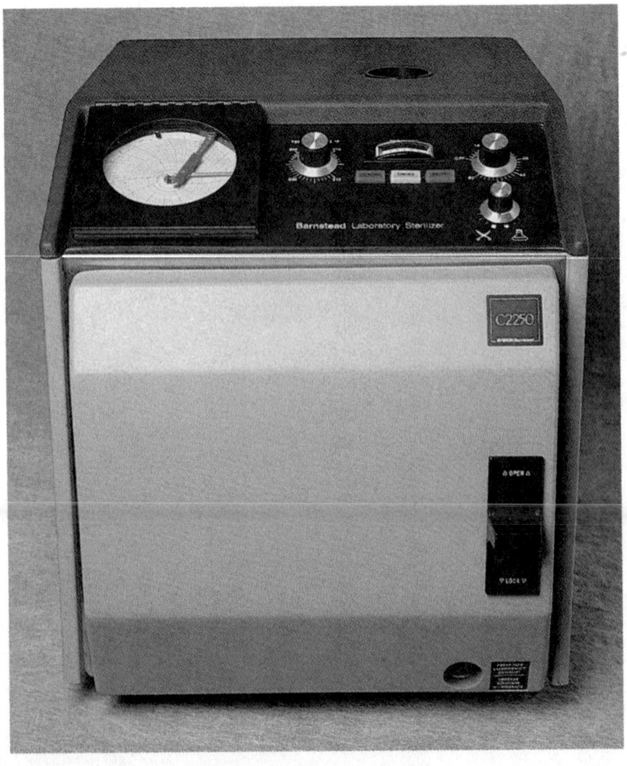

Figure 31-2 Small laboratory autoclave.

Safety Hood

Some laboratories, especially if they are culturing specimens with aerosols, will have a safety hood (Figure 31-3). **Aerosols** are airborne particles that can be released into the air when culturing. They are potentially dangerous if inhaled. By using the safety hood, the health care worker is separated from the specimen by a glass in front of the face, with fumes and aerosols suctioned into the hood. The use of a safety hood is mandatory when performing a culture on a specimen with a potential aerosol. Aerosols are particularly dangerous in fungus and mycobacterium cultures. It is a good idea to use the safety hood with foul-smelling specimens to minimize odors. Tuberculosis is an example of bacteria that travels by aerosol from person to person.

Incubator

The incubator is a cabinet that has a constant temperature of 35 to 37°C. Most organisms, whether **aerobic** (grow well in oxygen) or **anaerobic** (will not grow well or at all in oxygen), grow at these temperatures. Some bacteria, such as Yersina, grow at a lower temperature (26°C). A bacterium called Campylobacter requires a higher temperature (42°C). When working with these organisms, temperature requirements must be met for adequate growth.

Anaerobic Equipment

Certain types of cultures, such as deep-wound cultures, could contain anaerobic pathogens. At the time of culturing, the medical assistant sets up some cultures in an oxygenated environment, as well as an oxygen-reduced

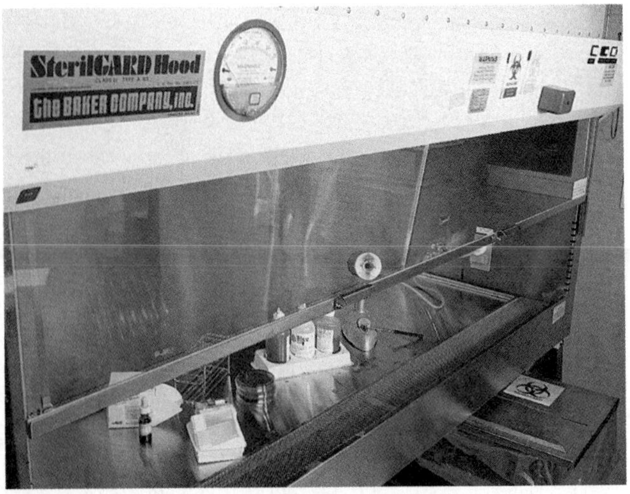

Figure 31-3 Laboratory safety hood.

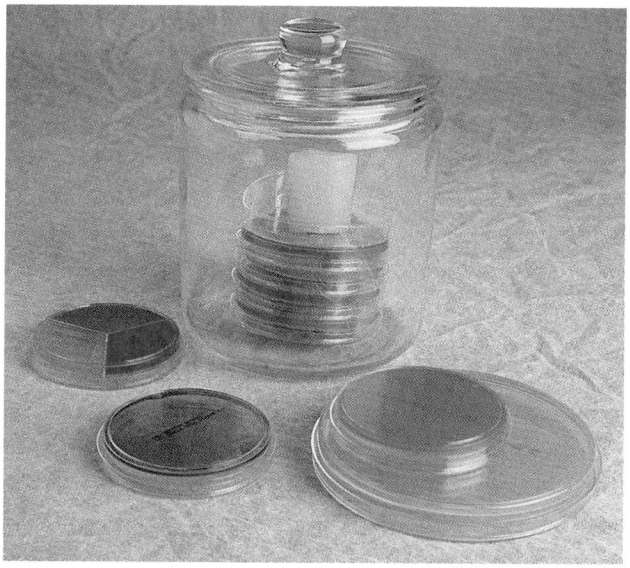

Figure 31-4 Candle jar with media for high CO_2 conditions.

environment. Most laboratories post lists of cultures that need an anaerobic setup.

To grow anaerobic bacteria, the absence of oxygen is achieved by using something as simple as a candle jar (Figure 31-4) containing a lighted candle into which the inoculated petri dish is placed. When the cover is put on the jar, the burning of the candle will use up the available oxygen and generate carbon dioxide. Organisms, such as *Neisseria gonorrhoeae*, which causes gonorrhea, need a high carbon dioxide atmosphere to survive. The use of a candle jar allows an easy collection and transport system that maximizes the recovery rate of certain microorganisms.

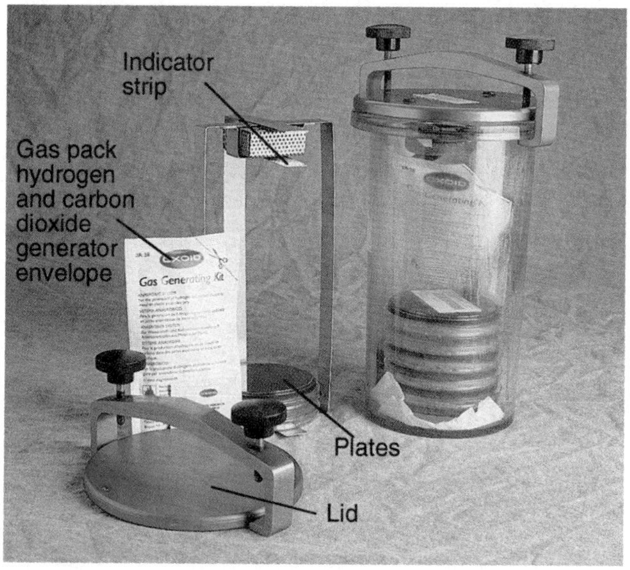

Figure 31-5 Gas pack anaerobic system.

Another method of maintaining an anaerobic condition is a specialized jar called a gas pack jar (Figure 31-5). This jar contains a foil pack that, when activated, gives off carbon dioxide, decreasing the oxygen in the jar. Extensive culturing of anaerobes often is not performed by smaller laboratories. Anaerobic specimens are sent to reference laboratories better equipped to process them. Some small laboratories will perform a Gram stain on the suspected anaerobic cultures. The **Gram stain** is the most common stain used to observe the gross morphologic features of bacteria and is discussed later in this chapter.

Inoculating Equipment

An *inoculating loop* (Figure 31-6) is a piece of wire with a rounded end and a handle at the other end. The loop is used to **inoculate** organisms onto a culture medium in a plate or broth. If it is made of wire, the loop can be flamed to sterilize it before and after use. As an alternative, sterile plastic disposable loops can be used. These are one-time use and are disposed of in the biohazardous waste.

An *inoculating needle* (Figure 31-7) is similar to the loop but has a straight end. The needle is used when performing a **stab culture** also known as "deep" inoculation. The needle is flamed, and the culture material is "stabbed" on the needle into medium in a tube. This technique is used for certain **biochemical tests** used for identification.

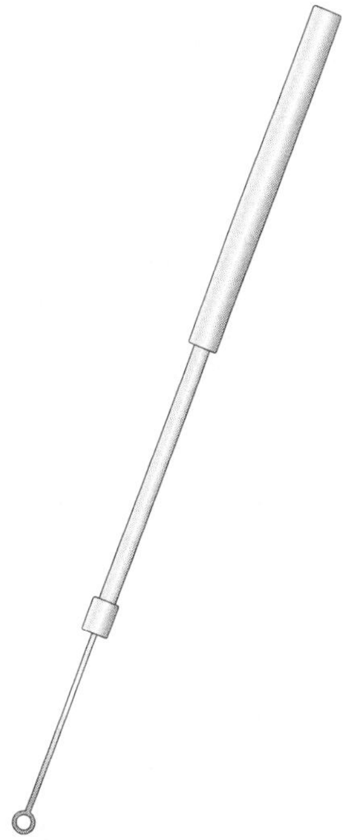

Figure 31-6 Inoculating loop.

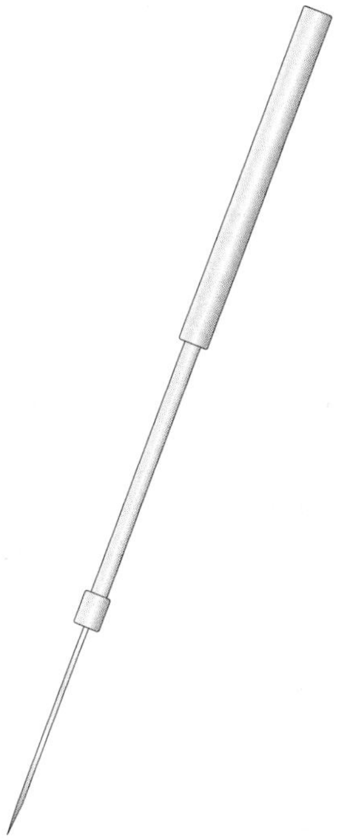

Figure 31-7 Inoculating needle.

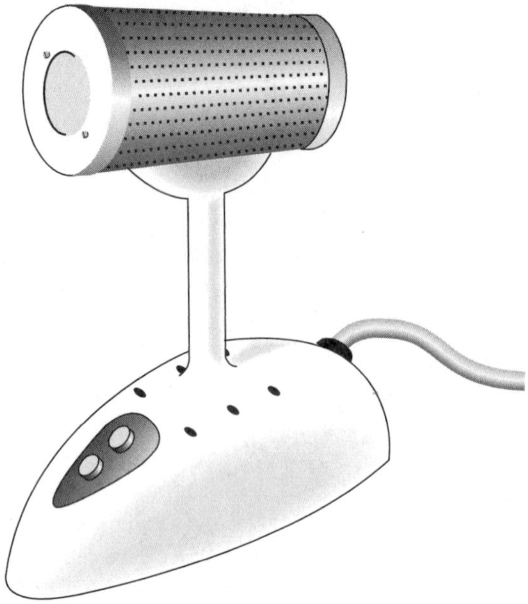

Figure 31-8 Electrical incinerator.

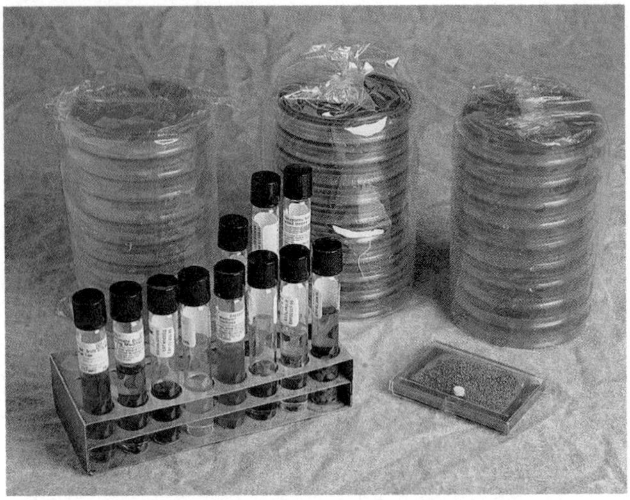

Figure 31-9 Various types of media tubes and plates.

Incinerator

Incineration is the quickest method of sterilizing the inoculating loop and needle. This can be accomplished by using an electrical incinerator (Figure 31-8) or a Bunsen burner (less popular today because of the open flame danger). When doing cultures, the inoculating needle or loop must be sterilized before and after it is used. This is done by placing the loop in the incinerator or passing through the flame of the Bunsen burner.

Media

Media in the microbiology laboratory refers to a host of substances used to foster the growth of bacteria. It is listed in this section of basic equipment (Figure 31-9) but is explained in detail in the section about media.

Refrigerator

A refrigerator is needed to store certain materials, such as media and testing kits that need a temperature of 2 to 8°C. Food or drink should never be stored in the refrigerator with any specimens, kits, or media.

SAFETY WHEN HANDLING MICROBIOLOGY SPECIMENS

Safety should be practiced in every area of the clinical laboratory at all times. Microbiology specimens can be dangerous because of potential pathogens. Following safety rules will reduce danger to all personnel concerned. Some important safety measures follow. Detailed discussions can be found in Chapters 10 and 26.

Personal Protective Equipment

Personal protective equipment should be worn at all times when processing microbiology specimens. It should be removed when leaving the work area. When processing microbiology specimens, the medical assistant wears a buttoned laboratory coat or apron, safety goggles, and gloves. At times, personnel performing microbiology testing will work behind a shield or use a safety hood to avoid inhalation of aerosol pathogens and to avoid splashes and spatters of blood and body fluids.

There is never any eating, smoking, drinking, or putting objects into the mouth while working with microbiology specimens or in the laboratory area itself. Contact lenses should not be touched nor should makeup be applied. The practice of washing hands several times should be a habit. Washing hands after glove removal is important.

Work Area

The counters where specimens are processed and set up should be cleaned with a strong germicide before and after daily use or immediately after a spill. Pathogens could be present where microbiology specimens are cultivated. This area should be dust-free and clean at all times.

Care should be taken not to have a cluttered work area. If using burners or incinerators, caution should be practiced to avoid body burns or fires.

Specimen Handling

Some microbiology specimens will be brought to the POL or clinic to be processed, so the medical assistant should look for leaks and contamination on the outside of the transporting containers. It is a good practice always to wear gloves when receiving specimens. Most specimens will arrive in an "outside" plastic bag to avoid danger to laboratory personnel. When sending specimens to an outside laboratory to be cultured, it is important to use the appropriate container to avoid contamination of others. Remember, if there is a possibility of an aerosol specimen, the specimen must be cultured under a safety hood. All specimens should be handled as if they were contaminated. (Refer to Chapter 10 for more information on Standard Precautions.)

Disposal of Waste and Spills

Most facilities will have a plan for disposal of dangerous biohazardous waste that should be strictly followed. Biohazardous waste generally is placed in red bags marked with the universal biohazard symbol (Figure 31-10). Most clinics or POLs employ an outside agency to dispose of waste. It is extremely important that biohazardous waste is not placed with the regular waste and disposal guidelines are followed.

If a spill should occur, follow the agency's or employer's rules. Remember to disinfect with a 5% phenol or a 10% bleach solution.

QUALITY CONTROL

Although **quality control** is practiced in all areas of the clinical laboratory, the microbiology department has equipment, media, and reagents that need quality-control checks with almost every test. The following list details some measures that are a part of a quality-control program in microbiology:

- All equipment with temperature controls should be monitored daily.
- The microscopes should be cleaned and kept dust-free.
- Testing for microorganism identification is often accomplished with the use of a special kit. When using kits for different tests, the positive and negative controls must be run at all times. Before use, the expiration date should be checked.
- Media of all types should not be used past the shelf life and should be stored at the proper temperatures. Your POL should have a specific list of bacteria to use on various media to test for growth. This list can be found in your laboratory manual.
- The laboratory manual should be updated periodically.
- All chemicals or reagents with Material Safety Data Sheets (MSDSs) should be available to reference when working with a chemical that is not familiar to you.

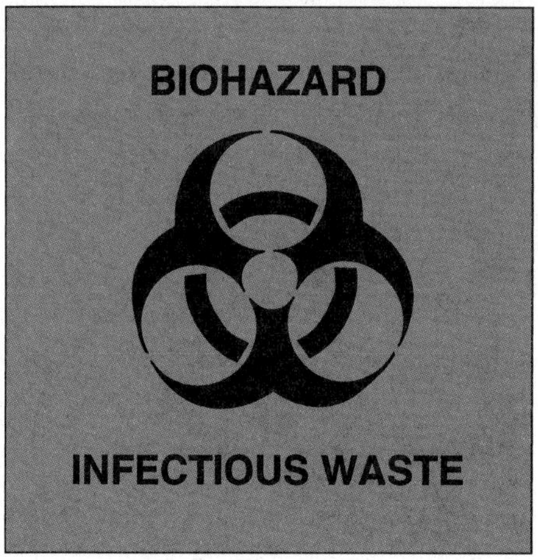

Figure 31-10 Biohazard symbol.

COLLECTION PROCEDURES

When a physician needs identification of an organism that is causing infection, he or she orders a culture from that site. The culture specimen should be collected properly, delivered within a reasonable period, and collected in sufficient quantity. The results of the culture will depend on the quality of the original specimen. All specimens obtained for identification of infectious organisms must be taken from the site of the infection, not the surrounding area.

Once the specimen is collected correctly, it should be placed in the appropriate container and delivered to the laboratory soon after collection. Many organisms will die if not kept moist. Transport media can have a moistening agent to keep the specimen from drying out.

If a specimen comes into the laboratory in an improper container or has not been delivered within a reasonable period soon after collection, it must be rejected and another specimen obtained. The container in which the specimen has been placed should be sterile, and the right type should be used for a specific culture (Figure 31-11). Sterile containers are used for most collections, with the exception of stool collection containers, which do not have to be sterile. Culturette cultures

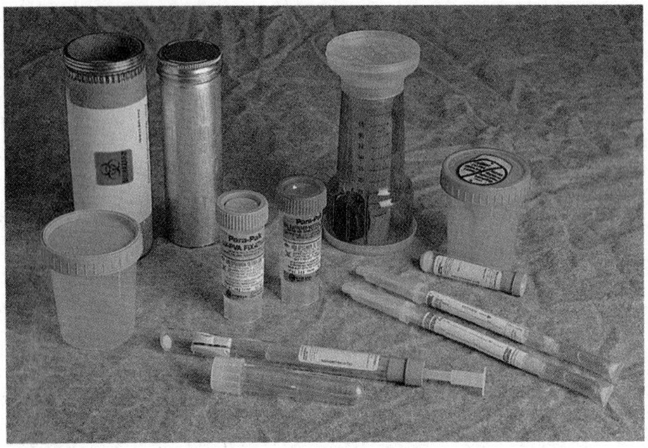

Figure 31-11 Various collection and transport containers for bacteriologic specimens.

are from swabs and should be kept moist. This system is a plastic tube that has a sterile swab used to collect the specimen and then is placed back into the tube. The tube contains a medium which keeps the swab moist and preserves the specimen.

The laboratory's success in isolating the causative pathogens depends on the following factors:

1. Proper collection from infection site
2. Collection of specimen during infection period
3. Sufficient amount of specimen
4. Appropriate specimen container
5. Appropriate transport medium
6. Specimen labeled properly
7. Specimen delivered to the laboratory in a minimal amount of time
8. Specimen collected before the administration of antibiotics
9. Specimen inoculated onto proper media and placed in correct atmosphere to ensure growth

When collecting specimens, it is important that the medical assistant carefully follow the instructions as designated in the laboratory manual. Standard Precautions must be strictly adhered to while obtaining and processing specimens and everyone (including couriers, receptionists, and laboratory assistants) handling specimens should wear gloves to protect themselves from leakage of the container and contamination with a pathogenic organism.

Specific Collection Requirements for Cultures

Urine. Patients should be instructed to obtain a clean-catch urine specimen in a sterile container. A clean-catch midstream specimen is obtained by first cleaning the genital area and then urinating midstream into a specimen container. Details of this procedure are found in Chapter 30. Patients should be given strict instructions so that a quality specimen for culturing can be obtained.

Sometimes a catheterization is done to collect a sterile urine specimen for culture. The urine must be collected into a sterile container.

Throat. When taking a throat specimen for culture, explain to the patient that a throat culture is necessary to identify certain organisms. Be sure to tell the patient that there may be some momentary discomfort in obtaining the specimen, especially if his or her throat is sore. Answer all questions about the process of obtaining the specimen. Throat culture specimens are taken using the culturette. As mentioned in the previous section, the culturette contains a sterile swab and growth medium for moisture to keep the bacteria viable.

Once you have gathered all the necessary supplies (see Procedure 31-1) and put on gloves and a face shield, have the patient open his or her mouth and say "ah." This will lower the back of the tongue for better viewing (Figure 31-12A). Be sure to have a good light source available. Use a sterile tongue depressor to help hold the tongue down. While avoiding the tongue and inside of the cheeks, take the specimen directly from the affected area with the sterile swab. Once the specimen is obtained on the swab, place the swab back into the culturette (see Figure 31-12B). The culturette is now ready for labeling and transport to the laboratory for testing (see Figure 31-12C). As with any culture test ordered, a requisition stating the site from which the specimen was obtained is required.

Throat swabs for the detection of Group A Streptococcus infection (strep throat) usually are tested in the POL using a self-contained kit that produces quick results (see Procedure 31-3). Performing the rapid strep tests are well within the medical assistant's scope under CLIA's waived test category. More information about performing rapid strep tests is provided later in this chapter in the Streptococcus Screening section. CLIA waived rapid strep tests are listed in Table 31-7.

Nose. A nasal-pharyngeal swab may be requested with a throat culture. This is collected with a swab on a thin wire. A separate swab may be used for each nostril. The patient tilts back the head, and each swab is gently inserted into each of the nostrils. The swab is then placed into a sterile tube and kept at room temperature for transport to the laboratory.

Patient Education

As you obtain throat cultures from patients, you may want to give them some helpful advice concerning their condition. Generally when a person has a sore throat, it is associated with other respiratory symptoms as well. The following suggestions may provide some relief from discomfort and help patients toward better health.

1. Advise patients to drink plenty of liquids, especially water, and to eat sensibly from the basic food groups.
2. Urge patients to get extra rest and dress comfortably (according to the weather/temperature outside).
3. Suggest use of gargles or throat lozenges (or both) to relieve painful sore throat.
4. Remind them to avoid tobacco/smoking.
5. Instruct them to cough/sneeze into tissue and discard into proper waste container wherever they are to prevent the spread of microorganisms. Because sewer waste is treated and disinfected, flushing a contaminated tissue is an effective method of disposal.
6. Remind patients to refrain from sharing drinking glasses and tableware and from intimate contact such as kissing while they are infected and still contagious. All eating utensils should be sanitized in hot water after use to avoid the spread of contagious diseases. Perhaps the most important educational advice is reminding patients to wash their hands frequently.

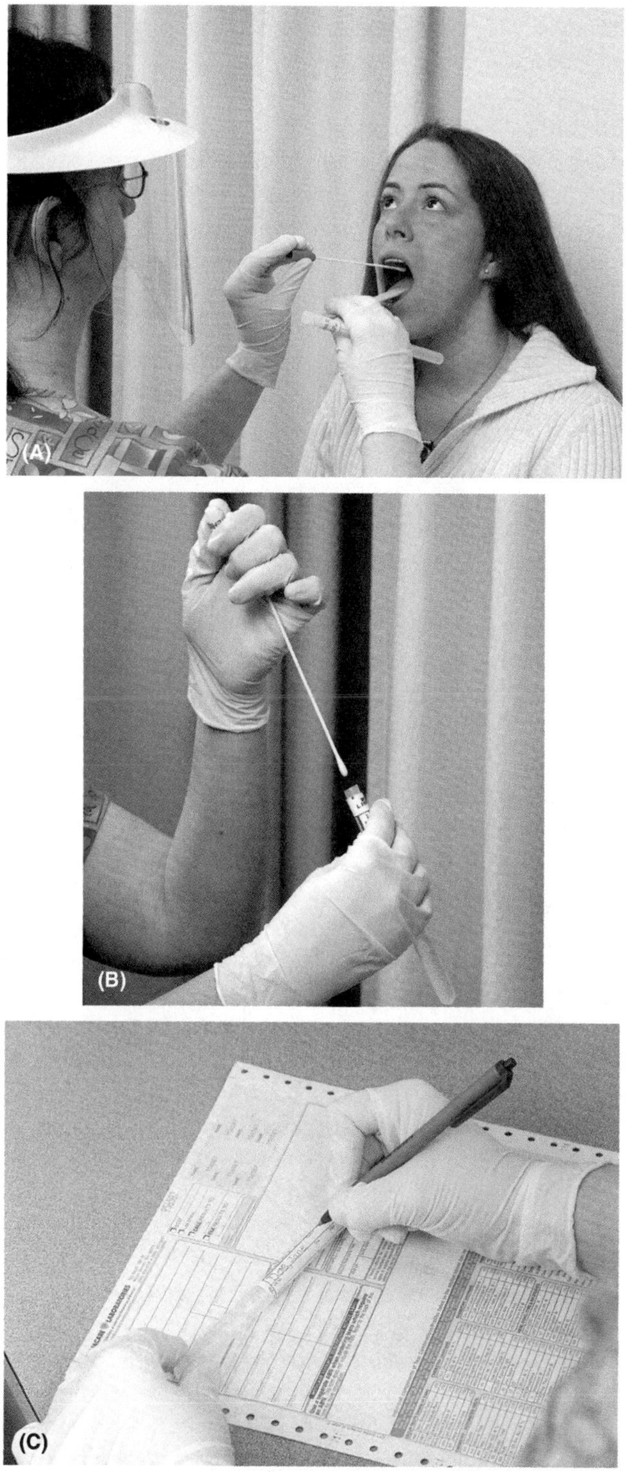

Figure 31-12 (A) The medical assistant obtains a throat culture using a culturette, taking care to not touch the cheeks or tongue. (B) After swabbing the patient's throat, the medical assistant returns the swab to the culturette, which contains the moist media. (C) The culturette is labeled and a requisition is completed in preparation for transport to the regional laboratory for testing.

Wound. When culturing a wound, a sterile needle might be used to aspirate pus-filled fluid from the wound, or a swab is used. It is important to get the swab deep into the wound without touching the surrounding skin. Specimens for wound cultures often are placed in anaerobic transport medium, especially if the wound is not superficial.

Sputum. To collect this specimen correctly, the patient should cough deeply and **expectorate** into the sterile container. The specimen should be a first morning specimen and placed into a sterile container designed to protect all who handle the specimen from contamination.

Stool. Stool specimens are brought to the laboratory for various tests. If the stool is to be examined for **ova** (eggs) or parasites, the specimen should be as fresh as possible. Special containers often are used for ova and parasites. Stool specimens must be kept at between room temperature and body temperature. Refrigeration may destroy the parasites within the specimen.

For bacterial cultures of stool (as well as for ova and parasites), several different specimens may be sent for testing at different times. The collection containers for stool cultures do not have to be sterile, but they must be clean and have a tight-fitting lid.

Cerebrospinal Fluid (CSF). The physician obtains CSF by doing a **lumbar puncture.** See Procedure 18-23. The fluid generally is dispersed in several departments of the clinical laboratory. Generally, the fluid goes first to the microbiology laboratory for a culture before it becomes contaminated by doing other tests. Before the culture set up, the tube should be placed in an incubator or left at room temperature. Refrigeration of spinal fluid can kill two common meningitis-causing bacteria, *Haemophilus influenzae* and *Neisseria meningitidis*. CSF culture is a STAT order for processing, and the medical assistant is responsible for calling the laboratory for immediate pickup.

Blood. Human blood is free from bacteria in a healthy human. If blood does become contaminated with bacteria, septicemia (septic blood infection) can result. Blood cultures are collected by the same means as regular blood collection, with special considerations to avoid any contamination of the blood. A variety of collection devices are available for collecting blood cultures, all requiring careful sterile techniques. See Procedure 29-4 for blood culture.

MICROSCOPIC EXAMINATION OF BACTERIA

There are usually two procedures involved in properly identifying bacteria: the microscopic examination and the culture. The microscopic examination involves viewing stained or unstained bacteria through the microscope.

Culturing is a means of isolating a disease-causing microorganism for identification. A specimen is obtained and placed in a culture medium, which contains nutrients comparable to human tissue to encourage growth of microorganisms. The medium is **agar,** a gelatin-like substance, mixed with nutrients. The nutrients mixed in the agar will vary according to what each particular bacterium prefers. The section Culture Media later in this chapter discusses in detail the types of nutrients each type of bacterium prefers. See also Table 31-4 for a list of some of the more common bacteria and their growth requirements.

Microscopically identifying bacteria is not in CLIA's waived categories; therefore, although the medical assistant will not actually be performing these tests, the staining information is included here to aid in understanding the staining and examination processes that culture specimens go through. It is important for medical assistants to be familiar with the processes and the terminology related to staining and microscopic identification of bacteria to better serve their patients, physician–employer, and colleagues.

Bacterial Shapes

Each genus of bacteria has a characteristic shape. A knowledge of the shapes of bacteria helps in identification (Figure 31-13). Bacteria have three basic shapes:

1. *Cocci*. Cocci are round in shape, occurring in clusters, pairs, singles, and tetrads (groups of three). They are nonmotile microorganisms. (They do not move on their own accord.)
2. *Bacilli*. Bacilli are rod-shaped and can have rounded, straight, or pointed ends. Some bacilli have flagella that give bacteria motility (movement). Most bacteria are the shape of bacilli.
3. *Spirilla*. Spirilla are spiral-shaped bacteria that have one too many turns. Most spirilla are motile.

The microscopic examination produces information that is often needed to identify bacteria. However, biochemical reactions and the sensitivity pattern (how the organisms respond to antibiotics) are also needed to make the full identification.

Dyes (Stains)

The dyes used in microbiology are derived from coal tar. These dyes are acidic or basic and impart a color to the microorganism. Basic dyes carry a positive ion and stain structures that are acidic in nature. An acid dye carries a negative ion and stains structures that are basic (alkaline) in nature such as cytoplasmic structures. Several different types of stains are used depending on what test is ordered. (Table 31-3 lists stains and their uses.)

Simple Stain

A simple stain uses a single stain on a fixed slide for a given period of time. A simple stain will show the arrangement and structure of the bacterial cell. It is fast, taking no more than three minutes to stain, but does not give much information.

Differential Stain

A differential stain is more complex than a simple stain. It is known as a differential stain because the stain result varies. A common differential stain is the Gram stain.

The Gram stain was developed in 1884 by Dr. Hans Christian Gram. More than 100 years later, this famous stain is still in use with little variation. This staining procedure differentiates bacteria by their Gram stain ability of being either negative or positive. A bacterium is Gram negative or positive by the nature of the cell wall and the ability of it either to retain or lose color through decolorization. This identification of Gram-positive or Gram-negative bacteria aids in identification of an organism. Gram-positive bacteria have a lower lipid (fat) content and are not decolorized as compared with Gram-negative bacteria, which have a higher lipid content and are readily decolorized.

The **reagents** used in the Gram stain are gentian or crystal violet, a purple stain that is the primary stain. Iodine, which acts as a **mordant,** holds the purple stain. Alcohol-acetone is the decolorizer that removes the purple color. Safranin is the red counterstain. When

TABLE 31-3 STAINS AND THEIR USES

Stain	Example
Simple	Carbolfuchsin Gentian violet Methylene blue Safranin
Differential	Gram Acid-fast (Ziehl-Neelsen, Kinyoun)
Special	Capsule (Welch negative) Flagella (Leifson) Nuclei (Feulgen) Spore (Doerner)

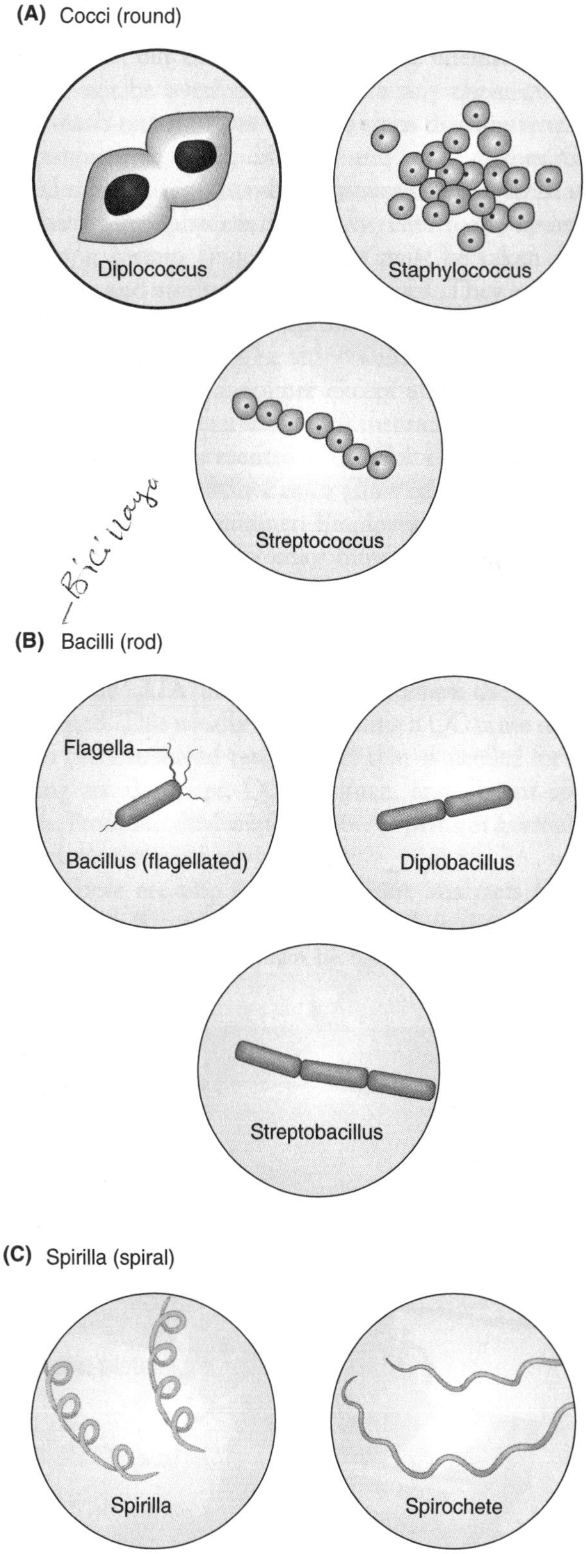

Figure 31-13 Three types of bacteria.

stained according to the manufacturer's directions, the Gram-positive bacteria stain purple, and the Gram-negative bacteria stain pink. Sometimes an organism will appear Gram-variable. This is found with Gram-positive organisms that have been exposed to acidic media, that are often old and lose their ability to retain the gentian violet, or the proper procedure has not been followed. See Procedure 31-3 and Figure 31-14.

The Gram stain is one of the most important procedures in the microbiology laboratory, giving valuable information by identifying Gram-positive bacteria such as *Staphylococcus* and *Streptococcus* or Gram-negative bacteria such as *Escherichia coli* and Proteus.

The morphologic arrangement, shape, and Gram stain characteristic will begin to help identify the bacteria. Sometimes this is all the physician needs to know to start treatment for a pathogenic organism. For example, the bacteria causing gonorrhea (*Neisseria gonorrhoeae*) is a distinctive organism, having a characteristic diplococci shape that resembles a coffee or kidney bean. These organisms are found in and outside of white blood cells and can be identified by a Gram stain.

Acid-Fast Stain

Another differential stain, which is often referred to as a specific stain, is the acid-fast stain. This stain is either differential or specific in that it allows microscopic examination of acid-fast organisms. This group of organisms does not respond well to the Gram stain and is difficult to stain under ordinary circumstances because of a waxy capsule cell wall that resists staining.

To stain these organisms, heat or a powerful dye is used in the procedure to stain the bacteria. The bacteria, once stained, resist decolorization with an acid alcohol, giving them the acid-fast name. The bacteria that causes tuberculosis is an acid-fast organism.

Two methods commonly used to stain acid-fast organisms are the Ziehl–Neelsen stain, which uses heat, and the Kinyoun stain, a cold method that does not include a heating process. Either of these stains is satisfactory.

Special Techniques

There are several special situations when more than the Gram stain or the shape and arrangement of an organism is needed to aid in the identification. Such situations would be the demonstration of the presence of flagella, spore, capsule, or nuclei of cells.

There also are microscopic examinations of organisms in a living state, without staining. Characteristics that can be studied by this method include motility, shape, and arrangement of organisms. This technique

Step	Time	Procedure	Result
1	one minute	Primary stain: Apply crystal violet stain (purple) ↓ Rinse slide	All bacteria stain purple 
2	one minute	Mordant: Apply Gram's iodine ↓ Rinse slide	All bacteria remain purple 
3	three to five seconds	Decolorize: Apply alcohol ↓ Rinse slide	Purple stain is removed from Gram-negative cells 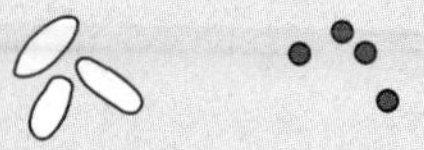
4	one minute	Counterstain: Apply safranin stain (red) ↓ Rinse slide	Gram-negative cells appear pink-red; Gram-positive cells appear purple 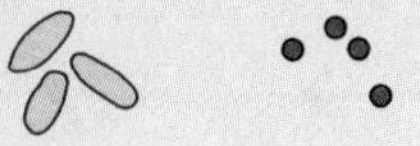

Figure 31-14 Steps in the Gram stain procedure.

requires the microorganisms to be in a liquid suspension. The medical assistant often is responsible for setting up the slide for microscopic examination by the physician. Although microscopy is not a CLIA waived test, the medical assistant can certainly view the slides microscopically and discuss the finding with the physician as a learning exercise.

For vaginal secretions, a swab of the vaginal discharge is placed in a sterile tube containing 1 ml normal saline and mixed. Then the suspension is viewed under a microscope. For stool or other bacterial specimens, a small amount of specimen is mixed with a drop of normal saline, then viewed under a microscope. These methods are known as the **wet-mount** preparation and the hanging drop preparation. Refer to Procedure 31-2.

The wet-mount preparation is a valuable diagnostic tool in determining the cause of vaginosis. Bacterial vaginosis is identified by the presence of "clue cells," epithelial cells covered by coccobacillary bacteria. Motile trichomonads are seen with *Trichomonas vaginalis*. The presence of pseudohyphae indicates a yeast infection. In many cases, an accurate diagnosis can be made from the wet-mount preparation, thus making more complex techniques unnecessary.

Potassium Hydroxide Preparation

Another type of wet preparation is using 10% solution of **potassium hydroxide (KOH)** in a wet preparation for the study of fungi and spores. The slide is prepared by using fragments of human hair, skin, or nails that could have fungus. KOH wet mounts are also useful for examining other body fluids such as vaginal swabs. These specimens are placed on a slide with a drop of 10% KOH and a coverslip on top. The KOH will clear debris. The slide should sit at room temperature for about a half hour before examination for debris settlement.

The direct examination of specimens is best viewed with a phase or dark-field microscope rather than a bright-field microscope because of reduced illumination. If using a bright-field microscope, lower the condenser to reduce transmitted light. Proper disposal of these specimens is important because the organisms are alive and possibly pathogenic.

CULTURE MEDIA

After the proper collection of the specimen, the material collected must be inoculated on a proper culture medium. This is necessary for growth and eventual identification of an organism.

The results of culture, the growing of an organism on special media in the laboratory, are only as reliable as the method used in collecting the specimen. In addition, growth requirements of different organisms must be considered, such as moisture, temperature, oxygen, carbon dioxide, and essential nutrients. Organisms that are sensitive to drying must be put into transport medium immediately after collection to prevent loss of viability. Some bacteria require a specialized medium to grow and multiply. Aerobic bacteria grow only in the presence of oxygen. Anaerobic bacteria live and grow in the absence of oxygen. Examples of some common bacteria and their growth requirements are illustrated in Table 31-4.

When specimens are collected for the laboratory, the microorganism's growth requirements must be considered. No matter how good the specimen, if an anaerobic organism is kept in an aerobic atmosphere while being transported to the reference laboratory, it will probably not survive. Special anaerobic transport systems must be used.

Neisseria gonorrhoeae, the causative agent of the sexually transmitted disease (STD) gonorrhea, requires special media and an atmosphere of reduced oxygen and increased carbon dioxide. Therefore, the specimen must be collected from the patient and immediately placed on a special media in a reduced oxygen atmosphere.

Medical assistants who send bacterial specimens to a reference laboratory must be familiar with the transport media the reference laboratory provides. Your laboratory manual explains how and when to use the various microbiology transport systems.

Media can be a solid, liquid, or semisolid substance that has the required nutrients to support the growth of

TABLE 31-4 SOME COMMON BACTERIA AND THEIR GROWTH REQUIREMENTS

Organism	Disease	Medium	Oxygen Requirements
Streptococcus	Strep Throat	Blood agar	$\downarrow O_2$, $\uparrow CO_2$
Neisseria gonorrhoeae	Gonorrhea	Chocolate agar, modified Thayer–Martin (MTM)	$\downarrow O_2$, $\uparrow CO_2$
Staphylococcus	Infections, boils	Blood agar	O_2
Escherichia coli	Urinary tract infections	Blood agar, eosin methylene blue (EMB), MacConkey's	O_2

bacteria. Such ingredients include vitamins, sugar, salt, minerals, and amino acids. Some media have the addition of special products such as egg, potato, meat, milk, blood, and dyes.

The solid form of media is called agar. Agar has an appearance similar to gelatin and is made of seaweed. When heated, agar is a liquid; when cooled, it solidifies. Agar is poured into a **petri dish** (a plastic dish used to grow bacteria) so the bacteria can be studied for gross **morphology** (form and structure). Agar can also be placed in tubes.

Semisolid media is made by adding less agar. Media in a liquid broth form is stored in tubes called **broth tubes** and allows for the observation of gas production, change in pH, and odor. Figure 31-5 shows many different types of media that can be used to identify bacteria. Media can be purchased already prepared, or it can be produced from ingredients in the laboratory. Charts listing the proper media to set up for specific types of cultures generally are prominently displayed in the setup area of most microbiology laboratories.

Media Classification

There are several classifications of media, including:

- *Basic*. Basic media are used for general purposes and do not contain added nutrients. They will support the growth of many Gram-negative and Gram-positive organisms.
- *Differential*. Differential media contain substances that alter the appearance of some types of organisms and not other types. An eosin methylene blue (EMB) plate for lactose and nonlactose fermenters is an example of differential media. The lactose fermenter can use lactose and looks different on the agar.
- *Selective*. Selective media support the growth of one type of organism, whereas inhibiting the growth of another. This is done by the addition of either a salt, dye, chemical, or antibiotic. A hektoen enteric (HE) plate for the growth of salmonella and shigella is a selective type of medium.
- *Enriched*. This type of medium contains substances that inhibit certain bacteria from growing. These media work well with cultures from sites that possess normal flora, such as the throat. The normal flora is inhibited and pathogenic bacteria are encouraged to grow. Blood agar and chocolate agar are examples of enriched media.

All media that are used should first be checked with known organisms for quality control and for contaminants. The manufacturer will usually suggest a list of organisms for a quality-control check. A check for contaminants involves a thorough visual check of the plate before using it. It is also important to store media according to the manufacturer's direction. *Never use outdated media*.

Table 31-5 lists common media by classification and use, and Table 31-6 is a listing of media that might be selected for specific sources. All laboratories vary slightly in their recommendations of media to set up on specimens.

TABLE 31-5 COMMON MICROBIOLOGY MEDIA BY CLASSIFICATION AND USE

Type	Name	Use
Basic	Trypticase agar Trypticase broth	Supports the growth of most organisms
Differential	Blood agar	Supports the growth of *Streptococcus* and *Staphylococcus;* demonstrates hemolysis
	MacConkey	Certain Gram-negative organisms
	Eosin methylene blue (EMB)	*Escherichia coli*
Selective	Salmonella and Shigella (SS)	Gram-negative Salmonella and Shigella
	Hektoen	Enteric organisms
	Phenylethyl alcohol	Inhibits Gram-negative growth
	Mannitol salt	Promotes growth of *Staphylococcus*
	Selenite (GN) broth	Promotes growth of enteric organisms
	Thayer–Martin	Promotes growth of *Neisseria* species
	Thioglycollate broth	Promotes growth of anaerobes
Enriched	Loefflers	Promotes growth of *Corynebacterium*
	Chocolate	Promotes growth of *Haemophilus* species
	Lowenstein–Jensen	Promotes growth of mycobacteria

TABLE 31-6 COMMON SPECIMENS, SUSPECTED PATHOGENS, AND MEDIA RECOMMENDATIONS

Specimen Source	Potential Pathogens	Blood agar	Chocolate	Eosin Mthylene Blue	MacConkey	Salmonella and Shigella Hektoen Enteric	Selenite	Thayer-Martin	Thioglycollate	CO_2
Eye/Ear	*Neisseria gonorrhoeae* *Haemophilus* species *Staphylococcus aureus* *Streptococcus pyogenes* *Pseudomonas aeruginosa* *Moraxella* species	x	x	x	x			x	x	x
Cerebrospinal fluid	*Neisseria meningitidis* *Streptococcus pneumoniae* *Haemophilus influenzae*	x	x						x	x
Throat	*Streptococcus pyogenes*	x								x
Sputum	*Streptococcus pneumoniae*	x								
Urine	*Escherichia coli* *Klebsiella* *Proteus* *Pseudomonas aeruginosa* *Enterococcus*	x		x	x					
Wounds	*Staphylococcus* *Streptococcus* *Enterobactericae* Anaerobic bacteria	x	x	x	x				x	x
Stool	*Salmonella* *Shigella*			x	x	x	x			
Stool	Pathogenic *E. coli* *Yersinia* species									
Vaginal	*Neisseria gonorrhoeae*	x	x					x		x

MICROBIOLOGY CULTURE

Inoculating the Media

After selecting the right medium for the culture and observing the specimen to make sure it is properly collected, the specimen is then inoculated onto the medium. If the specimen is on a swab, the swab is rolled directly onto the upper quadrant of the agar plate. If the specimen is a sputum or liquid, it is inoculated onto the plate with a loop.

The inoculum is spread back and forth in a sweeping motion with a flamed loop or needle.

After the agar plate has been inoculated and properly labeled, it should be turned upside down and placed in the proper environment for growth. By turning the agar upside down, any condensation that forms from bacterial growth will be on the inside lid.

Liquid broths and agar slant tubes have screw caps. These caps must not be screwed on too tightly because of gas production by some organisms that can break the tube.

Other Types of Streaking

Other types of streaking include the lawn streak. This streaking technique is used to place an organism over an entire area of an agar plate for sensitivity testing. The bacteria is spread over the entire plate using a swab (Figure 31-15), streaking over the entire area several times from different angles. After the streaking has been completed, disks saturated with different antibiotics are placed equidistant throughout the streaked area.

The colony count is a streaking technique much like the lawn technique. This technique is used to plate urine cultures. A special calibrated urine loop is used to make the first streak, followed by a second streak that goes across the entire length of the initial streak. Then another complete streaking is placed over the original streaks after

Figure 31-15 Lawn or spread streak.

rotating the plate (Figure 31-16). This method of using a calibrated loop to get a more accurate inoculation gives the physician an idea of how many colonies of bacteria are present.

Every laboratory will use slightly different ways of performing the basic streaks. The important factor is to use good aseptic techniques so there is no contamination from outside organisms, and all organisms that are streaked out are isolated enough to test further if necessary.

Primary Culture

After the media has been incubated for 24 to 48 hours, the initial or primary culture is read.

Subculture

When working with bacterial cultures, there can be more than one pathogen growing in the culture. For instance, a wound culture may have both Gram-positive and Gram-negative organisms growing. To identify each organism, you must separate these bacteria to other media (see Figure 31-17). It is also necessary at times to separate the pathogenic bacteria from the normal flora, as in the throat and sputum cultures. Some initial cultures do achieve excellent isolation without having to subculture.

RAPID IDENTIFICATION SYSTEMS

The age of high technology and computerized equipment has also made inroads into microbiology laboratories, clinics, and POLs. Many traditional methods of identifying bacteria have been replaced by rapid identification test kits.

Rapid test systems, which are CLIA waived, give a quick identification, are economical, and allow physicians to start treatment sooner. Rapid tests allow the physician to receive results while the patient is still in the office.

Streptococcus Screening (Rapid Strep Testing)

There are a number of instant or rapid test kits on the market to identify Group A Streptococcus (also known as Beta-Hemolytic Streptococcus Group A), the causative agent of a serious sore (strep) throat. It is important to identify this Gram-positive Streptococcus as soon as possible because the bacteria can do serious damage (i.e., kidney and heart valve damage) if not treated with antibiotics immediately.

This test is sensitive and eliminates false-positive results. The directions should be followed strictly to produce an accurate test result. The results are based on color development of a spot on the test filter. Test results are available in minutes.

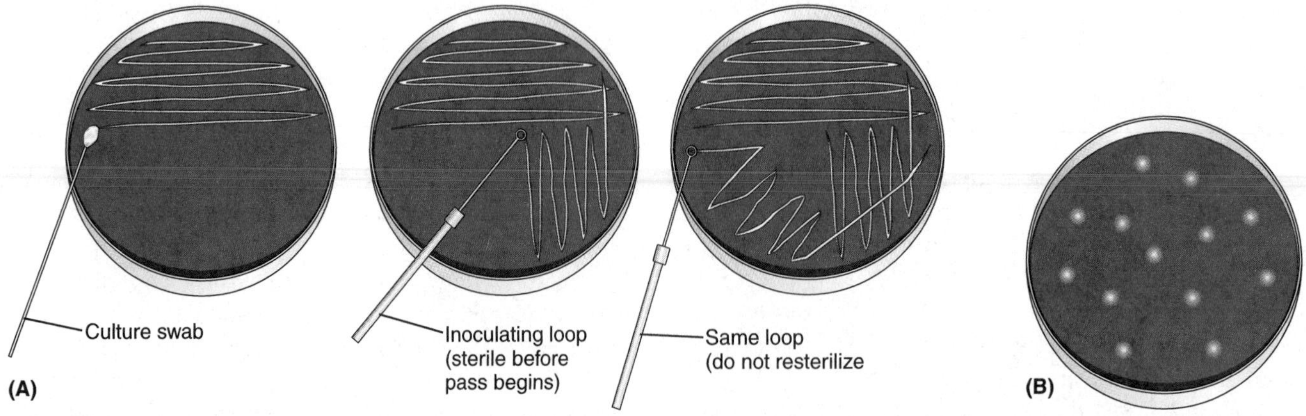

Figure 31-16 Colony count streak.

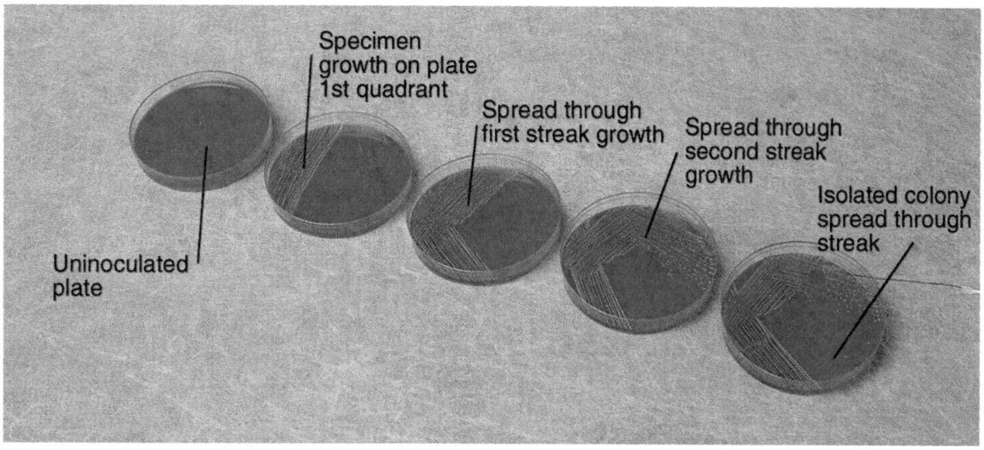

Figure 31-17 Stages of spreading out the bacteria to isolate colonies.

A latex agglutination test for Group A Streptococcus is based on an antigen and antibody agglutination. A throat swab is placed directly on the antibody-coated slide, and the presence of a positive test is seen by the appearance of agglutination (clumping). Although these tests are quick and convenient, the following rules should be followed strictly:

- Read and understand the manufacturer's instructions and directions before starting the test.
- Never use outdated materials.
- Observe all safety guidelines and precautions.
- Use the correct swab in taking the throat culture. Some cottons and chemicals on swab will interfere with the test reagents. If possible, use the swabs provided with the kit.
- Always run the positive and negative control together with the patient's actual test.

If a patient has symptoms of an infected throat and the slide test is negative, the physician will also order a regular throat culture to make sure there is no infection present. Latex agglutination kits can give false readings, and it is best to follow up with the throat culture. Table 31-7 lists Rapid Strep kits approved for CLIA '88 waived testing.

SENSITIVITY TESTING

Antibiotic sensitivity testing often is ordered on the pathogenic organisms recovered from the culturing process. By setting up an antibiotic sensitivity test, the laboratory can identify which antibiotics destroy the pathogen, and the physician will be able to set up antibiotic treatment for the patient. Today's health care environment demands that this information be made available to the physician as soon as possible.

When a patient has had multiple bacterial infections and the physician is concerned with prescribing an ineffective antibiotic, or when the bacterial infection is not responding to the currently prescribed antibiotic, the physician will order a culture and sensitivity (C & S). The antibiotic that is effective against the culture bacteria is reported as "sensitive to," and the antibiotics that are not effective will be reported as "resistant to," meaning that the bacteria will be sensitive to some antibiotics and resistant to others.

To determine which antibiotic will destroy the culture bacteria, the technician places small discs on the culture plate. The discs contain various antibiotics. The antibiotic to which the bacteria is sensitive will eventually become surrounded by an area of no growth (Figure 31-18).

PARASITOLOGY

With the age of travel and more public awareness, we are beginning to see more parasitic infections. The field of parasitology is a vast one with many different types of parasites. They range from extremely small microscopic ones to those that are large and macroscopic in size. Parasites have varying life cycles. The degree of severity of illness depends on which parasite enters the human body and infects it. Parasites can be found in the blood, urine, or feces. The more common ones are found in the feces.

Different geographic areas have different types of parasites that are seen. Resettled immigrant populations may be infected with a parasite previously unseen in a geographic area. World travelers can also bring back rare parasitic infections from their adventures.

TABLE 31-7 LIST OF WAIVED TESTS FOR STREPTOCOCCUS, GROUP A (STREP A)

Kit Name	Manufacturer
Abbott—Signify Strep A Test	Wyntek Diagnostics, Inc.
Acon Strep A Rapid Strip Test	Acon Laboratories, Inc.
Acon Strep A Twist Rapid Test	Acon Laboratories, Inc.
Applied Biotech SureStep Strep A (II) (direct from throat swab)	Applied Biotech, Inc.
Beckman Coulter Primary Care Diagnostics ICON DS Strep A	Acon Laboratories, Inc.
Beckman Coulter ICON SC Strep A	Acon Laboratories, Inc.
Beckman Coulter Primary Care Diagnostics ICON FX Strep A Immunochemical Strep A Test	Beckman Coulter
Becton Dickinson Link 2 Strep A Rapid Test (direct from throat swab)	Applied Biotech, Inc.
Binax NOW Strep A Test	Binax
BioStar Acceava Step A Test (direct from throat swab)	Wyntech Diagnostics, Inc.
DE Healthcare Products, TruView Strep A Test	DE Healthcare Products
Fisher HealthCare Sure-Vue Strep A (direct from throat swab)	Applied Biotech, Inc.
Genzyme Contrast Strep A (direct from throat swab)	Genzyme Diagnostics
Genzyme OSOM Strep A Ultra Test	Genzyme Diagnostics
Germain Laboratories StrepAim Rapid Dipstick Test	Germaine Laboratories
Germain Laboratories Strep AIM Tower	Germaine Laboratories
Henry Schein One Step + Strep A Test	Henry Schein
Immunostics Immuno/Strep A Detector	Acon Laboratories
Instant Technologies iStrep Strep A	Acon Laboratories
Jant Pharmacal AccuStrip Strep A II (direct from throat swab)	Applied Biotech, Inc.
LifeSign LLC Status Strep A	Princeton BioMeditech
Mainline Confirms Strep A Dots Test (direct from throat swab)	Applied Biotech, Inc.
Meridian Diagnostics ImmunoCard STAT Strep A (direct from throat swab)	Applied Biotech, Inc.
Polymedco, Inc. Poly stat A (II)	Applied Biotech, Inc.
QuickVue In-Line One-Step Strep A Test	Quidel Corporation
QuickVue Dipstick Strep A	Quidel Corporation
Quidel QuickVue In-Line Strep A	Quidel Corporation
Remel RIM A.R.C. Strep A Test	Applied Biotech, Inc
SmithKline ICON Fx Strep A Test (from throat swab only)	Binax
Stanbio QuStick Strep A	Stanbio Laboratory
Wyntek Diagnostics OSOM Strep A Test	Wyntek Diagnostics, Inc.
Wyntek OSOM Ultra Strep A Test	Wyntek Diagnostics, Inc

Source: Clinical Laboratory Improvement Amendments of 1988 categorized list as of June 17, 2004. See the Centers for Disease Control and Prevention Web site (www.cdc.gov) for the most current listing.

Examination Methods

The most common methods of fecal specimen examination for parasitic identification in a clinic or POL is the direct wet-mount slide.

Specimen Collection

Fecal specimens for identification of ova and parasites should be collected in wide-mouth containers with a tight lid to prevent leakage. The container should be put in a biohazard transport bag to avoid contamination and sent for examination immediately. The patient should be instructed not to contaminate the specimen with urine because it could interfere with testing. Special vials containing formalin are also available for ova and parasite testing that are preferred by some laboratories. Refer to the laboratory users manual for specific instructions.

The laboratory procedure for collection and processing of the parasite specimen should be strictly followed to provide an accurate testing of the specimen. The collection time of the specimen should be followed as directed by the physician. Three specimens may be ordered over a specified period. Physician's offices will have specific instructions and containers with a preservative in them when an ova and parasite examination is requested.

When the specimen is sent for testing, it should be labeled correctly with the patient's name, date, and time of the specimen. It is important to know if the patient has been traveling, to what area of the world, and what is suspected by the physician to help aid in identification.

Common Parasites

Some of the more common parasites identified in the POL are *Enterobius vermicularis*, the causative organism of pinworm infection, and *Trichomonas vaginalis*, a parasite that infects the urogenital tracts of men and women.

Enterobius vermicularis. This **nematode** (round worm) is found worldwide, predominantly in children. The adult worm is shaped like a pin, wide at one end and

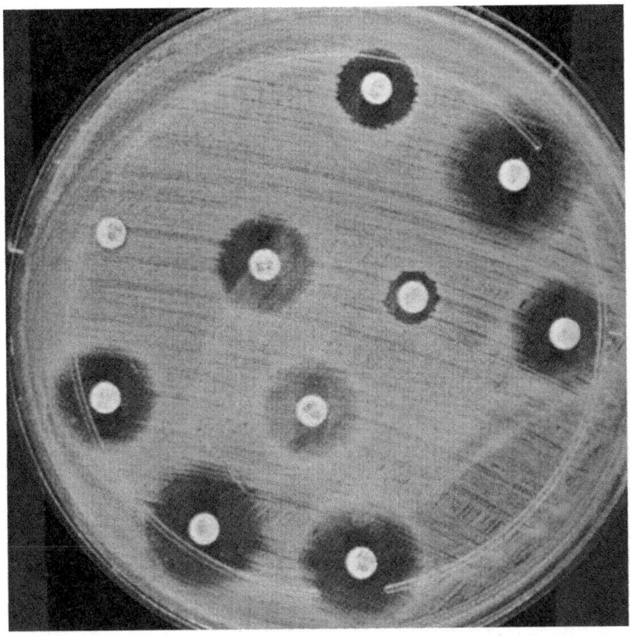

Figure 31-18 Culture plate showing antibiotic discs on bacteria. Note the one antibiotic disc in the top left area that the bacteria are totally "resistant to." Most of the other antibiotics have varying degrees of effectiveness and would be labeled "sensitive to." The one just right of the center area is barely effective. This one would be reported as "intermediate."

pointed at the other end. The female worm is larger than the male. Infection with pinworm can cause severe itching, irritability, and insomnia, depending on the severity of the infection. The adult female worm migrates to the anus at night, depositing ova (eggs) that cause itching during hatching. At times, the adult worm can be found around the anus and on the stool. The adult worm measures approximately 7 to 12 mm long (Figure 31-19A). The egg is the infectious stage of the parasite (see Figure 31-19B).

To diagnose the presence of the parasite, either the adult worm or ova has to be located in the specimen. A negative test should be confirmed by as many as six negative tests performed. The test is performed by taking a cellophane tape swab and placing the sticky side down to the skin around the anal area. The tape is placed on a slide and brought to the laboratory for examination (Figure 31-20).

Trichomonas vaginalis. This parasite is found in both men and women, but its presence is five times higher in women (men can harbor the organism for years without symptoms). Because men can harbor this parasite and have no symptoms, it is recommended that both partners be treated. This will prevent the ongoing reinfection of

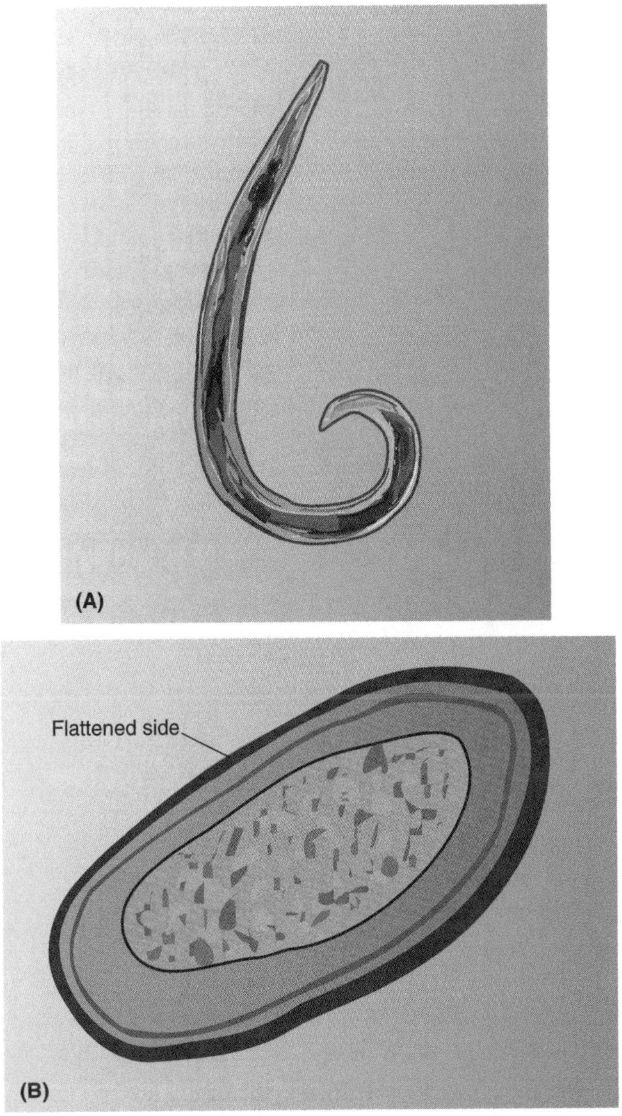

Figure 31-19 (A) Adult pinworm, *Enterobius vermicularis.* (B) *Enterobius vermicularis* egg (pinworm egg) at the infectious stage.

Online Images and Information about Parasites

The Centers for Disease Control and Prevention (CDC) has an extensive Web site with a wealth of information about many health issues. Of particular interest to medical assistants and other health care professionals interested in parasites is its section on Parasitic Diseases and Prevention. This section of the CDC's Web site can be located via the http://www.cdc.gov address, or an easier, more direct route is using the keywords "cdc pdp" while accessing your favorite search engine. Be sure to visit the "Professional" pages and "PDx Lab Assistance" for a great image library and even some video clips that allow you to watch these parasites in action.

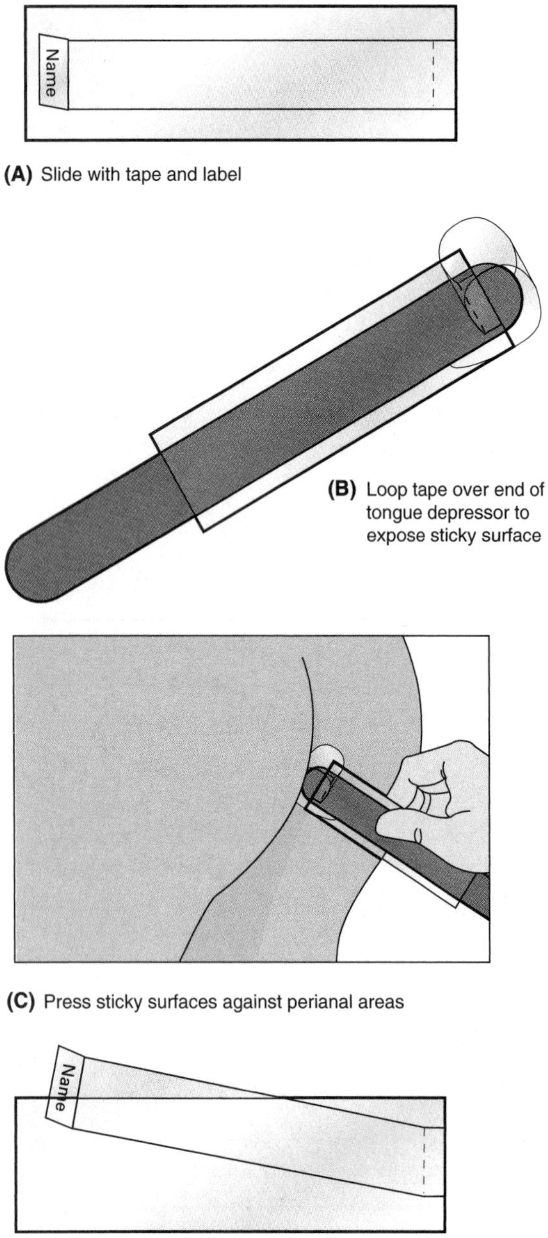

(A) Slide with tape and label

(B) Loop tape over end of tongue depressor to expose sticky surface

(C) Press sticky surfaces against perianal areas

(D) Replace tape

Figure 31-20 Technique for preparing and using a cellophane tape swab.

the female patient. The organism belongs to the flagellate (possesses flagella) class and is extremely motile. Infection with this flagellate causes a purulent yellowish green discharge and dysuria. The organism is recovered from the discharge or urine and is transmitted sexually.

The trichomonad is recovered in a wet preparation slide of spun urine or vaginal secretion mixed with a drop of saline. (See Procedure 31-2.) The specimen should not be contaminated with fecal material that could contain *Trichomonas hominis*, another flagellate. The prepared slide is examined under the low and high objectives of the microscope to observe the motility and morphology of the parasite (see Figure 30-14). There are also test kits and fluorescent stains used to diagnose this parasite.

MYCOLOGY

The field of mycology and the infections that cause fungi are extensive. Most identification and sensitivities testing for fungal organisms take place in larger laboratories and specific reference laboratories. Identification of two of the common fungal infections can be made quickly in the clinic or POL.

The genus *Candida* has several species that cause yeast infections in the body. *Candida* species are also present in the environment around us. They present a particular problem in the health care setting where they can cause serious nosocomial infections. Equipment can be easily contaminated with *Candida* organisms.

Yeast infections commonly are found on the moist areas of the body and in the subcutaneous tissue. An infection with yeast can range from mild to serious. *Candida albicans* is the causative agent of vaginal yeast infections. The specimen is examined microscopically for the characteristic budding yeast forms. (See Procedure 31-2.) If the specimen is fluid and clear, it is placed on a slide with a drop of saline. If the specimen is thick, it should be mixed with 10% KOH (one drop) on the slide to clear away debris. Once the specimen is prepared, it is examined microscopically.

Another group of significant fungi that sometimes can be generally identified are the **dermatophytes.** These fungi cause infections on the hair, skin, and nails. The microscopic structure of these fungi is detailed. Some of the fungi that cause dermatophytic infections can be diagnosed using a **Wood's lamp.** This is a lamp with an ultraviolet light. Some dermatophytes will fluoresce (glow brightly) under this light.

Mycotic infections can also be identified through culture and kit identification systems. Fungi can produce heavy aerosols and should be processed and observed under a safety hood.

Procedure 31-1 Procedure for Obtaining a Throat Specimen for Culture

STANDARD PRECAUTIONS:

PURPOSE:

To obtain secretions from the nasopharnyx and tonsillar area for means of identifying a pathogenic microorganism.

EQUIPMENT/SUPPLIES:

Tongue depressor
Culture tube with applicator stick or commercially prepared culture collection system (culturette)
Label and requisition form
Gloves and face shield
Good light source

PROCEDURE STEPS:

1. Identify yourself and explain the procedure to the patient. RATIONALE: Identifying yourself helps establish professional trust and rapport with the patient. Explaining the procedure allows the patient to understand the process and encourages cooperation.
2. Have an emesis basin and tissues ready. RATIONALE: You will want to be prepared in case the patient spits up or vomits.
3. Have the patient in a sitting position. RATIONALE: The patient in a sitting position will facilitate better visualization of the throat area.
4. Wash hands, gather supplies, and apply gloves and face shield. RATIONALE: Washing hands before any patient contact will eliminate contamination. Gathering equipment before beginning the procedure assures less chance of errors caused by missing supplies. Gloves and a face shield will offer personal protection in case the patient coughs, spits up, or vomits.
5. Ask the patient to open his or her mouth wide and then adjust the light source. RATIONALE: A widely opened mouth and properly adjusted light source will facilitate better visualization of the throat area.
6. Remove the swab from the culturette using sterile technique. RATIONALE: Using sterile technique maintains the sterility of the swab, which results in a quality specimen for culture.
7. Ask the patient to say "ah." Depress the tongue with the tongue depressor and swab the back of the throat and tonsillar area. Concentrate primarily on any red, raw areas and pustules. Take care to not touch the swab on the inside of the cheeks or on the tongue. RATIONALE: Having the patient say "ah" lowers the back of the tongue. Depressing the tongue reminds the patient to keep the mouth opened and assists in keeping the back of the tongue down. Swabbing only the tonsillar area and the back of the throat without touching the inside of the cheeks or the tongue assures that the specimen will contain mostly the bacterial infectious agent (streptococci), if present, and not normal mouth flora or other contaminants. The red, raw areas and pustules will most likely contain the greatest concentration of streptococci.
8. Place the swab back into the culturette using sterile technique and crush the glass capsule containing the culture media. (NOTE: Some culturettes require a puncturing action to release the media. Follow the manufacturer's instructions.) RATIONALE: Using sterile technique avoids contaminating the specimen and having the specimen contaminate any other area. Crushing the glass capsule (or piercing the culture membrane) releases the culture medium, which will maintain the optimum environment for the specimen until it is tested at the regional laboratory.
9. Label the culturette according the POL policy and requirements. RATIONALE: Proper and timely labeling of all specimens assures that samples will not be mixed up with other patient samples.
10. Ensure patient comfort and answer any questions related to the testing. RATIONALE: Ensuring patient comfort and answering questions will establish professional rapport.
11. Discard contaminated supplies into a biohazard waste container. Disinfect all work surfaces.

(continues)

Procedure 31-1 (continued)

Properly remove gloves and face shield and discard appropriately. RATIONALE: Following Standard Precautions when disposing of contaminated supplies and disinfecting work surfaces will eliminate biohazard contaminations.

12. Wash hands. RATIONALE: Gloves will protect hands from most but not all infectious microorganisms. Washing hands will also remove residual powders and latex.
13. Complete the laboratory requisition and record the procedure in the patient's medical record/chart. RATIONALE: Completing the laboratory requisition properly and in a timely manner will give the regional laboratory accurate information regarding the patient and the specimen. Charting the procedure will establish a timeline and document the procedure.

DOCUMENTATION

1/12/XX 10:11 AM Throat culture specimen obtained and sent to Inner City Laboratory for C & S. Patient tolerated the procedure well and will return for a follow-up visit and medication reevaluation in two days per Dr. King's request. Appt scheduled 1/14 at 3:30 PM. Joe Guerrero, CMA

Procedure 31-2 Wet Mount and Hanging Drop Slide Preparations

STANDARD PRECAUTIONS:

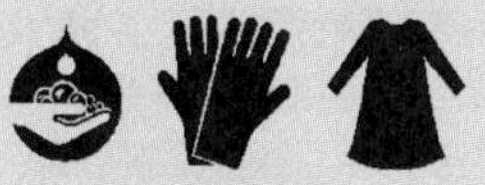

PURPOSE:

Prepare a slide for viewing live organisms for motility and identifying characteristics.

EQUIPMENT/SUPPLIES:

Gloves
Laboratory coat
Clean glass slide
Glass slide with concave well
Coverslips
Petroleum jelly
Dropper
Bacterial suspension

PROCEDURE STEPS:

1. Wash hands and apply gloves. RATIONALE: Washing hands before any procedure helps to eliminate contamination. Gloves will offer personal protection.
2. Assemble equipment and supplies. RATIONALE: Gathering equipment before beginning the procedure assures less chance of errors caused by missing supplies.
3. For wet-mount slide preparation:
   a. Place a drop of the bacterial suspension onto a clean glass slide (Figure 31-21A). RATIONALE: The suspension of bacteria in a drop facilitates viewing.
   b. Place petroleum jelly around the edges of the coverslip (Figure 31-21B) and place the coverslip on top of the bacterial suspension (Figure 31-21C). RATIONALE: The petroleum jelly cuts down on the air currents and keeps the slide from drying out.

(continues)

Procedure 31-2 (continued)

4. For hanging drop slide preparation:
   a. Place the bacterial specimen (in suspension) in the center of the coverslip with petroleum jelly around the edges (Figure 31-22A). RATIONALE: For the suspended drop to be formed properly, this technique is used.
   b. Invert the slide and place the concave well of the slide over the specimen drop on the cover slip (Figure 31-22B). RATIONALE: This method allows the slide well to protect the drop.
   c. The slide is then carefully turned right side up for microscopic examination (Figure 31-22C). RATIONALE: The slide must be handled carefully to avoid slippage and disruption of the drop.

NOTE: After the smear is prepared properly, it can be observed microscopically at any power. Viewing the slide is considered by CLIA to be a physician-performed microscopy procedure.

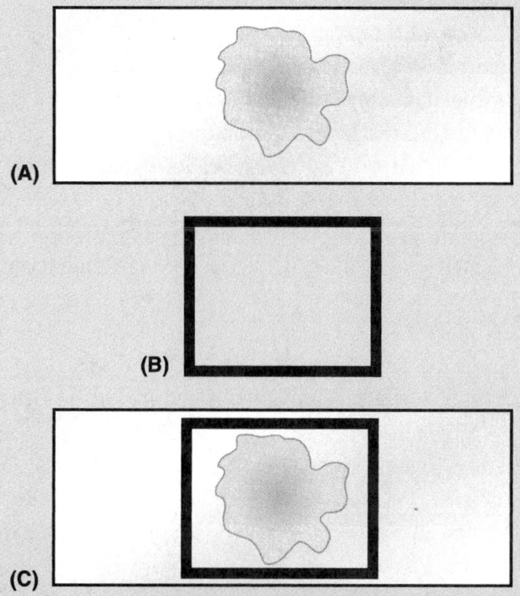

Figure 31-21 Wet-mount slide. (A) Specimen placed on a glass slide. (B) Coverslip with petroleum jelly on edges. (C) Coverslip placed directly on top of slide with specimen.

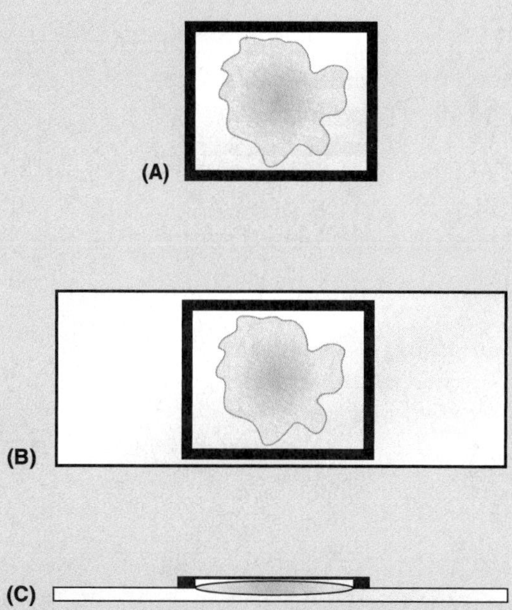

Figure 31-22 Hanging drop slide. (A) Specimen placed on coverslip. (B) Slide placed over coverslip. (C) Slide turned right side up for examination.

Procedure 31-3 Performing Strep Throat Testing

STANDARD PRECAUTIONS:

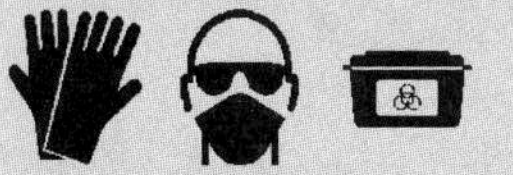

PURPOSE:

To test for streptococcus infection of the throat for diagnostic purposes. The following steps are intentionally general, so a variety of kits can be used.

EQUIPMENT/SUPPLIES:

Gloves
Commercial (CLIA waived) strep throat testing kit:
- Controls and reagents
- Sterile cotton tipped swabs
- Test tubes and holder or receptacles (depending on the kit used)

Tongue blade
Adjustable light source

PROCEDURE STEPS:

1. Wash hands and apply PPE. RATIONALE: Hands should always be washed prior to working with patients to avoid transferring pathogens. The PPEs are to protect you from the patient in case he or she coughs or vomits during the procedure.
2. Assemble and organize equipment and supplies. RATIONALE: Organization always presents a more professional image.
3. Introduce yourself, identify the patient, and explain the procedure. RATIONALE: Introducing yourself and explaining the procedure to the patient will gain their cooperation and establish a good rapport. Identifying the patient assures that the right patient will receive the test.
4. Using the tongue blade and light source, obtain the specimen from the patient's throat on the cotton tipped applicator. RATIONALE: The tongue blade will assist in keeping the mouth opened for ease in obtaining the specimen without contaminating it on the tongue, cheek, or roof of the mouth.
5. Follow the manufacturer's instructions exactly to perform the strep throat test. Be sure to also run the controls tests. RATIONALE: Each manufacturer's kit varies slightly in the method used. The controls are to ensure quality results.
6. Properly dispose of all waste in biohazard container. Disinfect the equipment and the area. RATIONALE: Standard precautions are used to prevent disease transmission.
7. Complete the laboratory report form and notify the physician of the results. RATIONALE: The physician will treat the disease as soon as it is confirmed.
8. Document the procedure in the patient's medical record. RATIONALE: Proper documentation assures good recordkeeping for quality medical.

Case Study 31-1

Mary O'Keefe has brought her 3-year-old son Chris to the office of Drs. Lewis and King with a temperature of 102°F and an extremely sore and red throat. He is irritable and crying. After examining Chris, Dr. King orders a quick test for Group A Streptococcus. Medical assistant Joe Guerrero has a difficult time acquiring the throat swab for the test because of Chris's condition. The test is run, and the results are negative.

CASE STUDY REVIEW

1. What are some reasons the test is negative?
2. What other procedure can be done to diagnose strep throat?
3. How would the test in question 2 be set up?

SUMMARY

The field of microbiology is vast. There are many microorganisms that are pathogenic and can cause serious infection in patients. The successful culturing and identification of such organisms is an important aspect of the successful treatment of patients. All specimens that are processed in the POL should be handled carefully, and all safety guidelines should be followed.

For the pathogen to be identified correctly, the utmost care must be taken in obtaining the culture. Sterile equipment must be used. When the culture is processed, the correct microscopic examination, media, incubation, and confirmatory tests must be used correctly to identify the pathogen.

Often a sensitivity test will be requested together with the culture. The information from this test will guide the physician in selecting the appropriate treatment for the patient.

POLs vary in the type and number of cultures that are performed on the premises and those that are sent out to be performed in a reference laboratory. It is important to provide the best care for the patient by doing only those tests that a POL can reasonably handle given equipment, personnel limitations, and CLIA regulations.

In addition to performing bacterial identification, some POLs perform parasitology and mycology tests on a limited basis. When performing parasitology tests, it is important to obtain the proper specimen in the correct manner. When performing mycology tests, it is important to work under a safety hood to minimize the risk for exposure to spores from the fungal specimens.

Of utmost importance is the careful adherence to Quality Control guidelines. These procedures ensure the integrity of test results.

STUDY FOR SUCCESS

To reinforce your knowledge and skills of information presented in this chapter:

- ❑ Review the Key Terms
- ❑ Practice the Procedures
- ❑ Consider the Case Study and discuss your conclusions
- ❑ Answer the Review Questions
  - ❑ Multiple Choice
  - ❑ Critical Thinking
- ❑ Navigate the Internet by completing the Web Activities
- ❑ Practice the StudyWARE activities on the CD
- ❑ Apply your knowledge in the Student Workbook activities
- ❑ Complete the Web Tutor sections
- ❑ View and discuss the DVD situations

REVIEW QUESTIONS

Multiple Choice

1. A structure that is *not* part of all bacterial cells is the:
   a. nucleus
   b. ribosome
   c. spore
   d. cell wall
2. An example of nonselective media would be media that:
   a. contain a substance that alters the appearance of some organisms
   b. will support the growth of all organisms and does not alter their appearance
   c. support the growth of one type of organism and inhibit the growth of other types of organisms
   d. identify the biochemical activity of some organisms

3. When a CSF culture cannot be set up immediately, it should be placed in the incubator or remain at room temperature as opposed to being placed in the refrigerator because some organisms are affected by a low temperature. An example of this type of organism would be:
   a. *Beta streptococci*
   b. *Neisseria meningitidis*
   c. *Streptococcus pneumoniae*
   d. *Staphylococcus aureus*
4. The enterobacteriaceae are:
   a. Gram-positive organisms that include *staphylococcus* and *streptococcus* species
   b. fungal organisms that are easily identified in the laboratory
   c. Gram-negative organisms that commonly reside as normal flora in the intestinal tract but can cause infection
   d. common agents of sore throats
5. The best method of taking a specimen for the recovery of anaerobic organisms is to:
   a. swab deep and place into an anaerobic container
   b. aspirate purulent fluid and place into a test tube
   c. swab around the wound and place into an anaerobic container
   d. take as any other specimen for culture

Critical Thinking

1. Name two ways to identify whether an organism is motile.
2. Define an aerosol and explain how protection is provided when working with an aerosol.
3. Identify one potential pathogen and list the specimen source, media for culture, microscopic appearance, and the disease it causes.
4. A patient is given a requisition slip for a stool culture, ova, and parasite examination. How would you instruct this patient to collect the specimen?
5. Explain why pinworm specimens are collected at a certain time of the day.

WEB ACTIVITIES

Visit the Centers for Disease Control and Prevention's Web site and other Web sites to review guidelines on reportable diseases for your state.

REFERENCES/BIBLIOGRAPHY

Department of Health and Human Services, Centers for Disease Control and Prevention. (2004). Diseases and Conditions. Retrieved from http://www.cdc.gov. Accessed June 27, 2005.

U.S. Food and Drug Administration. (2004). Databases on the FDA Website. Retrieved from http://www.fda.gov/search/databases.html. Accessed June 27, 2005.

Walters, N. J., Estridge, B. H., & Reynold, A. P. (2000). *Basic medical laboratory techniques* (4th ed.). Clifton Park, NY: Thomson Delmar Learning.

Wedding, M. E., & Toenjes, S. A. (1998). *Medical laboratory procedures* (2nd ed.). Philadelphia: FA Davis.

THE DVD HOOK-UP

DVD Series	Program Number
Skills Based Series	**12**

Chapter/Scene Reference
- *Administer Fecal Collection and Performing Occult Blood Test*
- *Administering Sputum Collection*
- *Administering Throat Culture and Performing Rapid Strep Test*

This chapter discusses basic microbiology procedures. The selected scenes in this program demonstrate how to educate patients in collecting more sensitive specimens.

1. Do you think that Mr. Turell was a little embarrassed about discussing the proper technique for collecting a stool sample with the medical assistant? Why?
2. In the scene about collecting a sputum specimen, the medical assistant waited in the room while the patient collected the specimen. Did that scene bother you? Do you think that you will be able to stay in the room with the patient when you are responsible for collecting a sputum sample?
3. Why should you not touch the tongue when collecting a throat specimen?

DVD Journal Summary

Write a paragraph that summarizes what you learned from watching the selected scenes from today's DVD program. Are you worried about collecting specimens that may cause you or the patient to gag? What if you suddenly become sick yourself and have to run out of the patient's room? How would you handle such an episode with the patient?

CHAPTER 32

Specialty Laboratory Tests

OUTLINE

KEY TERMS

- ABO Blood Group
- Agglutination
- Antibody
- Antigen
- Antiserum
- Bilirubin
- Blood Urea Nitrogen (BUN)
- Cholesterol
- Choriocarcinoma
- Cushing's Syndrome
- Diabetes Mellitus
- Ectopic Pregnancy
- Enzyme Immunoassay
- Epstein–Barr Virus (EBV)
- Guthrie Screening Test
- Heterophile Antibodies
- High-Density Lipoprotein (HDL)
- Human Chorionic Gonadotropin (hCG)
- Hydatidiform Mole
- Hyperglycemia
- Hypoglycemia
- Infectious Mononucleosis
- Insulin
- Latex Beads
- Low-Density Lipoprotein (LDL)
- Mantoux Test
- Phenylketonuria (PKU)
- Purified Protein Derivative (PPD)
- Rh Factor
- Semen
- Triglycerides
- Tuberculosis (TB)
- Wheal

FEATURED COMPETENCIES

CAAHEP—ENTRY-LEVEL COMPETENCIES

Clinical Competencies

Fundamental Procedures

- Perform handwashing
- Dispose of biohazard materials
- Practice Standard Precautions

Specimen Collection

- Perform capillary puncture

Diagnostic Testing

- CLIA waived tests
- Perform hematology testing
- Perform chemistry testing
- Perform immunology testing

General Competencies

Legal Concepts

- Perform within legal and ethical boundaries
- Document appropriately
- Demonstrate knowledge of federal and state health care legislation and regulations

Operational Functions

- Use methods of quality control

ABHES STANDARDS—ENTRY-LEVEL COMPETENCIES

Professionalism

- Conduct work within scope of education, training, and ability

Clinical Duties

- Apply principles of aseptic techniques and infection control
- Use quality control

(continues)

OBJECTIVES

The student should strive to meet the following performance objectives and demonstrate an understanding of the facts and principles presented in this chapter through written and oral communication.

1. Define the key terms as presented in the glossary.
2. List the three main precautions to be observed during all tests and the collection of samples included in this chapter.
3. Collect samples and perform and interpret all tests included in this chapter.
4. Discuss factors to be considered when evaluating test results.
5. Discuss transmission, incubation period, and symptoms of Epstein–Barr virus/infectious mononucleosis.
6. List the blood group antigens and antibodies found in each of the four ABO groups and the Rh factors.
7. Explain the cause of phenylketonuria (PKU) and the symptoms caused by untreated PKU.
8. Indicate normal and increased levels of phenylalanine and the dietary restrictions to be observed by PKU patients.
9. Discuss the cause of tuberculosis and some major characteristics of *Mycobacterium tuberculosis.*
10. Discuss the role of insulin in the regulation of blood glucose levels.
11. List and discuss differences among the normal values for fasting blood glucose, two-hour postprandial glucose, and the glucose tolerance test.
12. Explain the importance of cholesterol and triglyceride testing to identify patients at high risk for coronary heart disease.
13. Give the desirable values of cholesterol for adults.
14. Give the acceptable level of low-density lipoprotein (LDL) in persons with or without coronary heart disease, and discuss the role of high-density lipoprotein and LDL in coronary heart disease.
15. Give the normal values of urea nitrogen for adults, children, infants, and newborns, and discuss the significance of increased blood urea levels.

SCENARIO

Audrey Jones, CMA, has worked at Drs. Lewis and King's office for more than five years. In that time, Audrey has become proficient in obtaining specimens from patients for various laboratory tests. Audrey enjoys the work and finds it extremely challenging. She also realizes that communicating with patients to help them understand why their specimens are necessary for testing is just as important as being skillful in collecting and testing the specimens. Audrey has found that when she explains the reason the specimen is needed in terms patients can understand, they are often less fearful, which helps them relax. This can be especially helpful when collecting blood specimens.

FEATURED COMPETENCIES (continued)

- Collect and process specimens
- Perform selected tests that assist with diagnosis and treatment
- Dispose of biohazard materials
- Practice Standard Precautions
- Perform capillary puncture (heelstick)
- Obtain throat culture for microbiological testing
- Perform chemistry testing
- Perform immunology testing

Legal Concepts

- Document accurately

Spotlight on Certification

RMA Content Outline

- Medical law
- Patient education
- Laboratory procedures

CMA Content Outline

- Patient instruction
- Medicolegal guidelines and requirements
- Collecting and processing specimens; diagnostic testing

CMAS Content Outline

- Legal and ethical considerations
- Communication

INTRODUCTION

An increasing number of tests are performed in the ambulatory care setting, many of them by the medical assistant. To meet these new demands, the medical assistant must have a strong background in a variety of areas including medical terminology, Clinical Laboratory Improvement Amendments (CLIA) Regulations, laboratory safety procedures, and specimen collection. Because many procedures require collection of a blood specimen, the medical assistant must also be an excellent phlebotomist. Good recordkeeping and communications skills round out the requirements. A quality-control program is necessary to assure that the results are accurate and reliable. This will require a commitment on the part of the medical assistant to maintain the highest standards throughout the process.

A variety of specialty tests are covered in this chapter, including testing for pregnancy, infectious mononucleosis, tuberculosis (TB), and PKU (phenylketonuria), as well as blood types, hemoglobin A1c, and protime. This chapter also discusses the chemistry of blood, including chemistry panels, blood glucose, cholesterol, triglycerides, and other specialty laboratory tests such as semen analysis.

PREGNANCY TESTS

Pregnancy tests are used when pregnancy is suspected. Pregnancy tests may also be used to rule out pregnancy before prescribing birth control pills, radiograph studies, certain antibiotics or other drugs, and for female patients who are to undergo surgery.

Pregnancy testing is based on detection of **human chorionic gonadotropin (hCG),** a hormone secreted by the placenta that can be detected in the serum or urine of pregnant women as early as five days after conception. During pregnancy, hCG levels peak at about eight weeks, then decrease to lower but detectable levels for the remainder of the pregnancy.

Commercial/Home Pregnancy Tests

A variety of accurate and easy-to-use commercial tests are available for use in the medical office. Manufacturers of pregnancy test kits have designed them to be sensitive, to be easy to perform and interpret, and to give rapid results. Pregnancy tests are one of many tests available for purchase as an over-the-counter product. However, results of tests performed at home should be confirmed by a laboratory test using appropriate quality-control measures and properly trained personnel. CLIA has granted waived status to all urine pregnancy tests that use visual color comparison and specifically to the Bayer Corporations Clinitek 50 Urine Chemistry Analyzer for hCG in urine. Medical assistants qualify for the waived test category within the physicians' office laboratory (POL).

Testing Methods

Two testing methods using urine are discussed in this section: the slide test or agglutination inhibition test and the modified enzyme immunoassay. Diagnosis of pregnancy is made using these test results in conjunction with a physical examination including a pelvic examination by a physician.

A positive reaction to any pregnancy test does not necessarily indicate a normal pregnancy. Detection of hCG can also indicate such abnormal conditions as an **ectopic pregnancy,** a developing **hydatidiform mole** of the uterus, **choriocarcinoma,** or cancer of the lung, stomach, pancreas, colon, or breast.

Quality Control. Kits must be stored and used at the temperature directed by the manufacturer. Most kits contain a built-in control; however, appropriate positive and negative urine controls must always be run with patient specimens. Kits and reagents must not be used after the expiration date. Manufacturer's instructions must be followed precisely for the particular test used.

Precautions for Pregnancy Testing

1. Use a clean container for collection of the urine specimen. Disposable containers are preferred. Detergent residue on nondisposable containers may interfere with test results.
2. The first-voided morning urine has the highest concentration of hCG and is the preferred specimen. If this is not available, a urine specimen with a specific gravity of at least 1.010 is acceptable.
3. Although it is always best to run tests on fresh specimens, if the urine specimen cannot be tested immediately, it may be stored at 4°C for up to 24 hours. Both urine and serum specimens may be used with some test kits; other kits use only one or the other.
4. Allow refrigerated urine specimens and test reagents to come to room temperature before starting test procedures.
5. If using the slide test procedure:
   a. Avoid cross contamination with other urine specimens.
   b. Use a new stirrer for each test.

Slide Test or Agglutination Inhibition Test

The slide test is based on inhibition of **agglutination** (clumping) of hCG-coated **latex beads.** The hCG **antiserum** (**antibody** against hCG) is added to urine on a microscope slide. If hCG is present in the urine, an hCG/anti-hCG complex forms between the antiserum and the patient's hCG. Next, an **antigen** reagent containing latex beads coated with hCG is added to the mixture. If the hcG/anti-hCG complex formed, then there is no hCG antiserum available to react with the latex beads, and agglutination will *not* occur. No agglutination indicates positive pregnancy. Agglutination of the latex beads indicates negative pregnancy.

Enzyme Immunoassay Test

The **enzyme immunoassay** (EIA) is a more complex procedure than agglutination. The test can be designed in several different ways, but it always involves an antigen, an antibody specific for the antigen, and a second antibody. The test may be designed to detect a particular antibody in a patient's serum or to detect an antigen in a patient specimen.

Numerous tests are based on variations of the EIA. New technologies have been developed called membrane EIAs. In these tests, most of the reagents are incorporated into an absorbent membrane, which is enclosed in plastic. When the sample (serum or urine) is added, it migrates through the membrane, reacting with the reagents and forming a color. Many of these tests are simple to set up and interpret even though the technology is complex. Examples of membrane EIAs include over-the-counter pregnancy test kits and tests for Group A Streptococcus.

Enzyme immunoassays for hCG vary in design but have some features in common. Most have the reagents incorporated into an absorbent membrane within a self-contained test unit, which may look like a plastic slide, a reagent strip, or a test cylinder. Tests may require the addition of the sample only or the addition of the sample and reagents to the test unit. Procedure 32-1 shows the general steps for pregnancy testing.

INFECTIOUS MONONUCLEOSIS

Infectious mononucleosis (IM) is a contagious disease that may have vague clinical symptoms and can mimic other diseases. Serologic tests are often the basis for an early diagnosis of the disease and may also be used to follow the course of the disease.

IM is commonly called "mono" or "kissing disease." The disease is a result of infection of the lymphocytes by the **Epstein–Barr virus (EBV).** EBV is common in our population. By 5 years of age, approximately 50% of the population are infected, increasing to 90% to 95% in adults. After the primary infection, the virus establishes a lifelong latency. The infectious virus may be isolated from saliva from several months, whereas antigens may be detected for life. In addition to causing IM, EBV has been implicated in other diseases such as nasopharyngeal carcinoma (NPC) and chronic fatigue syndrome.

Transmission of EBV

Transmission of EBV IM is primarily by saliva, which is why it is often referred to as "the kissing disease." EBV may also be spread by the sharing of drinking glasses, and less often by blood transfusion. The disease is moderately contagious and is transmitted approximately 10% to 38% of the time in close social groups. In the home or in the hospital, careful handwashing will help prevent transmission of the virus.

Symptoms of IM

Mononucleosis is seen most often in children and young adults. Incubation may vary from 4 to 50 days; however, 7 to 14 days is the average. Infection in younger children is usually asymptomatic or manifests minor symptoms such as pharyngitis, otitis media, bronchitis, and other upper respiratory discomforts.

Classic symptoms usually occur when the primary infection is delayed until the second decade of life. It is the 15- to 25-year-old age group in which IM is most often observed. Symptoms usually begin with a fever and swollen glands lasting for three to five days. Over the next 7 to 20 days, the patient may develop a headache, malaise, chest pain, a cough, tonsillitis, a rash, soft, swollen lymph nodes, and a swollen spleen. While the spleen is enlarged, the patient is advised to curtail activity, especially contact sports and rough activities, to prevent the rare, but serious, rupture of the spleen. Symptoms usually persist for two to four weeks and in more serious cases may last for more than a month.

Treatment of IM

Because there are currently no effective drugs available for EBV IM treatment is primarily palative, or supportive. Although a vaccine is not yet available, some important work in that direction is ongoing.

Diagnosis of IM

To properly diagnose IM, the physician must consider blood and serology test results together with the patient's symptoms.

Blood Test for IM. The hematologic tests for IM include white blood cell count and evaluation of the patient's lymphocytes. In IM, a lymphocytosis, or increase in lymphocytes, usually occurs, and large numbers of lymphocytes (greater than 20%) have an unusual or atypical appearance.

Serologic Test for IM. Persons with IM produce antibodies called **heterophile antibodies** by the sixth to tenth day of the illness. Heterophile antibodies are antibodies that react with similar antigens in more than one species. They are usually of the IgM class.

Detection of heterophile antibodies combined with the blood tests and patient sypmtoms provide the basis for the diagnosis of IM. The serologic test is usually positive after the first week of illness. However, if test results are negative, the test should be repeated after a week if clinical symptoms are still present.

CLIA Waived IM Tests

Several manufacturers have produced Clinical Laboratory Improvement Amendments (CLIA) waived test kits suitable for use by the medical assistant in the POL. See Table 32-1 for a listing of test kits.

Kits for IM usually provide all the necessary reagents, materials, and controls. The laboratory must obtain only the specimen to be tested, which is usually a small sample of the patient's plasma or serum or a drop of capillary blood.

Prothrombin Time/ProTime/INR

Prothrombin time, which is also called protime, PT, and international normalized ratio (INR), is a test for blood's clotting ability. It is used often for people who are taking anticoagulant medications such as Coumadin (warfarin). There is a careful balance that must be monitored between the blood clotting too readily or being so thin it will not clot. The desired levels of INR are 2.0 to 3.0.

BLOOD TYPING

Blood typing is based on the presence or absence of certain antigens on the surface of red blood cells (RBC). These antigens are carbohydrate molecules that react with antibodies specific to them to cause agglutination of the RBCs. Antibodies are protein molecules that are found in serum; they are also referred to as immunoglobulins (Ig). When RBC antigens and antibodies react, they cause the RBCs to agglutinate. This process is called hemagglutination. Hemagglutination reactions are used in the typing of blood. The two major categories of blood

TABLE 32-1 LIST OF WAIVED TESTS FOR HETEROPHILE ANTIBODIES (INFECTIOUS MONONUCLEOSIS/EPSTEIN–BARR VIRUS)

Kit Name	Manufacturer
Applied Biotech SureStep Mono Test (whole blood)	Applied Biotech, Inc.
BioStar Acceava Mono Test (whole blood)	Wynteck Diagnostics, Inc.
Genzyme Contrast Mono (whole blood)	Genzyme Diagnostics
Genzyme OSOM Mono Test	Wyntek Diagnostics, Inc.
Jant Accutest Infectious Mononucleosis Test (whole blood)	Applied Biotech, Inc.
LifeSign UniStep Mono Test (whole blood)	Princeton BioMeditech Corp
Meridian ImmunoCard STAT Mono (for whole blood)	Applied Biotech, Inc.
Polymedco, Inc. Poly STAT Mono	Applied Biotech, Inc.
Quidel Cards O.S. Mono (for whole blood)	Quidel Corporation
Quidel QuickVue+ Infectious Mononucleosis (whole blood)	Quidel Corporation
Remel RIM A.R.C. Mono Test	Applied Biotech, Inc.
Seradyn Color Q Mono (whole blood)	Genzyme Diagnostics
Wampole Mono-Plus WB	Wampole Laboratories
Wyntek Diagnostics OSOM Mono Test (whole blood)	Wyntek Diagnostics

Source: Clinical Laboratory Improvement Amendments of 1988 Categorized List as of June 2004. See the Centers for Disease Control and Prevention's Web site (http:www.cdc.gov) for the most current listing.

typing are for the **ABO blood group** and the **Rh factor.** What is meant by ABO blood groups is type A, type B, type AB, or type O. Within each of those types are the Rh factors, either Rh-positive (factor present) or Rh-negative (no factor). Figure 32-1 illustrates how RBCs are tested for blood type. In that example, type O blood would have no reaction to either anti-A or anti-B, whereas type AB blood would have a reaction to both. By process of elimination, one can determine which type the specimen is.

The ABO and Rh systems place certain restrictions on how blood may be transfused from one individual to another. Depending on their blood type, individuals with a particular RBC antigen may have antibodies against the other types (Table 32-2). An incompatible blood transfusion results when the antigens of the donor RBCs react with the antibodies of the recipient RBCs. This is a potentially life-threatening situation, varying in severity from mild fever to anaphylaxis with severe intravascular hemolysis. Although ABO and Rh typing does not completely rule out the possibility of reaction, it greatly reduces the chances.

ABO Blood Typing

ABO blood typing is determined by the presence or absence of two major antigens, A and B. All people have one of the four blood group categories: A, B, AB, or O. People with group A RBCs have A antigens, group B RBCs have B antigens, group AB RBCs have antigens for both A and B, and group O RBCs lack both A and B antigens. Naturally occurring antibodies to the other antigen types are found in the serum.

ABO type may be determined by the slide or tube method. The tube method is now most often used for blood typing. Neither method is considered in the waived category by CLIA, thus they usually are not performed in the POL. Before any transfusion, the blood type is retested for "blood cross and match" as a precaution rather than accepting any previously performed and recorded result. Nevertheless, it is a good idea to know your individual blood type and Rh factor.

Rh Blood Typing

Rh typing is routinely performed together with ABO typing. The Rh system is named for the rhesus monkey used in experiments that led to its discovery. The Rh factor is found on the surface of RBCs. People possessing the Rh factor are said to have Rh-positive (Rh+) blood. Those without the Rh factor have Rh-negative (Rh–) blood.

About 85% of North Americans are Rh-positive; 15% are Rh-negative. Neither Rh-negative nor Rh-positive people have naturally occuring Rh antibodies in their blood. However, if an Rh-negative individual receives a transfusion of Rh-positive blood, he or she will develop antibodies to it. The antibodies take two weeks to develop. Both blood type and Rh factor must be taken into account for safe and successful transfusions.

Rh blood typing is also performed on pregnant patients to determine the mother's Rh blood type. During the patient's initial prenatal care examination, the blood typing is usually performed as part of the prenatal panel. In situations where the mother is Rh-negative, the mother's blood is tested for the presence of Rh antibodies. If the test is negative, then there is no risk to the fetus. A negative test should be repeated at weeks 30 and 36. If the test is positive, then the mother has been exposed to Rh-positive blood and has produced antibodies. A positive reaction also means that maternal hemolysis of fetal RBCs can occur. This condition is also called hemolytic disease of the newborn (HDN) (also known as erythroblastosis fetalis). When the mother's antibodies attack the baby's RBCs, the RBCs are destroyed. This will make the baby anemic, which limits the amount of oxygen to his or her tissues and organs. The baby responds by trying to make more RBCs in his or her liver and spleen. This overuse can cause these two organs to become enlarged. The new RBCs are usually immature (called erythroblasts) and are not able to do the work of the mature RBC. Also, when the RBCs are destroyed, **bilirubin** is formed. Babies cannot get rid of bilirubin, and it can build up in the blood and tissues and body fluids of the baby. This condition is called hyperbilirubinuremia (too much bilirubin in the blood). Bilirubin is pigmented and causes a yellowing or jaundice of the newborn's skin and tissues.

This jaundice is not to be confused with the jaundice many newborns have, which is caused by a similar process but to a much less degree and with mild consequences. Hemolytic disease can be determined by evaluating the quantity of bilirubin in the amniotic fluid and in the newborn's blood.

HDN can cause severe complications for the newborn, ranging from the enlarged liver and anemia to seizures, brain damage, and even death.

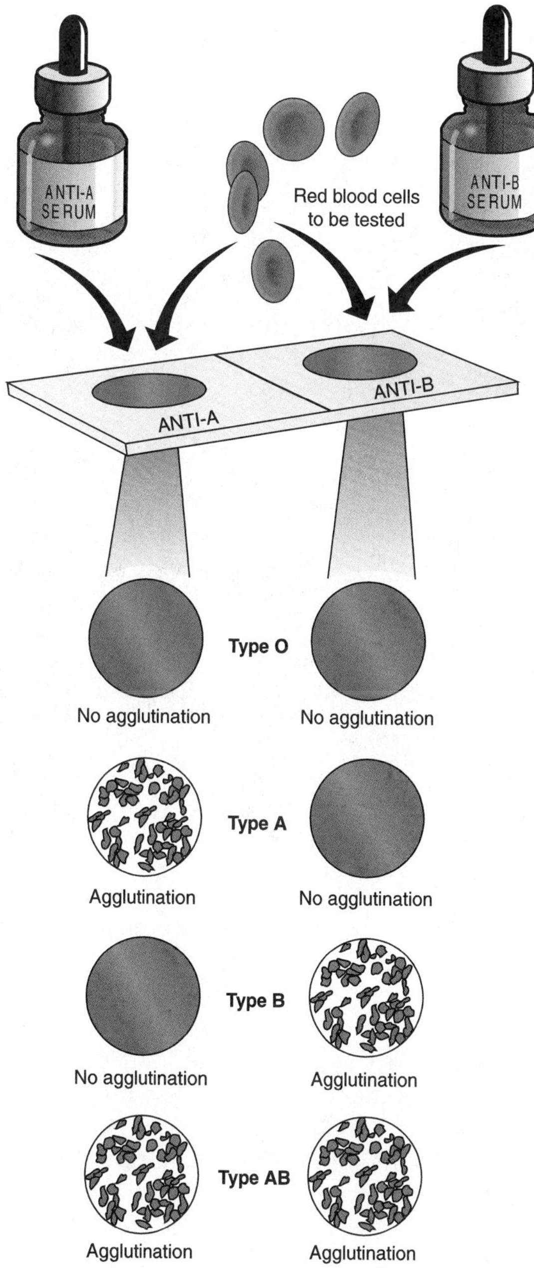

Figure 32-1 Blood typing the ABO groups.

TABLE 32-2 ANTIGENS AND ANTIBODIES IN ABO AND RH BLOOD SYSTEMS

Blood Group/Type	Antigen on RBC	Serum Antibodies
O (universal donor)	None	Anti-A and Anti-B
A	A	Anti-B
B	B	Anti-A
AB	A and B	None
Rh+	D	No anti-D*
Rh–	D	No anti-D*

*There are no naturally occurring antibodies to the Rh system.

Patient Education

When a woman gives birth (or has a miscarriage or abortion), some of the fetal blood can mix with the mother's as the placenta tears away from the uterus. When the Rh-negative woman is exposed to the baby's Rh positive blood (there is an 85% chance that the baby is Rh-positive), she builds antibodies against the Rh factor. Consequently, during the next pregnancy, her antibodies (which cross the placental barrier) would attack the next Rh-positive baby's RBCs. By giving the woman an injection of RhoGAM after each exposure to the Rh antigens, we prevent her from building the antibodies. Rh-negative women will need RhoGAM each time they are exposed to the Rh factor.

Treatment before the baby is born can include intrauterine blood transfusions and early delivery if the baby is mature enough to survive. After the baby is born, blood transfusions, intravenous fluids, and help with respiration and oxygen intake may be necessary.

Fortunately, most cases of HDN can be prevented by administering RhoGAM to the Rh-negative mother. When injected into the mother, RhoGAM will prevent her from producing the RhD antibody. The injection must be administered at the 28th week of pregnancy and within 72 hours after delivery of an Rh-positive baby, miscarriage, or termination of pregnancy.

SEMEN ANALYSIS

With the progression of managed health care, more primary care physicians are performing **semen** analysis in their offices to determine sperm cell counts before referring patients to fertility specialists. Examination of semen is also performed as part of a complete fertility work-up, to evaluate the effectiveness of a vasectomy, to determine paternity, and to substantiate rape cases.

When semen analysis is performed as part of a fertility work-up, the procedure involves macroscopic and microscopic analysis of seminal fluid for determination of total sperm count, percentage of motility, presence of agglutination, and percentage of normally formed sperm cells (Table 32-3). All male individuals will have variable sperm counts; therefore, a single analysis is insufficient. To achieve a reasonable estimate of these factors, the seminal analysis should be repeated at least three times over a two-month period. A complete analysis will also include an evaluation of the partner's cervical secretions and sperm survival. This involves determining the ability of sperm to penetrate the mucus and maintain motility.

TABLE 32-3 REFERENCE VALUES FOR SEMEN ANALYSIS

Parameter	Normal Range
Appearance	White, viscid, opaque
Volume	1.5–5 ml
pH	7.12–8.00
Total count	50–200 million
% normal sperm	At least 80%
% motility	At least 60%

Post vasectomy semen analysis is evaluated a few weeks after surgery. If sperm are seen at that time, then follow-up analysis is required. The patient is not considered sterile until he has returned *two* samples, at least one week apart, that demonstrate no sperm, viable or dead. This typically will take several weeks. Until that time, an alternative method of birth control must be used.

Semen Composition

Semen is a composite solution produced by the testes and the accessory male reproductive organs. It consists primarily of spermatozoa suspended in seminal plasma. Because there is considerable variation in composition between different portions of the fluid as ejaculated, it is important to collect the entire sample. Refer to the Patient Education box on page 891 for instructions to give to the patient before semen analysis.

Altering Factors in Semen Analysis

Many factors can alter the results of semen analysis. Several drugs such as cyclophosphamide (Cytoxan) and nitrogen mustard reduce sperm count, as well as orchitis (inflammation of the testes), testicular atrophy, testicular failure, and obstruction of the vas deferens. Cigarette smoking is associated with a decrease in the volume of semen, whereas coffee drinking results in increased sperm density and an increase in the percentage of cells with abnormal morphology. Fever may temporarily suppress the count. Although research suggests that consumption

Patient Education

The following instructions should be given to male patients when a semen sample is required for analysis:

1. Advise the patient to avoid consumption of alcohol for several days before the test. He should also avoid ejaculation for three days before collection of the semen sample.
2. Provide the patient with instructions and a container. The entire sample should be collected in a clean, dry, glass bottle that has been labeled, dated, and timed. The sample is collected by masturbation or interrupted coitus at home, or it may be collected at the medical office of the laboratory. A condom should never be used to collect a semen specimen due to the spermide content.
3. Specimens for complete fertility analysis collected outside the laboratory must be brought to the laboratory within 30 minutes. Postvasectomy specimens should be brought to the laboratory within one hour of collection.
4. The sample must be transported to the laboratory at 37°C (98.6°F). Low temperature during transport will decrease the motility of sperm. Temperature that is too warm could destroy the sperm. Keeping the sample close to his body during transport might be the best advice.

of alcohol does not affect sperm function as measured by semen analysis, the patient is instructed to avoid alcohol for several days before testing as a precaution.

Although research suggests that fertility is most closely correlated with motility and morphology, men with very high (>200 million/ml) or very low (≤20 million/ml) counts are likely to be infertile. Patients with aspermia (no sperm) or oligospermia (low sperm count, ≤20 million/ml) should be endocrinologically evaluated for pituitary, testicular, adrenal, or thyroid abnormalities.

PHENYLKETONURIA TEST

Phenylketonuria (PKU) is an inherited condition in which the baby is lacking an enzyme, phenylalanine, necessary to metabolize amino acids (protein molecules). Phenylalanine is present in milk and other dairy proteins. If the baby is missing this enzyme, the phenylalanine can build up in his or her brain and other organs and cause irreversible mental retardation, loss of muscle coordination, and other serious disorders. Diagnosis should be made early so the baby can be put on a diet low in proteins. The baby should be tested at about 2 days old and again at 7 to 14 days old. Although a phenylalanine-restricted diet will prevent mental retardation, it will not cure the underlying condition. Routine screening of newborns for PKU is mandatory in all states and may be performed in the hospital or the medical office. The medical assistant's role is to properly explain the procedure to the infant's parents and collect the blood specimen for analysis.

Many other tests can be performed using the blood sample sent on the PKU card, including tests for congenital hypothyroidism (CH), congenital adrenal hyperplasia (CAH), galactosemia, sickle cell disease, and others. The tests that are performed depend on individual state requirements.

Excess phenylalanine can be detected in blood or in urine. Normal levels of phenylalanine are less than 2 mg/deciliter (dl); more than 4 mg/dl is considered elevated. The **Guthrie screening test** is used to evaluate blood and is considered more accurate than urine tests. Phenylalanine can be detected in the blood of infants with PKU after three to four days on a breast milk or formula milk diet. Testing of breast-fed infants is delayed a few days because of the lack of phenylalanine in colostrum, the first breast milk. Colostrum is produced for the first two to three days after birth and is rich in antibodies, protein, and calories. True breast milk production begins after this time. Positive results from blood testing are confirmed by measuring serum phenylalanine and tyrosine levels. Infants with PKU have increasing phenylalanine levels (>4 mg/dl) and decreasing tyrosine levels <0.6 mg/dl).

Blood Testing for PKU

The Guthrie test was developed to screen for phenylalanine in the blood, and the first test is usually performed before the discharge of infants from the hospital. However, with managed care and the trend toward very short hospital stays for newborns, many pediatrician offices are now performing this first test. Capillary blood is collected from a heel stick onto a "filter paper" test card and sent to the laboratory for testing. Patient, physician, and test information, together with the blood samples, are placed directly on the laboratory test card, which is typically

> **Patient Education**
>
> Infants who test positive for PKU require a restricted phenylalanine diet for normal development to occur. Parents will need to have an appointment with a dietician to understand fully what foods the baby can and cannot eat. The diet will include a suitable milk substitute such as Lofenalac. Blood and urine tests will be necessary periodically to monitor the special diet.
>
> Women who have PKU and become pregnant must be especially careful to avoid phenylalanines during pregnancy.

provided by most State Departments of Health (Figure 32-2). See Procedure 32-3. Refer to Chapter 40 for proper capillary puncture technique.

Factors That May Influence the Guthrie Test. The following factors may influence the Guthrie test:

- Feeding problems such as vomiting may result in a false-negative reaction.
- Failure to ingest sufficient phenylalanine—testing before three to four days of the beginning of a milk diet—will result in a false-negative reaction.
- Premature infants may give false-positive test results because of a delay in the development of certain liver enzymes.
- If either the mother (if breast-feeding) or the child is taking drugs such as salicylates, aspirin, or antibiotics, they may interfere with the test results.

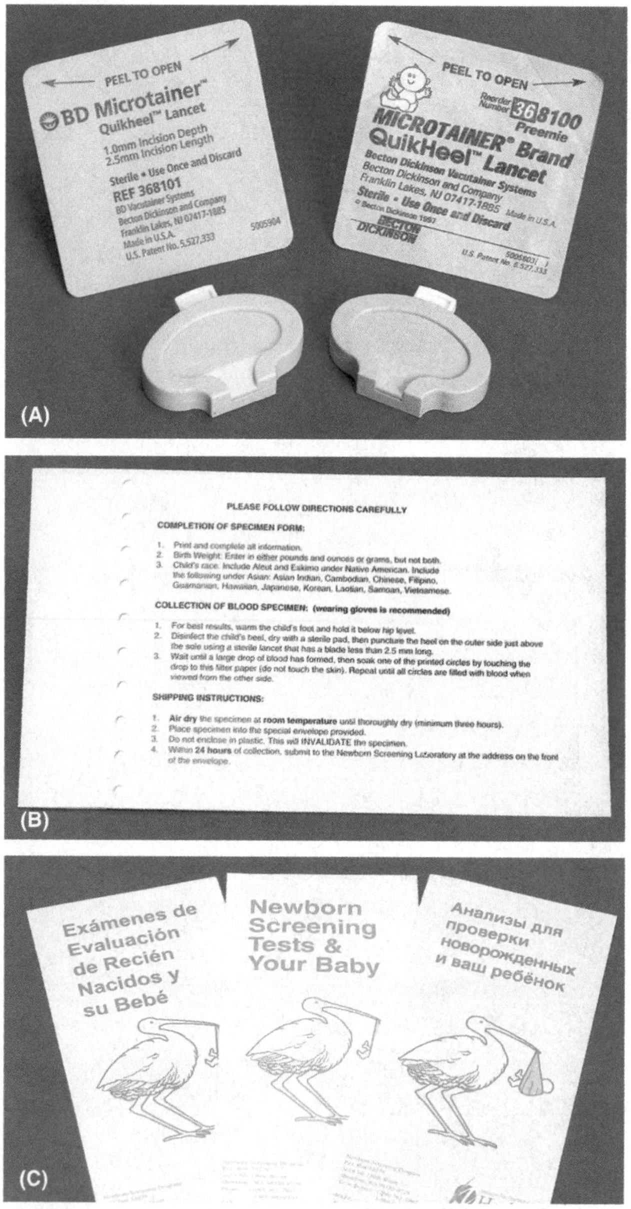

Figure 32-2 (A) Pediatric size safety lancets are available to limit the depth of the puncture. (B) The back of the PKU test card provides detailed instructions on performing the test and completing the card correctly. (C) Patient information and permission forms.

TUBERCULOSIS

Despite efforts to control its spread, **tuberculosis (TB)** infections are on the increase in the United States and around the world. Because tuberculosis morbidity is on the rise, increasing 14% from 1985 to 1997, more patients are screened now for the disease than ever before. The Advisory Council for Elimination of Tuberculosis, an independent group of TB-control experts, recommends screening all patients who fall into high-risk groups, or those who associate with high-risk groups, such as health care workers, including medical assistants. See the Current Family Practice Recommendations for TB Testing text box for a more complete list.

Cause of TB

Infectious TB is caused by the small, rod-shaped bacterium, *Mycobacterium tuberculosis*. This aerobic bacterium is nonmotile and has a high content of lipid in its cell wall making it difficult to stain using basic aniline dyes. For this reason, the Ziehl–Neelsen method was developed and is used as a tool for identification of mycobacteria.

Patient Education

Current Family Practice Recommendations for TB Testing

TB screening is recommended for:

- Close contacts of those with known or suspected TB.
- Persons infected with HIV.
- Intravenous drug users or users of other illicit drugs.
- Chronically ill patients with conditions or diseases that increase the risk for progressing from latent to active TB. Risk factors include diabetes, high-dose steroids, immunosuppressive therapy, chronic renal failure, lymphoma, leukemia, other cancer, weight loss to more than 10% below ideal weight, silicosis, gastrectomy, and jejunoileal bypass.
- Foreign-born persons and those arriving within the last five years from countries that have had a high incidence of TB.
- Residents and employees of high-risk institutions, such as correctional facilities, nursing homes, mental institutions, and homeless shelters.
- Health care workers, especially those caring for patients at high risk.
- Medically underserved and low-income populations.
- Infants, children, and adolescents exposed adults at high risk.

Mycobacteria will retain the red stain in the presence of acid alcohol and are therefore referred to as acid-fast. Other bacterial species stain blue.

Resistance in Mycobacteria

Mycobacteria exhibit an unusual degree of resistance on many fronts. They are able to tolerate drying and the effects of many disinfectants. Mycobacteria also show resistance to most antibiotics, making these infections difficult to treat. To help overcome bacterial resistance to antimicrobial agents, patients take two or three drugs for a period of six to nine months. The most common drug used to fight TB is isoniazid (INH). Other drugs used are rifampin, pyrazinamide, ethambutol, and streptomycin.

Transmission of Infectious TB

Infectious TB is highly contagious. Seventy-five percent of new cases occur by inhalation of cough-produced airborne droplets from symptomatic or asymptomatic persons. Crowded conditions contribute to this transmission. TB often is associated with poverty, poor nutrition, and crowded conditions such as what is often seen in prisons and mental health hospitals. A recent increase in TB is related to the increase in AIDS cases.

Diagnosis of TB

TB diagnosis will differentiate between active and inactive TB, and the treatments will differ. Active TB is a serious and contagious condition that requires isolation of the patient and aggressive treatment with several drugs over several months.

Patients exhibiting a positive or questionable **purified protein derivative (PPD)** reaction should have a chest x-ray to examine for tubercles, and a sputum sample should be stained to search for acid-fast rods. The presence of acid-fast rods in the sputum confirms active TB. Reasons for a positive reaction to PPD are varied. First and most obvious is that the patient has been exposed to TB or has an active case of TB. Persons with an old, inactive case will also give a positive skin test, as will persons who have been vaccinated with BCG. BCG (the bacille of Calmette and Guerin) is a vaccine made from live, avirulent *Mycobacterium bovis*. The vaccine is used in Europe and South America to help prevent childhood cases of TB. Persons who receive BCG will give a positive skin reaction for a minimum of four years, and much longer in many cases. Many immigrants will show positive PPD because of a BCG vaccination. The chest x-ray is an important second step for those individuals.

Screening for TB: Skin Testing

Screening for TB may be performed as part of a routine medical examination or as a prerequisite for school or employment. In states where medical assistants can legally perform injections, they may be responsible for administration and interpretation of the skin test. The most accurate method used is the **Mantoux test.** The tine test, which is a multiple-puncture test, may still be used in some areas but is no longer recommended by the American Academy of Pediatrics. Both the Mantoux and the tine methods use tuberculin, also referred to as PPD, which is a filtrate of tuberculin cultures that are used for skin testing. Persons who have been exposed to TB will develop a hypersensitive response to PPD resulting in the formation of an induration. An induration is a hard, red spot on the skin that is the result of sensitized lymphocytes migrating to the site of the injection. It is important to keep in mind that a positive skin test does not distinguish between active or inactive cases of TB. Again, a positive skin test will require further diagnostic testing including an x-ray for lung lesions and an acid-fast stain of sputum to examine for the presence of *Mycobacterium tuberculosis*. Because of the severity of the reaction, do not administer the skin test to persons who have had a positive reaction in the past.

The Mantoux Test

In the Mantoux test, 0.1 ml of 5 TU (toxin unit) strength PPD is injected intradermally using a 1 ml tuberculin syringe. A short (⅜–½ inch), 26 or 27 gauge needle is used. Care must be taken to inject the PPD so that a **wheal** forms (Figure 32-3). If the injection is too deep, it will be impossible to form the wheal. If the injection is too shallow, the PPD may leak onto the skin. Either of these two errors would invalidate the test results. It is also important to draw exactly 0.1 ml of the PPD, because too much or too little would also lead to erroneous test results.

Choosing a Site to Administer the Mantoux Test. To select a site for the Mantoux test, locate a site approximately 3 to 4 inches down from the bend of the arm on the anterior side. Avoid areas with excess hair, visible blood vessels, or scar tissue. The chosen site should be cleaned with alcohol and allowed to dry before administering the PPD. The left arm is the standard arm.

Reading the Results of the Mantoux TB Test. Have the patient return in 48 to 72 hours for examination of the injection site. Gently feel the induration—the hard, raised area. Do not include the area of redness or erythema in your assessment. See Procedure 24-7 for the complete injection procedure and Figures 32-4 and 32-5 for measuring the induration.

Proper patient instructions should be given both verbally and in written form to help ensure patient compliance. If the patient delays more than 72 hours in returning to the clinic for the test reading, the test cannot be accepted.

Some patients many show swelling, itching, or localized, raised hives when injected with the PPD. This is not a true induration, but rather an allergic reaction to the protein derivative, and should not be misinterpreted as a positive response. Do not repeat the Mantoux if an

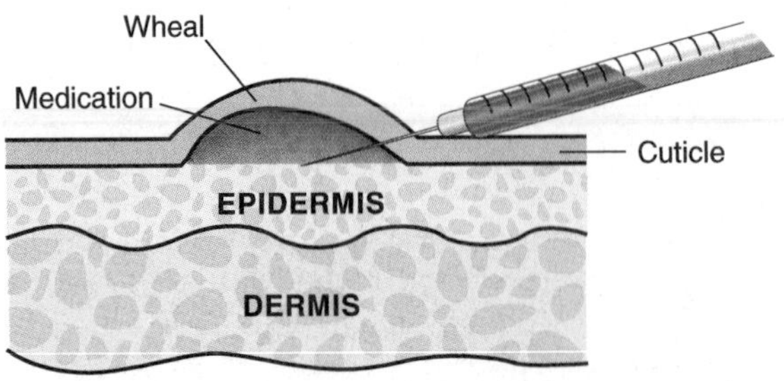

Figure 32-3 A raised wheal will form when the purified protein derivative is properly administered with an epidermal injection.

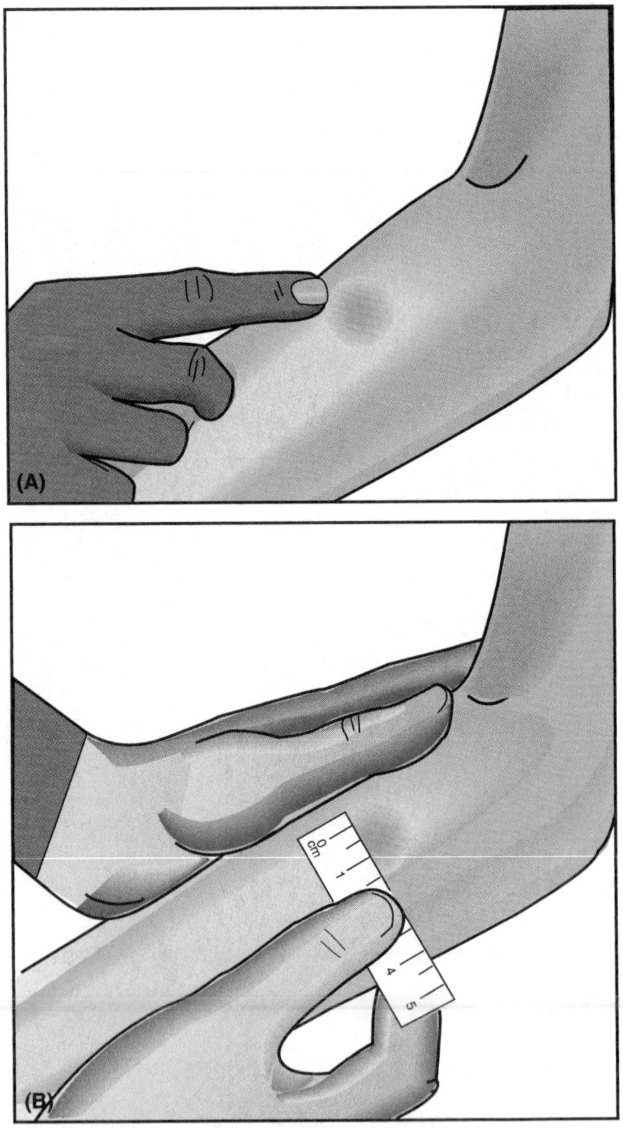

Figure 32-4 Gently inspect and measure the induration (the elevated and firm area, not the area of redness or erythema) in response to the tuberculin test within 48–72 hours after administration.

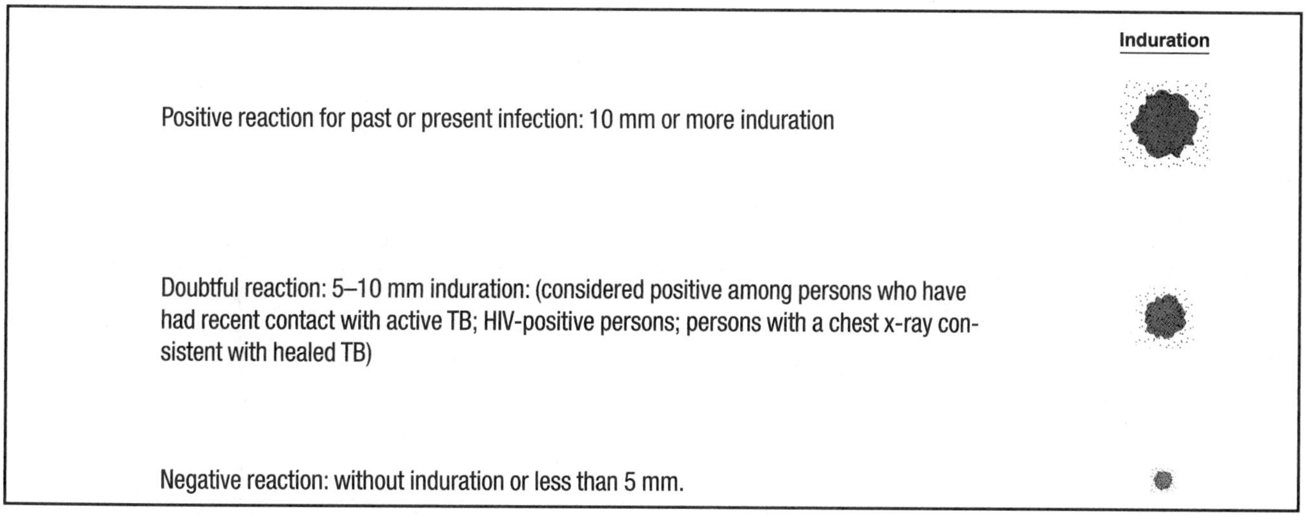
Induration
Positive reaction for past or present infection: 10 mm or more induration
Doubtful reaction: 5–10 mm induration: (considered positive among persons who have had recent contact with active TB; HIV-positive persons; persons with a chest x-ray consistent with healed TB)
Negative reaction: without induration or less than 5 mm.

Figure 32-5 The results of an induration are read and recorded as shown. Some patients will show no trace of induration.

allergic reaction occurs. If you are unable to get a wheal, repeat the test at least 2 inches from the first attempt.

BLOOD GLUCOSE

Glucose is the principal and almost exclusive carbohydrate found circulating in blood. It may also be detected in urine, cerebrospinal fluid, and semen. Glucose serves as an energy source for the body. Excess glucose is converted into glycogen for short-term storage in the liver and muscle cells, and as adipose tissue for long-term storage. Tests for blood glucose levels are commonly performed in the medical office. The results are used to screen for carbohydrate disorders such as **hypoglycemia** (low blood glucose level), **hyperglycemia** (high blood glucose level, which occurs in **diabetes mellitus**), and liver dysfunction. A variety of testing methods have been developed to diagnose, evaluate, and monitor abnormalities in carbohydrate metabolism. They include the fasting blood glucose (FBG), the two-hour postprandial blood glucose, and the glucose tolerance test (GTT). All tests are discussed here, but the FBG is preferred as the first step in the clinical setting because it is easier and faster to perform, more convenient and acceptable to patients, and less expensive.

Blood glucose concentrations rise after a meal and are regulated by the action of several hormones including **insulin** and glucagon. Both insulin and glucagon are produced by the pancreas. Insulin is secreted by pancreatic cells in response to increased glucose levels and aids with the entry of glucose into cells for conversion into energy. Insulin is also required for proper storage of glucose (which is first converted into glycogen) in the liver and in muscle cells. Glucagon is secreted by the pancreas when blood sugar levels decrease and triggers the breakdown of glycogen to help increase and regulate blood sugar levels.

Fasting Blood Glucose

Evaluation of FBG levels is commonly used to screen for diabetes mellitus. Diabetes mellitus is a type of carbohydrate disorder characterized by insulin deficiency (or no insulin) and a state of hyperglycemia (*hyper* means "too much," *glyc* means "sugar," and *emia* means "blood").

The normal fasting value of glucose ranges from 70 to 110 mg/100 ml (mg/dl). Refer to Table 32-4 for reference glucose values. A value of 120 mg/dl glucose is

> **Patient Education**
>
> In preparation for the test, the patient should be instructed to fast for 12 hours (except for water). A fasting blood sample is usually collected in the morning to minimize inconvenience to the patient. Certain drugs such as oral contraceptives, salicylates, diuretics, and steroids may alter the results so the physician may restrict their use for two to three days before the test. The patient should receive both verbal and written instructions for the testing requirements and preparation.

TABLE 32-4 REFERENCE VALUES FOR BLOOD GLUCOSE LEVELS

Test	Glucose Concentration (mg/dl)
Fasting	
Serum	70–110
Whole blood	60–100
Two-hour postprandial	≤110
Glucose tolerance (oral, serum)	
Fasting	70–110
1 hour	20–50 above fasting
2 hour	5–15 above fasting
3 hour	Fasting level or below

Values vary slightly between laboratories depending on testing method used.

the dividing point between healthy and hyperglycemic individuals. Generally, truly increased glucose levels indicate diabetes mellitus. Other causes of hyperglycemia include **Cushing's syndrome** and acute stress response. Increased blood glucose levels should be further evaluated using the glucose tolerance test.

Two-Hour Postprandial Blood Glucose

The two-hour postprandial (after eating) evaluation of blood glucose levels is used to screen for diabetes and to monitor insulin dosage. After fasting from midnight the night before, the patient eats a prescribed meal containing 75 to 100 g carbohydrate or consumes a 75 to 100-gram glucose test load solution such as Glucola®. Two hours later, a blood specimen is collected and tested for glucose concentration. Glucose levels will return to or fall below the fasting level within two hours in individu-

Patient Education

Let your patient know there are more than 25 glucose meters available for them to choose from. All of them use the typical process of a drop of blood applied to a disposable "test strip" and inserted into the meter. The unit measures how much glucose is in the sample. All the meters display the result. Some meters allow a much smaller sample to be used and allow the sample to be taken from sites other than the fingertip (alternate site testing). Some meters record and store a number of test results, and some meters can connect to a personal computer to store results and print them out. Some new models have automatic timing, error codes and signals, or barcode readers to help with calibration. Some meters have a large display screen or spoken instructions for people with visual impairments. In choosing a meter, the patient should consider the following:

- Cost per strip
- Number of tests required per day
- Amount of blood needed for testing
- Testing speed
- Overall size and portability
- Cost of the meter
- Ability to store test results in memory
- Ability to test sites other than fingertip
- Other personal preferences

Many manufacturers offer free meters with the purchase of the test strips. Your clinic may be given free meters to give to patients together with a few sample strips in hopes the patient will continue to use that meter and purchase the strips. Unfortunately, the meters given to patients might not be the best choice for them, but they will continue to use it because their doctor gave it to them. Be sure to let patients know that there are many choices, and that the free meter you are giving them is *not necessarily an endorsement* of one meter over another.

als without diabetes. Increased glucose levels should be further examined using the GTT.

According to the standards of the American Diabetes Association, a normal blood glucose is defined as less than 100 mg/dl in a fasting plasma glucose test and a two-hour postload (75 g glucose load solution) value of less than 140 mg/dl.

A fasting plasma glucose test of 126 mg/dl or greater indicates a need for further testing, a two-hour post load value of 140 mg/dl or greater is a diagnosis of having "pre-diabetes" indicating a relatively high risk for development of diabetes.

A two-hour postload value of 200 mg/dl or greater is a positive test for diabetes and should be confirmed on another day.

Glucose Tolerance Test

The GTT provides more detailed information used to assess insulin response to glucose and to diagnose diabetes.

When the patient arrives, he or she should be fasting (nothing but water) for at least 10 hours. A capillary specimen is drawn to determine the fasting blood sugar (FBS) level. If the FBS level is less than 200 mg/dl, then a venous specimen and urine specimen are obtained. These are labeled as fasting specimens with the date and time noted. If the results of the capillary test shows the FBS level greater than 200 mg/dl, the physician should be notified immediately. Hyperglycemia after fasting is abnormal and not an appropriate condition for further loading with additional glucose and may be dangerous to the patient.

After providing the fasting urine and blood specimens, the patient consumes a glucose test solution containing 1.75 g glucose/kilogram of body weight, or the standard adult dose of 75 to 100 g. The patient must consume the entire glucose solution within a five-minute time frame. The test timing starts immediately after the patient has finished drinking the solution. If the patient should vomit within the first 30 minutes after drinking the solutions, the test will be stopped and rescheduled on a different day. It is probably best not to mention this to the patient, though, because it is a rare occurrence and it is best not to have the patient worried about the possibility of vomiting. Blood and urine specimens are typically collected at 30 minutes, 1 hour, 2 hours, 3 hours (and sometimes 6 hours) after ingestion of the glucose solution and are tested for glucose level. These measurements help determine the patient's ability to deal with increased glucose. During the test, the patient must not ingest anything (other than the solution) except water. The patient must also abstain from smoking, because smoking acts as a stimulant and increases blood glucose levels. The patient must also refrain from chewing gum, which stimulates the digestive process and also may add sugar to his or her system. Physical activity should be strongly discouraged because activity can activate sugar utilization in the body and affect the test results. Sedentary activity level is suggested.

During the second and third hours of the test, the patient may experience weakness, slight faintness, and perspire. These are all normal symptoms. If, however, the patient develops a headache, faints, or displays irrational speech or behavior, he or she may be experiencing hypoglycemic shock and the physician should be notified immediately.

The blood glucose level of patients without diabetes usually peaks 30 to 60 minutes after consumption of the test load at 160 to 180 mg/dl and returns to the fasting level after 2 to 3 hours. Patients with diabetes will still have increased glucose levels at the end of the test.

Automated Methods of Glucose Analysis

Several types of glucose analyzers are available that are suitable for POLs or small clinical laboratories. Many of these operate on the principle of reflectance photometry and use adaptations of the enzymatic methods of glucose analysis. One example of an instrument suitable for small laboratories is the HemoCue® blood glucose analyzer. See Table 32-5 for a listing of CLIA waived glucose test kits and analyzers.

Dozens of small, inexpensive, handheld glucose meters are also made and are designed for home use by patients with diabetes. See the Patient Education box on page 896 for some criteria for patients to consider when purchasing an at-home testing method. Most of these are suitable for use in point-of-care (POC) testing or in physician's offices (Figure 32-6).

Glucose controls may be purchased to check instrument performance. It is always necessary to use test materials that are made for a particular instrument only with that instrument.

All of these analyzers are designed to be easy to use and to give rapid results. With all instruments, it is necessary to use consistent proper specimen collection and testing technique to avoid variations in results.

The medical assistant often is responsible for providing education to patients on how to use glucometers, including maintenance and calibration of the meter. It is important that the medical assistant who works with patients with diabetes become familiar with a variety of meters and their differences and similarities.

Photometry Analyzers. The HemoCue® Blood-Glucose system is a compact glucose analyzer based on the principle of photometry. The system consists of a compact

TABLE 32-5 LIST OF WAIVED BLOOD TESTS FOR DIABETIC TESTING AND MONITORING

Kit Name	Manufacturer
Any blood glucose monitoring device cleared by the FDA for home use (*see Patient Education box for a list)	Various manufacturers
Abbott Laboratories, Medisense Products Precision Xtra Advance Diabetes Management System	Abbott Laboratories, Inc
Cholestech LDX (measures total cholesterol, HDL, cholesterol, triglycerides and glucose)	Cholestech
HemoCue B-Glucose Photometer	HemoCue, Inc.
HemoCue Glucose 201 Microcuvettes and Analyzer	HemoCue, Inc.
LXN Fructosamine Test System (two- to three-week control test)	LXN Corporation
LXN Duet Glucose Control Monitoring System (two- to three-week control test)	LXN Corporation
LXN IN CHARGE Diabetes Control System (two- to three-week control test)	LXN Corporation
Bayer DCA 2000—glycosylated hemoglobin (Hgb A1c)	Bayer Corporation
Bayer DCA 2000+—glycosylated hemoglobin (Hgb A1c)	Bayer Corporation
Bio-Rad Micromat II Hemoglobin A1c Prescription Home Use Test	Bio-Rad Laboratories
Cholestech GDX A1c Test (Prescription Home Use)	Cholestech Corporation
Metrika A1c Now—Professional Use	Metrika, Inc.
Metrika A1c Now—for Prescription Home Use	Metrika, Inc.

Source: Clinical Laboratory Improvement Amendments of 1988 Categorized List as of June 2004. See the Centers for Disease Control and Prevention's Web site (http://www.cdc.gov) for the most current listing.

photometer and disposable microcuvettes. The self-filling microcuvette automatically draws up 5 μl blood from a capillary puncture into its reaction chamber. The microcuvette is then placed into the holder and pushed into the photometer. The glucose concentration in milligrams per deciliter (mg/dl) is displayed within 45 to 240 seconds (Figure 32-7). This system is ideal for POLs and POC testing because of the stability of calibration and the minimum operator training required.

Reflectance Photometry Analyzers. Several glucose analyzers are available that are based on reflectance photometry. Blood from a fingerstick, serum, or plasma is applied to the reagent area of a test strip. The glucose in the sample reacts with the reagents in the pad(s) causing a color to form. The more glucose present in the sample, the darker or more intense the color. At the appropriate time, the strip is inserted into the test chamber and light is directed onto the test area. The amount of light reflected from the colored test area is measured by the photometer and converted to a digital readout showing the glucose concentration in milligrams per deciliter (or mmol/L). Most instruments give results in one to three minutes. Instructions included with the test strips must be followed carefully for reliable test results. See Procedure 32-5.

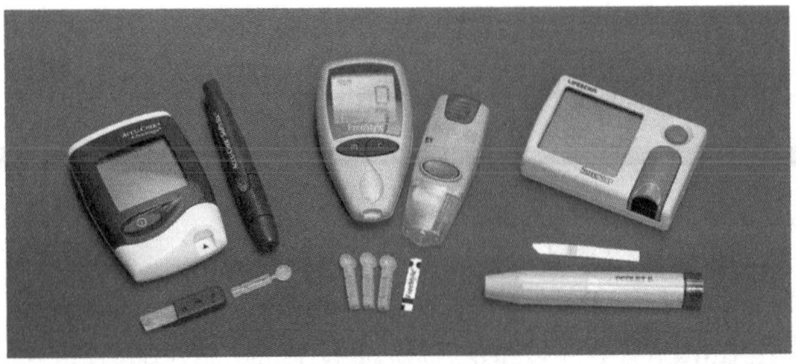

Figure 32-6 A variety of hand-held glucose analyzers are available for home and office use.

Testing Profiles

Glucose testing may be part of a general profile chemistry test that can be useful in giving an overall view of an individual's state of health, especially when used in conjunction with other tests. Glucose testing may also be performed as part of a specific chemistry panel (renal panel) to determine the function of a particular biologic system (Figure 32-8). The renal panel helps determine normal or abnormal function of the kidney.

Glycosylated Hemoglobin

Glycosylated hemoglobin or hemoglobin A1c (Hb A1c) determination is a blood test that measures how well the glucose level has been controlled over the past four to six weeks versus the conventional blood test that shows only current day status. Physicians can use this test to determine if patients with diabetes are consistently adhering to their diet and health guidelines or are adhering to their diet only for a day before their office visit.

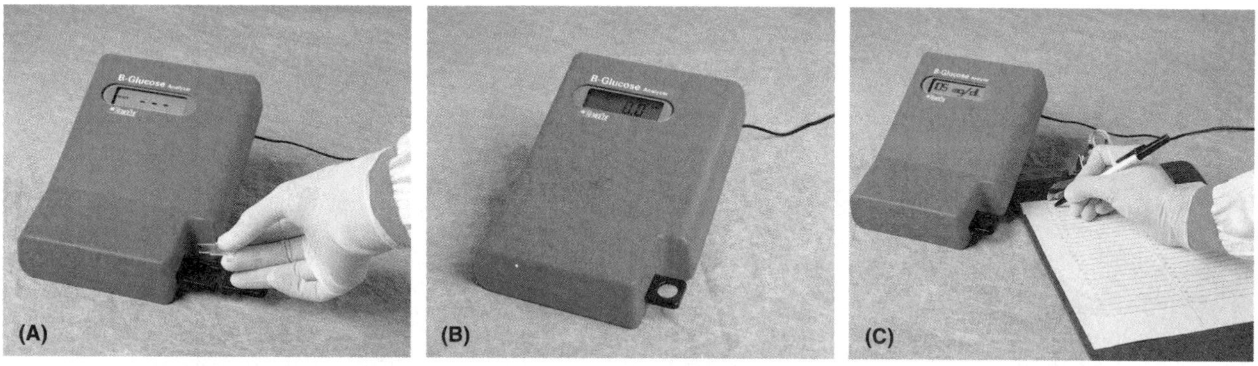

Figure 32-7 HemoCue Blood Glucose System: (A) A blood specimen is placed on the microcuvette, inserted into its holder, and pushed into the photometer. (B) Specimen is allowed to remain in the analyzer until test is completed. (C) Glucose concentration is displayed in mg/dl after more than 45 seconds.

Glycosylated hemoglobin is a stable molecule formed when sugar and hemoglobin bind together on the RBC. An increased finding of glycosylated hemoglobin indicates poor glucose control in the assessment of glucose in the diabetic patient.

When the RBC is first formed, it contains no glucose. If there are increased glucose levels in the blood, the excess enters the RBC and attaches (glycates) to the hemoglobin. The more glucose, the more hemoglobin gets glycated.

Patient Education

Following are some of the many over-the-counter (OTC or without a prescription) glucose meters available that have been approved by the Food and Drug Administration (FDA) for at home use (in alphabetical order):

- Accu-Chek Advantage meter
- Accu-Chek VoiceMate meter (voiced result)
- Ascensia Breeze
- Ascensia Contour (alternate site testing and memory)
- BD Logic monitoring system (very small sample needed)
- BD Latitude (combines test and calculates injection)
- Bioscanner Beyond Glucose Analyzer and Test Strip
- Bioscanner Plus
- Evencare Blood Glucose Monitoring System
- FreeStyle Blood Glucose Monitoring System (alternate site testing)
- Glucometer Dex Blood Glucose System
- Glucometer Elite Diabetes Care System
- Liberty Blood Glucose Monitoring System
- One Touch Induo Blood Glucose Meter (monitors and calculates injection)
- One Touch SureStep
- Optimum monitor
- Prestige IQ Meter
- Prestige TrueTrack
- Quicktek Blood Glucose System
- Precision Xtra Advantage (easy to see)
- Sof-Tact Diabetes Management System (very small sample)

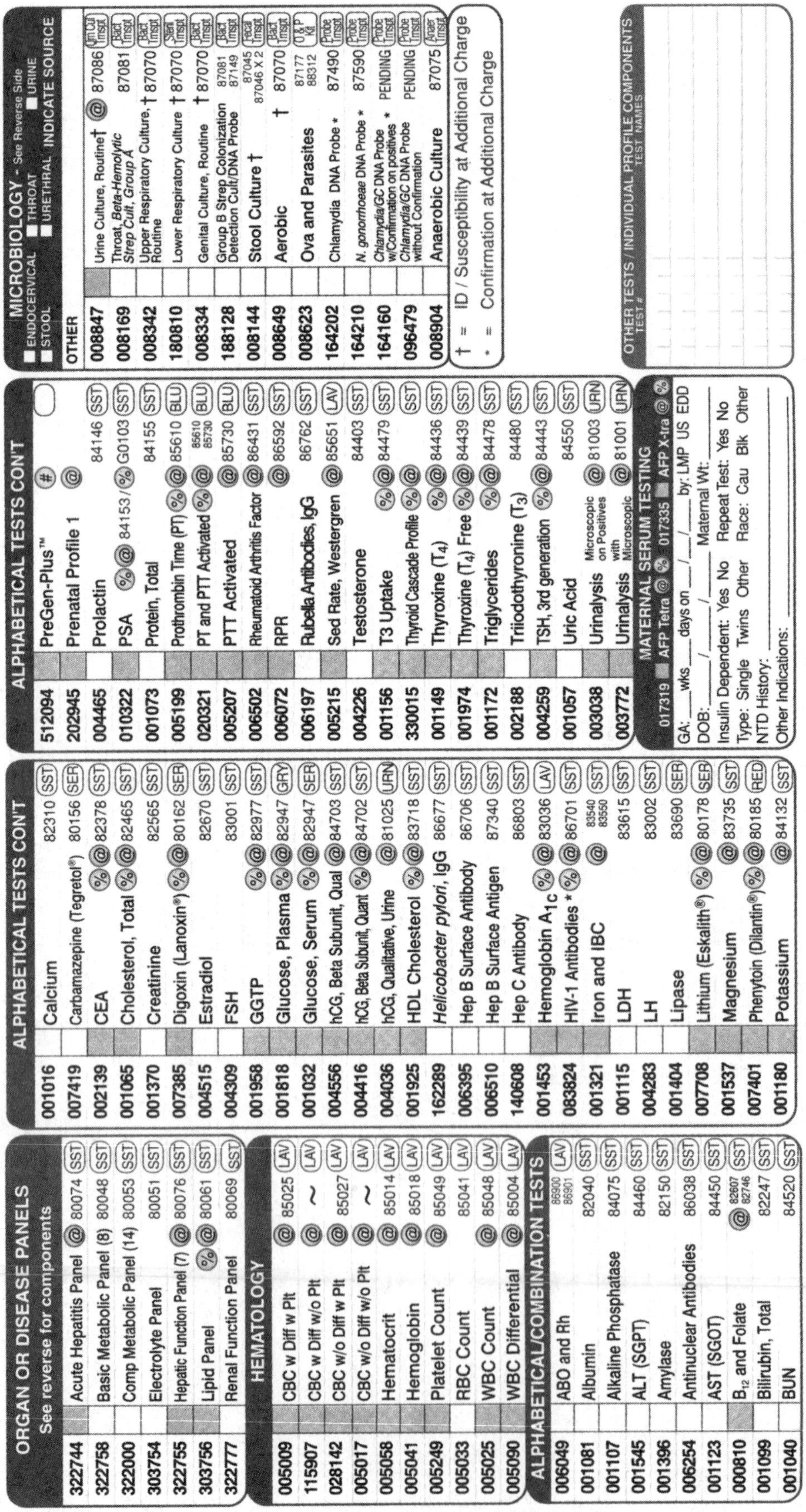

ORGAN OR DISEASE PANELS See reverse for components				
322744	■	Acute Hepatitis Panel	@ 80074	SST
322758		Basic Metabolic Panel (8)	80048	SST
322000		Comp Metabolic Panel (14)	80053	SST
303754		Electrolyte Panel	80051	SST
322755	■	Hepatic Function Panel (7)	@ 80076	SST
303756	■	Lipid Panel	% @ 80061	SST
322777		Renal Function Panel	80069	SST

HEMATOLOGY				
005009	■	CBC w Diff w Plt	@ 85025	LAV
115907	■	CBC w Diff w/o Plt	@ ~	LAV
028142	■	CBC w/o Diff w Plt	@ 85027	LAV
005017	■	CBC w/o Diff w/o Plt	@ ~	LAV
005058	■	Hematocrit	@ 85014	LAV
005041	■	Hemoglobin	@ 85018	LAV
005249	■	Platelet Count	@ 85049	LAV
005033		RBC Count	85041	LAV
005025	■	WBC Count	@ 85048	LAV
005090	■	WBC Differential	@ 85004	LAV

ALPHABETICAL/COMBINATION TESTS				
006049		ABO and Rh	86900 86901	LAV
001081		Albumin	82040	SST
001107		Alkaline Phosphatase	84075	SST
001545		ALT (SGPT)	84460	SST
001396		Amylase	82150	SST
006254		Antinuclear Antibodies	86038	SST
001123		AST (SGOT)	84450	SST
000810	■	B_{12} and Folate	@ 82607 82746	SST
001099		Bilirubin, Total	82247	SST
001040		BUN	84520	SST

ALPHABETICAL TESTS CON'T				
001016		Calcium	82310	SST
007419		Carbamazepine (Tegretol®)	80156	SER
002139	■	CEA	% @ 82378	SST
001065	■	Cholesterol, Total	% @ 82465	SST
001370		Creatinine	82565	SST
007385	■	Digoxin (Lanoxin®)	% @ 80162	SER
004515		Estradiol	82670	SST
004309		FSH	83001	SST
001958	■	GGTP	% @ 82977	SST
001818	■	Glucose, Plasma	% @ 82947	GRY
001032	■	Glucose, Serum	% @ 82947	SER
004556	■	hCG, Beta Subunit, Qual	@ 84703	SST
004416	■	hCG, Beta Subunit, Quant	% @ 84702	SST
004036	■	hCG, Qualitative, Urine	@ 81025	URN
001925	■	HDL Cholesterol	% @ 83718	SST
162289		*Helicobacter pylori*, IgG	86677	SST
006395		Hep B Surface Antibody	86706	SST
006510		Hep B Surface Antigen	87340	SST
140608		Hep C Antibody	86803	SST
001453	■	Hemoglobin A_{1c}	% @ 83036	LAV
083824	■	HIV-1 Antibodies *	% @ 86701	SST
001321	■	Iron and IBC	@ 83540 83550	SST
001115		LDH	83615	SST
004283		LH	83002	SST
001404		Lipase	83690	SER
007708	■	Lithium (Eskalith®)	% @ 80178	SER
001537	■	Magnesium	@ 83735	SST
007401	■	Phenytoin (Dilantin®)	% @ 80185	RED
001180	■	Potassium	@ 84132	SST

ALPHABETICAL TESTS CON'T				
512094	■	PreGen-Plus™	#	
202945	■	Prenatal Profile 1	@	
004465		Prolactin	84146	SST
010322	■	PSA	% @ 84153 / % G0103	SST
001073		Protein, Total	84155	SST
005199	■	Prothrombin Time (PT)	% @ 85610	BLU
020321	■	PT and PTT Activated	% @ 85610 85730	BLU
005207	■	PTT Activated	@ 85730	BLU
006502	■	Rheumatoid Arthritis Factor	@ 86431	SST
006072	■	RPR	@ 86592	SST
006197		Rubella Antibodies, IgG	86762	SST
005215	■	Sed Rate, Westergren	@ 85651	LAV
004226		Testosterone	84403	SST
001156	■	T3 Uptake	% @ 84479	SST
330015	■	Thyroid Cascade Profile	% @	SST
001149	■	Thyroxine (T_4)	% @ 84436	SST
001974	■	Thyroxine (T_4) Free	% @ 84439	SST
001172	■	Triglycerides	% @ 84478	SST
002188		Triiodothyronine (T_3)	84480	SST
004259	■	TSH, 3rd generation	% @ 84443	SST
001057		Uric Acid	84550	SST
003038	■	Urinalysis Microscopic on Positives	@ 81003	URN
003772	■	Urinalysis with Microscopic	@ 81001	URN

MATERNAL SERUM TESTING

017319 ■ AFP Tetra @ % 017335 ■ AFP X-tra @ %

GA: ____wks____days on ___/___/____ by: LMP US EDD
DOB: ______/______/______ Maternal Wt: ________
Insulin Dependent: Yes No Repeat Test: Yes No
Type: Single Twins Other Race: Cau Blk Other
NTD History: ______________________
Other Indications: ______________________

MICROBIOLOGY - See Reverse Side ■ ENDOCERVICAL ■ THROAT ■ URINE ■ STOOL ■ URETHRAL INDICATE SOURCE				
OTHER				
008847	■	Urine Culture, Routine †	@ 87086	Urn Cul Trnspt
008169		Throat, *Beta-Hemolytic Strep Cult, Group A*	87081	Bact Trnspt
008342		Upper Respiratory Culture, Routine	† 87070	Bact Trnspt
180810		Lower Respiratory Culture	† 87070	Steril Trnspt
008334		Genital Culture, Routine	† 87070	Bact Trnspt
188128		Group B Strep Colonization Detection Cult/DNA Probe	87081 87149	Bact Trnspt
008144		Stool Culture †	87045 87046 X 2	Fecal Trnspt
008649		Aerobic †	87070	Bact Trnspt
008623		Ova and Parasites	87177 88312	O & P Kit
164202		Chlamydia DNA Probe *	87490	Probe Trnspt
164210		*N. gonorrhoeae* DNA Probe *	87590	Probe Trnspt
164160		*Chlamydia/GC* DNA Probe w/Confirmation on positives *	PENDING	Probe Trnspt
096479		*Chlamydia/GC* DNA Probe without Confirmation	PENDING	Probe Trnspt
008904		Anaerobic Culture	87075	Anaer Trnspt

† = ID / Susceptibility at Additional Charge
* = Confirmation at Additional Charge

OTHER TESTS / INDIVIDUAL PROFILE COMPONENTS TEST #	TEST NAMES

Figure 32-8 Laboratory panels are combinations of tests related to a specific function or body organ or system.

The A1c measures the percentage of the glycated hemoglobin. This offers us an average of the glucose in the blood over about three months. Most RBCs live about 120 days and maintain the glycated state.

What hemoglobin A1c does not do is indicate whether the patient has experienced hyperglycemia or hypoglycemia over that time frame, because day-to-day readings of glucose levels are not provided, thus it is not useful in adjusting insulin. Having the patient monitor his or her blood glucose level with a meter and keep a daily diary is a good way to look at his or her day-to-day blood glucose levels. Both tests are useful tools in helping manage diabetes.

The advantage of hemoglobin A1c not being affected by day-to-day variations in blood glucose levels is that the patient does not need to be fasting for this test.

Patient Education

Let your patients know that several factors can influence their blood cholesterol levels:

- *Age and sex:* Cholesterol levels naturally increase as we age, and women experiencing menopause often will experience an increase in their LDL levels.
- *Heredity and family history:* High cholesterol often runs in families. Studies are still in process about the role genetics play in cholesterol levels.
- *Weight:* Gaining weight increases cholesterol levels in the blood, and losing weight helps to reduce cholesterol levels.
- *Exercise:* Regular physical exercise may reduce the LDL level, as well as increase the HDL levels.

CHOLESTEROL AND LIPIDS

Cholesterol is a fatty compound that is essential for many vital life functions and is a normal constituent of blood. Although it is required for life, excess cholesterol is not a necessary part of the diet, except in babies and children. Sufficient quantities are manufactured by the body from carbohydrates and other fats. Cholesterol has been linked to coronary artery disease. According to the American Heart Association and the National Institutes of Health, cholesterol should not be restricted in babies and toddlers. Fats and cholesterol are important for normal growth and development. Babies and very young children should be on healthy diets, though, not a lot of fried foods, and so on. From about 4 or 5 years old, they can be transitioned to heart-healthy foods such as nonfat milk. To help reduce the risk for coronary artery disease, nutritionists and agencies such as the American Heart Association and the National Cholesterol Education Program advise that fats make up no more than 30% of the total intake of calories daily, and that the concentration of cholesterol in blood not exceed 200 mg/dl. Cholesterol of 240 mg/dl or greater is considered to present a high risk for heart disease. Cholesterol levels between 200 and 239 mg/dl are considered borderline.

The Chemistry of Cholesterol

The cholesterol molecule consists of carbon, hydrogen, and oxygen. Cholesterol is a saturated, fatty acid. Saturated refers to the number of hydrogen atoms attached to the molecule. The more saturated the fat, the harder it is at room temperature. Fats of animal origin, for example, butter and animal fat, are saturated and are solid at room temperature. Monounsaturated and polyunsaturated fats are liquid at room temperature. Research into coronary artery disease has shown that saturated fats tend to increase levels of blood cholesterol. Monounsaturated fats (olive and peanut oils) do not change blood cholesterol levels, and polyunsaturated fats (corn, safflower, sunflower, and many fish oils) tend to reduce those levels.

Functions of Cholesterol

The human body is efficient at manufacturing cholesterol. Most cells are capable of doing so, especially the liver, the adrenal cortex, the testes, and the ovaries. All of the preceding cells, with the exception of the liver, use cholesterol to manufacture steroid hormones. In addition, cholesterol is an important component of bile and cellular membranes. Although the body is efficient at making cholesterol, it is not as easily degraded and may accumulate in the body and reach dangerous levels.

In addition to what the body produces, humans take in additional cholesterol through the ingestion of meat, eggs, and dairy products (Figure 32-9). The liver metabolizes cholesterol to its free form, which is then bound to lipoprotein and transported through the blood. Over

Patient Education

The Simple Scoop on Cholesterol

Cholesterol can be a confusing subject to try to explain to patients. Here is a very basic explanation that may help them:

Our bodies need cholesterol and we get it in two ways. We eat it and our liver manufactures it. Our liver manufactures plenty of cholesterol, so we do not need to eat it (except as babies and young children). There is only one source of cholesterol in our food: animal products (meat, eggs, and dairy). Vegetables, fruits, and grains naturally contain no cholesterol, although they may contain oils.

Our bodies have cholesterol transporters called high-density lipoproteins (HDLs) and low-density lipoproteins (LDLs).

HDLs (sometimes called "healthy lipoprotein") carry cholesterol to the liver where it can be released into the stool as bile. We want high levels of HDLs so we can get rid of excess cholesterol.

LDLs (sometimes referred to as the "lousy lipoprotein") carry cholesterol to our tissues and blood vessels where it is stored and can cause problems such as blocked arteries, fatty liver, and obesity. We want low levels of the LDLs so we can have less risk for heart disease and arterial disease.

Fats and oils can also be confusing. Saturated fats are solid at room temperature and come from animal fats and butter and from manufactured products such as hydrogenated fats. These are the worst fats. Unsaturated fats, which are liquid at room temperature, may be in two forms: monounsaturated fats (*mono* means "single") and polyunsaturated fats (*poly* means "many"). Monounsaturated fats such as olive and peanut oils do not affect blood cholesterol levels, whereas polyunsaturated fats such as corn, safflower, sunflower, and fish oils will actually reduce blood cholesterol levels.

Triglycerides are a type of lipid found in our blood that provides energy. If we have too much in our blood, it is also stored in our tissues as fat. The liver converts some of our foods (fatty acids and glycerol) into triglycerides.

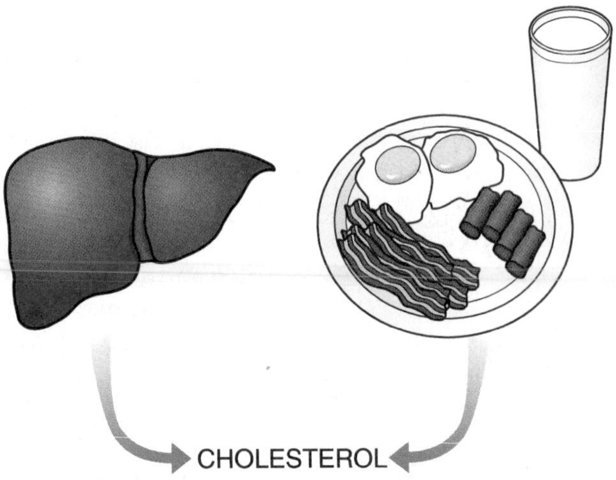

Figure 32-9 Cholesterol is created by the liver or obtained through meat, eggs, and dairy products.

time, excess cholesterol in the diet can result in a gradual increase of cholesterol concentration in the plasma. Increased concentrations of cholesterol in the plasma can increase to pathogenic levels. Some of the excess is stored in the liver, whereas some is deposited on the walls of blood vessels (atherosclerosis). Atherosclerosis of the coronary arteries is the most common cause of acute myocardial infarction (heart attack).

Lipoproteins and Cholesterol Transport

Two kinds of lipoprotein are involved in the transport of cholesterol through the body: **high-density lipoprotein (HDL)** and **low-density lipoprotein (LDL).** Cholesterol bound to HDL is transported to the liver where it is excreted in the form of bile. HDL is sometimes referred to

TABLE 32-6 DESIRABLE VALUES FOR CHOLESTEROL, HIGH-DENSITY AND LOW-DENSITY LIPOPROTEINS, AND TRIGLYCERIDES

Total Cholesterol	
Desirable	<200
Less desirable	200–239
At risk	>240
High-density lipoprotein	
Removes one risk factor	>60
Adds a risk factor	<40
Low-density lipoprotein	
With multiple known risk factors	Below 100
With one known risk factor	<130
With no known risk factors	<160
Triglycerides	
Desirable	< 150

All values are measured in milligrams per deciliter (mg/dl).

as good cholesterol. LDL cholesterol is deposited in the tissues as fat and inside the walls of blood vessels, and it is referred to as bad cholesterol. High levels of LDL are associated with an increased risk for coronary artery disease. Persons with coronary artery disease should have levels of less than 100 mg/dl LDL, whereas those without the disease should have levels of less than 160 mg/dl. Desirable values for HDL and LDL are shown in Table 32-6. Levels of HDL and LDL are influenced by many factors, both genetic and environmental. It is possible to increase HDL levels through a combination of weight loss, a diet low in saturated fats, exercise, and cessation of smoking.

Blood cholesterol may be reported as total cholesterol or as total cholesterol and the HDL and LDL fractions. Cholesterol screening is used to help identify patients that are at a high risk for heart disease.

Cholesterol testing is part of a lipid profile that also evaluates lipoproteins and triglycerides to help identify patients at a high risk for heart disease. Refer back to Figure 32-8, which shows tests performed for lipid profiles on the laboratory form.

Triglycerides

Triglycerides are a type of lipid found in the blood that serve as a source of energy. Fatty acids and glycerol from the diet are converted into triglycerides by the liver. When triglyceride levels in the blood are excessive, they are deposited in tissues as adipose tissue. Triglycerides are transported within the bloodstream by LDL and very low-density lipoproteins (VLDLs).

TABLE 32-7 FACTORS THAT INFLUENCE SERUM TRIGLYCERIDE LEVELS

Factors That Increase Concentration	Factors That Decrease Concentration
Pregnancy	Fasting
Estrogens, oral contraceptives	Ascorbic acid, clofibrate
Ingestion of fatty food	Uncontrolled diabetes mellitus
Ingestion of alcohol	Hyperthyroidism
Gout	Malnutrition

Many factors influence serum triglyceride levels; several of these are listed in Table 32-7. Serum triglyceride concentration will increase moderately after ingesting a meal containing fat, peaking four to five hours later. Increased concentrations of triglycerides are associated with an increased risk for coronary and vascular disease.

BLOOD CHEMISTRY TESTS

There are many natural chemicals in blood. The amounts of those chemicals are controlled by the efficiency of the body's organs and organ systems and certainly by environmental factors such as diet, smoking, drugs, and activity, as well as genetic composition.

The physician can order a general chemistry panel or specific panels. A panel is a series of tests related to a body system, organ, or function. In interpreting a chemistry panel, the physician can determine pathology within the organ or malfunctions.

This chapter discusses each of the components briefly and explains some of the conditions and diseases that can cause these chemical tests to be abnormal. Keep in mind that all laboratory chemistry tests can vary slightly from laboratory to laboratory. Also remember, no one test, just like no one symptom will make a diagnosis independent of other clues. The physician is considering laboratory tests together with the clinical picture, patient symptoms, and many other data in finalizing a diagnosis or diagnoses.

Alanine AminoTransferase (ALT)

ALT is an enzyme. It is found in liver tissue. A high level would indicate liver damage. A normal ALT level is less than 45 U/L.

Albumin

Most of the protein in plasma is albumin. It is responsible for transporting many small molecules (such as calcium, drugs, and bilirubin). It is synthesized in the liver, thus low levels of albumin may indicate liver disease. It may also result from kidney disease, because the kidney is allowing too much albumin to spill into the urine. Low albumin may also be caused by malnutrition or a low-protein diet. A normal albumin level is 3.4 to 5.4 mg/dl.

Alkaline Phosphatase (ALP)

ALP is an enzyme. It is in all our body tissues, but mostly in the liver and bone. When levels are high in the blood, liver or bone disease must be suspected. A normal ALP level is 44 to 147 IU/L.

Aspartate Aminotransferase (AST)

AST is found in the muscle cells (heart and skeletal muscles) and in the liver. High levels cannot indicate specifically liver disease, but it is considered together with other liver enzymes. It is also used to monitor patients who have had heart muscle damage (such as heart attacks), but it is not the best or only enzyme for that purpose either. A normal AST level is 10 to 34 IU/L.

Bilirubin, Total and Direct

Bilirubin is a yellow–orange substance that comes from the breakdown of hemoglobin. Hemoglobin is contained within our RBCs. Because individual RBCs live for only 120 days, they are constantly breaking down and being replaced. When the RBCs "die," the "heme" part of the hemoglobin circulates in the blood until the liver filters it out. The liver is responsible for changing the "heme" into a water-soluble substance called bilirubin. Before it gets to the liver, it is called "indirect" or "free" bilirubin. After it leaves the liver, it is called "direct" or "conjugated" bilirubin. The liver sends the conjugated bilirubin to the gall bladder where it is released with bile into the small intestine. When there is a blockage in the liver/gall bladder ducts or a disorder/disease of the liver, the bilirubin cannot get past the gall bladder to the small intestine so it continues to circulate in the blood. This excess of bilirubin in the blood can lead to a yellow–orange coloring of the skin called jaundice. The body will try to get rid of extra bilirubin through the urine. Hence, any detection of bilirubin in the urine (bilirubinuria) can be indicative of a problem in the liver or gall bladder. When the bilirubin level increases, it causes the skin and whites of the eyes to become yellow. This change to yellow is called jaundice. Newborn babies can be jaundiced because their systems are not sophisticated enough to get rid of the bile. Because bilirubin breaks down in sunlight, babies with jaundice are treated with special "bili-lights" to help them break down the bilirubin in their skin. The total bilirubin test will indicate problems in the liver and the hepatic system. Notice the total bilirubin test is in the general panel and the direct bilirubin test is part of the hepatic panel. Some types of general blood problems can cause high levels of bilirubin because more blood cells are breaking down than usual. Normal bilirubin ranges are as follows:

Total bilirubin	0.1–0.2 mg/dl
Indirect bilirubin	0.1–0.7 mg/dl
Direct bilirubin	0.1–0.3 mg/dl
Newborn total bilirubin	1–12 mg/dl

Blood Urea Nitrogen Test

The **blood urea nitrogen (BUN)** test measures the concentration of urea in blood. The amount of urea in blood reflects the metabolic function of the liver and the excretory function of the kidneys. Most renal diseases result in inadequate excretion of urea from the body; therefore, increased concentrations of urea appear in the blood. BUN is one of several tests that are used to screen for renal disease and is especially useful for evaluating glomerular function.

Excess protein in the diet is not stored in the body but is metabolized (catalyzed) for energy production. Urea is the nitrogenous end product of protein catabolism and is produced in the liver. It is deposited in the blood and carried to the kidneys for excretion. Surplus urea is measured as BUN. Normal values of urea vary but in adults range between 8 and 25 mg/dl; concentrations greater than 100 mg/dl indicate serious impairment of renal function.

Calcium

All the cells in the human body need calcium for many functions. It is a critical element for bones, muscles, and the nervous system. Too much calcium can cause the muscles and nerves to become hyperactive, whereas too little calcium can cause the muscles and nerves not to function at all.

Muscle cramps (Charlie Horses) are often caused by low calcium. Calcium needs to be maintained in our blood within certain levels. If we eat more calcium than we need, the excess is stored in our bones. If our diets are low in calcium, the needed amount is pulled from our bones. The storage of excess calcium becomes less efficient as women lose estrogen, hence the need to take in adequate daily calcium to avoid osteoporosis as we age. A normal calcium level is 8.5 to 10.2 mg/dl.

Chloride

Chloride is an electrolyte. Its main function is to help with the electrical impulses of the cells. Chloride works closely with sodium. Changes in either sodium or chloride levels usually affect each other. A normal chloride level is 96 to 106 mEq/L.

Carbon Dioxide (CO_2)

Measuring CO_2 actually is measuring bicarbonate. This test is part of an arterial blood gas analysis. The kidneys are the main organs responsible for balancing CO_2. Anything that throws off the body's metabolic balance (excessive vomiting and diarrhea) can affect the CO_2 levels. The CO_2 levels in the blood are influenced by kidney and lung function. Normal CO_2 is 20 to 29 mEq/L.

Creatinine

Creatinine forms when muscle (creatine) breaks down. Logically, these levels will vary depending on the patient's size and muscularity. This test is used to determine kidney function. A normal creatinine level is 0.8 to 1.4 mg/dl.

Gamma Glutamyltransferase (GGT)

The highest concentrations of GGT are in the liver and kidney. Abnormal levels usually indicate diseases of the liver, kidney, or bone. It is used in conjunction with other enzymes, especially ALP, to diagnose diseases. A normal GGT level is 0 to 51 IU/L.

Lactate Dehydrogenase (LDH)

LDH is an enzyme found in many organs, especially the liver, heart, kidneys, brain, skeletal muscles, and lungs. Abnormal levels indicate tissue damage but are not specific by themselves. Like all enzymes, LDH is examined in conjunction with other tests. A normal LDH level is 105 to 133 IU/L.

Phosphorus (Phosphate)

Phosphorus works closely with calcium, another electrolyte. It is used to assist in the proper assessment of calcium levels and to detect endocrine disorders. A normal phosphorus level is 2.4 to 4.1 mg/dl.

Potassium (K)

K is an electrolyte and is critical to muscle and nerve function and for the transportation of nutrients and cellular wastes across cellular membrans. Abnormal levels of K can cause heart muscle irregularities and, if severe, can lead to cardiac arrest. K is controlled by aldosterone, a hormone. Uncontrolled diabetes or excessive vomitting/diarrhea can cause abnormal K levels. Patients taking certain diuretics (such as Lasix) should be observed for low K. A normal K level is 3.7 to 5.2 mEq/L.

Sodium

Sodium is an electrolyte and works closely with chloride. Dietary intake of sodium is usually sufficient, and the kidney can excrete the excess. Sodium is closely related to fluid balance and retention. Normal sodium is 135 to 145 mEq/L.

Total Protein

Total protein is a measurement of protein in the blood serum and can reflect the nutritional state of the body, liver, kidneys, and many other conditions. If the total protein is abnormal, then further, more specific tests will need to be performed to find out exactly the source of the problem. Of course, if the total protein is abnormal, other tests might show some abnormal levels, too. A normal total protein level is 6.0 to 8.3 mg/dl.

Uric Acid

Uric acid is created when purine is metabolized. It is usually secreted by the kidneys, but too much can build up as crystals in the body and seem to settle in the largest dependent joint, the great toe. This is known as gout. A normal uric acid level is 3.0 to 7.0 mg/dl.

Procedure 32-1 Pregnancy Test

STANDARD PRECAUTIONS:

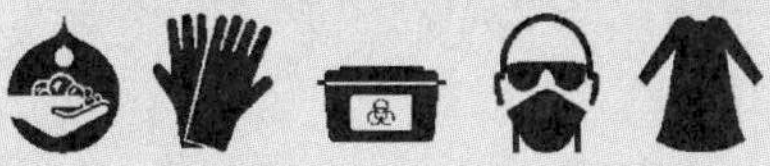

PURPOSE:

To perform the enzyme immunoassay or agglutination inhibition test to detect hCG in urine to determine positive or negative pregnancy results.

EQUIPMENT/SUPPLIES:

Gloves
Urine specimen
Stopwatch
Disinfectant (10% chlorine bleach solution)
Biohazard container
hCG negative and positive urine control
Pregnancy test kit

PROCEDURE STEPS:

1. Wash hands and put on gloves. RATIONALE: While working with body fluids, such as urine, gloves should be worn as personal protection.
2. Assemble all equipment and supplies. RATIONALE: Organizing all equipment and supplies before running the test will eliminate errors caused by missing supplies.
3. Perform the test following the manufacturer's instructions. The following steps are intentionally general so a variety of kits can be used. RATIONALE: The manufacturer's instructions will differ from kit to kit. It is important, as a quality-assurance measure, for the instructions to be read and understood thoroughly. Any questions must be directed to the manufacturer.
   a. Determine materials are at room temperature.
   b. Apply urine to the test unit using dispenser provided (Figure 32-10).
   c. Wait appropriate time interval (use stopwatch to time test).
   d. Apply first reagent/antibody to test unit using dispenser provided.
   e. Observe color development after appropriate time interval.
   f. Stop reaction.
   g. Consult manufacturer's package insert to interpret test results (Figure 32-11).
4. Record the results of the test on a laboratory report form following laboratory policy. RATIONALE: Interpretation of results may differ from kit to kit according to the manufacturer's design, and even though laboratory processes are the same, policies and forms will differ from laboratory to laboratory.
5. Repeat steps with both positive and negative urine controls (Figure 32-12). RATIONALE: Controls are performed to assure the quality of the reagents and testing supplies. If a positive control test does not show a positive result, then

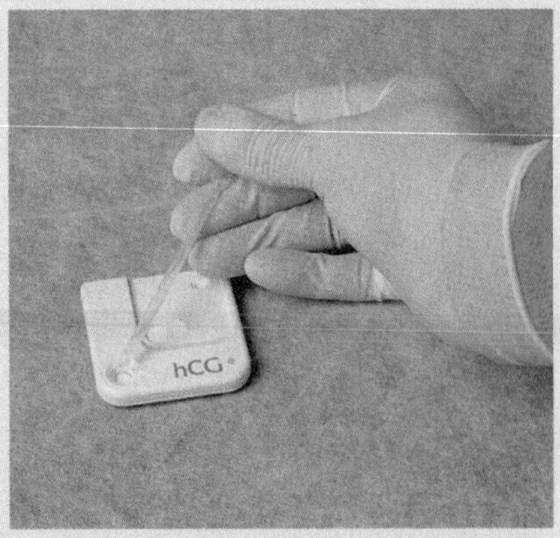

Figure 32-10 Urine is placed in the test unit according to package instructions.

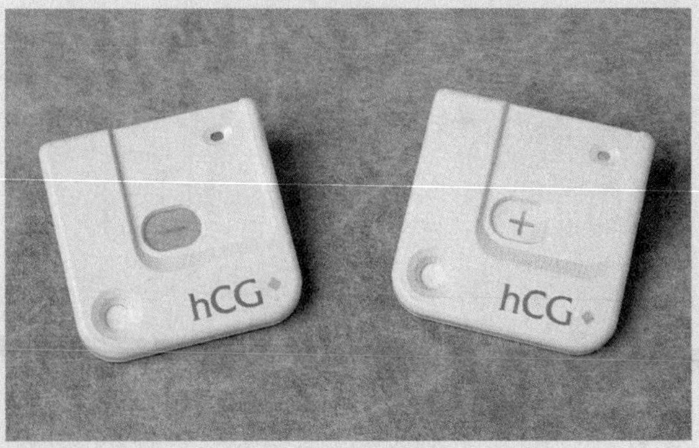

Figure 32-11 The package instructions will specify how the test is to be interpreted. A common interpretation is with a negative sign (left) and a positive sign (right).

(continues)

Procedure 32-1 (continued)

something is wrong with the reagent or the testing supplies. If the control test is not accurate, the patient's test will not be accurate either.

6. Disinfect reusable equipment. Discard disposable supplies into biohazard container. Dispose of specimen per laboratory policy. Clean work area with disinfectant. RATIONALE: Follow Standard Precautions and laboratory policies for disposal of biohazard substances and disinfection of supplies/equipment.
7. Remove gloves and discard into biohazard container. Wash hands. RATIONALE: Gloves protect hands from most but not all microorganisms. Hands should always be washed after removal of gloves to assure complete protection and also to remove glove powders and latex residue.
8. Document procedure in patient chart. RATIONALE: Documentation should refer the reader to the test result in the laboratory section of the medical record and document any patient reactions to the test, as well as any patient education/instructions given.

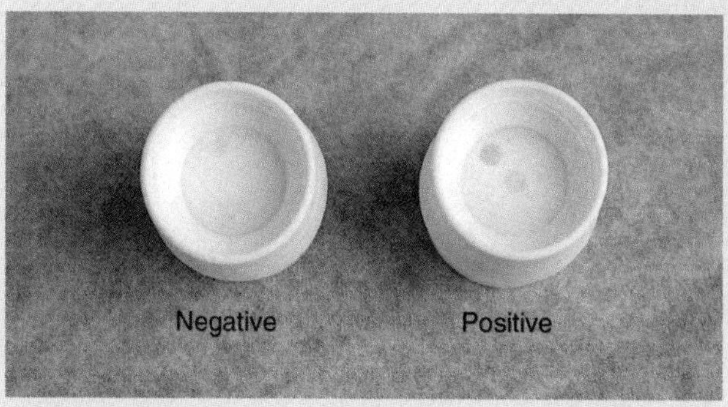

Figure 32-12 Control tests must be performed according the manufacturer's instructions. This illustration shows the results of the positive and negative controls test.

DOCUMENTATION

11/17/XX 8:14 AM Urine pregnancy test performed. Results forwarded to physician and form filed in laboratory section of medical record. Joe Guerrero, CMA

Procedure 32-2 Performing Infectious Mononucleosis Test

STANDARD PRECAUTIONS:

PURPOSE:

To perform an accurate test of serum or plasma to detect the presence or absence of antibodies of infectious mononucleosis (IM).

EQUIPMENT/SUPPLIES:

Gloves
Serum or plasma specimen
Stopwatch or lab timer
Surface disinfectant (10% chlorine bleach solution)
Test kit for IM
Biohazard container

(continues)

Procedure 32-2 (continued)

PROCEDURE STEPS:

NOTE: These instructions are intentionally general so a variety of test kits may be used. The manufacturer's instructions will differ from kit to kit. It is important, as a quality-assurance measure, for the instructions to be thoroughly read and understood before performing the test. Any instructions not clearly understood should be clarified with the manufacturer.

1. Wash hands and put on gloves. RATIONALE: While working with body fluids, such as urine, gloves should be worn as personal protection.
2. Assemble all equipment and supplies. RATIONALE: Organizing all equipment and supplies before running the test will eliminate errors caused by missing supplies.
3. Perform the test according to the manufacturer's instructions exactly. RATIONALE: The manufacturer's instructions will vary with each specific kit. Quality results are assured only when instructions are followed precisely.
4. Record the results on a laboratory report form following laboratory policy. RATIONALE: Even though laboratory processes are the same, policies and forms will differ from laboratory to laboratory.
5. Repeat the test procedure using positive and negative controls. RATIONALE: Controls are performed to assure the quality of the reagents and testing supplies. If a positive control test does not show a positive result, then something is wrong with the reagent or the testing supplies. If the control test is not accurate, the patient's test will not be accurate either.
6. Discard contaminated materials into biohazard container. Dispose of specimen appropriately and disinfect reusable materials. Clean work area with disinfectant. RATIONALE: Follow Standard Precautions and laboratory policies for disposal of biohazard substances and disinfection of supplies/equipment.
7. Remove gloves and discard into biohazard container. Wash hands. RATIONALE: Gloves protect hands from most but not all microorganisms. Hands should always be washed after removal of gloves to assure complete protection and also to remove glove powders and latex residue.
8. Document results. RATIONALE: Documentation should refer the reader to the test result in the laboratory section of the medical record and document any patient reactions to the test, as well as any patient education/instructions given.

DOCUMENTATION

4/27/XX 2:54 PM Mononucleosis test performed. Results forwarded to physician and form filed in laboratory section of medical record. Joe Guerrero, CMA

Procedure 32-3 Obtaining Blood Specimen for Phenylketonuria (PKU) Test

STANDARD PRECAUTIONS:

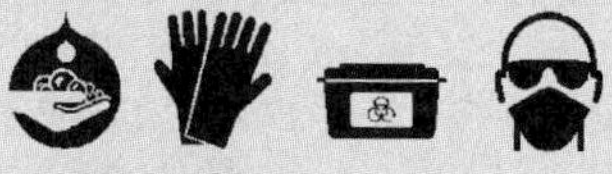

PURPOSE:

To obtain a blood specimen using a PKU test card or "filter paper" to determine phenylalanine levels in newborns who are at least three days old.

EQUIPMENT/SUPPLIES:

Gloves
PKU filter paper test card and mailing envelope
Alcohol swabs
Cotton balls/gauze pad
Sterile pediatric-sized lancet
Biohazard waste container

PROCEDURE STEPS:

1. Wash hands and put on gloves. RATIONALE: While working with body fluids, gloves should be worn as personal protection.
2. Identify the infant. Explain the purpose of the test and the procedure to the parents. Discuss the current health of the infant before beginning the procedure. RATIONALE: Certain antibiotics, medications, or vomiting problems may cause false results.
3. Select and clean an appropriate puncture site (Figure 32-13). Allow the alcohol to dry before the puncture. RATIONALE: Cleaning the site before puncture will remove any powders, oils, lotions, and contaminates. Allowing the alcohol to dry prevents the stick from stinging.
4. Grasp the infant's foot, taking care not to touch the cleansed area. Make a puncture approximately 2 to 3 mm deep in the infant's heel, making sure the infant's lateral, or side, portion of the heel pad is used. A pediatric-sized lancet, which limits the depth of puncture, should be used (Figure 32-14). If possible, recent puncture sites should always be avoided. See Procedure 28-5, Capillary Puncture.
5. Wipe away the first drop of blood with a gauze pad. RATIONALE: The first drop is diluted with alcohol and should not be collected for the test. Using a gauze pad rather than a cotton ball is preferred because the cotton ball may leave tiny fibers on the puncture site. The fibers may encourage clotting which will interfere with obtaining sufficient specimen for the test.
6. To collect blood for the test, press the back side of the filter paper test card against the infant's heel while exerting gentle pressure on the heel (Figure 32-15). The drop of blood should be large enough to completely fill and soak through the circle. *Do not* layer the multiple blood drops within a single circle. Completely fill all of the circles on the test card. RATIONALE: Failure to do so will require a retest.

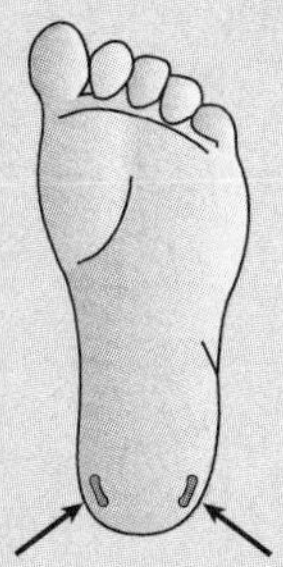

Figure 32-13 Capillary blood collection sites on an infant's heel pad.

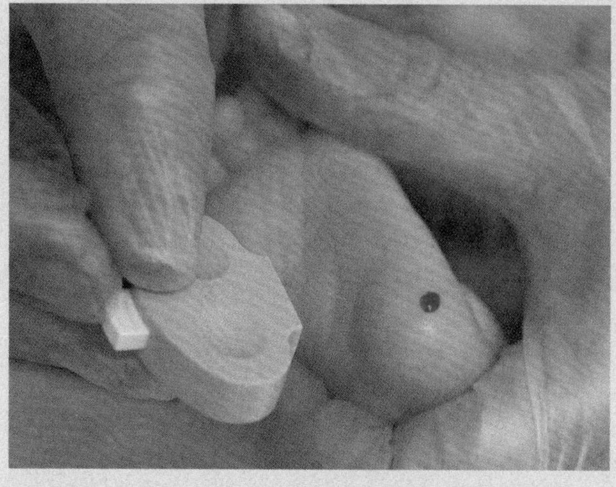

Figure 32-14 The infant's leg should be held securely with the non-dominant hand and arm while the dominant hand uses a pediatric lancet to perform a capillary heel stick.

(continues)

Procedure 32-3 (continued)

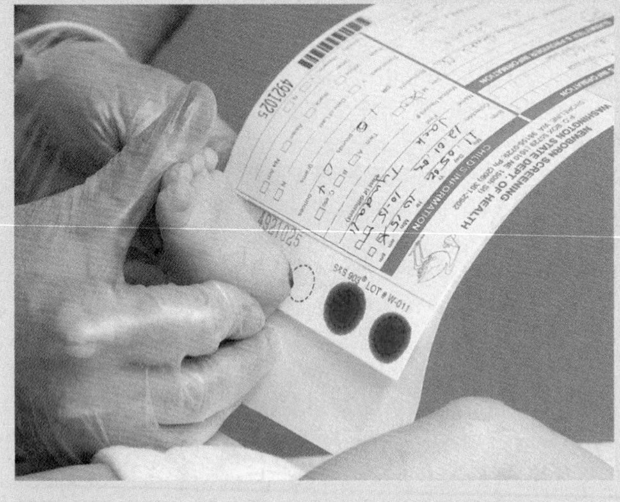

Figure 32-15 Drops of blood are transferred from the capillary heel stick puncture to the phenylketonuria filter card, completely filling all the circles on the filter test card.

7. Hold a cotton ball over the puncture and apply gentle pressure until the bleeding stops. Do not apply a bandage. RATIONALE: The bleeding should be stopped before the patient is released from your care. Bandages are discouraged because they can be a choking hazard for infants and toddlers.
8. Properly dispose of all waste in biohazard container. RATIONALE: Follow Standard Precautions and laboratory policies for disposal of biohazard substances and disinfection of supplies/equipment.
9. Remove the gloves and wash hands. RATIONALE: Gloves protect hands from most but not all microorganisms. Hands should always be washed after removal of gloves to assure complete protection and also to remove glove powders and latex residue.
10. Allow the PKU test card to completely dry on a nonabsorbent surface at room temperature. This will take about two hours. If collecting more than one card, *do not* lay one card on another when drying. RATIONALE: This could cause cross contamination of blood between the cards.
11. After the test card is dry, complete the PKU test card with all patient and physician information. RATIONALE: Allowing the blood to dry thoroughly before further handling lessens the chances of contaminating other parts of the form.
12. Place the test card in the mailer envelope and send it to the laboratory within two days. RATIONALE: It is important that the completed card be mailed as soon as possible to eliminate the breakdown of the contents within the specimen and to obtain the results as soon as possible to begin treatment if necessary.
13. Dispose of contaminated supplies into biohazard container and disinfect work area. RATIONALE: Follow Standard Precautions and laboratory policies for disposal of biohazard substances and disinfection of supplies/equipment.
14. Remove gloves and wash hands. RATIONALE: Gloves protect hands from most but not all microorganisms. Hands should always be washed after removal of gloves to assure complete protection and also to remove glove powders and latex residue.
15. Document the procedure in the patient's medical record. When test results are returned, these should be initialed by the physician and be placed in the patient's medical record. RATIONALE: Documentation should refer the reader to the test result in the laboratory section of the medical record and document any patient reactions to the test, as well as any patient education/instructions given.

DOCUMENTATION

6/27/XX 10:54 AM Capillary puncture performed on lateral aspect of left heel for PKU testing. Patient is 12 days old, currently taking no medication, and is not ill. Patient tolerated the procedure well and adequate specimen was obtained. PKU card completed and mailed. Joe Guerrero, CMA

7/10/XX PKU test results received and initialed by Dr. King and filed in the laboratory section of the patient's medical record. The patients parents were notified of the negative results per Dr. King's instructions. Joe Guerrero, CMA

Procedure 32-4 Screening Test for PKU

STANDARD PRECAUTIONS:

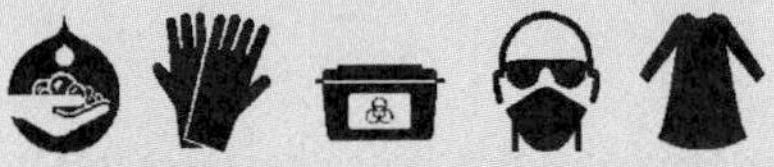

PURPOSE:

Test a urine specimen using the diaper test or the Phenistik test to determine phenylalanine levels in newborns who are at least six weeks old. This is a quick screening test only.

EQUIPMENT/SUPPLIES:

Gloves
10% ferric chloride for the diaper test
or
Phenistik for the Phenistik Method Test
Biohazard waste container

PROCEDURE STEPS:

1. Identify the infant. Verify that the infant is at least six weeks of age. Explain the purpose of the test and the procedure to the parents.
2. Wash hands and apply gloves.
3. Follow one of the two following procedures:
   a. *Diaper test:* Apply several drops of 10% ferric chloride to a diaper that contains fresh urine. Development of a green color indicates a positive test.
   b. *Phenistik test:* Dip the Phenistik test strip into fresh urine or press it against a diaper containing fresh urine. Development of a green color indicates a positive test.
4. A positive urine test should be followed up with a blood test.
5. Properly dispose of all waste in a biohazard waste container.
6. Remove gloves and wash hands.
7. Document the procedure and results in the patient's medical record.

Procedure 32-5 Measurement of Blood Glucose Using an Automated Analyzer

STANDARD PRECAUTIONS:

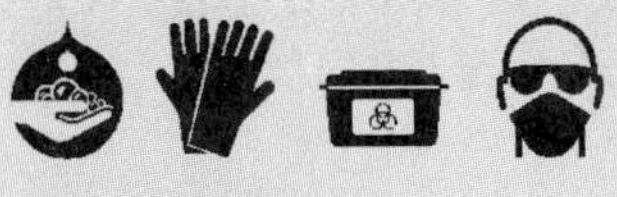

PURPOSE:

To measure blood glucose at timed intervals after the patient's ingestion of a standard glucose dose.

EQUIPMENT/SUPPLIES:

Gloves
Goggles
Safety lancet
Alcohol swabs
Glucose analyzer
Adhesive strip
Gauze
Control solutions for glucose analyzer
Test strips for glucose analyzer
Laboratory tissue
Cotton balls

PROCEDURE STEPS:

1. Review the manufacturer's manual for the specific glucose analyzer being used. Turn on the analyzer. RATIONALE: Always read and follow the manufacturer's instructions exactly for your particular analyzer to ensure accurate results.
2. Clean the work area and assemble all materials and supplies. RATIONALE: Organizing all equipment and supplies before running the test will eliminate errors caused by missing supplies.
3. Wash hands. Put on gloves and goggles. RATIONALE: Washing your hands assures that your skin is clean before gloving and decreases contaminants. Applying personal protection equipment when working with body fluids will lessen

(continues)

Procedure 32-5 (continued)

the chances of exposure to dangerous biohazard substances.

4. Record the control ranges, control lot number, and test strip lot number. RATIONALE: Recording the lot numbers and control ranges is another type of quality-assurance measure and is required by CLIA for many automated tests.
5. Perform the check test and the control test according to the manufacturer's instructions. If both tests are within range, proceed to the glucose test. Repeat both tests if either is out of acceptable range. RATIONALE: Controls are performed to assure the quality of the reagents and testing supplies. If a positive control test does not show a positive result, then something is wrong with the reagent or the testing supplies. If the control test is not accurate, the patient's test will not be accurate either.

To perform the glucose test:

1. Remove a test strip from the bottle and replace the lid.
2. Insert the test strip into the test chamber.
3. Perform a capillary puncture (see Procedure 28-5). Wipe first drop with gauze.
4. Apply a large drop of blood to the test strip.
5. After the appropriate time interval has passed, read the glucose concentration. Check the puncture site and apply adhesive strip.
6. Document the results.
7. Remove gloves and wash hands.
8. Properly dispose of all waste in a biohazard waste container.

Procedure 32-6 Cholesterol Testing

STANDARD PRECAUTIONS:

PURPOSE:

To measure cholesterol and triglyceride for monitoring purposes. For cholesterol, HDL, or triglyceride monitoring. NOTE: The following steps are intentionally general so a variety of kits can be used. The manufacturer's instructions will differ from kit to kit. It is important, as a quality-assurance measure, for the instructions to be read and understood thoroughly. Any questions must be directed to the manufacturer.

EQUIPMENT/SUPPLIES:

Gloves
Blood collecting equipment
Pipettes with disposable tips
Chlorine bleach
Commercial kit for manual determination of cholesterol
Controls and standards
Marking pen
Biohazard container

PROCEDURE STEPS:

1. Assemble all necessary equipment and materials. RATIONALE: Organizing all equipment and supplies before running the test will eliminate errors caused by missing supplies and will show the patient a more professional process.
2. Wash hands; apply gloves. RATIONALE: Washing your hands assures that your skin is clean before gloving and decreases contaminants. Applying personal protection equipment when working with body fluids will lessen the chances of exposure to dangerous biohazard substances.
3. Obtain a blood sample from the patient, either by fingerstick or venipuncture, depending on the manufacturer's instructions (see Chapter 28). Always read and follow the manufacturer's instructions to assure accurate results.

(continues)

Procedure 32-6 (continued)

4. Follow the manufacturer's instructions to perform the cholesterol test. Be sure to run the controls also. RATIONALE: Following all manufacturer's instructions will assure accurate test results. Controls are performed to assure the quality of the reagents and testing supplies. If a positive control test does not show a positive result, then something is wrong with the reagent or the testing supplies. If the control test is not accurate, the patient's test will not be accurate either.
5. Properly dispose of all waste in biohazard container. RATIONALE: Follow Standard Precautions when disposing of sharps and biohazard and contaminated waste.
6. Document results. Record the results of the test on a laboratory report form and document the procedure in the patient's chart. After the physician has initialed the report, file it in the patient's chart. RATIONALE: The chart note should refer the reader to the laboratory section of the medical record/chart. No laboratory reports should be filed without the physician's approval.

Case Study 32-1

Anna Preciado, CMA, a clinical medical assistant with Drs. Lewis and King, has performed many venipunctures during her training at college, throughout her externship, and since her employment with Drs. Lewis and King. She has not, however, performed a heelstick capillary draw since she was in college and even then she practiced on a doll. Until now another medical assistant in the clinic was doing all the heelstick capillary draws for PKU testing, but Anna is ready to start performing them herself. She is concerned and understandably nervous about performing this procedure on an infant.

CASE STUDY REVIEW

1. What course of action should Anna take to prepare herself for performing a procedure that she has not done in several years?
2. Once Anna feels she is technically ready to perform the PKU blood test, what should she do to assure that the procedure goes well?

SUMMARY

CLIA has identified many rapid test kits and automated methods for use in the ambulatory care setting in the waived category. For all of the tests discussed in this chapter, it is important for the medical assistant to have a basic understanding of the principles involved and the proper sampling procedures required. Safety procedures and Standard Precautions must be observed at all times and include the proper disposal of infectious materials and reagents. Gloves and goggles are always used when obtaining samples and while performing the actual test. Careful documentation by the medical assistant will help the physician in the diagnosis of the patient.

STUDY FOR SUCCESS

To reinforce your knowledge and skills of information presented in this chapter:

- ❑ Review the Key Terms
- ❑ Practice the Procedures
- ❑ Consider the Case Study and discuss your conclusions
- ❑ Answer the Review Questions
  - ❑ Multiple Choice
  - ❑ Critical Thinking
- ❑ Navigate the Internet by completing the Web Activities
- ❑ Practice the StudyWARE activities on the CD
- ❑ Apply your knowledge in the Student Workbook activities
- ❑ Complete the Web Tutor sections
- ❑ View and discuss the DVD situations

REVIEW QUESTIONS

Multiple Choice

1. In addition to pregnancy, a positive hCG test can be found in the following pathologic conditions *except*:
   a. ectopic pregnancy
   b. hydatidiform mole of the uterus
   c. pelvic inflammatory disease
   d. cancer of the lung
2. If a urine sample for a pregnancy test cannot be tested immediately, it may be stored in the following way for 24 hours:
   a. room temperature, 25°C
   b. body temperature, 37°C
   c. frozen
   d. refrigerated at 4°C
3. The kissing disease is synonymous with the disease:
   a. tuberculosis
   b. infectious mononucleosis
   c. hemolytic anemia
   d. hypoglycemia
4. Serum or blood would be the *specimen of choice* for all but the following test:
   a. ABO typing
   b. testing for EBV
   c. cholesterol
   d. hCG hormone
5. Which of the following statements is incorrect regarding blood type:
   a. Type A RBCs have A antigens on the cell.
   b. Type B RBCs have B antigens on the cell.
   c. Type O RBCs have A and B antigens on the cell.
   d. Type AB RBCs have both A and B antigens on the cell.
6. Which of the following is a *true* statement about the Rh factor?
   a. Rh factor is a rare blood type.
   b. Rh factor is present on all RBCs.
   c. Rh factor was discovered from rhesus monkeys.
   d. People without the Rh factor on their RBCs have naturally occurring antibodies called anti-D in their plasma.

7. When instructing a patient in the correct collection of a specimen for semen analysis, all of the following should be considered *except:*
   a. avoid the consumption of alcohol several days before the test
   b. collection of semen into a condom is unacceptable
   c. specimen should be transported to the laboratory at 37°C within 30 minutes of collection
   d. avoid the consumption of fats several days before the test
8. Testing for PKU is done on:
   a. newborns
   b. children 1 to 3 years of age
   c. teenagers
   d. adults older than 40 years
9. The best site location for a tuberculin Mantoux test is:
   a. back of the hand
   b. forearm 3 to 4 inches from bend of arm
   c. ½ inch above the back of the knee
   d. upper part of the arm in the deltoid muscle
10. A patient with hypoglycemia would have a blood glucose level of:
   a. 50–70 mg/dl
   b. 70–110 mg/dl
   c. 110–150 mg/dl
   d. 150–200 mg/dl

Critical Thinking

1. Why is the first-voided morning urine the preferred specimen for a pregnancy test?
2. Why is it necessary to repeat the seminal analysis three times over a two-month period?
3. What factors may alter the results of a blood glucose measurement?
4. How can you distinguish between the diabetic and nondiabetic patient based on the results of the two-hour postprandial glucose evaluation?
5. Discuss the relation between saturated fats and coronary artery disease.
6. What is the function of triglycerides in the body?
7. What instructions should the patient be given in preparation for a triglyceride evaluation?
8. What is the source of urea in the blood?

WEB ACTIVITIES

1. Search the CDC's and other government Web sites for information on infectious diseases such as mononucleosis.
2. Use search engines to research some of the conditions discussed in this chapter, such as PKU and TB.

THE DVD HOOK-UP

DVD Series	Program Number
Skills Based Series	**11, 12**

Chapter/Scene Reference

- *Performing Blood Sugar Test*
- *Performing Mononucleosis Test*
- *Performing Pregnancy Test*

This chapter discusses specialty tests that may be performed in the medical office.

1. This program illustrated the technique for performing a blood glucose test. The medical assistant ran a control before performing the test. Why is it important to run a control before performing the test?
2. What should you do if a patient asks you for his or her laboratory results before the doctor has had a chance to review them?

DVD Journal Summary

Write a paragraph that summarizes what you learned from watching the selected scenes from today's DVD programs. When viewing the scene from program 12, you saw a medical assistant give a testimonial about giving out a test result without checking with the physician first. The patient was traumatized and the physician was furious with the medical assistant for giving out the test results without checking with him first. Why is it best for the physician to communicate test results to the patient? Is it ever acceptable for the medical assistant to communicate test results to a patient?

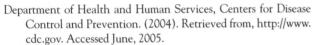

REFERENCES/BIBLIOGRAPHY

Department of Health and Human Services, Centers for Disease Control and Prevention. (2004). Retrieved from, http://www.cdc.gov. Accessed June, 2005.

Walters, N. J., Estridge, B. H., & Reynold, A. P. (2000). *Basic medical laboratory techniques* (4th ed.). Clifton Park, NY: Thomson Delmar Learning.

U.S. Food and Drug Administration. (2004). *Databases on the FDA Web site*. Retrieved from http://www.fda.gov/search/databases.html. Accessed June, 2005.

UNIT 8
Office and Human Resources Management

CHAPTER 33

The Medical Assistant as Office Manager

OUTLINE

KEY TERMS

Agenda
Ancillary Services
Authoritarian Manager
Benchmark
Benefit
Bond
Brainstorming
Conflict Resolution
Embezzle
Externship
Fringe Benefit
"Going Bare"
Internet
Involuntary Dismissal
Itinerary
Liability
Malpractice
Management by Walking Around (MBWA)
Marketing
Mentor
Minutes
Negligence
Participatory Manager
Practicum
Procedure Manual
Professional Liability Insurance
Profit Sharing
Risk Management
Salary Review
Search Engine
Self-actualization
Shadow
Subordinate
Teamwork
Web Site
Work Statement

FEATURED COMPETENCIES

CAAHEP—ENTRY-LEVEL COMPETENCIES

Professional Communication

- Respond to and initiate written communications
- Recognize and respond to verbal communications
- Recognize and respond to nonverbal communications

Legal Concepts

- Identify and respond to issues of confidentiality
- Perform within legal and ethical boundaries
- Document appropriately
- Demonstrate knowledge of federal and state health care legislation and regulations

Patient Instruction

- Explain general office policies
- Identify community resources

Operational Function

- Perform an inventory of supplies and equipment
- Perform routine maintenance of administrative and clinical equipment

ABHES—ENTRY-LEVEL COMPETENCIES

Professionalism

- Project a positive attitude
- Maintain confidentiality at all times
- Be a "team player"
- Be cognizant of ethical boundaries

(continues)

OBJECTIVES

The student should strive to meet the following performance objectives and demonstrate an understanding of the facts and principles presented in this chapter through written and oral communication.

1. Define the key terms as presented in the glossary.
2. Describe the qualities of a manager.
3. Discuss characteristics of managers and leaders.
4. Differentiate between authoritarian and participatory management styles.
5. Describe management by walking around and its usefulness in ambulatory care settings.
6. Recall a minimum of four common risks and risk-control measures.
7. List three benefits of a teamwork approach.
8. Discuss the importance of a meeting agenda.
9. Describe appropriate evaluation tools for employees.
10. Recall effective methods of resolving conflict.
11. Identify the steps required to make travel arrangements.
12. Define the term itinerary and list important information the itinerary should contain.
13. List three methods of increasing productivity and efficient time management.
14. Describe the purpose of a procedure manual.
15. Discuss the impact of HIPAA's privacy policy in ambulatory care settings.
16. Describe the general concept of marketing and recall at least three marketing tools.
17. Describe the purpose and benefit of marketing.
18. Define records management, financial management, facility and equipment management, and risk management.
19. Describe the steps involved in payroll processing.
20. Describe liability coverage and what bonding means.

SCENARIO

Marilyn Johnson has been employed by Drs. Lewis and King's office for the past eight years. Three years ago, she was promoted to the position of office manager when the facility added the second office for its associates in the next suburb. Marilyn has a baccalaureate degree in business administration. Her responsibilities at Drs. Lewis and King's office include various duties involving personnel, finances, and office efficiency.

FEATURED COMPETENCIES (continued)

- Evidence a responsible attitude
- Be courteous and diplomatic

Communication

- Serve as liaison between physician and others
- Interview effectively
- Recognize and respond to verbal and nonverbal communications
- Professional components

Administrative Duties

- Locate resources and information for patients and employers
- Manage physician's professional schedule and travel

Legal Concepts

- Determine needs for documentation and reporting
- Document accurately
- Use appropriate guidelines when releasing records or information
- Follow established policy in initiating or terminating medical treatment
- Dispose of controlled substances in compliance with government regulations
- Maintain licenses and accreditation
- Monitor legislation related to current healthcare issues and practices
- Perform risk management procedures

(continues)

INTRODUCTION

The drive to improve the productivity of the medical office, precipitated by managed care, Medicare and insurance limits placed on fees, have broadened the scope of employment options and job marketability for medical assistants. This has created an opportunity for medical assistants to advance to the position of office manager.

In small offices, the position of office manager may include the duties of the human resources (HR) representative; in larger clinics, these positions will be independent. This book treats them as separate positions (see Chapter 34). In the larger facilities, the office manager and HR representative must coordinate their personnel-related functions into a seamless organization.

Spotlight on Certification

RMA Content Outline

- Medical law
- Medical ethics
- Human relations

CMA Content Outline

- Basic principles (Psychology)
- Working as a team member to achieve goals
- Evaluating and understanding communication
- Medicolegal guidelines & requirements
- Resource information and community services
- Managing physician's professional schedule and travel
- Managing the office
- Office policies and procedures
- Employee payroll

CMAS Content Outline

- Legal and ethical considerations
- Professionalism
- Patient information and community resources
- Medical records management
- Medical office financial management
- Medical office management

FEATURED COMPETENCIES (continued)

Office Management

- Maintain physical plant
- Operate and maintain facilities and perform routine maintenance of administrative and clinical equipment safely
- Inventory equipment and supplies
- Evaluate and recommend equipment and supplies for practice
- Maintain liability coverage
- Exercise efficient time management

Instruction

- Orient patients to office policies and procedures
- Orient and train personnel

Financial Management

- Process employee payroll

THE MEDICAL ASSISTANT AS OFFICE MANAGER

The office manager of a medical office or ambulatory care facility is a role that can have vast and diverse responsibilities. This chapter covers the following office manager duties:

1. Arrange and maintain practice insurance and develop risk management strategies
2. Supervise office personnel
3. Prepare staff meeting agenda, conduct the meeting, and record minutes
4. Make travel arrangements and prepare an itinerary
5. Assist in improving work flow and office efficiencies (time management)
6. Create and update the office procedure manual, Material Safety Data Sheets (MSDSs), and Health Insurance Portability and Accountability Act (HIPAA) manual.
7. Prepare patient education materials and arrange patient/community education workshops as needed
8. Approve financial transactions and account disposition; generate financial reports as needed
9. Supervise the purchase and storage of office supplies
10. Supervise the purchase, repair, and maintenance of office equipment

QUALITIES OF A MANAGER

An office manager should not feel the need to be superior to employees. The best manager is like an orchestra conductor. He or she constructively blends together the skills and abilities of diverse people to produce a smooth and efficient team. The result is an organization having greater capability than would be achievable by the individuals acting independently.

The office manager should have two overarching goals:

- Get the job done.
- Make the process enjoyable.

This does not mean work should be one big party. It means developing ownership for the work, pride in doing the job well, and a sense of teamwork. There will be times when employees will not like having to stay late to meet important deadlines, but through developed self-actualization, they will take enjoyment from even the most undesirable task.

A good office manager needs to be two persons in one body: leader and manager. The two functions are different, and the good manager will use some of each characteristic in meeting objectives. Table 33-1 illustrates the differences between an authoritarian style manager and a leader/manager.

Good managers are leaders, providing their coworkers with vision, guidance, and a feeling of ownership in the process. They do these things without threats, usually through the power of their personal charisma. It is also important that managers clearly convey their expectations to their employees. Possibly nothing leads to ill feeling between the manager and an employee more than failure to let the employee know what is expected of him or her. Furthermore, a lack of expectations stifles career growth and organizational vitality. Good leaders need to blend many admirable personality traits of leadership to be successful and still control the resources entrusted to them.

Before proceeding with a listing of qualities of a leader/manager, a rule that defines almost all of the ethical qualities needs to be mentioned (Figure 33-1). Some texts call it the Golden Rule; this rule will make the difference between a manager who is successful and one who fails miserably. The rule needs no explanation, and will serve any manager well in any circumstance.

TABLE 33-1 DIFFERENCES BETWEEN AN AUTHORITARIAN STYLE MANAGER AND A LEADER/MANAGER

Manager	Leader
• Establishes and adheres to written procedures	• Empower people
• Focused on short-range goals	• Inspires by example
• Authoritarian style of management	• Vision and long range goals
• Bottom line all important	• Consensus or team style of management
• Does things right	• Does the right thing
• Annual raises	• Pay for performance
• Reluctant to change	• Not afraid of change

The following bulleted items list most of the qualities needed by a leader/manager:

- *Effective communication skills*. Communication skills include written and oral methods. The manager must communicate clearly, diplomatically, tactfully, and with respect for the feelings of others.
- *Fairmindedness*. It is important to always be fair with coworkers. Decisions that impact one fellow employee create a ripple effect. That is, you may have to make the same decision for another employee at another time. Decisions should be based, as much as possible, on the assumption that what is granted to one employee will be granted to others in similar situations. This approach will decrease the risk for being accused of playing favorites or being unfair.
- *Objectivity*. The office manager must be able to view challenges without bias or prejudice. For example, when promotions are made, the office manager must be able to focus on the job description criteria and individual qualifications without introducing personal preference.
- *Organizational skills*. Being organized includes being able to prioritize tasks, working efficiently and methodically. Know when and be willing to delegate tasks when others have the expertise and time to complete the task within the time lines.
- *People skills*. The office manager must like people in general and enjoy working with them. Building confidence and self-esteem in others and being interested in promoting constructive relationships are essential qualities of the office manager. The ability to function as an effective team leader provides a role model for other staff members to emulate.
- *Problem-solving skills*. The office manager must be a problem solver. This may include being creative and doing away with old paradigms and traditional approaches to solving a problem. When difficult issues arise, focus on the situation, issue, or behavior, not on the person. A discussion about solving the problem without laying blame is much more productive. Positive solutions may be more readily attained when discussing what was observed rather than what was told by someone else.
- *Technical expertise*. Have a working knowledge of each procedure performed in the office, although it is not necessary to be the acknowledged technical expert. A good office manager is continually learning and encourages **subordinates** to seek opportunities to continue their education and advance their technical skills.
- *Truthfulness*. Lead by example! If an honest mistake is made, be the first to admit to the error and seek the best solution for preventing it from happening again. Respond honestly to requests. For example, two staff members ask for the same day off. The office manager will make the decision that only one member may have the day off and will review the policy manual to determine the appropriate criteria for designating who will have the request granted.

Office Manager Attitude

Many managers share a common enemy—themselves. The part of ourselves that is our enemy is our mind and the outlook we have on the world. People who succeed attribute positive results to their own actions. People who underachieve or fail usually attribute negative results to someone else or to chance, over which they have no control. Because underachievers feel helpless to affect results, psychologists conclude that their motivation to succeed

TREAT OTHERS, AS YOU WOULD LIKE TO BE TREATED!

Figure 33-1 The Golden Rule.

is diminished. A low achiever would be unlikely to have a personal risk management system in place. They would feel they could not affect events. The more positive person could easily take steps to avoid these problems.

The effect of a negative mindset does not stop with failure to accept responsibility for the things that happen to each of us, it continues on. Unless we change our outlook, we lower our expectations and begin accepting the mediocre. Individuals who feel they are helpless to affect events become afraid of success, as well as failure, and subconsciously find a way to fail to avoid the challenges success will bring.

How do you change your mindset? Following are a few suggestions considered helpful:

- Come to terms with what you would have to change if you are to be successful and be ready for the change.
- Identify what you really want to achieve.
- Put your goals in writing using positive terms (say "I will" not "I'll try").
- Begin with small, achievable goals.
- Eliminate poor habits such as procrastination.
- Tune out negative thoughts and focus on positive thoughts.

We are what we think we are. Be careful of your mindset, it can derail you and your job as a manager.

Professionalism

The medical assistant as office manager must exhibit professional behavior at all times. He or she must be courteous and diplomatic and demonstrate a responsible and positive attitude. All verbal and written communications should be accurate, correct, and follow appropriate guidelines. The office manager should demonstrate knowledge of federal and state health care legislation and regulations and must perform within legal and ethical boundaries. All documentation must be performed appropriately.

The office manager serves as a liaison between the physician, patient, and other professionals. Therefore, professional demeanor in all respects must be followed. It is not uncommon to be called on to locate community resources and information for patients and employers. Review Procedure 4-1 for specific information on how this is done. A good working relationship with other community service organizations fosters the sharing of information vital to your patient's health care needs and promotes quality public relations.

> In many offices, the office manager is also designated to fill the role of Security Officer. The responsibilities of the Security Officer include coordinating and overseeing the various impacts of HIPAA on each department and assisting with compliance issues related to HIPAA regulations. The Security Officer must also keep abreast of any changes and rulings and how they may apply to their particular office environment. Some online resources are available at: http://www.cms.hhs.gov; or e-mail questions to askhipaa@cms.hhs.gov.

> **Critical Thinking**
>
> How does the office manager begin to develop good working relationships with other community service organizations to better serve and provide for the patient's health care needs? How would this improve the quality of public relations?

MANAGEMENT STYLES

There are many books written on management styles; however, it is possible to break all of them down into only two basic styles, each with an infinite number of variations. Because this is not a management text, we will take a simplistic view and look at only the fundamental styles: authoritarian and participatory. We will also examine a third management style, managing by walking around, which, although not a people interaction style, is an effective management technique for keeping abreast of what is going on in an organization.

Authoritarian Style

Authoritarian managers operate on the premise that most workers cannot make a contribution without being directed, sometimes in the minutest detail, and even if they could, they would not be inclined to do so. This type of manager believes in the carrot and the stick approach to motivate people to work. The carrot is monetary reward, and the stick is docked pay or being reprimanded or fired. The personality of the manager tends to influence natural tendencies of style. Individuals who are task or procedure oriented tend to be authoritarian. Authority control is easily accomplished in the case of simple tasks that can readily be structured and defined. Authoritarian managers try to control work to the maximum extent possible, for example, micro-management. Complex jobs, however, are difficult for the authoritarian manager to control.

Sometimes a manager may need to use the authoritarian style. It should be used quite sparingly, because it may destroy morale and personal incentive. An assumption regarding the character of an employee frequently becomes a self-fulfilling prophecy. Workers with an authoritarian manager either give up and quit, or they become mindless robots asking "how high" when told to jump. As a manager, you will use the authoritarian style in the case of new employees until you have a chance to determine their capabilities, in the case of a worker who has proved to be without self-motivation, or in supervising short-term temporary labor.

Can an authoritarian manager style work in the twenty-first century? Yes. It has worked for a few well-respected, large companies in the United States, but this occurred only because management had unlimited resources to use as a carrot for rewarding employees. Most managers will not have these resources.

Participatory Style

The **participatory management** style is based on the premise that the worker is capable and wants to do a good job. The best known form of participatory management is the use of teams to do work tasks. This type of management is well suited to complex tasks where each member can contribute his specialty to the job at hand. The manager's function in this type of system is to communicate direction and vision to the team and to sell the team on the importance of the task. Managers using this type of style need to be comfortable teaching, coaching, communicating, inspiring, and motivating. Workers engaged in a participatory management style are motivated by much more than monetary reward and develop an ownership for the work in which they are involved. Although the carrot is still important, their reward comes from teamwork, peer recognition, and self-actualization, that is, the pleasure from doing a job well and being recognized for it. Competition between teams is sometimes used as a motivation technique.

Management by Walking Around

Management by walking around (MBWA) is not really a management style, but rather a technique for keeping the manager informed about the health of his or her organization. This style consists of just what the title says, the manager walks around looking at what is going on in the organization and talks with employees to get their opinion on how things could be done better. The manager collects data on new ideas; in a participatory system, a team would be assigned to study and come up with a better way of doing the work. The manager must be careful to make sure his or her motives are not to micro-manage and to convey this to the workers.

RISK MANAGEMENT

The office manager should formulate a **risk management** procedure that assesses risks to which he or she and the organization is exposed and takes steps to develop contingencies that minimize probable risks. Some common risks and risk-control measures are:

- *Loss of a critical employee.* Have cross training of employees to permit them to assume the duties of an employee who is ill or terminates his or her employment.
- *Failure of a supplier or contractor.* Maintain sufficient inventory to permit contracting with a secondary supplier before having critical shortages. Monitor the status of orders so you are aware of any failures in delivery before they have a negative impact and so supplies can be obtained from a second source. Have a list of secondary sources.
- *Accidental disclosure of confidential information through error or unauthorized entry.* Have protocols in place regarding breach of confidentiality and defining steps to be taken in the event information is compromised. Define protocols to patients alerting them to the unlikely but potential possibility of accidental disclosure. Notify patients immediately if confidential information is compromised, and work with them for resolution.
- *Computer failure.* Back up the system regularly. Have a secondary system that could permit the office to operate until repairs are effected. Have a maintenance contract in place with a reputable firm permitting overnight repair.
- *Injury to a staff member or nonemployee.* Continually review safety procedures and conduct safety surveys. Have adequate liability insurance for the medical office.

> **Critical Thinking**
>
> How would you make the medical office (front- and back-office space) safe for employees and nonemployees (e.g., patients, venders, visitors)? List as many considerations as possible.

- *Managerial position change*. Continuously network with friends and associates to permit you to rapidly seek a new position before experiencing a job loss. It's always easier to get a job while you still have a job.

IMPORTANCE OF TEAMWORK

The use of **teamwork** to improve the efficiency of the office at first may seem incongruent to your desire to improve office efficiency, because it seems that several people are now involved in solving a problem that you as the manager should solve and explain. Teamwork builds morale and actually results in getting more accomplished with the resources you have because the team members develop ownership of the solution to a problem and want to make it work. When it works, it flatters them and builds their esteem.

Efficiency of a team results from the collective working together to plan how to "work smarter" and how to dovetail tasks and support each other so that wasted effort is avoided. To achieve all of these things, a team must not only be given the responsibility and the authority to plan and execute their plan to solve a problem, but they must know your expectations for them. Sometimes this means that you, the office manager, must stick your neck out for them. They will reward you handsomely for doing so.

Getting the Team Started

A successful teamwork approach is not a mysterious event that just happens, it is the result of clear vision, specific goals, and a well-planned strategy on the part of the team leader. For teamwork to be successful, individual team members must understand and support the specifics of the problem they are being asked to solve. This is probably the most significant task of the team leader or the office manager. It is helpful in taking this important step to let the team develop its own **work statement,** for in this way they assume ownership of the goals and objectives you want them to achieve. The work statement frequently outlines specific tasks and their sequential order of accomplishment. Its purpose is to ensure that everyone is working toward the team goals and objectives.

A major pitfall at this stage may be diverse opinions that can lead to a work statement that does not meet the manager's goals and objectives for the team. It is your job as office manager to try to direct the team back to what you want them to work on without undermining their team spirit. Take care at this stage not to begin making assignments or to let team members start solving the problem until the work statement is complete. Under some circumstances, it may be necessary for you, the office manager, to exercise your authority in defining the work statement, but be careful, because this approach could harm the team's collective spirit.

The next step in team development is to establish a timetable for achieving results and identifying the standards that must be maintained. Without a timetable a team feels no sense of urgency and tends to lose direction. You also have to paint a clear picture of the standards that must be maintained as you attempt to solve the problem. You should let the team develop both the standards and the timetable, but with your leadership and support.

Using a Team to Solve a Problem

Problem solution is the next step in team development. Some people call this stage **brainstorming** a solution. Brainstorming is fun, but unless it is controlled by the leader, it will bog down into needless arguments and hurt feelings. In a successful brainstorming session everyone should feel free to contribute solutions to the problem without any consideration for practicality or flaws in the proposal. Only after everyone has had a chance to speak are the solutions looked at in terms of practicality and for technical correctness. At this point the team should not look at what is wrong with the solution, but what needs to be done to make it a workable solution.

Prioritization of the solutions comes next. To do this, it is helpful to assign scores for impact on solving the problem and for changeability, or the difficulty in implementing a particular solution in your office environment. The result will be a list of solutions to the problem in descending order from the greatest impact on the problem with the least cost or difficulty in implementation. Do a needs assessment, remove oneself from the issue, and look at it from a different perspective. **Benchmark** (compare) your facility to other facilities and organizations to see how they accomplish tasks, compensate employees, and so on.

Planning and Implementing a Solution

The team should work out a detailed plan for implementation of the solution selected, including a schedule. Assignments should be made, resources of equipment and funds available to the team should be defined, and any remaining problems assigned to subteams that will function just as the primary team did in solving them. The team should continue to meet to discuss progress and to resolve additional problems that may occur.

Recognition

A successful team should not be disbanded until it is acknowledged for its efforts and physical recognition is given in the case of an important problem that was solved. In some cases, a dinner or luncheon is in order. This is the most important phase of team development, because it is responsible for developing a team spirit or sense of **self-actualization** within the organization. Once this spirit is implanted into an organization, it becomes infectious.

SUPERVISING PERSONNEL

Creating an atmosphere in which open and honest communication can take place is critical to supervising personnel. This type of communication may be encouraged through the establishment of regular staff meetings, with each staff member sharing ideas for improvement and areas of concern. Eliciting the help of others in problem-solving strategies will promote harmony (Figure 33-2).

Staff and Team Meetings

The office manager usually initiates the staff and team meeting idea and should officiate at such meetings. Failure of the office manager to be present may convey a message that the meeting is an event not worthy of attention. It is important that the office manager be familiar with basic parliamentary procedures. The purchase of books such as *Robert's Rules of Order* or *Parliamentary Procedure at a Glance* is an excellent investment.

Successful staff and team meetings are announced well in advance or on established time lines to enable the majority of office personnel to attend. An **agenda** identifying the subjects to be covered during a given meeting should be issued before the meeting so that each attendee arrives prepared with input or questions relevant to the topics. Procedure 33-1 outlines the procedural steps for creating a meeting agenda. Figure 33-3 is a sample agenda. Each meeting should end with opportunity for non-agenda items to be discussed or suggested for inclusion in the next meeting. The meeting should have a fixed time to end.

A written record in the form of **minutes** should be maintained and sent to all team members regardless of whether they attended the meeting. This policy will keep all members informed about policy changes and decisions that impact the office operations. The minutes also trigger a reminder for any new procedures or revisions to be made in the procedure manual.

The minutes for a staff and team meeting should record action plans under each agenda topic. Summarize all action items agreed to in the meeting in one section of the minutes. This will facilitate easy access to information at a later date should it be required.

The date, time, and place of the next meeting should be included. The person preparing the minutes should always sign them. A copy of the minutes should always be maintained in a book for easy reference.

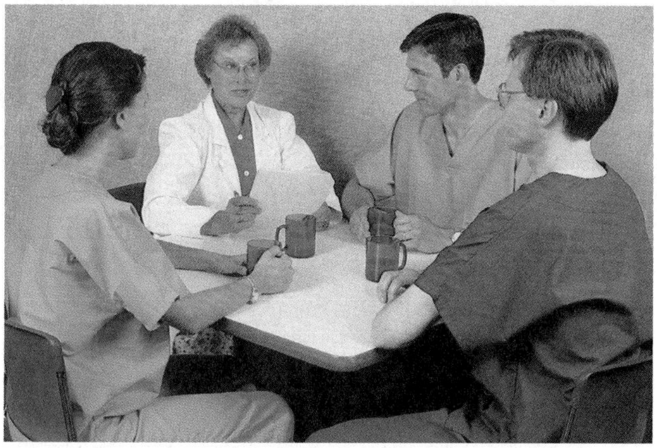

Figure 33-2 Consistently scheduled staff meetings promote communication and harmony among the health care team.

AGENDA

STAFF MEETING Wednesday, February 16, 20XX
2:00 PM — Conference Room

1. Read and approve minutes of last meeting
2. Reports
   A. Satellite facility — Marilyn Johnson
   B. Patient flow — Joe Guerrero
   C.
3. Discussion of new telephone system
4. Unfinished Business
   A. Review new procedure manual pages
   B.
5. New Business
   A. Appoint committee for design of new marketing brochure
   B.
6. Open discussion and/or topics for next meeting's agenda
7. Set next meeting time
8. Adjourn

Figure 33-3 Sample meeting agenda.

Assimilating New Personnel

The goal in the assimilation of new personnel into the workplace is to make it happen as seamlessly as possible. The office manager and HR representative usually assume this task jointly, with the office manager being responsible for orientation in medical protocols and procedures, and the HR representative handling orientation regarding medical practice rules and regulations and any legal implications.

New Personnel Orientation. The new personnel orientation process consists of orienting and training new employees in the medical protocols and procedures unique to the practice. If the procedure manual is detailed and accurate, this manual now becomes a guide for new employees.

It is important to introduce new employees to other staff members and to assign a **mentor** who can respond to questions that new employees may encounter. Sometimes the individual leaving a position may still be present and is asked to assist in the orientation process. This is especially beneficial if there is a good working relationship between the employee who is leaving and the management of the practice. Depending on the responsibilities of the new employee, a supervisor may be asked to monitor all procedures for a period for accuracy, safety, and patient protection.

The orientation should clearly present what is expected of the new employee and explain that at the end of their probationary period, their performance will be evaluated to determine if full-time employment will be offered. The same procedures followed for new employees should be followed for student practicums, with the exception that expectations and the evaluation process may vary.

Probation and Evaluation. It is common for a new employee to be placed on probation for 60 to 90 days. During this period, both the employee and supervisory personnel determine if the position is a suitable match for both employer and employee. Near the end of the probation period, the employee should be officially evaluated to determine how competently they are performing their assigned tasks/duties. The employee should also be given an opportunity to express their personal thoughts relative to job satisfaction. Figure 33-4 illustrates a sample probationary employee evaluation form. The evaluation becomes part of the employee's personnel record at the end of the probation period.

PROBATIONARY EMPLOYEE EVALUATION FORM

Name ____________________

Hire Date ____________________

Job Title ____________________

Pay Rate __________ Supervisor __________

Do you recommend the employee continue in employment?

_______ Yes _______ No

Please state your reasons for whatever action you recommend. Use the guidelines below to make your decision.

1. Has the employee required more training than is normally needed for the job?
2. Has the employee grasped this job with very little training?
3. Is the employee performing at, above, or below (circle one) the standard for this job?
4. If below, when do you expect the employee to reach the standard?
5. Does the employee get along well with all staff members?
6. Has the employee maintained a good attendance record and a good work attitude?
7. Has the employee expressed any dissatisfactions?

____________________ __________

Supervisor's Signature Date

Figure 33-4 Sample probationary employee evaluation.

Supervising Student Practicums. The student **practicum** is a transitional stage that provides opportunity for the student to apply theory learned in the classroom to a health care setting through practical, hands-on experience. Some institutions may use the term **externship** or *internship* and still others may operate through a cooperative education program. The number of hours for the practicum are predetermined together with criteria for site selection and tasks to be performed by the student.

The office manager should schedule an information interview with the student before the practicum begins. During this time, a discussion of the expectations of the office manager and the student may be established. A tour of the facility and introductions to key personnel aid the student in feeling more comfortable the first day of "work."

Because the student will be writing in medical records where correct spelling is mandatory or may be scheduling appointments and must write telephone numbers without transposition, some pretesting may be offered. By giving a spelling test of 10 commonly used medical terms or verbally stating five telephone numbers for the student to write down, an immediate evaluation is attained.

The office manager should directly supervise or identify someone else to supervise the student. During the first few days of the practicum, the student may simply **shadow** the supervisor, learning the routine, physician preference, and protocols for that particular office. As the student begins to feel comfortable in the new environment, minimal tasks should be assigned. Based on the student's ability to follow directions and perform tasks, increased skill-level tasks may be added.

The supervisor will direct and evaluate the student's progress; schedule activities that will provide experience in all aspects of medical assisting, including administrative, clinical, and laboratory procedures; maintain accurate records of attendance and hours "worked"; and communicate the student's progress to the medical assisting supervisor from the educational institution. Procedure 33-2 provides steps for supervising a student practicum.

When working with students, it is important to remember that they still have much to learn and will need lots of reassuring guidance. When you take time to explain each step and to provide the rationale for each, students will learn more quickly. Demonstrating new or different techniques and approaches helps students by providing them with options that they may find more comfortable.

Remember that this type of learning is stressful. The student is not yet accustomed to communication with a "real" patient, let alone working with a physician. Your role as office manager is to reduce as much stress as possible for everyone concerned. Introduce the student to the patient and ask the patient's permission to allow the student to perform a procedure. Many patients will be tolerant when they realize the circumstances and will be quite cooperative.

Employees with Chemical Dependencies or Emotional Problems

Employees with chemical dependencies or emotional problems are ill and are to be treated as such. Approach the situation constructively rather than punitively. Make a commitment to the employee, to the rest of the staff, and to the patients that at no time will patient care be put at risk. Help an employee with a problem to find the support and counseling necessary. No staff member should be permitted to remain on the premise with impaired judgment while under the influence of alcohol or controlled substances. If chemical dependency treatment is necessary, make accommodation as seems appropriate or is warranted. Everyone occasionally feels discouraged and distressed. Hopefully, the physician–employer and the manager are able to recognize problems before they become too serious.

It has been said that one in four individuals will experience some form of mental health problem during the course of a year. Work-related stress is the base cause of a significant degree of mental ill health. Plan for and create a work environment that reduces as much stress as possible. Actions to consider may include the following:

1. Properly educate and train all employees for their positions.
2. Encourage teamwork and reward those who help each other.
3. Mandate "break periods" in the day for each employee.
4. Create a pleasant work environment (plants, water, music, and so on).
5. Establish a blowing off steam place for when employees are especially frustrated.
6. Take everyone out for lunch at least once a quarter.
7. Have regular staff meetings to discuss employee concerns and office improvements.
8. Celebrate birthdays and special occasions (i.e., length of service).

Keep in mind that a happy employee who feels valued in his or her position will stay much longer than someone who is unhappy and does not feel valued.

Evaluating Employees and Planning Salary Review

It is important that all employees know whether they are performing their job as expected and know how they can improve their performance if necessary.

Performance Evaluation. Not only is evaluation of employees necessary during the probation period, but it is necessary for current employees as well. Evaluations should be performed no less than once a year on the anniversary of the hire date. Some office managers may wish to evaluate an employee more often, especially if a problem has surfaced in an evaluation.

The evaluation may take many forms; it can be formal or informal; it may involve more than one person. The results of the evaluation, however, must be a part of the employee's personnel record. For that reason, a formal evaluation is preferred. Many practices use a written evaluation that requires that the employee evaluate himself before meeting with the office manager (Figure 33-5). The office manager uses the same form for evaluation.

PERFORMANCE REVIEW FORM

______________________________ Employee Name

______________________________ Title

______________________________ Supervisor

______________________________ Department

TYPE OF REVIEW (Check One)

_______ Quarterly

_______ Annual

_______ Probation

_______ Other _______________

Review Period Covered ____________ to ____________

PERFORMANCE DEFINITIONS

5 = Outstanding — Performance that is clearly superior, beyond the call of duty, or substantially above standard level. Seldom attained level of performance but achievable.

4 = Above Standard — Very commendable performance; exceeds the norm for the job.

3 = Standard — Competent and consistent performance; expected level of activity and performance for the job. Most often rating received.

2 = Below Standard — Performance needs improvement. This level of performance is unacceptable; needs improvement to meet the standards for the job.

Employee new to the job: Performance might receive below standard rating due to lack of job knowledge and is expected to improve with experience.

Experienced Employee: Performance is below acceptable level and requires direction and/or counsel.

1 = Unsatisfactory — Performance is unacceptable. Job activity is clearly and substantially lacking in quality, quantity, or timeliness. May also not be meeting cost or budget constraints. Needs much improvement to meet the standards for the job.

(office use only)	FINAL RATING: CHECK ONE (office use only)
EVALUATION SUMMARY	______ Merit Increase Recommended
Total I ______	______ No Merit Increase—Satisfactory Performance/No Growth
+ Total II _____	______ No Merit Increase (Probationary/Special Evaluation)
	______ No Merit Increase (Performance Probation)
	Re-evaluate in 90 Days for Unsatisfactory or in 180 Days for Needed Improvement

GENERAL PERFORMANCE RATING (PART I)

General Criteria	*Rating*	*Comments Supporting Rating*
1. Patient Relations: How well does the employee communicate a "we care" image to the patients, visitors, physicians, and fellow employees?		
2. Work Responsibilities: What is the quality of the employee's work relative to quality, quantity, and timeliness?		
3. Teamwork: Does the employee have a team spirit? Does the employee interact well with co-workers/supervisor/manager?		

(continues)

Figure 33-5 Sample performance review form.

General Criteria	*Rating*	*Comments Supporting Rating*
4. Adaptability: Is the employee open to change and new ideas? Does the employee remain flexible to changes in routine, workload, and assignments?		
5. Personal Appearance: How well does the employee maintain appropriate personal appearance, including proper attire, hygiene?		
6. Communication: Does the employee communicate well? Is information given and received clearly? Does he/she have good verbal and written skills?		
7. Dependability: Can the employee be relied upon for good attendance? Does the employee perform and follow through on work without supervisory intervention or assistance?		

Subtotal I ____________ + 7 General Criteria = ____________

JOB-SPECIFIC CRITERIA RATING (PART II) (To be used with Job Description attached)

Responsibility and Standard	*Rating*	*Comments Supporting Rating*
Complete a section for each responsibility listed on the employee's job description.		

Subtotal II ____________ + ____________ = ____________
job duties

Contributions made since last review:

____

____

____

Education or training received since last review:

____

____

____

Action to be taken based on performance:

____

____

____

Comments:

____

____

____

______________________________ ____________
Employee Signature Date

______________________________ ____________
Supervisor Signature Date

______________________________ ____________
Physician Signature Date

Figure 33-5 (continued)

During the meeting, notes are compared as the evaluation is conducted.

The climate of the performance evaluation should be comfortable and provide privacy (Figure 33-6). The meeting should be friendly, but the employee must sense the importance of the evaluation. Do not allow any disagreements to escalate into arguments during the evaluation. Without reading the employee's self-evaluation, ask the employee to tell about the self-assessment. Acknowledge the employee's point of view and identify when you agree or differ from the self-assessment. Be prepared to describe specific examples of positive performance and negative performance.

When negative performance is identified, ask the employee for possible solutions. Then a plan can be determined to alter the negative performance. In this way, a trusting atmosphere is established in that both of you are working together for a solution that will benefit the medical practice. Always look for and seek a win-win situation whenever possible. The action plan determined should then be evaluated at the next performance evaluation.

At the close of the evaluation, always express your confidence in the individual to make any changes necessary, offer assistance where needed, and thank the employee for participating. End any evaluation with a positive statement about some portion of the employee's performance.

There are occasions when reviews are performed more frequently than annually. A review would occur two to three months after a significant promotion to measure how things are progressing. Reviews occur more often when general performance falls well short of past efforts or a serious error in judgment has been made. This type of review may end with a reprimand, a warning to correct the problem by a given date, or possibly, immediate dismissal. Document any steps to be taken to correct a problem and any reason that is cause for dismissal.

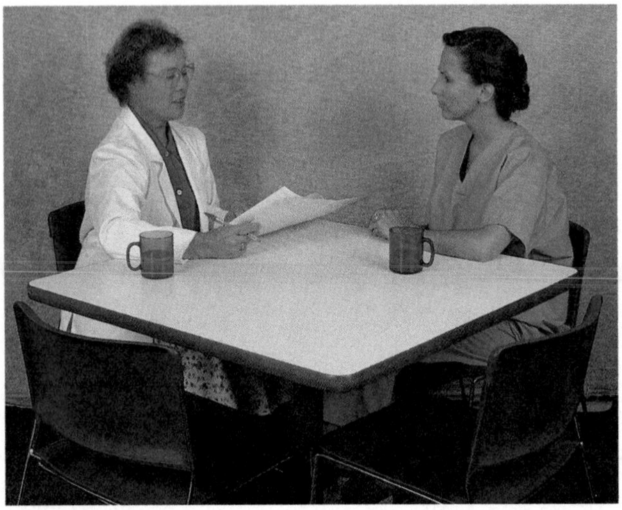

Figure 33-6 A comfortable, private setting encourages discussion during an employee performance review.

Salary Review. Although the practice is common in some areas, it may be better not to tie salary increases or bonuses with the annual performance evaluation. Conduct the **salary review** at the beginning of the new year separate from performance evaluations.

Salary review is important. Unfortunately, in smaller medical offices and ambulatory care settings, the review of salary may have to be raised by the employee. Physician–employers tend to forget that their employees have been with them for over a year without a raise or a discussion of financial reimbursement. If this is the case, it is perfectly acceptable for the employee to raise the issue on a yearly basis. However, the best approach is for the office manager to conduct salary reviews at the beginning or end of each calendar year.

Data should be collected before a salary review. The office manager should network with other office managers to determine wages and salaries for comparable individuals with comparable skills. Remember, also, that it is far more cost-effective to reward good employees with a salary increase than it is to train a new employee who commands a lesser salary than current employees. Reward employees well and provide benefits that encourage them to stay with the practice. Employees who stay with the practice for a long time not only fully understand how best to serve their physician–employers, they have established a relationship with patients that is beneficial.

How much of a raise is to be awarded at the time of salary review is difficult to determine and will depend on many factors that might include the profits of the year, the patient load, the workload, and the current cost of living.

The critical shortage of health care employees today is reflected in the shortage of medical assistants across the country. Newspapers advertising for individuals to work in the ambulatory care setting tell the story. A consideration worth mentioning is that often the salary does not match the education, experience, and special training required of someone working in the health care field. Educators often hear, "Why would I spend a year or more in education to be paid what I would make working in a fast food restaurant?" Because it is costly in time and resources to replace employees, it is best to invest that cost into a fair and just salary increase for valued employees.

Conflict Resolution

A good human resources manager will be a master at **conflict resolution,** solving problems between any two parties. The most difficult task is to prevent or solve conflicts that occur between employees or between employees and supervisors or physician–employers. Most conflict occurs because of poor communication or a misunderstanding, thus effective communication is a goal for any manager.

Volumes of materials have been written about successful conflict management. One can probably never get enough material on the subject. Some guidelines that may be helpful in preventing and resolving conflicts follow:

- Listen to your employees. What do they say? What do they communicate nonverbally?
- Be prepared to temporarily assist an employee having a difficult time.
- Create a safe environment for an employee to admit a mistake.
- Manage by walking around and talking to your employees.
- Acknowledge the stressors of the job and compensate employees.
- Give ample verbal positive comments and pats on the back.
- Be honest with employees at all times.
- Provide office staff meetings in which employees can express their concerns.
- Treat employees fairly.
- Do not tolerate negative comments or actions among employees.
- Remember birthdays and special occasions with cards or small gifts.
- Provide small rewards when possible.
- Expect to work longer and harder than any employee.
- Have the physician–employer host a social lunch every 60 days.
- Keep employees informed of changes impacting them.
- Encourage an open-door policy for concerns and complaints.
- Be a role model for all employees.
- Keep confidences.
- Encourage continuing education through workshops and seminars.

There is no end to such a list. An office manager who cares about each employee, who "carries water for the workers in the trenches," and who administers fairly and honestly creates an environment where conflict will be at a minimum.

Dismissing Employees

Most human resources managers do not enjoy rating the performance of other employees particularly when difficult topics are involved and it may be necessary to dismiss an employee. However, the written performance evaluation actually establishes the format for such a dismissal when necessary and is more likely to remove the emotion from the situation. **Involuntary dismissal** is still difficult when it is necessary.

Involuntary Dismissal. Involuntary dismissal results from two primary causes: poor performance or serious violation of office policies or job descriptions. When it becomes apparent to the office manager that the effectiveness of an employee is dropping well below expectations, it will be known in the review or a performance review may be called. The review allows the employee to be informed of the shortcomings, to explain any reasons for the present situation, and to determine a plan to alleviate the problem. If the problem is a serious one, probation is usually invoked and any lack of significant improvement in the time provided results in immediate dismissal.

When the problem is a violation of either office policy or procedures, both a verbal and a written warning are given to the employee. Involuntary dismissal follows if the situation persists. Dismissal may be immediate if the action is a serious violation of policy. Serious violations will depend on the office practice, but some causes for immediate dismissal include theft, making fraudulent claims against insurance, placing the patient in jeopardy by not practicing safe techniques, and breach of patient confidentiality.

Some key points to keep in mind when dismissal is necessary are:

1. The dismissal should be made in privacy.
2. Take no longer than 10 minutes for the dismissal.
3. Be direct, firm, and to the point in identifying reasons.
4. Do not engage in an in-depth discussion of performance.
5. Explain terms of dismissal (keys, clearing out area of personal items, final paperwork).
6. Listen to employee's opinion and emotions; it is not necessary to agree.
7. Accompany the employee to his or her desk to pack his or her belongings.
8. Escort the employee out of the facility; do not allow him or her to finish the work of the day.

Voluntary Dismissal. Other reasons for dismissal may be more pleasant. Changes in personnel occur for many good reasons and people voluntarily leave their jobs. They may relocate, seek advancement in another facility, or simply have personal reasons for leaving. These employees will give their manager proper notice and will be able to turn their current projects and duties over to their replacements. They have time to say good-bye to their friends and leave with a good feeling about their employment.

PROCEDURE MANUAL

The **procedure manual** provides detailed information relative to the performance of tasks within the facility in which one is employed. Each procedure manual should be designed for that specific office setting and should satisfy its requirements.

The procedure manual serves as a guide to the employee assigned a specific task and may also be useful in evaluating the employee's performance. If a temporary employee is assigned the task, the procedure manual will be invaluable in assuring that each procedure is completed as outlined.

The physician(s) and the office manager should have copies of the procedure manual and it should also be accessible to all employees. Copies of individual sections may be given to the employee responsible for the task; the employee should be instructed to follow these guidelines and told that they may be used as employee evaluation tools.

Organization of the Procedure Manual

It is best to use a loose-leaf binder with separator pages denoting each procedure. Many office managers find it helpful to divide the binder into administrative and clinical sections with subdivisions for each primary task performed (Figure 33-7).

Administrative Section	Clinical Section
Personnel Management	Physical Examinations
Communication (oral and written)	Infection Control
Patient Scheduling	Collecting Specimens
Records Management	Laboratory Procedures
Financial Management	Surgical Asepsis
Facility and Equipment Management	Emergencies
	Material Safety Data Sheets (MSDS)
	OSHA
	CLIA '88

Figure 33-7 Many offices find that dividing the procedure manual into tabbed sections helps organize the material. A table of contents with page numbers helps locate information easily.

To facilitate using the procedure manual, a consistent format should be developed and used throughout the manual. Each procedure should be a step-by-step outline or list of steps to be taken to complete a task as desired in that facility. Providing the rationale for a step, when appropriate, enhances the learning process, especially for new staff members. Material Safety Data Sheets (MSDSs) are required to be maintained in the clinic and available for personnel to reference at any time. MSDS must be compiled for all chemicals considered hazardous and maintained in an appropriate manual. Some offices opt to maintain these records in a separate tabbed section of the procedure manual. Others choose to maintain a separate MSDS manual. The information must be reviewed and updated on a regular basis. See Chapter 26 for detailed information regarding MSDS. Procedure 33-5 provides steps for developing and maintaining a procedure manual.

Updating and Reviewing the Procedure Manual

When new procedures are added to the office routine, a new procedure page should be developed immediately. The new page is then useful as an educational tool or job aid while team members are learning new techniques.

An annual page-by-page review should be done to ascertain if each procedure is still being used and assure that each page is correct in each detail and satisfies all criteria established by the staff personnel. This contributes to an efficient office and gives all employees a sense of pride and satisfaction that they are performing within the scope of their training and to their greatest potential. The procedure manual should be reviewed by personnel performing the various tasks and their suggestions should be evaluated and incorporated into the revisions when appropriate. All new procedure pages and revisions should be dated (Rev. 02/15/XX).

HIPAA IMPLICATIONS

The new HIPAA regulations require each office to develop a separate HIPAA manual that is to be either an electronic form or paper manual. It is to spell out all policies and procedures of the practice and security management measures; identify the security officer; address workforce security issues, information access concerns, security awareness and training, security incidents, and contingency plans; evaluate security effectiveness; and contain copies of all business associate contracts.

The HIPAA manual must be available to all employees and is to be updated on a regular basis. During an audit, the office manager will be asked to produce the HIPAA manual for review and to establish compliance with all regulations. All documentation of policies and procedures are to be kept for six years even though the wording has changed or been eliminated. If an incident is under investigation, this allows an investigator to go back to what a policy said six years ago.

TRAVEL ARRANGEMENTS

The office manager may be asked to make travel arrangements for physicians going on vacation or to conventions, symposiums, or out-of-town seminars and Continuing Medical Education (CME) courses. If the physicians do a fair amount of travel or if they live in a metropolitan area, they may use the services of a travel agent. Attention to detail is extremely important in preventing travel disruptions.

Read carefully the instructions for completing registration forms, complete them, and mail them as quickly as possible to secure reservations to conventions and so forth. Next make hotel and travel arrangements. General information regarding the physician's travel preferences should be maintained in a file folder and be referred to when making travel arrangements. Helpful information to maintain in this file includes:

- Name of travel agents used in the past (ranked by reputation and recommendation)
- Physician's or office credit card numbers
- Car rental preference
- Preferred airline, class of travel, seating choice
- Hotel/motel accommodations (bed size, suite, studio, connecting rooms, price range, amenities)
- Shuttle service

Next, contact the travel agent and identify the destination, date and time for departure and return, number traveling in party, and seating preference. A travel agent can also assist with rental car and hotel accommodations if needed. Take your time and pay attention to details. When tickets are received, always check to see that all departure and arrival times match what is needed and that a confirmation number has been provided for car rentals and hotel arrangements. Procedure 33-3 outlines the procedural steps involved in making travel arrangements through a travel agent.

The Internet may be used to search for the lowest cost air, auto, and lodging reservations. The procedures do not require extensive knowledge of travel and airline reservation protocols. Searching for information on the **Internet** requires the use of a search engine if you do not already have a list of favorite travel **Web sites.** A **search engine** is a special computer program available through your Internet service provider. With a search engine, you enter only the subject of your search, and the Web will provide a list of Web sites related to your subject. For example, if you are making travel arrangements, you might access a search engine such as Google.com and enter the key words "air fares." The engine will return either a list of Web sites or ask you to further refine your subject with suggestions such as cheap air fares, international travel, and so on. Once you have refined your search, you may have choices such as Travelocity.com, Expedia.com, or Priceline.com. Select the appropriate Web site and follow its instructions.

Priceline.com and similar Web sites are services that allow you to name the price you want to pay; Priceline finds a major airline willing to release seats on flights where they have unsold space. You need to have a reasonable idea of the price of the service you are trying to purchase; unreasonably low bids will just waste your time and effort. Procedure 33-4 outlines the steps for making travel arrangements via the Internet.

Itinerary

If you have used a travel agent in making the travel arrangements, the agency will most likely provide several copies of the **itinerary.** An itinerary is a detailed plan for a proposed trip. The office should maintain one copy of the itinerary in case the physician must be reached for emergencies. The physician should have one copy to carry with him or her and a copy to leave with family members. You may need to develop the itinerary if you have made the travel arrangements via computer. Figure 33-8 shows a sample travel itinerary.

Important information to be included on any itinerary includes:

- *Air travel:* departure and arrival date and time, meals, airline name and telephone number, airport
- *Car rental:* name of provider, telephone number, confirmation number
- *Hotel/motel:* name, confirmation number, dates, telephone number
- *Meeting location:* name, address, room number, telephone number

TRAVEL ITINERARY

James Whitney, MD
Inner City Health Care
400 Inner City Way
Seattle, WA 98400

15 Sept 20XX INVOICE: 880133795

29 Sept Friday					
USAIR	630	Coach Class	Equip-Boeing 757 Jet		
LV: Seattle		11:55P	Nonstop	Miles-2125	Confirmed
AR: Pittsburgh		7:23A	Elapsed time-4:28	Arrival Date-30Sept	
			Seat-31C		

30 Sept-Saturday					
Alamo			1 Compact 2/4 DR	Drop-101CT	Confirmed
Pickup-Pittsburgh			Pittsburgh Airport	Chg-USD .00	
Rate-	59.98	Baserate	Guaranteed		Extra Hr 10.00-UN
Phone-412-472-5060					
		Confirmation-1870649			

01 Oct Sunday				
USAIR	1419 Coach Class	Equip-Boeing 737 Jet		
LV: Pittsburgh	3:05P	Nonstop	Miles-2125	Confirmed
AR: Seattle	5:27P	Elapsed time-5:22		
Lunch		Seat-20A		

Ticket Number/s:					
Whitney/James	3570933		BA Card		$461.00
Air Transportation	$416.36	Tax	44.64	TOTAL	$461.00
		Sub Total			$461.00
		Credit Card Payment			$461.00-
		Amount Due			0.00

TICKET IS NON REFUNDABLE. TRIP INSURANCE IS AVAILABLE. RECONFIRM ALL FLTS 24 HRS PRIOR TO DEPARTURE

Figure 33-8 Sample travel itinerary.

TIME MANAGEMENT

Time management is an item of critical importance to the manager. You may have upward of 20 staff members putting demands on your time, and added to this are vendors, your superiors, business associates, and a host of others. A manager has not a moment to lose in the day, so managing time makes the difference between a normal 8- or 10-hour day and a 15-hour or more day. The following suggestions are some proven means of managing your time:

- *Handle items once.* Once the mail is opened, sorted, and prioritized, try to handle it only once more, when action is taken with it. Picking it up, reading it, and setting it down again without taking action is a real waste of time.
- *Develop a to-do list.* At the end of each day prepare a list of things you plan to complete the next day and try to work down this list. Prioritize the list by importance or by practical order.
- *Guard your time.* Schedule meetings with personnel and vendors so that it does not fragment your time, making you have to restart a task and get up to speed over and over again. Although modern management practice is to have an open-door policy with employees, this does not mean you should allow them to come into your office whenever they

think about it. Have them schedule time with you. Make them think about what they want to discuss and do not let them monopolize your time. This is also true of meeting with vendors; require vendors to schedule ahead a time to meet with you.

- *Delegate work*. Assign others or a team to perform some of the functions discussed in this chapter. Having a team prepare weekly work schedules and vacation schedules results in less bickering and feelings of favoritism that you would have to spend time defusing if you made the schedules yourself. This does not mean that you do not have to approve them and, in some instances, make the hard decisions, but it results in your people having ownership in the decisions.

MARKETING FUNCTIONS

Effective communication skills are essential in the management of the ambulatory care setting. These skills are used by the office manager inside the ambulatory care setting to establish friendly, professional relationships with colleagues and patients. Communication is just as critical when relating to external audiences, such as other organizations, potential new patients, and community members. Developing relationships outside the office is often called marketing, a concept that office managers may use to enhance the image and visibility of an ambulatory care setting while also providing benefits to patients, potential patients, and the neighboring community.

In its broadest sense, **marketing** can be defined as the process by which the provider of services makes the consumer aware of the scope and quality of these services. Although marketing is a tool traditionally used by for-profit organizations to promote and sell products and services, it has become increasingly acceptable among health care organizations, whether they are for- or not-for-profit.

Marketing functions and materials are diverse and can include seminars and workshops, patient education brochures, brochures that describe the ambulatory care setting and its scope of services, HIPAA policies, newsletters, press releases, and special events such as open houses or participation in community health care events. Depending on the size and resources of the medical office, the manager may choose to use all or some of these tools (Figure 33-9).

Marketing Tool	**Potential Uses and Value**
Seminars	Can educate patients and provide good will in the community. All staff—administrative and clinical—can work as a team to organize, publicize, and deliver the seminars.
Brochures	Brochures are typically of two types: patient education brochures and brochures on office services. Can be simple 8-1/2" x 11" fact sheets, with text only, or more elaborate brochures folded to 4" x 9" that incorporate both text and graphics or photos. Both types of brochures are informative for patients and present a professional image of the ambulatory care setting.
Practice Web site and E-zines	The practice Web site is an excellent means of promoting the practice. Personnel can be introduced, and procedures and technologies can be discussed. The E-zine approach is rapidly catching on as a promotional tool. It can be e-mailed to patients so it saves time and money. The patient may choose to view, delete, or save to read at a later time.
Newsletters	Newsletters can be produced on a biannual or quarterly basis and can form the nucleus of a marketing program. Because they are versatile tools, they can include a wide range of information from health-related articles to staff introductions to insurance updates. They should be sent to individuals on the office's mailing list and be available in the reception area.
Press Releases	Periodic press releases on new equipment, new staff, and expanded or remodeled office space can be a vital link to the local community.
Special Events	Special events are an effective way to join with other community organizations to promote wellness. They can include participation in health fairs, cosponsorship of a charity event, or an open house on the premises to acquaint the community with new services or equipment.

Figure 33-9 Marketing tools and their use in a medical environment.

When producing written material and organizing events, it is essential that ethical guidelines be respected at all times. Marketing tools should be appropriate, in good taste, and designed to quietly enhance the reputation of the office. Cultural issues should always be considered. For example, patient education brochures for a practice with many Spanish-speaking patients should be produced in bilingual editions, with English on one side and Spanish on the other. Legal issues are important as well; when presenting material of a medical nature, it is extremely important that information be accurate and up to date.

Effective marketing is a valuable tool for the office manager, especially as managed care calls on all health care professionals to become more competitive to survive. Marketing can increase visibility and credibility. The effective manager will enlist the talents and skills of the entire team in developing a marketing plan.

Seminars

As consumers become increasingly aware of lifestyle choices, they look to health care professionals for information and guidance. Seminars and workshops are useful vehicles for presenting health-related information; while expert advice can be given, there is also the opportunity for patients and health care professionals to interact.

Seminars can be organized to meet patient and community needs. Some popular seminar topics include hypertension, diabetes, eating disorders, and exercise and weight management programs.

No matter what the topic area, the content should be oriented to the lay person's level of understanding, with a focused message and a delivery designed to maintain attention. Interactive seminars, which encourage audience participation, can be productive and enjoyable. Audiovisuals, such as projected slides, will provide visual reinforcement. Handouts, either from professional organizations or those produced by office staff, can elaborate on seminar content and help the participant review and remember what was said.

Brochures

Despite the promise of a paperless society, brochures continue to be valuable sources of information. In the health care setting, patients welcome a rack of brochures as a source of current, accurate background on medical issues. New patients also find that a brochure on office services will answer many questions about the practice, its philosophy, and its scope of services, and will provide physician profiles.

Today, it is possible to produce a professional-looking brochure in the office using one of the computer programs that integrate text and graphics. If a brochure is produced in-house, it is important to consider writing, design, and production. Writing should be clear, to the point, and grammatically correct. Always proofread carefully before printing. Design should be kept simple. Avoid the use of too many typefaces; choose a typeface and size for readability, and, if using artwork or photography, consider its reproduction qualities. Black or another dark ink against a light background is best for readability.

Often, a local printer will be able to advise the office manager on how to prepare a brochure or handout for printing. The simplest handouts can be quick-copied (a high-speed photocopy) on a white or lightly colored or textured stock. After printing, brochures should be made accessible to patients and other visitors in a rack or neatly arranged in piles (Figure 33-10). Occasionally, a brochure will be mailed; one that folds to 4 × 9 inches will fit into a standard #10 business envelope.

Patient Education Brochures. Like seminars, patient education brochures can address a variety of topics, including hypertension, diabetes, eating disorders, and exercise and weight management programs. When writing these brochures, always research material carefully, request permission for copyrighted materials, and present the information in a manner that is accessible to your patient population.

Office Brochures. A brochure on the practice can provide a wide range of information and will orient the new patient to the practice. One way to determine what information to include is to develop a list of frequently asked patient questions. Once this list is compiled, it can serve as the beginning of the brochure outline. Issues to consider might include:

- Brief history of the practice
- Brief résumés or credentials of physicians

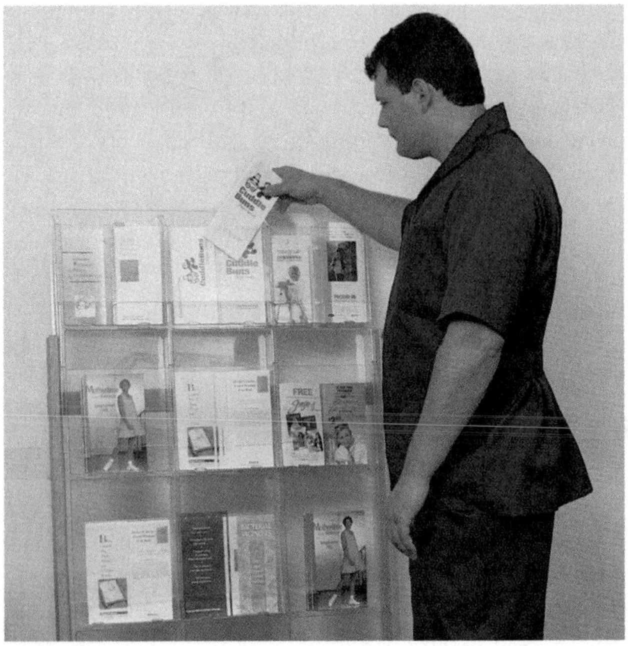

Figure 33-10 Brochures and handouts should be accessible and inviting to patients and office visitors.

- Philosophy of the practice
- Scope of services
- How to reach the practice in case of emergency
- Insurances accepted
- Rights of patients
- Policies regarding the release of information
- Scheduling information: how to schedule an appointment, cancellation policies
- Amenities on the premises such as parking, pharmacy, laboratory
- Location, map if necessary, and location of satellite offices

Newsletters

Newsletters are effective communication tools because they encourage regular contact with patients and other readers. Newsletters are a versatile medium, too; they can contain patient education articles, updates on staff changes, awards, information on insurance carriers, calendars of events, even recipes that are consistent with a healthful lifestyle.

Most newsletters can be written and produced in the office. Like brochures, they should be simple in design and format. An additional factor in newsletter production is mailing; an up-to-date database must be maintained, postal regulations must be followed, and the costs of mailing considered.

Press Releases

Press releases are simple, inexpensive marketing tools. Use them to announce new staff, promote a new service, or publicize a series of seminars. If a professional, courteous relationship is developed with the local press, most will be happy to receive and publish releases. When writing releases, always follow proper format, which includes a date of release, a contact person's name and telephone number, and a short headline. Releases are best kept to one double-spaced typed page. At the end of the release, type "30" or a number sign (#). Maintain an active list of local newspapers and editors' names so that you can mail or fax the release to the appropriate editor.

Special Events

Although they can be time-consuming to organize and participate in, special events are rewarding, for they present an opportunity to interact with the community. They have high visibility, for often a group of community organizations will collaborate to cosponsor an event such as a walk-a-thon, blood pressure clinic, health fair for seniors, or wellness day for children and families. Sponsorship can be as simple as a donation to the cause; other times, staffing a booth or offering a service such as blood pressure checks is appropriate.

Like all marketing efforts, special events require organizational skills and teamwork, but they often result in heightened communication with the community and provide an educational service to patients and their families.

RECORDS AND FINANCIAL MANAGEMENT

Physicians entrust a great deal of responsibility to their medical office managers. The daily payments received through the mail and office visits must be processed and prepared for banking. Office expenses must be processed and paid in a timely fashion to capitalize on any discounts available. Employee requirements and records such as Social Security records, Withholding Allowance Certificates (W-4 forms) (Figure 33-11) indicating the number of exemptions claimed, and Employment Eligibility Verification Forms (I-9) ensuring that all persons employed are either United States citizens, lawfully admitted aliens, or aliens authorized to work in the United States must be completed and filed with the appropriate federal agencies. Also, state and local tax records must be maintained for each employee.

Payroll Processing

In some cases, it is the office manager's responsibility to prepare payroll checks for each employee and record all deductions withheld. A W-2 form (Figure 33-12) summarizing all earnings and deductions for the year must be prepared for each employee by January 31 of each year. The Social Security Administration must receive a summary report of W-2 forms each year.

To comply with all governmental regulations, federal, state, and local, it is important that the office manager who processes payroll maintain complete, up-to-date records on every employee. This information should be gathered from new employees and updated every year and on any change in employee status. For more specific information regarding printed and electronic filing forms, go to the Internal Revenue Service Web site (http://www.irs.gov) for detailed instructions. It is a good idea to have employees update their W-4 form each year in case they want to adjust their deductions or make any other change. To accomplish this, many payroll managers include a new W-4 form with the first paycheck at the beginning of each year. Every employee file should contain Social

Form W-4 (2005)

Purpose. Complete Form W-4 so that your employer can withhold the correct federal income tax from your pay. Because your tax situation may change, you may want to refigure your withholding each year.

Exemption from withholding. If you are exempt, complete only lines 1, 2, 3, 4, and 7 and sign the form to validate it. Your exemption for 2005 expires February 16, 2006. See Pub. 505, Tax Withholding and Estimated Tax.

Note. You cannot claim exemption from withholding if (a) your income exceeds $800 and includes more than $250 of unearned income (for example, interest and dividends) and (b) another person can claim you as a dependent on their tax return.

Basic instructions. If you are not exempt, complete the **Personal Allowances Worksheet** below. The worksheets on page 2 adjust your withholding allowances based on itemized deductions, certain credits, adjustments to income, or two-earner/two-job situations. Complete all worksheets that apply. However, you may claim fewer (or zero) allowances.

Head of household. Generally, you may claim head of household filing status on your tax return only if you are unmarried and pay more than 50% of the costs of keeping up a home for yourself and your dependent(s) or other qualifying individuals. See line **E** below.

Tax credits. You can take projected tax credits into account in figuring your allowable number of withholding allowances. Credits for child or dependent care expenses and the child tax credit may be claimed using the **Personal Allowances Worksheet** below. See Pub. 919, How Do I Adjust My Tax Withholding? for information on converting your other credits into withholding allowances.

Nonwage income. If you have a large amount of nonwage income, such as interest or dividends, consider making estimated tax payments using Form 1040-ES, Estimated Tax for Individuals. Otherwise, you may owe additional tax.

Two earners/two jobs. If you have a working spouse or more than one job, figure the total number of allowances you are entitled to claim on all jobs using worksheets from only one Form W-4. Your withholding usually will be most accurate when all allowances are claimed on the Form W-4 for the highest paying job and zero allowances are claimed on the others.

Nonresident alien. If you are a nonresident alien, see the Instructions for Form 8233 before completing this Form W-4.

Check your withholding. After your Form W-4 takes effect, use Pub. 919 to see how the dollar amount you are having withheld compares to your projected total tax for 2005. See Pub. 919, especially if your earnings exceed $125,000 (Single) or $175,000 (Married).

Recent name change? If your name on line 1 differs from that shown on your social security card, call 1-800-772-1213 to initiate a name change and obtain a social security card showing your correct name.

Personal Allowances Worksheet (Keep for your records.)

A Enter "1" for **yourself** if no one else can claim you as a dependent . . . . **A** ______

B Enter "1" if: { • You are single and have only one job; or • You are married, have only one job, and your spouse does not work; or • Your wages from a second job or your spouse's wages (or the total of both) are $1,000 or less. } . . **B** ______

C Enter "1" for your **spouse**. But, you may choose to enter "-0-" if you are married and have either a working spouse or more than one job. (Entering "-0-" may help you avoid having too little tax withheld.) . . . . **C** ______

D Enter number of **dependents** (other than your spouse or yourself) you will claim on your tax return . . . . . . **D** ______

E Enter "1" if you will file as **head of household** on your tax return (see conditions under **Head of household** above) . **E** ______

F Enter "1" if you have at least $1,500 of **child or dependent care expenses** for which you plan to claim a credit . . **F** ______
(**Note.** Do **not** include child support payments. See **Pub. 503,** Child and Dependent Care Expenses, for details.)

G **Child Tax Credit** (including additional child tax credit):
- If your total income will be less than $54,000 ($79,000 if married), enter "2" for each eligible child.
- If your total income will be between $54,000 and $84,000 ($79,000 and $119,000 if married), enter "1" for each eligible child plus "1" **additional** if you have four or more eligible children. **G** ______

H Add lines A through G and enter total here. (**Note.** This may be different from the number of exemptions you claim on your tax return.) ▶ **H** ______

For accuracy, complete all worksheets that apply. {
- If you plan to **itemize or claim adjustments to income** and want to reduce your withholding, see the **Deductions and Adjustments Worksheet** on page 2.
- If you have **more than one job** or are **married and you and your spouse both work** and the combined earnings from all jobs exceed $35,000 ($25,000 if married) see the **Two-Earner/Two-Job Worksheet** on page 2 to avoid having too little tax withheld.
- If **neither** of the above situations applies, **stop here** and enter the number from line H on line 5 of Form W-4 below. }

Cut here and give Form W-4 to your employer. Keep the top part for your records.

Form **W-4** — Department of the Treasury, Internal Revenue Service

Employee's Withholding Allowance Certificate

▶ **Whether you are entitled to claim a certain number of allowances or exemption from withholding is subject to review by the IRS. Your employer may be required to send a copy of this form to the IRS.**

OMB No. 1545-0010 — **2005**

1 Type or print your first name and middle initial	Last name	2 Your social security number
Home address (number and street or rural route)		3 ☐ Single ☐ Married ☐ Married, but withhold at higher Single rate. **Note.** If married, but legally separated, or spouse is a nonresident alien, check the "Single" box.
City or town, state, and ZIP code		4 **If your last name differs from that shown on your social security card, check here. You must call 1-800-772-1213 for a new card.** ▶ ☐

5 Total number of allowances you are claiming (from line **H** above **or** from the applicable worksheet on page 2) **5** ______

6 Additional amount, if any, you want withheld from each paycheck . . . . **6** $ ______

7 I claim exemption from withholding for 2005, and I certify that I meet **both** of the following conditions for exemption.
- Last year I had a right to a refund of **all** federal income tax withheld because I had **no** tax liability **and**
- This year I expect a refund of **all** federal income tax withheld because I expect to have **no** tax liability.

If you meet both conditions, write "Exempt" here . . . . ▶ **7** ______

Under penalties of perjury, I declare that I have examined this certificate and to the best of my knowledge and belief, it is true, correct, and complete.

Employee's signature
(Form is not valid unless you sign it.) ▶ **Date** ▶

8 Employer's name and address (Employer: Complete lines 8 and 10 only if sending to the IRS.)	9 Office code (optional)	10 Employer identification number (EIN)

For Privacy Act and Paperwork Reduction Act Notice, see page 2. Cat. No. 10220Q Form **W-4** (2005)

Form W-4 (2005) Page **2**

Deductions and Adjustments Worksheet

Note. Use this worksheet *only* if you plan to itemize deductions, claim certain credits, or claim adjustments to income on your 2005 tax return.

1 Enter an estimate of your 2005 itemized deductions. These include qualifying home mortgage interest, charitable contributions, state and local taxes, medical expenses in excess of 7.5% of your income, and miscellaneous deductions. (For 2005, you may have to reduce your itemized deductions if your income is over $145,950 ($72,975 if married filing separately). See *Worksheet 3* in Pub. 919 for details.) . . . **1** $ ______

2 Enter: { $10,000 if married filing jointly or qualifying widow(er); $ 7,300 if head of household; $ 5,000 if single or married filing separately } . . . . **2** $ ______

3 **Subtract** line 2 from line 1. If line 2 is greater than line 1, enter "-0-" . . . . **3** $ ______

4 Enter an estimate of your 2005 adjustments to income, including alimony, deductible IRA contributions, and student loan interest **4** $ ______

5 **Add** lines 3 and 4 and enter the total. (Include any amount for credits from *Worksheet 7* in Pub. 919) . **5** $ ______

6 Enter an estimate of your 2005 nonwage income (such as dividends or interest) . . . . **6** $ ______

7 **Subtract** line 6 from line 5. Enter the result, but not less than "-0-" . . . . **7** $ ______

8 **Divide** the amount on line 7 by $3,200 and enter the result here. Drop any fraction . . . . **8** ______

9 Enter the number from the **Personal Allowances Worksheet,** line H, page 1 . . . . **9** ______

10 **Add** lines 8 and 9 and enter the total here. If you plan to use the **Two-Earner/Two-Job Worksheet,** also enter this total on line 1 below. Otherwise, **stop here** and enter this total on Form W-4, line 5, page 1 . **10** ______

Two-Earner/Two-Job Worksheet (See *Two earners/two jobs* on page 1.)

Note. Use this worksheet *only* if the instructions under line H on page 1 direct you here.

1 Enter the number from line H, page 1 (or from line 10 above if you used the **Deductions and Adjustments Worksheet**) **1** ______

2 Find the number in **Table 1** below that applies to the **LOWEST** paying job and enter it here . . . . **2** ______

3 If line 1 is **more than or equal to** line 2, subtract line 2 from line 1. Enter the result here (if zero, enter "-0-") and on Form W-4, line 5, page 1. **Do not** use the rest of this worksheet . . . . **3** ______

Note. If line 1 is *less than* line 2, enter "-0-" on Form W-4, line 5, page 1. Complete lines 4–9 below to calculate the additional withholding amount necessary to avoid a year-end tax bill.

4 Enter the number from line 2 of this worksheet . . . . **4** ______

5 Enter the number from line 1 of this worksheet . . . . **5** ______

6 **Subtract** line 5 from line 4 . . . . **6** ______

7 Find the amount in **Table 2** below that applies to the **HIGHEST** paying job and enter it here . . . . **7** $ ______

8 **Multiply** line 7 by line 6 and enter the result here. This is the additional annual withholding needed . . **8** $ ______

9 Divide line 8 by the number of pay periods remaining in 2005. For example, divide by 26 if you are paid every two weeks and you complete this form in December 2004. Enter the result here and on Form W-4, line 6, page 1. This is the additional amount to be withheld from each paycheck . . . . **9** $ ______

Table 1: Two-Earner/Two-Job Worksheet

Married Filing Jointly

If wages from **HIGHEST** paying job are—	AND, wages from **LOWEST** paying job are—	Enter on line 2 above
$0 - $40,000	$0 - $4,000	0
	4,001 - 8,000	1
	8,001 - 18,000	2
	18,001 and over	3
$40,001 and over	$0 - $4,000	0
	4,001 - 8,000	1
	8,001 - 18,000	2
	18,001 - 22,000	3
	22,001 - 25,000	4
	25,001 - 30,000	5

If wages from **HIGHEST** paying job are—	AND, wages from **LOWEST** paying job are—	Enter on line 2 above
$40,001 and over	30,001 - 36,000	6
	36,001 - 45,000	7
	45,001 - 50,000	8
	50,001 - 60,000	9
	60,001 - 65,000	10
	65,001 - 75,000	11
	75,001 - 90,000	12
	90,001 - 100,000	13
	100,001 - 115,000	14
	115,001 and over	15

All Others

If wages from **LOWEST** paying job are—	Enter on line 2 above
$0 - $6,000	0
6,001 - 12,000	1
12,001 - 18,000	2
18,001 - 24,000	3
24,001 - 31,000	4
31,001 - 45,000	5
45,001 - 60,000	6
60,001 - 75,000	7
75,001 - 80,000	8
80,001 - 100,000	9
100,001 and over	10

Table 2: Two-Earner/Two-Job Worksheet

Married Filing Jointly		All Others	
If wages from **HIGHEST** paying job are—	Enter on line 7 above	If wages from **HIGHEST** paying job are—	Enter on line 7 above
$0 - $60,000	$480	$0 - $30,000	$480
60,001 - 110,000	800	30,001 - 70,000	800
110,001 - 160,000	900	70,001 - 140,000	900
160,001 - 280,000	1,060	140,001 - 320,000	1,060
280,001 and over	1,120	320,001 and over	1,120

Privacy Act and Paperwork Reduction Act Notice. We ask for the information on this form to carry out the Internal Revenue laws of the United States. The Internal Revenue Code requires this information under sections 3402(f)(2)(A) and 6109 and their regulations. Failure to provide a properly completed form will result in your being treated as a single person who claims no withholding allowances; providing fraudulent information may also subject you to penalties. Routine uses of this information include giving it to the Department of Justice for civil and criminal litigation, to cities, states, and the District of Columbia for use in administering their tax laws, and using it in the National Directory of New Hires. We may also disclose this information to other countries under a tax treaty, to federal and state agencies to enforce federal nontax criminal laws, or to federal law enforcement and intelligence agencies to combat terrorism.

You are not required to provide the information requested on a form that is subject to the Paperwork Reduction Act unless the form displays a valid OMB control number. Books or records relating to a form or its instructions must be retained as long as their contents may become material in the administration of any Internal Revenue law. Generally, tax returns and return information are confidential, as required by Code section 6103.

The time needed to complete this form will vary depending on individual circumstances. The estimated average time is: Recordkeeping, 45 min.; Learning about the law or the form, 12 min.; Preparing the form, 58 min. If you have comments concerning the accuracy of these time estimates or suggestions for making this form simpler, we would be happy to hear from you. You can write to: Internal Revenue Service, Tax Products Coordinating Committee, SE:W:CAR:MP:T:T:SP, 1111 Constitution Ave. NW, IR-6406, Washington, DC 20224. **Do not** send Form W-4 to this address. Instead, give it to your employer.

Figure 33-11 The Form W-4 indicates the number of exemptions claimed by the employee for income tax purposes.

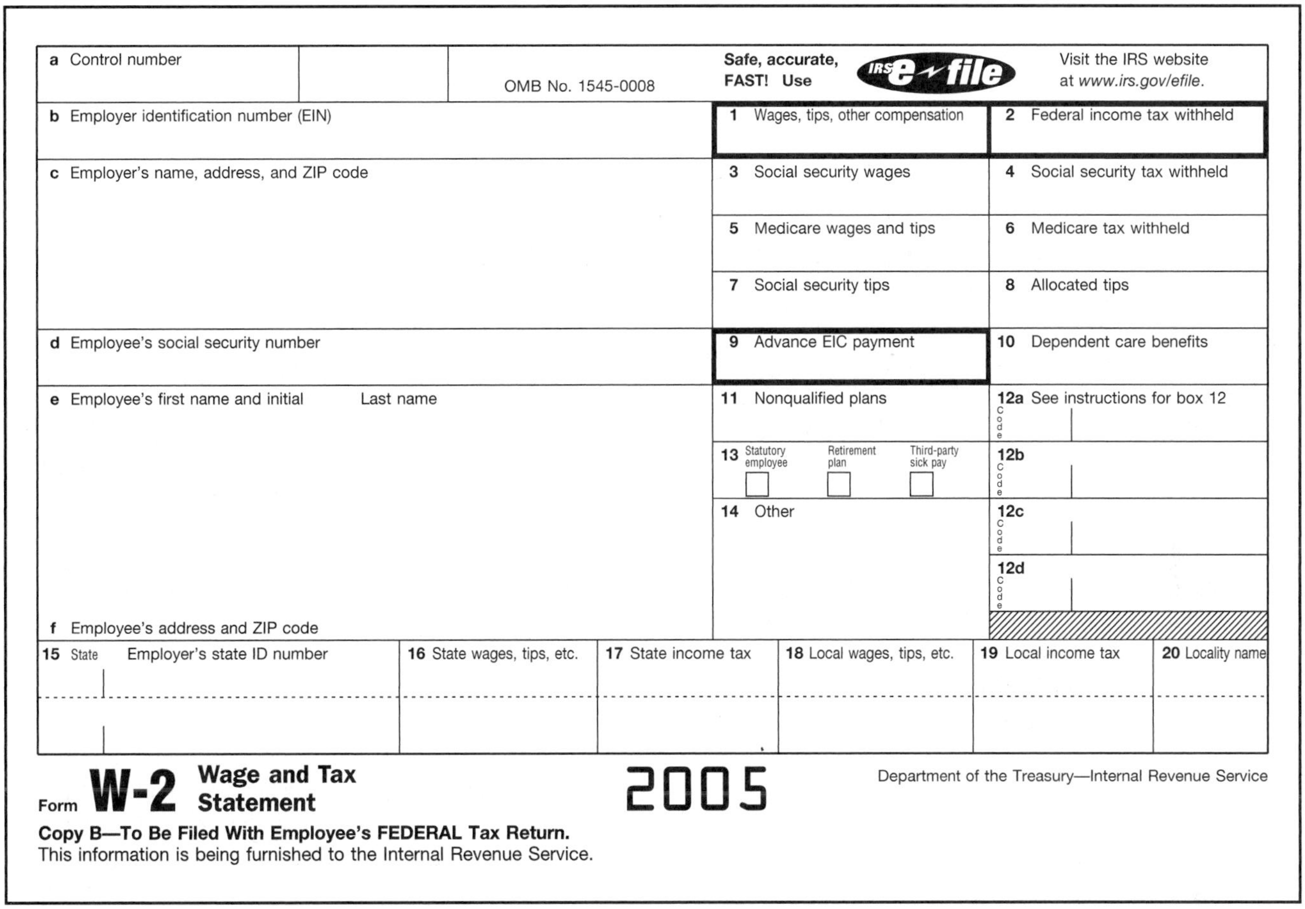

a Control number			OMB No. 1545-0008	Safe, accurate, FAST! Use **IRS e~file**	Visit the IRS website at *www.irs.gov/efile*.

b Employer identification number (EIN)	1 Wages, tips, other compensation	2 Federal income tax withheld

c Employer's name, address, and ZIP code	3 Social security wages	4 Social security tax withheld
	5 Medicare wages and tips	6 Medicare tax withheld
	7 Social security tips	8 Allocated tips

d Employee's social security number	9 Advance EIC payment	10 Dependent care benefits

e Employee's first name and initial Last name	11 Nonqualified plans	12a See instructions for box 12
	13 Statutory employee ☐ Retirement plan ☐ Third-party sick pay ☐	12b
	14 Other	12c
		12d
f Employee's address and ZIP code		

15 State Employer's state ID number	16 State wages, tips, etc.	17 State income tax	18 Local wages, tips, etc.	19 Local income tax	20 Locality name

Form **W-2** Wage and Tax Statement **2005** Department of the Treasury—Internal Revenue Service

Copy B—To Be Filed With Employee's FEDERAL Tax Return.
This information is being furnished to the Internal Revenue Service.

Figure 33-12 The Form W-2 summarizes all earnings and deductions for the year and must be prepared for each employee by January 31.

Security number, number of exemptions claimed on the W-4 Form, the employee's gross salary, and all deductions withheld for all taxes, including Social Security, federal, state, local, plus unemployment tax (where applicable), and disability insurance (where applicable).

To process payroll, the physician's office must have a federal tax reporting number, obtained from the Internal Revenue Service. In some states, a state employer number also is needed.

Preparing Payroll Checks. When preparing payroll checks, it is important to keep a record of all tax and insurance amounts deducted from an employee's earnings. Many ambulatory care settings that operate on a manual bookkeeping system find that the write-it-once system is the most efficient way to accurately maintain these records. Payroll records should include:

- Employee name, address, and telephone number
- Social Security number
- Date of employment

Each paycheck stub should contain:

- Number of hours worked, including regular and overtime (if hourly)
- Date of pay periods
- Date of check
- Gross salary
- Itemized deductions for federal income tax, Social Security (FICA) tax, state taxes, city or local taxes
- Itemized deductions for health insurance and disability insurance
- Other deductions such as uniforms, loan payments, and so on
- Net salary (gross earnings minus taxes and deductions)

Figuring Employee Taxes. When figuring federal income taxes and Social Security taxes, use the "Circular E" tables provided by the Internal Revenue Service.

Federal tax is based on amount earned, marital status, number of exemptions claimed, and length of pay period. State and city or local taxes are typically a percentage of the gross earnings.

All federal and state taxes withheld must be paid on a quarterly basis to the appropriate government offices. These monies should be accompanied by the required reporting forms. It is important to observe deposit requirements for withheld income tax and Social Security and Medicare taxes. These requirements, which change frequently, are listed in the Federal Employer's Tax Guide, available from the U.S. Government Printing Office, Internal Revenue Service (or online at: http://www.irs.gov).

Managing Benefits and Other Responsibilities. **Benefits,** or additional remuneration to the salary earned by full-time employees, must also be managed and records maintained for each employee. Examples of benefits may include paid vacation, paid holidays, health/dental insurance, disability, **profit-sharing** options, and complimentary health care. Some ambulatory care settings may refer to all or some of these benefits as **fringe benefits.**

Other responsibilities of the office manager include maintaining a personal file for each employee providing their history with the facility, application for their current position, evaluations, promotions, problems, awards, entitlements, legal forms required by state and federal agencies, and so on. All Occupational Safety and Health Administration (OSHA) data, hazard material training and documentation, HIPAA training documentation, cardiopulmonary resuscitation (CPR) certifications, immunization records, AIDS education, and confidential agreement must be recorded and maintained.

FACILITY AND EQUIPMENT MANAGEMENT

The physical plant or building must be observed and maintained with safety being a key ingredient. It should be the responsibility of each staff member to report to the office manager any facility repairs that require attention and suggest replacement or recommend new pieces of equipment as required by the practice to support the health care needs of its population.

The office manager is usually responsible for the maintenance of the office and may hire **ancillary services** to provide janitorial and laundry services, dispose of hazardous materials, and maintain aquariums or plants that may enhance the environment of the facility. The office manager must be cognitive of the importance of patient confidentiality when ancillary services are present. Ancillary services must not view confidential material. A signed Business Associate agreement must be on file for each ancillary service contracted.

Magazine subscriptions and health-related literature for the reception area are the responsibility of the office manager. Selections should be made carefully, keeping in mind the interests of the patients and their cultures. These materials should not be kept once they become dog-eared, torn, and outdated. The use of plastic protectors and appropriate storage shelving aid in keeping the area and materials tidy.

The office manager, together with the physician, is also responsible for facility improvements including any necessary repairs, decorating and color scheme, and floor plan suggestions. The wise office manager does not make these decisions independently, but asks for suggestions from staff members. Remember, the team-building approach adds a cohesive element to any office environment.

Inventories

All administrative and clinical equipment in the facility must be inventoried and maintained. Documented files should be maintained for each piece of equipment. These files may be maintained in a separate reference looseleaf binder and may be divided into administrative and clinical categories. The binder may contain pocket pages in which copies of any warranties, service agreements/contracts, and instructions for use and maintenance may be placed. This binder should be accessible to anyone who may need to refer to its pages. It is also important that as new items or updated service agreements/contracts are purchased, the old ones are removed from the binder and replaced with the new items. Equipment must be routinely evaluated and recommendations for new purchases be made to keep the practice efficient.

The office manager is also responsible for overseeing the inventory and storage of controlled substances and sample medications. See Chapter 23 for specific guidelines regarding these responsibilities.

Equipment and Supplies Maintenance

The office storage areas should be well maintained, and each item should always be put back in its place with lids replaced properly to prevent any accidents. Medication storage requires special attention. Many medications must be stored at certain temperatures, kept dry, or stored in dark, airtight containers. All medications, including samples, must be kept out of patient access areas. Narcotics should always be stored in a separate locked cabinet. Dispensing requires two individuals to sign off when narcotic supplies are used and maintain a daily inventory.

Laboratory equipment must be maintained and quality-control measures utilized. Calibration checks are required for a number of pieces of equipment: sphygmomanometers and centrifuges to name two. Microscopes and various types of scopes used during physical examinations and specialty procedures contain light sources that must be checked before each use. A replacement supply of bulbs should be available. See Chapter 26 for more information on quality control and safety in the medical laboratory. Assigning a clinical laboratory manager to oversee the equipment is a good idea.

LIABILITY COVERAGE AND BONDING

Negligence is performing an act that a reasonable and prudent physician would not perform or failure to perform an act that a reasonable and prudent physician would perform. The common term used to describe professional **liability** or legal responsibility today is **malpractice.** It is much easier to prevent malpractice than to defend it in litigation, therefore every effort should be taken to prevent negligence.

Insurance policies specifically designed to protect the physician's assets in the event a liability claim is filed and awarded in the patient's favor are available. Any physician not carrying such insurance is said to be **"going bare"** and would personally be responsible for any court costs, damages, and attorney fees if a malpractice suit were lost.

Practicing medical assistants should carry **professional liability insurance** for protection. Medical assistants who are members of the American Association of Medical Assistants (AAMA) have the option of purchasing personal and professional insurance through the organization at corporate rates.

Some physicians will carry the names of their employees on their policies. If this is the case, always ask to see the policy and verify that your name is printed on the policy—no name indicates no coverage. The manager may need to see that professional liability insurance has been purchased, all appropriate names are listed, and the premiums are paid in a timely fashion.

Professional liability insurance is important if the physician–employer is sued. In this event, the physician and the medical assistant could be named in the suit. If the case were lost, both the physician and the medical assistant could be liable.

Individuals who are responsible for handling financial records and money in the medical office may be bonded. A **bond** is purchased for a cash value in an employee's name that insures that the physician will recover the amount of loss in the event that an employee **embezzles** funds. It is the office manager or the HR manager's responsibility to ask prospective employees if they are bondable. Individuals who are not bondable may not be the best candidates for the position.

LEGAL ISSUES

The office manager must be aware of and follow all State and Federal regulations impacting the practice. Information related to Clinical Laboratory Improvement Amendments of 1988 (CLIA '88) and Occupational Safety and Health Administration (OSHA) may be found in Chapter 14. Federal regulations related to physician office laboratories (POLs) are discussed in Chapter 15. The Centers for Medicare and Medicaid Services Web site is also helpful: http://www.cms.hhs.gov/suppliers/acs/.

Procedure 33-1 Preparing a Meeting Agenda

PURPOSE:
To prepare a meeting agenda, a list of specific items to be discussed or acted on, to maintain the focus of the group and allow business to be transacted in a timely fashion.

EQUIPMENT/SUPPLIES:
List of participants
Order of business
Names of individuals giving reports
Names of any guest speakers
Computer and paper to print agendas

PROCEDURE STEPS:

1. Reserve proposed date, time, and place of meeting. RATIONALE: Ensure that the facilities are available for the meeting.
2. Collect information for meeting agenda by previewing the previous meeting's minutes for old business items, checking with others for report items, and determining any new business items. RATIONALE: Ensure that all old and new business items have been identified.
3. Prepare a hard copy of the agenda and have it approved by chair of the meeting. RATIONALE: Confirmation by the chair of the agenda content ensures that agenda is correct and complete.
4. Send agenda to meeting participants a few days in advance of the meeting. RATIONALE: Permits participants to prepare for the meeting by completing any tasks required and preparing any necessary documentation.

Procedure 33-2 Supervising a Student Practicum

PURPOSE:
To prepare a training path for a student extern being assigned to the office. To make the involved office personnel aware of their responsibilities. To preplan which jobs the student extern performs and in what sequence they will be assigned. To make the externship successful by providing as much supervision and assistance as necessary.

EQUIPMENT/SUPPLIES:
None needed

PROCEDURE STEPS:

1. Review the clinical externship contract or agreement between your agency and the educational institution. RATIONALE: Guidelines and procedures are reviewed and refreshed in your mind.
2. Determine the amount of supervision the student will require. RATIONALE: Prepares you to speak with the student and site supervisor regarding supervision.
3. Identify the supervisor who will be immediately responsible for the student. RATIONALE: Establishes a person who knows he or she is to supervise the student and be responsible for the externship procedures.
4. Plan what tasks the student will be allowed or encouraged to perform. RATIONALE: The office may or may not permit the student to perform invasive procedures. Determining tasks the student can and can not perform beforehand promotes a better relationship.
5. Create a schedule outlining the time the student will be assigned to each unit. RATIONALE: Establishing a schedule keeps everyone appraised of what is happening and when.
6. Begin orientation for the student as soon as he or she arrives at the office. Include a tour of the office and introduction to the staff. RATIONALE: Orients student and staff to each other and establishes guidelines for procedures.

(continues)

Procedure 33-2 (continued)

7. Give the student a copy of the Office Policy Manual and the work schedule for the entire externship. Answer any questions the student might have. RATIONALE: Orients student and staff to each other and establishes guidelines for procedures.
8. Maintain an accurate record of the hours the student works. Also log the date and reason for any missed days, late arrivals, or early dismissals. RATIONALE: Provides necessary documentation for the hours completed by the student.
9. Check with the student frequently to be sure the student is receiving meaningful training from the work experience. RATIONALE: Verifies that necessary training is being provided.
10. Consult physicians and staff members with whom the student has worked for their opinion of the student's capabilities. Follow up on any problems that might be identified. RATIONALE: Verifies that necessary training is being provided.
11. Report the student's progress to the medical assisting supervisor from the educational institution. This person usually visits once or twice each rotation. RATIONALE: Verifies that necessary training is being provided.
12. Prepare the student an evaluation report from comments provided by the supervisor assigned and each employee who worked with the student. RATIONALE: Provides necessary documentation for the externship experience.

Procedure 33-3 Making Travel Arrangements

PURPOSE:
To make travel arrangements for the physician.

EQUIPMENT/SUPPLIES:
Travel plan
Telephone and telephone directory
Computer
Physician's or office credit card to pay for reservations

PROCEDURE STEPS:

1. Confirm the details of the planned trip: dates, time, and place for departure and arrival; preferred mode of transportation (plane, train, bus, car); number of travelers; preferred lodging type and price range; and whether travelers checks are required. RATIONALE: Confirming pertinent travel details ensures that correct arrangements will be made.
2. Make travel and lodging reservations by calling travel agent or using the computer for online ticket services. RATIONALE: Ensure that space for physician is reserved at desired times.
3. Pick up tickets or arrange for their delivery.
4. Check to see that ticket arrangements are accurate (dates, times, places).
5. Check to see that car rental and lodging accommodations are accurate and confirmed. RATIONALE: Avoid inaccuracies and confusion with schedule.
6. Make additional copies of the itinerary or create the itinerary if making arrangements via computer. The itinerary should list date and time of departures and arrivals, including flight numbers and seat assignments. Note mode of transportation to lodging (shuttle, bus, car, taxi). Include name, address, and telephone number of lodgings and meeting places.
7. Maintain one copy of the itinerary in the office file.
8. Give several copies of the itinerary to the physician. RATIONALE: Ensure that a copy is on file with the office and that there are sufficient copies for the traveler(s) and their families.

Procedure 33-4 Making Travel Arrangements via the Internet

PURPOSE:

To make travel arrangements for the physician using the Internet.

EQUIPMENT/SUPPLIES:

Travel plan
Computer
Physician's or office credit card to pay for reservations.

PROCEDURE STEPS:

1. Confirm the details of the planned trip: dates, time, and place for departure and arrival; preferred mode of transportation (plane, train, bus, car); number of travelers; preferred lodging type and price range; and whether travelers checks are required. RATIONALE: Confirming pertinent travel details ensures that correct arrangements will be made.
2. Go to the computer and access the Internet.
3. Select a search engine to locate Web pages using the key term "air fares." Web pages may provide links to air fares, auto reservations, and hotel/motel reservations. Follow Web page instructions for making arrangements. Review and copy confirmation of your transaction. RATIONALE: The Internet can be a time saver and a cost-effective way of securing travel arrangements.
4. Pick up tickets or arrange for their delivery, if necessary. Tickets purchased on the Internet may be mailed or picked up at an airport, or they may be electronic tickets.
5. Make additional copies of the itinerary or create the itinerary. The itinerary should list date and time of departures and arrivals, including flight numbers and seat assignments. Note the mode of transportation to lodging (shuttle, bus, car, taxi). Include name, address, and telephone number of lodgings and meeting places.
6. Maintain one copy of the itinerary in the office file.
7. Give several copies of the itinerary to the physician. RATIONALE: Ensure that a copy is on file with the office and that there are sufficient copies for the traveler(s) and their families.

Procedure 33-5 Developing and Maintaining a Procedure Manual

PURPOSE:

To develop and maintain a comprehensive, up-to-date procedure manual covering each medical, technical, and administrative procedure in the office, with step-by-step directions and rationale for performing each task.

EQUIPMENT/SUPPLIES:

Computer or electronic typewriter (electronic storage allows changes and revisions to be made easily)
Binder, such as a three-ring binder
Paper
Standard procedure manual format

PROCEDURE STEPS:

1. Write detailed, step-by-step procedures and rationales for each medical, technical, and administrative function. Each procedure is written by experienced employees close to the function and then reviewed by a supervisor and office manager. Rationales help employees understand *why* something is done. RATIONALE: Establishes consistent guidelines to be followed.
2. Include regular maintenance instructions and a flow sheets for cleaning, servicing, and calibrating of all office equipment, both in the clinical

(continues)

Procedure 33-5 (continued)

area and in the office/business areas. RATIONALE: Equipment will need to be cleaned and maintained on a regular basis to assure it is working properly and that it lasts as long as needed. Some manufacturer guarantees and service contracts require regular cleaning and maintenance, especially on new and leased equipment. Instructions are necessary so the task can be performed properly. The flow sheets provide documentation of dates the equipment was cleaned, serviced, and/or calibrated and the person who performed the task.

3. Include step-by-step instruction on how to accomplish each task in the office/clinic in both the clinical area and in the office/business areas. RATIONALE: Clear and concise instructions assure that each task is consistently performed to the clinic standards.
4. Include local and out-of-the-area resources for clinical staff, office/business staff, physicians/providers, and patients. Provide a listing in each area with contact information and services provided. RATIONALE: The procedures and instructions listed in the Procedure Manual should provide supporting documentation needed for accomplishing each task. An example would be if the clinic requires that local public transportation resources be given to each patient who needs transportation, the Procedure Manual would have a listing of all transportation available in the area with numbers and schedules. This document could either be printed from the computer or photocopied from the Manual and provided to the patient.
5. Include basic rules and regulations, state and federal, which are related to processes performed in both clinical and office/business areas. RATIONALE: Having a listing of the rules and regulations will assist in performing those regulated duties correctly and legally.
6. Include the clinic procedures and flow sheets for taking inventory in each of the areas and instructions on ordering procedures. RATIONALE: When a clinic has processes clearly written for managing inventory and ordering of equipment and supplies, the clinic is less likely to run out of needed items and may even be able to take advantage of discounts offered by the manufacturers.
7. Collect the procedures into the Office Procedure Manual. RATIONALE: Provides a reference guide with step-by-step instruction and examples where appropriate.
8. Store one complete manual in a common library area. Provide a completed copy to the physician–employer and the office manager. Distribute appropriate sections to the various departments. RATIONALE: Provides a reference guide with step-by-step instruction and examples where appropriate.
9. Review the procedure manual annually and add any new procedures, delete or modify as necessary, and indicate the revision date (Rev. 10/12/XX). RATIONALE: Maintains current office protocols.

Case Study 33-1

Drs. Lewis and King have requested sigmoidoscopy procedures to be scheduled for two different patients. The patients are scheduled. Both patients are put on a strict diet and pretest protocol for several days to prepare for the procedures. The day of the appointments, it is discovered that the two sigmoidoscopy procedures have been scheduled at the same time. The problem is that the office has only one sigmoidoscope available.

CASE STUDY REVIEW

1. Divide the class into two groups to discuss problem-solving solutions. Assume that rescheduling a patient is not an acceptable solution because of the patient's pretest protocol. The patients would be upset if the procedure could not be performed due to a scheduling problem.
2. How could this problem have been avoided?
3. Both patients have been told about the scheduling problem and one is upset and argumentative. What role should the office manager assume in this predicament?

Case Study 33-2

Anita Juarez, the office receptionist, speaks privately with Jane O'Hara, the office manager and the person responsible for personnel. Anita has a suspicious lump in her breast. She has seen both her internist and a surgeon for evaluation. Next week, she will have the lump removed, perhaps even a complete mastectomy. Anita is concerned about the time she will need to be away from the office.

CASE STUDY REVIEW

1. Identify the first and immediate concerns to be addressed.
2. What action might be taken to help both Anita and the office manager address these concerns?
3. Is it helpful to plan for the best results, the worst results, or both?

SUMMARY

The office manager is the glue that holds the office together and keeps it running smoothly. When the manager sets a positive example for others, is considerate and aware of the diversity of others, a positive environment is created for teamwork. A teamwork approach enables the entire office to be more productive, provide the best health care, and foster an enjoyable work relationship.

The role of office manager varies greatly depending on the size of the medical practice, the physician's trust in the manager's competency level, and the physician's comfort in delegating authority to others. An effective office manager is a tremendous asset to physicians. The personal and financial rewards are worthwhile to the medical assistant who desires a new dimension to explore and enjoys a challenge.

STUDY FOR SUCCESS

To reinforce your knowledge and skills of information presented in this chapter:

- ❑ Review the Key Terms
- ❑ Practice the Procedures
- ❑ Consider the Case Studies and discuss your conclusions
- ❑ Answer the Review Questions
  - ❑ Multiple Choice
  - ❑ Critical Thinking
- ❑ Navigate the Internet by completing the Web Activities
- ❑ Practice the StudyWARE activities on the textbook CD
- ❑ Apply your knowledge in the Student Workbook activities
- ❑ Complete the Web Tutor sections

REVIEW QUESTIONS

Multiple Choice

1. For teamwork to be successful, individual team members must:
   a. do as they are told by the office manager
   b. not ask why they are doing something a certain way
   c. understand and support the task
   d. think independently and solve the problem on their own
2. Meeting minutes:
   a. should address each agenda topic and include a brief summary of discussions, actions taken, name of each person making a motion, the exact wording of motions, and motion approval or defeat
   b. are a detailed plan for a proposed trip
   c. include information regarding mode of transportation and lodging reservations
   d. must follow parliamentary procedures
3. When working with externship students, it is important to remember that:
   a. they should have expert knowledge about their field
   b. they do not need supervision when working with a patient
   c. they are experienced with working on real patients
   d. they have much to learn
4. Which of the following statements is *not* correct regarding a student practicum?
   a. It is a transitional stage that provides opportunity for students to apply theory learned in the classroom to a health care setting through hands-on experience.
   b. It assumes that the student is an employee who does not need to be introduced to patients.
   c. It may require the student to shadow another medical assistant for a few days.
   d. It involves an evaluation of the student's progress.

5. The procedure manual:
   a. is a detailed plan for a proposed trip
   b. provides detailed information regarding mode of transportation and lodging reservations
   c. provides detailed information relative to the performance of tasks within the health care facility
   d. summarizes action details of staff meetings
6. Developing relationships outside the office is often called:
   a. marketing
   b. benchmarking
   c. advertising
   d. sales
7. Record and financial management involves all of the following *except:*
   a. payroll processing
   b. preparing payroll checks
   c. figuring taxes
   d. equipment and supplies maintenance
8. Controlled substances must:
   a. be kept separate from other drugs
   b. be stored in a double locked cabinet
   c. be recorded in a book that is maintained daily
   d. all of the above

Critical Thinking

1. How would you, as the office manager, handle someone who is spreading a harmful rumor about another employee in the office?
2. How can the office manager promote open and honest communication?
3. The student practicum can be a stressful time for the extern. As an office manager, how can you help the extern feel more at ease the first day of "work"?
4. Describe how a procedure manual for a single-physician practice would differ from a procedure manual for a multiphysician practice.
5. Describe how a procedure manual could become outdated and need revision.

WEB ACTIVITIES

Use the Web sites described in the text, or alternative sites you know about, to plan a trip between two cities within the United States. Compare the fares for Sunday departure and Friday return dates with the fares for low volume days as obtained from the Priceline.com site. Also compare fares on flights purchased within one week of departure with fares on flights purchased a month before departure. Follow the instructor's instructions on completing and turning in your results.

REFERENCES/BIBLIOGRAPHY

Colbert, B. J. (2000). *Workplace readiness for health occupations*. Clifton Park, NY: Thomson Delmar Learning.

ingenix. (2003, December). HIPAA Tool Kit. Salt Lake City, UT: St. Anthony Publishing/Medicode.

Institute for Management Excellence (2004, June). *Linking personality with management style*. Retrieved from http://itstime.com/jun98.htm. Accessed May 16, 2005.

Krager, D., & Krager, C. (2005). *HIPAA for Medical Office Personnel*. Clifton Park, NY: Thomson Delmar Learning.

Pyzdek, T. (2004). *Management styles: Participatory management style*. Retrieved from http://www.qualityamerica.com/knowledgecente/articles/CQMStyle2.html. Accessed May 16, 2005.

CHAPTER 34

The Medical Assistant as Human Resources Manager

KEY TERMS

Exit Interview
Involuntary Dismissal
Job Description
Letter of Reference
Letter of Resignation
Networking
Overtime
Probation

OUTLINE

Tasks Performed by the Human Resources Manager
The Office Policy Manual
Recruiting and Hiring Office Personnel
- Job Descriptions
- Recruiting
- Preparing to Interview Applicants
- The Interview
- Selecting the Finalists

Orienting New Personnel
Dismissing Employees
- Exit Interview

Maintaining Personnel Records
Complying with Personnel Laws
Special Policy Considerations
- Temporary Employees
- Smoking Policy
- Discrimination

Providing/Planning Employee Training and Education

OBJECTIVES

The student should strive to meet the following performance objectives and demonstrate an understanding of the facts and principles presented in this chapter through written and oral communication.

1. Define the key terms as presented in the glossary.
2. Describe the role of the human resources manager.
3. Explain the function of the office policy manual.
4. Identify methods of recruiting employees for a medical practice.
5. Discuss the interview process.
6. Identify items to keep in an employee's personnel record.
7. List and define a minimum of four laws related to personnel management.

FEATURED COMPETENCIES

CAAHEP—ENTRY-LEVEL COMPETENCIES

Legal Concepts

- Document properly
- Demonstrate knowledge of federal and state health care legislation and regulations

ABHES—ENTRY-LEVEL COMPETENCIES

Professionalism

- Evidence a responsible attitude
- Be courteous and diplomatic

Communication

- Interview effectively
- Recognize and respond to verbal and non-verbal communication

Administrative Duties

Legal Concepts

- Document accurately
- Monitor legislation related to current healthcare issues and practices

Instruction

- Orient and train personnel

SCENARIO

Jane O'Hara, CMA, is the officer manager at Inner City Health Care. She also functions in the role of the human resources manager. Part of her responsibilities includes recruiting, hiring, and orienting employees.

In one day Jane may meet with Dr. Rice to update the policy manual; begin the hiring process for a new medical assistant; welcome a new physician to the practice, being sure she completes all of the necessary employment forms; and meet with another staff member to evaluate her continuing education.

INTRODUCTION

The medical assistant's employment responsibilities are many and varied. As you learned in Chapter 33, often they become office managers and assume a quite different function in the medical setting. The size of the ambulatory care setting and the number of employees likely determines if a human resources (HR) manager is a part of the practice. Whether the HR manager heads an HR department in a large, corporate medical setting with the title Human Resources Manager or is a medical assistant/office manager who serves as the HR representative, there are some common tasks assigned as specific HR duties.

TASKS PERFORMED BY THE HUMAN RESOURCES MANAGER

Tasks usually assigned to the HR manager include determining job descriptions, hiring, and orienting employees, and maintaining employee personnel records that include credentials and continuing education units (CEUs). With today's quest for greater office efficiency and the tremendous increase in federal and state regulatory requirements, the skills required of an HR manager have greatly broadened. Former responsibilities have been expanded to include preparing the policy manual, scheduling employee evaluations, preventing and inves-

Spotlight on Certification

RMA Content Outline
- Medical law
- Medical ethics
- Human relations

CMA Content Outline
- Basic principles (Psychology)
- Interview techniques
- Medicolegal guidelines & requirements
- Maintaining the physical plant
- Office policies and procedures

CMAS Content Outline
- Legal and ethical considerations
- Professionalism
- Human resources

tigating discrimination and harassment claims, and complying with regulatory agencies. The HR manager also assists in providing training and educational opportunities for employees so they are up to date in all aspects of quality patient care.

Increasingly, HR managers are expected to be able to support the organization's efforts that focus on productivity, service, and quality. In a climate in which there are too few persons for the positions to be filled, and the delivery methods for health care are changing almost daily, productivity, service, and quality are essential to a successful practice. It becomes the responsibility of the HR manager to see that every employee's productivity level is high, that the service is A+, and that quality is at the highest level. Today's customers, the patients, often choose their health care provider on the basis of service and quality.

The position of HR manager now requires a higher level of education and experience to better grasp the legal and regulatory aspects of personnel management. The HR manager also must have excellent people skills, a strong sense of fairness, and the ability to resolve conflicts. None of this is accomplished in a vacuum. It requires working in close cooperation with the office manager and the physician–employer(s).

This chapter discusses these responsibilities in the following separate but overlapping functions:

1. Creating and updating the office policy manual
2. Recruiting and hiring office personnel
3. Orienting new personnel
4. Scheduling salary reviews
5. Conducting exit interviews
6. Maintaining personnel records
7. Complying with all state and federal regulations regarding personnel
8. Planning/providing employee training and education
9. Maintaining records of credentials, CEUs, and certificates such as cardiopulmonary resuscitation (CPR)

THE OFFICE POLICY MANUAL

The procedure manual described in Chapter 33 identifies specific methods of performing tasks. The policy manual provides more general guidelines for office practices.

Possible Content of Policy and Procedure Manual

Policy Manual	Procedure Manual
General practices and policies of an office	Daily guide; step-by-step instructions for procedures

The policy manual will identify clear guidelines and directions required of all employees, as well as define appropriate expectations and boundaries of the employment relationship. Having written policies means not having to determine a policy on a case-by-case basis. Policy manuals will vary by the size of the practice or problems to be addressed, but some topics include the mission statement of the practice, biographic data on each physician, employment policies, wage and salary policies, benefits to be awarded, and employee conduct expectations.

Establishing and stating the mission of the practice clearly identifies for employees the goals and objectives to be sought by each employee. Having biographic data of each physician helps employees to respond to queries from patients about a physician's experience, education, and interests.

Employment policies might include statements on equal employment opportunity, job requirements for particular positions and to whom the person reports, recruitment and selection procedures, orientation of new employees, probation, and dismissal. Wage and salary policies should be in writing. How are employees classified, what are the working hours, how is overtime compensated, how are salary increases determined, what benefits (medical, retirement, vacation, holidays, sick leave, profit sharing) does the practice have? The answers to such questions are part of the policy manual. Employee conduct is another piece of the policy manual. Guidelines should be established about uniforms, dress codes, appearance, and personal hygiene. Can an employee hold a second job outside the practice? Is smoking allowed? Are staff members responsible for housekeeping duties? A statement regarding the confidentiality of all information received in the practice is essential in this area of the policy manual.

Having a policy manual with clearly written directives helps employees understand the expectations and boundaries of the employment relationship. The policy manual should be reviewed with each new employee and updated on a regular basis. See Procedure 34-1 for details on developing and maintaining a policy manual.

RECRUITING AND HIRING OFFICE PERSONNEL

Before recruiting and hiring personnel to fill positions within the medical office, the HR manager and physician–employer must know exactly what the role and responsibilities of the position are by having a current job description for the position and following a recruiting policy that is effective, fair, and observes all appropriate laws and regulations.

Job Descriptions

Before any position is filled, a **job description** must be in place. This usually is created cooperatively by the office manager and the physician–employer. Once the job qualifications are defined, the lead personnel and HR manager can begin efforts to fill the position.

In daily operations most job descriptions are on file, but if the situation involves a new or greatly expanded office, a complete set of job descriptions is needed before recruiting can begin. Even when a written description is on file, it should be reviewed when a new employee is to be hired. The person who is leaving the position is often an excellent resource for the accuracy of the current job description and any changes that should be made.

The job description must include basic qualifications for the position and have enough information to provide both the supervisor and the employee with a clear outline of what the job entails (Figure 34-1). Necessary work experience, skills, education, and any special certification or licensure that is expected is to be identified in the job description. See Procedure 34-2 for details on preparing job descriptions.

Another important point with respect to the job description is that a review and update of the description should be done every year. Most jobs change constantly whether from a minor shifting of duties or the addition of some new technical procedure or device. Without updating a job description, a person with the wrong qualifications may be recruited to fill a vacancy.

JOB DESCRIPTION

POSITION TITLE:
Administrative Medical Assistant

REPORTS TO:
Office Manager and Physician–Employer

RESPONSIBILITIES AND DUTIES:
- Being a therapeutic and helpful receptionist
  1. Answer telephone as quickly as possible, hopefully by the second ring
  2. Greet all patients warmly and with a helpful attitude
- Efficiently managing time with appropriate scheduling for patients and professional staff
  1. Schedule patients according to their needs, office scheduling guidelines, staff availability, and equipment readiness
  2. Call to remind patients of their visit the day before appointment
- Responding to patient requests on the telephone and in person
  1. Ascertain reason for request
  2. Satisfy patient request or refer patient to one who can
- Preparing patient charts for professional staff
  1. Print out schedules and encounter forms
  2. Pull patient charts late afternoon on the day before appointment
  3. Check charts for completeness
  4. Attach encounter form when patient arrives to check in

AUTHORITY BOUNDARIES:
The office manager will assist in answering questions. Remember that it is better to ask than to make an error. Triage concerns not identified in a policy/procedure manual also can be directed to the clinical medical assisting staff.

POSITION REQUIREMENTS:
Two years experience and/or graduate of a medical assistant program. CMA, RMA, or CMAS preferred.

Figure 34-1 Sample job description for administrative medical assistant.

Critical Thinking

Identify proper qualifications for a front-office medical assistant or receptionist in a fairly large ambulatory care setting. Determine what work experience might qualify versus what work experience is preferred.

Recruiting

A major challenge facing the HR manager today is recruitment. Medical assistants are listed in the top 10 occupations with the fastest employment growth through 2012 according to the U.S. Department of Labor, Bureau of Labor Statistics. One reason for this demand is the aging of the U.S. population. It is estimated that more than 80% of jobs are in the service industry, and all health care positions fit into that category. When physician–employers have been unsuccessful in recruiting qualified medical assistants, they have turned to contracting out some work, such as transcription and billing.

Once the hiring need is determined, the HR manager begins the recruitment process. Often a process called networking is a highly effective method of finding employees. **Networking** is a process in which people of similar interests exchange information in social, business, or professional relationships. For instance, the HR manager may network with members of the American Association of Medical Assistants and express an interest in a new employee for a position that is open. Current employees are often an excellent resource because they may know of a qualified person who is looking for a position.

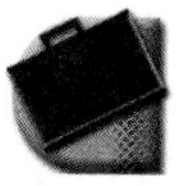

Checking with nearby colleges' medical assistant departments is another good resource. Employing a private or state placement agency is another possibility. Although newspaper advertisements may generate many résumés, they are only marginally effective as a search tool. It is often far too time consuming to review the large volume of applications generated by this approach. Online options may be beneficial. There are a number of medical Web sites that identify positions for medical assistant personnel, often in specific localities.

Critical Thinking

Is there ever a time when physicians are considered recruiters for their medical practice's personnel? When and how?

Preparing to Interview Applicants

Once several applicants have expressed interest in the position, preparation for the interview begins. The HR manager should have a number of résumés to consider. Some may have already filled out a job application when they dropped off a résumé. The résumés and applications can be reviewed together. Some important points to remember in reading résumés and applications follow.

When considering education, look beyond the degree earned. Look for a good performance record at school and the kinds of supplemental education achieved. Does attendance at seminars and short-course training programs relate to your position needs? When reading a person's work history, make note of unexplained gaps in employment. You may want to ask specific questions in the interview. Has advancement been gained in each new position? Are the responsibilities and duties of the applicant's positions explained, or will questions need to be asked of the prospective employee?

Look for information that indicates if this candidate really enjoys the kind of work setting you have. Is the applicant comfortable serving the infirm? Can you truly identify the level of skill from the descriptions, or are the skills vague? The cover letter, if one is included, should address the specifics required of your position. Does the person display a negative or a positive attitude? Do not excuse any errors or unprofessional appearance in the job application or the résumé. Each should be letter perfect. An individual who is careless in this respect is likely to be careless on the job.

Some applications will be discarded after using the preceding guidelines. With the remaining candidates, determine who is to be interviewed and make telephone calls to establish interviews. You may make note of the quality of speaking skills, especially if this person will be using the telephone on the job. Make an interview appointment date with only those who seem truly interested in the position during your telephone conversation.

The Interview

The interview is usually conducted by only one person if second interviews are anticipated. The physician–employer, office manager, or another employee may be present in either the first or the second interview, however (Figure 34-2). The interviewer(s) will want to review the application and résumé before the interview for particular points to ask the candidate. Before the interview, those doing the interviews should establish a set of questions for the applicants. These predetermined questions will help alleviate one applicant being given privileges over another and will help assure continuity throughout

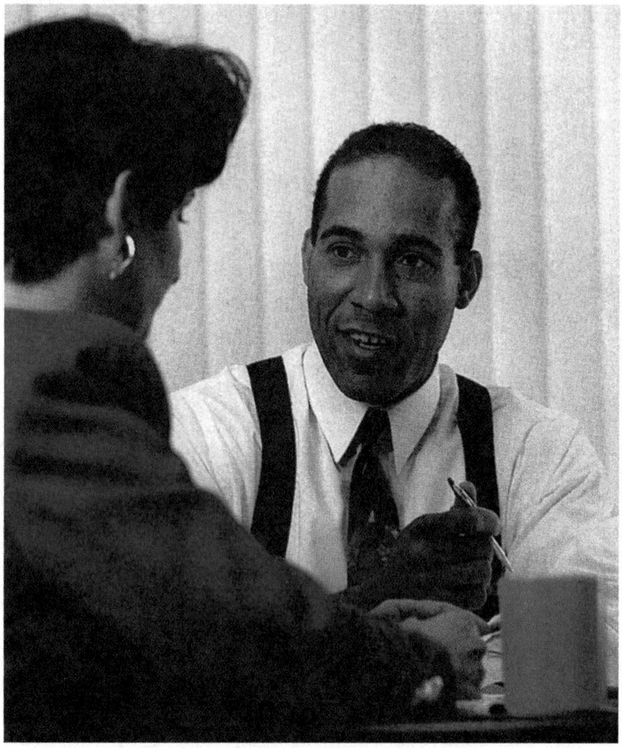

Figure 34-2 The interview can be conducted on a one-to-one basis with only the applicant and one staff member or with several staff members meeting with the applicant at once.

General Questions
- What are your strengths and weaknesses?
- Why did you leave your last job?
- Identify what is most important to you in a job.

Questions Related to Work Relationships
- Describe an individual you have enjoyed working with.
- Explain how a conflict with a coworker was resolved.
- How would a coworker describe you?

Questions Related to Problem Solving
- Describe a work-related decision that made you very proud.
- Identify a task/procedure/assignment you could not do, and explain why.
- How do you approach a task when it seems mundane or boring?

Questions Related to Integrity
- If asked to do something illegal or unethical, what would you do?
- Tell us about a time when you broke a confidence.
- If you saw a coworker put a patient at risk, what would you do?

Figure 34-3 Common interview questions.

all the interviews. An interview worksheet is an excellent tool to use to make certain that you are fair and equitable with each candidate. The worksheet should provide enough room for notes taken during the interview.

Suggested items for the interview worksheet are:

- Applicant's name
- Telephone number
- Education and training
- Work experience
- Special skills
- Professional demeanor
- Voice and mannerisms specific to position
- Questions and responses
- Ability to problem solve when given a scenario
- Any health-related or work-related problems applicant discloses
- Interviewer's personal impressions and recommendations

Conduct interviews in a quiet and private setting. Do not schedule interviews back to back without time to collect your thoughts or to allow you to compare notes with others participating in the interview. Ask job-related questions. For example, Describe your last job. What did you like best about it? What did you like least? What is most important to you about a job? Describe your administrative and clinical skills. Figure 34-3 shows some sample questions. Let the applicant do the most of the talking.

Any questions related to age, sex, race, religion, or national origin are inappropriate. Inquiries about medical history, drug use, or arrest records may not be made. Keep your questions related to performance on the job. If you may want to bond this employee, you may ask candidates if they have been bonded before or are willing to be bonded. It may be best to leave salary discussions for a second interview, but it can also be helpful to determine if applicants' salary expectations are in line with what you can offer. A question such as What salary are you expecting? is appropriate. Do not make a job offer until all the candidates selected for interview have been interviewed, and do not prejudge someone on any factor during or after the interview, except the person's qualifications.

At the close of the interview, let the applicant know when a decision will be made or whether a second interview will be conducted and how notification will be made. A tour of the facility and introduction to key staff members may be offered but are not necessary at the time of the first interview. Finally, thank the applicant for participating in the interview and being interested in the position.

Selecting the Finalists

Shortly after the final interview is completed, the HR manager should compare notes with all the others involved in the interview to select the top candidates. This is done by comparing notes and impressions from the interviews and by taking into consideration the ability of a candidate to work with patients and colleagues who might have a variety of problems and cultural backgrounds. The next step is to check references from former employers, supervisors, coworkers, and instructors. A large corporate medical practice may even have a consent form each candidate is asked to sign that gives permission to check references and call former employers and instructors. You may need to recognize, however, that even with a release from a potential new employee, many organizations and businesses restrict the release of reference information to only name, dates of employment, and title of position served. Telephone checks for references are an excellent strategy before you receive an immediate response. If you stress confidentiality when you make the contact, it will be easier for the person to respond to your questions. Always check with more than one reference and former employer to get an accurate assessment of the candidate. All reference information is to be kept confidential. A sample telephone reference check form is shown in Figure 34-4.

A checklist of questions to ask might include:

1. What were the dates of employment of (name of applicant) in your firm?
2. Describe the job performed.
3. Reason for leaving the job?
4. Strong points of the employee?
5. Limitations of the employee?
6. Can you comment on attendance and dependability?
7. Would you rehire?
8. Anything else we should know about this candidate?

TELEPHONE REFERENCE

Name of Applicant ____________________

Person Contacted ____________________

Position and Name of Business ____________________

____

Telephone Number ____________________

Relationship to Applicant ____________________

- May I verify the employment history of (applicant's name) who is applying for a position with our medical clinic?

  __________, 20____ to __________, 20____
- Describe the responsibilities held by this individual.
- Identify the salary ____________________
- What are this individual's strong points?
- What are this individual's weak points?
- Describe this individual's overall attitude toward the job and toward patients.
- Please comment on dependability and attendance.
- Given the opportunity, would you rehire? Why or why not?
- Why did this individual leave the job?
- Describe personal and professional growth this individual made while in your firm.
- Is there anything else you would like to tell us?

Reference call made by ____________________

Date ____________________

Figure 34-4 Sample form to use for telephone references.

Offer the position when a first-choice candidate has been determined and indicate when a response is needed. Be prepared with a second-choice candidate should the preferred candidate respond negatively. At the time of the offer, the candidate should understand the salary offered, the starting date, the practice policies, and the benefits. When a candidate has accepted the position, a confirmation letter should be written that clearly spells out details discussed earlier. Give specific instructions on when and where the new employee should report the first day on the job. If practical, the employee should be given the policy and procedure manuals to read.

For the unsuccessful applicants, send a letter explaining that "we have selected another candidate whose qualifications and experience more closely meets our needs at this time. We would like to keep your résumé on file should another suitable position become available." Copies of these letters, as well as the interview checklists, should be kept for a minimum of six months should any questions arise regarding your choice of candidates. See Procedure 34-3 for details on interviewing.

ORIENTING NEW PERSONNEL

Orienting new employees is usually the responsibility of both the office manager and lead personnel who are most likely to work the closest with the new employee. It is common for a new employee to be placed on **probation** for 60 to 90 days during which time both the employee and supervisory personnel may determine if the environment and the position are satisfactory for the employee. Procedure 34-4 outlines how to orient personnel.

Important elements to orientation include the introduction of the new employee to other staff members, assigning a mentor who can respond to questions, and making the employee aware of the procedures to be performed in this new position. If the procedure manual is detailed and accurate, this manual now becomes the daily guide for the new employee. Sometimes the individual leaving a position may still be present and is asked to assist in the orientation process. This is especially beneficial if there is a good working relationship between the employee who is leaving and the management of the practice. Depending on the responsibilities of the new employee, a supervisor may be asked to monitor all procedures for a period for accuracy, safety, and patient protection. During the probation period, the employee should be officially evaluated by the office manager.

DISMISSING EMPLOYEES

The function of employee dismissal falls mostly to the office manager; however, in a large facility with an HR representative, discussing dismissal with that individual can be quite beneficial. Such a discussion assures that all the information necessary is in place before a dismissal. There are voluntary and involuntary dismissals.

Voluntary dismissals usually occur when an employee is relocating, advancing to another position elsewhere, retiring, or leaving for personal reasons. A letter of resignation is usually submitted to both the office manager and the HR representative. These employees will give their manager proper notice and may be able to turn current projects and duties over to their replacement. There is also time to say good-bye to their colleagues and have a good feeling about their employment.

Involuntary dismissals usually occur when an employee's performance is poor or there has been a serious violation of the office policies or job description. The office manager is aware of poor performance through the probationary reviews. Verbal and written warnings must be given to the employee and be well documented. Dismissal can be immediate if there is a serious breach of office policy. The HR director can provide necessary detail to the office manager regarding when and if immediate dismissal is recommended. If an office manager expects any serious difficulties with an employee during an immediate dismissal, the HR director should be present when the employee is notified. See Chapter 33 for a more detailed discussion.

Exit Interview

An **exit interview** is an excellent opportunity for the employee who voluntarily leaves a practice and the HR manager to discuss the positive and negative aspects of the job and what changes might be made for a new person coming into the facility. A sample exit interview form is shown in Figure 34-5. It also allows the opportunity for the employee to ask for a **letter of reference** or to view the personnel file before leaving. In a voluntary dismissal, a **letter of resignation** for the personnel file is necessary.

Any dismissal process, voluntary or involuntary, must include a statement in the personnel file. For involuntary dismissal, be certain that the reasons for the dismissal are well documented in an honest, nonjudgmental statement. State only the facts in the personnel file; do not state opinion. Remember that employees have the right to view their personnel file at any time.

The physician–employer should always be informed of any dismissal as quickly as possible. Some may be involved in the actual dismissal process.

MAINTAINING PERSONNEL RECORDS

An important aspect of the responsibilities of the HR manager is maintaining personnel records. All documentation and correspondence related to each employee from

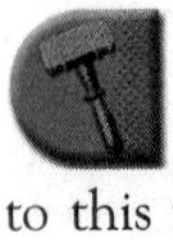

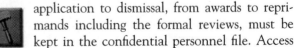

application to dismissal, from awards to reprimands including the formal reviews, must be kept in the confidential personnel file. Access to this file is limited to certain management personnel and the employee. Not all of these people are allowed to

EXIT INTERVIEW FORM

1. What did you like and dislike about the work you have been doing?
   (Including: support on the job; opportunity for personal growth; recognition and rewards)
2. What kind of people have you found the doctors, your immediate supervisor, and co-workers to be?
   (Including: attitude; fairness; scheduling and assignment of work; work expectations; technical competence; assistance and guidance available; team spirit)
3. What is your view of our management practices and policies?
   (Including: clarity and fairness of practice policies; communications; management and staff)
4. How have you felt about performance appraisals, your salary and benefits?
   (Including: adequacy of salary; regularity and fairness of appraisals)
5. What are your principal reasons for leaving the practice?
   (Including: primary dissatisfactions; job or personal changes)
6. In what areas do you feel we need to improve?

Interviewer signature: ______________ Date ________

Employee signature: ______________ Date ________

Figure 34-5 Sample exit interview form. (From *Personnel Management Handbook,* 2nd ed., by Maryann Ricardo, The McGraw-Hill Companies, Inc. Copyright 1992. Reprinted with permission.)

see the entire file. These files are usually kept for a period of three to five years after employees leave the practice.

This file also includes the kind of information normally maintained for payroll and business practices. That information includes name, address, and sex of employee. The position title, date of beginning employment, rate of pay (hourly or otherwise), total overtime pay, deductions or additions to wages, wages paid each pay period, and date employee leaves the practice also are included.

COMPLYING WITH PERSONNEL LAWS

This text is not meant to be a legal guide for an HR manager. The practice attorney should always be contacted if there is any question regarding personnel laws, which may vary in some states depending on the size of the practice. Only a brief introduction of the laws related to the ambulatory care setting are given.

Overtime must be addressed in each practice. Who is reimbursed for overtime and how is that reimbursement determined? Typically, medical receptionists and secretaries, insurance billers, medical transcriptionists, and medical assistants are likely to be paid overtime. Overtime pay at a rate of not less than one and one-half times the regular rate of pay after a 40-hour work week is standard. Each week stands alone and one week cannot compensate for another. If the practice does not want to be involved in overtime situations, require that any overtime be preauthorized in advance.

The Equal Pay Act of 1963 prevents wage discrimination for jobs that require equal skill, effort, and responsibility. The Civil Rights Act of 1964 prevents employers from discriminating against individuals on the basis of race, color, religion, sex, age, or national origin.

Sexual harassment violates Title VII of the Civil Rights Act. Steps must be taken to ensure that all employees are working in an atmosphere that is not hostile, where sexual gestures, the presence of pornographic or offensive materials, or obscene language are not allowed.

Employees have a right to expect safe working conditions. The Occupational Safety and Health Act (OSHA) was established to prevent injuries and illnesses resulting from unsafe or unhealthy working conditions. (Refer to Chapter 10 for detailed discussion of the standards and requirements, especially the section on bloodborne pathogens, which went into effect in 1992.) Compliance with this law requires that each employee be aware of possible risks associated with chemical hazards and how to protect themselves. Because there are many of these hazards in a medical practice, compliance and protection for employees are extremely important, and training sessions should be held in this area.

The Immigration Reform Act requires employers to verify the right of employees to work in the United States. Documentation acceptable for verification is a Social Security card or birth certificate. The U.S. Department of Justice Immigration and Naturalization Service will provide instructions and a form for employees and employers to complete, commonly referred to as the I-9 or Employment Eligibility Verification form.

Employers cannot discriminate or condemn any full-time employee for jury duty. Although the employer does not have to continue pay during jury duty, the employee cannot lose seniority, insurance, or other benefits. Many employers continue an employee's full pay during the time of service on a jury because the reimbursement for jury service is so small. This is a way to benefit your employees and encourage good citizenship.

This list is by no means comprehensive but does include personnel regulations most likely to affect the medical practice. Any concerns should be directed to the practice's attorney.

SPECIAL POLICY CONSIDERATIONS

There are several other managerial issues that may arise in a medical setting for which the office manager and the HR manager will have to plan. These can include policies for temporary employees, smoking, avoiding discrimination, and having a support system in place for employees who need physical or emotional help.

Temporary Employees

Temporary employees who may be employed for 90 days or less include students who are serving an internship or externship from a local college practicing their skills for when they will be on the job. They should be reviewed on a regular basis in cooperation with their college supervisor. Give them as much actual hands-on experience as possible; they are your future employees. Accommodating students in the practice is a two-way benefit. Students learn what reality is in the ambulatory care setting and are able to practice newly developed skills. Current staff members in the facility are "sharpened" by the students' presence. Teaching and monitoring someone's actions always results in sharpening and rethinking the skills of the current staff. Many HR directors and managers depend on these programs for future job applicants.

Smoking Policy

Smoking on the premises has become a greater concern in the last decade or so. Many places of employment do not allow smoking at all. Some states and cities have laws that may govern this issue for you. When a policy is established, it should cover everyone—employers, employees, and patients. The objective is to have a policy that is workable and enforceable, promotes health, encourages employee morale and productivity, and sets examples for patients. A designated place for smoking may be considered.

Discrimination

The Americans with Disabilities Act (ADA) prohibits discrimination by all private employers with 15 or more employees. Some states may further prohibit discrimination in facilities regardless of the size of their workforce. *All* public entities are prohibited from discrimination against qualified individuals with disabilities. The ADA establishes guidelines prohibiting discrimination against a "qualified individual with a disability" in regard to employment. Someone with a disability who satisfies the skills necessary for the job; has the experience, education, and any other job requirements; and who, with reasonable accommodation, can perform the job cannot be discriminated against. Employers often find that persons with disabilities are their finest employees.

Persons who are HIV-positive or have AIDS are included in the guidelines set forth by the ADA. Persons with HIV/AIDS cannot be discriminated against. It can be assumed that if you are providing a safe working environment and all employees follow the rules for Standard Precautions then reasonable accommodation has been made for the person with HIV or AIDS.

An employer cannot refuse the job to a qualified person on the belief that in the future the employee may become too ill to work. The hiring decision must be based on the individual's ability to perform the functions of the position at the present time. If a current employee reveals to the manager that he or she is HIV positive or has AIDS, that information must be kept confidential and must be kept apart from the general personnel file. The manager may choose to hold a discussion at that time of what accommodations might be needed in the future.

PROVIDING/PLANNING EMPLOYEE TRAINING AND EDUCATION

Health care changes daily; new procedures are established, a better technique is discovered for performing a particular task. Major changes regularly occur in medical insurance. Computer systems are updated or new software is added. A more sophisticated telephone system is installed to make certain patients are responded to promptly. New state or federal regulations mandate additional training or compliance in safety. New medications become available that physicians may prescribe and employees must understand. All this demands that employees receive a continuing and constant update in their area of employment.

Training and education may be accomplished within the practice or outside the practice. When an employee is a member of a professional organization such as the American Association of Medical Assistants, many monthly meetings will include continuing education opportunities. Numerous seminars and conferences held throughout the country may be beneficial to employees. Local hospitals often have continuing education opportunities that might be beneficial. Managers will keep abreast of these opportunities and encourage employees to attend. Any continuing education opportunity that may benefit the employee on the job and the medical practice itself should ideally be paid for by the physician–employer(s). Credentialed employees will always need to update skills and earn CEUs to maintain their credentials in active status. An important function of HR is to make opportunities available to employees for CEUs.

It is often best to provide training and education within the facility when the training necessary is specific to the medical practice. For instance, training on new computer software is apt to be specific to the particular setting. When sophisticated new equipment is purchased, companies often provide in-house training for the individuals who will be using the equipment. Take advantage of as many of those opportunities as are available and for as many of your employees as possible. When the training is quite expensive or time consuming, make certain one person receives the training. Then have that individual train others. Whenever possible, provide training outside of regular hours when patients are not being seen—before or after the office closes or during a lunch period. Always pay employees for any time served over their regular working hours. Offer certificates for any inservices.

Careful attention to continuing education and training for employees will pay for itself many times over again. The more confident and secure employees feel in the skills they are expected to perform, the more satisfied the practice's patients will be.

Procedure 34-1 Develop and Maintain a Policy Manual

PURPOSE:

To develop and maintain a comprehensive, up-to-date policy manual of all office policies relating to employee practices, benefits, office conduct, and so on.

EQUIPMENT/SUPPLIES:

Computer
Binder, such as a three-ring binder
Paper
Standard policy manual format

PROCEDURE STEPS:

1. Following office format, develop precise, written office policies detailing all necessary information pertaining to the staff and their positions. The information should include benefits, vacation, sick leave, hours, dress codes, evaluations, rules of-conduct, and grounds for dismissal. RATIONALE: Well-defined policies clearly outlined for each employee are necessary for efficient and effective staff operations.
2. Identify procedures for reimbursing overtime, preventing discrimination and harassment, creating a safe working environment, and allowing for jury duty.
3. Include a policy statement related to smoking.
4. Identify steps to follow should an employee become disabled during employment.
5. Determine what employee opportunities for continuing education, if any, will be reimbursed; include requirements for recertification or licensure.
6. Provide a copy of the policy manual for each employee.
7. Review and update the policy manual regularly. Add or delete items as necessary, dating each revised page.

Procedure 34-2 Prepare a Job Description

PURPOSE:

To provide a precise definition of the tasks assigned to a job, to determine the expectations and level of competency required, and to specify the experience, training, and education needed to perform the job for purposes of recruiting and performance evaluation.

EQUIPMENT/SUPPLIES:

Computer
Paper
Standard job description format

PROCEDURE STEPS:

1. Detail each task that creates the job. RATIONALE: A detailed job description identifies clear expectations for each employee.
2. List special medical, technical, or clerical skills required.
3. Determine the level of education, training, and experience required for the position.
4. Determine where the job fits in the overall structure of the office.
5. Specify any unusual working conditions (hours, locations, and so on) that may apply.
6. Describe career path opportunities.

Procedure 34-3 Conduct Interviews

PURPOSE:

To screen applicants for training, experience, and characteristics to select the best candidate to fill the position vacancy.

PROCEDURE STEPS:

1. Review résumés and applications received.
2. Select candidates who most closely match the education and experience being sought.
3. Create an interview worksheet for each candidate listing points to cover.
4. Select an interview team; this team should always include the HR or office manager and the immediate supervisor to whom the candidate will report.
5. Call personally to schedule interviews; this allows you to judge the applicant's telephone manners and voice.
6. Remind the interviewers of various legal restrictions concerning questions to be asked.
7. Conduct interviews in a private, quiet setting. RATIONALE: Careful interviewing of potential employees is an important step in hiring the best candidate for the position.
8. Put the applicant at ease by beginning with an overview about the practice and staff, briefly describing the job, and answering preliminary questions.
9. Ask questions about the applicant's work experience and educational background using the résumé and interview worksheet as a guide.
10. Provide the most promising applicants additional information on benefits and a tour of the office if practical.
11. Applicant's general salary requirements may be discussed, but avoid discussion of a specific salary until a formal offer is tendered.
12. Inform the applicants when a decision will be made and thank each for participating in the interview.
13. Do not make a job offer until all the candidates have been interviewed.
14. Check references of all prospective employees.
15. Establish a second interview between the physician–employer(s) and the qualified candidate if necessary.
16. Confirm accepted job offers in writing, specifying details of the offer and acceptance.
17. Notify all unsuccessful applicants by letter when the position has been filled.

Procedure 34-4 Orient Personnel

PURPOSE:
To acquaint new employees with office policies, staff, what the job encompasses, procedures to be performed, and job performance expectations.

PROCEDURE STEPS:

1. Tour the facilities and introduce the office staff.
2. Complete employee-related documents and explain their purpose.
3. Explain the benefits programs.
4. Present the office policy manual and discuss its key elements.
5. Review federal and state regulatory precautions for medical facilities.
6. Review the job description.
7. Explain and demonstrate procedures to be performed and the use of procedure manuals supporting these procedures.
8. Demonstrate the use of any specialized equipment.
9. Assign a mentor from the staff to help with the orientation. RATIONALE: Without proper orientation and training, the best new employee can fail.

Case Study 34-1

Daly Jacobsen, RMA, is an administrative medical assistant at Inner City Health Care. The HR manager has suggested that she might expand her skills and learn some of the procedures in the hiring process. A new medical assistant who specializes in nutrition is coming on board. Daly has been asked to make certain the I-9 form is completed appropriately. The HR manager tells Daly that she will need to download the latest form before completion.

CASE STUDY REVIEW

1. Daly knows that the I-9 is a government form verifying employment eligibility. What keywords might she use in her Inernet search to find the form?
2. Once the form has been located, identify the specific rules necessary in completion of the form. What document in List A might a number of prospective employees likely have?
3. In what area of the office might you post the lists of acceptable documents for the I-9 form?
4. With what agency is the form filed on successful completion?

Case Study 34-2

Charles Kensington has just been hired as the HR manager in a large metropolitan clinic. In studying the policy manual, he notes that there is no defined policy for sick leave or bereavement leave. Describe the steps he might take to write such a policy.

CASE STUDY REVIEW

1. To whom should he speak regarding what currently occurs when an employee is ill or when there is a death in the family?
2. What might Charles consider in writing this policy?
3. How should a policy be approved once it is written?
4. What parameters would you suggest for the policy?

SUMMARY

As shown in this discussion, HR management is a challenge. It is, however, a rewarding one. While physician–employers are responsible for patients' physical care, the management team is responsible for hiring and maintaining the employees in the organization. The HR manager who is successful will hire the right people for the jobs and monitor employees in a way that enables and encourages them to give the best patient care possible. The medical assistant who has good communication skills and acquires additional training in HR management will always have variety on the job and will have the satisfaction of watching a health care team run smoothly and efficiently.

STUDY FOR SUCCESS

To reinforce your knowledge and skills of information presented in this chapter:

- ❑ Review the Key Terms
- ❑ Practice the Procedures
- ❑ Consider the Case Studies and discuss your conclusions
- ❑ Answer the Review Questions
  - ❑ Multiple Choice
  - ❑ Critical Thinking
- ❑ Navigate the Internet and complete the Web Activities
- ❑ Practice the StudyWARE activities on the textbook CD
- ❑ Apply your knowledge in the Student Workbook activities
- ❑ Complete the Web Tutor sections

REVIEW QUESTIONS

Multiple Choice

1. HR managers:
   a. need no special training for the job
   b. are responsible for hiring and orienting personnel
   c. usually work harder and longer hours than other employees
   d. both b and c
2. The following questions may be asked in an interview:
   a. How old are you?
   b. Have you ever been arrested?
   c. Can you supply a birth certificate or a Social Security card?
   d. Do you plan to start a family soon?
3. When a candidate has been accepted for a position, the HR manager should:
   a. call the candidate to determine what salary is preferred
   b. write a letter defining the position details
   c. check references listed by the candidate
   d. notify patients of a staff change
4. Overtime hours in the medical setting:
   a. are to be expected as part of the job
   b. do not require prior authorization
   c. are usually paid at no less than one and one-half times the regular pay rate
   d. are paid only to managers
5. The HR manager will work closely with:
   a. the physician–employer
   b. the office manager
   c. all employees
   d. all the above
6. OSHA:
   a. requires employers to verify an employee's right to work in the United States
   b. protects employees who have disabilities from employment discrimination
   c. protects employees with chemical dependencies or emotional problems
   d. protects employees from unsafe or unhealthy working conditions

7. The best area for hiring medical employees comes from:
   a. students in a business college
   b. newspaper advertisements
   c. networking sources
   d. the state's unemployment office
8. Employees receiving training or education necessary to the job:
   a. will seek that training after hours and not expect reimbursement
   b. will be continuous and constant in the health care field
   c. should always be paid for any time served over regular working hours
   d. both b and c
9. Personnel records:
   a. are usually kept for three to five years after employment ends and may include payroll data
   b. are not available for everyone to view and must be kept confidential
   c. include all papers related to employment and personal data
   d. all the above
10. Dismissal:
   a. may be voluntary or involuntary
   b. should always be documented
   c. is a good time for an exit interview
   d. all the above

Critical Thinking

1. You have just accepted a position to work in a larger, more specialized clinic where you will be able to use skills you are not currently able to exercise. Identify two or three main points for a letter of resignation you will prepare.
2. An employee approaches you, the HR manager, identifying that he or she has just become responsible for the care of an aging parent and may require occasional time away from work. You have no policy about how this absence should be treated. What kind of policy might be helpful? Where would you look for suggestions?
3. An exit interview form has been introduced in this chapter. Another simple form for an exit interview is to use the ABCs. A stands for "awesome." What do we do that is really good? B stands for "better." What could we do better in our organization? C stands for "change." What would you recommend we change? Discuss the merits of both forms for an exit interview.
4. Do a simple comparison of salaries in your community. Compare the hourly wages of a secretary, a medical assistant, a plumber, your automobile mechanic, and a person working in a fast-food restaurant. How might you use this material when seeking salary increases?
5. What might physician–employers and HR managers do to make certain they keep valued employees? Is salary really the most important issue?

WEB ACTIVITIES

1. Research the Centers for Medicare & Medicaid Services Web site (http://www.cms.hhs.gov) for information related to the prohibition of discrimination on the basis of sexual orientation. What do you find? Are there other sources on this subject that are helpful? Can the manager choose not to hire a person who is otherwise qualified on the basis that he or she is gay? Why or why not?
2. "NOLO Law for All" has a helpful Web site with many topics in their encyclopedia. Research the area related to personnel policies and practices. What suggestions do they make for establishing goals and standards for employee evaluations? Do they identify any helpful evaluation tips? If so, outline them for your instructor.
3. Research the ADA Web site to determine if there are any examples of accommodations made in the medical setting. If yes, describe them. Are all physician–employers covered by the ADA? If not, how might discrimination be prevented?

REFERENCES/BIBLIOGRAPHY

Mathis, R. L., & Jackson, J. H. (2000). *Human resource management* (9th ed.). Cincinnati, OH: South-Western College Publishing.

Ricardo, M. (1992). *Personnel management handbook* (2nd ed.). New York: McGraw-Hill, Inc.

UNIT 9
Entry into the Profession

CHAPTER 35

Preparing for Medical Assisting Credentials

OUTLINE

OBJECTIVES

The student should strive to meet the following performance objectives and demonstrate an understanding of the facts and principles presented in this chapter through written and oral communication.

1. Define the key terms as presented in the glossary.
2. List the necessary qualifications to sit for the CMA certification examination.
3. State when the CMA certification examination is offered and the registration deadlines.
4. List the necessary qualifications to sit for the RMA examination.
5. State when the RMA examination is offered and the registration protocols.
6. Differentiate between being certified and being registered.
7. Identify the benefits of certification and registration.
8. Describe several methods for continuing education opportunities.
9. Explain when recertification must take place for the CMA.
10. Describe the procedure for recertification for the RMA.

KEY TERMS

Accrediting Bureau of Health Education Schools (ABHES)
American Association of Medical Assistants (AAMA)
American Medical Technologists (AMT)
Certification Examination
Certified Medical Assistant (CMA)
Commission on Accreditation of Allied Health Education Programs (CAAHEP)
Continuing Education Units (CEUs)
Recertification
Registered Medical Assistant (RMA)
Task Force for Test Construction (TFTC)

FEATURED COMPETENCIES

CAAHEP—ENTRY-LEVEL COMPETENCIES

Legal Concepts

- Perform within legal and ethical boundaries
- Demonstrate knowledge of federal and state health care legislation and regulations

ABHES—ENTRY-LEVEL COMPETENCIES

Professionalism

- Allied health professions and credentialing

SCENARIO

Dr. Ray Reynolds currently is the senior physician at Inner City Health Care, a multi-physician urgent care center. When he began his practice 32 years ago, however, he had a private practice and employed one full-time and two part-time medical assistants. Dr. Reynolds felt the office ran smoothly, except when an assistant had to be replaced. Retraining a new person consumed a great deal of valuable time. Even if the new employee came with experience from another medical office, the procedures still required retraining.

Dr. Reynolds finds that when he needs to replace a medical assistant now, he looks at the applicants' résumés and interviews only those candidates who are Certified Medical Assistants or Registered Medical Assistants. The office is too busy to spend time training and retraining new people.

INTRODUCTION

Thirty years ago, medical assistants were trained on the job by the practitioner with whom they were employed. Quality control of training varied because there were no established criteria for evaluating such training.

Hence, the ***Certified Medical Assistant (CMA)*** *certification examination was developed by the* ***American Association of Medical Assistants (AAMA),*** *and the* ***Registered Medical Assistant (RMA)*** *examination was developed by the* ***American Medical Technologists (AMT).*** *Both examinations, together with methods of continuing education and recertification establish criteria for evaluating training.*

PURPOSE OF CERTIFICATION

Certification is intended to set a consistent minimum standard for evaluating an individual's professional competence as a medical assistant. The CMA is awarded to those candidates who successfully pass the **certification examination** offered by the Certifying Board of the AAMA or administered by the National Board of Medical Examiners. Only graduates of **Commission on Accreditation of Allied Health Education Programs (CAAHEP)** and **Accrediting Bureau of Health Education Schools (ABHES)** accredited medical assistant (MA) programs may sit for the CMA and RMA examinations.

The American Medical Technologists (AMT), a national certifying body for health professionals, established the Registered Medical Assistant (RMA) credential for those students graduating from schools accredited by the ABHES. To be eligible for the RMA examination, on-the-job training with five years' experience may qualify, or a student must graduate from an approved training program. Approved programs include either a CAAHEP- or ABHES-accredited MA program, a postsecondary MA program with regional accreditation, or medical training from the armed forces.

Hiring physicians view these credentials as professional and an indication of proficiency in entry-level skills. Maintaining the credential demonstrates a lifelong commitment to continuing education. The graduate medical assistant has a goal and challenge to which to aspire, first by earning the credential, and second by maintaining the credential through recertification.

Critical Thinking

Take time to think through your personal medical assisting career goals. Will credentialing be an important consideration? Why or why not?

Spotlight on Certification

RMA Content Outline
- Medical law
- Oral and written communication

CMA Content Outline
- Displaying a professional attitude
- Professional communication and behavior

CMAS Content Outline
- Legal and ethical considerations
- Communication

Formal medical assistant programs are offered throughout the country in vocation-technical colleges, proprietary schools, postsecondary vocational schools, community and junior colleges, and four-year colleges. Medical assistants may be trained on the job; however, physicians recognize that their offices operate more efficiently with professionally educated personnel.

PREPARING FOR THE EXAMINATION

Preparation for the examination requires planning, scheduling, and discipline. It is important to plan well in advance to ensure confidence and a passing score to earn your credential. If you are sitting for the examination immediately on graduation, your preparation time for the examination may only allow two to three months. If you have been out of school for some time or your work experience has been very specialized, you may need longer to prepare for the examination.

During the planning stage, determine the date you want to sit for the examination. Check with the appropriate Web site or call the appropriate examination department to obtain the current application form. The application form will contain information such as dates, times, and locations of test sites; policies regarding deadlines; incomplete applications; examination verification information; and information regarding study guides.

It is also important to consider looking for a study group or partner. The right study environment can be invaluable to your success for several reasons. First, it is important to select a study partner or group who shares your commitment to a successful outcome and who plans to sit for the examination on or near the same date you have selected. A study partner can also give you some accountability for keeping to the planned schedule.

Once it has been determined when and where you will sit for the examination and who your study partner(s), if any, will be, a meeting should be scheduled to discuss the review/study approach. It may be that your group will decide to review/study each subject provided in the Curriculum Content Outline accompanying the application. Other groups review/study only those areas in which they feel less confident. A plan that meets the needs of each group member and that all can agree to works best.

Meeting once or twice a week helps the group stay focused and on task. Independent study should be done throughout the week. During the independent study time, each group member may be asked to write 10 multiple choice questions relevant to the weeks' study topic. Answers to these questions should be on a separate page. Some find it helpful to also provide the rationale or textbook page number that supports their answer. When the group meets, a discussion of the study topic could take place and copies of the questions could be distributed for answering. The questions could then be corrected and discussion of any questionable or missed answers could take place.

Once a schedule has been established and agreed on, discipline is required. It is critical that each group member spend time individually preparing for the next group meeting. Someone should be put in charge of each group meeting to keep the event from turning into a social time. To help with this, it is a good idea to set a specific time limit for the study/review session. If individuals want to visit after the session, they are free to do that without disrupting the purpose of the session. All members should be committed to being prepared and attending each scheduled review/study session.

CMA

The AAMA offers the CMA certification examination. After successfully passing the certification examination, the CMA credential is awarded. The credential appears after your name and distinguishes you as a professional signifying achievement in a demanding career field.

CMAs are recognized by peers for their commitment to continued professional development. Survey results indicate that many employers recognize the value of this credential by paying higher salaries and offering more benefits to CMAs. Broader career advancement opportunities and enhanced job security represent other benefits of certification. The CMA credential is a national credential, and therefore is valid wherever the practitioner is employed within the United States.

The AAMA requires current CMA status for MAs to use the CMA registered trademarked credentials after their name in their place of employment. CEU requirements must be satisfied to qualify and apply for **recertification.** Individuals not having current status as a CMA can be charged with fraudulent use and be denied access to recertification. For more information, contact the AAMA at 1-800-228-2262.

Examination Format and Content

The CMA certification examination is a comprehensive test of the knowledge actually used in today's medical office. The content is drawn from an in-depth analysis of the numerous tasks medical assistants perform on a daily basis.

Examination questions are formulated by the Certifying Board's **Task Force for Test Construction (TFTC).** This group is composed of practicing medical assistants, physicians, and medical assisting educators from across the United States. The TFTC updates the CMA examination annually to reflect changes in medical assistants' day-to-day responsibilities, as well as the latest developments in medical knowledge and technology.

The three major areas tested include:

1. *General (Transdisciplinary)*: anatomy and physiology, medical terminology, medical law and ethics, psychology, and communication.
2. *Administrative*: data entry, equipment, computer concepts, records management, screening and processing mail, scheduling and monitoring appointments, resource information and community services, managing physician's professional schedule and travel, managing the office, office policies, and procedures, and managing practice finances.
3. *Clinical*: principles of infection control, treatment area, patient preparation and assisting the physician, patient history interview, collecting and processing specimens, diagnostic tests, preparing and administering medications, emergencies, and nutrition.

Students must enroll as an AAMA member before their graduation date to be eligible for the reduced student rate. Once they are a student member they may stay at the student rate for one year after graduation if they do not choose to be an active or associate member and pay the higher dues amount. The additional year of membership at the reduced rate helps the recent graduate maintain membership while finding a job and getting established in a career.

Application Process

Candidates should read all instructions carefully before completing the application form. Incomplete or incorrect applications will not be processed and will be returned to the candidate. Postmark deadlines for applications, cancellations, and examination location changes are strictly enforced.

The examination is offered at more than 260 test sites nationwide and in Guam. A complete listing of the locations is included in the application. Applications are available from the AAMA Certification Department, 20 North Wacker Drive, Suite 1575, Chicago, IL 60606-2903; telephone: 312-424-3100; or e-mail: certification@aama.ntl.org. The application may also be downloaded from the AAMA Web site (http://www.aama-ntl.org.)

The appropriate application form must be completed and postmarked by October 1 for the January examination and by March 1 for the June examination.

The certification examination is scheduled from 9:00 AM to 1:00 PM the last Friday of January and the last Saturday in June. An admission card will be mailed to the applicant on verification of information and approval by the AAMA approximately one to two weeks before the examination date. Photo identification is required for admission to the examination and candidates are not permitted to use any supplies other than #2 soft-leaded pencils and erasers. No electronic devices (e.g., cellular phones, pagers, and calculators) are allowed in the examination area.

It is recommended that the application be sent by certified mail, return receipt requested to verify delivery. The application must be typewritten or printed using black ink only. Be sure the application is signed and dated properly and the eligibility category section is completed appropriately.

Tear off the application page from the instruction pamphlet. Do not mail the instructions back with the application. Keep this information for future reference together with a copy of everything submitted, including a copy of your completed payment check or money order.

Critical Thinking

You will graduate from a CAAHEP-accredited program in June and want to sit for the CMA examination the last Saturday of June (the same month in which you graduate). When must your application be postmarked for acceptance for this test date?

If you are paying by VISA or MasterCard, provide the requested information at the top of the application.

A guide for the certification examination entitled *A Candidate's Guide to the AAMA Certification Examination* provides explanations of how to approach the types of questions used on the examination and tips on how to study for the content that will be tested. A sample 120-question examination is included to help assess your knowledge of the categories tested and the format used to formulate the questions.

Eligibility Categories and Requirements

You must fulfill one of the four eligibility categories to apply for the CMA examination.

Grounds for Denial of Eligibility

The following are grounds for denial of eligibility for the CMA credential, or for discipline of CMAs:

- Obtaining or attempting to obtain certification, or recertification of the CMA credential, by fraud or deception
- Knowingly assisting another to obtain or attempt to obtain certification or recertification by fraud or deception
- Misstatement of material fact or failure to make a statement of material fact in application for certification or recertification
- Falsifying information required for admission to the CMA examination, impersonating another examinee, or falsifying education or credentials
- Copying answers, permitting another to copy answers, or providing or receiving unauthorized advice about examination content during the CMA examination
- Unauthorized possession or distribution of examination materials, including copying and reproducing examination questions and problems

Individuals who have been found guilty of a felony, or pleaded guilty to a felony, are not eligible to take the CMA examination. However, the Certifying Board may grant a waiver based on mitigating circumstances, which may include, but need not be limited to the following:

- The age at which the crime was committed
- The circumstances surrounding the crime
- The nature of the crime committed
- The length of time since the conviction
- The individual's criminal history since the conviction
- The individual's current employment references
- The individual's character references
- Other evidence demonstrating the ability of the individual to perform the professional responsibilities competently, and evidence that the individual does not pose a threat to the health or safety of patients

How to Recertify

Effective January 2005, all newly certified and recertifying CMAs will be current through the last day of their birth month in the 6th calendar year following their last certification/recertification. In other words, if you were born on August 6th and certified in June 2000, you would be due to recertify by the end of August 2006.

This process may be achieved by either reexamination or by the continuing education method. Recertification credits are evaluated on supportive documentation and on their relevancy to medical assisting as defined by the AAMA Medical Assistant Role Delineation Study or the Content Outline for the Certification/Recertification Examination.

A total of 60 points is necessary to recertify the CMA credential. A minimum of 15 points is required in each category: general, administrative, and clinical. The remaining 15 points may be accumulated in any of the three content areas or from any combination of the three categories. At least 20 of the required 60 recertification points must be accumulated from AAMA-approved **continuing education units (CEUs).** If desired, all 60 points may be AAMA CEUs.

On successfully passing the Certification Examination and earning the CMA credential, one should begin to document all CEUs earned. It is important to have the following information for CEU documentation:

- Complete date of the activity
- Sponsor (group or organization issuing the credit for the continuing education activity)
- Program title
- Amount and type of credit earned (e.g., CEU, CME, contact hour or college credit)
- Recertification points (AAMA CEUs or other credit)
- Points per content area (general, administrative, clinical)

CMAs applying for recertification must also provide documentation of current cardiopulmonary resuscitation (CPR) certification for health care professionals or providers. Acceptable courses of CPR include the American Red Cross, the American Heart Association, or the National Safety Council. The components of certification must include adult and pediatric CPR and obstructed airway training and Automated External Defibrillator (AED) instruction.

Applicants who accumulate all 60 points through AAMA CEUs, and in the correct content areas, may order a recertification over the telephone. Application fees still apply, however an application form is not required. All CMAs employed or seeking employment must have current certified status to use the CMA credential.

Continuing education courses are offered by local, state, and national AAMA groups. Guided study programs are also available through AAMA's "Quest for Excellence" program. CMA *Today*, the official bimonthly publication of AAMA, provides articles designated for CEUs.

A CMA need not be a member of the AAMA, nor currently employed, to recertify. The entire recertification by continuing education instructions and application can be downloaded from AAMA's Web site (http://www.aama-ntl.org). Review of recertification applications can take up to 90 days. If all criteria are met, recertification is granted. The date that the application is postmarked to the AAMA Executive Office will be the date of recertification.

On meeting recertification requirements, the applicant receives a seal to affix to the original certificate. A Recertification Certificate is also available for purchase.

RMA

The AMT, a national certifying body for health professionals, established the RMA credential in 1976. The RMA/AMT has its own bylaws, officers, local, state, and national organizations. Applicants for the RMA examination may have graduated from an accredited program, an accredited school, a U.S. Armed Forces program, or have 5 years employment in the field of medical assisting. Currently, there are more then 52,000 RMAs certified by AMT.

Examination Format and Content

AMT certification examinations are intended to evaluate the competence of entry-level practitioners. The Education, Qualifications, and Standards Committee of American Medical Technologists develop RMA examinations. The MA committee writes test questions and reviews questions submitted from other sources (e.g., instructors, experts, practitioners, and other individuals associated with the MA profession). The MA committee also determines certification requirements and addresses standard-setting issues related to the credential. Once test construction has been completed, the examination is reviewed and approved by the AMT Board of Directors.

The AMT registration examination consists of 200 to 210 four-option multiple-choice questions. Examinees are required to select the single best answer; multiple answers for a single item are scored as incorrect. Test questions may require examinees to recall facts, interpret graphic illustrations, interpret information presented in case studies, analyze situations, or solve problems. The approximate percentages of questions in content areas are as follows:

1. General Medical Assisting Knowledge—42.5%
   - anatomy and physiology
   - medical terminology
   - medical law
   - medical ethics
   - human relations
   - patient education
2. Administrative Medical Assisting—22.5%
   - insurance
   - financial bookkeeping
   - medical secretarial-receptionist
3. Clinical Medical Assisting—35.0%
   - asepsis
   - sterilization
   - instruments
   - vital signs
   - physical examinations
   - clinical pharmacology
   - minor surgery
   - therapeutic modalities
   - laboratory procedures
   - electrocardiography
   - first aid

All AMT registration examination tests are available in paper-and-pencil format or computerized formats at over 200 locations in the United States, its territories, and Canada. Tests may be scheduled daily except Sundays and holidays. Both formats are identical in length; however, experience has shown the computerized test takes less time to complete. Your computerized test score is displayed moments after completing your test. A paper copy of your result letter is provided to you before leaving the testing center.

Application Process

The following criteria have been established for applicants sitting for the RMA examination:

1. Applicant shall be of good moral character and at least 18 years of age.
2. Applicant shall be a graduate of an accredited high school or acceptable equivalent.
3. Applicant must meet one of the following requirements:
   a. Applicant shall be a graduate of a(n):
      - MA program that holds programmatic accreditation by (or is in a post-secondary school or college that holds institutional accredition by) the ABHES or the CAAHEP.
      - MA program in a postsecondary school or college that has institutional accreditation by a Regional Accrediting Commission or by a national accrediting organization approved by the U.S. Department of Education. That program must include a minimum of 720 clock hours (or equivalent) of training in medical assisting skills (including a clinical externship).
      - Formal medical services training program of the U.S. Armed Forces.

   b. Applicant shall have been employed in the profession of medical assisting for a minimum of five years, no more than two years of which may have been as an instructor in a postsecondary MA program.
4. Applicants applying under 3 A or B *must* take and pass the AMT certification examination for RMA.
5. The AMT Board of Directors has further determined that applicants who have passed generalist MA certification examination offered by another medical assisting certification body (provided that examination has been approved for this purpose by the AMT Board of Directors), who have been working in the medical assisting field for the past three of five years, and who meet all other AMT training and experience requirements may be considered for the RMA (AMT) certification without further examination.

Applications may be downloaded from AMT's Web site (http://www.amt1.com) either in print and fill-in format or as online fill-in format.

Application Completion and Test Administration Scheduling

All applications must be completed online or printed clearly except for the signatures required. All ancillary documentation must also be submitted (e.g., application fee; proof of high school graduation or equivalent; official final transcripts stating graduation from MA school, college, or training program [with school seal affixed or notarized]).

When the AMT Registrar has received the application and all required information, an authorization letter containing a toll-free number is mailed to you. You may then contact Prometric, through AMT, to schedule a date and time to take the examination. Two forms of valid identification are required both bearing your signature and at least one bearing your photo. Photo identification is limited to a driver's license, state-issued identification card, military identification, or passport.

The RMA credential is granted in conjunction with other indicators of training and experience because test results provide only one source of information regarding examinee competence. The credential remains current as long as membership is maintained in the AMT organization. Recertification of the RMA credential requires an annual fee of $48 every December.

PROFESSIONAL ORGANIZATIONS

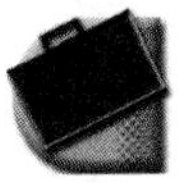

Professional organizations have evolved to establish standards by which MAs and MA programs may be evaluated. Programs accredited by agencies must meet criterion, and students must pass national examinations to become certified. MAs are not licensed and need not be certified to meet employment requirements; however, those certified are viewed as professionals with entry-level skills and a commitment to continued education.

AAMA

The AAMA was recognized by the U.S. Department of Education in 1978 working solely for the profession of medical assisting. They were instrumental in defining the scope of training required for the profession and developed standards and guidelines by which programs could become accredited and MA credentialed.

The AAMA Endowment is a not-for-profit corporation that provides funding for two purposes:

- Awarding of scholarships to students in CAAHEP-accredited medical assisting education programs
- Accreditation of medical assisting education programs through CAAHEP

The Curriculum Review Board (CRB) operates under the authority of the endowment and evaluates medical assisting programs according to standards adopted by the endowment and the CAAHEP. The CRB recommends programs to CAAHEP for accreditation. The CRB also reviews standards for medical assisting curricula, conducts accreditation workshops for educators, and provides medical assisting educators with current information about CAAHEP, accreditation laws, policies, and practices. CAAHEP's purpose is to accredit entry-level, allied health education programs.

Some of the benefits of AAMA membership include:

- Medical assisting news and health care information through the bimonthly magazine CMA *Today*
- CEUs for AAMA activities entered in the Continuing Education Registry and access to your transcript online
- Educational events provided by local chapters, state societies, and national meetings
- Answers to legal questions regarding job-related issues
- If eligible, application for the prestigious CMA examination at a reduced fee
- Discounts on car rentals, conventions, workshop and seminar fees, and self-study courses
- Opportunity to network with other practicing MAs

AMT

The AMT is another nonprofit certification agency and professional membership association representing allied health care individuals. It began in the 1970s and certifies MAs by awarding the RMA national credential to those candidates successfully satisfying requirements. AMT has many local chapters, 38 State Societies, and a Uniform Services Committee. Each of these societies meets regularly and annually for a national convention.

AMT benefits and services include:

- Continuing education through the *Journal of Continuing Education Topics & Issues* published three times a year
- AMT's Institute for Education (AMTIE), which monitors your continued education credits and sends a "report card" to you each year
- Four scholarships available to members who want to return to school, and five scholarships for current students enrolled in allied health care programs
- State Societies that offer opportunities for continued education, activities, and networking
- Peer recognition through AMT's prestigious RMA credential
- Personal discount programs

Case Study 35-1

It is February, and Juan Estaban is beginning to research the procedures and requirements for taking the CMA examination. Juan is enrolled in a CAAHEP-accredited program.

CASE STUDY REVIEW

1. If Juan wants to take the examination in June, what is the procedure for applying?
2. Juan is setting up a study schedule. He plans to review course textbooks and tests, purchase a certification review study guide, and set up a study group. Set up a sample study schedule.
3. What criteria should Juan use when asking people to join his study group?

Case Study 35-2

It is May, and Nancy McFarland, who graduated from an ABHES-accredited program four-and-a-half years ago, is beginning to research the procedures and requirements for taking the RMA examination. Nancy completed her internship at Inner City Health Care and was hired to work there full-time (35 hours per week) when she graduated.

CASE STUDY REVIEW

1. If Nancy wants to take the examination in January, what is the procedure for applying?
2. Nancy is setting up a study schedule. She plans to review course textbooks and tests, purchase a study guide, and set up a study group. Develop a simple study schedule.
3. What criteria should Nancy use when asking people to join her study group?

SUMMARY

Many advantages for certification/recertification and registration have been discussed in this chapter. Although certification examinations are not legally required for practicing MAs, it is the goal of CAAHEP-accredited and ABHES-accredited institutions to encourage graduates to sit for and maintain their credentials. Membership in the AAMA or in the AMT is also encouraged.

With nearly 400 local AAMA chapters and 51 affiliate state societies, there is the benefit of networking with others in the profession. As an information source for both professional and association issues, the executive staff at the AAMA's national headquarters is available to answer questions at a toll-free number (1-800-228-2262).

AMT currently has 38 chapters that meet regularly and allow networking with other RMAs plus other allied health professionals registered through the AMT, including phlebotomists, medical laboratory technicians, and dental assistants.

STUDY FOR SUCCESS

To reinforce your knowledge and skills of information presented in this chapter:

- ❑ Review the Key Terms
- ❑ Consider the Case Studies and discuss your conclusions
- ❑ Answer the Review Questions
  - ❑ Multiple Choice
  - ❑ Critical Thinking
- ❑ Navigate the Internet and complete the Web Activities
- ❑ Practice the StudyWARE activities on the textbook CD
- ❑ Apply your knowledge in the Student Workbook activities
- ❑ Complete the Web Tutor sections
- ❑ View and discuss the DVD situations

REVIEW QUESTIONS

1. The goal and challenge of each graduating medical assistant should be to:
   a. find employment
   b. have a good benefit package
   c. possess entry-level skills
   d. earn the CMA/RMA credential and maintain it
2. The certification examination is:
   a. a comprehensive test based on tasks medical assistants perform daily
   b. all true/false questions
   c. developed by the AMTIE
   d. developed by the NBME
3. Benefits from membership in a professional organization such as AAMA or AMT include all of the following *except*:
   a. discounted rates on legal representation
   b. legal advice
   c. nationwide networking opportunities
   d. professional journal publications
4. Recertification of the CMA credential options include:
   a. submit work experience
   b. reexamination or CEU method
   c. submit on-the-job training
   d. submit military training
5. Applications for the CMA examination must be postmarked by:
   a. October 1 for January examination and March 1 for June examination
   b. October 31 for January examination and March 31 for June examination
   c. September 30 for January exam and April 30 for June examination
   d. September 1 for January examination and April 1 for June examination
6. The RMA was established by the:
   a. ABHES
   b. CAAHEP
   c. AMT
   d. AAMA
7. Candidates who graduate from a medical assisting program that is not CAAHEP-accredited on the date of graduation, but is accredited by CAAHEP within 36 months of that date, are eligible to apply for the CMA examination under which category(ies)?
   a. Category 1
   b. Category 4
   c. Categories 3 or 4
   d. Categories 1 or 2
8. RMA examinations:
   a. are offered at Prometric testing center locations
   b. are offered twice a year
   c. are offered three times a year
   d. are offered six times a year

Critical Thinking

1. You are a recent high school graduate and have decided to pursue medical assisting as a career. What will you do to find a school offering an accredited program? Is accreditation important? How might your school selection impact your future as a professional MA?
2. After graduation you plan to sit for the certification examination. How will you prepare for the examination to assure a positive outcome and earn your CMA/RMA credential?
3. After graduating from an accredited program, you immediately went to work as an MA. Now that you have been working several years you decide to become credentialed. How will you achieve this?

WEB ACTIVITIES

Using the World Wide Web, search your local and state AAMA or AMT Web sites. Print and turn in to your instructor the location, meeting schedules, and any upcoming events planned for your state. Review the certification process that applies to your program.

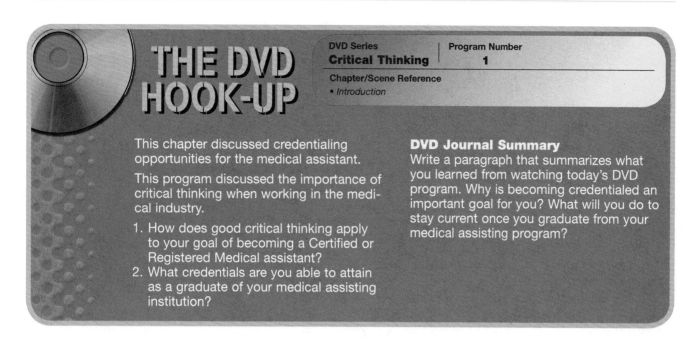

THE DVD HOOK-UP

DVD Series	Program Number
Critical Thinking	1

Chapter/Scene Reference
- *Introduction*

This chapter discussed credentialing opportunities for the medical assistant.

This program discussed the importance of critical thinking when working in the medical industry.

1. How does good critical thinking apply to your goal of becoming a Certified or Registered Medical assistant?
2. What credentials are you able to attain as a graduate of your medical assisting institution?

DVD Journal Summary
Write a paragraph that summarizes what you learned from watching today's DVD program. Why is becoming credentialed an important goal for you? What will you do to stay current once you graduate from your medical assisting program?

REFERENCES/BIBLIOGRAPHY

American Association of Medical Assistants. (2004–2005). AAMA *certification/recertification examination for medical assistants;* January and June 2005 application instructions. Retrieved from http://www.aama-ntl.org. Accessed May 16, 2005.

American Medical Technologists. Retrieved from http://www.amt1.com. Accessed May 16, 2005.

Fordney, M.T., French, L.L., Follis, J.J. (2004). *Administrative medical assisting* (5th ed.). Clifton Park, NY: Thomson Delmar Learning.

CHAPTER 36

Employment Strategies

OUTLINE

Developing a Strategy
- Attitude and Mindset
- Self-Assessment

Job Search Analysis and Research

Résumé Preparation
- Résumé Specifications
- Clear and Concise Résumés
- Accomplishments
- References
- Accuracy
- Résumé Styles
- Vital Résumé Information

Application/Cover Letters

Completing the Application Form

The Interview Process
- The Look of Success
- Preparing for the Interview
- The Actual Interview
- Closing the Interview

Interview Follow-Up
- Follow-Up Letter
- Follow Up by Telephone

Professionalism and Employment Strategies

OBJECTIVES

The student should strive to meet the following performance objectives and demonstrate an understanding of the facts and principles presented in this chapter through written and oral communication.

1. Define the key terms as presented in the glossary.
2. List the steps involved in job analysis and research.
3. Describe a contact tracker and its usefulness.
4. Give three examples of accomplishment statements.
5. Differentiate chronologic, functional, and targeted résumés.
6. Identify the purpose and content of a cover letter.
7. Demonstrate effective ways to anticipate and respond to an interviewer's questions.
8. Describe appropriate overall appearance and dress for an interview.
9. Identify the benefits of writing a follow-up letter.
10. Discuss professionalism as it relates to employment strategies.

KEY TERMS

Accomplishment Statements
Application/Cover Letter
Application Form
Benefits
Bullet Point
Career Objective
Chronologic Résumé
Contact Tracker
Direct Skills
E-résumé
Functional Résumé
Interview
Keywords
Power Verbs
References
Résumé
Targeted Résumé
Transferable Skills

FEATURED COMPETENCIES

CAAHEP—ENTRY-LEVEL COMPETENCIES

General Competencies

- Respond to and initiate written communication
- Recognize and respond to verbal communication
- Recognize and respond to nonverbal communication

Legal Concepts

- Identify and respond to issues of confidentiality
- Document appropriately

ABHES—ENTRY-LEVEL COMPETENCIES

Professionalism

- Be cognizant of ethical boundaries
- Exhibit initiative
- Evidence a responsible attitude
- Be courteous and diplomatic

Communications

- Interview effectively
- Fundamental writing skills
- Professional components

SCENARIO

Eun Mee Soo is a graduate of an accredited medical assisting program and recently passed the certification examination. She is now preparing her résumé and beginning her job search. Eun Mee plans to move out of state (she always dreamed of moving north), so she will also be looking for a new apartment. All of these changes are a bit unsettling for Eun Mee. She is beginning to wonder if she should defer relocating at this time and stay close to home until she feels more secure.

INTRODUCTION

So you are about to graduate from the medical assistant program! This time is often unsettling because many changes are occurring; the loss of security the classroom environment provided, loss of contact with fellow classmates, and loss of a structured schedule are just a few changes. Questions such as: Am I ready for my first job? How do I find a job? What do I say at the interview? begin to surface.

The focus on employment may represent apprehension and doubt or be sparked with anticipation and a sense of fulfillment. This chapter has been included to provide direction and to help answer some of the questions related to the job search.

DEVELOPING A STRATEGY

It is best to begin developing your job search strategy early in your training as a medical assistant. If you have not started this phase, determine to begin today.

Spotlight on Certification

Content Outline
- Medical law
- Human relations
- Oral and written communications

CMA Content Outline
- Displaying professional attitude
- Job readiness and seeking employment

CMAS Content Outline
- Legal and ethical considerations
- Professionalism
- Communication

Attitude and Mindset

One important quality an employer will look for in employees is their attitude. Your attitude is not something you turn on and off or learn in school. It is the result of your innate personality combined with the events that mold you during your life. Your instructors and acquaintances have a significant impact over who you are. Your attitude is reflected by how you react to:

1. taking direction
2. seeking excellence or doing just enough to get by
3. meeting employer's needs, not just looking forward to payday
4. assuming responsibility for your actions and considering your problems to be someone else's fault

If you find yourself having a negative attitude in any of the ways mentioned in the preceding list, you need to make an effort to change while you are still in training. An employer will zero in on a negative attitude and eliminate you as a candidate almost immediately. Your formal training is important and you can be retrained to do things the way a new employer desires, but your attitude takes time to change and requires a willingness to make the change. Develop a strategy to evolve a positive attitude while you are still in school because this is a time when you will have professional guidance and resources, as well as excellent models.

Beyond a positive attitude, being successful in your search for a job requires positive thinking on your part. There is a good position out there for you. Finding it is your first job. Those individuals who are successful at finding that first job devote many hours per week at job strategy tactics. You should not become discouraged by rejection, but rather seek to learn from it and apply what you have learned to the next interview opportunity.

Self-Assessment

As you begin your job search campaign, you should identify what you want in a job. It is always better to do work you enjoy in the type of practice you find most interesting. Take a moment now to complete the self-evaluation work sheet in Figure 36-1. When you have finished, you will have some idea of the type of practice you would like to work in and what position you would find most satisfying.

As part of the self-assessment you should also evaluate what direct and transferable skills you have that will make you a contributing member of the medical team. **Direct skills** are the medical procedures you have acquired in school and in which you are proficient. **Transferable skills** are those skills that would be useful in a wide variety of professions and may have been perfected during the education process or learned in other employment settings. Leadership, communication, writing, computer literacy, keyboarding, linguistics, and spelling are some examples of transferable skills.

When you have completed this portion of the self-assessment, you will be in a better position to determining what type of job to seek. You will also have identified the skills that you can highlight as you prepare your application/cover letter and résumé.

The final part of your self-assessment is conducting a budgetary need analysis to determine how much income you need to make per month to meet your living expenses.

The budgetary analysis should include listing the **benefits** you will find necessary; that is, medical, dental, and vision insurance, 401K program, stock options, and so forth. You might also need to consider work schedule, location/travel, medical benefits, childcare leave policies, and so on.

To accomplish this, begin to keep a diary of all purchases and payments. By reviewing your checkbook register, you should be able to itemize basic expenditures; that is, rent, utilities, payments (car, credit card), food, clothing, insurance, taxes, and so on. Once a monthly expenditure record is established, an estimate of the money required to live on may be calculated.

JOB SEARCH ANALYSIS AND RESEARCH

The job analysis and research phase of your job search should also start before graduation. Telephoning or visiting various clinics and asking questions to determine what the duties of a medical assistant are in different types

SELF-EVALUATION WORK SHEET

Respond to the following questions honestly and sincerely. They are meant to assist you in self-assessment.

1. List your three strongest attributes as related to people, data, or things.

   i.e., Interpersonal skills related to people

   Accuracy related to data

   Mechanical ability related to things

   ______________________ related to ______________________

   ______________________ related to ______________________

   ______________________ related to ______________________

2. List your three weakest attributes as related to people, data, or things.

   ______________________ related to ______________________

   ______________________ related to ______________________

   ______________________ related to ______________________

3. How do you express yourself? Excellent, Good, Fair, Poor

   Orally ______________________ In writing ______________________

4. Do you work well as a leader of a group or team? Yes _____ No _____
5. Do you prefer to work alone? Yes _____ No _____
6. Can you work under stress/pressure? Yes _____ No _____
7. Do you enjoy new ideas and situations? Yes _____ No _____
8. Are you comfortable with routines/schedules? Yes _____ No _____
9. Which work environment do you prefer?

   Single-physician setting _____ Multiple-physician setting _____

   Small clinic setting _____ Large clinic setting _____

10. Which type of practice do you prefer?

    Pediatrics _____ Obstetrics/Gynecology _____

    Geriatrics _____ General Medicine _____

    Internal Medicine _____ Other ______________

11. Which work setting do you prefer?

    Front office, (reception) _____ Back office, (assisting physician) _____

    Laboratory (phlebotomy) _____ Administrative (coding/billing) _____

Figure 36-1 Self-evaluation work sheets can help determine a person's strengths, weaknesses, and preferences before the job search begins.

of practices will help to further clarify where you would like to work and will help you become acquainted with a potential employer or identify a possible site for externship. If you visit the facility, dress appropriately just as you would for an interview. You want to impress the clinic personnel just as if it were a formal interview. Remember to send a letter thanking the person taking time on the telephone or authorizing the visit.

Based on the self-assessment you have completed and preliminary job analysis, you know what type of clinic or practice you want to work in, so now is the time to compile a list of potential employers in the geographic area where you want to work. Compile a list from the Yellow Pages, Job Expositions, the Internet, Want Ads for your specialty in the local papers, American Association of Medical Assistants/American Medical Technologists

(AAMA/AMT) publications, and contacts acquired through attending state and local meetings. Other sources include your program director and instructors and the network of contacts at the site where you did your externship. An externship site is frequently your best prospect because they will know your capabilities and your attitude and have expended time and resources in your training. If the site is hiring and you performed well, experience has shown that most sites will frequently hire the extern.

Candidate job sites can also be found through employment agencies. These agencies usually charge a fee, although sometimes the employer will pay the fee. Extreme caution should be exercised in dealing with agencies because fees are sometimes excessive. Fees should only be paid after successfully obtaining a job and never for getting an interview.

Prioritize the list based on your assessment of chances of employment. Sites where you have personal contacts or where you have done your externship should be at the top of the list, with sites advertising for help wanted next. Further down the list should be sites that, in sales parlance, would be called cold prospecting. You can further prioritize the list by putting your personal choices at the top each category.

Now is the time to complete detailed homework or research on each prospective employer. Start collecting information on each prospective site, identifying their services, policies, fees and insurance protocol, hours of service, number of physicians, and very importantly their mission statement and philosophy of practice criteria. Brochures may be available in their offices, on the Internet, and in wellness publications for patients. Pamphlets on new procedures are also sources of this information. You can use this information in preparation of the cover letter for your résumé and to brief yourself should you be invited for an interview.

> Copy or design your own contact tracker form and document all pertinent information regarding your job search contacts.

As part of a serious job search, you should contact many individuals and will need some means of recording the contacts, their responses, and your actions. The table presented in Figure 36-2 is a helpful sample **contact tracker.** It should be used to prevent confusion and to keep track of valuable information and action items.

RÉSUMÉ PREPARATION

A **résumé** is a summary data sheet or a brief account of your qualifications and progress in the career you have chosen and should include both direct and transferable skills. The purpose of your résumé is to sell you. It provides opportunity to describe your education, what you have done, and what you can do, and lists those who can vouch for your integrity and experience. A résumé that is well thought out and written in such a way as to create interest in what you have to contribute to the employer may reward you with many interviews. During the interview your résumé serves as a reference from which the interviewer may be prompted to ask questions.

CONTACT TRACKER

Company Name/Address	Telephone Number	Contact's Name	Resume Sent	Application/ Cover Letter	Application Form Sent	Follow-Up Phone	Follow-Up Letter	Result
1.								
2.								
3.								
4.								
5.								
6.								

Figure 36-2 A simple contact tracker such as this can help organize all communication you may have with potential employers.

Résumé Specifications

The résumé should be limited to one page in length whenever possible. Each page should contain your name and the page number. Keep a 1- to 1½-inch margin on all four sides of the page to create a picture-like frame. Capitalize major headings and single space between lines. Double space between sections. The use of **bullet point** lists instead of paragraphs aids the interviewer in gleaning key points quickly.

Select a high-quality bond stationery that is standard 8½ × 11 inches with a weight of between 16 and 25 pounds. This paper weight provides aesthetic benefit and will also accept the ink better resulting in a clean, sharp print resolution. Buff or ivory paper with matching envelope has great eye appeal and helps distinguish your résumé from others.

Use a word processing program to produce your résumé. It allows you the freedom to experiment with placement to create a picture-perfect résumé or to individualize the résumé for a particular position or facility.

Clear and Concise Résumés

Your résumé must be concise and easy to read and understand. Use statements that are positive, reflect confidence, and portray you as a problem solver. Be sure that any information given within your résumé or application form is not misleading or exaggerated. Leave out the word *I* when writing your résumé. This is your personal résumé and it is understood that you are referring to yourself.

Accomplishments

Use **accomplishment statements** if you have them from your externship or work experience. Accomplishment statements begin with **power verbs** and give a brief description of what you did, and the demonstrable results that were produced. Figure 36-3 provides a list of sample power verbs. Some accomplishment statement examples are: "Utilized computer skills to schedule and reschedule patient appointments" and "Demonstrated skills in setting up sterile trays and assisting with sterile procedures."

Accompanied	Changed	Corrected	Entertained	Implemented	Listed
Accumulated	Charged	Corresponded	Enumerated	Improved	Listened
Achieved	Charted	Counseled	Established	Improvised	Loaded
Acquired	Classified	Created	Estimated	Increased	Located
Administered	Cleaned	Debated	Evaluated	Indexed	Logged
Admitted	Cleared	Decided	Examined	Indicated	Mailed
Advised	Closed	Delegated	Exchanged	Influenced	Maintained
Allowed	Coded	Delivered	Exhibited	Informed	Managed
Analyzed	Collated	Demonstrated	Expanded	Initiated	Manufactured
Answered	Collected	Deposited	Expedited	Inspected	Marked
Applied	Commanded	Described	Experienced	Installed	Marketed
Appointed	Communicated	Detailed	Fabricated	Instructed	Measured
Appraised	Compiled	Determined	Facilitated	Insured	Met
Arranged	Completed	Developed	Figured	Integrated	Modified
Assembled	Composed	Devised	Filled	Interpreted	Monitored
Assessed	Computed	Diagnosed	Financed	Interviewed	Motivated
Assigned	Conducted	Directed	Finished	Introduced	Negotiated
Attached	Conferred	Discovered	Fitted	Inspected	Nominated
Attained	Constructed	Dismantled	Fixed	Inventoried	Noted
Attended	Consulted	Dispatched	Formalized	Investigated	Notified
Authorized	Contacted	Distributed	Formulated	Invoiced	Observed
Balanced	Contracted	Documented	Fulfilled	Issued	Obtained
Billed	Contrasted	Drew	Generated	Judged	Opened
Bought	Contributed	Drove	Graded	Justified	Operated
Budgeted	Controlled	Earned	Graphed	Kept	Ordered
Built	Converted	Educated	Greeted	Learned	Organized
Calculated	Convinced	Employed	Headed	Lectured	Outlined
Cashed	Coordinated	Encouraged	Hired	Led	
Catalogued	Copied	Engineered	Identified	Licensed	(continues)

Figure 36-3 These sample power verbs may help you define your previous job responsibilities.

Overcame	Priced	Ran	Related	Secured	Summarized
Packaged	Printed	Rated	Relayed	Selected	Supervised
Packed	Processed	Read	Renewed	Sent	Supplied
Paid	Procured	Rearranged	Reorganized	Separated	Taught
Participated	Produced	Rebuilt	Repaired	Served as	Telephoned
Patrolled	Programmed	Recalled	Replaced	Serviced	Tested
Perfected	Promoted	Received	Reported	Set up	Trained
Piloted	Prompted	Recommended	Requested	Showed	Transferred
Placed	Proofread	Reconciled	Researched	Sold	Transported
Planned	Proposed	Recorded	Responsible for	Solicited	Typed
Posted	Proved	Reduced	Retrieved	Sorted	Verified
Prepared	Provided	Referred	Revised	Stocked	
Prescribed	Published	Registered	Routed	Stored	
Presented	Purchased	Regulated	Scheduled	Straightened	

Figure 36-3 (continued)

References

Select a variety of **references** to be included with your résumé. References should be listed on a separate sheet of paper that matches your résumé. Remember to include the same letterhead as on your résumé on the references page. An individual who knows you or has worked with you long enough to make an honest assessment and recommendation regarding your background history is an excellent reference person. Use only nonrelated persons as references unless the work relationship has been formalized.

Choose references who are well-respected and are clear speakers and writers. No matter how much someone likes you and your work, they may not be helpful to you if they cannot convey the information in a business-like manner. Professional references such as a former instructor, physician, externship supervisor, or fellow coworkers are excellent reference choices.

Always ask permission to use someone as a reference *before* the name is printed on the reference list. You will want to verify the correct spelling of the reference's name, title, place of employment and position, and telephone number for prospective employers.

Help your references aid you in obtaining an interview and employment. A personal visit or telephone call to discuss your career objectives and how you plan to conduct your job search will be helpful. Ask for any suggestions they may have to offer. Provide them with a copy of your résumé and cover letter. This helps them visualize the position for which you are applying and picture how you may benefit that employer.

Keep in touch with references. Check back to see who has called and how things went. Knowing what employers ask may produce some valuable pointers for your next letter, résumé, or interview.

Finally, thank your references. They will appreciate knowing how you are doing and that you value their assistance.

Leave out "References Upon Request" if necessary to shorten your résumé to save space. Employers know they can ask for references at a later date.

Accuracy

Proofread, proofread, and proofread your résumé. Ask someone who is a good speller or your references to edit your résumé. Then proofread it again yourself. Do not rely on your computer spell check; it does not differentiate between words such as to, too, two or here and hear. Eliminate repetition of information such as task descriptions. Summarize employment before 10 years ago or leave it off entirely if not relevant to the position you are seeking.

Résumé Styles

Various résumé styles have been developed, each having specific résumé and disadvantages. You will want to choose the style or combination of styles that best describes your strengths and ability to do the job. It may be to your advantage to check with the human resources department of the facility to which you are applying to see if there is a résumé style preference.

Chronologic Résumé. Your **chronologic résumé** should be organized so the most important information you want to share is the first thing the reader sees. If your job experience is your greatest asset and may set you apart from other applicants, put your work history and job skills first. If your education and training is your best professional feature, put your education and training first. Some medical managers and human resources directors only take 10 seconds to scan

ASHLEY JACKSON, CMA
2031 Craig Street ~ Renton, Washington 98055

Work: 206-878-1545 Cell: 206-835-9879
Home: 253-838-6690 e-mail: asjack@pinetree.com

WORK EXPERIENCE

September, 1999-Present GROUP HEALTH COOPERATIVE
Directed support for a dermatology/surgery practice.
Patient preparation.
Medical and surgical asepsis.
Assist with sterile procedures.
Patient follow-up.

June, 1997-August, 1999 VALLEY INTERNAL MEDICINE
Clinical responsibilities.
Assisted with surgeries in ambulatory care setting.
Patient preparation.
Medical and surgical asepsis.
Assisted with sterile procedures.

March, 1997-June, 1997 VALLEY INTERNAL MEDICINE
Medical Assistant Externship
Administrative duties and clinical responsibilities utilizing all medical assisting skills, including patient induction, chief complaint, vital signs, patient preparation, EKGs, medical and surgical asepsis, and sterile procedures.

EDUCATION/CERTIFICATION

Associate in Applied Science degree, June, 1997, Highline Community College, Des Moines, Washington, 98198-9800.

Certified Medical Assistant, June, 1997.

Figure 36-4 Sample chronological résumé.

a résumé. You want them to see clearly and quickly what you have to offer.

The chronologic résumé is advantageous when:

- The position is in a highly traditional field, such as teaching, law, or health care, where specific employers are of paramount interest
- You are staying in the same field as prior jobs
- Job history shows real growth and development
- Prior titles are impressive

The chronologic résumé is *not* advantageous when:

- Your work history is spotty
- You are changing career goals
- You have been in the same job for many years
- You are looking for your first job

Figure 36-4 is an illustration of a chronologic résumé.

Functional Résumé. The **functional résumé** highlights specialty areas of accomplishment and strengths. It allows you to organize these in an order that supports your work objective.

The functional résumé is advantageous when:

- Your experience can be sorted into areas of function; i.e., administrative, clinical, supervisory
- You are changing careers

- You are reentering the job market after an absence
- Your career path or growth is not clear from a chronologic listing
- You have had a variety of different, apparently unconnected work experiences
- Much of your work has been volunteer, freelance, or temporary
- You want to eliminate repetition of descriptions of job duties
- You have extensive specialized experience

The functional résumé is *not* advantageous when:

- You want to emphasize a management growth pattern
- Your most recent employers have been highly prestigious and the specific employers are of paramount interest

A sample of a functional résumé for a person reentering the job market is shown in Figure 36-5.

Targeted Résumé. The **targeted résumé** is best for focusing on a clear, specific job target. It should contain a

JOAN BISHOP, RMA
4320 Sprig Street
Renton, Washington 98055

Work: 206-878-1545 | Cell: 206-835-9879
Home: 253-838-6690 | e-mail: jbishop@abc.net

TEACHING:

Instructed community groups on issues related to child abuse.

Taught volunteers how to set up community program for victims of domestic violence.

Conducted workshops for parents of abused children.

Instructed public school teachers on signs and symptoms of potential and actual child abuse.

COUNSELING:

Consulted with parents for probable child abuse and suggested courses of action.

Worked with social workers on individual cases, in both urban and suburban settings.

Counseled single parents on appropriate coping behaviors.

Handled pre-take interviewing of many individual abused children.

ORGANIZATION/COORDINATION:

Coordinated transition of children between original home and foster home.

Served as liaison between community health agencies and schools.

Wrote proposal to state for county funds to educate single parents and teachers.

WORK HISTORY:

1998–2000 Community Mental Health Center, Tacoma, Washington
Volunteer Coordinator—Child Abuse Program

2000–2003 C.A.R.E.—Child-Abuse Rescue-Education, Trenton, New Jersey
County Representative

EDUCATION:

1998 B.S. Sociology, Douglass College, New Brunswick, New Jersey

Figure 36-5 Sample functional résumé; this style is useful for a person reentering the job market.

career objective and list your skills, capabilities, and any supporting accomplishments related to that objective. Graduating students will find this résumé style enables them to list classes related to their career objective, grade point average, student awards, and achievements. This information adds substance to a résumé when work experience is minimal and should be at the beginning of the résumé because it is your most significant asset.

The targeted résumé is advantageous when:

- You are very clear about your job target
- You have had a variety of experiences that appear unrelated to each other, but that include skills that you can use in a skills list related to your job target
- You can go in several directions and want a different résumé for each
- You are just starting your career and have little experience, but know what you want and are clear about your capabilities
- You are able to keep your résumé on a computer disk

The targeted résumé is *not* advantageous when:

- You want to use one résumé for several different applications
- You are not clear about your abilities and accomplishments

Figure 36-6 provides a sample of a targeted résumé.

ASHLEY JACKSON, CMA
2031 Craig Street ~ Renton, Washington 98055

Work: 206-878-1545 Cell: 206-835-9879
Home: 253-838-6690 e-mail: asjack@pinetree.com

CAREER OBJECTIVES: To obtain a challenging position as a medical assistant in an ambulatory care/surgery facility.

ACHIEVEMENTS:
Certified Medical Assistant.
Graduate of an Accredited Medical Assistant Program.
Experienced in providing assistance with surgeries in an ambulatory care setting.
Excellent communication and interpersonal skills.

SKILLS AND CAPABILITIES:
Post-surgery patient follow-up.
Patient induction.
Vital Signs.
Patient preparation.
EKGs.
Medical and surgical asepsis.
Sterile procedures.

WORK HISTORY:

September, 1996 to present	Group Health Cooperative, Seattle, WA Surgical Medical Assistant.
June, 1994-August, 1996	Valley Internal Medicine, Renton, WA Clinical Medical Assistant.
March 1994-June, 1994	Valley Internal Medicine, Renton, WA Externship Student/Trainee.

EDUCATION/CERTIFICATION:
Associate in Applied Science Degree, Highline Community College.
Certified Medical Assistant.

AFFILIATIONS:
American Association of Medical Assistants.

Figure 36-6 Sample targeted résumé; this style is useful when focusing on a specific job target.

E-Résumé. An electronic résumé, also known as an **e-résumé,** may be electronically delivered via e-mail, submitted to Internet job boards, or placed on Web pages. When employers post jobs on their own Web sites, they generally expect job seekers to respond electronically.

Special care must be taken when preparing the e-résumé because many employers place résumés directly into searchable databases. The following are some points to consider:

- Formatting must be removed before the résumé can be placed in a database. Submitting a formatted résumé may cause it to be eliminated.
- Submit a text résumé, also known as a text-based résumé, plain-text résumé, or ASCII text résumé. These variations are preferred when submitting résumés electronically.
- The e-résumé is not visually appealing. Eye appeal is not required because its main purpose is to be placed into one of the keyword-searchable databases.
- The text résumé is not vulnerable to viruses and is compatible across computer programs and platforms.
- The text résumé is versatile and may be used for:
  - Posting on job boards
  - Pasting piece-by-piece into the profile forms of job boards, such as Monster.com
  - Pasting into the body of an e-mail to be sent to prospective employers
  - Converting to a Web-based HTML résumé
  - Sending as an attachment to prospective employers
  - Conversion to a scannable résumé

Employers are often inundated with résumés from job seekers each time they advertise a position opening. Therefore, in an effort to save time and to determine the best-qualified candidates for the position, employers digitize the résumés to create an electronic résumé. Using software to search for specific **keywords** that relate to the position, the numbers of candidates can quickly be narrowed. If you apply for a job with a company that searches databases for keywords and your résumé does not conform, you may not be considered for the position.

How do you determine keywords? Begin scrutinizing employment ads and list keywords repeatedly mentioned in association with jobs that interest you. Nouns that relate to the skills and experience the employer is looking for will quickly surface. Keywords may include:

- Job specific skills/profession-specific words (e.g., specialty experience, bilingual, scheduling, data entry, insurance verification, telephone and communication skills, laboratory/X-ray experience)
- Technologic terms and descriptions of technical expertise (including hardware and software in which you are proficient; e.g., PRISM, DEXA experience)
- Job titles, certifications (e.g., MA, CMA, RMA, CMAS, Biller, Coder)
- Types of degrees, names of colleges (e.g., AAS, BA)
- Awards received, professional organization memberships (e.g., Dean's list, scholarships, certificates, AAMA or AMT member)

Keywords should be used throughout the résumé, however it should be front loaded. Front loaded means to use as many keywords as possible in the first 100 words of the résumé. A good goal is to aim for 25 to 35 keywords. This may be achieved by using synonyms, various forms of the keyword, and using both the spelled-out and acronym versions of common terms. If a person reviews the résumé, he or she will see enough keywords to process it through the software search.

Vital Résumé Information

All résumé styles must contain certain vital information about the job applicant. Essential information includes:

- Your full name and credential, address including street number, city, state, and zip code.
- Your telephone number or a number where a message may be left. The telephone selected should be one you are confident will be answered in a professional manner. Always include the area code with the number.
- Your e-mail address.
- Your education. Begin with the most recent school attended and include the name, address, and graduation date with the diploma, certificate, or degree earned.
- Work experience. List company name and address. Do not underestimate the value of any job; relate transferable skills to your career objective.

- Skills that are necessary for the job. The list may be completed from your program curriculum. Be careful not to list course titles that have no meaning to the reader. It is much better to list the skills obtained in courses.

APPLICATION/COVER LETTERS

The **application/cover letter** is a means of introducing yourself and submitting your résumé to a potential employer with the goal of obtaining an interview. A well-written cover letter will highlight your qualifications and experience for employment and will enhance the information contained within your résumé. The letter should follow a standard business style and should not be more than one page in length. It should be printed on the same paper as the résumé.

Because this may be your first contact with a potential employer, the letter should sell you and describe your intentions regarding employment, display your personality, and create an interest in reading your enclosed résumé.

Some guidelines to follow in writing the application/cover letter include:

1. Address your letter to a specific individual whenever possible. You may need to make a telephone call to obtain the name, title, and correct spelling.
2. Keep the letter concise, use correct grammar and spelling, and follow standard business letter format.
3. The first paragraph should state your reason for writing and focus the reader's attention. It should not give as a reason "in response to a help wanted ad."
4. The second paragraph should identify how your education, experience, and qualifications relate to the job and refer to the enclosed résumé.
5. The last paragraph should close with a request for an interview.
6. Do not reproduce cover letters. An original letter should be sent to each individual.
7. The cover letter should be placed on top of the résumé and mailed in a business size envelope that matches its contents or in an $8\frac{1}{2} \times 11$ manila envelope containing your return address.
8. Do not staple the cover letter to the résumé.

A sample of an application/cover letter is shown in Figure 36-7A.

An alternate example of an application/cover letter using Information Mapping® to highlight and draw attention to specific information in your letter is shown in Figure 36-7B. This format is considered easier to read because the focus is on specific blocks of information. In addition, its uniqueness draws attention to your letter and may result in your being selected when competition is keen.

COMPLETING THE APPLICATION FORM

Sooner or later during the job search you will be asked to complete an **application form.** How well you complete this task may be a key factor in obtaining an interview and that first job.

Reading through the application form questions, you may be tempted to write in "See résumé" rather than repeat pertinent information already contained within your résumé. Do not fall into this pitfall. Answer every item completely. The application is organized in the manner that suites the clinic, whereas individual résumés are organized in a variety of ways. Finding specific information on a résumé is more time consuming for the clinic, whereas finding the same information on the job application is easy and quick because they know where to look for it. Read all the directions carefully. Look for seemingly insignificant directions placed at the top or-bottom of the page that state "Print Carefully," "Complete in Your Own Handwriting," or "Please Type." Employers may use this to assess your ability to read and follow directions and pay attention to detail.

If the application is to be handwritten, use black ink to complete the form. Black ink is considered legal and often is an indelible (permanent) ink and is more legible if the form must be duplicated. Concentrate when completing the form and be sure to print clearly and make no errors. When possible, copy the application before beginning in case an error is made.

The current trend is toward on-line application forms. These forms are prepared by keying information into the appropriate spaces or blocks by using a computer. The completed forms may then be printed and mailed to the perspective employer or sent electronically. Sending electronically is increasingly the preferred method. All of the concerns relative to care in following instructions, providing complete and accurate information, and proofing the application for any errors before sending are applicable.

If you are asked to list experience but the application does not specify "paid experience," be sure to list any volunteer or externship experience that relates to the position you are seeking. Part-time employment can be important as an indicator of your willingness to work, your ability to serve the public, and your organizational skills.

You may be asked to complete the application form "on the spot." Plan ahead for this event and

2031 Craig Street
Renton, Washington 98055
August 22, 20XX

Sarah Molles, Manager
Seattle Group Health Cooperative
304 Fourth Avenue
Seattle, Washington 98124-1716

Dear Ms. Molles:

I am interested in the medical assistant position to assist in a dermatology surgery practice. I meet the qualifications and would like to be considered for the position.

I am currently a certified medical assistant graduated from a two-year accredited program. I have experience as a clinical assistant in an internal medicine clinic and have excellent communication and interpersonal skills.

I will be available Tuesday and Thursday afternoon from 1:00 p.m. to 4:00 p.m. I will call you next Thursday to set up an appointment for an interview.

Yours truly,

Ashley Jackson, CMA

Enclosure, Résumé

Figure 36-7A Sample application/cover letter.

carry a completed copy of your résumé, reference list, and application/cover letter with you. Information not included in your résumé, such as which years you attended high school and your salary history, should also be carried with you. These documents should provide all the information needed to complete the application form and may be submitted with the application form. This demonstrates to the potential employer your seriousness and preparedness for finding a job.

THE INTERVIEW PROCESS

If your application/cover letter, résumé, and application have made a favorable impression with the organization, you may be invited for an interview. An **interview** is a meeting in which you and the interviewer discuss the employment opportunities within that particular organization. It will be the interviewer's responsibility to determine if you have the personality, education, and skills to perform the job. The interviewer will use the interview process to access appearance, attitude, and dependability. They will also try to verify that you have been honest in the skills you claim to have mastered. You, on the other hand, will be selling your qualifications and assessing if this is an organization in which you want to be employed.

Being well prepared for the interview will increase your self-confidence and ability to focus during the actual interview. Knowing that your application/cover letter, résumé, and references all support your career goal and objectives allows you time to concentrate on interview preparation and presentation.

2031 Craig Street
Renton, Washington 98055
August 22, 2005

Sarah Molles, Manager
Seattle Group Health Cooperative
304 Fourth Avenue
Seattle, Washington 98124-1716

SUBJECT: SURGICAL MEDICAL ASSISTANT POSITION

Background	I am interested in the medical assistant position to assist in a dermatology surgery practice. I meet the qualifications and would like to be considered for the position.
Qualifications	I am currently a certified medical assistant graduated from a two-year accredited program. I have experience as a clinical assistant in an internal medicine clinic and have excellent communication and interpersonal skills.
Requested Action	I will be available Tuesday and Thursday afternoon from 1:00 p.m. to 4:00 p.m. I will call you next Thursday to set up an appointment for an interview.

Yours truly,

Ashley Jackson, CMA

Enclosure, Résumé

Figure 36-7B Sample information mapped letter.

The Look of Success

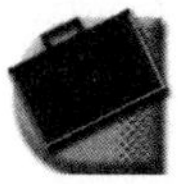

The look of success begins with the outward appearance. First impressions are lasting, so strive for a favorable, professional look from head to toe. Appropriate conservative attire is important. Remember, your goal is to sell your professional abilities.

Hair should be clean, and healthy looking, and worn in an appropriate style for the ambulatory care setting. Long hair should be worn off the collar in perhaps a French braid or twist. Strive for a neat, professional style.

The skin should have a healthy glow. Consultation with a cosmetician may prove helpful in solving skin problems or provide opportunity for trying new products. A basic understanding of your personal skin type and selection of cosmetics that complement your skin tone aid in the presentation of a professional appearance. The natural look is most appropriate for the medical office.

A daily shower and use of personal hygiene products is advised. Remember to use caution where perfumes and scents are concerned because many magnify when the body is under stress and the scent may be offensive or cause allergic reactions in others. Smokers should be aware that smoke odor carries in their hair, skin, and clothing. This odor may not be accaptable in health care settings.

Fingernails should be short and oval shaped or have rounded corners. Only clear nail polish should be worn in the ambulatory care setting if you are not working in the clinical area. Nail polish that is chipped or cracked must be removed or replaced immediately because it creates crevices in which pathogens may hide, multiply, and spread.

First impressions are lasting, so make yours professional in all respects. Conservative business attire is appropriate. A tailored suit for both men and women is effective in portraying a professional image. Pay attention to details such as your accessories and shoe selection. Accessories should be small and tasteful. Shoes should be clean, polished, and in good repair. They should fit properly and be comfortable and easy to walk in (Figure 36-8).

The purse should be neat and small; the briefcase should be of a slip-in type that does not require a flat surface to open. Both should be in good repair. A portfolio is recommended in which to keep an extra copy of your résumé, reference list, application, and cover letter. A pen should be handy. Do not plan to search in either a purse or a briefcase for a pen or papers, keys, and so forth. Also, be sure that your cell phone has been turned off before entering the clinic.

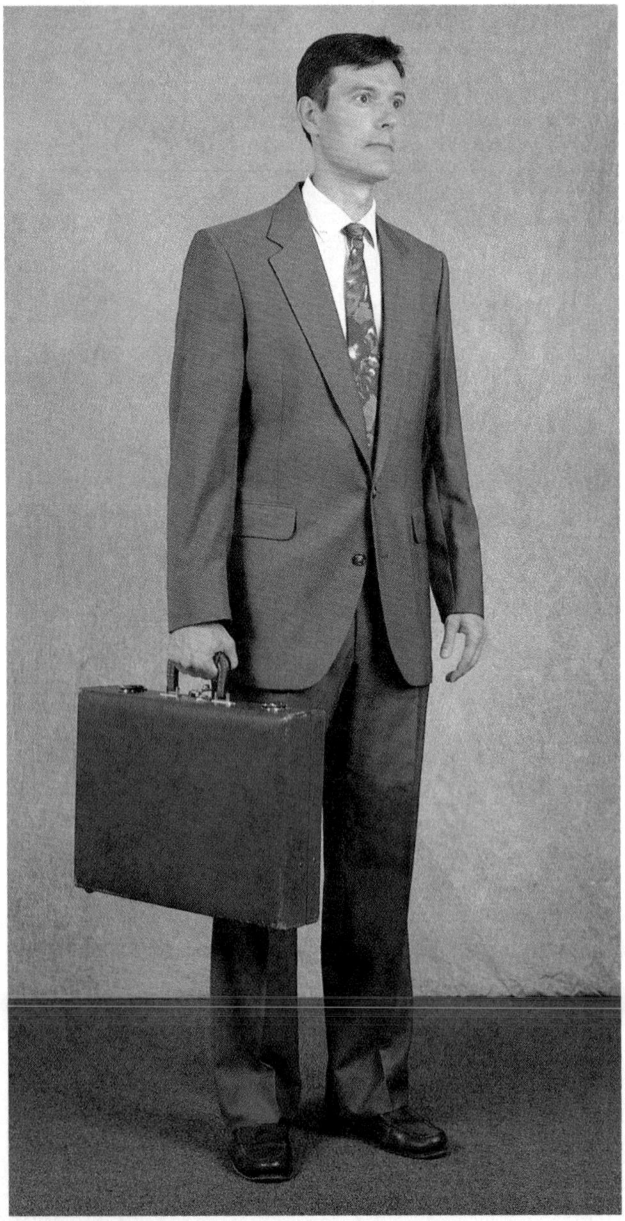

Figure 36-8 Medical assistant appropriately dressed and prepared for the interview.

Critical Thinking

If you are a smoker, how can you minimize the smoke odor carried on your person before you go on a job interview? Make a list and prioritize each suggestion into a plan of action.

When you feel well and know that you look good, you project a confident and professional appearance. In other words, you are professionally poised. Webster's dictionary defines *poise* as balance and stability; ease and dignity of manner. Personal poise combines all of the previously mentioned body appearances plus smoothness of movement and physical flexibility.

Preparing for the Interview

Before the interview takes place, you will want to study carefully the organization for which you are interviewing. Be prepared to relate your skills and interests to the needs of this organization. In other words, what can you contribute and why should they hire you? The interview is your opportunity to sell yourself and identify ways in which you can benefit the employer.

A copy of your résumé and cover letter should be brought to the interview just in case the interviewer can not locate the original or wants another copy. You should also have copies of letters of recommendation, a list of references, a copy of your transcript from the schools you attended, and copies of any certificates such as AIDS training, First Aid, and CPR. These items should not be presented unless dictated by events that take place during the interview. You might also have with you the name of the interviewer and a copy of any questions you plan to ask the interviewer. A last-minute review will refocus your thoughts before you go into the interview. You could also keep your list available for quick reference in the event that your mind goes blank when you are asked if you have questions.

To arrive 5 to 10 minutes early, you may need to check a map for directions or make a trip the day before your interview. Try to travel about the same time as you would for the interview so you have an idea of the time it takes, traffic flow, construction areas encountered, and parking availability. Plan for inclement weather (raincoat, umbrella, shoes, and so forth). It is a good idea to make a quick trip to the restroom on arrival to change shoes or recheck your appearance.

Introduce yourself confidently to the receptionist and identify by name the person you wish to see and the time of your appointment. Always arrive alone. The employer wants to see you and sense your self-reliance and responsibility. While you wait, try to relax and observe the office setting, other employees, what they are wearing, and their manner of conducting business. This may be helpful to you during the interview and in making a decision to work there.

Review Figure 36-9 for reasons employers do not hire applicants.

The Actual Interview

When you enter an interviewer's office, think of yourself as a guest and take your cues from him or her. Most interviewers will introduce themselves and extend a hand. A firm handshake, responding by introducing yourself, and smiling confidently convey a positive professional image. Remain standing until you are invited to be seated. Keep your personal items on your lap or place them on the floor near your chair. Do not invade the interviewer's territory by placing your things on the desk.

Sit erect in the chair with your feet flat on the floor or cross only your ankles. Avoid nervous mannerisms while you speak and maintain good eye contact, but do not stare the interviewer down. Be natural and positive about the position, organization, and yourself. Present a professional image by using medical terminology when responding to questions or providing information. Observe the interviewer carefully for cues. Respond to questions completely, trying not to repeat yourself or give more information than was requested.

Be prepared for the kinds of questions that may be asked during the interview process. Ask yourself, "If I were the employer, what would I want to know about the applicant?" Figure 36-10 contains examples of standard questions asked by most employers. Consider how you would respond to each question.

Remember that the interviewer is asking questions to determine if you are qualified for the position and if

REASONS FOR EMPLOYERS NOT HIRING

Employers in business were asked to list reasons for not hiring a job seeker. Given in rank order (from most unwanted to least unwanted), the 15 biggest gripes are as follows:

1. Poor appearance (not dressed properly, poorly groomed).
2. Acting like a know-it-all.
3. Cannot express self clearly; poor voice, diction, grammar.
4. Lack of planning for work—no purpose or goals.
5. Lack of confidence or poise.
6. No interest in or enthusiasm for the job.
7. Not active in school extracurricular programs.
8. Interested only in the best dollar offer.
9. Poor school record (academic, attendance).
10. Unwilling to start at the bottom.
11. Making excuses, hedges on unfavorable record.
12. No tact.
13. Not mature.
14. No curiosity about the job.
15. Critical of past employers.

Figure 36-9 Reasons for employers not hiring. (Courtesy of Highline Community College, Counseling/Career Center, Des Moines, WA).

TYPICAL QUESTIONS ASKED DURING AN INTERVIEW

1. I see from your résumé you graduated from ______________ college. What did that college have to offer that others didn't?
2. What subjects did you enjoy the most and why?
3. What do you see yourself doing five years from now?
4. What salary do you expect and what do you think it will be in five or ten years?
5. What do you consider to be your greatest strengths and weaknesses?
6. How do you think a friend or professor who knows you well would describe you?
7. What qualifications do you have that make you think you would be successful in this position?
8. In what ways do you think you can make a contribution to our organization?
9. What two or three accomplishments have given you the most satisfaction?
10. What didn't you like about your last employer?
11. How well do you work under pressure?
12. Will you be able to work overtime occasionally?
13. How do you respond to criticism?
14. How would you respond if a patient or co-worker made advances toward you?
15. How would you handle following procedures with which you do not agree?
16. Describe a specific medical procedure.
17. Do you have any questions you would like to ask?

Figure 36-10 Knowing how you would answer some of these typical questions can prepare you for your interview.

you are the kind of person that will fit into the organization. *Think* before answering questions; try to provide the information requested in a positive and professional manner. *Listen* carefully so that you understand what information the question is requesting. *Ask* for clarification if you are uncertain. This demonstrates your ability to be open enough to ask questions when in doubt.

Closing the Interview

By observing the interviewer and listening carefully, you will be able to determine when the interviewer feels he or she has enough information about you to make a decision. Usually during the closing the interviewer will ask if you have any additional questions. This is your opportunity to collect information helpful in making a decision to accept or decline an offer. Your questions provide another opportunity to sell yourself, show that you have done your homework about the organization, and have listened carefully during the interview. Select three or four questions that will help you the most.

Questions about the organization are excellent choices. Examples might be:

- "What are the opportunities for advancement with this organization?"
- "I read that your organization has educational benefits. Could you explain briefly how that program works?"
- "You mentioned in-house training programs for employees. Could you give one or two examples?"

You may also have some questions about the job itself. Examples of these types of questions are:

- "Is this a newly created position? If so, what results are you hoping to see?"
- "Was the last person in this position promoted? What contributed to their advancement?"
- "What do you consider the most difficult task on this job?"
- "What are the lines of authority for this position?"

Do not use this question time to ask about salary, sick leave, vacations, or retirement benefits. At this point, your focus should be on the value and skills you can contribute to the organization. These questions may be asked during a second interview or when a position is offered.

Before you leave, thank the interviewer for taking time to discuss the position with you. If you definitely are interested in the position, ask to be considered as a candidate for the position. If follow-up procedures have not been explained, now is the time to ask when the final selection will be made and how you will be notified. A firm handshake as you leave, a pleasant smile, and confidence as you exit will leave a professional picture in the interviewer's mind.

INTERVIEW FOLLOW-UP

Following up after the interview is essential. This is the time to telephone your references to let them know the name of the organization and the person's name with whom you interviewed, something about the position, and your qualifications. Share any information that will help your references support you in obtaining the position.

Follow-Up Letter

Take time to write a follow-up letter or handwritten note to the interviewer a day or two after your interview to thank them for the time spent interviewing you. The letter should be written in standard business format and printed on the same paper as your application/cover letter and résumé. Be sure that all spelling and grammar are correct.

The follow-up letter provides another opportunity to express your interest in the organization and the position. You can briefly emphasize the experience and skills you have to offer and again request being considered a candidate for the position.

Record the mailing date on your contact tracker and keep a copy of the letter in a file with other information about the organization. Figure 36-11 is a sample follow-up letter.

Follow Up by Telephone

Allow a few days for your follow-up letter to reach the interviewer. If you do not hear from the interviewer within a week or by the designated time established during the interview, you may telephone to ask if you are still being considered for the position or if a decision has been made.

Speak directly into the mouthpiece of the telephone using good diction and voice volume. Identify yourself and provide some information to aid the interviewer in recalling who you are. Perhaps mentioning the date you interviewed will suffice. Be polite and professional and remember to thank the individual for speaking with you. At the end of the conversation say good-bye and wait until the other person hangs up before you break the connection. Log the telephone call and its response on your contact tracker for future reference.

2031 Craig Street
Renton, Washington 98055
August 28, 20XX

Sarah Molles, Manager
Seattle Group Health Cooperative
304 Fourth Avenue
Seattle, Washington 98124-1716

Dear Ms. Molles,

Thank you for scheduling a personal interview with me last Wednesday, August 26, at 9:45 AM. I enjoyed discussing the medical assistant position open in one of your dermatology surgery practices. I would like to be considered for the position.

After talking with you, I feel my qualifications match closely with those you requested. My communication and interpersonal skills are excellent and a necessary ingredient for any medical assistant.

I look forward to hearing from you September 5 as you mentioned during the interview. If there are any questions I may answer, please telephone me.

Sincerely,

Ashley Jackson

Ashley Jackson, CMA
(206) 255-1365

Figure 36-11 Sample follow-up letter.

PROFESSIONALISM AND EMPLOYMENT STRATEGIES

Areas of professionalism directly related to the medical office may include:

- Display a professional manner and image. The chapter content stresses the importance of having a positive attitude, taking pride in doing the best you can, being prepared, and dressing appropriately for job interviews.
- Promote your CMA/RMA or CMAS credential. On graduation from an accredited school, you will be ready to sit for the national certification examination. On notification of passing the examination, you will be awarded the appropriate credential. When signing your name, include your credential as well and educate others regarding its significance.

Critical Thinking

As you begin to prepare for a job interview, how can you prepare yourself to reflect a professional image, attitude, demeanor, verbal and nonverbal communication skills, as well as articulately describe your skills and abilities to fit the position to which you are applying? Develop a complete written checklist and review it before an interview.

Case Study 36-1

Eun Mee Soo is a recent graduate of an accredited medical assisting program and has no medical work experience except her externship at Inner City Health Care. Eun Mee has been employed part-time as a sales representative (clerk) in one of the city's prestigious clothing stores while she attended school.

CASE STUDY REVIEW

1. Which résumé style would represent Eun Mee best and why?
2. What information should Eun Mee provide in the vital information section of the résumé?
3. What is the purpose of an accomplishment statement? Provide an example of one that Eun Mee might use.

Case Study 36-2

Drs. Lewis and King maintain a two-doctor family physicians' office. They are in need of a new medical assistant to take the place of one who will be leaving at the end of the month. They have established interviews with five applicants. Eun Mee Soo is the first candidate to be interviewed.

CASE STUDY REVIEW

1. Eun Mee enters the interview with some papers in her hand. What paperwork should she have brought with her?
2. Why should Eun Mee arrive 5 to 10 minutes early for the interview?
3. How should Eun Mee enter the room?

SUMMARY

Finding your first job is your first job. How well you research, plan, prepare, and implement your tasks will make the difference between being hired or not being hired. Learn from each interview session. Listen to the questions that were asked and formulate answers that you feel would be appropriate for your next interview. Tell everyone you are looking for a job and solicit their help. Follow up on all leads and do not become discouraged.

Once you have been hired at that first job, continue your learning experience. Ask appropriate questions and try not to ask the same question a second or third time. Pay attention to details and learn individual preferences. Become a team player and look for ways you can help others. Carry your share of responsibility and do not be afraid to admit you are unfamiliar with certain aspects of the office. Employers need to know you can be trusted to work within the scope of your education and not beyond. Practice being an asset to your employer.

STUDY FOR SUCCESS

To reinforce your knowledge and skills of information presented in this chapter:

- ❑ Review the Key Terms
- ❑ Consider the Case Studies and discuss your conclusions
- ❑ Answer the Review Questions
  - ❑ Multiple Choice
  - ❑ Critical Thinking
- ❑ Navigate the Internet by completing the Web Activities
- ❑ Practice the StudyWARE activities on the textbook CD
- ❑ Apply your knowledge in the Student Workbook activities
- ❑ Complete the Web Tutor sections
- ❑ View and discuss the DVD situations

REVIEW QUESTIONS

Multiple Choice

1. The résumé:
   a. is a summary data sheet or brief account of your qualifications and progress in your career
   b. is also known as a contact tracker
   c. always includes references
   d. is used to introduce yourself and identify qualifications
2. References:
   a. must always be listed on the résumé
   b. should be a relative
   c. should be someone who likes you and your work but may not be a good communicator
   d. should be someone who knows you or has worked with you long enough to make an honest assessment of your capabilities and integrity
3. The targeted résumé is advantageous:
   a. when prior titles are impressive
   b. when reentering the job market after an absence
   c. when you are just starting your career and have little experience
   d. when you have extensive specialized experience
4. The application/cover letter is:
   a. a detailed data sheet describing your vital information, education, and experience
   b. introduces you to a prospective employer and captures their interest in you as a candidate for the position
   c. lists individuals who can vouch for you
   d. should be lengthy and detailed

5. The interview:
   a. does not require much thought or preparation
   b. requires you to think before answering questions, listen carefully, and ask for clarification if uncertain of the question
   c. provides time to ask questions about salary, vacation, and benefits
   d. does not require any follow-up
6. Preparing for the interview:
   a. bathe yourself, groom your hair and fingernails, and wear clean and pressed conservative business attire
   b. allow adequate time to get to the interview
   c. prepare a packet to give the interviewer containing certificates, letters of recommendation, a list of references, and your list of questions
   d. a, b, and c
7. Job analysis should include:
   a. compiling a list of potential employers
   b. gathering information about employers in whom you have interest
   c. preparing a budgetary needs analysis
   d. all of the above
8. The best source for job search data is:
   a. the Internet
   b. friends and acquaintances
   c. the yellow pages and classified ads
   d. all of the above

Critical Thinking

1. Discuss the various résumé styles with a classmate and how to determine which style will best present your knowledge and skills to a prospective employer?
2. After reading the section discussing methods of researching a prospective employer, how will you proceed with your research?
3. Review Figure 36-9, which lists reasons for employers not hiring, with a classmate. How will you prevent the 15 biggest gripes from being an employment stumbling block for you personally?
4. How will you prepare a budget for living expenses to determine job salary requirements?
5. Sometimes employers may ask illegal or inappropriate questions during an interview in true innocence, or true ignorance. Give a legal reason why an employer might need the following information once you have been hired.
   a. Are you married?
   b. How many kids do you have?
   c. How old are you?
   d. Where were you born?

WEB ACTIVITIES

1. Being prepared to answer and discuss interview questions is critical in the selection for the position opening. Using Google.com, or your favorite search engine, search job interview questions. Many sites will provide sample questions and appropriate answers. Study these and prepare a list of questions with personal responses you feel are appropriate.
2. There are some illegal interview questions based on Federal Discrimination Laws enforced by the Equal Employment Opportunity Commission. They are questions that specifically discriminate against you on the basis of:
   - Age
   - Color
   - Disability
   - Sex
   - National origin
   - Race, religion, or creed

   Using your favorite search engine, research these inappropriate questions and ways in which you might handle them appropriately. Compile a list of questions and your personal appropriate response to each. Discuss these with a classmate and role-play responding to the questions.

REFERENCES/BIBLIOGRAPHY

Farr, M. (2000). *Quick resume & cover letter book*. Indianapolis, IN: JIST Works, Inc.

Noble, D. F. (2000). *Gallery of best resumes for people without a four-year degree*. Indianapolis, IN: JIST Works, Inc.

Washington, T. (2000). *Resume power selling yourself on paper in the new millennium*. Indianapolis, IN: JIST Works, Inc.

THE DVD HOOK-UP

DVD Series
Critical Thinking

Program Number
1

Chapter/Scene Reference
- *Preparing for a Job*

This chapter discusses strategies that you can use to help gain employment.

One of the first testimonials in this scene showed Paula talking about the fact that she can determine a person's professionalism within five minutes of the interview.

1. Do you really think that it is possible to gauge a person's professionalism within five minutes of an interview?
2. What do you think about the outfit that Dee was wearing for her interview? Do you think it was professional?
3. What will you wear for your interviews when you apply for a medical assisting position?

DVD Journal Summary
Write a paragraph that summarizes what you learned from watching the selected scenes from today's DVD program. Using a scale of 1 to 10, how would you have rated your professionalism skills when you started the program? How would you rate your professional skills now that you have almost completed with the program? What improvements do you need to make to be the best possible medical assistant you can be?

Glossary of Terms

abduction motion away from the midline of the body (Ch. 21).

ABO blood group genetically determined system of antigens found on the surface of erythrocytes. The population can be divided into four ABO blood groups: A, B, AB, and O (Ch. 32).

abortion expulsion of the products of conception before viability (Ch. 14).

abuse misuse; excessive or improper use, especially of narcotics or psychoactive drugs (Ch. 35).

accomplishment statements statements that begin with a power verb and give a brief description of what you did, and the demonstrable results that were produced (Ch. 36).

accreditation process whereby recognition is granted to an educational program for maintaining standards that qualify its graduates for professional practice; to provide with credentials (Ch. 1).

Accrediting Bureau of Health Education Schools (ABHES) entity accrediting institutions for the American Medical Technologists (Ch. 35).

Acetest® product used to test for the presence of abnormal amounts of acetone (ketones) in urine (Ch. 30).

acetone colorless, inflammable liquid. Found in the blood and urine of diabetics as a result of the breakdown of fatty acids (Ch. 26).

acid/base balance condition that occurs when the net rate at which the body produces acids or bases is equal to the net rate at which acids or bases are excreted (Ch. 30).

acquired immunodeficiency syndrome (AIDS) disorder of the immune system caused by a human immunodeficiency virus (HIV), a retrovirus that destroys the body's ability to fight infection. As the disease progresses, the individual becomes overcome by disorders, including cancers and opportunistic infections. There is no known cure for AIDS (Ch. 10).

active listening received message is paraphrased back to the sender to verify the correct message was decoded (Ch. 4).

activities of daily living (ADL) activities usually performed during a typical day that involve caring for oneself, such as eating and brushing teeth (Ch. 21).

acupuncture treatment to relieve pain and disease by puncturing the skin with thin needles at specific points (Ch. 2).

acyclovir antiviral drug used in some herpes infections (Ch. 10).

additive any material placed in a tube that maintains or facilitates the integrity and function of the specimen (Ch. 28).

adduction motion toward the midline of the body (Ch. 21).

administer to give a medication (Ch. 7, 23, 24).

administrative law establishes agencies that are given the power to make laws and enact regulations (Ch. 7).

aegis sponsorship or protection (Ch. 26).

aerobic organism that requires oxygen for growth (Ch. 31).

aerosols particles from potentially infectious materials that may be released in the air (Ch. 31).

afebrile without fever (Ch. 12).

agar a gelatin-like substance extracted from red algae that contains nutrients and moisture for bacteria growth (Ch. 31).

agenda printed list of topics to be discussed during a meeting, sometimes giving time allocation (Ch. 33).

agent person representing another (Ch. 7).

agglutination antigen–antibody reaction in which a solid antigen clumps with a solid antibody (Ch. 32).

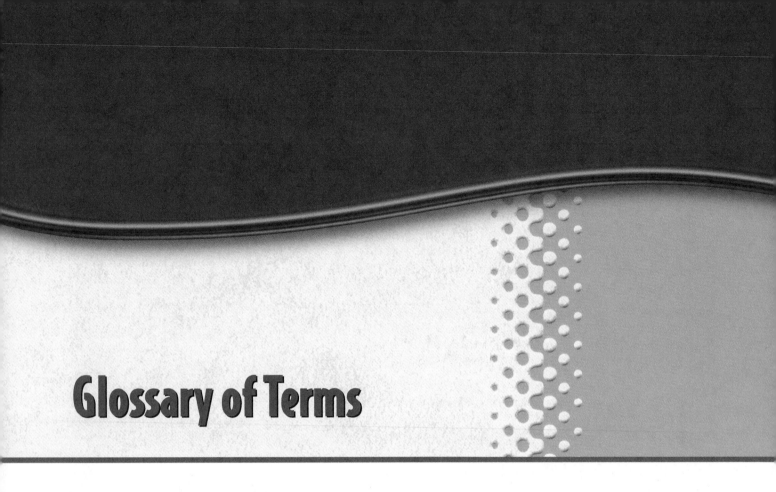

airborne transmission spread of disease-causing microorganisms over long distances through the air (Ch. 10).

alimentary canal digestive tract, made up of all the organs through which food passes throughout the body, from mouth to anus (Ch. 18).

aliquot part of the whole specimen that has been taken off for use or storage (Ch. 28).

allergen any substance that causes signs of allergy; examples are inhalants such as dust, pollen, foods such as wheat and strawberries, drugs, penicillin, chemicals, heat, bacteria (Ch. 18).

allergy acquired hypersensitivity to a substance (allergen) that does not normally cause a reaction (Ch. 11, 19).

allopathic method of treating disease with remedies that produce effects different from those caused by the disease itself. Most traditional physicians today are considered allopathic physicians (Ch. 3).

alternative dispute resolution (ADR) an alternative to trial that encourages the parties to settle their differences out of court (Ch. 7).

alveoli air sacs of the lungs that exchange carbon dioxide and oxygen (Ch. 18).

amblyopia disorder of the eye characterized by dimness of vision (Ch. 18).

Ambu Bag™ a brand name for a bag placed over nose and mouth to assist in providing artificial ventilation to the lungs (Ch. 9).

ambulation ability to walk (Ch. 21).

ambulatory care setting health care environment where services are provided on an outpatient basis. Ambulatory is from the Latin and means "capable of walking." Examples include the solo-physician's office, the group practice, the urgent care center, and the health maintenance organization (Ch. 1, 2).

American Association of Medical Assistants (AAMA) professional organization dedicated to serving the interests of Certified Medical Assistants (Ch. 35).

American Medical Technologists (AMT) national organization which certifies health care professionals, including Registered Medical Assistants and Certified Medical Administrative Specialists (Ch. 35).

amino acid basic structural unit of protein (Ch. 22).

amniocentesis surgical puncture of the amniotic sac to remove fluid for laboratory analysis (Ch. 10, 14).

amniotomy artificial rupture of the amniotic sac (Ch. 14).

amoebic dysentery infectious intestinal disease caused by amebas and characterized by inflammation of the mucous membrane of the colon (Ch. 10).

amorphous shapeless; possessing no definite form (Ch. 30).

amplified made larger or enlarged. The amplifier of the electrocardiograph enlarges the electrical impulse activity and the recording can be read more easily (Ch. 25).

amplitude amount, extent, size abundance, or fullness (Ch. 25).

Amsler grid a grid of lines used in testing for macular degeneration (Ch. 18).

anaerobic organism that needs little or no oxygen for growth (Ch. 31).

anaphylaxis hypersensitive state of the body to a foreign protein or drug (Ch. 9, 23).

ancillary services professional occupational companies hired to complete a specific job (Ch. 33).

andropause midlife changes in a male (Ch. 17).

anesthesia loss of feeling or sensation; an anesthetic is any mechanism that causes anesthesia (Ch. 19).

angiogram series of X-rays of a blood vessel(s) after injection of a radiopaque substance (Ch. 25).

anisocytosis marked variation in the size of cells (Ch. 29).

anorexia loss of appetite (Ch. 10).

antibacterial capable of destroying bacteria, often applied to a wound in the form of an ointment or cream (Ch. 19).

antibody specific chemical produced by B cells of the immune system in response to an antigen (Ch. 10, 32).

anticoagulant chemical in a blood tube that prevents the clotting of the blood by removing the calcium from the blood or by stopping the formation of thrombin (Ch. 28).

antigen substance such as bacteria or other agents that the body recognizes as foreign; the stimulus for antibody production (Ch. 10, 22).

antioxidant something that prevents oxidation (Ch. 22).

antiserum serum containing antibodies (Ch. 32).

aphasia inability to communicate through speech or other methods. Often caused by brain dysfunction (Ch. 18).

apical pertaining to the apex of the heart. A site for measuring heart rate with a stethoscope (Ch. 12).

apnea cessation or absence of normal spontaneous breathing (Ch. 12, 24).

appendicular skeleton skeleton that consists of the pectoral and pelvic girdles and the upper and lower extremities. The pelvic girdle attaches the upper extremities to the trunk (Ch. 18).

application/cover letter letter used to introduce yourself and your résumé to a prospective employer with the goal of obtaining an interview (Ch. 36).

application form form devised by a prospective employer to collect information relative to qualifications, education, and experience in employment (Ch. 36).

approximate to bring together the edges of a wound (Ch. 19).

arbitration a form of dispute resolution that allows a neutral party to settle the dispute (Ch. 7).

arrhythmia deviation from the normal pattern or rhythm of the heartbeat (Ch. 12, 25).

arteriosclerosis hardening of the arteries caused by buildup of plaque, a deposit of fatty substances on the artery lining (Ch. 17).

artifact anything artificially produced (Ch. 25).

ascorbic acid vitamin C (Ch. 22).

asepsis protecting against infection caused by pathogenic microorganisms (Ch. 3).

aseptic freedom from any infectious material; absence of microorganisms (Ch. 10, 18).

aspirate to remove by suction (Ch. 10).

assay analysis of a substance to determine constituents and relative proportion of each (Ch. 27).

assistive device any device used to help patients to walk (Ch. 21).

asymptomatic without symptoms (Ch. 27).

ataxia defective muscular coordination, primarily seen when attempting voluntary muscular movements (Ch. 13).

atrophy decrease in size or ability of a part of the body due to disease, inactivity, or other condition (Ch. 21).

attribute inherent characteristic (Ch. 1).

augment to add or increase (Ch. 25).

auricle the external ear, also called pinna (Ch. 18).

authoritarian manager operates on the premise that most workers cannot make a contribution without being directed (Ch. 33).

automated external defibrillator (AED) portable, self-contained, automatic device with voice instructions on use for individuals in cardiac arrest. It is used externally to electronically "shock" the myocardium into contracting again. Same as cardioversion (Ch. 9).

avascularization expulsions of blood from tissues. Leaves the tissues with no blood supply (Ch. 19).

axial skeleton consists of bones that lie around the center of the body (Ch. 18).

bachelor's degree degree of bachelor conferred by colleges and universities (Ch. 1).

bandage nonsterile gauze or other material applied over a sterile dressing to protect and immobilize (Ch. 9, 19).

barrier obstacle that exists to protect an individual from contact with blood or other potentially infected materials. Called personal protective equipment (PPE), barriers include gloves, masks, face shields, laboratory coats, protective eyewear, and gowns (Ch. 10).

Bartholin gland one of two small mucous glands located near the vaginal opening at base of labia majora (Ch. 14).

basal metabolic rate (BMR) level of energy required when the body is at rest (Ch. 22).

baseline known or initial measurement against which future measurements are compared (Ch. 12, 27); also, flat, horizontal line that separates the various waves of the ECG cycle (Ch. 25).

basophil granulocytic white blood cell with dark purple cytoplasmic granules. It is the least common of the white blood cells (Ch. 29).

benchmark making a comparison among different organizations relative to how they accomplish tasks, such as office computerization, organizing file systems, and employee remuneration (Ch. 33).

benefit remuneration that is in addition to the salary (Ch. 33, 36).

beriberi deficiency in vitamin B (thiamin) causes this disease characterized by headaches, depression, anorexia, constipation, tachycardia, edema, and heart failure (Ch. 22).

Betadine® brand of povidone-iodine solution used as a skin antiseptic. Betadine® is also available in a scrub (soap) solution (Ch. 19).

bias slant toward a particular belief (Ch. 4).

bilirubin orange–yellow pigment that forms from the breakdown of hemoglobin in broken down red blood cells. Bilirubin usually travels in the bloodstream to the liver, where it is converted to a water-soluble form and is excreted into the bile (Ch. 30, 32).

bilirubinuria the presence of bilirubin in urine (Ch. 30).

bimanual examination an examination performed by the physician using two hands to examine the internal pelvic organs. Two fingers of one hand are inserted into the vagina and the other hand presses on the outside of the abdominal wall. Shape, consistency, and position of the pelvic organs can be determined (Ch. 14).

biochemical tests tests that show biochemical properties and reactions of bacteria to achieve identification of microorganisms; often performed in solid and liquid media (Ch. 31).

bioethics branch of medical ethics concerned with moral issues resulting from high technology and sophisticated medical research. Social issues such as genetic engineering, abortion, and fetal tissue research raise important bioethical questions (Ch. 8).

biohazard material that has been in contact with body fluid and is capable of transmitting disease (Ch. 10).

biopsy removal of a small piece of living tissue from an organ or other part of the body for microscopic examination to confirm or establish a diagnosis (Ch. 18, 27).

bipolar having two poles or processes (Ch. 27).

bloodborne means of transmission of an infectious disease (such as HIV and HBV) via human blood (Ch. 10).

bloodborne pathogen microorganism capable of causing disease found in blood or components of blood (Ch. 10).

blood urea nitrogen (BUN) nitrogen in the blood in the form of urea. The level of nitrogen in the blood is an indicator of kidney function (Ch. 32).

body fluid any secretion or excretion from the human body such as vaginal, cerebrospinal, synovial, pleural, pericardial, peritoneal, amniotic, sputum, and saliva (Ch. 26).

body language nonverbal communication that includes unconscious body movements, gestures, and facial expressions that accompany verbal messages (Ch. 4).

body mechanics practice of using certain key muscle groups together with correct body alignment to avoid injury when lifting or moving heavy or awkward objects (Ch. 21).

body surface area (BSA) a highly accurate method for calculating medication dosages for infants and children up to 12 years of age (Ch. 24).

bond binding agreement with an employee ensuring recovery of financial loss should funds be stolen or embezzled (Ch. 33).

bradycardia (sinus) slow (less than 60 beats per minute), but regular heartbeat (Ch. 12, 25).

bradypnea abnormally slowed respiratory rate (Ch. 12).

brainstorming process of developing ideas through a synergistic interaction among participants in an environment free of criticism (Ch. 33).

Braxton–Hicks irregular, intermittent, and painless uterine contractions; also known as false labor (Ch. 14).

bronchi bifurcates from the trachea into each lung that terminate in the bronchial tubes (Ch. 18).

bronchodilator a drug that expands the bronchial tubes (Ch. 18).

broth tubes tubes filled with a broth substance that will support the growth of certain microorganisms (Ch. 31).

bruits sound of venous or arterial origin heard on auscultation (Ch. 13).

bubonic plague infectious disease with a high fatality rate transmitted to humans from infected rats and ground squirrels by the bite of the rat flea (Ch. 3).

buffer words expendable words used while answering the telephone (Ch. 4).

buffy coat layer of white blood cells and platelets that forms at the interface between the plasma and red blood cells in a tube of blood containing an anticoagulant (Ch. 28).

bullet point asterisk or dot followed by a descriptive phrase; helps the reader identify important points easily (Ch. 36).

burnout a state of fatigue or frustration brought about by a devotion to a cause, a way of life, or a relationship that failed to produce the expected reward (Ch. 5).

calculi stones found in the urethra, bladder, ureters, or kidneys; an abnormality (Ch. 28).

calibration determination of the accuracy of an instrument by comparing the information provided with an accepted standard known to be accurate (Ch. 25, 26).

calorie unit of heat. The large Calorie (which is always capitalized) is used in discussion of human nutrition. The large Calorie is also expressed as the kilogram calorie (kcal), equal to 1,000 small calories (Ch. 22).

candidiasis infection of the skin or mucous membrane with any species of *Candida* (Ch. 24).

cannula the blunting member in a Bio-Plexus Punctur-Guard® needle (Ch. 28).

carbuncle necrotizing infection of skin and tissue composed of a cluster of boils (Ch. 18).

carcinoma in situ cancer that does not extend beyond the basement membrane (Ch. 14).

cardiac catheterization passage of a catheter into the heart through an arm or leg vein and blood vessels leading into the heart. The purpose is to obtain cardiac blood samples, detect abnormalities, and determine intracardiac pressure. Contrast medium can be injected and a coronary artery angiogram can be performed (Ch. 25).

cardiac cycle period from the beginning of one heartbeat to the beginning of the next succeeding beat, including systole and diastole. One complete heartbeat (Ch. 25).

cardiopulmonary resuscitation (CPR) combination of rescue breathing and chest compressions performed by a trained individual on a patient experiencing cardiac arrest (Ch. 9).

cardioversion conversion of a pathological cardiac rhythm (arrhythmia), such as ventricular fibrillation, to normal sinus rhythm (Ch. 9, 25).

career objective expresses your career goal and the position for which you are applying (Ch. 36).

carotene vitamin A (Ch. 22).

carrier person who harbors a pathogenic organism and who is capable of transmitting the organism to others (Ch. 10).

casts tiny structures usually formed by deposits of protein or other substances on the walls of renal tubules; in urine, they can indicate kidney disease (Ch. 30).

catalyst substance that allows a chemical reaction to proceed at a much quicker rate and without as much energy input (Ch. 22).

catheterization insertion of a catheter tube into the body for evacuating fluids or injecting fluids into body cavities. In urinary catheterization, the tube is inserted through the urethra into the bladder for withdrawal of urine (Ch. 13, 18).

cathode a negative electrode from which electrons are emitted (Ch. 20).

caustic corrosive and burning; destructive to living tissue (Ch. 10, 19).

cauterized to destroy tissue through application of a caustic agent, a hot instrument, an electric current, or other agent (Ch. 9).

cautery destruction of tissue by burning (Ch. 19).

cell-mediated immunity the regulatory activities of T cells during the specific immune response (Ch. 10).

cellulose type of indigestible fiber made of carbohydrates found in plants (Ch. 22).

centrifuge device that spins tubes using centrifugal force to separate the fluid portion of blood from the formed elements (Ch. 28).

certification guarantees as being true or as represented by or as meeting a standard (Ch. 1).

certification examination standardized means of evaluating medical assistant competency (Ch. 35).

Certified Medical Assistant (CMA) a medical assistant who has successfully completed the AAMA's national certification examination (Ch. 1, 35).

cervical punch biopsy a biopsy of the uterine cervix using an instrument, the end of which is a punch (Ch. 14).

cesarean section delivery of fetus through surgical incision into the uterus (Ch. 14).

cheilosis caused by a deficiency of vitamin B_2 (riboflavin) and characterized by sores on the lips and cracks in the corners of the mouth (Ch. 22).

chemotherapeutic agents agents used in the treatment of diseases; the application of chemical reagents that are toxic to pathogenic microorganisms. Commonly used to describe agents (chemicals) used in the treatment of certain malignancies (Ch. 24).

Cheyne–Stokes regular pattern of irregular breathing rate often seen in children or may be seen in brain dysfunction (Ch. 12).

chief complaint (CC) specific symptom or problem for which the patient is seeing the physician today (Ch. 11).

chlamydia a bacteria that causes one of the most prevalent sexually transmitted disease (Ch. 14).

cholecalciferol vitamin D (Ch. 22).

cholesterol sterol lipid that is widely distributed in animal tissues. Cholesterol is produced in the liver and is a component of bile (Ch. 32).

choriocarcinoma rare malignant neoplasm, usually of the uterus or of an ectopic pregnancy. The exact cause is unknown (Ch. 32).

chronologic résumé résumé format used when you have employment experience (Ch. 36).

circadian rhythm pattern based on a 24-hour cycle emphasizing the repetition of certain physiologic phenomena such as eating and sleeping (Ch. 30).

circumduction circular motion of a body part (Ch. 21).

cirrhosis a chronic liver disease in which normal functioning liver tissue is replaced with nonfunctioning scar tissue (Ch. 10).

civil law law related to actions between individuals (Ch. 7).

claustrophobia fear of being confined in any space (Ch. 20).

clinical chemistry analysis and study of blood, body fluids, excreta, and tissues in the diagnosis and treatment of disease (Ch. 27).

clinical diagnosis identification of a disease by history, laboratory studies, and symptoms (Ch. 11, 27).

Clinitest® reagent tablet test that confirms the presence of reducing sugars in the urine (Ch. 30).

closed fracture uncomplicated fracture in which the bone does not break the skin (Ch. 18).

closed questions questions answered with a yes or no (Ch. 4).

clustering a grouping together of nonverbal messages into statements or conclusions. Can also be used to describe a scheduling system where patients with similar complaint/conditions are scheduled consecutively (example is scheduling all the allergy injections for 3:00 PM to 4:00 PM every Tuesday and Thursday) (Ch. 4).

cobalamin vitamin B_{12} (Ch. 22).

cochlear implantation an electrical device that receives sounds and transmits the resulting signal to electrodes implanted in the cochlea. The signal stimulates the cochlea and the individual is able to perceive sound (Ch. 15).

coenzyme substance that enhances a catalyst (Ch. 22).

cognitive functioning awareness with perception, reasoning, judgment, intuition, and memory (Ch. 17).

colonoscopy visual examination of the colon with a lighted scope (Ch. 18).

colposcopy visual examination of vaginal and cervical tissues using a colposcope following abnormal Pap smear. A magnifying lens and powerful lights are used (Ch. 14).

comedone blackhead; usually the result of blocked sebaceous glands caused by acne (Ch. 18).

Commission on Accreditation of Allied Health Education Programs (CAAHEP) entity accrediting institutions for the American Association of Medical Assistants (Ch. 35).

common law refers to laws developed in England and France and brought to the United States by the early settlers; sometimes referred to as judge-made law (Ch. 7).

communicable contagious. Capable of being transmitted from one person to another either directly or indirectly (Ch. 10, 26).

compensation overemphasizing of characteristics to make up for a real or imagined failure or handicap (Ch. 4).

competency legally qualified or adequate (Ch. 1).

complete blood count (CBC) battery of hematologic tests consisting of hemoglobin, hematocrit, total white blood cell and red blood cell counts, differential white blood cell count, and the erythrocyte indices (Ch. 29).

compliance conformity in fulfilling official requirements (Ch. 1).

compounding combining two or more substances in definite proportions (Ch. 24).

condenser directs the beam of light from the source to the specimen (Ch. 27).

condylomata a wartlike lesion of viral origin found on external genitalia or perianal region (Ch. 14).

conflict resolution solving problems between coworkers or any two parties (Ch. 33).

congenital anomalies being born with; existing at time of birth (Ch. 14).

congruency the verbal message and the nonverbal message must agree (Ch. 4).

constitutional law consists of laws that are made by constitutions of the United States or individual states (Ch. 7).

constrict to become smaller in diameter (Ch. 28).

constriction band term used to replace tourniquet (no longer used) in emergencies. A band of material used to control severe bleeding in an extremity that has been injured due to trauma. The band is applied above the source of bleeding, but not so tight that it restricts the flow of blood completely. Some slight trickling of blood should be evident. This action avoids loss of an extremity because of complete blood flow restriction. Complete blood flow restriction results in no blood flow to the extremity's cells and tissues; therefore, the cells, tissues and body part receive no oxygen and die (Ch. 9).

contact tracker form used to keep track of employment contact information such as name of employer, name of contact person, address and telephone number, date of first contact, résumé sent, interview date, follow-up information, and dates (Ch. 36).

contact transmission spread of disease-causing microorganisms by directly or indirectly touching the source of the infection or by touching an object or environmental surface (Ch. 10).

contaminate to make something unclean; often used to describe a sterile area being made "unsterile" or exposing a clean area to a pathogenic substance (Ch. 10, 19).

continuing education units (CEU) method for earning points toward recertification (Ch. 35).

contract law law that refers to agreements between individuals and entities that are binding (Ch. 7).

contracting acquiring an infection from pathogens (Ch. 10).

contracture fibrosis of connective tissue in skin, fascia, muscle, or joint that prevents normal mobility of the related tissue or joint (Ch. 21).

contraindication any symptom or circumstance that indicates that the use of a particular drug is inappropriate when it would otherwise be advisable. For example, the use of alcoholic beverages is a contraindication when the drug Flagyl® is prescribed (Ch. 23).

control test test of a sample of known results to be used to compare with the results of a patient's sample (Ch. 27).

coryza acute inflammation of the membranes of the nose accompanied by profuse drainage (Ch. 10).

countershock application of an electric current to the heart directly or indirectly to alter a disturbance in cardiac rhythm (Ch. 25).

coupling agent an agent used when ultrasonography is used; enhances penetration of sound waves through tissue (Ch. 14).

crash tray or cart tray or portable cart that contains medications and supplies needed for emergency and first aid procedures (Ch. 9).

creatinine waste product formed in muscle that is excreted by the kidneys; increased in blood and urine when kidney function is abnormal (Ch. 30).

credentialed testimonials showing that a person is entitled to credit or has a right to exercise official power (Ch. 1).

crepitation grating sound heard on movement of ends of a broken bone (Ch. 9).

criminal law law related to wrongs committed against the welfare and safety of society as a whole (Ch. 7).

critical values test results that indicate a potentially life-threatening or greatly debilitating situation that must be reported to the physician immediately (Ch. 30).

cryopreservation storage of biologic materials (sperm, embryo, tissue, plasma) at extremely cold temperature for use at a later time (Ch. 8).

cryosurgery the destruction of tissue by application of extreme cold, silver nitrate, and carbon dioxide (Ch. 14).

cryotherapy use of cold to treat a physical condition (Ch. 21).

cryptorchidism undescended testicle (Ch. 16).

crystals found in normal urine sediment having no particular significance; a few should be noted because they may indicate disease states (Ch. 30).

cultivate to foster the growth of (Ch. 1).

cultural brokering the act of bridging, linking, or mediating between groups or persons through the process of reducing conflict or producing change (Ch. 4).

culture and sensitivity often referred to as C & S. The sample is cultured for bacteria, and then is exposed to various antibiotics to determine what the bacteria is sensitive (and resistant) to (Ch. 27, 30).

cultures microorganisms cultivated in a nutrient medium (Ch. 30, 31).

Cushing's syndrome hypersecretion of the adrenal cortex producing excessive glucocorticoids. The condition may be caused by a tumor or hyperfunction of the anterior pituitary (Ch. 32).

cyanosis discoloration of the skin due to abnormal amounts of reduced hemoglobin in the blood caused by decreased oxygen and increased carbon dioxide in the blood (Ch. 13).

cystitis inflammation of the bladder (Ch. 17).

cytology science that deals with the formation, structure, and function of cells (Ch. 27).

cytoscopy visual examination of the urethra and bladder after insertion of a cytoscope, a lighted scope especially designed for the examination of these areas (Ch. 18).

debris remains of broken down or damaged cells or tissues (Ch. 10).

declination form written formal refusal (Ch. 10).

decode to translate into language that is easily understood; to interpret (Ch. 4).

defendant person who defends action brought in litigation (Ch. 7).

defense mechanism behavior that protects the psyche from guilt, anxiety, or shame (Ch. 4).

defibrillation stopping fibrillation of the heart by use of drugs or by physical means (Ch. 25).

defibrillator a machine that delivers an electric current to alter a disturbance in cardiac rhythm (Ch. 25).

dementia impairment of intellectual function that is progressive and interferes with normal activities (Ch. 17).

demyelination destruction of the myelin sheath; often a factor in multiple sclerosis (Ch. 18).

denial rejection of or refusal to acknowledge (Ch. 4).

deoxygenated blood that is high in carbon dioxide, low in oxygen, and pumped through the heart to the lungs where the carbon dioxide is exchanged for oxygen (Ch. 25).

depolarize process of reducing to a nonpolarized condition. Generation of an electrical current is enhanced. Electrical activity generated when the atria or ventricles contract (Ch. 25).

deposition oral testimony given by an individual with a court reporter and attorneys for both sides present; often used as part of the discovery process (Ch. 7).

dermatophytes category of fungi causing infections of hair, skin, and nails (Ch. 21).

dexterity skill and ease in using the hands (Ch. 1).

diabetes mellitus chronic disorder of carbohydrate metabolism characterized by hyperglycemia and resulting from inadequate production or utilization of insulin (Ch. 32).

diagnosis determination of disease or condition (Ch. 27).

diaphragm a lens or other object that opens and closes to increase or decrease the amount of light on the object being illuminated (Ch. 27).

diastole one component of blood pressure measurement representing the lowest amount of pressure exerted during the cardiac cycle; the force exerted on the arterial walls during cardiac relaxation (Ch. 12, 25).

diethylstilbestrol (DES) a synthetic hormone used therapeutically in menopausal disturbances. It should not be given during pregnancy. It has been related to cervicovaginal malignances in daughters of mothers who had it prescribed for them to treat a threatened abortion (Ch. 14).

differential diagnosis diagnosis based on comparison of symptoms of similar diseases (Ch. 27).

digestion breaking down of food into smaller particles. It can be either physical or chemical (Ch. 22).

dilate to enlarge in diameter (Ch. 28).

dilation expansion of an orifice or organ (Ch. 14).

diploma a document bearing record of graduation from or of a degree conferred by an educational institution (Ch. 1).

direct skills skills that are job specific. Skill in taking a blood pressure reading would be specific to the medical field (Ch. 36).

discovery the time in which both parties are allowed access to all information and evidence related to a case; follows the subpoena process (Ch. 7).

disinfection use of chemicals or boiling water to free an item from infectious materials but not its spores (Ch. 10).

dislocation displacement of a bone or joint from its normal position (Ch. 18).

dispense prepare and give out a medication to be taken at a later time (Ch. 7, 23, 24).

displacement displacing negative feelings onto something or someone else with no significance to the situation (Ch. 4).

disposition temperament, character, personality (Ch. 1).

diuretic substance that causes less water to be reabsorbed by the kidney, and therefore causes water to be excreted from the body (Ch. 22).

DNA deoxyribonucleic acid; important nucleus material that carries genetic codes (Ch. 27, 31).

doctrine principle of law established through past decisions (Ch. 7).

documentation providing factual support through written information; also, written material that accompanies purchased software containing the information necessary for using the software appropriately; sometimes known as the manual (Ch. 10).

dorsiflexion moving the foot upward at the ankle joint (Ch. 21).

dosimeter a device for measuring X-ray output (Ch. 20).

dressing sterile gauze or other material applied directly to a wound to absorb secretions and to protect (Ch. 9, 19).

droplet transmission method of spreading disease from respiratory secretions through the air. Spread is usually confined to within three feet of the infected patient (Ch. 10).

durable power of attorney for health care legal form that allows a designated person to act on another's behalf in regard to health care choices (Ch. 6, 7).

dysmenorrhea painful menses (Ch. 14).

dyspareunia painful intercourse (Ch. 14).

dysplasia abnormal development of tissue (Ch. 14).

dyspnea shortness of breath or labored/difficult breathing (Ch. 12).

dysuria painful or difficult urination (Ch. 18).

e-résumé electronic résumés may be delivered electronically via e-mail, submitted to Internet job boards, or placed on Web pages (Ch. 36).

echocardiogram noninvasive diagnostic method that uses ultrasound to visualize internal cardiac structure, including valves (Ch. 20).

eclampsia complication of pregnancy that includes general edema, hypertension, proteinuria, and convulsions (Ch. 14).

ectopic pregnancy pregnancy outside the uterus (Ch. 14, 22).

edematous abnormal accumulation of fluid in the tissues resulting in swelling (Ch. 28).

effacement thinning and shortening of the cervical canal during labor to permit passage of fetus (Ch. 14).

electrocardiogram record of the electrical activity of the heart; showing P, QRS, and T waves (Ch. 25).

electrocardiograph instrument for recording the electrical activity of the heart (Ch. 25).

electrocardiography process of recording the electrical activity originating in the heart (Ch. 25).

electrode also known as a sensor. Used to conduct electricity from the body to the electrocardiograph (Ch. 25).

electrolyte conductor of electricity whose components are important in maintaining fluid and acid–base balance (Ch. 22, 25, 27).

emaciation state of being extremely lean (Ch. 18).

emancipated minor persons under age 18 years who are financially responsible for themselves and free of parental care (Ch. 7).

embezzle to appropriate fraudulently to one's own use (Ch. 33).

Emergency Medical Services (EMS) Emergency Medical Services (EMS) system is a local network of police, fire, and medical personnel trained to respond to emergency situations. In many communities, the system is activated by calling 911 (Ch. 9).

empathy ability to be objectively aware of and have insight into another's feelings, emotions, and behaviors, and to be aware of the significance and meaning of these to the other person (Ch. 1, 17).

emphysema chronic pulmonary disease characterized by dilated and damaged alveoli (Ch. 12).

encode (encoding) creating a message to be sent (Ch. 4).

endemic disease that occurs continuously or in cycles with a certain number of cases expected for a given period (Ch. 10).

endometriosis tissue that resembles the endometrium invades various locations in the pelvic cavity and elsewhere (Ch. 14).

endoscopy visual examination of body cavities with a lighted scope (Ch. 10, 18).

engineering controls physical or mechanical devices that isolate or remove health hazards from the workplace (Ch. 10).

enzyme immunoassay measurement of reaction of antigen with specific antibody (Ch. 32).

eosinophil granulocytic white blood cell with red eosin-stained granules in the cytoplasm. It is elevated in cases of allergies (Ch. 29).

epidemic an infectious disease that attacks many persons at the same time in the same location (Ch. 10).

epidemiology field of science that studies the history, cause, and patterns of infectious diseases (Ch. 10).

epinephrine hormone also known as adrenaline. Epinephrine is manufactured as a chemical (pharmaceutical preparation) and is often mixed with local anesthetics for use as a vasoconstrictor in minor surgery (Ch. 19).

epistaxis nosebleed (Ch. 10).

Epstein–Barr virus (EBV) virus that is believed to be the cause of infectious mononucleosis and is implicated in such conditions as African Burkitt's lymphoma and nasopharyngeal carcinoma (Ch. 32).

equilibrium state of balance between opposing forces (Ch. 18).

erosion an eating away of tissues, destruction of a surface layer by physical or inflammatory processes (Ch. 14, 18).

erythema redness or inflammation of the skin or mucous membranes that is the result of dilatation and congestion of superficial capillaries (Ch. 18).

erythrocyte red blood cell, one of the formed elements of the blood (Ch. 28, 29).

erythrocyte indices three equations that provide information about the sizes and hemoglobin content of red blood cells. These include the mean corpuscular cell volume, mean corpuscular hemoglobin, and mean corpuscular hemoglobin volume (Ch. 29).

erythrocyte sedimentation rate measurement of how far the red cells in a sample of blood decrease in one hour (Ch. 29).

erythropoietin hormone that causes production of new red blood cells (Ch. 29).

esophageal varices tortuous dilation of the esophageal vein associated with any condition that causes obstruction of drainage from the esophageal veins into the portal vein of the liver. Seen in cirrhosis of the liver and alcoholism (Ch. 20).

ethics defined in terms of what is morally right and wrong; ethics will differ from person to person; often defined by a code or creed as in the Code of Ethics from the American Association of Medical Assistants (AAMA) (Ch. 8).

ethyl alcohol alcohol, used to make a solution (Ch. 26).

eupnea normal breathing (Ch. 12).

evaluation assessment of an employee's job performance (Ch. 34).

eversion moving a body part outward (Ch. 21).

excoriated abrasion of the epidermis by trauma, chemicals, burns, or other causes (Ch. 10).

excretion waste matter. The elimination of waste products from the body (Ch. 10, 26).

exfoliated the shedding of something such as cervical cells (Ch. 14).

exit interview opportunity for departing employees to provide their positive and negative opinions of the position and facility (Ch. 34).

expectorate act of coughing up material from airways that lead to the lungs (Ch. 10, 31).

expert witness individual with highly specialized knowledge and skills in a particular area who testifies to a standard of care (Ch. 7).

explicit fully revealed or expressed without ambiguity or vagueness, leaving no question as to intent (Ch. 9).

expressed contract written or verbal contract that specifically describes what each party in the contract will do (Ch. 7).

extension straightening of a body part (Ch. 21).

external respiration ventilation of the lungs when the exchange of oxygen and carbon dioxide takes place (Ch. 18).

externship transition stage between the classroom and actual employment; may also be referred to as internship or practicum (Ch. 1, 33).

extracellular pertaining to the environment outside of a body cell (Ch. 22).

exudate accumulated fluid in a cavity; an oozing of pus; matter that penetrates through vessel walls into adjoining tissue (Ch. 10, 15, 19).

facilitate to make an action or process easier (Ch. 1).

fat-soluble pertaining to substances that are hydrophobic and therefore dissolve better in fat (Ch. 22).

febrile having a fever (Ch. 12).

Federal Register federal government agency from which written CLIA '88 documents may be obtained (Ch. 26).

felony a serious crime such as murder, larceny, or thefts of large sums of money, assault, and rape (Ch. 7).

fenestrated having openings. A sterile, fenestrated drape is used in surgery. It has an opening (round) in it to expose only the operative site. The remainder of the drape covers the patient and is a sterile area (Ch. 19).

fenestrated drape a type of drape with an opening, usually round, that can be placed with the opening over a particular body area; used in surgery and for proctologic examinations (Ch. 13).

first aid immediate (or first) care provided to persons who are suddenly ill or injured; first aid is typically followed by more comprehensive care and treatment (Ch. 9).

flexion bending of a body part (Ch. 21).

fluoroscope a device consisting of a screen; mounts separately or with an X-ray tube that shows the images of objects interposed between the table and the screen (Ch. 20).

folic acid one of the B-complex vitamins (Ch. 22).

fomite substance that absorbs and transmits infectious material; for example, contaminated items such as equipment (Ch. 10).

fontanel soft spot lying between the cranial bones of the skull of a fetus, newborn, and infant (Ch. 15).

forensic pertaining to the law (Ch. 26).

formaldehyde colorless gas combined with methanol and used as a solution, such as a disinfectant, astringent, or a preservative for histologic specimen (Ch. 26).

formalin an aqueous solution of 37% formaldehyde (Ch. 14).

fracture break in a bone. There are several types of fractures, but all are classified as either open or closed fractures (Ch. 9).

frenulum of the tongue, a fold of mucus membrane located under the tongue attaching the tongue to the floor of the mouth (Ch. 12).

frequency urinating frequently (Ch. 18).

friable easily broken (Ch. 19).

fringe benefit benefit above and beyond salary to which an employee may be entitled. Examples include health and life insurance, paid vacation, sick days, personal days, and tuition reimbursement for courses related to employment (Ch. 2, 33).

fulgarated destroyed by electric current (Ch. 14).

fume hood type of hood or barrier used in the laboratory to capture chemical vapors and fumes and move them away from health care workers and into a building's exhaust fan system (Ch. 26).

functional résumé résumé format used to highlight specialty areas of accomplishment and strengths (Ch. 36).

furuncle localized, suppurative staphylococcal skin infection originating in a gland or hair follicle (Ch. 18).

gait manner or style of walking including rhythm and speed (Ch. 18, 21).

gait belt safety belt worn by the patient around the waist that provides a firm handhold for the caregiver when transferring the patient or when assisting in ambulation (Ch. 21).

gallium a nontoxic metal, similar to mercury in appearance, that can be used in place of mercury for fever thermometers. It is not yet widely available for use (Ch. 12).

galvanometer mechanism in the electrocardiograph that changes the voltage into a mechanical motion for recording purposes (Ch. 25).

genetic engineering alteration, manipulation, replacement, or repair of genetic material (Ch. 8).

genitalia the reproductive organs, internal and external (Ch. 14).

genus first Greek or Latin name given to a microorganism; always capitalized (Ch. 31).

geriatrics the branch of medicine concerned with the problems of aging (Ch. 17).

gerontology the scientific study of the problems associated with aging (Ch. 17).

gestation period of development from fertilization to birth (Ch. 14).

gestational diabetes diabetes that first manifests clinically during pregnancy. It usually subsides after delivery (Ch. 14).

gestures/mannerisms movement of various body parts while communicating (Ch. 4).

glucose simple sugar that is a major source of energy in the human body; monitoring of blood glucose levels in urine and blood is a vital diagnostic test in diabetes and other disorders; also a test on a reagent strip (Ch. 27, 30).

glucosuria the presence of glucose in urine (also correct is glycosuria) (Ch. 30).

glycogen carbohydrate form used for storage of sugar in the body (Ch. 22).

goal result or achievement toward which effort is directed (Ch. 5).

"going bare" said of a physician who does not carry professional liability insurance (Ch. 33).

goniometer instrument used to measure the angle of a joint's range of motion (Ch. 21).

goniometry measurement of joint motion (Ch. 21).

Gram stain most common stain used in microbiology to observe gross morphologic features of bacteria; a differential stain, allowing differentiation between Gram-negative and Gram-positive organisms (Ch. 31).

gravidity total number of pregnancies a woman has had regardless of duration, including a present one (Ch. 14).

gross contamination highly infectious material present (Ch. 10).

Guthrie screening test diagnostic test for the detection of phenylketonuria (PKU) (Ch. 22).

health maintenance organization (HMO) type of managed care operation that is typically set up as a for-profit corporation with salaried employees. HMOs "with walls" offer a range of medical services under one roof; HMOs "without walls" typically contract with physicians in the community to provide patient services for an agreed-upon fee (Ch. 2).

Heimlich maneuver abdominal thrusts designed to overcome breathing difficulties in patients who are choking (Ch. 9).

hematemesis vomiting blood (Ch. 18).

hematochezia presence of bright red blood in feces (Ch. 18).

hematocrit percentage of red blood cells within a specimen of anticoagulated whole blood (Ch. 29).

hematology study of blood and the blood-forming tissues (Ch. 27, 29).

hematoma accumulation of blood around the venipuncture site during or after venipuncture caused by the leakage of blood from where the needle punctured the vein (Ch. 28).

hematopoiesis formation of blood cells (Ch. 29).

hematuria abnormal presence of blood in urine, symptomatic of many disorders of the genitourinary system and renal diseases (Ch. 18, 30).

hemiplegia paralysis of one side of the body (Ch. 21).

hemoconcentration pooling of blood at the location of the venipuncture caused by leaving the tourniquet on the arm longer than one minute, resulting in inaccurate blood samples (Ch. 28).

hemoglobin molecule with the red blood cell that transports oxygen (Ch. 29).

hemoglobinopathy inherited disease resulting from the formation of an abnormal hemoglobin molecule (Ch. 29).

hemolysis rupturing of the red blood cells during the process of blood collection. The serum or plasma becomes contaminated and has a reddish color (Ch. 28).

hemoptysis spitting up of blood arising from the mouth, larynx, trachea, bronchi, or lungs characterized by a sudden attack of coughing with production of bloody sputum (Ch. 18).

heterophile antibody antibody that reacts with other than the specific antigens as seen in infectious mononucleosis (Ch. 32).

Hibeclens® brand of antiseptic soap solution (Ch. 19).

hierarchy of needs needs that are arranged in a specific order or rank; sequential arrangement. Associated with Abraham Maslow (Ch. 4).

high-density lipoprotein (HDL) lipoprotein in the blood composed primarily of protein; removes cholesterol from peripheral tissues and transports them to the liver for excretion (Ch. 32).

histology study of biopsy results of tissue samples for the determination of disease (Ch. 27).

holding media specific media used in the transport of microorganisms to support the life of the organisms until they can be put on nutrient medium in the laboratory (Ch. 31).

homeopathy a healing modality that uses diluted doses of certain substances to create an "energy imprint" in the body to bring about a cure (Ch. 2).

homeostasis state of equilibrium of internal environment (Ch. 22).

hormone replacement therapy (HRT) the replacement of hormones lacking from the patient's system. In this case, HRT refers to the replacement of varying levels of estrogen and progesterone in perimenopausal or postmenopausal women (Ch. 27).

hospital-based laboratories hospital-owned laboratories that perform most tests required by the hospital and local communities (Ch. 27).

human chorionic gonadotropin (hCG) hormone secreted by the trophoblast after fertilization of the ovum. It may be detected in the blood and urine of pregnant women (Ch. 14, 32).

human immunodeficiency virus (HIV) AIDS virus; it is a retrovirus that ultimately destroys immune system cells (Ch. 10).

humoral immunity immunity mediated by antibodies in body fluids such as plasma and lymph (Ch. 10).

hyaline transparent, clear; hyaline casts are transparent and often hard to see in urine (Ch. 30).

hydatidiform mole development of cysts and rapid growth of the uterus with bleeding (Ch. 32).

hydrogen peroxide antibacterial solution that has a mechanical cleansing action (Ch. 19).

hydronephrosis collection of urine in renal pelvis. This is caused by an obstruction and may result in a cyst (Ch. 18).

hyperemesis gravidarum severe nausea and vomiting during pregnancy with inability to eat; may lead to severe dehydration (Ch. 14).

hyperextension position of maximum extension, or extending a body part beyond its normal limits (Ch. 21).

hyperglycemia increased levels of blood glucose. Hyperglycemia does not necessarily mean that the patient is diabetic but may be an indication of prediabetes (Ch. 32).

hyperpnea increased respiratory rate and depth as seen in exercise pain, fever, and hysteria (Ch. 12).

hypertension blood pressure that is consistently greater than 140/90 mm Hg (Ch. 12).

hyperthermia body temperature above normal range; an unusually high fever (Ch. 17).

hyperventilation ventilation rate that is greater than metabolically necessary, potentially leading to alkalosis (Ch. 12).

hypochromic less color than normal (Ch. 29).

hypoglycemia state of having a lower than normal blood glucose level (Ch. 28, 32).

hypotension abnormally low blood pressure resulting in inadequate tissue profusion and oxygenation (Ch. 12).

hypothermia extremely dangerous cold-related condition that can result in death if the individual does not receive care and if the progression of hypothermia is not reversed. Symptoms include shivering, cold skin, and confusion (Ch. 9, 17).

hypoventilation decrease in respiration rate with shallow depth of respiration (Ch. 12).

hypoxemia lack of oxygen in the blood (Ch. 24).

hypoxia oxygen deficiency (Ch. 14).

hysterosalpingogram X-ray of uterus and fallopian tubes using a contrast medium (Ch. 14).

Ictotest® confirmatory test for bilirubin (Ch. 30).

immune system body's strong line of defense against invading microorganisms. The body recognizes foreign substances such as microorganisms and produces substances to fight them off. Antibodies, white blood cells, digestive enzymes, and resistance of the skin are some examples (Ch. 10).

immunity ability of the body to resist specific pathogens and their toxins (Ch. 10).

immunoglobulins family of proteins capable of acting as antibodies, thereby protecting individuals from pathogenic microorganisms; also, antibodies produced by the cells of the immune system (Ch. 10).

immunohematology study of blood group antigens and antibodies; blood banking (Ch. 27).

immunology the study of the components of the immune system and their function (Ch. 27).

immunosuppressed referring to a patient whose immune system is unhealthy because of disease, medication, genetics, and so on; these patients can be particularly susceptible to attack by microorganisms (Ch. 10, 31).

implicit capable of being understood from something else though unexpressed; implied (Ch. 9).

implied consent consent assumed by the health care provider, typically in an emergency that threatens the patient's life. Implied consent also occurs in more subtle ways in the health care environment; for example, when a patient willingly rolls up the sleeve to receive an injection (Ch. 7).

implied contract contract indicated by actions rather than words (Ch. 7).

improvise to make, invent, or arrange in an unplanned or spontaneous manner (Ch. 1).

incinerate to destroy by fire (Ch. 10).

incompetence legally, a person who is insane, inadequate, or not an adult (Ch. 7).

incontinence uncontrollable loss of urine (Ch. 17).

increment an increase or addition in number, size, or extent (Ch. 12).

independent physician association (IPA) independent network of physicians in private practice who contract with the association to treat patients for an agreed-upon fee (Ch. 2).

indirect statements means of eliciting a response from a patient by turning a question into a statement of interest (Ch. 4).

infarction area of tissue in an organ or part that becomes necrotic (dead) after cessation of blood supply (Ch. 25).

infection invasion of pathogens into living tissue (Ch. 19).

infection control methods to eliminate or reduce the transmission of infectious microorganisms (Ch. 10).

infectious agent pathogen responsible for a specific infectious disease (Ch. 10).

infectious mononucleosis acute infectious disease primarily affecting the lymphoid tissue caused by the Epstein–Barr virus (Ch. 32).

infectious waste items that have come in contact with patient blood or body fluids. Contaminated items (Ch. 10).

inflammation the normal nonspecific immune response by the body to any type of injury (trauma, bacterial, viral, temperature extremes, and so on) (Ch. 19).

inflammatory response body's defense against the threat of infection or trauma. Characterized by redness, pain, heat, and swelling (Ch. 10).

informed consent consent given by the patient who is made aware of any procedure to be performed, its risks, expected outcomes, and alternatives (Ch. 7, 19).

ingestion taking in of food, drugs, and so forth into the body by mouth (Ch. 18).

inner-directed people people who decide for themselves what they want to do with their lives (Ch. 5).

inoculate to place colonies of microorganisms onto nutrient media (Ch. 31).

instrument tray see **Mayo stand** (Ch. 19).

insulin hormone secreted by beta cells of the islets of Langerhans of the pancreas essential for the proper metabolism of glucose (Ch. 32).

integrate to incorporate into a larger unit; to form or blend into a whole (Ch. 1).

integrative medicine bringing together of two or more treatment modalities so they function as a harmonious whole; as seen in alternative forms of health care (Ch. 2).

internal respiration passage of oxygen from the blood into the cells (Ch. 18).

Internet worldwide computer network available via modem that connects universities, government laboratories, companies, and individuals around the world (Ch. 33).

internship transition stage between classroom and employment (Ch. 1).

interrogatory a written set of questions that must be answered, under oath, within a specific time period; part of the discovery process (Ch. 7).

interview meeting in which you and the interviewer discuss employment opportunities and strengths you can contribute to the organization (Ch. 36).

interview techniques methods of encouraging the best communication between the applicant and the interviewer (Ch. 4).

intraepithelium within the epithelium (Ch. 14).

intravenous pyelogram radiograph studies of the kidneys, ureters, and bladder using a contrast medium (Ch. 16).

invasive procedure surgical technique or procedure that penetrates healthy tissue. The potential for pathogenic microorganisms to enter the body exists (Ch. 10, 27).

inversion moving a body part inward (Ch. 21).

involuntary dismissal termination of employment based on poor job performance or violation of office policies (Ch. 33, 34).

involution return of the uterus to normal size and shape after childbirth (Ch. 14).

ionizing radiation X-ray beams (Ch. 20).

ischemia local and temporary lack of blood to an organ or part caused by obstruction of circulation (Ch. 25).

isoelectric having equal electrical potentials. It is represented on the ECG as the flat horizontal line, the baseline (Ch. 25).

isolation separating a patient with certain infections or communicable diseases from other individuals (Ch. 10).

isolation categories system of seven categories developed by the Centers for Disease Control (CDC) that isolates patients according to known infections. These categories have been condensed into three Transmission-Based Precautions based on air, contact, and droplet routes of transmission (Ch. 10).

isopropyl alcohol 70% alcohol solution commonly used as a disinfectant (Ch. 19).

isotope a chemical element (Ch. 20).

itinerary detailed written plan of a proposed trip (Ch. 33).

jaundice yellow discolorization of the skin and sclera caused by excess bilirubin in the blood (Ch. 10, 13).

jet injection an injection given under the skin without a needle, using the force of the liquid under pressure to pierce the skin (Ch. 10).

job description outline of tasks, duties, and responsibilities for every position in the office (Ch. 34).

ketoacidosis accumulation of ketones in the body, occurring primarily as a complication of diabetes mellitus; if left untreated, it could cause coma (Ch. 30).

ketone chemical compound produced during an increased metabolism of fat; also, test on a reagent strip (Ch. 30).

ketonuria having ketones in urine (Ch. 30).

ketosis a condition of the body burning fatty acids for energy in the absence of appropriate glucose/carbohydrates; may be referred to as lipolysis (Ch. 30).

keywords words that relate to a job specific position. Keywords may be job-specific skills or profession-specific words (Ch. 36).

kinesics study of body language (Ch. 4).

labyrinthitis inflammation of inner ear or labyrinth (Ch. 13).

lackluster dull, lacking in sheen (Ch. 9).

Lamaze technique consisting of breathing exercises to facilitate delivery (Ch. 14).

latex beads tiny latex beads coated with antibodies or antigens that react with antigens or antibodies in the test sample in an agglutination reaction. The latex beads may be colored to make the reaction easier to visualize (Ch. 32).

lead wire a conductor attached to an electrocardiograph. Consists of limb leads and chest leads (Ch. 25).

lesion injury or wound. A circumscribed area of tissue that has been altered pathologically (Ch. 10, 18).

letter of reference letter usually written by an employee's past employer describing the employee's performance, attitude, or qualifications. This letter is presented to a potential employer when applying for a new job (Ch. 34).

letter of resignation letter informing the current employer of the employee's decision to resign from a current position (Ch. 34).

leukocyte white blood cell, one of the formed elements of blood (Ch. 28, 29).

leukocyte esterase test on a reagent strip that indicates the presence of white blood cells in the urinary tract (Ch. 30).

leukorrhea whitish or yellowish mucous discharged from the cervical canal or vagina. Usually normal unless there is an increase in amount or variation in color (Ch. 10).

liability legal responsibility (Ch. 33).

libel false and malicious writing about another constituting a defamation of character (Ch. 7).

libido sexual drive (Ch. 16).

license permission by competent authority (the state) to engage in a profession; permission to act (Ch. 1).

licensure granting of licenses to practice a profession (Ch. 1).

ligature length of suture thread without a needle, used for tying off vessels during surgery (Ch. 19).

lipemia excessive amount of fat (lipids) in the blood, resulting in a blood sample that has a milky appearance (Ch. 28).

liquid nitrogen commonly and incorrectly referred to as dry ice, liquid nitrogen is a volatile freezing agent used to destroy unwanted tissue such as warts (Ch. 19).

lithotripsy procedure using shock waves directed at calculi to crush them (Ch. 18).

litigation court action (Ch. 7).

litigious prone to engage in lawsuits (Ch. 1).

living will document allowing a person to make choices related to treatment in a life-threatening illness (Ch. 6).

lochia discharge from the uterus of blood, mucus, and tissue during the period after childbirth (Ch. 10, 14).

long-range goals achievements that may take three to five years to accomplish (Ch. 5).

low-density lipoprotein (LDL) lipoprotein in the blood composed primarily of cholesterol. The cholesterol carried by LDL may be deposited in peripheral tissues and is associated with an increased risk for heart disease (Ch. 32).

lumbar puncture surgical puncture of the lumbar area of the intervertebral spaces to aspirate cerebrospinal fluid for laboratory analysis (Ch. 10, 31).

lumen the space within an artery, vein, intestine, needles, and catheter or tube (Ch. 12).

lymphadenopathy a disease of the lymph nodes (Ch. 10).

lymphocyte white blood cell with a dense nonsegmented nucleus and lacking granules in the cytoplasm (Ch. 29).

macroallocation of scarce medical resources; decisions are made by congress, health systems agencies, and insurance companies (Ch. 8).

macrocytic term that describes a larger than normal cell (Ch. 29).

macular pertaining to a discoloration of a patch of skin, neither elevated nor depressed, of various colors, sizes, and shapes (Ch. 10).

macular degeneration degeneration of the macula area of the retina caused by aging; a leading cause of visual impairment in people older than 50 years, making it difficult to do fine work (Ch. 17).

major mineral mineral that is required in large amounts by the body (Ch. 22).

malabsorption inadequate absorption of nutrients from the intestinal tract (Ch. 18).

malaise discomfort, uneasiness, or indisposition, often indicative of infection (Ch. 10, 18).

malaria acute infectious disease caused by the presence of protozoan parasites within the red blood cells; usually comes from the bite of a female mosquito (Ch. 3, 10).

malfeasance conduct that is illegal or contrary to an official's obligations (Ch. 7).

malpractice professional negligence (Ch. 7, 33).

managed care operation any health care setting or delivery system that is designed to reduce the cost of care while still providing access to care (Ch. 2).

management by walking around (MBWA) a technique for keeping managers informed about the health of their organization (Ch. 33).

mandate formal order to obey certain rules and regulations (Ch. 26).

manifest to reveal in an obvious way (Ch. 10).

manometer device for measuring a liquid or gaseous pressure. The measurement is expressed in millimeters of mercury or water (Ch. 12).

Mantoux test test for tuberculosis involving the intracutaneous injection of purified protein derivative (Ch. 32).

marketing process by which the provider of services makes the consumer aware of the scope and quality of those services. Marketing tools might include public relations, brochures, patient education seminars, and newsletters (Ch. 33).

masking attempt to conceal or repress true feelings or the message (Ch. 4).

mature minor a person, usually younger than 18 years, who is able to understand and appreciate the consequences of treatment despite their young age (Ch. 7).

Mayo stand portable metal tray table used for setting up small sterile fields for minor surgery and procedures (Ch. 19).

meconium first feces of newborn (Ch. 14).

mediation dispute resolution that allows a facilitator to help the two parties settle their differences and come to an acceptable solution (Ch. 7).

medical asepsis clean and free from infection (Ch. 10, 26).

medically indigent refers to those individuals unable to pay for their own medical coverage (Ch. 7).

melena tarry stools caused by blood in feces (Ch. 18).

meniscus curvature appearing in a liquid's upper surface when a liquid is placed in a container (Ch. 24).

menses menstruation (Ch. 10).

mentor person assigned or requested to assist in training, guiding, or coaching another (Ch. 33).

metabolism total of all changes, chemical and physical, that take place in the body (Ch. 22).

metastasis in cancer, malignant cells spread from the primary growth to a new location (Ch. 16).

metrorrhagia uterine bleeding at irregular intervals (Ch. 14).

microallocation of scarce medical resources; decisions are made by physicians and individual members of the health care team (Ch. 8).

microbiology branch of biology dealing with the study of microscopic forms of life (Ch. 27, 31).

microcytic term describing a smaller than normal cell (Ch. 29).

microorganism microscopic living creature capable of transmission and reproduction in specific circumstances (Ch. 10).

microscopy inspection with a microscope (Ch. 26).

midstream collection urine sample collected in the middle of a flow of urine (Ch. 30).

minor person who has not reached the age of majority, usually 18 years (Ch. 7).

minutes written record of topics discussed and actions taken during meeting sessions (Ch. 33).

misdemeanor a lesser crime; misdemeanors vary from state to state in their definition. Punishment is usually probation or a time of public service and a fine (Ch. 7).

misfeasance is a civil law term referring to a lawful act that is improperly or unlawfully executed (Ch. 7).

modalities physical agents such as heat, cold, light, water, and electricity used to treat muscular or joint malfunction (Ch. 21).

monocyte white blood cell without cytoplasmic granules that has a large convoluted nonsegmented nucleus (Ch. 29).

morbidity number of cases of disease in a specific population (Ch. 10).

mordant substance that causes dye to adhere to an object; iodine is a mordant in Gram stain (Ch. 31).

morphology form and structure of an organism (Ch. 10, 31).

mortality the ratio of the number of deaths to a given population (Ch. 10).

mounting process of applying in sequence a portion of each of the 12 leads of the ECG recording onto a commercially prepared mounting form or plain sheet of paper as part of the patient's permanent record (Ch. 25).

moxibustion ancient Chinese method of treatment that uses a powdered plant substance on the skin to raise a blister (Ch. 3).

multigravida a woman who has been pregnant more than once (Ch. 14).

muscle testing method of testing the motion, strength, and task potential of a muscle or group of muscles, their tendons, and associated tissues (Ch. 21).

mycology study of fungi (Ch. 27, 31).

myringotomy incision into the tympanic membrane; part of the treatment for otitis media (Ch. 15).

Nägele's rule usual method for calculating expected date of birth (Ch. 14).

nebulizer instrument used to produce a fine spray of medication (Ch. 18).

negligence failure to exercise a certain standard of care (Ch. 7, 33).

nematode round worm (Ch. 31).

neonatal pertaining to newborn (Ch. 14).

nephrolithotomy incision into the kidney to remove stones (Ch. 18).

networking process in which people of similar interests exchange information in social, business, or professional relationships (Ch. 34).

neutrophil the most common type of granulocytic white blood cell (Ch. 29).

nevus a mole (Ch. 17).

niacin one of the B-complex vitamins (Ch. 22).

nitrogenous waste products in the blood indicating kidney disease (Ch. 18).

nocturia excessive urination during the night (Ch. 16, 18).

nomogram graph that shows the relation among numeric values. Body surface area (BSA) of a patient can be estimated by its use (Ch. 24).

noncompliant failure to follow a required command or instruction (Ch. 7).

nonfeasance a civil law term referring to the failure to perform an act, official duty, or legal requirement (Ch. 7).

noninvasive procedures that do not require entering the body or puncturing the skin (Ch. 20, 25).

normal flora microorganisms that are normally present in a specific site (Ch. 10, 31).

normal saline a solution of sodium chloride (salt) and distilled water. It has the same osmotic pressure as blood serum. It is also known as isotonic or physiologic saline (Ch. 9).

normal sinus rhythm term used to describe the heart's rhythm when it is within the normal range (Ch. 25).

normochromic of normal color, in this case, when referring to red blood cells (Ch. 29).

normocytic term that describes a normal-sized cell (Ch. 29).

nosocomial hospital acquired (Ch. 31).

nullipara a woman who has not carried a pregnancy to the stage of viability (Ch. 14).

nutrient ingested substance that helps the body stay in its homeostatic state (Ch. 22).

nutrition study of the bringing of nutrients into the body and how the body uses these nutrients (Ch. 22).

nystagmus continuous involuntary movement of the eyes (Ch. 18).

objective a patient sign that is visible, palpable, or measurable by an observer (Ch. 11); also, magnifying lens that is closest to the object being viewed with a microscope (Ch. 27).

obturator tool that obstructs or closes a cavity or opening. The internal portion of an examination instrument that facilitates the entry of the instrument into the body; it is then withdrawn, permitting visualization of the internal area (Ch. 18).

occluder instrument used to obstruct or close off an eye (Ch. 18).

occlusion closure of a passage (Ch. 9).

oliguria decrease in urine output (Ch. 18).

open-ended questions questions that encourage verbalization and response; questions that seek a response beyond a simple yes or no (Ch. 4).

ophthalmoscope instrument for examination of the interior of the eye (Ch. 18).

opportunistic infection an infection that results from a defective immune system that cannot defend itself from pathogens normally found in the environment (Ch. 10).

opticokinetic drum test test used to help diagnose nystagmus (Ch. 18).

orchidectomy surgical excision of a testicle (Ch. 16).

orthopnea difficulty breathing in any position other than an upright position (Ch. 12).

oscilloscope an electronic device used for recording electrical activity of the heart, brain, and muscular tissues (Ch. 20, 25).

otoscope instrument used to examine the external ear canal and tympanic membrane (Ch. 18).

outer-directed people people who let events, other people, or environmental factors dictate their behavior (Ch. 5).

ova eggs of parasites (Ch. 31).

overtime money paid at a rate of not less than one and one-half times the regular rate of pay after a 40-hour work week is completed (Ch. 34).

oxidation process of a substance combining with oxygen (Ch. 22).

oxygenated containing high levels of oxygen (Ch. 28).

oxytocin a pituitary hormone that stimulates the muscles of the uterus to contract, thus inducing labor (Ch. 14).

palliative measures taken to relieve symptoms of disease (Ch. 10, 20).

pallor lack of color, paleness (Ch. 13).

palpate to search for a vein using the fingertips with a pressure and release touch (Ch. 28).

pandemic a disease affecting the majority of the population of a large region; is epidemic at same time in many parts of the world (Ch. 10).

panel a series of tests related to a particular organ or organ system of body function. For example, a liver panel would check many different functions of the liver. Previously called a "profile" (Ch. 27).

papular pertaining to a small, red elevated area of the skin, solid and circumscribed (Ch. 10).

paracentesis puncture of a cavity for removal of fluid (Ch. 10).

parasitology study of organisms (parasites and their eggs) that live within or on another organism and at the expense of that organism (Ch. 27, 31).

parasympathetic nervous system part of the autonomic nervous system that returns the body to its normal state after stress has subsided (Ch. 5).

parenteral injection of a liquid substance into the body via a route other than the alimentary canal (Ch. 10, 24).

paresthesia a sensation of numbness, prickling, or heightened sensitivity (Ch. 18).

parity carrying a pregnancy to the point of viability regardless of the outcome (Ch. 14).

participatory manager operates on the premise that the worker is capable and wants to do a good job (Ch. 33).

parturition the process of giving birth (Ch. 14).

patent open, not blocked (Ch. 14).

pathogen disease-producing microorganism (Ch. 10, 31).

Patient Self-Determination Act (PSDA) the Act that includes the Advance Directive giving patients the rights to be involved in their health care decisions (Ch. 7).

patient service centers satellite laboratory facilities located in convenient areas for patients where specimens can be collected or dropped off (Ch. 27).

peak the opposite of "trough," this is the point at which a drug is at its highest level in the body. Usually this occurs about 30 minutes after administration. In lab tests, the peak would tell the physician the strongest influence the drug would have on the body at that particular dose (Ch. 27).

pellagra disease caused by a deficiency in vitamin B_3 (nicotinic acid) characterized by sores on the skin, diarrhea, anxiety, confusion, and death if not treated (Ch. 22).

pelvic inflammatory disease infection of uterus, fallopian tubes, and adjacent pelvic structures; most common causes are gonorrhea and chlamydia; spread as sexually transmitted diseases (Ch. 14).

perception conscious awareness of one's own feelings and the feelings of others (Ch. 4).

perforation a hole caused by ulceration (Ch. 18).

peripheral nerve nerves and ganglia away from the spinal cord (Ch. 18).

peritonitis inflammation of the peritoneum (Ch. 18).

pernicious anemia chronic anemia caused by lack of hydrochloric acid in the stomach; weakness, fatigue, tingling of extremities, and even heart failure can result; vitamin B_{12} injections are the treatment for this condition (Ch. 17).

petri dish plastic dish into which agar is placed for the purpose of growing bacteria (Ch. 31).

pH scale that indicates the relative alkalinity or acidity of a solution; measurement of hydrogen ion concentration (Ch. 30).

phacoemulsification treatment for cataracts. An ultrasonic devise is used to disintegrate the cataract of the lens of the eye, which is then aspirated and removed (Ch. 18).

pharmacology study of drugs; the science concerned with the history, origin, sources, physical and chemical properties, and uses of drugs and their effects on living organisms (Ch. 23).

pharmacopoeia book describing drugs and their preparation or a collection or stock of drugs (Ch. 3).

phenylketonuria (PKU) a hereditary disease caused by the body's inability to oxidize an amino acid (phenylalanine). If not discovered and treated early, brain damage can occur, causing severe mental retardation (Ch. 15, 32).

phlebotomy process of collecting blood (Ch. 10, 28).

physician's directive another name for a living will (Ch. 6).

physicians' office laboratories (POLs) laboratories within physicians' offices where common office laboratory tests are performed (Ch. 27).

phytomedicines herbs used as medicinal plants. They contain plant material as their active ingredient (Ch. 24).

placenta abruptio sudden and abrupt separation of the placenta from uterine wall (Ch. 14).

placenta previa placenta lies low in uterus and can partially or completely cover the cervical os (Ch. 14).

plaintiff person bringing charges in litigation (Ch. 7).

plantar flexion moving the foot downward at the ankle (Ch. 21).

plasma fluid portion of blood from a tube containing anticoagulant. This fluid contains fibrinogen (Ch. 28).

pluralistic (pluralism) society where there are several distinct ethnic, religious, or cultural groups that coexist with one another (Ch. 3).

polycystic situation of many (poly) or multiple cysts (Ch. 18).

polyp tumor with a stem found in nose, uterus, bladder, colon, or rectum (Ch. 18).

potassium hydroxide (KOH) 10% solution is placed on vaginal smears, as well as skin scrapings, hair, and other dry substances to dissolve excess debris. This clears the vision field for better viewing of fungi and spores (Ch. 31).

power verbs action words used to describe your attributes and strengths (Ch. 36).

practicum transitional stage providing opportunity to apply theory learned in the classroom to a health care setting through practical, hands-on experience (Ch. 1, 33).

precedents refers to rulings made at an earlier time and include decisions made in a court, interpretations of a constitution, and statutory law decisions (Ch. 7).

precipitate substance in the form of fine particles that separates from a solution if allowed to stand for a time (Ch. 24).

precordial pertaining to the area on the anterior surface of the body overlying the heart (Ch. 25).

preeclampsia a complication of pregnancy characterized by generalized edema, hypertension, and proteinuria (Ch. 14).

preexisting injury or disease that occurs before a certain date (Ch. 10).

preferred provider organization (PPO) organization of physicians who network together to offer discounts to purchasers of heath care insurance (Ch. 2).

prejudice opinion or judgment that is formed before all the facts are known (Ch. 4).

prenatal time period between fertilization and birth (Ch. 14).

presbycusis progressive loss of hearing caused by the normal aging process (Ch. 17).

prescribe to order or recommend the use of a drug, diet, or other form of therapy (Ch. 7, 23).

preservative chemical added to food to keep it fresh longer (Ch. 22).

primary container container that directly contains the specimen (Ch. 28).

primigravida a woman pregnant for the first time (Ch. 14).

probation period during which the employee and supervisory personnel may determine if both the environment and the position are satisfactory for the employee (Ch. 24).

problem-oriented medical record (POMR) a type of patient chart recordkeeping that uses a sheet at a prominent location in the chart to list vital identification data. Patient medical problems are identified by a number that corresponds to the charting; for example, bronchitis is #1, a broken wrist is #2, and so forth (Ch. 11).

procedure manual manual providing detailed information relative to the performance of tasks within the job description (Ch. 33).

processed food food that is no longer in a whole, natural state; cooked or packaged with parts removed or ingredients added (Ch. 22).

professional liability insurance insurance policy designed to protect assets in the event a claim for damages resulting from negligence is filed and awarded (Ch. 33).

professionalism the qualities that characterize or distinguish a professional person who conforms to the technical and ethical standards of the profession (Ch. 1).

proficiency testing sample tests performed in a clinical laboratory to determine with what degree of accuracy tests are being performed. Testing samples are checked in the same manner as patient specimens (Ch. 26).

profit sharing sharing in the financial profits, gains, and benefits of an organization (Ch. 33).

projection act of placing one's own feelings on another (Ch. 4).

pronation moving the arm so the palm is down (Ch. 21).

proprietary privately owned and managed facility, a profit-making organization (Ch. 1).

prostaglandin modulator of biochemical activity in tissues (Ch. 14).

proteinuria protein in the urine (Ch. 18).

protozoa one-celled animals divided into four groups: amoebae, flagellates, ciliates, and coccidia (Ch. 31).

provider performed microscopy (PPM) also called PPMP, which stands for provider performed microscopy procedure. This is a CLIA term for those microscopic examinations that require the expertise of a physician or second level provider qualified in microscopic examinations. The PPM is part of the CLIA's moderately complex category of tests (Ch. 26).

pruritis itchiness (Ch. 23).

psychomotor retardation slowing of physical and mental responses; may be seen in depression (Ch. 6).

puerperium the period from the end of the third stage of labor until involution of uterus is complete, usually three to six weeks (Ch. 14).

pulmonary edema accumulation of serous fluid in the air vesicles and interstitial tissues of the lungs (Ch. 26).

purified protein derivative (PPD) filtrate obtained from Mycobacterium cultures used for intradermal testing for tuberculosis (Ch. 32).

purulent forming or containing pus (Ch. 10).

pyorrhea discharge of pus from the gums, around the teeth (Ch. 13).

pyrexia fever (Ch. 12).

pyridoxine vitamin B_6 (Ch. 22).

pyuria pus in the urine (Ch. 18).

qualitative test analysis to identify quality or characteristics of components, such as size, shape, and maturity of cells (Ch. 27).

quality assurance (QA) process to provide accurate, complete, consistent health care documentation in a timely manner while making every reasonable effort to resolve inconsistencies, inaccuracies, risk management issues, and other problems (Ch. 26).

quality control measures used to monitor the processing of laboratory specimens. Includes proper use, storage, handling, stability, expiration dates, and indications for measuring precision and accuracy of analytic processes (Ch. 26, 30, 31).

quantitative test analysis that can identify quantity or actual number counts such as counting the number of blood cells (Ch. 27).

radioactive emits rays or particles from nucleus (Ch. 20).

radiograph the film on which an image is produced through exposure to X-rays (Ch. 20).

radiolucent allowing X-rays to pass through. A dark area appears on the radiograph (Ch. 20).

radionuclides atoms that disintegrate by emitting electromagnetic radiation (Ch. 20).

radiopaque impenetrable to X-rays. A light area appears on the radiograph (Ch. 20).

radiopharmaceuticals radioactive chemicals used in testing the location, size, outline, or function of tissue, organs, vessels, or body fluids (Ch. 20).

rales abnormal bubbling or crackling sound heard by auscultation during the inspiratory phase of respiration (Ch. 12).

range of motion (ROM) amount of movement that is present in a joint (Ch. 21).

ratchets locking mechanisms on the handles of many surgical instruments (Ch. 19).

rationalization act of justification, usually illogically, that one uses to keep from facing the truth of the situation (Ch. 4).

reagent chemical substance that detects or synthesizes other substances in a chemical reaction; used in laboratory analyses because it is known to react in a specific way (Ch. 27, 30, 31).

reagent test strip narrow strip of plastic on which pads containing reagents are attached; used in the urinalysis chemical examination to detect glucose, bilirubin, ketones, specific gravity, blood, pH, urobilinogen, nitrites, and leukocyte esterase (Ch. 30).

recertification documentation admitted to support continued education for maintaining a professional credential (Ch. 35).

reference laboratories independent, regionally located laboratories used by hospitals for complex, expensive, or specialized tests (Ch. 27).

references individuals who have known or worked with a person long enough to make an honest assessment and recommendation regarding your background history (Ch. 36).

reference values also referred to as normal value, normal range, or reference range; range of values that includes 95% of test results for a normal healthy population (Ch. 27).

refractometer instrument that measures the refractive index of a substance or solution; used in the urinalysis physical examination to measure the urine specimen's specific gravity (Ch. 30).

Registered Medical Assistant (RMA) credential awarded for successfully passing the AMT examination (Ch. 1, 35).

regression moving back to a former stage to escape conflict or fear (Ch. 4).

regulated waste any waste that contains infectious material that would pose a threat due to possible transmission of pathogenic microorganisms (Ch. 10).

rehabilitation medicine field of medical disciplines that seeks to restore an individual or body part to normal or near-normal function after an illness or injury using physical and mechanical agents (Ch. 21).

reimbursement payment (Ch. 26).

repolarization reestablishment of a polarized state in a muscle after contraction (Ch. 25).

repression coping with an overwhelming situation by temporarily forgetting it; temporary amnesia (Ch. 4).

requisition request form sent with a specimen specifying tests to be performed on the specimen; most common tests are separated into logical categories with additional space for writing special requests (Ch. 26, 27).

rescue breathing performed on individuals in respiratory arrest, rescue breathing is a mouth-to-mouth (using appropriate protective equipment) or mouth-to-nose procedure that provides oxygen to the patient until emergency personnel arrive (Ch. 9).

residual urine amount of urine remaining in bladder immediately after voiding; seen with hyperplasia of prostate (Ch. 26, 27).

resistance ability of the immune system to resist or withstand an infectious disease (Ch. 10).

résumé written summary data sheet or brief account of qualifications and progress in your chosen career (Ch. 36).

retention urine held in the bladder; inability to empty the bladder (Ch. 16).

retrolental fibroplasia disease of blood vessels of retina in newborns (Ch. 24).

Rh factor blood factor indicating the presence or absence of the Rh antigen on the surface of human erythrocytes (Ch. 32).

rhythm strip ECG recording of a single lead, usually lead II, that is used to determine the rhythm of the heart beat. An arrhythmia can more easily be seen in a rhythm strip because it is run longer per physician's request (Ch. 25).

riboflavin vitamin B_2 (Ch. 22).

risk management techniques adhered to in the ambulatory care setting that keep the practice, its environment, and its procedures as safe for the patient as possible. Proper risk management also reduces the possibility of negligence that leads to torts and malpractice suits (Ch. 7, 9, 33).

roadblocks verbal or nonverbal messages that block communication (Ch. 4).

rosacea a chronic skin condition characterized by pustules, papules, erythema, and hyperplasia. Its cause is unknown (Ch. 18).

rotation turning a body part around its axis (Ch. 21); also, opportunity to spend two or three weeks in a variety of health care settings (Ch. 28).

salary review informing the employee of their revised base pay rate (Ch. 33).

salicylates aspirin-type drugs that can cause ulcers because of their irritation of the gastrointestinal tract (Ch. 18).

sanitization cleaning or scrubbing contaminated instruments or fomites to remove tissue, debris, or other contaminants (Ch. 10).

saturated fat fat that comes from an animal source and that contains more cholesterol than unsaturated fat, which comes from vegetable sources (Ch. 22).

scabies infectious skin disease caused by the itch mite (Sarcoptes scabiei), which is transmitted by direct contact with infected persons (Ch. 10).

scleroderma slowly progressing disease characterized by deposition of fibrous connective tissue in the skin and in internal organs (Ch. 13).

scoop technique a one-handed technique used to "scoop" up and cover a used needle only if a sharp's container is not immediately available, the covering (cap) over the needle is not manipulated in any way; it is then carried to the nearest sharps container for disposal (Ch. 10).

scope of practice the range of clinical procedures and activities that are allowed by law for a profession (Ch. 1).

screening preliminary examination used to detect the most characteristic signs of a disorder that may entail further investigation (Ch. 30).

scurvy a deficiency in vitamin C characterized by the abnormal formation of bones and teeth. Signs of hemorrhage can appear such as bruising (Ch. 22).

search engine specialized computer program designed to find specific information on the Internet (Ch. 33).

secretion substance produced by the cells of glandular organs from materials in the blood (Ch. 10, 26).

sediment insoluble material that settles to the bottom of a liquid; material examined in the urinalysis microscopic examination (Ch. 30).

self-actualization being all that you can be; developing your full potential and experiencing fulfillment (Ch. 5, 33).

semen thick, viscid secretion discharged from the urethra of males at orgasm. It is a mixed product containing various fluids and spermatozoa (Ch. 32).

senile mental and physical weakness sometimes associated with aging (Ch. 17).

sensitivity test in which an organism is placed with antibiotics to determine which antibiotic will effectively kill the organism with the smallest dose (Ch. 31).

sensor term used to describe a metallic-coated paper tab that is applied to the patient's body in preparation for an ECG (also known as electrode). Sensors are placed on specific locations on the skin, then attached to the ECG with wires. The sensors conduct electricity from the patient to the ECG machine (Ch. 25).

sensorineural permanent hearing loss that results from damage or malformation of the middle ear and auditory nerve (Ch. 15).

septicemia invasion of pathogenic bacteria into the bloodstream (Ch. 3).

serum liquid portion of blood obtained after blood has been allowed to clot (Ch. 27, 28).

severe acute respiratory syndrome (SARS) a viral outbreak of a respiratory illness first reported in Asia in 2003; spread by close person-to-person contact and characterized by fever and respiratory symptoms (Ch. 10).

shadow follow a supervisor or delegated subordinate to learn facility protocol (Ch. 33).

sharps needles or scalpels or other sharp instruments that are capable of causing a penetrating or puncture wound of the skin (Ch. 10).

shock potentially serious condition in which the circulatory system is not providing enough blood to all parts of the body, causing the body's organs to fail to function properly (Ch. 9).

short-range goals long-range goals are dissected and reassembled into smaller, more manageable time segments (Ch. 5).

sickle cell anemia an inherited blood disorder that may shorten life span (Ch. 14).

silver nitrate caustic astringent antiseptic. As a weak liquid, it is applied to the eyes of newborns to prevent infections at birth. In the medical office, it is most often seen as a solid substance impregnated onto the end of a wooden applicator. Silver nitrate applicator sticks contain hydrochloric acid and other chemicals and are commonly used to cauterize small blood vessels in the nose or other mucous membranes (Ch. 19).

sitz bath a warm water bath, in which only the hips and buttocks are immersed (Ch. 19).

slander false and malicious words about another constituting a defamation of character (Ch. 7).

SOAP acronym for patient progress notes based on subjective impressions (S), objective clinical evidence (O), assessment or diagnosis (A), and plans for further studies (P) (Ch. 11).

sodium hydroxide chemical used to chemically burn and destroy tissue; usually in a liquid state when used in minor surgery (Ch. 19).

sodium hypochlorite household bleach (Ch. 10).

solvent producing a solution, dissolving (Ch. 10).

sonographer professionally trained individual capable of performing the ultrasound examination (Ch. 25).

source-oriented medical record (SOMR) a type of patient chart record keeping that includes separate sections for different sources of patient information, such as laboratory reports, pathology reports, and progress notes (Ch. 11).

species second Greek or Latin name given to microorganisms; the species name is not capitalized (Ch. 31).

specific gravity ratio of weight of a given volume of a substance to the weight of the same volume of distilled water at the same temperature; test often performed during the urinalysis physical examination (can also appear on the reagent strip) (Ch. 30).

spermatogenesis the formation of mature sperm (Ch. 16).

spill kit commercially packaged materials containing supplies and equipment needed to clean up a spill of a biohazardous substance (Ch. 10).

spirometry test to measure the air capacity of the lungs (Ch. 18).

splint any device used to immobilize a body part. Often used by EMS personnel (Ch. 9).

spores an inactive state of some bacteria in which they are capsulated in protein. The encapsulation protects them from heat, chemicals, freezing, desiccation, and radiation. Spores can live for tens of thousands of years with no nutrient. When they are placed onto fertile soil (such as human tissue), they can become activated and grow. Tetanus is one type of bacteria that creates spores (Ch. 31).

sprain injury to a joint, often an ankle, knee, or wrist, that involves a tearing of the ligaments. Most sprains are minor and heal quickly; others are more severe, include swelling, and may not heal properly if the patient continues to put stress on the sprained joint (Ch. 9).

sputum substance from the respiratory tract expelled by coughing (Ch. 10).

stab culture culture where the microorganism is stabbed into tubed solid media (Ch. 31).

standard rules established to measure quality, weight, extent, or value (Ch. 10, 26).

Standard Precautions precautions developed in 1996 by the Centers for Disease Control and Prevention (CDC) that augment universal precautions and body substance isolation practices. They provide a wider range of protection and are used any time there is contact with blood, moist body fluid (except perspiration), mucous membranes, or nonintact skin. They are designed to protect all health care providers, patients, and visitors (Ch. 9, 10).

status asthmaticus severe episode of asthma that does not respond to ordinary treatment (Ch. 24).

statutory law refers to the body of laws established by states (Ch. 7).

sterile field area that immediately surrounds and is prepared exclusively for surgery for a particular patient. All items necessary for the surgical procedure are sterile (Ch. 19).

stertorous snoring sound heard with labored breathing (Ch. 12).

stigma a social condition marked by attitudinal devaluing or demeaning of persons who, because of disfigurement or disability, are not viewed as being capable of fulfilling valued social roles (Ch. 14).

stomatitis inflammation of the mouth associated with radiation therapy. Can include swelling, redness, halitosis, ulcerations (Ch. 20).

strabismus disorder of the eye in which optic axes cannot be directed to the same object (cross-eye) (Ch. 18).

strain injury to the soft tissue between joints that involves the tearing of muscles or tendons. Strains often occur in the neck, back, or thigh muscles (Ch. 9).

stratum corneum horny, outermost layer of the skin, epidermis, composed of dead cells converted to keratin that continually flakes away (Ch. 18).

stress body's response to change; can be manifested in a variety of ways, including changes in blood pressure, heart rate, and onset of headache (Ch. 5).

stressors demands to change that cause stress (Ch. 5).

strictures narrowing of a tubelike structure such as the esophagus or urethra (Ch. 19).

stridor crowing sound heard on inspiration, the result of an upper airway obstruction (Ch. 12).

stylus heated slender wire of the electrocardiograph that melts the wax off of the ECG paper during the recording (Ch. 25).

subjective symptom that is felt by the patient but not observable by others (Ch. 11).

sublimation redirecting a socially unacceptable impulse into one that is socially acceptable (Ch. 4).

subordinate in an organization, a person under the direction of (reporting to) a person of greater authority (Ch. 33).

subpoena written command designating a person to appear in court under penalty for failure to appear (Ch. 7).

supernatant urine that appears above the sediment when centrifuged; poured off before sediment is examined in the urinalysis microscopic examination (Ch. 30).

supination moving the arm so the palm is up (Ch. 21).

suppressed immune system term used to describe an immune system unable to function normally due to the presence of a disease such as AIDS (Ch. 26).

suppurant an agent causing pus formation (Ch. 19).

suppurative producing or associated with the generation of pus (Ch. 15).

surgery cards written reference for surgeries and procedures (Ch. 19).

surgical asepsis procedures that render objects sterile; techniques to maintain sterile conditions during invasive procedures (Ch. 10, 19).

surrogate substitute; someone who substitutes for another (Ch. 8).

suture surgical material or thread; may describe the act of sewing with the surgical thread and needle (Ch. 19).

swaged a surgical needle attached to a length of suture material (Ch. 19).

symmetry correspondence in shape, size, and position of body parts on opposites of the body (Ch. 13).

sympathetic nervous system large part of the autonomic nervous system that prepares the body for fight-or-flight (Ch. 5).

syncope fainting (Ch. 9, 25).

systemic pertaining to the whole body (Ch. 9).

systole one component of blood pressure measurement representing the highest amount of pressure exerted during the cardiac cycle; the force exerted on the arterial walls during cardiac contraction (Ch. 12, 25).

tachycardia, sinus abnormally rapid heartbeat greater than 100 beats/minute. A type of cardiac arrhythmia (Ch. 12, 25).

tachypnea abnormal increased rate of breathing (Ch. 12).

targeted résumé résumé format utilized when focusing on a clear, specific job target (Ch. 36).

Task Force for Test Construction (TFTC) committee of professionals whose responsibility is to update the CMA examination annually to reflect changes in medical assistants' responsibilities and to include new developments in medical knowledge and technology (Ch. 35).

taut to pull or draw tight a surface, such as skin (Ch. 24).

taxonomy classification of organisms into appropriate categories (Ch. 31).

Tay–Sachs an inherited disease that is usually fatal (Ch. 14).

teamwork persons synergistically working together (Ch. 33).

test cable accessory device that attaches between the Holter monitor and the electrocardiograph to check for correct waveform and lack of artifact (Ch. 25).

thalassemia a hereditary anemia that may be fatal (Ch. 14).

thallium scan chemical element given intravenously and used in cardiac stress tests. The radioisotope localizes in the myocardium, and a scanning device picks up the distribution of the thallium and can identify blockages in the coronary arteries. An accurate test for coronary artery disease (Ch. 25).

therapeutic communication use of specific and well-defined professional communication skills to create a feeling of comfort for patients even when difficult or unpleasant information must be exchanged (Ch. 4).

therapeutic drug monitoring (TDM) periodic blood tests to determine the effectiveness of a particular drug. Drugs will have a therapeutic level that must be attained in order for the drug to be therapeutic or effective. If the blood level of the drug is below the range of therapeutic effectiveness, the physician will probably increase the dosage. Likewise, if the drug is above the therapeutic range, the physician will probably lower it (Ch. 27).

thermolabile easily affected by heat (Ch. 10).

thermotherapy use of heat to treat a physical condition (Ch. 21).

thiamin vitamin B_1 (Ch. 23).

thixotropic separator gel gel material capable of forming an interface between the cells and fluid portion of the blood as a result of centrifugation (Ch. 28).

thoracentesis surgical puncture of the thoracic cavity to aspirate fluid (Ch. 10).

thrombocyte (platelet) cellular fragment of megataryocyte; plays an important role in blood coagulation, hemostasis, and clot formation (Ch. 28, 29).

tinnitus ringing or buzzing sound in the ear (Ch. 13).

titer measurement of amount of antibody present against a particular antigen (Ch. 14).

tocopherol vitamin E (Ch. 22).

tort wrongful act that results in injury to one person by another (Ch. 7).

tort law laws that stem from torts, or wrongful acts that cause harm to one person, by another (Ch. 7).

tourniquet device used to facilitate vein prominence (Ch. 28).

toxicity the level at which a drug or chemical becomes poisonous or toxic. Some substances, such as some metals are considered toxic at any level of accidental exposure (Ch. 27).

trace mineral mineral required by the body in small amounts (Ch. 22).

tracing graphic record usually of an event that changes with time as with the electrical activity of the heart (Ch. 25).

transducer device that converts one form of energy to another. During an ultrasound procedure, the transducer picks up echoes and converts them to electrical energy. The energy is transformed into a picture on a television monitor or printed on paper. Photographs of the image can be taken (Ch. 20, 25).

transferable skills skills that would be used in a host of different and unrelated occupations. Keyboarding skill is an example of a transferable skill. It could be used by a secretary, data entry clerk, medical assistant, or clothing manufacturer (Ch. 36).

transient ischemic attack temporary interference with blood flow to brain; may last only a few moments or several hours; neurological symptoms occur (Ch. 17).

transilluminator instrument used to inspect a cavity or organ by passing a light through the walls (Ch. 16).

transmission spread of infectious disease by direct contact, indirect contact, inhalation, ingestion, or bloodborne contact (Ch. 10).

Transmission-Based Precautions second tier of Centers for Disease Control and Prevention (CDC) guidelines that applies to specific categories of patients and that include air, contact, and droplet precautions. Transmission-Based Precautions are always used in addition to Standard Precautions (Ch. 10).

transurethral resection removal of prostate tissue using a device inserted through the urethra (Ch. 16).

triage process to determine and prioritize patients' needs and the likely benefit from immediate medical attention. From the French *trier,* meaning "to sort" (Ch. 2, 9).

trichomoniasis infestation with a Trichomonas parasite which may be transmitted through sexual intercourse (Ch. 10, 14).

triglycerides form of fat in the bloodstream that functions to store energy (Ch. 32).

trimester three months; one-third of the gestational period of pregnancy (Ch. 14).

trough the opposite of "peak," this is the point at which the drug is at its lowest level in the body. Usually this occurs just before the next dose is administered. In lab tests, the trough will tell the physician the weakest influence the drug would have on the body at that particular dose (Ch. 27).

tuberculosis (TB) infectious disease caused by the bacterium, *Mycobacterium tuberculosis* (Ch. 32).

turbid opaque, lacking clarity (Ch. 30).

tympanostomy placement of a tube through the tympanic membrane to allow ventilation of the middle ear; part of the treatment for otitis media (Ch. 15).

typhus (typhoid) acute infectious disease that causes severe headache, rash, high fever, and progressive neurologic involvement. Prevalent where conditions are unsanitary and congested (Ch. 3).

ultrasonic cleaner machine that uses the energy of high-frequency sound waves that agitate to sanitize instruments before sterilization (Ch. 10).

ultrasonography process of placing a handheld transducer against a body area to be tested. The transducer sends sound waves through the skin and the various internal organs. When echoes are formed and sent back the transducer converts them into electrical energy. This energy is transformed into a picture for a monitor, or printed on paper. Photographs of the images can be taken and become part of the patient's permanent record (Ch. 14, 25).

ultrasound use of high-frequency sound waves for therapeutic reasons to generate heat in deep tissue (Ch. 21).

undifferentiated a change in the character of a cell(s) toward a malignant state (Ch. 10).

undoing actions designed to make amends to cancel out inappropriate behavior (Ch. 4).

unipolar having or pertaining to one pole process (Ch. 25).

unit dose premeasured amount of medication, individually packaged on a per-dose basis (Ch. 24).

universal emergency medical identification symbol identification sometimes carried by individuals to identify health problems they may have (Ch. 9).

Universal Precautions guidelines established by the Centers for Disease Control and Prevention (CDC) for the protection of health care workers from infectious diseases (Ch. 10).

unsterile field area that is adjacent to the sterile field where items needed can be accessed, opened, and supplied by an individual who does not wear sterile garb (Ch. 19).

urea principal end product of protein metabolism (Ch. 30).

uremia toxic condition of the blood caused by the kidneys' inability to filter waste products from the blood (Ch. 18).

urgency the need to urinate immediately (Ch. 18).

urinalysis examination of the physical, chemical, and microscopic properties of urine (Ch. 27, 30).

urinary tract infection (UTI) also referred to as a bladder infection (Ch. 30).

urobilinogen colorless compound produced in the intestine after the breakdown by bacteria of bilirubin (Ch. 30).

urticaria hives (Ch. 23).

vaccine pharmacologic agent capable of producing artificial active immunity (Ch. 10).

vasoconstriction narrowing or constricting of blood vessels (Ch. 21).

vasodilation widening or dilating of blood vessels (Ch. 21).

vector a carrier of disease, usually an insect, that is the causative organism of disease from infected to noninfected individuals (Ch. 10).

venipuncture opening a vein to obtain a blood sample (Ch. 28).

vertigo the sensation of moving around in space; dizziness, lightheadedness (Ch. 13).

vesicular characterized by the presence of vesicles. Vesicles are blisters or other elevations on the skin (Ch. 10, 14).

viable able to live, grow, and develop after birth; usually 24 weeks or greater than 1 pound (Ch. 14).

virology study of viruses (Ch. 27, 31).

virulence an organism's relative power and degree of pathogenicity (Ch. 10).

viscosity degree of thickness of a liquid (Ch. 28).

vitiligo skin disorder characterized by smooth white spots on various areas of the body (Ch. 13).

volatile easily evaporated (Ch. 19).

waived used to describe a category of clinical laboratory tests that are simple, unvarying, and require a minimum of judgment and interpretation (Ch. 26).

water-soluble pertaining to substances that are hydrophilic and therefore dissolve better in water (Ch. 22).

Web site a remote computer that stores World Wide Web documents consisting of Web pages (Ch. 33).

wet mount a method of adding liquid, usually saline or formalin, to a specimen on a slide for examination and preservation. The specimen is placed on a slide and one drop of saline (for trichomonas vaginalis) or potassium hydroxide (for diagnosis vaginal yeast infections) is applied and mixes with the specimen. It is then covered with a coverslip and examined microscopically (Ch. 14, 31).

wheal slight elevation of skin that can be produced as a result of an intradermal injection (Ch. 18, 32).

wheezes high-pitched musical sound heard on expiration, often the result of an obstruction or narrowing of respiratory passages (Ch. 12).

Wood's lamp light source used to fluoresce certain fungal cultures; used to aid in the identification of dermatophytes (Ch. 31).

work practice controls measures used in the workplace that consist of physical equipment and mechanical devices to control employee exposure to bloodborne pathogens and other potentially infectious materials. Examples are sharps disposal containers, handwashing facilities, PPE, eyewash stations, and so on (Ch. 10).

work statement concise description of the work you plan to accomplish (Ch. 33).

wound a break in the continuity of soft parts of body structures caused by violence or trauma to tissues. In an open wound, skin is broken as in a laceration, abrasion, avulsion, or incision. In a closed wound, skin is not broken as in contusion, ecchymosis, or hematoma (Ch. 9).

xerophthalmia dry, lusterless mucous membranes of the eyes (Ch. 22).

yellow fever acute infectious disease where a person develops jaundice, vomits, hemorrhages, and has a fever; caused mostly by mosquitoes (Ch. 3).

APPENDIX A

Common Medical Abbreviations and Symbols

$\overline{aa}$	of each
AAMA	American Association of Medical Assistants
AAMT	American Association of Medical Transcription
AAPC	American Academy of Professional Coders
ab	abortion
abd	abdomen
ABE	acute bacterial endocarditis
ABG	arterial blood gases
ABHES	Accrediting Bureau of Health Education Schools
ABO	blood groups
abs	absent
ac	before meals (ante cibum)
ac	acute
ACAP	Alliance of Claims Assistance Professionals
ACTH	adrenocorticotropic hormone
ADA	Americans with Disabilities Act
ADL	activities of daily living
ad lib	as desired
adm	admission
AED	automated electronic defibrillator
AFP	alpha fetal protein
AHD	arteriosclerotic heart disease
	atherosclerotic heart disease
AHIMA	American Health Information Management Association
AIDS	acquired immunodeficiency syndrome
alb	albumin
AM	before noon (ante meridiem)
AMA	against medical advice
	American Medical Association
AMI	acute myocardial infarction
amt	amount
AMT	American Medical Technologists
AMTIE	American Medical Technologists Institute for Education
ant	anterior
ante	before
A&P	anterior and posterior
	auscultation and palpation
	auscultation and percussion
APC	ambulatory payment classifications
aq	water
A/R	accounts receivable
ARDS	acute (or adult) respiratory disease syndrome
ARU	automated routing unit
ASA	acetylsalicylic acid
ASAP	as soon as possible
ASCAD	arteriosclerotic coronary artery disease
ASCVD	arteriosclerotic cardiovascular disease
	atherosclerotic cardiovascular disease
A&W	alive and well
Ba	barium
BaE	barium enema
BBB	bundle branch block
BC	birth control
BCP	birth control pills
BC/BS	Blue Cross/Blue Shield
BE	bacterial endocarditis
bid	twice a day
bil	bilateral
BM	basal metabolism
	bowel movement
BMR	basal metabolism rate
BP	blood pressure
BPH	benign prostatic hypertrophy

BS	blood sugar
	bowel sounds
	breath sounds
BSA	body surface area
BSL	blood sugar level
BSN	bowel sounds normal
BSO	bilateral salpingo-oophorectomy
BSR	blood sedimentation rate
BUN	blood urea nitrogen
BW	below waist
	birth weight
	body weight
Bx	biopsy
C	Celsius
	centigrade
c̄	with
C1	first cervical vertebra
CA	cancer
	carcinoma
Ca	calcium
CAAHEP	Commission on Accreditation of Allied Health Education Programs
CAD	coronary artery disease
CAHD	coronary arteriosclerotic heart disease
caps	capsules
CAT	computerized axial tomography
CBC	complete blood count
CC	chief complaint
CCA	Certified Coding Associate
CCR	continuity of care record
CCS	Certified Coding Specialist
CCS-P	Certified Coding Specialist-Physician-Based
CCU	coronary care unit
C&D	cystoscopy and dilation
CDC	U.S. Centers for Disease Control and Prevention
CE	continuing education
cerv	cervical
	cervix
CEU	continuing education unit
CF	conversion factor
CHAMPVA	Civilian Health and Medical Program of the Veterans Administration
CHD	childhood disease
	congenital heart disease
	congestive heart disease
	coronary heart disease
CHF	congestive heart failure
CHO	carbohydrate
CIN	cervical intraepithelial neoplasia
ck	check
Cl	chlorine
cldy	cloudy
CLIA	Clinical Laboratory Improvement Amendments
cm	centimeter
CMA	Certified Medical Assistant
CMAS	Certified Medical Administrative Specialist
CME	continuing medical education
CMS	Centers for Medicare and Medicaid Services
CMT	Certified Medical Transcriptionist
CNS	central nervous system
C/O	complains of
CO_2	carbon dioxide
COB	coordination of benefits
COPD	chronic obstructive pulmonary disease
CPC	Certified Professional Coders
CPC-A	Certified Professional Coders-Apprentice
CPC-H	Certified Professional Coders-Hospital
CPC-HA	Certified Professional Coders-Hospital Apprentice
CPR	cardiopulmonary resuscitation
CPT	Current Procedural Code
CPU	central processing unit
CRB	Curriculum Review Board
crit	hematocrit
CS	cerebrospinal
	cesarean section
C&S	culture and sensitivity
CSF	cerebrospinal fluid
CT	computerized tomography
CVA	cerebrovascular accident
CVP	central venous pressure
CVS	chorionic villus sampling
cx	cervix
CXR	chest X-ray
cysto	cystoscopic examination
	cystoscopy
DACUM	developing a curriculum
DC	doctor of chiropracty
D&C	dilation and curettage
DDS	doctor of dentistry
DEA	U.S. Drug Enforcement Agency
dec	decrease
del	delivery
DHHS	U.S. Department of Health and Human Services
diab	diabetic
diag	diagnosis
diff	differential white blood cell count
dil	dilute
disc	discontinue
disp	dispense
DM	diabetes mellitus
DNA	deoxyribonucleic acid
	does not apply
DNR	do not resuscitate
DO	doctor of osteopathy
DOA	dead on arrival
DOB	date of birth
DOD	date of death
DOE	dyspnea on exertion
dos	dosage
DPM	doctor of podiatric medicine
DPT	diphtheria, pertussis, and tetanus
DR	delivery room
Dr	doctor
dr	dram
DRGs	diagnosis-related groups
DS	discharge summary
DSD	dry sterile dressing
dsg	dressing

DSS	digital speech standard
DT	delirium tremens
DTR	deep tendon reflex
D&V	diarrhea and vomiting
DW	distilled water
D/W	dextrose in water
dx	diagnosis
ea	each
EBV	Epstein–Barr virus
ECG	electrocardiogram
Echo	echocardiogram
	echoencephalogram
E. coli	*Escherichia coli*
ECT	electroconvulsive therapy
	electronic claims transmission
EDC	estimated date of confinement or expected date of confinement
EDD	estimated date of delivery or expected date of delivery
EEG	electroencephalogram
EENT	eyes, ears, nose, and throat
e.g.	for example
EKG	electrocardiogram
elix	elixir
e-mail	electronic mail
EMG	electromyography
EMR	electronic medical record
EMS	emergency medical service
ENT	ear, nose, and throat
EOB	explanation of benefits
eos	eosinophil
EPA	Environmental Protection Agency
EPO	exclusive provider organization
eq	equivalent
ER	emergency room
ERT	estrogen replacement therapy
ESR	erythrocyte sedimentation rate
EST	electroshock therapy
exam	examination
ext	extract
F	Fahrenheit
	female
fax	facsimile
FBS	fasting blood sugar
FDA	U.S. Food and Drug Administration
FECA	Federal Employees Compensation Act Program
FH	family history
FHR	fetal heart rate
FHS	fetal heart sound
fl	fluid
fl dr	fluid dram
fl oz	fluid ounce
FMP	first menstrual period
FP	family practice
freq	frequent
FSH	follicle-stimulating hormone
ft	foot
FTA	fluorescent treponemal antibody
FTP	file transfer protocol
fx	fracture
G	gravida
g	gram
GB	gallbladder
GC	gonococcus
	gonorrhea
GI	gastrointestinal
gm	gram
GP	general practice
GPCI	Geographic Practice Cost Index
gr	grain
grav	pregnancy
GTH	gonadotropic hormone
GTT	glucose tolerance test
gtt(s)	drop (drops)
GU	genitourinary
GYN	gynecology
h	hour
HBP	high blood pressure
HCFA	U.S. Health Care Financing Administration
hCG	human chorionic gonadotropin
HCl	hydrochloric acid
HCPCS	Healthcare Common Procedure Coding System
Hct	hematocrit
HCVD	hypertensive cardiovascular disease
HEENT	head, eyes, ears, nose, and throat
Hgb	hemoglobin
H&H	hemoglobin and hematocrit
HIPAA	Health Insurance Portability and Accountability Act
HMO	health maintenance organization
H/O	history of
H_2O	water
H&P	history and physical
HPI	history of present illness
HPV	human papillomavirus
HR	human resources
HRS	Healthcare Reimbursement Specialist
HRT	hormone replacement therapy
ht	height
hx	history
Hz	hertz
ICCU	intensive coronary care unit
ICD	International Classification of Diseases, Adapted
ICD-9-CM	International Classification of Diseases, 9th revision, Clinical Modification
ICU	intensive care unit
ID	intradermal
I&D	incision and drainage
IM	instant messaging
	internal medicine
	intramuscular
imp	impression
inf	infusion

inj	injection
I&O	intake and output
IPPB	intermittent positive pressure breathing
IPPS	inpatient prospective payment systems
ISP	Internet service provider
IUD	intrauterine device
IV	intravenous
IVP	intravenous pyelogram
JAAMT	*Journal of the American Association for Medical Transcription*
JAMA	*Journal of the American Medical Association*
JCAHO	Joint Commission on Accreditation of Healthcare Organizations
jt	joint
K	potassium
kg	kilogram
KOH	potassium hydroxide
KUB	kidney, ureter, and bladder
kV	kilovolt
L	left
	liter
l	length
LA	left atrium
	lactic acid
L&A	light and accommodation
lab	laboratory
lac	laceration
LAN	local area network
lap	laparotomy
lat	lateral
lb	pound
LBBB	left bundle branch block
LDL	low-density lipoprotein
LE	lupus erythematosus
liq	liquid
LLQ	lower left quadrant
LMP	last menstrual period
LP	lumbar puncture
LRQ	lower right quadrant
LUQ	left upper quadrant
L&W	living and well
lymphs	lymphocytes
M	male
m	meter
ʒ	minim
MBCD	management by coaching and development
MBCE	management by competitive edge
MBDM	management by decision models
MBP	management by performance
MBS	management by styles
MBWA	management by wandering around
MBWS	management by work simplification
MCHC	mean corpuscular hemoglobin and red cell indices
MCO	managed care organization
MCV	mean corpuscular volume and red cell indices
MD	doctor of medicine
	muscular dystrophy
MDR	minimum daily requirement
med	medicine
mEq/L	milliequivalents per liter
MFS	Medicare fee schedule
mg	milligram
MH	marital history
	medical history
	menstrual history
MHx	medical history
MI	maturation index
	myocardial infarction
ml	milliliter
mm	millimeter
mm^3	cubic millimeter
mm Hg	millimeters of mercury
MMR	measles, mumps, and rubella
MOM	milk of magnesia
mono	mononucleosis
MP	menstrual period
MRI	magnetic resonance imaging
MS	mitral stenosis
	multiple sclerosis
MSDS	material safety data sheets
MSHA	Mine Safety and Health Administration
MT	medical technologist
	medical transcriptionist
MTCC	Medical Transcriptionist Certification Commission
multip	multipara
MVP	mitral valve prolapse
NA	not applicable
NaCl	sodium chloride
narc	narcotic
NB	newborn
N/C	no complaints
ND	doctor of naturopathy
NEBA	National Electronic Billers Alliance
NEC	not elsewhere classified
neg	negative
NG	nasogastric
NGU	nongonococcal urethritis
NL	normal limits
NMP	normal menstrual period
noct	at night
Non-PAR	nonparticipating provider
non rep	do not repeat
NOS	not otherwise specified
NPI	national provider number
NPO	nothing by mouth
NR	no refill
	nonreactive
	normal range
NS	nonspecific
	normal saline
	not significant
	not sufficient
N&T	nose and throat

N&V	nausea and vomiting
NVD	nausea, vomiting, and diarrhea
O	oral
	oxygen
O_2	oxygen
OB	obstetrics
OB-GYN	obstetrics-gynecology
OC	office call
	on call
	oral contraceptive
occ	occasionally
OCR	Office of Civil Rights
	optical character reader
OGTT	oral glucose tolerance test
OM	office manager
OOB	out of bed
OP	outpatient
O&P	ova and parasites
OPIM	other potentially infectious material
OPPS	outpatient prospective payment systems
OPV	oral poliovaccine
OR	operating room
	operative report
ortho	orthopedics
os	mouth
OSHA	U.S. Occupational Safety and Health Administration
OT	occupational therapist
	occupational therapy
OTC	over the counter
OURQ	outer upper right quadrant
OV	office visit
OWCP	Office Workers' Compensation Programs
oz	ounce
P	phosphorus
	pulse
P&A	percussion and auscultation
PA	physician's assistant
	posteroanterior
PAC	phenacetin, aspirin, and codeine
	premature atrial contraction
Pap	Papanicolaou (smear, test)
PAR	participating provider
para	number of pregnancies
para I	primipara
PAT	paroxysmal atrial tachycardia
path	pathology
PBI	protein-bound iodine
pc	after meals
PC	personal computer
PCA	patient-controlled analgesic
PCC	Poison Control Center
PCN	penicillin
PCP	primary care physician
PCV	packed cell volume
PDA	personal digital assistant
PDR	*Physician's Desk Reference*
PE	physical examination

peds	pediatrics
PEG	pneumoencephalography
PERRLA	pupils equal, round, regular, react to light, and accommodation
PET	positron emission transmission or tomography
PH	past history
	personal history
	public health
pH	hydrogen in concentration
PHI	protected health information
PHO	physician-hospital organization
PI	present illness
	pulmonary infarction
PID	pelvic inflammatory disease
PKU	phenylketonuria
PM	after noon (post meridiem)
	post mortem (after death)
PMN	polymorphonuclear neutrophils
PMP	past menstrual period
PMS	premenstrual syndrome
PNC	penicillin
PO	postoperative
po	by mouth
POB	place of birth
POMR	problem-oriented medical record
POS	point-of-service plan
pos	positive
poss	possible
postop	postoperative
PP	postprandial
PPB	positive pressure breathing
PPBS	postprandial blood sugar
PPD	purified protein derivative
PPO	preferred provider organization
PPT	partial prothrombin time
preop	preoperative
PRERLA	pupils round, equal, react to light and accommodation
primip	woman bearing first child
prn	as the occasion arises, as necessary
procto	proctoscopy
prog	prognosis
PROM	premature rupture of membranes
pro-time	prothrombin time
PSA	prostate-specific antigen
PSRO	Professional Standards Review Organization
PT	physical therapy
	prothrombin time
pt	patient
PTA	prior to admission
pulv	powder
PVC	premature ventricular contraction
px	physical examination
	prognosis
q	each; every
q AM	every morning
QA	quality assurance
qh	every hour
q (2, 3, 4)h	every 2, 3, or 4 hours

qid	four times a day
QISMC	Quality Improvement System for Managed Care
qn	every night
qns	quantity not sufficient
qs	of sufficient quantity
qt	quart
R	registration
	right
RAM	random access memory
RBC	red blood cell
RBC/hpf	red blood cells per high power field
RBCM	red blood cell mass
RBCV	red blood cell volume
RBRVS	Resource-Based Relative Value Scale
REM	rapid eye movement
resp	respiration
Rh	rhesus (factor)
Rh-	rhesus negative
Rh+	rhesus positive
RHD	rheumatic heart disease
RLQ	right lower quadrant
RMA	Registered Medical Assistant
RNA	ribonucleic acid
R/O	rule out
ROA	received on account
ROM	range of motion
	read-only memory
ROS	review of systems
RT	radiation therapy
RUQ	right upper quadrant
RVUs	relative value units
Rx	prescription
S	subjective data (POMR)
$\bar{s}$	without
S&A	sugar and acetone (urine)
SA	sinoatrial
SARS	severe acute respiratory syndrome
SBE	shortness of breath on exertion
	subacute bacterial endocarditis
SE	standard error
sed rate	sedimentation rate
segs	segmented neutrophils
seq	sequela
SF	scarlet fever
	spinal fluid
SG	specific gravity
SH	social history
SIDS	sudden infant death syndrome
sig	instructions, directions
sigmoid	sigmoidoscopy
SMA 12/60	Sequential Multiple Analyzer (12-test serum profile)
SOAP	subjective data, objective data, assessment, and plan
SOB	shortness of breath
SOF	signature on file
sol	solution
solv	solvent
SOP	standard operating procedure
SOS	if necessary
spec	specimen
sp gr	secific gravity
spont ab	spontaneous abortion
SR	sedimentation rate
SS	signs and symptoms
$\overline{ss}$	one-half
SSI	Supplemental Security Income
Staph	Staphylococcus
stat	immediately
STD	sexually transmitted disease
Strep	Streptococcus
subcut	subcutaneous
supp	suppository
surg	surgery
sx	signs
	symptoms
sym	symptoms
syr	syrup
T	temperature
T_3	tri-iodothyronine
T_4	thyroxine
T&A	tonsillectomy and adenoidectomy
tab	tablet
TB	tuberculin
	tuberculosis
tbs	tablespoon
TC	throat culture
	tissue culture
	total capacity
	total cholesterol
TFTC	Task Force for Test Construction
ther	therapy
therap	therapeutic
TIA	transient ischemic attack
tid	three times a day
tinct	tincture
TLC	tender loving care
TMJ	temporomandibular joint
top	topically
TOPV	trivalent oral poliovirus vaccine
TP	total protein
TPI	treponema pallidum immobilization test
TPR	temperature, pulse, and respiration
tr	tincture
trig	triglycerides
TSH	thyroid-stimulating hormone
tsp	teaspoon
TUR	transurethral resection
tus	cough
T&X	type and cross match
UA	urinalysis
UB92	Uniform Bill 92
UCG	urinary chorionic gonadotropin
UCHD	usual childhood diseases
UCR	usual, customary, reasonable
ULQ	upper left quadrant

ung	ointment
UR	utilization review
urg	urgent
URI	upper respiratory infection
URL	Uniform Resource Locator
urol	urology
URQ	upper right quadrant
URT	upper respiratory tract
URTI	upper respiratory tract infection
USB	universal system bus port
USP	United States Pharmacopoeia
UT	urinary tract
UTI	urinary tract infection
UV	ultraviolet
vac	vaccine
vag	vagina
	vaginal
VD	venereal disease
VDRL	Venereal Disease Research Laboratory
vit	vitamin
vit cap	vital capacity
vol	volume
VS	vital signs
WAN	wide area network
WAV	waveform audio
WBC	white blood cell
WC	white cell
WDWN	well developed, well nourished
WHO	World Health Organization
WN	well nourished
WNF	well-nourished female
WNL	within normal limits
WNM	well-nourished male
WO	written order
w/o	without
wt	weight
x	multiply by
XR	X-ray
YOB	year of birth
yr	year

Symbols

*	birth
†	death
♂	male
♀	female
+	positive
–	negative
±	positive or negative, indefinite
÷	divide by
=	equal to
>	greater than
<	less than
×	multiply by
#	number, pound
′	foot, minute
″	inch, second
ʒ	dram
℥	ounce
μ	micron
@	at

APPENDIX B

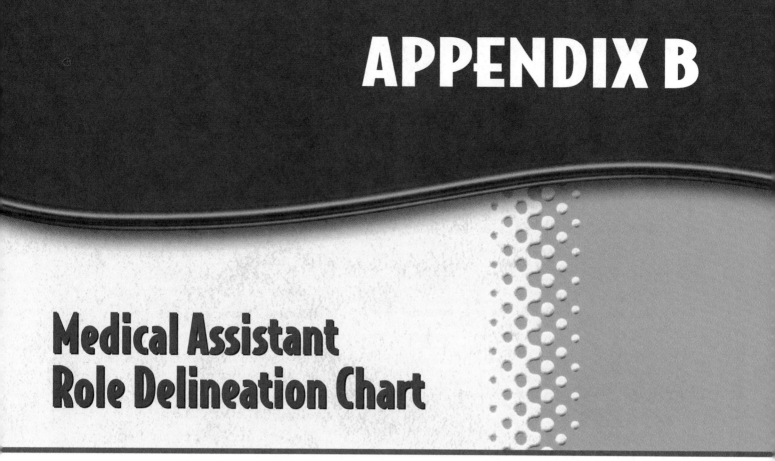

Medical Assistant Role Delineation Chart

ADMINISTRATIVE

Administrative Procedures

- Perform basic administrative medical assisting functions
- Schedule, coordinate, and monitor appointments
- Schedule inpatient/outpatient admissions and procedures
- Understand and apply third-party guidelines
- Obtain reimbursement through accurate claims submission
- Monitor third-party reimbursement
- Understand and adhere to managed care policies and procedures

* *Negotiate managed care contracts*

Practice Finances

- Perform procedural and diagnostic coding
- Apply bookeeping principles
- Manage accounts receivable

* *Manage accounts payable*
* *Process payroll*
* *Document and maintain accounting and banking records*
* *Develop and maintain fee schedules*
* *Manage renewals of business and professional insurance policies*
* *Manage personnel benefits and maintain records*
* *Perform marketing, financial, and strategic planning*

CLINICAL

Fundamental Principles

- Apply principles of aseptic technique and infection control
- Comply with quality assurance practices
- Screen and follow up patient test results

---

*Asterisk denotes advanced skill.

Diagnostic Orders

- Collect and process specimens
- Perform diagnostic tests

Patient Care

- Adhere to established patient screening procedures
- Obtain patient history and vital signs
- Prepare and maintain examination and treatment areas
- Prepare patient for examinations, procedures, and treatments
- Assist with examinations, procedures, and treatments
- Prepare and administer medications and immunizations
- Maintain medication and immunization records
- Recognize and respond to emergencies
- Coordinate patient care information with other health care providers
- Initiate IV and administer IV medications with appropriate training as permitted by state law

GENERAL

Professionalism

- Display a professional manner and image
- Demonstrate initiative and responsibility
- Work as a member of the health care team
- Prioritize and perform multiple tasks
- Adapt to change
- Promote the CMA credential
- Enhance skills through continuing education
- Treat all patients with compassion and empathy
- Promote the practice through positive public relations

Communication Skills

- Recognize and respect cultural diversity
- Adapt communications to individual's ability to understand
- Use professional telephone technique
- Recognize and respond to verbal, nonverbal, and written communications
- Use medical terminology appropriately
- Use electronic technology to receive, organize, prioritize, and transmit information
- Serve as liaison

Legal Concepts

- Perform within legal and ethical boundaries
- Prepare and maintain medical records
- Document accurately
- Follow employer's established policies dealing with the health care contract
- Implement and maintain federal and state health care legislation and regulations
- Comply with established risk management and safety procedures
- Recognize professional credentialing criteria

* *Develop and maintain personnel, policy and procedure manuals*

Instruction

- Instruct individuals according to their needs
- Explain office policies and procedures
- Teach methods of health promotion and disease prevention
- Locate community resources and disseminate information

* *Develop educational materials*

* *Conduct continuing education activities*

Operational Functions

- Perform inventory of supplies and equipment
- Perform routine maintenance of administative and clinical equipment
- Apply computer techniques to support office operations

* *Perform personnel management functions*

* *Negotiate leases and prices for equipment and supply contracts*

APPENDIX C

Top 50 Prescriptions for 2003 by Number of U.S. Prescriptions Dispensed

Brand Name	Generic Name
1. Lipitor	1. Atorvastatin calcium
2. Synthroid	2. Levothyroxine
3. Norvasc	3. Amlodipine
4. Toprol XL	4. Metoprolol succinate
5. Zoloft	5. Sertraline hydrochloride
6. Zocor	6. Simvastatin
7. Zithromax Z-pack	7. Azithromycin
8. Ambien	8. Zolpidem tartrate
9. Lexapro	9. Escitalopram
10. Prevacid	10. Lansoprazole
11. Nexium	11. Esomeprazole magnesium
12. Singulair	12. Montelukast sodium
13. Levoxyl	13. Levothyroxine sodium
14. Celebrex	14. Celecoxib
15. Fosamax	15. Alendronate sodium
16. Effexor LR	16. Venlafaxine hydrochloride
17. Premarin tabs	17. Estrogens conjugated
18. Allegra	18. Fexofenadine hydrochloride
19. Plavix	19. Clopidogrel bisulfate
20. Protonix	20. Pantoprazole sodium
21. Zyrtec	21. Cetirizine hydrochloride
22. Advair Diskus	22. Salmeterol/Fluticasone
23. Neurontin	23. Gabapentin
24. Flonase	24. Fluticasone
25. Viagra	25. Citalopram
26. Levaquin	26. Levofloxacin
27. Pravachol	27. Pravastatin
28. Lotrel	28. Amlodipine
29. Diovan	29. Valsartan
30. Vioxx	30. Rofecoxib
31. Altace	31. Ramipril
32. Klor-Con	32. Potassium chloride
33. Bextra	33. Valdecoxib
34. Celexa	34. Citalopram
35. Ortho-Evra	35. Norelgestromin ethinyl estradiol
36. Diovan HCT	36. Valsartan
37. Accupril	37. Quinapril hydrochloride
38. Paxil CR	38. Paroxetine
39. Actonel	39. Risedronate sodium
40. Actos	40. Pioglitazone hydrochloride
41. Wellbutrin XL	41. Bupropion hydrochloride
42. Cozaar	42. Losartan potassium
43. Zetia	43. Ezetimibe
44. Yasmin 28	44. Ethinyl estradiol/Drospirenone
45. Avandia	45. Rosiglitazone maleate
46. Aciphex	46. Rabeprazole sodium
47. Zithromax Susp	47. Azithromycin
48. Adderall XR	48. Amphetamine
49. Concerta	49. Methylphenidate hydrochloride
50. Flomax	50. Tamsulosin hydrochloride

Source: Drug Topics. *Top 200 brand-name drugs by retail dollars in 2004*. Retrieved from www.drugtopics.com/drugtopics/article/articleDetail. Accessed May 23, 2005.

Index

Note: Page references in **bold type** refer to boxes, procedures, figures, and tables.

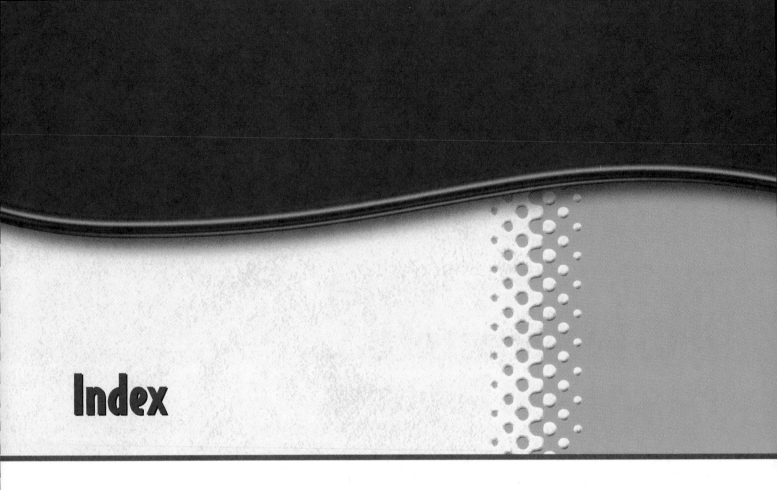

MinimumSystem Requirements for Student Software CD

- Operating System: Microsoft Windows (98 SE, 2000 or XP)
- Processor: Pentium PC 500 MHz or higher (750Mhz recommended)
- RAM: 64 MB of RAM (128 MB recommended)
- Free Drive Space: 120 MB • Screen Resolution: 800 x 600 pixels
- Color Depth: 16-bit color (thousands of colors)
- Sound Card: Yes • Macromedia Flash Player V7.x.

Free Macromedia Flash Player can be downloaded from http://www.macromedia.com

Installation Instructions for Student Software CD

1. Insert disc into CD-ROM player. The installation program should start up automatically. It will prompt you to install program on your hard drive. Follow each step. Leave the box for "Install icon on desktop" unchecked. Program should launch automatically. If program does not install, go to step 2.
2. From My Computer, double click the icon for the CD drive. Double click the setup.exe file to start the program.
3. When program is launched, a menu page will appear.
4. Click icon of program you want to open (Audio Library, Critical Thinking Challenge, or StudyWARE™) and it should launch immediately.

Technical Support

Telephone: 1-800-477-3692, 8:30 A.M.-5:30 P.M. Eastern Time
Fax: 1-518-881-1247 E-mail: delmarhelp@thomson.com

Thomson Delmar Learning End User License Agreement

IMPORTANT! READ CAREFULLY: This End User License Agreement ("Agreement") sets forth the conditions by which Thomson Delmar Learning, a division of Thomson Learning Inc. ("Thomson") will make electronic access to the Thomson Delmar Learning-owned licensed content and associated media, software, documentation, printed materials, and electronic documentation contained in this package and/or made available to you via this product (the "Licensed Content"), available to you (the "End User"). BY CLICKING THE "I ACCEPT" BUTTON AND/OR OPENING THIS PACKAGE, YOU ACKNOWLEDGE THAT YOU HAVE READ ALL OF THE TERMS AND CONDITIONS, AND THAT YOU AGREE TO BE BOUND BY ITS TERMS, CONDITIONS, AND ALL APPLICABLE LAWS AND REGULATIONS GOVERNING THE USE OF THE LICENSED CONTENT. **1.0 SCOPE OF LICENSE** 1.1 Licensed Content. The Licensed Content may contain portions of modifiable content ("Modifiable Content") and content which may not be modified or otherwise altered by the End User ("Non-Modifiable Content"). For purposes of this Agreement, Modifiable Content and Non-Modifiable Content may be collectively referred to herein as the "Licensed Content." All Licensed Content shall be considered Non-Modifiable Content, unless such Licensed Content is presented to the End User in a modifiable format and it is clearly indicated that modification of the Licensed Content is permitted. 1.2 Subject to the End User's compliance with the terms and conditions of this Agreement, Thomson Delmar Learning hereby grants the End User, a nontransferable, nonexclusive, limited right to access and view a single copy of the Licensed Content on a single personal computer system for noncommercial, internal, personal use only. The End User shall not (i) reproduce, copy, modify (except in the case of Modifiable Content), distribute, display, transfer, sublicense, prepare derivative work(s) based on, sell, exchange, barter or transfer, rent, lease, loan, resell, or in any other manner exploit the Licensed Content; (ii) remove, obscure, or alter any notice of Thomson Delmar Learning's intellectual property rights present on or in the Licensed Content, including, but not limited to, copyright, trademark, and/or patent notices; or (iii) disassemble, decompile, translate, reverse engineer, or otherwise reduce the Licensed Content. **2.0 TERMINATION** 2.1 Thomson Delmar Learning may at any time (without prejudice to its other rights or remedies) immediately terminate this Agreement and/or suspend access to some or all of the Licensed Content, in the event that the End User does not comply with any of the terms and conditions of this Agreement. In the event of such termination by Thomson Delmar Learning, the End User shall immediately return any and all copies of the Licensed Content to Thomson Delmar Learning. **3.0 PROPRIETARY RIGHTS** 3.1 The End User acknowledges that Thomson Delmar Learning owns all rights, title and interest, including, but not limited to all copyright rights therein, in and to the Licensed Content, and that the End User shall not take any action inconsistent with such ownership. The Licensed Content is protected by U.S., Canadian and other applicable copyright laws and by international treaties, including the Berne Convention and the Universal Copyright Convention. Nothing contained in this Agreement shall be construed as granting the End User any ownership rights in or to the Licensed Content. 3.2 Thomson Delmar Learning reserves the right at any time to withdraw from the Licensed Content any item or part of an item for which it no longer retains the right to publish, or which it has reasonable grounds to believe infringes copyright or is defamatory, unlawful, or otherwise objectionable. **4.0 PROTECTION AND SECURITY** 4.1 The End User shall use its best efforts and take all reasonable steps to safeguard its copy of the Licensed Content to ensure that no unauthorized reproduction, publication, disclosure, modification, or distribution of the Licensed Content, in whole or in part, is made. To the extent that the End User becomes aware of any such unauthorized use of the Licensed Content, the End User shall immediately notify Thomson Delmar Learning. Notification of such violations may be made by sending an e-mail to delmarhelp@thomson.com. **5.0 MISUSE OF THE LICENSED PRODUCT** 5.1 In the event that the End User uses the Licensed Content in violation of this Agreement, Thomson Delmar Learning shall have the option of electing liquidated damages, which shall include all profits generated by the End User's use of the Licensed Content plus interest computed at the maximum rate permitted by law and all legal fees and other expenses incurred by Thomson Delmar Learning in enforcing its rights, plus penalties. **6.0 FEDERAL GOVERNMENT CLIENTS** 6.1 Except as expressly authorized by Thomson Delmar Learning, Federal Government clients obtain only the rights specified in this Agreement and no other rights. The Government acknowledges that (i) all software and related documentation incorporated in the Licensed Content is existing commercial computer software within the meaning of FAR 27.405(b)(2); and (2) all other data delivered in whatever form, is limited rights data within the meaning of FAR 27.401. The restrictions in this section are acceptable as consistent with the Government's need for software and other data under this Agreement. **7.0 DISCLAIMER OF WARRANTIES AND LIABILITIES** 7.1 Although Thomson Delmar Learning believes the Licensed Content to be reliable, Thomson Delmar Learning does not guarantee or warrant (i) any information or materials contained in or produced by the Licensed Content, (ii) the accuracy, completeness or reliability of the Licensed Content, or (iii) that the Licensed Content is free from errors or other material defects. THE LICENSED PRODUCT IS PROVIDED "AS IS," WITHOUT ANY WARRANTY OF ANY KIND AND THOMSON DELMAR LEARNING DISCLAIMS ANY AND ALL WARRANTIES, EXPRESSED OR IMPLIED, INCLUDING, WITHOUT LIMITATION, WARRANTIES OF MERCHANTABILITY OR FITNESS OR A PARTICULAR PURPOSE. IN NO EVENT SHALL THOMSON DELMAR LEARNING BE LIABLE FOR: INDIRECT, SPECIAL, PUNITIVE OR CONSEQUENTIAL DAMAGES INCLUDING FOR LOST PROFITS, LOST DATA, OR OTHERWISE. IN NO EVENT SHALL THOMSON DELMAR LEARNING'S AGGREGATE LIABILITY HEREUNDER, WHETHER ARISING IN CONTRACT, TORT, STRICT LIABILITY OR OTHERWISE, EXCEED THE AMOUNT OF FEES PAID BY THE END USER HEREUNDER FOR THE LICENSE OF THE LICENSED CONTENT. **8.0 GENERAL** 8.1 Entire Agreement. This Agreement shall constitute the entire Agreement between the Parties and supercedes all prior Agreements and understandings oral or written relating to the subject matter hereof. 8.2 Enhancements/Modifications of Licensed Content. From time to time, and in Thomson Delmar Learning's sole discretion, Thomson Delmar Learning may advise the End User of updates, upgrades, enhancements and/or improvements to the Licensed Content, and may permit the End User to access and use, subject to the terms and conditions of this Agreement, such modifications, upon payment of prices as may be established by Thomson Delmar Learning. 8.3 No Export. The End User shall use the Licensed Content solely in the United States and shall not transfer or export, directly or indirectly, the Licensed Content outside the United States. 8.4 Severability. If any provision of this Agreement is invalid, illegal, or unenforceable under any applicable statute or rule of law, the provision shall be deemed omitted to the extent that it is invalid, illegal, or unenforceable. In such a case, the remainder of the Agreement shall be construed in a manner as to give greatest effect to the original intention of the parties hereto. 8.5 Waiver. The waiver of any right or failure of either party to exercise in any respect any right provided in this Agreement in any instance shall not be deemed to be a waiver of such right in the future or a waiver of any other right under this Agreement. 8.6 Choice of Law/Venue. This Agreement shall be interpreted, construed, and governed by and in accordance with the laws of the State of New York, applicable to contracts executed and to be wholly preformed therein, without regard to its principles governing conflicts of law. Each party agrees that any proceeding arising out of or relating to this Agreement or the breach or threatened breach of this Agreement may be commenced and prosecuted in a court in the State and County of New York. Each party consents and submits to the nonexclusive personal jurisdiction of any court in the State and County of New York in respect of any such proceeding. 8.7 Acknowledgment. By opening this package and/or by accessing the Licensed Content on this Web site, THE END USER ACKNOWLEDGES THAT IT HAS READ THIS AGREEMENT, UNDERSTANDS IT, AND AGREES TO BE BOUND BY ITS TERMS AND CONDITIONS. IF YOU DO NOT ACCEPT THESE TERMS AND CONDITIONS, YOU MUST NOT ACCESS THE LICENSED CONTENT AND RETURN THE LICENSED PRODUCT TO DELMAR LEARNING (WITHIN 30 CALENDAR DAYS OF THE END USER'S PURCHASE) WITH PROOF OF PAYMENT ACCEPTABLE TO THOMSON DELMAR LEARNING, FOR A CREDIT OR A REFUND. Should the End User have any questions/comments regarding this Agreement, please contact Thomson Delmar Learning at delmarhelp@thomson.com.